Recommended Dietary Allowances (RDA), 1980*

P9-DWY-044

Age (years)	Weight (kg)	Weight (lbs)	Height (cm)	Height (in)	Protein (g)	(RE) Vitamin A	(µg) Vitamin D	(mg) Vitamin E	(mg) Vitamin C	(mg) Thiamin	(mg) Riboflavin	(mg equiv.) Niacin	(mg) Vitamin B₆	(µg) Folacin	(µg) Vitamin B₁₂	(mg) Calcium	(mg) Phosphorus	(mg) Magnesium	(mg) Iron	(mg) Zinc	(µg) Iodine
Infants																					
0.0–0.5	6	13	60	24	kg × 2.2	420	10	3	35	0.3	0.4	6	0.3	30	0.5	360	240	50	10	3	40
0.5–1.0	9	20	71	28	kg × 2.0	400	10	4	35	0.5	0.6	8	0.6	45	1.5	540	360	70	15	5	50
Children																					
1–3	13	29	90	35	23	400	10	5	45	0.7	0.8	9	0.9	100	2.0	800	800	150	15	10	70
4–6	20	44	112	44	30	500	10	6	45	0.9	1.0	11	1.3	200	2.5	800	800	200	10	10	90
7–10	28	62	132	52	34	700	10	7	45	1.2	1.4	16	1.6	300	3.0	800	800	250	10	10	120
Males																					
11–14	45	99	157	62	45	1,000	10	8	50	1.4	1.6	18	1.8	400	3.0	1,200	1,200	350	18	15	150
15–18	66	145	176	69	56	1,000	10	10	60	1.4	1.7	18	2.0	400	3.0	1,200	1,200	400	18	15	150
19–22	70	154	177	70	56	1,000	7.5	10	60	1.5	1.7	19	2.2	400	3.0	800	800	350	10	15	150
23–50	70	154	178	70	56	1,000	5	10	60	1.4	1.6	18	2.2	400	3.0	800	800	350	10	15	150
51+	70	154	178	70	56	1,000	5	10	60	1.2	1.4	16	2.2	400	3.0	800	800	350	10	15	150
Females																					
11–14	46	101	157	62	46	800	10	8	50	1.1	1.3	15	1.8	400	3.0	1,200	1,200	300	18	15	150
15–18	55	120	163	64	46	800	10	8	60	1.1	1.3	14	2.0	400	3.0	1,200	1,200	300	18	15	150
19–22	55	120	163	64	44	800	7.5	8	60	1.1	1.3	14	2.0	400	3.0	800	800	300	18	15	150
23–50	55	120	163	64	44	800	5	8	60	1.0	1.2	13	2.0	400	3.0	800	800	300	18	15	150
51+	55	120	163	64	44	800	5	8	60	1.0	1.2	13	2.0	400	3.0	800	800	300	10	15	150
Pregnant					+30	+200	+5	+2	+20	+0.4	+0.3	+2	+0.6	+400	+1.0	+400	+400	+150	†	+5	+25
Lactating					+20	+400	+5	+3	+40	+0.5	+0.5	+5	+0.5	+100	+1.0	+400	+400	+150	†	+10	+50

*The allowances are intended to provide for individual variations among most normal, healthy people in the United States under usual environmental stresses. They were designed for the maintenance of good nutrition. Diets should be based on a variety of common foods in order to provide other nutrients for which human requirements have been less well defined. See the text for a more detailed discussion of the RDA and of nutrients not tabulated.

The Committee on RDA has published a separate table showing energy allowances in ranges for each age-sex group and another table for vitamins and minerals not previously covered by the recommendations. These tables appear in Appendix O. The FDA has published a special table of selected RDA values for use on food labels: these, the U.S. RDA, appear on p. 441.

Reproduced from *Recommended Dietary Allowances*, 9th ed. (1980), with the permission of the National Academy of Sciences, Washington, D.C.

†Supplemental iron is recommended.

UNDERSTANDING NORMAL AND CLINICAL NUTRITION

UNDERSTANDING NORMAL AND CLINICAL NUTRITION

Eleanor Noss Whitney

Corinne Balog Cataldo

West Publishing Company

St. Paul   New York   Los Angeles   San Francisco

QP
141
.W458
1983

COPYRIGHT ©1983 By WEST PUBLISHING CO.
50 West Kellogg Boulevard
P.O. Box 3526
St. Paul, Minnesota 55165

Printed in the United States of America

Library of Congress Cataloging in Publication Data

Whitney, Eleanor Noss.
  Understanding normal and clinical nutrition.

  Bibliography: p.
  Includes index.
  1. Nutrition.   2. Diet in disease.   3. Nutrition
disorders.   I. Cataldo, Corinne.   II. Title. [DNLM:
1. Nutrition.   2. Diet therapy.   QU 145 W618ua]
QP141.W458   1983   612′.3   82-17529
ISBN 0-314-69685-7

Copy editing: Beverly Peavler
Design: Janet Bollow
Text illustration: Brenda Booth
Cartoons: Barbara Clark
Composition: Innographics
Cover: Photomicrograph of Vitamin B_1.
        Tore Johnson from Woodfin Camp & Associates.

PHOTO CREDITS:

54 ©Janes Schen/Icon. **130** UNICEF photo. **262** Spring-Daytona/Stock, Boston, Inc. **291** upper left, Michael Keller/FPG; upper right, Dave Bartruff/FPG; lower right, R. Mackson/FPG; lower left, Delaforest/Alpha Photo. **312** Jim Garretson. **376** Ron Alexander/Stock, Boston, Inc. **408** Courtesy of Gjon Mili. **482** Anestis Diakopoulous/Stock, Boston, Inc. **522** Courtesy of Landrum B. Shettles. **529, 541** George Malave/Stock, Boston, Inc. **570** Lorraine Rorke/Icon. **576** Elizabeth Crews/Icon. **630** Frank Siteman/Stock, Boston, Inc. **672** Paul Crosby, with cooperation from Group Health, Inc. **794** Paul Crosby, with cooperation from Abbott-Northwestern Hospital. **940** Paul Crosby. **1004** United Press International Photo.

To the memory of Sam, who gave me the courage to begin writing about nutrition as I love to do, and to Lynn, Russell, Kara, and Roy, whose love and understanding sustains me as I work.

ELLIE WHITNEY

To Tony, Adam, Cory, Mom, Dad, and my sisters who gave me the support and motivation I needed to complete this project, and to Sara Hunt for inspiring my interest in nutrition.

CORKIE CATALDO

Acknowledgments

We are grateful to many people for many kinds of help.

To Annette Franklin for her patient labor over every page of the manuscript. To Delores Truesdell for her many research and organizing efforts and good ideas. To Lynn and Russell for their help on the computer. To Frances Sizer for her help, especially with Appendix P, and to Marie Boyle for her loving care of the index. To Marjorie Sparkman for her criticisms of the new Highlights in Parts One and Two, Phyllis Acosta for her review of Highlight 3, Sharon Rady and Linda DeBruyne for their review of Chapter and Highlight 15, and Stephanie Dalvit McPhillips for her insights on bulimia.

To our reviewers, whose thoughtful comments and criticisms on the manuscript have been most helpful: Jerry Rivers, Gayle Gess, Paula Howat, Rosa Poling, Martha Baker, Claire May, Mary Kupper, Jeanne Rackow, and Marguerite Walton. And lastly to our families and friends who gave us encouragement, listened to our complaints, and helped us in countless ways.

About the Authors

Eleanor Noss Whitney, Ph.D., R.D., received her B.A. in Biology and English from Radcliffe College in 1960 and her Ph.D. in Biology from Washington University, St. Louis, in 1970. Formerly on the faculty at the Florida State University, she now devotes full time to research and writing in nutrition and health. Her previous publications include articles in *Science*, the *Journal of Nutrition*, *Genetics*, and other journals, and the textbooks *Understanding Nutrition* and *Nutrition: Concepts and Controversies*.

Corinne Balog Cataldo, M.M.Sc., R.D., received her B.S. in community health nutrition from Georgia State University in 1976 and her M.M.Sc. in clinical dietetics from Emory University in 1979. She has worked as both a clinical dietitian and as a faculty member and dietetic internship coordinator at Emory University. She currently devotes full time to writing.

CONTENTS

Diets

APPENDIXES

PREFACE

This book is written in response to reader demand, and to our own sense that it was needed. Users of the text, *Understanding Nutrition*, have written to say, "If only we could use your book in our two-semester sequence . . ." "If only your book included a diet therapy section . . ." "If only our nurses could use this book . . ." This book is based on the original *Understanding Nutrition*, and it now has a diet therapy section. But it is not a pasted-together version of the earlier book. It is an integrated whole, born of the authors' convictions and experience in teaching nutrition to nurses and other allied health personnel.

Parts One and Two lay the foundation for an in-depth understanding of clinical nutrition by presenting the fundamentals of nutrition in **chapters** that are the same as those in *Understanding Nutrition*. The key innovation in these parts is the **highlights**, which have been entirely rewritten with allied health students in mind. They emphasize the normal *physiological* basis underlying nutritional health, so that the student will be well prepared to understand the *pathophysiology* of the disease states presented later. The chapters of Part Three are new, and center on clinical concerns through the life cycle in healthy people. Parts Four and Five are entirely new. They present, first, an overview of important aspects of clinical nutrition, and then concentrate on the nutrition problems associated with specific disease states.

The book takes a molecular approach — not because it is trying to be "hard" but because it is easier, in the end, to really understand health and disease on that basis. However, it assumes only a high school background in chemistry and biology. The needed chemistry facts are reviewed and explained in Appendix B for the reader who wants a brief refresher course; further chemical concepts that underlie nutrition are presented gradually in a logical sequence as they are needed, and they are fully and patiently explained.

To master the concepts, the student will find it helpful, first to read each chapter for the general ideas, and then to study the page margins where the technical terms are presented in formal **definitions**. Many people approach chemistry more easily by way of words than by equations and chemical symbols; we have used the "words" approach in the natural flow of the text.

At the end of each chapter in Parts One and Two is a **self-study** section. Taken together, these sections constitute a complete diet analysis and revision. In Parts Three, Four, and Five, where the emphasis shifts from "you" to "your patient," the self-study is replaced by a **case study** giving you the opportunity to apply what you have learned to actual clinical situations.

Nutrition is everyone's concern. Even if you are reading about it primarily in order to be able to help other people (hospital patients, for example), you are likely to be interested in knowing how the information you read applies in your own life, too. This book keeps in touch with your interest as a consumer of food products and of nutrition information. Remarks addressed especially to you about these matters are set off as **digressions** on a shaded background.

The digressions attempt to present a realistic picture of current nutrition research and applied nutrition. Nutrition is a science, and in science all conclusions are tentative, new answers are constantly being sought, and an honest person has to keep an open mind and be prepared to accept new evidence, even if it contradicts cherished beliefs. The digressions are intended to help you examine sources of nutrition information and to assess their validity. In them, we have identified the most common characteristics of fraudulent advertising with **flag signs** that will help you to recognize false claims, and **caution signs** to alert you to the most common misunderstandings that arise from reading about nutrition research. In Parts Three, Four, and Five, digressions also are used to alert you to everyday problems that occur in clinical practice.

The digressions are set off with color. You can skip over them without missing the main import of a chapter. But if you choose to read them we hope they deepen your understanding and strengthen your judgment about nutrition information.

A note about our style: We have a continuing problem with the use of the words *he* and *she*. Today's usage dictates that a writer play no favorites, but we dislike shifting to the plural *they*, because we want to encourage you, the reader, to think in terms of the individual's nutrition needs and the individual who delivers nutrition services. We have therefore alternated between *he* and *she*, showing an apparent prejudice in each instance. If you count the *he's* and *she's* and find either one to be dominant, let us know and we'll rectify the inequity in our next printing.

Another pair of words we have trouble with is *patient* and *client.* Some health professionals think lovingly of their patients as people to care for, and understand the term *client* to have a crass, commercial connotation. Others feel that *client* is a term that shows respect to the person who pays for the services rendered, and who therefore has rights. By this view, *patient* is a condescending term that implies the patient being served is passive, not a full-fledged member of the health-care team. We choose to use both terms, each in the positive sense. To us, both patients and clients are persons who are entitled to the best of care and respect.

In all health care settings, the physician is responsible for prescribing diets. In this book, though, we often address you as if you have full control over the client's diet. We feel that by temporarily shifting this responsibility to you, we are encouraging you to develop the skills and confidence you need to become an active participant in the diet planning process.

We hope you will find this book useful as you embark on your study of our favorite subject. We hope that your learnings will improve the quality of your life and of the lives of those you serve as a health professional.

UNDERSTANDING NORMAL AND CLINICAL NUTRITION

PART ONE

THE ENERGY NUTRIENTS:
Carbohydrate, Fat, and Protein

INTRODUCTION

CONTENTS

MOLECULES: The Unseen Actors

All things are in process and nothing stays still. . . . You would not step twice into the same river.

HERACLITUS

We

You are a collection of molecules that move. All these moving parts are arranged into patterns of extraordinary complexity and order—cells, tissues, and organs. The arrangement is constant, but its parts are continuously being replaced. Your skin, which has reliably covered you from the time you were born, is not the same skin that covered you seven years ago; it is made entirely of new cells. The fat beneath your skin is not the same fat that was there a year ago. Your oldest red blood cell is only 120 days old, and the entire lining of your digestive tract is renewed every three days. To maintain your "self," you must continually replace the pieces you lose.

All of these pieces have come from your food: You are made entirely of what you have eaten. This is not meant to imply, of course, that if you ate spaghetti last night, you are made of spaghetti now! Some complex events take place between your eating of food and its becoming "you." A bowl of spaghetti or a piece of apple pie must be entirely taken apart and

food: nutritive material taken into the body to keep it alive and to enable it to grow (**nutritive:** containing nutrients).

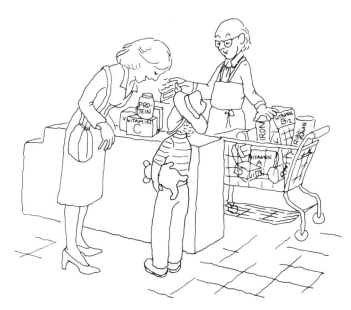

"Darling, would you go back to aisle 6 and get us another 40 milligrams of iron?"

nutrient: a substance obtained from food and used in the body to promote growth, maintenance, and/or repair.

adequate diet: a diet providing all the needed nutrients in the right total amounts. Such a diet is ideally also **balanced,** providing nutrients in the proportions that best meet the body's needs.

science of nutrition: the study of nutrients and of their digestion, absorption, transport, metabolism, interaction, storage, and excretion. A broader definition includes the study of the environment and of human behavior as it relates to nutrition.

Atoms, molecules, and compounds: Appendix B summarizes basic chemistry facts and provides definitions.

Organic: see the following pages.

ash: minerals that remain after a food is completely burned (oxidized).

rearranged before its pieces can be used to make the structures of your eye, brain, or skin. You eat foods, but what you obtain from them is nutrients, and these undergo many transformations and rearrangements in your body. If the spaghetti and the apple pie, together with the other foods you choose to eat, do not contain the nutrients you need, you lose a little. For optimum nutrition you need an adequate diet.

The science of nutrition is the study of the nutrients in food and the body's handling of these nutrients.

The Nutrients

Almost any food you eat is composed of dozens or even hundreds of different kinds of materials, tinier by far than the smallest things that can be seen with the most powerful microscope; they are atoms and molecules. The complete chemical analysis of a food such as spinach shows that it is composed mostly of water (95 percent) and that most of the solid materials are organic compounds: carbohydrate, fat, and protein. If you could remove these materials, you would find a tiny residue of minerals, vitamins, and other organic materials. Water, carbohydrate, fat, protein, vitamins, and some of the minerals are nutrients. Some of the other organic materials and minerals are not.

The six classes of nutrients:	
carbohydrate	vitamins
fat	minerals
protein	water

A complete chemical analysis of your body would show that it is made of very similar materials. If you weigh 150 pounds, your body contains about 90 pounds of water and (if 150 pounds is the proper weight for you) about 30 pounds of fat. The other 30 pounds are mostly protein, carbohydrate, and related organic compounds made from them, and the major minerals of your bones: calcium and phosphorus. Vitamins, other minerals, and incidental extras constitute a fraction of a pound. Thus you, like spinach, are composed largely of nutrients.

(This book is devoted mostly to the nutrients, but you should be aware that other constituents are found in foods and in your body—organic additives, both intentional and incidental, and trace minerals—of no recognized positive value to humans. Some may even be harmful. Later sections of the book focus on these and their significance.)

If you burn a food like spinach in air, it disappears. The water evaporates, and all of the organic compounds are oxidized to gas (carbon dioxide) and water vapor, leaving only a residue of ash. This leads us to a definition of the word *organic*.

Protein-rich
food (beef)
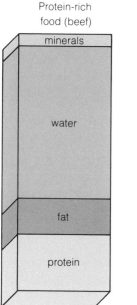

Human body
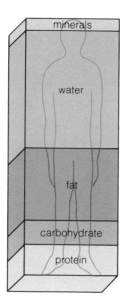

Carbohydrate-rich
food (corn)
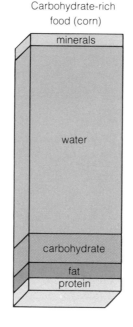

Figure 1   Food and the human body are made of the same classes of chemicals. (Vitamins are not shown because the amount is too small to be seen in a picture this size.)

The Meaning of Organic   An organic compound is one that contains carbon atoms. The first organic compounds known were natural products synthesized by plants or animals; indeed, it used to be thought that only living things contributed organic compounds to our world. The term has since been expanded to include all carbon compounds, whatever their origin. Actually, in a sense, all organic compounds are produced by living things. Some of them, like petroleum (which comes from the remains of microorganisms, plants, and animals that grew in prehistoric times), began life millions of years ago. Others are produced by plants and animals alive today. Still others come from the laboratories where chemists (who are also "living things") produce them in the test tube.

organic: containing carbon or, more strictly, containing carbon and hydrogen or carbon-carbon bonds. This definition excludes coal (which has no defined bonds); a few carbon-containing compounds, such as carbon dioxide (which contains only a single carbon and no hydrogen); and salts such as calcium carbonate ($CaCO_3$), magnesium carbonate ($MgCO_3$), and sodium cyanide ($NaCN$).

Labels on food products sometimes make the claim that the product is "organic," implying that it is therefore somehow superior to a chemically fertilized food. By the definition given above, any carbon compound is organic, even a synthetic vitamin preparation from the laboratory of a pharmaceutical company. Is there any reason to believe that "organic" or "natural" foods or nutrient preparations sold in "health food" stores are superior to grocery store foods or synthetic vitamins? Let us take vitamin C as an example.

Vitamin C, or ascorbic acid, is an organic compound with a certain chemical structure (see Chapter 10). Regardless of its source, it always has the same structure. One carbon atom (or hydrogen atom or oxygen atom) is exactly like all the others. They have no individuality; all molecules with this structure are identical. When a molecule of vitamin C enters your bloodstream, your body cannot tell where it came from. Hence the vitamin C from a chemist's lab is no different from the vitamin C in an orange fresh from a Florida citrus grove. An important point made by the American Dietetic Association is that:

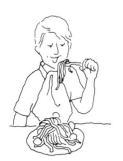

All foods are "organic," because they are all composed of organic compounds containing carbon.[1]

However, the orange may still be better for you, because the orange also contains carbohydrate, calcium, potassium, and other nutrients, as well as beneficial nonnutrient fiber. The pill contains only vitamin C—nothing more. In other words:

There is no advantage to eating an organic nutrient from one source as opposed to another, but there may be fringe benefits to eating that nutrient in a food as opposed to a purified nutrient preparation.

To interpret what you read on food labels you need two kinds of information. First, of course, you need to know the meanings of the terms that are used (an acquaintance with the definitions given throughout this book will help). Second—and this is especially important with "health food" products—you must be aware that a technical term may be misused by an industry to imply an inflated importance or value. The word *organic* is an example. As used on health food labels it is intended to imply superiority to ordinary foods. The product labeled organic has merely been organically grown; that is, in soil to which no "chemical fertilizer" has been added (only "natural fertilizer," such as manure and compost) and without the use of any insecticide sprays, such as DDT. The term *health food* is another example, implying that the food has extraordinary power to promote health. Actually, a food promotes health depending solely on the amounts and balance of nutrients it contains and on the response to it of the person who eats it.

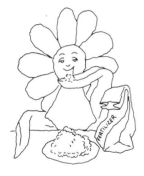

Your choice of what foods to buy is a personal choice. Insofar as it is based on your knowledge of the nutritional value of the foods, the information in this book may help you to choose wisely. The subject is a big one, and different aspects of it will be taken up in the series of

[1]Position paper on food and nutrition misinformation on selected topics, *Journal of the American Dietetic Association* 66 (1975):277-280.

digressions that follow. For the present, let us content ourselves with one additional important point—about fertilizers.

Plants take up minerals from the soil (including those from fertilizers) depending not on what is present in the soil but on what the plant needs. A tomato grown on synthetic fertilizer achieves the same chemical composition as one grown on decomposed organic material, such as compost. To put it most simply, the composition of a plant depends more on the plant than on the soil. Nutritionally, therefore, an "organically grown" plant is not superior to a "chemically fertilized" one, and a label that implies otherwise is misleading. All fertilizers are composed of chemicals.

> A FLAG SIGN OF A SPURIOUS CLAIM IS THE USE
> OF THESE WORDS:
>
> organic
> health food

spurious: false, fraudulent.

Pending legislation proposes forbidding the use of these words on labels.

Of course, if a needed element is absolutely lacking in the soil, the plant cannot select it. Plants grown on soil that lacks iodine, for example, will be iodine-poor. *Any* poorly (inadequately) fertilized soil is inferior to adequately fertilized soil. There are good and poor "organic" fertilizers, as well as good and poor "chemical" fertilizers. By the same token, there may be fringe benefits from the use of natural fertilizers like compost. For example, such a fertilizer has a beneficial effect on the structure (tilth) of the soil, which most chemical fertilizers do not have. This is not a nutritional but a mechanical advantage to the plant.

An "adequate diet" for a plant might be defined as any plant food (fertilizer) that supplies all the needed nutrients for the plant.

The only unequivocal statement about the nutritive quality of a fertilizer is a statement of the specific chemicals it contains and the amount of each; their source is irrelevant. The only unequivocal statement about the nutritive quality of a food is a statement of the specific nutrients it contains and the amount of each; their source is also irrelevant.

unequivocal: clear, unambiguous, leaving no doubt.

The Principal Actors: The Energy Nutrients

> The organic nutrients:
>
> carbohydrate   protein
> fat   vitamins

The distinction between organic and inorganic nutrients is important for several reasons. For one thing, in cooking foods you need to be aware that some organic nutrients are sensitive to and can be altered or destroyed by chemical and physical agents such as acids, air, heat, and light. This is especially important with respect to the vitamins. The minerals, however, are simple elements that cannot be destroyed.

Moreover, when organic nutrients are metabolized, waste materials (such as carbon dioxide) are produced. Everything has to go somewhere, and the metabolism of certain organic nutrients obligates the body to excrete these wastes.

Furthermore, organic nutrients can release heat or other kinds of energy. When oxidized, they break down; that is, their carbon atoms and others come apart and are combined with oxygen. If you burn a potful of food on the range, the same thing happens. Heat is released together with carbon dioxide and water vapor, and you are left with a ruined pot, blackened with the carbon and mineral residue from the food. But when you oxidize food in your body, the energy is not all released as heat. Some is transferred into other compounds (including fat) that compose the structures of your body cells, and some of the energy that holds the atoms of the energy nutrients together is used to power your activities, enabling you to move.

At the outset we stated that you are a collection of molecules that move. Now you can see a little more clearly what this means. Human beings are made of atoms taken from some of the molecules of food and rearranged into the molecules of their bodies. You move thanks to the energy released when other food molecules are taken apart.

You can metabolize all four classes of organic nutrients, but only three yield energy for the body's use. These three are the energy nutrients.

> The energy nutrients:
>
> carbohydrate
> fat
> protein

The amount of energy they release can be measured in "calories" (or, more properly, kilocalories), which no doubt are familiar to you as those things that make foods "fattening." The calorie content of a food thus depends on how much carbohydrate, fat, and protein it contains. If not used immediately, these nutrients and the energy contained in them are rearranged, mostly into body fat, and then stored. Thus an excess intake of any of the three energy nutrients can lead to overweight. Too much

Metabolism, the set of processes by which nutrients are rearranged into body structures or broken down to yield energy, is defined on page 199.

oxidation: a reaction in which atoms from a molecule are combined with oxygen, usually with the release of energy. Chemical oxidation of nutrients differs from oxidative combustion (burning) in that the energy released is largely chemical and mechanical, rather than heat and light energy. A further explanation is given in Appendix B.

calorie: a unit in which energy is measured. Technically, a calorie is the amount of heat necessary to raise the temperature of a gram of water one degree Centigrade. Food energy is measured in **kilocalories** (thousands of calories), abbreviated **kcalories** or **kcal**, or capitalized **Calories**. Most people, even nutritionists, speak of these units simply as calories, but on paper they should be prefaced by a "k." (The pronunciation of "kcalories" ignores the "k.") We will use this convention throughout this book.[2]

[2]Food energy can also be measured in kilojoules (kJ). A kilojoule is the amount of energy expended when a kilogram is moved one meter by a force of one newton. One kcalorie equals 4.2 kJ. The kilojoule is now the international unit of energy, and the United States and Canada will slowly be switching to it over the next decades, but it is not in popular use as yet. This book does not use the kilojoule.

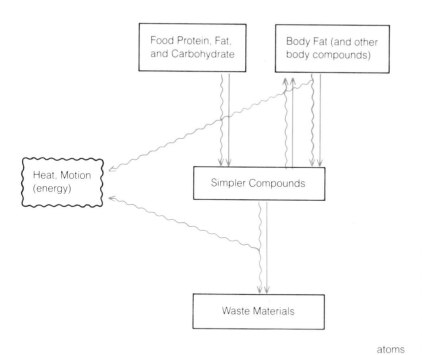

Figure 2 Metabolism of the energy nutrients. The atoms in a molecule are held together by energy in the form of chemical bonds. When a large molecule, such as a carbohydrate molecule, is broken apart, some of the chemical bonds are broken and energy is released. The atoms themselves are never broken apart in chemical reactions, only regrouped.

(We will use the convention throughout this book that arrows pointing downwards represent reactions in which molecules [groups of atoms] are being broken into smaller molecules and energy is being released. Arrows pointing upwards represent reactions in which larger molecules are being built with energy used for the bonding.)

meat (a protein-rich food) is just as fattening as too many potatoes (a carbohydrate-rich food).

It is important not to forget the organic compound found in alcoholic beverages: alcohol. This compound is not properly called a nutrient by the definition given on page 4, but it shares several characteristics with the energy nutrients. Like them, it is metabolized in the body to yield energy. When taken in excess of energy need, it, too, is converted to body fat and stored. But when alcohol contributes a substantial portion of the energy in a person's diet, its effects are damaging. (Highlight 9 is devoted to this compound.)

Practically all foods contain mixtures of all three energy nutrients, although they are sometimes classified by the predominant nutrient. Thus it is not correct to speak of meat as a protein or of bread as a carbohydrate; they are foods rich in these nutrients. A protein-rich food like beef actually contains a lot of fat as well as protein; a carbohydrate-rich food like corn also contains fat and protein (see Figure 1, page 5). Only a few foods are exceptions to this rule, the common ones being sugar (which is pure carbohydrate) and oil (which is almost pure fat).

The energy nutrients are the principal actors in the drama of nutrition and are the subject of Part One of this book. Figure 2 outlines very simply the flow of the energy nutrients into and through the body. The vitamins and the inorganic nutrients—minerals and water—serve functions other than providing energy and the direct building of body compounds; they are the subject of Part Two.

Summing Up

The six classes of nutrients found in foods are carbohydrate, fat, protein, vitamins, minerals, and water. The first four are organic compounds, the last two inorganic. The first three of these, the energy nutrients, are the subject of Part One.

After entering the body, the energy nutrients are metabolized to simpler compounds that may be reassembled into body compounds or may be oxidized, releasing energy. The energy they release may be used to help construct other body compounds, to move body parts, or to generate heat. The final products, after complete oxidation, are excreted from the body.

To Explore Further

People interested in nutrition often want to know where, in their own town or county, they can find reliable nutrition information. One place you are not likely to find it is the local library, where fad diet books sit side by side on the shelf with books of facts. However, wherever you live, there are several sources you can turn to:

- The Department of Health may have a nutrition expert.
- The local extension agent is often an expert.
- The food editor of your local paper may be well informed.
- The dietitian at the local hospital had to fulfill a set of qualifications before he or she became an R.D. (Registered Dietitian).
- There may be knowledgeable professors of nutrition or biochemistry at a nearby college or university.

In addition, you might want to accumulate a library of your own. Many references of a general nature are suggested in Appendix J, and references specific to the topics in the chapters that follow are suggested in the To Explore Further sections at the ends of those chapters.

SELF-STUDY

Food Intake Record

This is the first of a series of exercises you will find at the ends of the chapters throughout this book. Our purpose in including them is to encourage you to study your own diet. Your reaction to these exercises may be that they are both good news and bad news. The bad news is that they will slow you down, and filling out all the forms is tedious. Like income tax returns, they have to be done carefully, with frequent checking of arithmetic and in tidy handwriting, so that they will be accurate and meaningful.

The good news, however, may well outweigh these drawbacks. Most students who do these activities with thoughtful attention report that unlike income tax returns they are intriguing, informative, and often reassuring. In further contrast to tax returns, these exercises will reward you in direct proportion to your honesty.

In this first exercise you are to make a record of your typical food intake and analyze it for the nutrients it contains. It may seem premature to undertake this analysis before you have learned very much about the nutrients, but having the results in front of you as you read will make the reading more meaningful. As you learn about each nutrient and ask yourself how much of the nutrient you consume, you will already have the answer in front of you ready for interpretation and action.

Use Form 1 to record all the foods you eat for a three-day period. If, like most people, you eat differently on weekdays than on weekends, then to get a true average you should probably record for two weekdays and one weekend day—or, record your food intake for a week.

As you record each food, make careful note of the measure. Estimate the amount to the nearest ounce, quarter cup, tablespoon, or other common measure. In guessing at the sizes of meat portions, it helps to know that a piece of meat the size of the palm of your hand weighs about 3 or 4 oz. If you are unable to estimate serving sizes in cups, tablespoons, or teaspoons, try measuring out half-cup, tablespoon, and teaspoon size servings onto a plate or into a bowl to see how they look. It also helps to know that a slice of cheese (like sliced "American" cheese) or a 1 1/2-inch cube of cheese weighs about 1 oz.

You may have to break down mixed dishes to their ingredients. However, many mixed dishes, including soups, are listed in Appendix H, in the miscellaneous section at the end. Other mixtures are simple to analyze. A ham and cheese sandwich, for example, can be listed as 2 slices of bread, 1 tbsp mayonnaise, 2 oz ham, 1 oz cheese, and so on. If you can't discover all the ingredients, estimate the amounts of only the major ones, like the beef, tomatoes, and potatoes in a beef-vegetable soup.

You will, of course, make errors in estimating amounts. In calculations of this kind, errors are expected and tolerated. You can expect your calculations to be off by as much as 20 percent, or even more. Still, you will have a rough approximation that will enable you to compare your nutrient intakes with the recommended ones.

Using Appendix H, calculate for each day your total intakes of kcalories, protein, fat, fatty acids (saturated, oleic, and linoleic), carbohydrate, calcium, iron, vitamin A, thiamin, riboflavin, niacin, and vitamin C (ascorbic acid). If you wish, look up fiber in Appendix C, cholesterol in Appendix D, and sugar in Appendix F. If the foods you have eaten are not included in these appendixes, read the label on the

Form 1. Nutrient Intakes (use one form for each day)

| Food | Approximate measure or weight | Energy* (kcal) | Protein† (g) | Fat† (g) | Fatty acids†(g) | | | Carbo-hydrate† (g) | Cal-cium* (mg) | Iron‡ (mg) | Vitamin A* (IU) | Thia-min‡ (mg) | Ribo-flavin‡ (mg) | Niacin† (mg) | Vitamin C† (mg) |
					Saturated (total)	Oleic	Linoleic								
Total															

*Compute these values to the nearest whole number.
†Compute these values to one decimal place.
‡Compute these values to two decimal places.

package or use your ingenuity to guess their composition, using the most similar food you can find as a guide. For example, if you ate halibut (which is not listed in Appendix H), you would not be far off in using the values for haddock or perch. If you ate garbanzo beans, you might substitute the values for navy beans. As for fast foods, their composition is given in Appendix N.

Be careful in recording the nutrient amounts in odd-size portions. For example, if you used 1/4 c milk, then you will have to record a fourth of the amount of every nutrient listed for 1 c milk. And note the units in which the nutrients are measured:

● *Energy.* Food energy is measured in calories, as explained on page 8.

● *Protein, fat, fatty acids, and carbohydrate* are measured in grams (g). A gram is the weight of a cubic centimeter (cc) or milliliter (ml) of water under defined conditions of temperature and pressure. For example, 1 tsp salt weighs about 5 g.

● *Calcium, iron, thiamin, niacin, riboflavin, vitamin C (ascorbic acid), and cholesterol* are measured in milligrams (mg) — thousandths of a gram (0.001 g). A microgram (mcg or μg) is a thousandth of a milligram or a millionth of a gram (0.001 mg or 0.000001 g).

● *Vitamin A* is measured in international units (IU), an arbitrary unit that was agreed on by investigators before they had purified vitamin A and knew how much it really did weigh. The old IU of vitamin A now has a known value,[1] but food tables still present vitamin A contents in IU. Vitamin A values can also be expressed in RE (retinol equivalents); 1 RE equals 5 IU. (For more details, see Chapter 11.)

Now total the amount of each nutrient you've consumed for each day, and transfer your totals to Form

[1]One IU of vitamin A is equal to 0.344 μg of crystalline vitamin A acetate or 0.6 μg of all-*trans* beta-carotene.

2. Form 2 provides a convenient means of deriving and keeping on record an average intake for each nutrient.

As a final step, transfer your average intakes to Form 3 for future reference. For comparison, enter the intakes recommended for a person of your age and sex, using either the Recommended Dietary Allowance (the U.S. recommendations shown on the inside front cover) or the Canadian Dietary Standard (Table 1 in Appendix O), whichever you prefer. Note that no recommendations are made for intakes of fat or carbohydrate. Guidelines for these nutrients and for others, like cholesterol and fiber, will be presented and discussed in the chapters to come. Succeeding Self-Studies will guide you in focusing on each of the nutrients provided by your diet.

Suspend judgment about the adequacy of your diet for the moment. You have much to learn about your individuality, the nutrients, and the recommendations before you can reach any reasonable conclusions.

Form 2. Average Daily Energy and Nutrient Intakes

Day	Energy (kcal)	Protein (g)	Fat (g)	Fatty acids (g)			Carbo-hydrate (g)	Cal-cium (mg)	Iron (mg)	Vitamin A (IU)	Thia-min (mg)	Ribo-flavin (mg)	Niacin (mg)	Vitamin C (mg)
				Saturated (total)	Oleic	Linoleic								
1														
2														
3														
Total														
Average daily intake (divide 3-day total by 3)														

Form 3.   Comparison with a Standard Intake

| Day | Energy (kcal) | Protein (g) | Fat (g) | Fatty acids (g) | | | Carbo-hydrate (g) | Cal-cium (mg) | Iron (mg) | Vitamin A (IU) | Thia-min (mg) | Ribo-flavin (mg) | Niacin (mg) | Vitamin C (mg) |
				Saturated (total)	Oleic	Linoleic								
Average daily intake (from Form 2)														
*Standard**														
Intake as percentage of standard†														

*Taken from RDA tables (inside front cover) or Canadian Dietary Standard (Appendix O).

†For example, if your intake of protein was 50 g and the standard for a person your age and sex was 46 g, then you consumed (50 ÷ 46) × 100, or 109 percent of the standard.

CHAPTER 1

CONTENTS

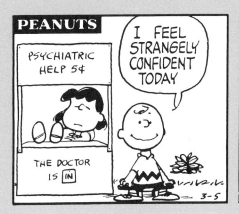
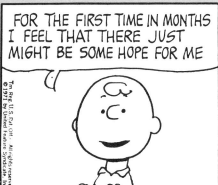
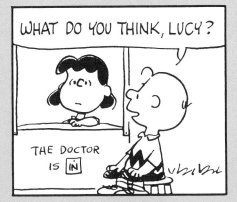
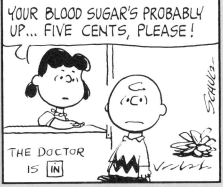

THE CARBOHYDRATES: Sugar, Starch, and Fiber

The Universe is not only queerer than we imagine—it is queerer than we can *imagine.*

J.B.S. HALDANE

Most of us would like to feel good all the time. The enjoyment available in a day, no matter what the day may bring, can be tremendous if your body and mind are tuned for it. The feeling of well-being that comes from being full of energy, alert, clear-thinking, and confident is so rewarding that if you know how to produce it, you will probably make the effort required.

It would be an exaggeration to say that good eating habits alone produce this feeling of well-being. If you try to think of what makes you feel good, you can come up with several answers. Being in love, for example, is certainly one. Facing and solving a personal problem is another. Being well rested helps too; when you wake up after a good night's sleep, you may feel bright-eyed and bushy-tailed, ready to take on the world, without having eaten a thing for 12 hours or more. Exercise helps too; the feeling of being physically tired after climbing a mountain or running a mile is a "good tired." Being clean is still another; a cold shower after heavy work or exercise can be bracing and exhilarating. Sparkling weather, clean air, beautiful scenery, pleasant company—all these play a part.

Even among the best of these pleasures, however, some limits are set by your nutritional state. You can feel really good only when your blood sugar (glucose) level is right. If that condition isn't met, neither the most beautiful mountaintop nor the most stimulating companion can compensate.

The health and functioning of every cell in your body depend on blood sugar to a greater or lesser extent. Ordinarily the cells of your brain and nervous system depend *solely* on this sugar for their energy. The brain cells are continually active, even while you're asleep, so they are continually drawing on the supply of sugar in the fluid surrounding them. They oxidize it for the energy they need to perform their functions. To maintain the supply, a continuous flow of blood moves past these cells, replenishing the sugar as the cells use it up.

Because your brain and other nerves ordinarily cannot make use of any other energy source, they are especially vulnerable to a temporary deficit in the blood sugar supply. This is why sugar is sometimes known

Glucose, a simple sugar, is often called blood sugar, because it is the principal carbohydrate found in mammalian blood (see also p. 26).

For the exception to this rule—ketosis—see p. 212.

Oxidation: see p. 8.

as brain food. When your brain is deprived of energy, your mental processes are affected. You may be unable to think clearly. Your brain controls your muscles, so you may feel weak and shaky. You are likely to miscalculate—perhaps by making an error in balancing your checkbook or by tripping while walking downstairs. Your mind resides in your brain, and so your attitude toward life, the world, and other people may also be distorted. You may become anxious, easily upset, depressed, or irritable. Your head may ache; you may feel dizzy or even nauseated. These are the signs of hypoglycemia, or too little glucose in the blood.

The body has an amazing ability to adapt to changing conditions by altering its own chemistry to maintain an internal balance. For example, when you get too hot, your blood circulation is routed closer to the skin surface so that the blood can be cooled; you perspire, and the evaporation of the secreted moisture cools you still further. When you are too cold, your circulation is rerouted inward so that heat will not be lost by exposure of the blood to the outside air. In the same way, when your blood sugar concentration rises too high or falls too low, your body makes internal adjustments to bring it back to normal. Still, human folly can defeat the body's best efforts to keep in balance. An awareness and understanding of how blood sugar is regulated can enable you to cooperate with your body in the best interest of both of you. The following paragraphs show how the body maintains its blood glucose level and what can be done to help.

hypoglycemia (HIGH-po-gligh-SEEM-ee-uh): an abnormally low blood glucose concentration. Hypoglycemia is a symptom of a number of disease conditions.

hypo = too little
glyce = glucose
emia = in the blood

The Constancy of the Blood Glucose Level

When you wake up in the morning, your blood probably contains between 80 and 120 milligrams (mg) of glucose in each 100 milliliters (ml) of blood (about half a cup). This range, which is known as the fasting blood glucose concentration, is normal and is accompanied by a feeling of alertness and well-being (provided that nothing else is wrong, of course—that you don't have the flu, for example). If you don't eat, the blood glucose level gradually falls as your cells draw on the supply. At 70 mg/100 ml, the low end of the normal range, a feeling of hunger is often experienced. The normal response to this sensation is to eat. If the meal includes some carbohydrate, your blood sugar level soon rises again.

If your meal has been unusually high in carbohydrate, and especially if it has consisted mostly of simple carbohydrate (ordinary, granulated sugar or syrup), your blood sugar concentration may threaten to rise too high. This too is an undesirable condition, known as hyperglycemia. A simple way for the body to contend with this imbalance would be to excrete the excess sugar in the urine. But the body is conservative; it stores the excess against a possible future need. The first organ to respond is the pancreas, which detects the excess and puts out a message about it; then liver, muscle, and fat cells receive the message, remove the sugar from the blood, and store it.

normoglycemia (NOR-mo-gligh-SEEM-ee-uh): a normal blood glucose concentration—80 to 120 mg/100 ml.

normo = normal

Milligrams and milliliters are metric measures of weight and volume. For definitions of these terms, see Appendix D.

hyperglycemia (HIGH-per-gligh-SEEM-ee-uh): an abnormally high blood glucose concentration.

hyper = too much

Chapter 5 describes some of the functions of the pancreas and liver. Their anatomical relationship to the digestive system is shown in Figure 1 in that chapter.

Special cells of the pancreas are sensitive to the blood glucose concentration. When it rises, they respond by secreting more of the hormone insulin into the blood. As the circulating insulin bathes the liver cells, they take up sugar from the blood, just as all cells in the body do. Within the liver cells, the small glucose units are assembled into long chains of glycogen and stored. Muscle and fat cells also participate in bringing blood glucose down to normal. In muscle, as in the liver, the glucose is stored as glycogen. In fat cells the glucose is used to make fat.

After you have eaten, then, your blood glucose level has returned to normal, and any excess glucose has been put in storage. During the hours that follow, before you eat again, the stored glycogen (but not the fat) can replenish the glucose supply as the brain and other body cells use it to meet their energy needs. Only glycogen from the liver, not from muscle, can return glucose units to the blood.

These special cells are the **beta cells** (BAY-tuh): one of the four types of cells in the pancreas. The beta cells secrete insulin in response to increased blood glucose concentration.

Hormone: see p. 82.

insulin (IN-suh-lin): a hormone secreted by the pancreas in response to increased blood glucose concentration.

glycogen (GLIGH-co-gen): a storage form of glucose in liver and muscle (see also p. 36).

glyco = glucose
gen = gives rise to

High blood glucose

1. High blood glucose stimulates pancrease to release insulin.

Pancreas

insulin

2. Insulin stimulates the uptake of glucose into cells and its storage as liver and muscle glycogen and as fat.

Muscle cells

Fat cells

Liver cells

glycogen

fat

glycogen

blood glucose

3. Later, low blood glucose is raised by reconverting liver glycogen to glucose and releasing it into the blood. (Other hormones are involved but not shown.)

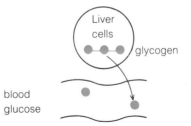

Liver cells

glycogen

blood glucose

epinephrine (epp-ih-NEF-rin): a hormone secreted by the adrenal glands in response to stress. Epinephrine used to be called **adrenaline** (uh-DREN-uh-lin).

adrenal glands: two small glands located on top of the kidneys.

ad = on
renal = kidney

One of the hormones that can call glucose out of the liver cells is the famous "fight-or-flight" hormone, epinephrine. Epinephrine is produced quickly when you are under stress, insuring that all your body cells have energy fuel in emergencies. At ordinary times other hormones guarantee that liver glycogen returns glucose to the blood whenever it is needed for maintenance.

Muscle glycogen, too, can be dismantled to glucose, but this glucose is used primarily within the muscle cells themselves, where it serves as an important fuel for muscle action. Long-distance runners know that adequate stores of muscle glycogen can make a crucial difference in their endurance toward the end of a race. Before an event, the athlete is well advised to eat a meal high in carbohydrate (see "The Teenage Athlete," Chapter 16). If there is an extraordinary need for blood glucose and the liver supply has run low, muscle glycogen can break down to an intermediate product, lactate, which can enter the blood. The liver can pick it up, convert it to glucose, and release it once again. Thus muscle glycogen can contribute indirectly to the blood glucose supply if necessary.

The maintenance of a normal blood glucose level thus depends on two types of safeguards. When the level gets too low, it can be replenished quickly either from liver glycogen stores or from a food source of glucose. When the level gets too high, insulin is secreted to siphon the excess into storage. (There is more to this story; insulin performs other roles too. This description is intended only to give you a sense of how the body maintains balance.)

If your blood glucose level reaches 70 mg/100 ml and you don't eat, the level may fall further still as the glycogen reserves are used up. Then you feel the undesirable symptoms associated with hypoglycemia. In addition to those already mentioned (weakness, mental confusion, dizziness), you may experience a craving for sweets. Some people succumb to this craving and eat a quick-energy food, such as a coke or a candy bar—and this is maladaptive behavior. The blood glucose level shoots up rapidly in response to pure simple carbohydrate of this type, and an insulin overreaction may occur. Then blood glucose rebounds to a too-low level, and hypoglycemia once again sets in. This alternation between extremes upsets the system, destroying the normal state of well-being.

maladaptive behavior: behavior intended to help an organism meet its needs that is not actually in its best interest.

reactive hypoglycemia: a temporary hypoglycemia that may be experienced by any normal person in response to an overload of sugar. Also called functional or **postprandial** hypoglycemia.

post = after
prandial = a meal

The hypoglycemia described here is the symptom of a temporary imbalance and is known as reactive hypoglycemia. It may be experienced briefly by any normal person. It has been reported, for example, in one out of every five women under the age of 45.[1]

[1]Y. Jung, R. C. Khurana, D. G. Corredor, A. Hastillo, R. F. Lain, D. Patrick, P. Turkeltaub, and T. S. Danowski, Reactive hypoglycemia in women: Results of a health survey, *Diabetes* 20 (June 1971): 428-434.

Spontaneous hypoglycemia, on the other hand, is an extremely rare disease condition in which the pancreas chronically oversecretes insulin, so that the person's blood glucose is constantly too low. Such a person must eat high-protein foods frequently and must exclude simple carbohydrates altogether. Among the quarter-million or so patients seen annually at the Mayo Clinic, fewer than a hundred have true, spontaneous hypoglycemia.[2]

The symptoms of anxiety, dizziness, weakness, and the rest can be caused by a number of conditions other than hypoglycemia, such as oxygen deprivation to the brain. In fact, eating concentrated sweets sometimes attracts large volumes of fluid from the bloodstream into the digestive tract, thus lowering the blood volume and causing reduced blood flow to the brain. The same symptoms may also be caused psychologically, by an anxiety state. Even such a serious condition as multiple sclerosis can be mistaken for hypoglycemia by the unwary diagnostician. Thus we laypersons, who are not trained in the diagnosis of conditions that present similar symptoms, are extremely unwise if we try to diagnose ourselves.

spontaneous hypoglycemia: a rare chronic hypoglycemia seen in people with abnormal carbohydrate metabolism; requires diagnosis, medical treatment, and a special diet. See Chapter 24.

CAUTION:

A little knowledge is a dangerous thing. Don't self-diagnose.

For maximum well-being, you need to eat in such a way as to avoid either extreme. This primarily means doing two things. First, when you are hungry you should eat, without waiting until you are famished. For most people, hunger is a reliable indicator of the appropriate time to eat (although in some—notably the intractably obese and diabetics—hunger is not necessarily a sign of physiological need for food). Second, when you do eat, you should eat a balanced meal, including some protein and fat as well as complex carbohydrate. The fat slows down the digestion and absorption of carbohydrate, so that it trickles gradually into the blood rather than flooding the system all at once. The protein elicits the secretion of a hormone antagonistic to insulin that damps its effect. The protein also provides a more slowly digested, alternative source of blood glucose for use in case the glycogen reserves are exhausted.

Hunger and appetite: see p. 269.

The hormone antagonistic to insulin is **glucagon** (GLOO-kuh-gon), produced by the alpha cells of the pancreas.

For a discussion of how fat slows down digestion and the absorption of carbohydrate, see Chapter 5. Chapter 6 tells how protein yields glucose.

[2]F. J. Service, Hypoglycemia, *Contemporary Nutrition* 2 (July 1977).

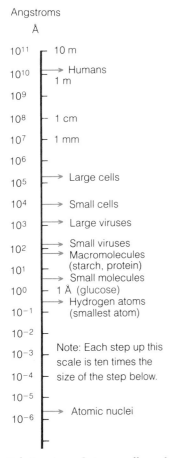

Relative sizes of atoms, cells, and organisms.

Compound and chemical formula: for basic chemistry, see Appendix B.

The Chemist's View of Sugars

Those who work with atoms and molecules—chemists, physicists, and other scientists—are people whose curiosity has impelled them to ask questions about everything. The answers they seek are explanations of substances in terms of the next smaller units of which they are made. These scientists also explain you in this way; that is, you are a bundle of a great many atoms (perhaps 3,000,000,000,000,000,000,000,000,000, give or take 1,000,000,000,000,000,000,000,000,000), held together and moved about by virtue of their associated energy.

If your mind boggles at such a thought, don't be dismayed. It staggers anyone's imagination to contemplate the ultimate realities of our universe. If you willingly go along with the chemists, all the way down to the atoms of which the carbohydrates are made, you may feel a little bit out of your depth, but you stand to gain much insight. An understanding of how energy is contained in glucose molecules and of how it is released when these molecules are metabolized in the body will help you achieve some desirable ends—to acquire the energy you need from your food at a minimum dollar cost, for example, or to balance your food energy sources for maximum health and efficiency without weight gain.

To promote an understanding of the carbohydrates, the remainder of this section is devoted to a discussion of the structures of glucose and the other single sugars (monosaccharides) and of the reactions by which glucose and similar molecules are put together to make the larger sugars (disaccharides) and complex carbohydrates (polysaccharides). (The release of energy from glucose and the ways the body uses this energy are the subjects of Highlight 7A.)

Glucose   A chemist views a glucose molecule as a compound composed of 24 atoms: 6 carbon, 12 hydrogen, and 6 oxygen atoms. These atoms are symbolized by the letters C, H, and O. Thus the chemical formula for glucose, which reflects the number of atoms it contains, is $C_6H_{12}O_6$.

Each type of atom has a characteristic amount of energy available for forming chemical bonds with other atoms. A carbon atom can form four such bonds; an oxygen atom two; and a hydrogen atom only one. One way to represent the number of bonds associated with each type of atom is to use lines radiating from the letters. The bond of a hydrogen atom is represented by one line radiating from the H; the bonds of an oxygen atom are represented by two such lines; and those of a carbon atom by four:

$$H- \qquad -O- \qquad -N- \qquad -\overset{|}{\underset{|}{C}}-$$

$$1 \qquad\quad 2 \qquad\quad 3 \qquad\quad 4$$

(Nitrogen — N — is included here because it comes up later.)

C, H, and O atoms may be put together in any way that satisfies their bonding requirements. The following drawing of the active ingredient of alcoholic beverages shows that each atom's bonding capabilities are fully used in its structure:

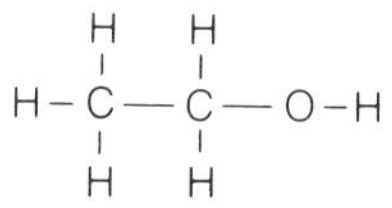

Chemical structure of ethyl alcohol.

The carbons both have four lines (bonds), the oxygen has two, and the hydrogens each have one to connect them to other atoms. In any drawing of a chemical structure these conditions must be met, not because a fussy scientist made up these rules but because this represents the way nature demands it.

Glucose is a larger and more complicated molecule than alcohol, but it obeys the same rules—as do all chemical compounds. The complete structure of a glucose molecule is:

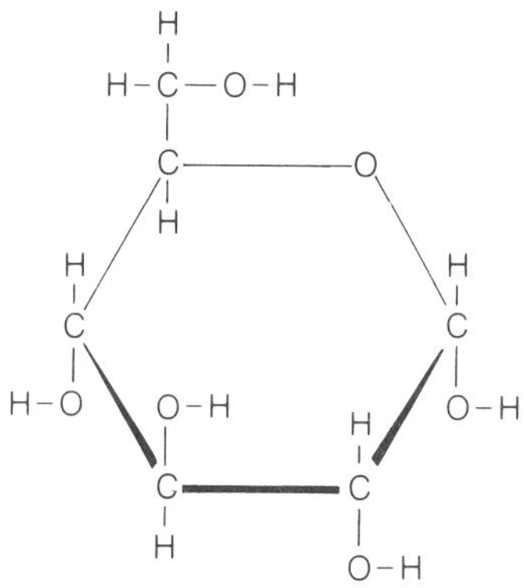

Chemical structure of glucose. On paper, it has to be drawn flat, but in nature the ring is on a plane and the attached structures extend above and below.

Again, each carbon atom has four bonds, each oxygen two, and each hydrogen one bond connecting it to other atoms.

The diagram of a glucose molecule may look formidable, but it shows all the relationships between the parts and proves simple on examination. Since you will be viewing other complex structures (not necessarily to memorize them but rather to understand certain things about them), let us adopt a simpler way to depict them—one that shows fewer details. In the following drawing, the corners where lines intersect represent carbon atoms; thus many of the bonds need not be shown. Wherever a carbon atom needs Hs to complete its four bonds, the Hs can be dropped from the diagram and can be assumed to be present. Knowing the rules of chemical structure, it is possible to reconstruct the complete structure, with all its details, from such a picture:

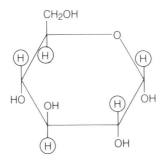

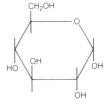

Future drawings of the glucose structure will be made simpler still, by omitting the circled Hs:

Another way to look at glucose is to notice that its six carbon atoms are all connected:

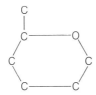

In the simplest diagrams of all, when the number of carbon atoms is the only concern, glucose is symbolized this way:

$$C-C-C-C-C-C$$

carbohydrate: a compound composed of carbon, hydrogen, and oxygen, arranged as monosaccharides or multiples of monosaccharides.

carbo = carbon (C)
hydrate = water (H_2O)

monosaccharide (mon-oh-SACK-uh-ride): a carbohydrate of the general formula $C_nH_{2n}O_n$; *n* may be any number, but the monosaccharides important in nutrition are all **hexoses** (monosaccharides containing 6 carbon atoms—$C_6H_{12}O_6$).

mono = one
saccharide, ose = sugar
hex = six

disaccharide: a pair of monosaccharides bonded together.

di = two

All carbohydrates are composed of glucose and other C-H-O compounds very much like glucose in structure. They come in three main sizes: single molecules, like glucose; pairs (for example, two glucose molecules bonded together); and chains (for example, 300 glucose molecules strung in a line). The chemist's terms for these three types of carbohydrates are mono-, di-, and polysaccharides.

With this information, the chemist's terms defining the carbohydrates are understandable, and the common terms we use to describe them—sugars and starches—can be understood more precisely. The sugars are the mono- and disaccharides; starch, glycogen, and some fibers are the polysaccharides. Store-bought cane or beet sugar is one of the disaccharides.

It remains to be seen how these units are put together and taken apart in the continuous flow of matter and energy through living things.

Making and Breaking Pairs: Chemical Reactions When a disaccharide is formed from two monosaccharides, a chemical reaction known as a condensation reaction takes place. In a condensation reaction, a hydrogen atom is removed from one monosaccharide and an oxygen-hydrogen (OH) group is removed from the other, leaving the two molecules bonded by a single O:

polysaccharide: many monosaccharides bonded together.

poly = many

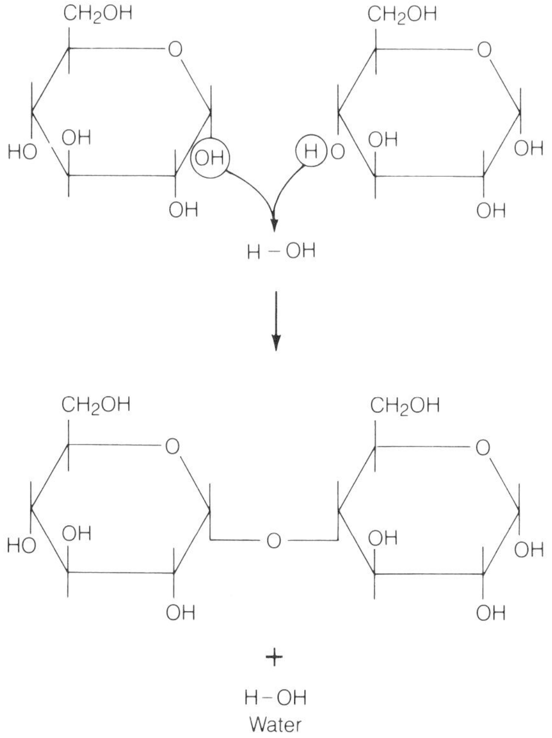

Two glucoses, water being removed

Chemical reaction: See Appendix B.

The disaccharide maltose (new bond between the two glucoses)

+

H – OH
Water

Condensation.

The H and OH that were removed from the monosaccharides in this reaction also bond to form a molecule of water (H_2O).

When a disaccharide is taken apart to form two monosaccharides again, as during digestion in the human body, a molecule of water participates in the reaction. H is added to one monosaccharide and OH to the other to reform the original structures. This reaction is called a hydrolysis reaction:

condensation: a chemical reaction in which two reactants combine to yield a major product, with the elimination of water or a similar small molecule.

hydrolysis (high-DROL-uh-sis): a chemical reaction in which a major reactant is split into two products, with the addition of H to one and OH to the other (from water).

hydro = water
lysis = breaking

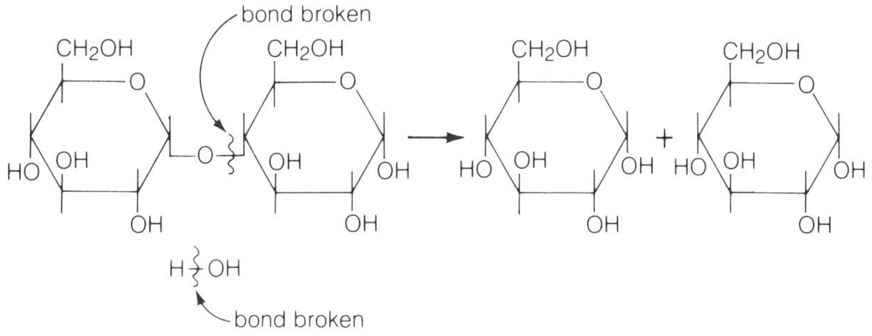

bond broken

H – OH
bond broken

The disaccharide maltose

Two glucose units

Hydrolysis.

It is by condensation and hydrolysis reactions that all of the carbohydrates are put together and taken apart. For this reason among many others, water is of tremendous importance to living things like yourself; without it, literally nothing would happen. (Chapter 14 is devoted to this extraordinary substance.) As you read, notice that water is involved in every process that is described.

Enzyme: see also p. 98.

The enzymes, the facilitators of condensation and hydrolysis reactions, are also of great importance. (They are described fully in Chapter 3.) For the moment, however, let us adopt a simple definition: An enzyme is a giant molecule (about the size of a molecule of starch) that provides a surface on which other molecules (such as glucose) may come together and react with one another. Since the making and breaking of chemical bonds tells the whole story of growth, maintenance, and change in living creatures, the enzymes that facilitate these reactions are indispensable to life.

But enough about chemical bonds. You know now that glucose is the predominant energy source for all the body's cells and can appreciate the importance of having a constant energy supply if you are to feel well. So let's return to the more familiar chemical mixtures called foods, which are the sources of glucose in the diet.

The Sugars in Foods

One exception: Alcohol also contributes energy (kcalories). See Highlight 9.

complex carbohydrates: the polysaccharides (starch, glycogen, and cellulose).

simple carbohydrates: the monosaccharides (glucose, fructose, and galactose) and the disaccharides (sucrose, lactose, and maltose); also called the sugars.

glucose: a monosaccharide; sometimes known as blood sugar or grape sugar. Labs and hospitals often refer to glucose as **dextrose**; see Chapter 20, for example.

 = glucose

Practically all your energy comes from the food you eat, about half from carbohydrate and half from fat and protein. In fact, one of the principal roles of carbohydrate in the diet is to supply energy in the form of blood glucose. A look at the carbohydrates found in foods and at the way they are put together will show why this is so.

The carbohydrates are conveniently divided into two classes: the complex carbohydrates, of which starch is the most familiar example, and the simple carbohydrates, exemplified by ordinary table sugar. All carbohydrates are composed of monosaccharides, and by far the most common is glucose. Starch is the most significant contributor of glucose to people's diets, but let us first consider the simple carbohydrates. There are actually six common sugars found in foods: glucose, fructose, galactose, sucrose, lactose, and maltose.

Glucose This monosaccharide is one of the sugars. Glucose is not especially sweet tasting; a pinch of the purified sugar on your tongue gives only the faintest taste sensation. However, it is absorbed with extraordinary rapidity into the bloodstream. If a diabetic has gone into a hypoglycemic coma (for example, from an overdose of insulin), a quick way to supply the needed blood glucose is to tip the head to one side and to drip a water solution of glucose into the cheek pocket. The glucose will be absorbed directly into the bloodstream.

Fructose   When you bite into a ripe peach or plum and savor the natural sweetness of its juice, the sugar you are enjoying is fructose. Curiously, fructose has exactly the same chemical formula as glucose—$C_6H_{12}O_6$—but its structure is quite different:

CH₂OH

Glucose   Fructose

(If you learned the rules on p. 24, you will be able to "see" 6 Cs, 12 Hs, and 6 Os in both these compounds.)

The different arrangements of the atoms in these two sugars stimulate the taste buds on your tongue in different ways. The next time you sit down to a plate of pancakes dripping with pure Vermont maple syrup, give thanks to the way nature has arranged the carbon, hydrogen, and oxygen atoms in fructose to make it the sweetest of the sugars.

Fructose can be absorbed directly into your bloodstream. When the blood circulates past the liver, the fructose is taken up into the liver cells, where enzymes rearrange the C, H, and O atoms to make compounds indistinguishable from those derived from glucose and sometimes glucose itself. Thus the effect of fructose on the body is very similar to the effect of glucose.

Food chemists have studied the exact arrangement of the atoms in sweet-tasting substances, such as fructose, and have identified the structures in them that stimulate your sweetness taste buds. They have developed a number of artificial, nonnutritive sweeteners, such as saccharin and the cyclamates, that stimulate your taste receptors in the same way but cannot be oxidized by the body to yield energy. Thus they are noncaloric.

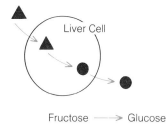

Liver Cell

Fructose ⟶ Glucose

(Sometimes fructose breaks down to intermediates, which are used for other purposes.)

For the advantages and disadvantages of these additives, see Highlight 13.

Galactose   Glucose and fructose are the only two monosaccharides of importance in foods; a third, galactose, is seldom found free in nature but is instead found as part of the disaccharide lactose. Like glucose and fructose, galactose is a hexose with the formula $C_6H_{12}O_6$. It is shown here beside a molecule of glucose for comparison:

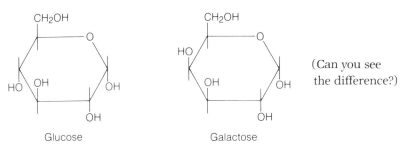

(Can you see the difference?)

Glucose   Galactose

sucrose: a disaccharide composed of glucose and fructose; commonly known as table sugar, beet sugar, or cane sugar.

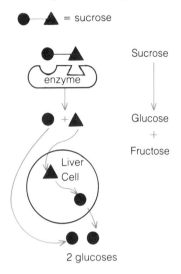

= sucrose

Sucrose

↓

Glucose
+
Fructose

2 glucoses

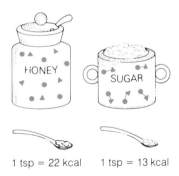

1 tsp = 22 kcal   1 tsp = 13 kcal

Sucrose The other three common sugars are disaccharides—pairs of monosaccharides linked together. Glucose is found in all three; the second member of the pair is either fructose, galactose, or another glucose.

Sucrose (*sucro* means sugar)—table sugar—is the most familiar of the disaccharides. It is the sugar found in sugar cane and sugar beets; it is purified and granulated to various extents to provide the brown, white, and powdered sugars available in the supermarket. Because it contains fructose, it is a very sweet sugar.

When you eat a food containing sucrose, enzymes in your digestive tract hydrolyze the sucrose to yield glucose and fructose. These monosaccharides are absorbed, and the fructose may be converted to glucose in the liver. (Alternatively, the fructose may be broken down to smaller compounds identical to those derived from glucose.) Thus one molecule of sucrose can ultimately yield two of glucose.

You can see from this description that it makes no difference whether you eat these monosaccharides hitched together as table sugar or already broken apart. In either case they will end up as monosaccharides in the body. People who think that the "natural sugar," honey, is somehow superior to purified table sugar fail to understand this point.

It so happens that honey, like table sugar, contains glucose and fructose. Like table sugar, honey is concentrated to the point where it contains very few impurities, even such desirable ones as vitamins and minerals. In fact, being a liquid, honey is more dense than its crystalline sister and so contains more kcalories per spoonful. Table 1 shows that honey is not significantly more nutritious than sugar:

Table 1. Vitamins and Minerals Supplied by Sugar Sources

Sugar source (1 tbsp)	Cal- cium (mg)	Iron (mg)	Vita- min A (IU)	Thia- min (mg)	Ribo- flavin (mg)	Vita- min C (mg)
Sugar (white granulated)	0	trace*	0	0	0	0
Honey (strained or extracted)	1	0.1	0	trace*	0.01	trace*
Possible daily nutrient need†	1,000	18	5,000	1.5	1.7	60

*A trace is an amount large enough to be detectable in chemical analysis but too small to be significant in comparison to the amounts recorded in these tables.

†These are amounts that an adult might typically need in a day. Not all the vitamins and minerals are listed.

To say that honey is no more nutritious than sugar, however, is not to say that there are no differences among sugar sources. Consider a piece of fruit, like an orange. From the fruit you would receive the same monosaccharides and the same kcalories as from the sugar. But the packaging is different. The fruit's sugars are diluted in a large volume of water which contains valuable trace minerals and vitamins, and the flesh and skin of the fruit are supported by fibers that also offer health value.

From these two comparisons, you may see that the really significant difference between sugar sources is not between "natural" and "purified" sugar but between concentrated sweets and the dilute, naturally occurring sugars that sweeten nutritious foods.

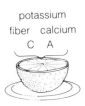
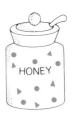

potassium
fiber   calcium
    C   A

1 tsp = 22 kcal

1 tsp = 2 kcal
with vitamins,
minerals,
and fiber

A FLAG SIGN OF A SPURIOUS CLAIM
IS THE ASSERTION THAT:

Added honey makes a product more nutritious.

A newcomer on the fad diet scene is the fructose diet, whose advocates claim that it is a wonderfully effective means of losing weight. Purified fructose, they say, is a "natural sugar" that gives you energy without accumulating as body fat. The diet plan requires that you buy bottles of purified fructose and use this sugar in place of the "unnatural sugar," sucrose, which causes ugly weight gain. In light of what has just been said about honey, it should be clear that there is nothing more natural about purified, crystalline fructose sold in bottles than about its cousin, sucrose.

A FLAG SIGN OF A SPURIOUS CLAIM
IS THE ASSERTION THAT:

Fructose (purified) is more natural than any other refined sugar.

Sucrose is the principal energy-nutrient ingredient of carbonated beverages, candy, cakes, frostings, cookies, and other concentrated sweets. Highlight 16 addresses the questions of whether sucrose is a threat to health and whether its intake, especially by children, should be limited.

Lactose   Lactose is the principal carbohydrate found in milk, comprising about 5 percent of its weight. A human baby is born with the digestive enzymes necessary to hydrolyze lactose into its two

lactose: a disaccharide composed of glucose and galactose; commonly known as milk sugar.

 = lactose

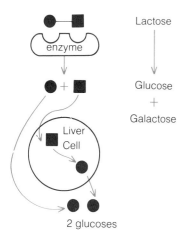

Digestion of lactose.

lactose intolerance: inherited or acquired inability to digest lactose, due to failure to produce the enzyme lactase. Lactose intolerance is prevalent in the majority of adult human population groups.[3] Highlight 15 offers help in finding milk substitutes for lactose-intolerant individuals.

maltose: a disaccharide composed of two glucose units; sometimes known as malt sugar.

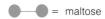 = maltose

fermentation: the breakdown of sugar in the absence of oxygen, yielding alcohol.

monosaccharide parts, glucose and galactose, so that they can be absorbed. The galactose is then converted to glucose in the liver, so each molecule of lactose yields two molecules of glucose to supply energy for the baby's growth and activity. Babies can digest lactose at birth, but they don't develop the ability to digest starch until they are several months old. This is one of the many reasons why milk is such a good food for babies; it provides a simple, easily digested carbohydrate in the right amount to supply energy to meet their needs.

Some individuals lose the ability to digest lactose as they grow older and become lactose-intolerant. They react badly to large doses of milk, feeling nauseated and sometimes having diarrhea when they drink it. Lactose intolerance arises at about the age of four and is especially common among American Indians, Orientals, and the black races; it is less frequently found in whites. It is not the same as the commonly observed milk allergy, which is caused by certain babies' hypersensitivity to the protein in cow's milk and sometimes to that in other milks.[4]

Maltose The third disaccharide is found at only one stage in the life of a plant. When the seed is formed, it is packed with starch—stored glucose—to be used as fuel for the germination process. When the seed begins to sprout, an enzyme cleaves the starch into maltose units. Another enzyme splits the maltose units into glucose units. Other enzymes degrade the units still further, releasing energy for the sprouting of the shoot and root of the plant. By the time the young plant is established and growing, all the starch in the seed has been used up, and the plant is able to capture the sun's light in its leaves. The plant then uses this light energy to put new molecules of glucose together and to elaborate chains of starch, cellulose, and other plant constituents from them. Thus the sugar maltose is present briefly during the early germination process, as the starch is being broken down. The malt found in beer contains maltose formed as the grains germinate (the alcohol is produced by yeast in a process known as fermentation).

As you might predict, when you eat or drink a food source of maltose, your digestive enzymes hydrolyze the maltose into two glucose units, which are then absorbed into the blood.

In summary, then, the simple carbohydrates or sugars are:

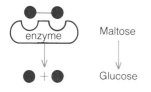

Digestion of maltose.

Monosaccharides	**Disaccharides**
glucose ●	maltose ●—●
fructose ▲	sucrose ●—▲
galactose ■	lactose ●—■
(found only in lactose)	

[3]N. Kretchmer, Lactose and lactase, *Scientific American* 227 (1972): 70-78.
[4]Kretchmer, 1972.

All of these are derived from a variety of plants except for lactose, which is the sugar of mammalian milk, and galactose, which is part of the lactose molecule.

Sugar, Starch, Fiber, and Your Health

For years people have learned that carbohydrates were "bad" for them. Sugar and starch have been accused of being fattening, and protein-rich foods like meat have been praised as being nutritious and nonfattening. It now comes as a surprise to learn that carbohydrate is not only not "bad" but is also the ideal fuel for most body functions. The educated consumer would probably choose carbohydrate as the principal kcalorie source in the diet. To convey this idea means trying to confront beliefs as deeply ingrained as people's religious faith. To persuade a person to act on it may be harder still, for food prejudices linger in the mouth.

Before this theme is developed further, the use of words like *good* and *bad* deserves a brief comment. Nutrition is a science, and science cannot make value judgments; only people can. Science involves finding out what happens under different sets of circumstances and experimenting to see how things happen. It can show, for example, that people with artery disease or cancer more often have diets high in fat or protein than diets high in carbohydrate. But science cannot pronounce these nutrients "bad" and certainly cannot prove that it is morally wrong to eat them, even though they may entail health disadvantages.

In this book we never mean to imply moral judgments, but we do have a prejudice in favor of health. When we say that something is "good" or "bad," we mean that it is "health-promoting" or "harmful to health." We use these terms because they are in common use and save space, but we have put them in quotation marks wherever they appear to remind you of what we really mean.

During the 1970s, public interest in nutrition grew tremendously. Earlier surveys in both the United States and Canada had shown that some people in these developed countries were inadequately nourished, despite the countries' wealth. Public and governmental inquiry into the significance of nutrition for health led to the development of programs to remedy nutritional deficiencies. Some of these programs are described in later chapters.

The concerns of the 1970s evolved into an interest in overnutrition—the consumption of too much food. Among the agencies inquiring into the consequences of being overfed was a committee of the United States Senate: the Select Committee on Nutrition and Human Needs. In 1977 this committee published a document titled *Dietary Goals for the United States*.

The publication of the *Dietary Goals* kicked up a whirlwind of conflicting opinions. Their proponents hailed them as long overdue and only regretted that they were understated and conservative. Their opponents criticized them as premature, exaggerated, and inappropriate for dissemination to the public. One of the objections to the *Goals* was that they had come out under the auspices of a political body—a powerful Senate committee—rather than a group of scientists. This criticism, among others, led to the disbanding of the Senate committee at the end of 1977, and the distribution of its responsibilities to two government departments whose charges include matters of nutrition and health: the Department of Agriculture (USDA) and the Department of Health, Education, and Welfare (USDHEW).

In 1979, after much more discussion and disagreement, representatives of these two departments produced a document entitled *Dietary Guidelines for Americans*, which included seven guidelines similar to the *Goals* but less specific and less controversial (see box).

Dietary Guidelines for Americans and Suggestions for Food Choices*

1. *Eat a Variety of Foods Daily.* Include these foods every day: fruits and vegetables; whole grain and enriched breads and cereals; milk and milk products; meats, fish, poultry, and eggs; dried peas and beans.

2. *Maintain Ideal Weight.* Increase physical activity; reduce kcalories by eating fewer fatty foods and sweets and less sugar, and by avoiding too much alcohol; lose weight gradually.

3. *Avoid Too Much Fat, Saturated Fat, and Cholesterol.* Choose low-fat protein sources such as lean meats, fish, poultry, dry peas and beans; use eggs and organ meats in moderation; limit intake of fats on and in foods; trim fats from meats; broil, bake, or boil—don't fry; read food labels for fat contents.

4. *Eat Foods with Adequate Starch and Fiber.* Substitute starches for fats and sugars; select whole grain breads and cereal, fruits and vegetables, dried beans and peas, and nuts to increase fiber and starch intake.

5. *Avoid Too Much Sugar.* Use less sugar, syrup, and honey; reduce concentrated sweets like candy, soft drinks, cookies, etc.; select fresh fruits or fruits canned in light syrup or their own juices; read food labels—sucrose, glucose, dextrose, maltose, lactose, fructose, syrups, and honey are all sugars; eat sugar less often to reduce dental caries.

6. *Avoid Too Much Sodium.* Reduce salt in cooking; add little or no salt at the table; limit salty foods like potato chips, pretzels, salted nuts, popcorn, condiments, cheese, pickled foods, and cured meats; read food labels for sodium or salt contents especially in processed and snack foods.

7. *If You Drink Alcohol, Do So in Moderation.* For individuals who drink—limit all alcoholic beverages (including wine, beer, liquors, etc.) to one or two drinks per day. NOTE: use of alcoholic beverages during pregnancy can result in the development of birth defects and mental retardation called Fetal Alcohol Syndrome.

*USDA, USDHEW, 1979

The publication of these two sets of recommendations—the *Goals* and *Guidelines*—so close together in time reveals the nation's increased interest in nutrition and especially its concern about overnutrition. Whichever document you look at, you will see the same general principles stressed: the *Goals* state them in terms of nutrients, the *Guidelines* translate them into foods.

Altogether the Select Committee listed seven goals.[5] The first was to avoid excess weight by consuming only as many kcalories as expended or to lose weight, if necessary, by reducing kcalorie intake and increasing energy expenditure. The next two goals dealt with carbohydrate. According to the Select Committee, people should:

- Increase the consumption of complex carbohydrates and "naturally occurring" sugars (mainly those from fruits).
- Reduce the consumption of refined and processed sugars.

In terms of foods, these goals translate into the practical recommendations of guidelines 4 and 5.

- Increase consumption of fruits and vegetables and whole grains.
- Decrease consumption of refined and other processed sugars and of foods high in such sugars.

[5] U.S. Senate, Select Committee on Nutrition and Human Needs, *Dietary Goals for the United States*, 2nd ed. (Washington, D.C.: Government Printing Office, December 1977).

The recommended changes in the diet are shown in Figure 1. The bottom part of each column deals with carbohydrate. As you can see, the Select Committee advised that we cut sugar intake in half and more than double the intake of complex carbohydrate and naturally occurring sugars.

This was startling news. It meant eating not only more fruits and vegetables but also more bread, pasta (spaghetti, macaroni, noodles, and the like), rice, and potatoes. How could you do this without getting fat?

For the definition of kcalories, see p. 8.

The secret is that carbohydrates by themselves are really not so fattening. A 3 1/2-oz baked potato is only about 90 kcal, far less than a

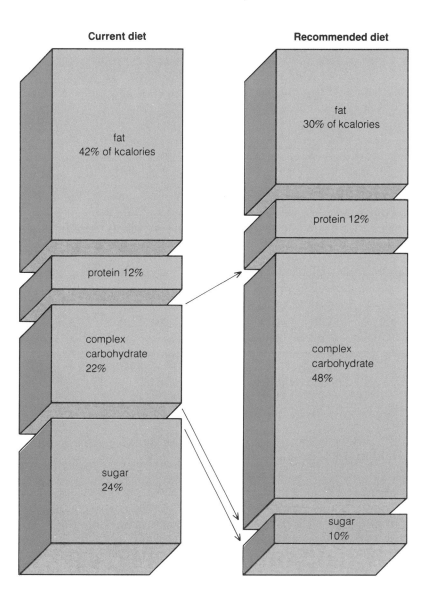

Figure 1   The U.S. Dietary Goals.

3 1/2-oz hamburger (about 285 kcal). What adds kcalories to starchy foods is not the starch itself so much as the fat—butter, margarine, sour cream, and so forth—that is often served with them. With two pats of butter, the 90-kcal potato becomes a 160-kcal potato. With a heaping tablespoon of sour cream on top of that, it becomes a 210-kcal potato. Butter and sour cream are fats, and fats are a much more concentrated source of kcalories than are carbohydrates. As you might expect, several of the dietary goals recommend reduced intake of fats (see Chapter 2). If you do cut back on fats, you can easily afford the extra kcalories you gain by eating more starchy foods.

For the composition of foods from which these numbers are calculated, see Appendix H.

The evidence that shows that complex carbohydrates and naturally occurring sugars are "good" for you is not presented here but will emerge at intervals throughout the book. But now it is time to deal with the complex carbohydrates. You should recall that these are polysaccharides—and the most important among them are starch, glycogen, and cellulose.

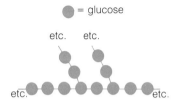

Portion of a starch molecule.

The Chemist's View of Complex Carbohydrates

Now that you know something about the structure and role of carbohydrates in the diet, you have a basis for understanding the importance of the complex carbohydrates—starch, glycogen, and cellulose.

starch: a plant polysaccharide composed of glucose and digestible by humans.

Starch   As the chemist sees it, starch is a branched chain of dozens of glucose units connected together. These units would have to be magnified more than 10 million times to appear at the size shown on this page. However, as molecules go, starches are rather large. A single starch molecule may contain from 300 to 1,000 or more glucose units linked together. These giant molecules are packed side by side in the rice grain or potato root—as many as a million in a cubic inch of food.

In the plant, starch serves a function similar to that of the glycogen in your liver. It is a storage form of glucose needed for the plant's first growth. (When you eat the plant, of course, you get the glucose to use for your own purposes.)

All starchy foods are in fact plant foods. Seeds are the richest food source; 70 percent of their weight is starch. Many human societies have a staple grain from which 50 to 80 percent of their food energy is derived. Rice is the staple grain of the Orient. In Canada, the United States, and Europe the staple grain is wheat. If you consider all the food products made from wheat—bread (and other baked goods made from wheat flour), cereals, and pasta—you will realize how all-pervasive this grain is in the food supply. Corn is the staple grain of much of South America and of the southern United States; the Mexicans use corn in their tacos and tortillas. The staple grains of other peoples

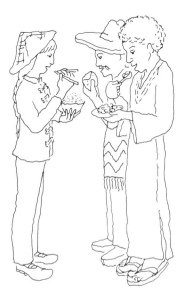

include millet, rye, barley, and oats. In each society a bread, meal, or flour is made from the grain, which is then used for many purposes.

A second important source of starch is the bean and pea family, including such dry beans found in the supermarket as lima beans, kidney beans, "baked" beans, black-eyed peas (cowpeas), chickpeas (garbanzo beans), and soybeans. These vegetables are about 40 percent starch by weight and also contain a significant amount of protein. A third major source of starch is the tubers such as the potato, yam, and cassava. One of these may serve as the primary starch source in many non-Western societies.

When you eat any of these foods, the starch molecules are taken apart by enzymes in your mouth and intestine. The enzymes hydrolyze the starch molecules to yield glucose units, which are absorbed across the intestinal wall into the blood. One to four hours after a meal, all the starch has been digested and is circulating to the cells as glucose.

Starch can be broken down to shorter chains of glucose units known as **dextrins**. These can be used as thickening agents in foods; the word sometimes appears on labels.

glycogen (GLIGH-co-gen): an animal polysaccharide composed of glucose, manufactured in the body, and stored in liver and muscle.

Glycogen Glycogen is not found in plants and is stored in animal meats only to a limited extent. It is not, therefore, of major importance as a nutrient, although it performs an important role in the metabolism of carbohydrates in the body, as already described. Glycogen is more complex and more highly branched in structure than starch.

cellulose (CELL-yoo-lose): a plant polysaccharide composed of glucose and indigestible by humans.

Cellulose The third polysaccharide of importance in nutrition is cellulose. Cellulose, like starch, is found abundantly in plants and is composed of glucose units connected in long chains. However, the bonds holding its glucose units together are different. This difference is of major importance for humans, because each type of bond requires a different enzyme to hydrolyze it. The human digestive tract is supplied with abundant enzymes to hydrolyze the bonds in starch but has none that can attack the bonds in cellulose. As a result, starch is digestible for humans and cellulose is not. Cellulose passes through the digestive tract largely unchanged, which explains the different roles of these two major plant polysaccharides: Starch is the most abundant energy source in the staple foods of the world, whereas cellulose provides no energy for humans at all.

fiber: a loose term denoting the indigestible substances in plant food. It would be best for this term to disappear from common use, to be replaced by the terms *crude fiber* and *dietary fiber*, which are more clearly defined (see p. 38).

pectin and **hemicellulose:** carbohydrates found in plant foods. Like cellulose, they are indigestible.

Cellulose is, however, one of the fibers, and these are as important to health as the energy nutrients are. During the last decade, cellulose and other plant fibers have received increasing attention as the public has learned of their health value. Researchers are still very actively trying to determine what they do and do not do, and there is much disagreement. But because some of the fibers are polysaccharides, it seems appropriate to present here the most important facts about the fibers as a group.

Besides cellulose, two other carbohydrates—pectin and hemicellulose—provide indigestible residue in the human digestive tract and so are classified as fiber. Another material classified as fiber because it is

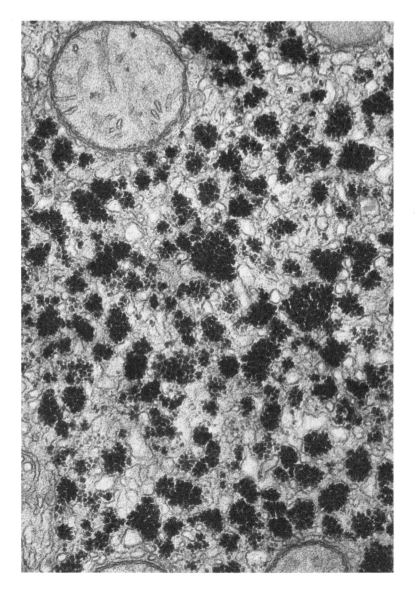

Glycogen in a liver cell. The black "rosettes" are aggregates of glycogen granules. The circular membrane-bound bodies, such as the one in the upper-left corner, are subcellular energy-producing organelles known as mitochondria. This cell was photographed under an electron microscope at a magnification of 65,000X.

From D. W. Fawcett, *An Atlas of Fine Structure* (Philadelphia: Saunders, 1966), Fig. 161. Courtesy of the author and publisher.

indigestible is lignin, a noncarbohydrate. Still others are the gums and mucilages often used as thickening agents in prepared foods.

Some of these food fibers may have beneficial effects on long- or short-term health:

● Attracting water into the digestive tract, thus softening the stools and preventing constipation.

● Exercising the muscles of the digestive tract so that they retain their health and tone and resist bulging out into the pouches characteristic of diverticulosis.

lignin: a noncarbohydrate fiber that occurs in plant foods.

Constipation: see also Chapter 5 and Chapter 23.

Diverticulosis: see Chapter 23.

● Speeding up the passage of food materials through the digestive tract, thus shortening the "transit time" and helping to prevent exposure of the tissue to cancer-causing agents in food.

● Binding lipids such as cholesterol and carrying them out of the body with the feces so that the blood lipid concentrations are lowered and possibly the risk of artery and heart disease as well.

bran: the fiber of wheat.

However, not all the fibers have similar effects. For example, the fiber of wheat—bran, which is composed mostly of cellulose—has no cholesterol-lowering effect, whereas the fiber of apples—pectin—does lower blood cholesterol. On the other hand, bran seems to be one of the most effective stool-softening fibers, especially if a certain particle size is used.

crude fiber (CF): the residue of plant food remaining after extraction with dilute acid followed by dilute alkali in a laboratory procedure.

Another problem for people trying to sort out the effects of fiber is that the amounts of fiber in food are hard to estimate. Food can be analyzed for fiber content in the laboratory by digesting it with acids and bases. Whatever remains is called crude fiber. But if you eat the same food, subjecting it to the action of your own enzymes, the undigested residue will be greater, because the body's enzymes are less harsh than the laboratory treatment. What we really need to know is how much fiber remains in the body after the normal human digestive process, but how can we measure that? One imprecise and unpleasant procedure involves collecting all the stools excreted over a 24-hour period and then drying and weighing them.

dietary fiber (DF): the residue of plant food resistant to hydrolysis by human digestive enzymes.

The fiber that remains in the human digestive tract after the body's normal action on food is known as dietary fiber. For every gram of crude fiber in a food, there are probably about 2 or 3 grams of dietary fiber.

Diets in the United States presently provide about 4 g of crude fiber a day, as compared with about 6 g in 1900. If foods such as fruits, vegetables, and whole-grain breads and cereals are used as the fiber sources, then 6 g is probably a safe intake. The wholesale addition of purified fiber (for example, bran) to foods is probably ill-advised, however, because it can cause dehydration and siphon off needed minerals with the lost water. (Appendix K presents what is known about the fiber contents of foods.)

Food Groups and the Carbohydrates

Most authorities agree that dietary carbohydrate is essential as a source of glucose. You must have some every day—but how much? One authority recommends intakes considerably above a minimum level of 50 to 100 grams a day,[6] so you might aim for at least 125 g carbohydrate a day for yourself. At 4 kcal per gram, that would be not less than 500 kcal. How can you be sure that you get at least that amount?

---

[6] Recommended Dietary Allowances, 9th ed. (Washington, D.C.: National Academy of Sciences, 1980), p. 33.

The number and variety of different foods that people eat is staggering. Appendix H lists 615 of the most common ones, and no two are exactly alike in nutritional value. Must you memorize the nutrient composition of all these foods in order to plan and assess your diet properly? This would be a formidable task. To avoid such a tedious undertaking, experts have devised various systems of grouping foods together. The two most useful kinds are exchange systems and food group systems. Some understanding of both will help you to get a feel for the composition of foods.

Exchange Systems   In an exchange system, foods are grouped so that their carbohydrate, fat, protein, and kcalorie contents are similar. For example, a slice of bread is similar to a small potato because both contain about 15 g carbohydrate, 2 g protein, and negligible fat. Both provide about 70 kcal of energy. A slice of bread could be exchanged (traded) for a potato without altering the amount of carbohydrate or protein or the number of kcalories served.

A typical exchange system divides foods into six classes, as shown in Table 2.

Exchange systems emphasize carbohydrate, fat, protein, and kcalories.

Foods containing carbohydrate:

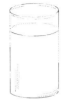

12 g in 1 c milk

(The variable amounts of fat in milk exchanges are explained fully in Chapter 2.)

Table 2.   **The Six Exchange Groups***

Exchange group	Serving size	Carbohydrate (g)	Protein (g)	Fat (g)	Energy (kcal)
(1) **Skim milk**	1 c	12	8	0	80
(2) **Vegetables**	1/2 c	5	2	0	25
(3) **Fruit**	varies†	10	0	0	40
(4) **Bread**	1 slice	15	2	0	70
(5) Lean meat	1 oz	0	7	3	55
(6) Fat	1 tsp	0	0	5	45

*Taken from the ADA Exchange System (see Appendix L).

†Serving sizes for fruits vary (see Appendix L).

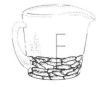

5 g in 1/2 c vegetables

Carbohydrate is found in four of the six types of food listed: milk, vegetables, fruits, and breads.

1 c skim milk (or any other serving of food in the milk list) provides 12 g carbohydrate as lactose, a naturally occurring sugar. Cheeses have negligible carbohydrate and so are not included with milk in this system.

1/2 c green beans (or any other serving of food on the vegetable list) provides 5 g carbohydrate, mostly as naturally occurring sugars. Starchy vegetables are not included on this list.

10 g in one fruit exchange

1 serving of fruit (serving sizes are shown on the fruit list) provides 10 g carbohydrate as naturally occurring sugars.

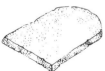

15 g in one slice bread

1 slice of bread (or any other serving of food on the bread list) provides 15 g carbohydrate, mostly in the form of starch. All grain foods, such as cereal and pasta, and such starchy vegetables as corn, lima beans, and potatoes are included on this list.

Exchange systems do not include sugary foods like candy, jam, and soft drinks, because they are not considered desirable in diet plans. But people do consume them. To estimate an accurate total of the carbohydrate you may consume, you may need a "sugar list," and we have invented one for the purpose:

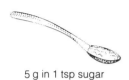

5 g in 1 tsp sugar

1 tsp white sugar (or any other concentrated sweet) provides 5 g carbohydrate.

Among the other concentrated sweets treated as equivalent to 1 tsp of white sugar are:

- 1 tsp brown sugar
- 1 tsp molasses
- 1 tsp corn syrup
- 1 tsp maple syrup
- 1 tsp honey
- 1 tsp jam
- 1 tsp jelly
- 1 tsp candy

1 tbsp catsup = 1 tsp sugar

8-oz can cola
  beverage = 6 tsp sugar

For a person who uses catsup (ketchup) liberally, it may help to remember that 1 tbsp catsup supplies about 1 tsp sugar. An 8-oz can of a cola beverage contains about 6 tsp sugar, or 30 g carbohydrate.

To sum up, all of the foods containing carbohydrate have been identified in these five boxes. A familiarity with the gram amounts gives you a command of the total carbohydrate content of any diet.

You can translate carbohydrate grams into kcalories if you multiply by 4. That is, a gram of any carbohydrate—sugar or starch—yields 4 kcal in the body. (A gram of protein also yields 4 kcal, but a gram of fat yields 9 kcal.) A study of Table 2 will reveal that the kcalorie amounts for each group of foods have been derived from these numbers and then rounded off. For example, a slice of bread contains 15 g carbohydrate (that's 60 kcal) and 2 g protein (that's another 8 kcal), or about 70 kcal

1 g carbohydrate = 4 kcal
1 g fat = 9 kcal
1 g protein = 4 kcal

in all. A half-cup of vegetables (not including starchy vegetables) contains 5 g carbohydrate (20 kcal) and 2 g protein (8 more) and has been rounded *down* to 25 kcal. (This slight understatement of the energy value of vegetables is probably intended to encourage people to use them in abundance. At 25 kcal a serving, you could consume eight servings of vegetables for less than the kcalorie cost of a single hamburger patty.)

The complete exchange systems used in the United States and Canada are presented in Appendix L. If you familiarize yourself with the specific foods in each list, you can become quite proficient at diet planning or diet evaluation.

Suppose that one day's meals consisted of the menus illustrated here. That day's meals contain the following carbohydrate exchanges:

Breakfast:	1 bread
Lunch:	2 bread
	2 tsp sugar[7]
	1 milk
Dinner:	2 bread[8]
	1 vegetable[9]
Snack:[10]	1 bread
	1 fruit
	6 tsp sugar

Thus your total carbohydrate consumption for the day is:

6 bread	= 90	g carbohydrate
8 tsp sugar	= 40	
1 milk	= 12	
1 vegetable	= 5	
1 fruit	= 10	
Total:	157	g carbohydrate

This is more than the recommended 125 g and so is adequate in carbohydrate.

This kind of calculation provides only an estimate but is close enough for most purposes. A more accurate way to determine the carbohydrate composition of foods is to refer to Appendix H, which lists individual foods rather than food groups. Adding the carbohydrate values obtained from Appendix H yields 138 g carbohydrate.

[7]The sandwich contains 2 tsp jelly.

[8]This is a 1 c serving of mashed potato.

[9]This is a 1/2 c serving of green beans.

[10]This is a 2-inch diameter biscuit with 3/4 c strawberries, 1 tbsp heavy cream, and 6 tsp sugar added in preparation.

Complete lists of the foods in each group appear in Appendix L.

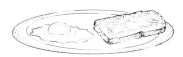

Breakfast:
fried egg
toast with margarine

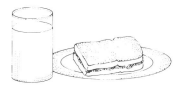

Lunch:
peanut butter and jelly sandwich
milk

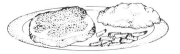

Dinner:
6-oz steak
green beans
mashed potato with margarine

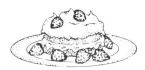

Evening snack:
strawberry shortcake
whipped cream

The difference between the 157-g estimate and the 138-g amount obtained by the more accurate calculation may be disconcerting. Rough estimates are often more valuable than close calculations, however, because of the time saved and because often only a "ballpark" figure is needed. In this example, we know that 50 g carbohydrate would be too little, but 260 would be more than twice the recommended amount (125 g). The numbers 157 and 138 both fall between these extremes; the difference between them becomes insignificant from this perspective.

Most estimates of the nutrient contents of foods are rough but serviceable approximations. In this book we refer repeatedly to a "90-kcal potato"; you should understand this to mean "90 plus-or-minus-about-20-percent," which makes it not significantly different from a 100-kcal potato. In general, for most purposes, a variation of about 20 percent is tolerable.

It takes only one or two calculations of this kind to get a feel for the carbohydrate content of your diet. Once you are aware of the major carbohydrate-contributing foods you eat, you can return to thinking in terms of these foods alone, developing a sense of how much of each is enough.

Food groups emphasize protein, vitamins, and minerals.

Food Group Plans   Food group plans emphasize the protein, vitamin, and mineral contents of foods and are quite inexact with respect to carbohydrate, fat, and kcalories. Still, they have their uses. The most familiar of them is the Four Food Group Plan. This plan separates nutritious foods into the four groups shown in Table 3. For an adequate diet, an adult should select a 2-2-4-4 pattern each day: two servings from the milk group, two from the meat group, four from the fruit/vegetable group, and four from the bread/cereal group.

This pattern ensures diet adequacy for several important nutrients. Two servings of milk or milk products (including cheese) provide some of the protein and most of the calcium needed by an adult in a day. Two servings of meat or meat substitutes complete the protein requirement and make a substantial contribution of iron. Four servings of fruits and vegetables (including starchy vegetables), if properly chosen, will meet the needs for vitamin A and vitamin C. These three groups also contribute B vitamins. Four servings of grain products (breads and cereals) add additional B vitamins and iron.

A complete presentation of the Four Food Group Plan, with its uses and limitations, is presented in Appendix M. For the remainder of Part

Table 3. Servings in the Four Food Group Plan*

Food group	Recommended number of servings (adult)	Serving size
Meat and meat substitutes	2	2-3 oz cooked meat, fish, or chicken; 1 c cooked legumes
Milk and milk products	2†	1 c (8 oz) milk; 1-2 oz cheese
Fruits and vegetables	4‡	1/2 c fruit, vegetable, or juice
Grains (bread and cereal products)	4§	1 slice bread; 1/2 c cooked cereal; 1 c ready-to-eat cereal

*For further details, see Appendix M.

†For children up to 9, 2-3 c; for children 9 to 12, 3-4 c; for teenagers and pregnant women, 3-4 c; for nursing mothers, 4 c or more.

‡One should be rich in vitamin C; at least one every other day should be rich in vitamin A.

§Enriched or whole-grain products only.

One, which deals with carbohydrate, fat, protein, and kcalories, the exchange system will be emphasized. In Part Two the uses of the Four Food Group Plan will become more apparent. With practice, you can use both to great advantage.

Before leaving this subject, however, you might look back at the day's meals just presented and ask whether they meet the recommendations of the Four Food Group Plan. Inspection will show that the foods chosen fall short because they include only one milk serving and poor choices in the fruit/vegetable group. A complete analysis would show that as a consequence the day's intakes of calcium and vitamin A were less than ideal.

This chapter began by showing you how important glucose is for the functioning of the brain and the body's other tissues. Then it went on to demonstrate how the body can derive glucose from all carbohydrates. Finally, it showed where the carbohydrates are in foods. Armed with this information, you can explode some of the myths perpetrated by television commercials advertising sweets. Sugar is brain food? True, but which sugar are we talking about? Not sucrose! When you need quick energy, what is the best source? A candy bar? A coke? No. Carbohydrate-containing *foods* are a better choice, for many reasons.

Summing Up

The world's people derive 50 to 80 percent of their food energy from carbohydrate, most of it from starch, although sugar (sucrose) can make a large contribution to their diet. The carbohydrates can be grouped into complex carbohydrates—the polysaccharides—and simple carbohydrates—the mono- and disaccharides.

Of the monosaccharides, fructose, or fruit sugar, is the sweetest; it gives honey, syrup, and many fruits their sweet flavor. Both fructose and glucose are found free in these and other plant foods. All three monosaccharides—glucose, fructose, and galactose—share the chemical formula $C_6H_{12}O_6$, but they differ in the arrangement of their atoms. This difference in arrangement gives each its particular character.

Each of the three disaccharides contains a molecule of glucose paired with another monosaccharide. The two disaccharides of importance in nutrition are lactose and sucrose. Lactose is the simple carbohydrate of milk. It is very digestible, except by those who lack the digestive enzyme to hydrolyze lactose and thus are lactose-intolerant. Sucrose, or table sugar, is the sugar of candies, sweets, and confections. (It is featured in Highlight 16.) Nutritionists are attempting to decide whether sucrose is innocent or guilty-as-charged in the rising incidence of diabetes and heart disease.

Of the polysaccharides, starch and cellulose are found in plants. Starch is found predominantly in grains and starchy vegetables; cellulose is found in all plants, especially as the bran in wheat. Cellulose, being an indigestible carbohydrate, provides the diet with fiber. Other fibers occurring in plant foods are pectin, hemicellulose, and lignin (a noncarbohydrate). Glycogen, or animal starch, is the polysaccharide synthesized in animal liver and muscle from temporary excess glucose. All three polysaccharides are chains of glucose units strung together. Cellulose is indigestible because of a difference in the character of the bonds holding the glucose units together.

People need about 125 grams of carbohydrate or more each day, preferably mostly as complex carbohydrate. Food grouping systems enable consumers to estimate the amounts of nutrients in foods; for carbohydrate the most useful system is the exchange system. The exchange system groups foods according to their carbohydrate, fat, and protein content and includes four groups of food containing carbohydrate: milk (12 g per cup), vegetable (5 g per half-cup serving), fruit (10 g per serving), and bread (15 g per serving). In addition to these four groups, a category that might be called the sugar group contributes 5 g per teaspoon; an 8-oz cola beverage contains 6 tsp. These five groups of food constitute a complete list of the carbohydrate-containing foods in the diet.

The more familiar Four Food Group Plan is not so useful for estimating carbohydrate and fat intakes as for estimating protein, vitamin, and mineral intakes, but it is introduced here for later use. The food groups and recommended servings are shown in Table 3.

To Explore Further

Recommended references on all nutrition topics are listed in Appendix J. In addition, the following specific references may be useful.

On the question of hypoglycemia—who actually experiences it, at what blood glucose level, and with what symptoms—a researcher in the area has published a monograph that the advanced student might find interesting:

● Danowski, T. S. The hypoglycemia syndromes. Pittsburgh, Pa. (15234): Harper Printing Service, 1978.

A subject not covered here in detail is that of the alternative sweeteners: fructose, the polyols, and the nonnutritive sweeteners. Complete treatment of this subject can be found in:

● Worthington-Roberts, B. S. *Contemporary Developments in Nutrition.* St. Louis: Mosby, 1981. Chapter 1. Carbohydrates in health and disease.

We also recommend our own book:

● *Nutrition: Concepts and Controversies*, 2d ed. St. Paul: West, 1981. Controversy 4A is on sugar; Controversy 11B is on saccharin.

No reliable popular reference on fiber is available, but for the more technically inclined we recommend:

● G. E. Inglett and S. I. Falkehag, eds. *Dietary Fibers: Chemistry and Nutrition.* New York: Academic Press, 1979.

Also, issues 1 and 2 of the *Journal of Plant Foods and Human Nutrition*, 1978, were devoted entirely to fiber.

For references on sugar, see Highlight 16.

The Mystery of the Body

Anyone entering a profession involving the health or medical treatment of the human body should acquire an in-depth understanding of how the body works. You especially need this understanding when you advise your patients or clients on nutrition. This Highlight introduces a principle that underlies all competent diet advice: the principle of homeostasis. To the diet advisor, this principle means that some things can't be fixed by eating differently, and that the body does its thing no matter what you feed it. Most misguided nutrition advice from well-meaning health professionals neglects this principle.

A few examples will illustrate misguided nutrition behavior, based on incorrect assumptions about the way the body works. Unfortunately, many people engage in these practices; they are not at all uncommon. The end of this Highlight reveals the more correct view of each situation.

1. A person with low blood sugar decides to eat a sugary snack. The blood sugar may rise briefly in response, but if this person has true, spontaneous hypoglycemia (and very few people do), then sugar is the poorest possible choice because it will evoke an insulin surge and a return to low blood sugar. This particular person's body has a

If conditions are such that there is a tendency to tip the organism in one direction, a series of processes are at once set at work which oppose that tendency. And if an opposite tendency develops, another series of processes promptly oppose it.

WALTER B. CANNON

low set-point for blood glucose, or a typical overreaction to the ingestion of sugar. The mistake? To think that a simple move like eating sugar would raise the blood sugar; to forget that eating sugar is followed by an adjustment made as the body does its thing. After adjusting, the body ends up with the low, but constant blood glucose level that it is set to maintain. This is homeostasis—the maintenance of constancy.

2. A middle-aged woman has read that women's bones lose calcium after the menopause. She decides to take calcium supplements. Her body, however, decides how much calcium to absorb, and if her bones are not much used (if she doesn't exercise much), or if a

number of other conditions are not met, the body's decision may be not to use the extra amounts of calcium she is eating. The money she spends on calcium supplements is wasted because she excretes their contents.

3. A young man wants bigger muscles and knows

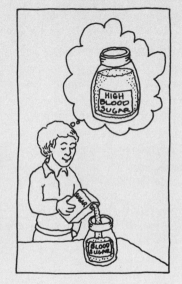

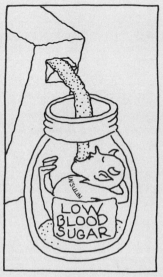

that muscle meat is high in protein. He eats large quantities of meat and supplements his diet with protein powders as well. In the body, however, the excess protein is rapidly converted to fuel and is either "burned up" (oxidized) or turned to stored fuel (fat) — the last thing the young man wants. What he doesn't know is that his body's rules, not his will, determine the fate of the protein he ingests. The body will build muscle only in response to muscle work, not to diet.

4. A world-class competitive runner has a checkup during her training season and learns she has low blood iron. She adopts a regime of iron supplements but after weeks of this a repeat check shows that her iron is still low. Her body is regulating, homeostatically, to achieve this iron level.

5. An ulcer patient experiences pain at mealtimes and fears that his foods are irritating his stomach lining. He adopts a strict, bland diet and eliminates all brightly colored, strongly flavored, coarse-textured foods and, unfortunately, excludes most of the foods he likes, too, as well as those containing nutrients and fiber that he needs. Then he begins to dread mealtimes and, ironically, his pain gets worse. His mistake: to think that the foods were irritating his

stomach, when in fact his stomach was irritating itself by secreting too much acid in response to stress. His body has its own set-point for acid secretion—too high, perhaps, but not primarily caused by diet.

6. A dieter wants to lose weight in the fastest way possible, so she chooses to fast. She has learned that fasting will induce degradation of her body's protein tissue as well as of its fat, however, so she decides to eat only protein to "spare" her body's protein. However, her body does not respond as she has planned; fat loss is no more, and may be less, than if she had eaten more kcalories;[1] she does lose lean tissue; and she also feels quite ill. Her mistake: to forget that her body would respond to this diet by altering its internal balances.

7. A man whose father has a debilitating heart disease learns that the lesions of his father's atherosclerosis are plaques in the arteries, made largely of cholesterol. He decides to stop eating all high-cholesterol foods, including eggs, shellfish, and other

[1]M. F. Ball, J. J. Canary, and L. H. Kyle, Comparative effects of caloric restriction and total starvation on body composition in obesity, *Annals of Internal Medicine* 67 (1967): 60-67

> **Miniglossary**
>
> **homeostasis** (HOME-ee-oh-STAY-sis): the maintenance of relatively constant internal conditions in body systems by corrective responses to forces that, unopposed, would cause unacceptably large changes in those conditions. A homeostatic system is not static. It is constantly changing, but within tolerable limits.
>
> *homeo* = the same
> *stasis* = staying

foods that he likes and enjoys, but the build-up of cholesterol in his own arteries proceeds unchecked.

8. A woman notices that she tends to accumulate fluid during the week before her period every month. So she cuts down on her fluid intake at that time, thinking that if she gives her body less water, it will swell less. To her dismay, it swells more, obeying some mysterious rules of its own.

In every one of these cases the body is behaving as it typically does, but its owner is misinterpreting that behavior. In every case the effect of the nutrient input is feeble or nonexistent in comparison with the powerful controls exerted by the body itself. Here — briefly — is what is happening in each case. What is important to learn here is not the individual facts (those are the subjects of chapters throughout the book) but the common thread that runs through all eight of them viewed together:

1. The person with "low blood sugar" secretes abnormally great amounts of insulin or abnormally small amounts of the opposing hormone, glucagon, in response to sugar ingestion. He has true, spontaneous hypoglycemia that has been diagnosed by his doctor's observing a blood glucose level of about 40 mg/100 ml after 24 hours of fasting. Hopefully his doctor, the dietitian, or the nurse will soon explain to him that he can take some dietary measures to help control his blood sugar level (see Chapter 24). It won't help to try to push sugar into his blood. He'll need to eat in such a way as to get the response from his body that he's after: to enhance secretion of the hormones that raise the blood glucose level.[2]

2. The woman who fears bone loss is entirely right: A woman's bones do lose calcium, sometimes great amounts of it, after the menopause and this is a major problem of the elderly, but she can't alter this by merely pushing calcium into her body. The hormones of menopause are a powerful factor influencing bone maintenance; the bone-building activity stimulated by exercise also has an important effect; and the hormonelike vitamin D is indispensable for the absorption of calcium. The woman may need to take more calcium, indeed (see Chapter 17), but to take that measure alone will not have the desired effect. Only a naive, misinformed, or malpracticing health professional would recommend to such a person that she just take calcium supplements. If you really wanted to help in such a situation you would advise the woman to create the circumstances that promote bone-building, rather than breakdown by her body.

3. The young man who wants bigger muscles is indeed providing the material they are made of when he eats meat, but this is having no effect. In fact, he almost certainly had enough building material for muscles in his diet before he made the change. What he needs is to set in motion the muscle-building activity that occurs in response to exercise. In other words, he needs an adequate, not high-protein, diet, and then he needs to work out as well.

4. The athlete who is trying to raise her blood iron by taking iron supplements is unaware that "athletes' anemia" may be a normal state of the body in a highly trained athlete and that there may be no way in which she can change this.[3] She should be checked, of course, because low blood values occurring in young women can reflect serious medical conditions, but she would be foolish to fight her body's natural adaptation to her way of life.

5. As for the ulcer patient, he has yielded to the widely held belief that foods are the cause of stomach irritation. Foods can irritate, it is true; almost everyone can identify particular foods that "disagree with" him or her. But a far more powerful factor in ulcer causation is the individual's particular nervous and hormonal system that responds to stress with enhanced stomach acid secretion. The health professional who advises someone with an ulcer to avoid eating particular foods may be adding a burden to an already heavy load. Except for coffee, alcohol, and possibly meat extracts and pepper, no specific

[2]The appropriate strategy is based on eating protein foods to stimulate glucagon secretion, and avoiding simple sugars to prevent oversecretion of insulin. See Hypoglycemia in Chapter 25.

[3]R. H. Dressendorfer, C. E. Wade, and E. A. Amsterdam, Development of pseudoanemia in marathon runners during a 20-day road race, *Journal of the American Medical Association* 246 (1981): 1215-1218.

foods deserve black marks in the ulcer patient's book. An understanding of the real dynamics of ulcer causation will enable the advisor to give truly helpful information (Chapters 4 and 23).

6. The dieter has been deceived, as have thousands of others, by some complicated, but logical-sounding reasoning in a book by someone with an impressive title. The diet advisor would compound the error by endorsing the book's advice. Diet frauds like this are among the most successful of all nutrition profiteering schemes, and are hard to see through because they are based on sophisticated-sounding descriptions of the body's metabolic processes. The public knows very little about these, so it can't see through the distortion. Nurses, doctors, and even dietitians are more often and easily tricked by these subtle persuasions than they would like to believe. Because there is a vital need for health professionals to prevent the damage done to people who follow these diets, there is heavy emphasis on the effects of different diets in the early chapters of this book (Chapters 7 and 8).

7. About the man who fears heart disease: Many people believe that cutting out dietary cholesterol will be enough to reduce inside-the-body cholesterol. Actu-

ally, the body makes cholesterol not from the cholesterol a person eats, but from other compounds he eats, according to the body's own rules and in response to other factors in that person's lifestyle — for example, his exercise habits. A long and complex sequence of events leads to the depositing of cholesterol in someone's arteries. The body's internal climate, including its chemical and hormonal balances, has much more to do with the narrowing of arteries than the eating of cholesterol does. Again, the diet advisor has to know more about the body; the cholesterol content of food is only a small part of the story.

8. What makes the body retain fluid and swell before menstruation is a series of events that readies the body for pregnancy. If fertilization doesn't occur, then the fluid is excreted at the same time as the menstrual blood is lost. The woman who tries to restrict her fluid intake at this time makes the body's task more difficult but doesn't prevent this important process from occurring. The body will obey the rule that fluid must accumulate prior to menstruation. The woman who restricts her water intake may not only hinder water excretion but make her swelling worse.

All of these examples show mistaken uses of diet tactics.

Choosing to eat a certain food or a certain kind of diet in the hope of having a special effect on the body is a hit-or-miss process. In all eight cases, the people described here guessed wrong.

In every case, however, the knowledgeable advisor can manipulate the diet to the subject's advantage, and profound health benefits can result. For each problem, researchers have learned what to do about diet by first studying the body's internal regulation and control systems. Then they design experiments to learn the effect that changes in diet will have, not on the body's end products (like "muscle" or "fluids" or "bones"), but on its regulatory systems (the hormones, enzymes, nervous systems). Managing these regulatory systems is the only way to get at the end products.

This is an exciting time to be studying nutrition, precisely because so much is being learned about the body's control systems. The more that is learned, the more effective diet advice can become. But because authorities are still in the process of learning how the body responds to different diet therapies, their conclusions have to be revised from time to time. Even advice from authorities can change, and it is important to keep up to date.

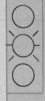

CAUTION WHEN YOU READ!

Keep alert for new knowledge about nutrition.

As described here, the human body is a homeostatic system that is regulated by a complex set of controls. An airport is a comparable system. Should you want to shift a single small plane onto a different runway, you might try to position yourself in its path and wave your arms wildly to persuade the pilot to change course in response.

If you use your head, however, you will seek to discover where and how the commands are given. You will get into the control tower and work from there. The next Highlight displays the control systems of the body. Effective therapies, including diet therapies, work by acting on these control systems.

Carbohydrate

After reading Chapter 1, you are in a position to study your carbohydrate consumption. From your Self-Study at the end of the Introduction, answer the following questions:

1. How many grams of carbohydrate do you consume in a day?

2. How many kcalories does this represent? (Remember, 1 gram of carbohydrate contributes 4 kcal.)

3. It is estimated that you should have considerably more than 100 grams of carbohydrate in a day. How does your intake compare with this minimum?

4. What percentage of your total kcalories is contributed by carbohydrate (carbohydrate kcalories ÷ total kcalories × 100)?

5. How does this figure compare with the dietary goal that states that 60 percent of the kcalories in your diet should come from carbohydrate? (Note: If you are on a diet to lose weight, then this goal does not apply to you. See the exercises in Self-Study: Diet Planning, at the end of Chapter 8.)

6. Sort the food items you ate that contained carbohydrate into three groups:

● foods containing complex carbohydrate (foods found on the bread and vegetable exchange lists in Appendix L)
● nutritious foods containing simple carbohydrate

(foods on the milk and fruit lists)
● foods containing mostly concentrated simple carbohydrate (sugar, honey, molasses, syrup, jam, jelly, candy, cakes, doughnuts, sweet rolls, cola beverages, and so on)

How much carbohydrate did you consume in each of these three categories? What percentage of your total kcalories comes from concentrated sugars? From other simple carbohydrates? Does your concentrated sugar intake fall within the recommended maximum of 10 percent of kcalories?

Optional Extras

7. Estimate how many pounds of sugar (concentrated simple carbohydrate) you eat in a year (1 lb = 454 g). How does your yearly sugar intake compare with the estimated U.S. average of about 125 pounds per person per year? (If you need additional information about the sugar in the foods you eat, look at Appendix F.)

8. Find the hidden sugar in the processed foods you buy.

Refer to Appendix F, which shows how many teaspoons of sugar are in many common processed foods, or read the labels and note the position of sugar in the list of ingredients. The ingredient in the largest amount appears first. Sugar is not the only word to look for; words that mean essentially the same thing as sugar include: brown sugar, corn sweeteners, corn syrup, dextrose, honey, invert sugar, levulose, natural sweeteners, raw sugar, sorbitol, mannitol, maltitol, xylitol, and sucrose. The next time you are purchasing sugar-containing processed foods, determine if you can buy the same item without sugar. For example, frozen strawberries can be bought with or without sugar.

9. The cereal section of a supermarket is a good place to go in pursuit of hidden sugar. (Appendix F lists about eighty cereals and shows the percentage of sucrose in each.) Make a list of the brand names of cereals in the store where you shop, and indicate if there is sugar in the list of ingredients and where in the list it is positioned. (Again, be sure to count sugar's sisters as well.) It will be interesting to see how many cereals are primarily sugar products, not grain products, and how many contain no sugar.

10. Notice your own serving sizes. Many people think that the spoon they use for sugar is a teaspoon, but when it is heaped high with sugar it is more nearly two. Using your sugar spoon as you usually do, spoon ten helpings of sugar into a bowl. Now measure this sugar with a measuring spoon, using level teaspoonfuls. How many teaspoons is a spoonful of sugar as you use it?

11. Visualize your intake of concentrated sweets. Calculate your intake of concentrated sweets as directed in 6. Now measure into a glass or jar the same amount of sugar. People often find this to be a surprising experience.

12. You may be interested in computing fiber intake as well. To get a rough idea of the amount of fiber you consume, turn to Appendix K. Then compare your fiber intake with the estimated 6 g (crude fiber) provided by the typical U.S. diet in about 1900 and with the estimated 4 g provided today. Some authorities believe that 6 or more grams per day is a desirable intake.[1]

[1]Chapter 23 in this book explains the role of fiber in various diseases of the GI tract. A more complete discussion of dietary fiber for the healthy person appeared in E. M. N. Hamilton and E. N. Whitney, Controversy 4B: Fiber, *Nutrition: Concepts and Controversies*, 2d ed. (St. Paul: West, 1982), pp. 107-110.

CHAPTER 2

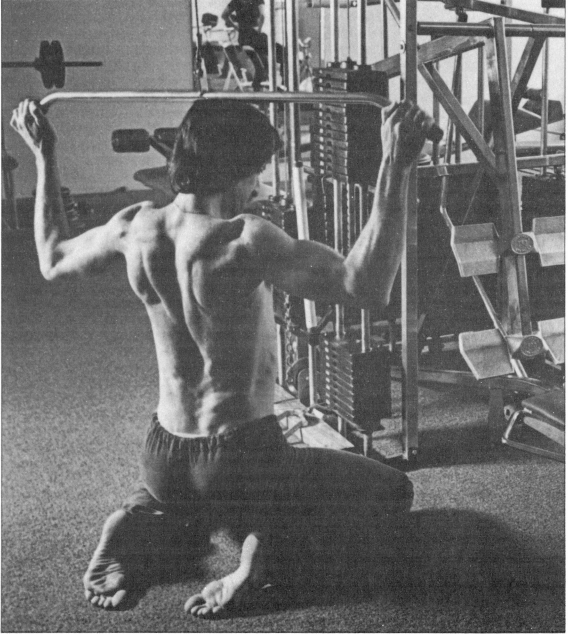

Body fat provides much of the energy for these muscles.

THE LIPIDS: Fats and Oils

The notion that matter is something inert and uninteresting is surely the veriest nonsense. If there is anything more wonderful than matter in the sheer versatility of its behavior, I have yet to hear tell of it.

FRED HOYLE

You have been conditioned to believe that slim is beautiful. The less fat you carry on your frame, the lovelier (sexier, healthier) you are thought to be. On the other hand, your body fat does things for you that you would be hard put to do without. If you carry neither too much nor too little body fat, you will enjoy the benefits nature intended in providing stores of this very important nutrient.

Although a third of the world's population is underfed, at least a third of our population is overfed. And indeed, overweight is a major health problem in the developed countries, contributing to the incidence of heart disease, diabetes, and many other ills.

Fat in the Body: Pros and Cons

The fats—more properly called the lipids—are actually a family of compounds that include both fats and oils. Both fats and oils occur in your body, and both help to keep it healthy. Natural oils in the skin provide a radiant complexion; in the scalp they help nourish the hair and make it glossy. The layer of fat beneath the skin, being a poor conductor of heat, insulates the body from extremes of temperature. A pad of hard fat beneath each kidney protects it from being jarred and damaged, even during a motorcycle ride on a bumpy road. The soft fat in the breasts of a woman protects her mammary glands from heat and cold and cushions them against shock. The fat that lies embedded in the muscle tissue shares with muscle glycogen the task of providing energy when the muscle cells are active.

An uninterrupted flow of energy is so vital to life that in a pinch any other function is sacrificed to maintain it. If a growing child is fed too little food, for example, the food she does consume will be used for energy to keep her heart and lungs going, but her growth will come to a standstill. To go totally without an energy supply, even for a few

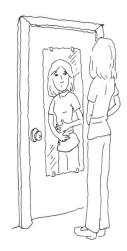

"I have *got* to go on a diet."

minutes, would be to die. The urgency of the need for energy has ensured, over the course of evolution, that all creatures have built-in reserves to protect themselves from ever being deprived of it. One provision against this sort of emergency has already been described in Chapter 1: the stores of glycogen—chains of sugar (glucose) units—in the liver that can be returned to circulation whenever the blood glucose supply runs short.

However, the liver cells can store only a limited amount of energy as glycogen; once this is depleted, the body must receive new food or turn to its backup reserve, the body fat. Unlike liver cells, fat cells have an unlimited storage capacity. During a prolonged period of food deprivation fat stores make an important contribution to energy needs.

The average 20-year-old woman needs about 2,000 kcal a day to fuel her body's maintenance and activities. If she fasts (drinking only water to flush out her metabolic wastes), she will rapidly oxidize her own body fat. A pound of body fat provides 3,500 kcal. In conditions of enforced starvation, say, during a siege or famine, the fatter person has a better chance of surviving.

If you happen to be acquainted with a polar bear, you will be aware that the same thing is true for him. As he lumbers about on his iceberg, great masses of fat ripple beneath his thick fur coat. When he hibernates, he oxidizes that fat, extracting tens of thousands of kcalories from it to maintain his body temperature and to fuel other metabolic processes while he sleeps. Come spring, he is several hundred pounds thinner than when he went to sleep.

Since we do not yet anticipate facing a famine in this country, the thinner person actually has most of the advantages. To lose 50 pounds, you would have to deprive yourself of all food for at least three months—and for much longer if you didn't elect total starvation. No one acquainted with the risks of this course would undertake such a program except under close medical supervision.

Living on body fat has other disadvantages. Fat can provide energy—but not as glucose, the form from which the brain and nerve cells can best extract energy. After a long period of glucose deprivation, these cells develop the ability to derive about half of their energy from a special form of fat known as ketones, but they still require glucose as

Fat cells are often called **adipose** (ADD-hi-poce) **cells.**

1 lb "body fat" = 3,500 kcal (but see p. 216).

ketones (KEE-tones): a condensation product of fat metabolism produced when carbohydrate is not available (see Chapter 7).

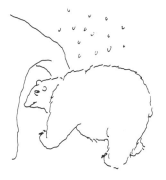
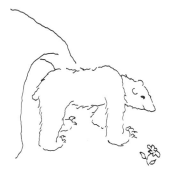

well. With the available glycogen long gone, they demand this glucose from the only alternative source—protein. And since no protein is coming in from food, the only supply is in the muscle and other lean tissues of the body. With the demand for body protein, these tissues atrophy, bringing on weakness, loss of function, and ultimately—when half the body protein has been used up—death. Death from loss of lean body mass will occur even in a fat person if a fast is too prolonged.

To sum up what's good about body fat: It helps maintain the health of the skin and hair, protects body organs from temperature extremes and mechanical shock, and provides a reserve fuel supply for use whenever body carbohydrate is depleted. As for what is bad about body fat: There can simply be too much of it. When fat is being oxidized for energy in the absence of glucose, ketones are formed to meet about half of the energy needs of the brain and nervous system. Protein released from wasting muscle and other lean tissue provides the other half.

atrophy (ATT-ro-fee): to waste away.

a = without
$trophy$ = growth

For more about the dangers of fasting, see Chapter 7.

Fat in Foods: More Pros and Cons

Many of the compounds that give foods their flavor and aroma are found in fats and oils; they are fat-soluble. Four vitamins—A, D, E, and K—are also soluble in fat. Understanding this fact provides insight into many different areas in nutrition, so let us spend a moment here considering the phenomenon of fat solubility.

As you know, fats and oils tend to separate from water and watery substances. The oil floats to the top when salad dressing stands. As hot meat drippings cool, the fat separates and hardens on top of the other juices. You can probably think of many other examples of this phenomenon. Whenever a mixture of a fatty liquid and a watery liquid separates in this manner, the other compounds in the mixture must go with either the fat or the water. The nutritional significance of this is evident if you think what happens when the fat is removed from a food.

In general, foods from which the fat or oil has been removed lack much of their original flavor, aroma, and fat-soluble vitamin content. If you skin chicken meat before cooking it, the layer of fat is removed with the skin. The result is a tasteless, odorless meat. Chicken meat without its fat is almost indistinguishable from defatted veal or lamb or water-packed tuna; many of the compounds that give the meat its flavor are removed with the fat. The aromatic nature of many fat-soluble compounds becomes obvious when foods are cooking. Meat fat, especially from bacon, ham, pork, and fatty beef (hamburgers), and the fat added to vegetables—onions smothered in butter, french fries—all contribute to a "good food" smell. Milk when skimmed loses much of its buttery flavor too, and more importantly, it loses all of the vitamins A and D that the cow secreted into the milk. To make skim milk nutritionally equivalent to whole milk, these vitamins must be

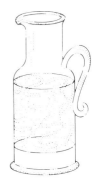

Fat solubility. Oil and water separate; fat-soluble compounds stay dissolved in the oil, water-soluble compounds in the water.

Fortification actually involves adding back more vitamin D than was in the whole milk originally.

Remember, fat is a more concentrated energy source than the other energy nutrients:

1 g carbohydrate = 4 kcal
1 g fat   = 9 kcal
1 g protein   = 4 kcal

mixed in; hence the "vitamin A & D fortified" label you see on skim milk.

An additional feature is lost when fat is removed: kcalories. A medium pork chop with the fat trimmed to within a half inch of the lean meat contains 260 kcal; with the fat trimmed off completely it contains 130 kcal. A baked potato with butter and sour cream (1 tbsp each) is 260 kcal; plain, it is 90 kcal. So it goes. The single most effective step you can take to reduce the energy (kcalorie) value of a food is to eat it without the fat.

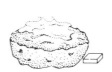

Pork chop with 1/2″ fat (260 kcal)   Potato with 1 tbsp butter and 1 tbsp sour cream (260 kcal)   Whole milk, 1 c (170 kcal)

Pork chop with fat trimmed off (130 kcal)   Plain potato (90 kcal)   Skim milk, 1 c (80 kcal)

The Chemist's View of Fats

For a precise definition of triglycerides, the major class of dietary lipids, see p. 60.

For a precise definition of phospholipids, a minor class of dietary lipids, and of sterols (including cholesterol), see pp. 69-70.

"Your blood triglycerides are up." If a doctor says this, the patient may be alarmed, perhaps rightly. Most of us are aware nowadays that there is a close relationship between the fats in the blood and the health of the heart. A closer look at the fats will lay the foundation for an understanding of this relationship.

When we speak of fats, we are usually speaking of triglycerides. Almost all (95 percent) of the lipids in the diet are triglycerides. The other two classes of dietary lipids are the phospholipids—of which lecithin is one—and the sterols, including cholesterol. Phospholipids and sterols amount to only 5 percent of the dietary lipids. Because the triglycerides predominate in the diet, the following section focuses on them.

Fats (lipids) in foods:

95 percent triglycerides (synonymous with fats and oils)

5 percent phospholipids (example: lecithin)
sterols (example: cholesterol)

The Triglycerides Triglycerides come in many sizes and several varieties, but they all share a common structure; they all have a "backbone" of glycerol to which three fatty acids are attached. All glycerol molecules are alike, but the fatty acids may vary in two ways: length and degree of saturation.

To understand the fats and the beneficial and harmful effects they have on your body, you must understand their molecular structure. It is not so complicated as it may seem at first. If you follow the few steps of reasoning presented here, you can reap an appreciation for the whole subject—and for its beauty—that you may never otherwise enjoy.

A fatty acid is a chain of carbon atoms with hydrogens attached and with an acid group (COOH) at one end. The fatty acid shown here is acetic acid, the compound that gives vinegar its sour taste:

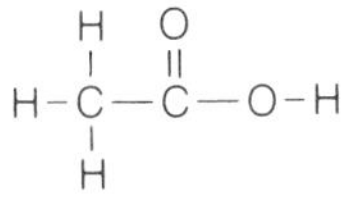

Acetic acid (a 2-carbon fatty acid)

This is the simplest of the fatty acids; the chain is only two carbon atoms long. A longer fatty acid may have four, six, eight (they mostly come in even numbers), or more carbon atoms. Among those common in dairy products are fatty acids that are six to ten carbons long. Butyric acid, which is present in butter, is a four-carbon fatty acid. Fatty acids that predominate in meat and fish are 14 or more carbon atoms long.

To illustrate the characteristics of these fatty acids, let us look at the 18-carbon series. Stearic acid is one of these:

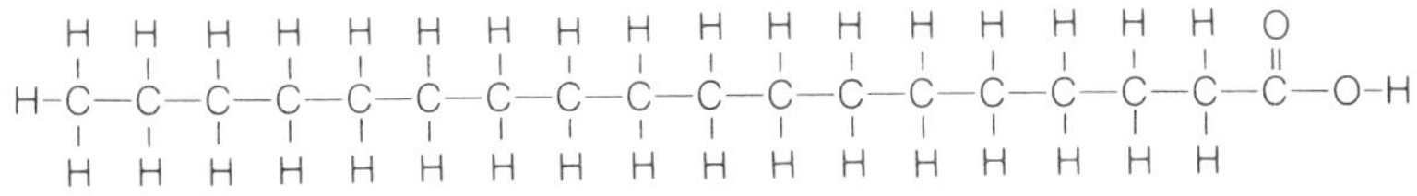

Stearic acid (an 18-carbon fatty acid)

A simpler way to depict this structure:

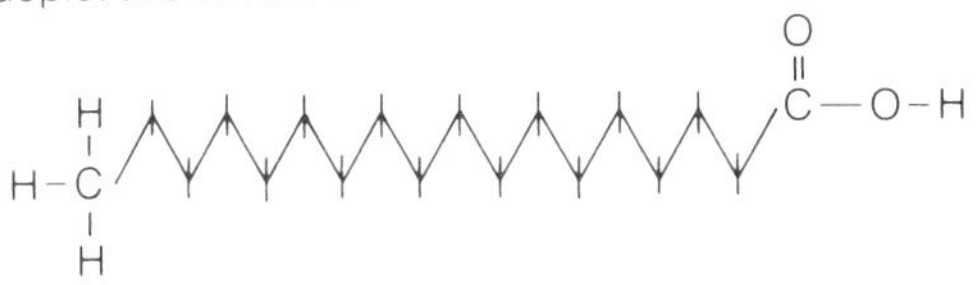

Each "corner" on the zigzag line represents a carbon atom with 2 attached Hs.

Still more simply, the lines representing bonds to the Hs can be left out:

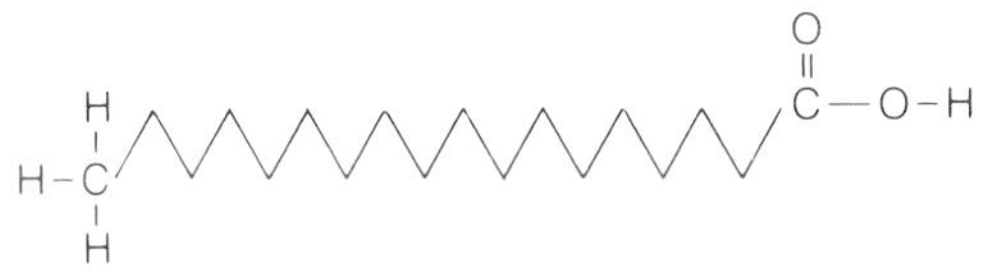

If you count the "corners," you will see that this still represents an 18-carbon fatty acid. This is the way fatty acids will be represented in many of the following diagrams.

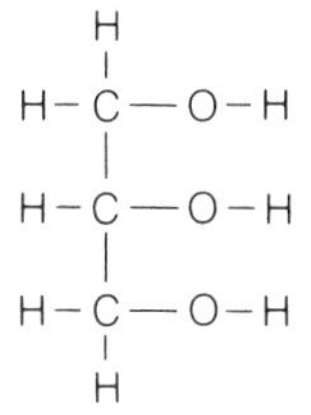

Glycerol

glycerol (GLIS-er-ol): a organic alcohol composed of a 3-carbon chain, each with an alcohol group attached. An alcohol is a compound containing a reactive OH group.

ol = alcohol

acid: a compound that tends to ionize in water solution, releasing H^+ ions. The more H^+ ions that are free in the water, the stronger the acid (see Appendix B).

acid group: the COOH group of an organic acid, which can also be represented

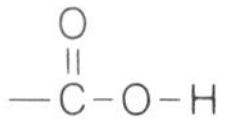

fatty acid: an organic compound composed of a carbon chain with hydrogens attached and an acid group at one end.

triglyceride (try-GLIS-uh-ride): a compound composed of carbon, hydrogen, and oxygen arranged as a molecule of glycerol with three fatty acids attached to it.

tri = three (fatty acids)
glyceride = a compound of glycerol

When a triglyceride forms, three fatty acids attach to a molecule of glycerol. A triglyceride composed of glycerol and three molecules of stearic acid is shown forming below. The resulting structure is called a fat (triglyceride).

1. The first fatty acid approaches the glycerol, a condensation reaction occurs (water is eliminated), and a bond forms between an O on the glycerol and the C at the acid end of the fatty acid.

2. Later, 2 more fatty acids attach themselves to the glycerol by the same means; the resulting structure is a triglyceride.

Formation of a fat (triglyceride).

A fat (triglyceride) that might be found in butter

saturated fatty acid: a fatty acid carrying the maximum possible number of hydrogen atoms—for example, stearic acid. Thus a **saturated fat** is composed of triglycerides in which a majority of the fatty acids are saturated.

fat: a mixture of mixed triglycerides.

impossible structure

People threatened with heart trouble may be told to reduce their intake of saturated fats and to increase their intake of polyunsaturated fats. Cutting out butter and using vegetable oil in its place is one way to do this. The triglyceride just shown is a saturated fat; it is loaded, or saturated, with all the hydrogen (H) atoms it can carry.

Some soft margarines are rich in polyunsaturated fats, triglycerides in which the fatty acids are carrying less than their full complement of hydrogens. To understand them, let us consider stearic acid once more. If we remove two Hs from the middle of the carbon chain, we are left with a compound that looks like this:

The two carbon atoms that formerly held the Hs are, in a sense, empty-handed. Each has a bond that is going unused. Such a compound cannot exist in nature. But an extra bond can be formed between the two carbons to satisfy nature's requirement that every carbon must have four bonds connecting it to other atoms. There is then a "double bond" between them:

Simplified diagram:

Oleic acid

(The same situation exists in the acid group at the end of the chain, where an O is double-bonded to the terminal C. That carbon has its full four bonds, and the oxygen meets its requirement of having two.) The resulting structure is an unsaturated (in this case *mono*unsaturated) fatty acid, oleic acid, which is found abundantly in the triglycerides in olive oil.

The heart patient is advised to eat *poly*unsaturated fats, because they seem to reduce the risk of artery disease. A polyunsaturated fat is a triglyceride in which the fatty acids have two or more points of unsaturation. An example is linoleic acid, which lacks four Hs and has two double bonds:

Simplified diagram:

Linoleic acid, the essential fatty acid

Linoleic acid is found in the triglycerides of most vegetable oils—corn oil, safflower oil, and the like. It is the most common of the polyunsaturated fatty acids in foods and the most important. In fact it is an *essential nutrient*. (We will discuss it further at the end of this section.)

Having looked at three of the most common fatty acids in foods, you can probably anticipate what the others look like. The fourth member of the family of 18-carbon fatty acids is linolenic acid, which has three

monounsaturated fatty acid: a fatty acid that lacks two hydrogen atoms and has one double bond between carbons—for example, oleic acid.

polyunsaturated fatty acid (PUFA): a fatty acid that lacks four or more hydrogen atoms and has two or more double bonds between carbons—for example, linoleic acid (2 double bonds) and linolenic acid (3 double bonds). Thus a **polyunsaturated fat** is composed of triglycerides containing a high percentage of PUFA.

Note: Linoleic acid (18 C, 2 double bonds) should not be confused with linolenic acid (18 C, 3 double bonds). The shorthand way of describing these two fatty acids is 18:2 and 18:3.

double bonds. A similar series of 20-carbon fatty acids exists, as well as a series of 22-carbon fatty acids. These are the long-chain fatty acids. In lesser amounts, medium-chain (14 to 16 Cs) and short-chain (8 to 12 Cs) fatty acids are also present in foods.

To repeat, the fats and oils in foods are mostly (95 percent) triglycerides: glycerol backbones with fatty acids attached. To complete the picture, it only remains to say that any combination of fatty acids is possible in a fat or oil. A mixed triglyceride, one that contains more than one type of fatty acid, is shown here:

A mixed triglyceride typical of those found in foods.

essential nutrient: a compound that cannot be synthesized in the body in amounts sufficient to meet physiological needs. Many nutrients are needed by the body, but the word *essential* refers only to those that must be supplied by eating food.

dermatitis (derm-uh-TIGHT-us): infection or inflammation of the skin evidenced by itching, redness, and various skin lesions.

derma = skin
itis = infection or inflammation

Acetic acid, or acetyl CoA, is formed from glucose (see Chapter 7 and Highlight 7).

Linoleic Acid: The Essential Nutrient   Because the concept of essential nutrients pervades much of nutrition science, let us devote our attention to it for a moment. Why is this fatty acid essential for health, whereas a lack of any of the others would produce no ill effects?

When polyunsaturated fatty acids are missing from the diet, the skin reddens and becomes irritated and the liver develops abnormalities. Adding the fatty acids back to the diet clears up these symptoms. It turns out that what the body cells need is arachidonic acid (20 Cs, four double bonds); you can make this compound for yourself if linoleic acid is supplied in your diet.

The body's cells are equipped with many enzymes that can convert one compound to another. To make body fat or oil—triglycerides—all the enzymes need is a usable food source containing the atoms that triglycerides are composed of: carbon, hydrogen, and oxygen. Glucose does perfectly well. In fact, given an excess of blood glucose (and a filled glycogen storage space), this is precisely what the enzymes do: They cleave the glucose to make the two-carbon compound acetic acid and then combine many acetic acid molecules, with the appropriate alterations, to make long-chain fatty acids. (This is why most fatty acid carbon chains come in even numbers.) But the cells do not possess an enzyme that can arrange the double-bonding of linoleic acid.

Linoleic acid has thus come to be considered "the essential fatty acid,"[1] although arachidonic acid alleviates the dermatitis and, to a

[1] R. B. Alfin-Slater and L. Aftergood, Fats and other lipids, in *Modern Nutrition in Health and Disease*, 5th ed., eds. R. S. Goodhart and M. E. Shils (Philadelphia: Lea and Febiger, 1973), pp. 117-141.

limited extent, linolenic acid also helps. Nearly all diets supply enough linoleic acid to meet the requirement. Deficiencies are usually seen only in infants fed a formula that lacks this nutrient and in hospital patients who have been fed through a vein for prolonged periods using a formula that provides no essential fatty acids. Even in a totally fat-free diet, only 1 tsp (5 g) of corn oil would be sufficient to supply the needed amount of linoleic acid.

A (linoleic acid) →
B (arachidonic acid)

Compound A is the **precursor** of compound B.

The relief of dermatitis by linoleic acid might suggest to the unwary observer that all cases of dermatitis indicate a deficiency of this nutrient. Not so! Dermatitis is, by definition, a skin condition; the word does not imply a single cause. Actually there are more than a hundred body compounds—including other oils, vitamins, minerals, and hormones—that are needed in certain proportions to ensure the health of the skin. A deficiency or imbalance of any of these, caused either by a dietary lack or by failure of the body to produce necessary compounds in the normal way, may create a dermatitis condition. Bacterial and viral infections, allergens, physical agents such as radiation, and chemical irritants also cause dermatitis. There may also be a "psychosomatic" cause, as when excessive nervous activity in the brain (*psyche* means "mind") generates a hormone imbalance that affects the skin (*soma* means "body"). For these reasons, you can't be sure that a symptom is necessarily the result of the one cause that may be familiar to you.

A distinction must be made between a symptom and a disease. A symptom can be alleviated (soothing oils can be applied to the skin to make it feel better, for example), but until you have identified the disease, you cannot achieve a cure. The rule is that if a certain nutrient clears up the symptom, then a deficiency of that nutrient may have been the cause.

allergen (AL-er-gen): an agent that provokes an allergic reaction.

symptom: the outward manifestation of a disease condition.

disease: the impairment or failure of a vital function, due to viral or bacterial infection, lack of an essential nutrient, genetic abnormality, or other causes.

A symptom is not a disease. Prescription of a cure depends on correct diagnosis of the disease.

diagnosis: identification.

You can also be fooled into thinking that a particular food—safflower oil, for example—is essential for healthy skin. Health food stores make millions of dollars a year promoting misconceptions like this. Actually, of course, safflower oil is not essential at all; you need never taste a drop of it all your life. All you need, to avoid a deficiency of linoleic acid, is to eat an ordinary mixed diet; it will inevitably include some polyunsaturated fat. The chance that you will then lack linoleic acid is virtually nil, since it is found in almost all oils (Appendix H).

The distinction between foods and nutrients has been emphasized once before (page 4). The implication that any specific food has magical, miraculous, or curative powers is false.

A FLAG SIGN OF A SPURIOUS CLAIM IS THE IMPLICATION THAT:

Any specific food is needed for any reason.

One way to determine the degree of unsaturation of a fat is to perform a chemical test using iodine to obtain the "iodine number." The higher the iodine number, the greater the degree of unsaturation:

safflower oil = about 140
other vegetable
oils (except
coconut and
palm) = about 110-120
soft
margarines = about 90
olive oil = about 75
hard
margarines = about 70
butter = about 25-40
coconut and
palm "oil" = about 10-15

Oxidation of a fatty acid.

aldehyde (AL-duh-hide): an organic compound containing a CHO group:

$$-\overset{\overset{\text{O}}{\|}}{\text{C}}-\text{H}$$

For more about these additives, see Highlight 13.

Processed Fat Ever since researchers first began to conclude that saturated fats were linked to heart disease and that polyunsaturated fats might be preventive, advertisers have been proclaiming the value of their margarines and oils as "high in polyunsaturates." Indeed, margarines made from vegetable oils and plant foods such as peanut butter do contain unsaturated fatty acids, and this is why they spread and melt more easily than foods that contain saturated fats. But virtually all margarines and all the leading peanut butters are at least partially hardened, and in the process they lose much of their polyunsaturated character.

Unfortunately, however, whatever you may gain in health from polyunsaturated fats, you lose in keeping quality. The more double bonds there are in a fatty acid, the more easily oxygen can destroy it.

Oxygen attacks an unsaturated fatty acid at the double bond.

Result: two aldehydes.

The oxidation of a fatty acid is shown above. An oxygen molecule attacks the double bond and combines with the carbons at that site to yield two aldehydes. Aldehydes smell bad, giving a clue that the product has spoiled. (Other types of spoilage, due to bacterial or mold growth, can occur too.) In general, unsaturated fatty acids are less stable than their saturated counterparts.

Marketers of fat-containing products have three alternatives, none perfect. They may keep the product tightly sealed and under refrigeration—an expensive storage system. The consumer will have to do the same, and most people prefer not to buy a product that spoils readily. Marketers may also protect the fat by adding preservatives and antioxidants, but there are disadvantages to this course too. Finally, they may increase the product's stability by extracting the unsaturated fat and replacing it with a more saturated one, or by chemically hydrogenating it. Either method makes it more solid, which is often desirable. Margarine made from vegetable oils is solid at room temperature because the oils have been partially hydrogenated, and this improves its usefulness for some purposes. Hydrogenation, however, diminishes the margarine's polyunsaturated fat content and possibly, therefore, its health value. Moreover, new evidence suggests that there may be other concerns about hydrogenated oils.

hydrogenation (high-dro-gen-AY-shun): a chemical process by which hydrogens are added to unsaturated or polyunsaturated fats to make them more solid and more resistant to oxidation.

The new evidence on the processed fats began surfacing in the late 1970s, when reports began to appear of an unexpected effect of fat processing. When vegetable oils are partially hydrogenated, some of the fatty acids that remain unsaturated may undergo a change at their double bonds. The significance of this change is still poorly understood and its occurrence would be of no interest to anyone other than the theoretical chemist except for one thing: There is an association between the consumption of processed vegetable fats and the incidence of certain kinds of cancer, and it is possible that the changed fatty acids are responsible for the connection.

At the outset we promised that the chapters of this book would deal with known facts and that the Highlights would take up current controversies. Notice how carefully the statements above are worded: "There is an association" and "it is possible that the changed fatty acids are responsible." These statements are tentative, and the rest is speculation. To learn more about the status of fat/cancer research, turn to Highlight 28.

Meanwhile, it is hoped that your curiosity about the shift in fatty acids has been sufficiently aroused to motivate you to read a little more chemistry. It is actually quite a simple matter.

The change that occurs at a double bond during processing can be understood by way of an analogy. A single bond is like a dowel stick between two blocks. The blocks attached by such a stick can rotate. A double bond is like two dowel sticks between the blocks; the blocks can't rotate. (You may remember discovering these rules while playing with your Tinker Toy set.) The double bond between carbons in an unsaturated fatty acid holds the carbons and hydrogens in a fixed position and determines the shape of the molecule.

Almost all unsaturated fatty acids occur in nature in the *cis* form; that is, the hydrogens on the carbons adjacent to the double bond stick out on the same side of the molecule. During processing, one of the two double bonds may be broken and reformed. As this happens, the groups may rotate so that they become fixed in the *trans* position— across from each other. This changes the shape of the molecule.

cis (sis): same side.

trans: opposite sides.

cis-fatty acid
The Hs are on the same side of the
double bond, forcing the molecule
to assume a horseshoe shape.

trans-fatty acid
The Hs are on opposite sides of
the double bond, forcing the
molecule into an extended position.

One effect of this change is to create a more solid product while still leaving double bonds in the fatty acids—so the manufacturer can still say his product is unsaturated or polyunsaturated. But *trans* fatty acids are not made by the body's cells, and they are rare in foods. It is not clear that our bodies are equipped to deal with large quantities of these *trans* fatty acids; the presence of these unusual molecules in our cells and tissues may create problems.[2] As yet this issue is poorly understood.

It is as frustrating for us to have to write the statement "we don't know" as it is for you to read it. This short discussion of a new finding in lipid research is intended to alert you to new developments that will occur after this book is in print and to help you understand what you read about them. You are urged to withhold judgment regarding the risks of using processed fats and not to jump to conclusions. If you are curious about the possible relationship of diet to cancer, read Highlight 28. It won't give you the answers, but it will help to give you an overview of the whole area and to put these few facts in perspective.

In the meantime, a prudent and practical course is doubtless one of moderation. A principle of wise diet planning is the principle of dilution. Almost any substance—even water, even "natural," unadulterated, unprocessed foods—could be harmful in large quantities. To minimize the probability of accumulating any single substance, choose from a wide variety of foods. In the process, you will maximize the likelihood of obtaining all the nutrients you need for optimum nutrition.

[2]M. G. Enig, R. J. Munn, and M. Keeney, Dietary fat and cancer trends: A critique, *Federation Proceedings* 37 (1978): 2215-2220.

If you wish to avoid using processed fats, you can adopt some additional strategies. Rather than margarine, for example, you can mix warm butter with vegetable oil in equal amounts, producing a spread that is cheaper than butter, spreads well, has the same degree of polyunsaturation as margarine but more linoleic acid, and contains no *trans* fatty acids. The only disadvantage of this spread is that it contains cholesterol (and the question of whether this is a disadvantage is still being debated). As for peanut butter, it is possible to find unhydrogenated varieties on the shelf. The peanut mash and the oil separate readily in these products, but you can stir them back together before using them or pour off the oil for a product lower in kcalories.

Ultimately, if fat processors wish to produce margarines that are free of *trans* fatty acids, they will use an alternative process that hydrogenates double bonds without producing the *cis-trans* change. But because this process is a little more expensive and technically more difficult than the one presently in use, it has not been employed on a wide scale.

How the Body Handles Fat

The body has a problem in digesting and using fats—how to get at them. Substances that are soluble in fat are called water-fearing, and among these substances are, of course, the fats themselves. Fats in any compartment of the digestive tract tend to float to the top of that compartment, clumping together and separating themselves as far as possible from the watery digestive juices. On the other hand, the enzymes that digest fats are water-loving. Water molecules tend to ionize, to separate into positively charged H^+ and negatively charged OH^- ions, both of which attract their opposites. Enzymes also have positively and negatively charged groups on their surfaces, and so they mix comfortably with the ions in water. What the body needs to help mix them together is a substance that is friendly with both water-fearing and water-loving substances. The bile acids meet that need.

Manufactured by the liver and stored in the gallbladder until needed, the bile acids are released into the intestine whenever fat arrives there. Not surprisingly, they are made largely from lipids themselves. The system seems to have been designed for maximum efficiency and balance. The more fat you eat, the more is available to manufacture the bile acids needed to prepare the fat for digestion.

Each molecule of bile acid has at one end an ionized group that is attracted to water and at the other end a fatty acid chain that has an affinity for fat. Just as a skilled hostess will take your hand, draw you away from the company of your old friends, and leave you shaking hands with a new acquaintance, so a molecule of bile acid will attach itself to a lipid molecule in a droplet and draw it into the surrounding water solution where it can meet an enzyme. The process is known as emulsification (see Figure 1).

Water-fearing substances are known to chemists as **hydrophobic**.

hydro = water
phobia = fear

They may also be called **lipophilic**.

lipo = lipid
phile = friend

Water-loving substances are known as **hydrophilic.**

Ionize: see Appendix B.

enzyme: a large protein molecule that facilitates the making or breaking of chemical bonds (in this case the digestion, or breaking). Enzymes are fully defined and described in Chapter 3.

bile: the emulsifying compound manufactured by the liver, stored in the gallbladder, and released into the small intestine when fat is present there. Bile contains no enzymes. Bile appears sometimes in acid form, sometimes in salt form; for our purposes these are interchangeable.

Figure 1   Emulsification of fat by bile. Detergents work the same way (they are also emulsifiers), which is why they are so effective in removing grease from clothes and dishes. Molecule by molecule, the grease is dissolved out of the spot and suspended in the water, where it can be rinsed away. You can guess where the manufacturers of "detergents with enzymes" got their idea.

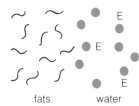
1. Fats and water separate; enzymes (E) are in water:

fats   water

2. Emulsifier has an affinity for both:

emulsifier with fat and water

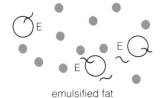
3. Emulsifier helps distribute fats in water, where enzymes can work on them:

emulsified fat

emulsify (ee-MULL-suh-fye): to disperse and stabilize fat droplets in a watery solution.

Now, after all of this preparation, the enzymes can get at the triglycerides. The enzymes digest each triglyceride by removing two of its fatty acids, leaving a monoglyceride, or by removing all three of them, leaving a molecule of glycerol. As with the carbohydrates, the digestive process requires the participation of water, as shown in Figure 2. Finally the monoglycerides, glycerol, and fatty acids pass into the cells of the intestinal wall.

The products of lipid digestion are then released for transport through the body. Some of the larger ones are packaged in protein for this purpose. The protein-wrapped packages, called lipoproteins, are the subject of intensive research as laboratory sleuths seek to detect their structure and their relationships to heart and artery disease. The lipoproteins will appear again later in this chapter and are fully described in Chapter 6.

Lipoproteins: see also pp. 71, 182.

The Phospholipids and Sterols

The preceding pages have been devoted to one of the three classes of lipids, the triglycerides. The other two classes, the phospholipids and sterols, comprise only 5 percent of the lipids in the diet, but they are interesting and important and receive a lot of attention in the press.

The Phospholipids   One of the "magical" nutrients that periodically receives much attention is lecithin. You are told that this nutrient is a major constituent of cell membranes (true), that the functioning of all cells depends on the integrity of their membranes (true, and on a great many other structures), and that you must therefore include large quantities of lecithin in your daily meals (false). You might as well believe that in order to grow healthy hair or to maintain the brain you must eat hair or brains! The enzyme lecithinase in the intestine takes lecithin apart before it passes into the body fluids anyway, so the lecithin you eat does not reach the body tissues intact. The lecithin you need for building cell membranes and for other functions is made from

lecithin (LESS-uh-thin): one of the phospholipids.

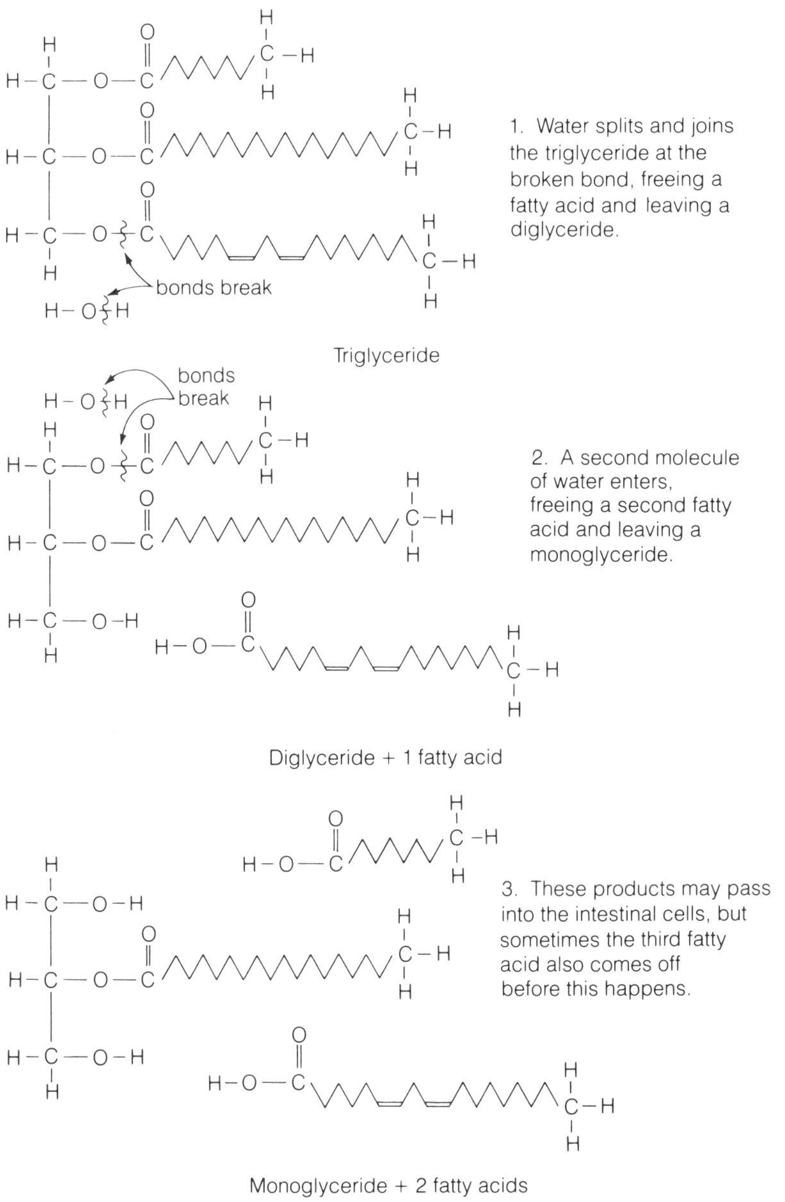

Figure 2   Digestion (hydrolysis) of a fat (triglyceride).

1. Water splits and joins the triglyceride at the broken bond, freeing a fatty acid and leaving a diglyceride.

bonds break

Triglyceride

bonds break

2. A second molecule of water enters, freeing a second fatty acid and leaving a monoglyceride.

Diglyceride + 1 fatty acid

3. These products may pass into the intestinal cells, but sometimes the third fatty acid also comes off before this happens.

Monoglyceride + 2 fatty acids

scratch by the liver. In other words, the lecithins are not essential nutrients.[3]

Like the triglycerides, the lecithins and the other phospholipids have a backbone of glycerol; they are different because they have only two fatty acids attached to them. In place of the third fatty acid is a molecule of choline or a similar compound containing phosphorus (P)

[3]D. C. Fletcher, Lecithin for hyperlipemia: Harmless but useless (questions and answers), *Journal of the American Medical Association* 238 (1977): 64.

phospholipid: a compound similar to a triglyceride but having choline or another phosphorus-containing acid in place of one of the fatty acids.

Choline: see also p. 334.

and nitrogen (N) atoms. A diagram of a lecithin molecule follows (others differ in the nature of the attached fatty acids):

Lecithin.

(The plus charge on the N is balanced by a negative ion—usually chloride—that stays nearby.)

sterol: a compound composed of C, H, and O atoms arranged in rings like those of cholesterol, with any of a variety of side chains attached.

The Sterols: Cholesterol A student observing the chemical structure of cholesterol for the first time once remarked, "Would you believe dimethyl dihydroxy chicken wire?" He was not far wrong; chemists do remarkable "terminologizing." According to them, cholesterol is a member of the cyclopentanoperhydrophenanthrene family, whose particular designation is 3-hydroxy-5,6-cholestene. Never mind. It is not necessary to memorize a structure as complex as this one. But once having viewed it, you can say, "I have seen the structure of cholesterol."

Cholesterol.

cholesterol: one of the sterols.

Cholesterol is not at all an unusual type of molecule. There are dozens of similar ones in the body; all are interesting and important. Among them are the bile acids, the sex hormones (such as testosterone), the adrenocortical hormones (such as cortisone), and vitamin D.

Like lecithins, cholesterol is needed metabolically but is not an essential nutrient. Your liver is manufacturing it now, as you read, at the rate of perhaps 50,000,000,000,000,000 molecules per second. The raw materials that the liver uses to make cholesterol can all be taken from glucose or saturated fatty acids.

All of the carbons in cholesterol come from acetyl CoA (see Chapter 7), which in turn can be derived from several different compounds in the body besides glucose and fatty acids.

After manufacture, cholesterol either is transformed into related compounds like the hormones just mentioned or leaves the liver. The cholesterol that leaves the liver has three possible destinations: (1) It may be excreted, (2) it may be deposited in body tissues, or (3) it may wind up accumulating in arteries and causing artery disease.

How Cholesterol Is Excreted   Most of the cholesterol that the liver makes becomes part of the bile salts, and these are released into the intestine to emulsify fat. After doing their job, some of the bile salts reenter the body with absorbed products of fat digestion. The cholesterol is thus recycled—back to the liver, once again into bile salts, back to the intestine, again into the body, and once more back to the liver.

The recycling of cholesterol and bile is diagramed on p. 185.

Once out in the intestine, however, some of the bile salts can be trapped by certain kinds of dietary fibers, which carry them out of the body with the feces. The excretion of bile salts reduces the total amount of cholesterol remaining in the body.

How Cholesterol Is Deposited in the Body   Some cholesterol leaves the liver packaged with other lipids for transport to the body tissues. These packages are the lipoproteins. The blood carries them through all the body's arteries, and any tissue can extract lipids from them.[4] To pass into the cells, lipids must first cross the artery walls, and it is here that they may be implicated in artery disease.

Both the intestine and the liver make lipoproteins to transport fat.

How Cholesterol Relates to Artery Disease   Artery disease often begins with a condition called atherosclerosis—hardening of the arteries. Atherosclerosis denotes the soft lipid accumulations called plaques on the inner wall of the arteries. As these plaques enlarge, the artery walls lose their elasticity, and the passage through them narrows.

atherosclerosis (ath-er-oh-scler-OH-sis): a type of artery disease characterized by patchy nodular thickenings of the inner walls of the arteries, especially at branch points.

athero = porridge
scleros = hard
osis = too much

Normally, blood surges through the arteries with each beat of the heart, and the arteries expand with each pulse to accommodate the flow. Arteries hardened and narrowed by plaques cannot expand, and so the blood pressure rises. The increased pressure can damage the artery walls further.

In addition to being elastic, the inner walls of the arteries must be glass-smooth so that the blood can move over the surface with as little friction as possible. Clotting of blood is an intricate series of events triggered when the blood moves past a rough surface, such as the edge of a cut. As long as the inner wall remains smooth, clotting will not occur inside the vessel, but if the plaques encroach on the bore of the vessel, the roughness of these plaques can cause the clotting reactions to begin.

plaques (PLACKS): mounds of lipid material mixed with smooth muscle cells and calcium, which are lodged in the artery walls. The same word is also used to describe an entirely different kind of accumulation of material on teeth, which causes dental caries.

[4]Some lipoproteins enter the body cells whole, as described in M. S. Brown and J. L. Goldstein, Receptor-mediated control of cholesterol metabolism, *Science* 191 (1976): 150-154.

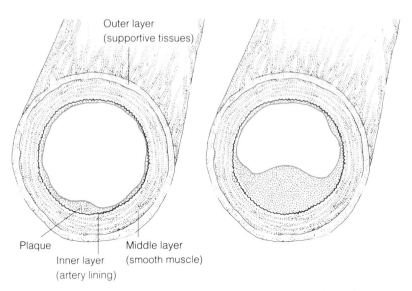

Outer layer
(supportive tissues)

Plaque

Inner layer
(artery lining)

Middle layer
(smooth muscle)

An artery (section) with plaque just beginning to form. Plaques could easily appear in a person as young as 15.

The same artery, years later, almost completely blocked by plaque.

Development of atherosclerosis.

A stationary clot is called a **thrombus**. When it has grown enough to close off a blood vessel, it is a **thrombosis**. A **coronary thrombosis** is the closing off of a vessel that feeds the heart muscle. A **cerebral thrombosis** is the closing off of a vessel that feeds the brain.

coronary = crowning (the heart)
thrombo = clot
cerebrum = part of the brain

A thrombus that breaks loose is an **embolus** (EM-boh-LUSS), and when it causes sudden closure of a blood vessel, it is an **embolism**.

embol = to insert

multifactorial: having many causes.

risk factors: factors known to be related to (or correlated with) a disease but not proven to be causal.

The clot thus formed may linger, attached to a plaque, and gradually grow until it shuts off the blood supply to that portion of the tissue supplied by the artery. That tissue may die slowly and be replaced by scar tissue. Or the clot may break loose and travel along the system until it reaches an artery too small to allow its passage. Then the tissues fed by this particular artery will be robbed of oxygen and nutrients and will die suddenly. Should such a clot lodge in an artery of the heart, we would say that the person had a heart attack. If the clot should lodge in an artery of the brain, we would call this event a stroke.

More than half of the people who die each year in the United States and Canada die of heart and blood vessel disease. The underlying condition that contributes to most of these deaths is atherosclerosis, which is now so widespread that it has been called an epidemic.[5] This disease, which takes its heaviest toll among men in the most productive period of their lives, has been called the number-one killer, and many health agencies have devoted millions of hours to the battle against it.

So far, all that can be said for sure about the causes of atherosclerosis is that it is multifactorial in origin. There are many risk factors—smoking, gender (being male), heredity (including diabetes), high blood pressure, lack of exercise, obesity, stress, high blood cholesterol and triglyceride concentrations, and some 30 others.[6] But it is not at all

[5] Alfin-Slater and Aftergood, 1973.

[6] E. M. N. Hamilton and E. N. Whitney, Controversy 5A: Atherosclerosis, in *Nutrition: Concepts and Controversies* 2d ed. (St. Paul: West, 1982), pp. 132-139.

clear which of these is caused by what; they are only correlations. Chapter 26 delves into the many lines of inquiry. We do not know whether reducing any of the risk factors will actually reduce the risk of dying of heart disease.

An analogy may help you to understand this important point. Suppose that there is an outbreak of crime in a certain city—arson, for example. Someone is setting fires, and the police are after him. It is observed that a certain person, Mr. A, is always seen in the neighborhoods when the fires start, and he is deemed guilty of the crimes. However, it may be that a very sneaky individual, Ms. B, is the real culprit and that Mr. A is only following her around. Mr. A is associated with but not a causal agent in the setting of the fires. The evidence against him is only circumstantial (correlational) unless we can show that whenever he is locked up there are no fires and that whenever he is let out the fires start again. Better yet, we will know for sure if we catch him pouring the gasoline and lighting the match. You may recall that this point has been made before: Correlation is not cause.

In light of all the evidence relating to plaque formation, it seems more than likely that dietary fat (triglycerides) and possibly cholesterol are among the contributing factors in atherosclerosis. Plaques are composed largely of cholesterol, and this cholesterol is manufactured largely from fragments derived from saturated fat. Thus limiting your consumption of fat will do no harm, and it may do some good. And on the assumption that some of the body's cholesterol may come from the diet, it may make sense to limit your cholesterol intake as well. It is on this reasoning that three of the U.S. Dietary Goals are based.

Fat: Goals and Guidelines

The U.S. Dietary Goals make three recommendations relating to lipids in the diet. According to the Goals, you should

● Reduce consumption of fat, so that it contributes only 30 percent of the kcalories in your diet (at present, the U.S. average is 42 percent).

● Reduce saturated fat intake, so that it contributes only 10 percent of total kcalories, letting the remaining fat come from mono- and polyunsaturated fat sources.

● Reduce cholesterol consumption to about 300 mg a day (the present U.S. average is about 600 mg).

When these goals were translated into the more moderate guidelines of 1979 (pp. 32-33), the resulting practical recommendation was simply to avoid excess fat, saturated fat, and cholesterol.

The Fats in Foods

The exchange system presented in Chapter 1 provides a useful means of learning where the fats are in foods. Three of the six lists in the exchange system—the milk list, the meat list, and the fat list—include foods containing appreciable amounts of fat. The items on the milk list contain protein, carbohydrate, and fat; those on the meat list contain protein and fat; and those on the fat list contain only fat. Table 1 shows the fat content of each of these groups of foods in the context of their overall energy-nutrient composition.

Milk List The foods on the milk list contain variable amounts of fat. A cup of skim milk has negligible fat, a cup of 2% fortified milk has 5 g, and a cup of whole milk has 10 g. Users of the exchange system think of this added fat as being equivalent to teaspoons of fat (fat "exchanges"). Thus, a cup of 2% milk is like skim milk plus 1 tsp fat, and a cup of whole milk is like skim milk plus 2 tsp fat.

Foods containing fat:

10 g in 1 c whole milk

1 c skim milk contains	0 g fat
1 c 2% milk contains	5
1 c whole milk contains	10

Table 1. Fat Content of the Six Exchange Groups

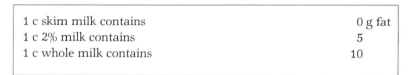

Exchange group	Serving size	Carbohydrate (g)	Protein (g)	Fat (g)	Energy (kcal)
(1) **Skim milk***	1 c	12	8	0	80
(2) Vegetables	1/2 c	5	2	0	25
(3) Fruit	varies	10	0	0	40
(4) **Bread†**	1 slice	15	2	0	70
(5) **Meat‡**	1 oz	0	7	3	55
(6) **Fat**	1 tsp	0	0	5	45

*Skim milk is the standard milk item in diet planning. Planners are encouraged to think of low-fat or whole milk as "milk with added fat." A cup of low-fat milk contains 5 g fat (1 fat exchange), and 1 c whole milk contains 10 g fat (2 fat exchanges).

†Ordinary bread items contain low or negligible fat, but some baked goods, such as baking powder biscuits, have enough added fat to count as an additional fat exchange (see the exchange lists in Appendix L).

‡An ounce of low-fat meat contains 3 g fat. An ounce of medium-fat meat contains 2 1/2 additional grams (1/2 fat exchange), or 5 1/2 g in all. An ounce of high-fat meat contains 5 g more than the lean, or 8 g in all. Peanut butter is included on the meat list because it is a protein-rich food, but it is higher in fat than any other item: 2 tbsp peanut butter are equivalent to 1 oz meat in protein but contain 13 g fat.

The fat in milk is mostly saturated fat; the cholesterol content is 25 mg per cup of whole milk or 7 mg per cup of skim milk. Thus choosing skim in place of whole milk reduces your intakes of both saturated fat and cholesterol.

Meat Lists   The meats have been sorted into three lists depending on their fat content. An ounce of lean meat has 3 g of fat, an ounce of medium-fat meat has about 2 1/2 g more or 5 1/2 g total, and an ounce of high-fat meat has 8 g of fat. Peanut butter, which is a protein-rich food grouped with meat, has 15 1/2 g of fat per 2-tbsp serving.

1 oz lean meat contains	3 g fat
1 oz medium-fat meat contains	5 1/2
1 oz high-fat meat contains	8
2 tbsp peanut butter contains	15 1/2

3 g in 1 oz lean meat

All of these items are equivalent in protein content, however. One can be exchanged or traded for another in a menu without changing the amount of protein that is delivered.

A person studying the meat list for the first time may be surprised to note how many fat kcalories are in meat. An ounce of lean meat supplies 28 kcal from its protein and 27 kcal from its fat. An ounce of high-fat meat supplies the same number—28 kcal—from protein but 72 kcal from fat. Two tablespoons of peanut butter, also with 28 kcal from protein, supply 117 kcal from fat! Thus meat, which is often thought of as a protein food, actually contains more fat energy than protein energy and is an unexpectedly fattening food, often accounting for the excess weight that meat eaters tend to gain.

1 oz = about 30 g
An ounce (30 g) of lean meat contains 5 g protein and 3 g fat. The rest, of course, is largely water.

Note that the unit by which meat is measured in this system is only an ounce. To use this system you need to be aware of serving sizes. An egg is like one ounce of meat. A hamburger is usually three or four ounces. A dinner steak may be six or eight ounces or even larger.

The fats in meats and eggs are mostly saturated; those in poultry and fish have a better balance between saturated and polyunsaturated fats. (A rank listing of fats from most to least saturated is presented in Appendix G.) As for cholesterol, the foods that contain the highest amounts are such organ meats as liver and kidneys and such shellfish as lobster, oysters, and shrimp. Lower but still significant levels of cholesterol are contained in beef, ham, lamb, veal, and pork, followed by poultry and fish. (The cholesterol contents of foods are also presented in Appendix G.) As a general rule, however, a person wishing to reduce cholesterol and saturated fat intake could accomplish both objectives by eating less meat and more poultry and fish (except shellfish).

Fat List   In addition to the obvious items (butter, margarine, and oil), this list includes bacon, olives, and avocados. These foods are grouped together because the amount of lipid they contain makes them essentially pure fat contributors. An eighth of an avocado or one slice of bacon contains as much fat as a pat of butter, and like butter, they contain negligible protein and carbohydrate. Hence when you eat bacon you are not eating a protein food; you are eating a fat food.

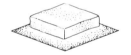

5 g in a pat of butter or margarine

1 tsp butter or margarine (or any other serving of food listed on the fat list) contributes:	5 g fat

Saturated fats have a high melting point and are solid at room or body temperature.

Polyunsaturated fats have a low melting point and are liquid at room or body temperature.

A rule of thumb in determining the degree of saturation of a fat is to observe how hard it is at room temperature. Chicken fat is softer than pork fat, which is softer than beef tallow. Of the three, beef tallow is the most and chicken fat the least saturated. The double bonds in polyunsaturated fats make them melt more readily. Generally speaking, vegetable and fish oils are rich in polyunsaturates, whereas the harder fats—animal fats—are more saturated.

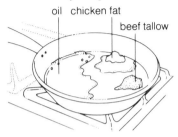

oil   chicken fat

beef tallow

The most polyunsaturated fat melts soonest.

If you wish to make choices consistent with the recent goals or guidelines, you should learn how to read food labels. But beware: Words like *vegetable fat* and *unsaturated fat* can be used to mislead you. Not all vegetable oils are polyunsaturated. Coconut oil, for example, is often used in nondairy creamers, and coconut oil is a saturated fat. Vegetable oils that are hydrogenated may have lost their polyunsaturated character. Another exception to the rule is olive oil, widely used in salad dressings and in Greek and Italian foods. The predominant fatty acid in olive oil is the *mono*unsaturated fatty acid oleic acid. Thus olive oil can claim to be *un*saturated but not to be *poly*unsaturated.

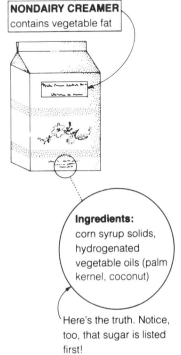

NONDAIRY CREAMER
contains vegetable fat

Ingredients:
corn syrup solids, hydrogenated vegetable oils (palm kernel, coconut)

Here's the truth. Notice, too, that sugar is listed first!

Estimating Fat with the Exchange System   The values presented above provide a way to estimate the amount of fat eaten at a meal or in a day. Two reminders are needed. First, fat is often hidden in cooked vegetables. As a rule of thumb, vegetables served with butter or margarine can be assumed to contain one fat exchange (1 tsp) per half-cup serving. Second, some baked goods also contain appreciable fat; these are listed on the bread list in Appendix L.

Using these values, let us see how much fat was provided by the day's meals described on page 41. Adding up the meat exchanges for the egg, peanut butter, and steak; taking into account the extra fat in these meats, the whole milk, and the shortcake biscuit; adding the fat used in frying the egg and flavoring the beans and potato; and finally adding a fat exchange for the heavy cream—we reach a total of 109 g fat for the day:

Breakfast	Exchanges	Grams fat
1 egg fried in 1 tsp fat	1 meat + 1/2 fat	5 1/2
1 piece toast with 1 tsp margarine	1 fat	5

Lunch		
2 slices bread		
2 tbsp peanut butter	1 meat + 2 1/2 fat	15 1/2
2 tsp jelly		
1 c milk	2 fat	10

Dinner		
6-oz steak	6 meat + 6 fat	48
1/2 c green beans served with		
1 tsp margarine	1 fat	5
1 c mashed potato served with		
1 tsp margarine	1 fat	5

Dessert		
2-inch diameter biscuit	1 fat	5
3/4 c strawberries		
1 tbsp heavy cream	1 fat	5
6 tsp sugar		
	Total	104 g fat

The day's meals thus supplied about 936 kcal from fat (9 times 104). The day's total from all these foods was about 1,930 kcal, so this eater consumed about 50 percent of her kcalories from fat.

In addition to facilitating calculations of this kind, the exchange lists divide fats into two classes—saturated and polyunsaturated—to aid in meal planning for the diabetic. The importance of being aware of the quality of dietary fat as well as its quantity must be abundantly evident by now.

Each culture has its own favorite food sources of fats and oils. In Canada, rapeseed oil is popular and is enjoying increasing use. The peoples of the Mediterranean (Greeks, Italians, and Spaniards) rely heavily on olive oil, which is high in monounsaturates, and the Orientals use the polyunsaturated oil of soybeans. Jewish cookery traditionally employs chicken fat, whereas U.S. Southerners rely heavily on pork fat—lard and bacon. The saturated fat consumption of blacks is cause for concern among health authorities who note a high incidence of hypertensive heart disease among these people. This high rate of heart disease may be diet-related, genetically caused, or both.

[7]Y. K. Seedat and J. Reddy, A study of 1000 South African nonwhite hypertensive patients, *South African Medical Journal* 48 (1974): 816-820.

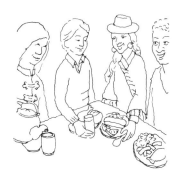

hypertension: high blood pressure. This problem may also be related to salt (sodium) intake;[7] thus the Dietary Goals and the Guidelines recommend limiting salt (see Chapter 14).

Summing Up

Lipids in the body serve as a major energy reserve and also provide structural material for many tissues; in specific locations body fat protects organs from heat, cold, and mechanical shock. The oxidation of a pound of human body fat supplies 3,500 kcal to meet energy needs.

The lipids are known familiarly as the fats and oils. In foods they are not soluble in water but serve as a solvent themselves for the fat-soluble vitamins and for the aromatic compounds that give foods their flavor and aroma. About 95 percent of them are triglycerides, compounds composed of glycerol with three fatty acids attached. The fatty acids may be long-, medium-, or short-chain fatty acids, and they may be saturated or mono- or polyunsaturated. Triglycerides are classed by the nature of the fatty acids they contain. For example, a triglyceride containing polyunsaturated fatty acids is a polyunsaturated fat. The other 5 percent of dietary lipids are the phospholipids and sterols, cholesterol being a member of the latter group.

During digestion, the triglycerides must be emulsified (dispersed in water) by bile before they can be hydrolyzed by enzymes to diglycerides and then to monoglycerides and fatty acids, which are absorbed into the intestinal cells. Phospholipids also undergo hydrolysis, but cholesterol is absorbed virtually as is. All three classes of lipid are carried in lipoproteins that circulate in the body fluids.

Deficiencies of essential fatty acids manifest themselves in dermatitis and liver abnormality. The symptoms can be cleared up by administering linoleic acid, which has therefore come to be called "the" essential fatty acid.

Food fats containing unsaturated fatty acids spoil easily but may be processed (hydrogenated) to make them less vulnerable to oxidation. In the processing, *trans* fatty acids may be formed, whose effects on health are as yet unknown.

Cholesterol is normally made in the body by the liver and is transported to all tissues, where it is picked up and used for cell functions. Abnormal deposition of cholesterol in artery walls, together with smooth-muscle cells and other constituents, forms plaques characteristic of atherosclerosis, the major killer disease of the developed countries. Research shows atherosclerosis to be multifactorial in origin, with smoking and high blood pressure among the major risk factors; a diet high in saturated fat and cholesterol is also implicated. The U.S. Dietary Goals and the Guidelines that evolved from them suggest limiting intakes of total fat, saturated fat, and cholesterol as a preventive measure.

In the exchange system, the foods that contribute fat to the diet are found mainly on the milk list, the meat list, and the fat list. The size of a milk exchange is a cup; an exchange of 2% milk contains 5 g fat, and an exchange of whole milk contains 10 g fat. For meat, the size of an exchange is an ounce or the equivalent; an exchange of lean meat contains 3 g, of medium-fat meat 5 1/2 g, and of high-fat meat 8 g of fat. An exchange (2 tbsp) of peanut butter contains 15 1/2 g fat. For fat itself, the exchange size is a teaspoon or the equivalent, and one fat exchange contains 5 g of fat. When fat is added to vegetables, the amount is usually 5 g per half-cup serving. Some baked goods also contain fat (see the bread list in Appendix L).

For the most part, meats and animal fats are the main contributors of saturated fat to the diet. Foods containing cholesterol include most notably the organ meats, shellfish, and eggs, with meats and other animal fats also containing significant amounts. Vegetable oils, with a few exceptions, contain more polyunsaturated fats, and no plant product contains cholesterol.

To Explore Further

Recommended references on all nutrition topics are listed in Appendix J. For practical guidelines on diet, useful in helping to control fat intake, we especially recommend this paperback:

● Mayer, J. *Fats, Diet and Your Heart.* Norwood, N.J.: Newspaperbooks, 1976.

The American Heart Association also puts out a multitude of useful and informative materials on both prevention and treatment of heart and artery disease. Check your phone book for the local office or write to the National Center, 7320 Greenville Avenue, Dallas, TX 75231.

The controversy over whether dietary fat and cholesterol affect heart disease deaths has been so noisy and lasted so long that it has a name of its own: the diet-heart controversy. Both sides are summed up in a pair of short articles, one by the editor of the *Journal of the American Medical Association* (he says diet has no effect) and the other by the American Heart Association (which says it does):

● Mann, G. V. Diet-heart: End of an era. In *Current Concepts in Nutrition.* Boston: Massachusetts Medical Society, 1979, pp. 104-121.

● Nutrition Committee, American Heart Association. Diet and coronary heart disease: Another view. In *Current Concepts*, 1979 (same as above), pp. 122-131.

Most of the May-June, 1980, issue of *Nutrition Today* was also devoted to this controversy. The cover bore a picture of the eruption of Mount St. Helens and suggested that the diet-heart debate was as violent as that famous volcano.

The interesting and optimistic view that people do respond to suggestions and make health-promoting changes in their lifestyle is presented in:

● Walker, W. J. Changing United States life-style and declining vascular mortality: Cause or coincidence? *New England Journal of Medicine* 297 (1977):163-165.

You may wish to read more about the relationship of exercise to heart attack risk:

● Paffenbarger, R. S., Wing, A. L., and Hyde, R. T., Current exercise and heart attack risk, *Cardiac Rehabilitation* 10 (2) (1979):1-4.

An entire issue of a monthly newsletter for physicians and nutritionists was devoted to an update on the diet-heart controversy: *Nutrition and the MD*, April 1979.

The following free pamphlet was recommended in the April 1979 issue of *Nutrition and the MD*:

● *Dietary Management of Hyperlipoproteinemia: A Handbook for Physicians and Dietitians*, DHEW publication no. 73-110, available from the Office of Information, National Heart and Lung Institute, Bethesda, MD 20014.

The following pamphlet on dietary management of hyperlipidemia can be obtained free from your local Heart Association office:

● *Dietary Modification to Control Hyperlipidemia*, Ad Hoc Committee for Medical and Community Programs, American Heart Association, reprinted from *Circulation* 58 (1978):381A.

Some 400 pages of controversy over the diet-heart issue were published in:

● *Proceedings of the Conference on the Decline in Coronary Heart Disease Mortality*, U.S. Department of Health, Education and Welfare (NIH publication no. 79-1610, May 1979).

HIGHLIGHT 2

AN OPTIONAL CHAPTER
The Wisdom of the Body

The full development and ample expression of the living organism are ... made possible by such automatic regulation of the routine necessities that the functions of the brain which subserve intelligence and imagination ... are set free for the use of these higher services.

WALTER B. CANNON

Highlight 1 showed that a person wishing to affect a nutrient in the body like blood glucose or bone calcium stores could not do it merely by adding glucose or calcium to the diet. The body's internal regulatory systems override outside influences. To achieve the desired effect, you can't simply push material into the body; rather, you have to find a way to affect the regulatory system. To give just one example, feeding glucose won't effectively raise blood glucose for long because the body responds with the hormone insulin, which lowers it again; but feeding protein may raise it because the body responds by producing the hormone glucagon, which acts to raise blood glucose.

This Highlight is offered as an optional chapter for readers who want to enhance their understanding of the body's ways of coordinating its activities. It presents a brief summary of the workings of the body's two major regulatory systems—the hormones and the nerves—as they are presently understood. Research into both systems is very active these days, and any of the information you read here may change in the future.

The Hormones

The hormones insulin and glucagon have already been introduced. Insulin lowers blood glucose by driving it into cells and promoting its conversion to glycogen and fat; glucagon raises it by enhancing the breakdown and release of stored glycogen and the conversion of amino acids to glucose. These hormones work rapidly and they work on cells all over the body as hormones typically do. They can do this because they are secreted directly into the blood by their producing organs—the endocrine glands—so they reach all cells without fail.

insulin, glucagon: see pages 19, 21.

hormone: a chemical messenger. Hormones are secreted in response to altered conditions by a variety of endocrine glands in the body. Each affects one or more specific target tissues or organs and elicits specific responses to restore normal conditions.

endocrine: with reference to a gland, one that secretes its product directly into (*endo*) the blood, like the pancreas cells that produce insulin. An **exocrine** gland secretes its product(s) out (*exo*) of the blood through a duct into a cavity; the sweat glands of the skin and the enzyme-producing glands of the pancreas are both examples. The pancreas is therefore both an endocrine and an exocrine gland.

Endocrinology is the study of hormones and their effects.

The **pituitary** gland in the brain has two parts — the **anterior** (front) and the **posterior** (hind) part.

adrenocorticotropin: so named because it stimulates (*trope*) the adrenal cortex.

follicle: that part of the female reproductive system where the ovary lies and eggs are produced.

luteinizing: so called because the follicle turns orange as it matures.
lutein = an orange pigment

prolactin: so named because it promotes (*pro*) the production of milk (*lacto*).

melanocyte (MEL-an-oh-cite): a cell containing the pigment melanin.
cyte = cell

cortex: The adrenal gland, like the pituitary, has two parts, in this case an outer portion (*cortex*) and an inner core (*medulla*).

The hormones, the glands they originate in, and their target organs and effects are described in the next sections. All the hormones you might be interested in are included, but only a few are discussed in detail. The object is not to present a long list to be memorized but to give you a general idea of the territory so you can begin to find your way around in it. (The study of physiology requires that you learn the details; the beginning study of nutrition requires knowing the details are there.)

The whole picture is of a complex system in which many of the parts interact with each other. Wherever you start, you will be led to many other places. For example, several hormones are produced in the anterior pituitary gland in the brain. All of these are regulated by hormones produced in another part of the brain, the hypothalamus. Furthermore, each of the pituitary gland hormones has effects on the production of compounds elsewhere in the body. Some of these compounds are also hormones that will affect still other body parts. Like an idea that originates in one person's mind and ends up altering the course of history, a hormone may travel far from its point of origin and ultimately have profound, even unexpected, effects. The reader who takes the time, now, to merely read through these sections will develop a "feel" for the way the body manages its affairs that no amount of guesswork could approximate.

Hormones of the Pituitary Gland and Hypothalamus The anterior pituitary gland produces the hormones:

- adrenocorticotropin (ACTH)
- thyroid-stimulating hormone (TSH)
- growth hormone (GH)
- follicle-stimulating hormone (FSH)
- luteinizing hormone (LH)
- prolactin
- melanocyte-stimulating hormone (MSH)

Each of these hormones acts on one or more target organs and elicits a characteristic response. ACTH acts on the adrenal cortex, promoting the making and release of its hormones. TSH acts on the thyroid gland, promoting the making and release of thyroid hormone. GH works on all tissues, promoting growth, fat breakdown, and the formation of antibodies. FSH works on the ovaries in the female, promoting their maturation, and on the testes in the male, promoting sperm formation. LH also acts on the ovaries, forwarding their maturation, the making of progesterone and estrogens, and ovulation; and on the testes, promoting the making and release of androgens (male hormones). Prolactin, secreted in the female after she has borne a baby, acts on the mammary glands to stimulate their growth and the making of milk. Finally, MSH acts on the pigment cells, promoting the making and dispersal of pigment.

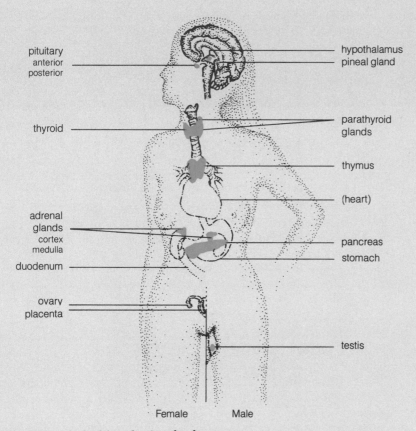

pituitary
anterior
posterior

hypothalamus
pineal gland

thyroid

parathyroid
glands

thymus

(heart)

adrenal
glands
cortex
medulla

duodenum

pancreas

stomach

ovary
placenta

testis

Female   Male

Figure 1 The body's endocrine glands.

The array of actions just described is impressive. Whatever controls them all had better be sensitive to the body's local needs so that only the appropriate actions will take place. The controls are sensitive and very specific: Each of the seven hormones itemized above has one or more signals that turn it on and another (or others) that turn it off.

Among the controlling signals are several hormones from the brain center known as the hypothalamus:

- corticotropin-releasing hormone (CRH), which promotes release of ACTH. This is itself turned on by stress and off by ACTH when enough has been released.

- TSH-releasing hormone (TRH), which promotes release of TSH. This is turned on by large meals or low body temperature.

- GH-releasing hormone (GRH), which is turned on by insulin.

- FSH/LH-releasing hormone (FSH/LH-RH), which is turned on in the female by nerve messages or low estrogen and in the male by low testosterone.

- GH-inhibiting hormone (GIH or somatostatin), which inhibits the release of GSH and interferes with the release of TSH. This is turned

somatostatin (GIH): the opposite of **somatotropin.**

somato = body
statin = keep the same
tropin = make more

hypothalamus: a brain region (see Figure 2) that is connected by a channel to the pituitary and can produce many hormones in response to signals from it or from other body conditions.

hypo = below
thalamus = another brain region

Hormones that are turned off by their own effects are said to be regulated by **negative feedback**. For example, when a pituitary gland hormone has caused the release of a substance from a target organ, that substance itself switches off the original hormone signal (that is, it feeds back, negatively).

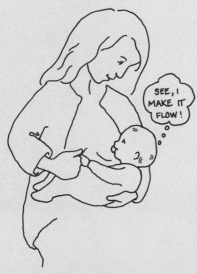

antidiuretic hormone (ADH): the hormone that prevents water loss in urine (also **vasopressin**).

anti = against
di = through
ure = urine
vaso = blood vessels
pressin = pressure

oxytocin: the hormone of childbirth.

oxy = quick
tocin = childbirth

on by hypoglycemia and/or exercise, and is rapidly destroyed by body tissues so that it does not accumulate.

● prolactin-release-inhibiting hormone (PIH), which is turned on by high prolactin levels and off by estrogen, testosterone, and suckling (by way of nerve messages).

● MSH-release-inhibiting hormone (MIH), which is turned on by melatonin.

Let's stop here a minute to examine some of these controls. PIH, for example, responds to high prolactin levels (remember, prolactin promotes the making of milk). High prolactin levels will ensure that milk is made and — by calling forth PIH — will ensure that they don't get too high. But when the infant is suckling — and creating a demand for milk — then PIH is not allowed to work (suckling turns off PIH). The consequence: Prolactin remains high and milk manufacture continues. Demand from the infant thus directly adjusts the infant's supply of milk. This example shows not only how the need is met but also illustrates the cooperation between nerves and hormones that achieves this effect.

As another example, take CRH. Stress, perceived in the brain and relayed to the hypothalamus, switches on CRH. CRH, on arriving at the pituitary, switches on ACTH. Then ACTH acts on its target organ, the adrenal cortex, which responds by producing and releasing stress hormones, and the stress response is under way. Events cascading from there involve every body cell and many other hormones (see Highlight 6).

You may wonder why so many steps are required to set the stress response in motion. Having many steps makes it possible for the body to fine-tune the stress response, because control can be exerted at each step.

The two examples just given provide the smallest hint of what the body can do in response to two different stimuli — producing milk in response to an infant's need, and gearing up for stress when under threat. Other examples will appear in later chapters, but the full array of hormones should be presented here to display the entire territory.

Two hormones produced by the posterior pituitary gland are:

● vasopressin, or antidiuretic hormone (ADH)

● oxytocin

Vasopressin promotes contraction of arteries and acts on the kidney to prevent water from being excreted. It is turned on whenever the blood volume is depleted, or the blood pressure is low, or the salt concentration in the blood is too high. It is turned off by correction of these deviations from normal. Oxytocin is produced in response to reduced progesterone levels, suckling, or the stretching of the cervix, and acts on two target organs. One, the uterus, contracts in response; the other, the mammary glands, eject milk. Oxytocin is turned off by raised progesterone.

So far, only one large group of hormones has been described, those of the pituitary and hypothalamus. A grand total of twenty-three more remain to be described here, and the descriptions will necessarily be brief.

Hormones that Regulate Energy Metabolism   Hormones produced by a number of different glands have effects on energy metabolism:

- insulin, from the pancreas beta cells
- glucagon, from the pancreas alpha cells
- thyroxin, from the thyroid gland
- norepinephrine and epinephrine, from the adrenal medulla
- growth hormone (GH), from the anterior pituitary (already mentioned)
- glucocorticoids, from the adrenal cortex

Insulin is turned on by many stimuli including raised blood glucose, high levels of its opposing hormone glucagon, and several other hormones; and acts on all cells to increase glucose and amino acid uptake into cells and to promote the secretion of GRH. Glucagon responds to low blood glucose and to its opposing hormone insulin and acts on the liver to promote the breakdown of glycogen to glucose, the conversion of amino acids to glucose, and the release of glucose. Thyroxin responds to TSH and acts on many cells to increase their metabolic rate, growth, and heat production. The hormones norepinephrine and epinephrine respond to stimulation by sympathetic nerves and produce reactions in many cells that facilitate the body's readiness for fight or flight: increased heart activity, blood vessel constriction, breakdown of glycogen and glucose, raised blood glucose levels, and fat breakdown; they also influence the secretion of the many hormones from the hypothalamus that exert control on the body's other systems.

Every body part is affected by these hormones. Different hormones each have unique effects, and hormones that oppose each other can be produced in carefully regulated amounts, so each part can respond to the exact degree that is appropriate to the occasion.

Hormones that Adjust Other Body Balances   Three hormones are involved in moving calcium in and out of the body's storage deposits in the bones:

- calcitonin (CT), from the thyroid gland
- parathyroid hormone (PTH), from the parathyroid gland
- vitamin D, from the kidney

One of calcitonin's target tissues is the bones, which respond by storing calcium from the bloodstream whenever blood calcium rises above the normal range. Calcitonin also acts on the kidney to increase excretion of

progesterone: see page 88.

Norepinephrine and epinephrine were formerly called noradrenaline and adrenaline; also known as the *catecholamines* or *stress hormones.*

glucocorticoid: hormone from the adrenal cortex affecting the body's management of glucose.

gluco = glucose
corticoid = from the cortex

calcitonin: so called because it regulates (tones) calcium level.

parathyroid: Named for their location, the four parathyroid glands nestle in the surface layers of the two thyroid lobes in the neck.

para = beside, next to

erythropoietin (eh-REE-throw-POY-eh-tin): named for its red-blood-cell-making function.

erythro = red (blood cell)
poiesis = creating (like poetry)

relaxin: the hormone of late pregnancy.

cervix: the circular muscle that guards the opening of the uterus. When a baby is about to be born, the cervix begins to stretch.

cervic = neck

renin (REEN-in): a blood-pressure-raising enzyme from the kidney, which works by activating angiotensin.

ren = kidney

aldosterone: a hormone from the adrenal gland, involved in blood pressure regulation.

aldo = aldehyde

angiotensin: a hormone involved in blood pressure regulation.

angio = blood vessels
tensin = pressure

Vitamin D, once thought to be a nutrient, is now viewed as a hormone, because it is produced in one body organ and regulates others. For details, see Chapter 11.

both calcium and phosphorus in the urine. Parathyroid hormone responds to the opposite condition—lowered blood calcium—and acts on three targets: the bones, which release stored calcium into the blood; the kidney, which slows its excretion of calcium; and the intestine, which increases its calcium absorption. Vitamin D acts with parathyroid hormone and is essential for the absorption of calcium in the intestine.

Another hormone has effects on blood-making activity:

● erythropoietin, from the kidney

Erythropoietin is responsive to oxygen depletion of the blood and to anemia, and acts on the bone marrow to stimulate its making of red blood cells.

Another hormone, special for pregnancy, is:

● relaxin, from the ovary

This hormone is secreted in response to the raised progesterone and estrogen levels of late pregnancy, and acts on the cervix and pelvic ligaments to allow them to stretch so that they can accommodate the birth process without strain.

Other agents also help regulate blood pressure:

● renin (enzyme), from the kidney, in cooperation with angiotensin in the blood
● aldosterone, a hormone from the adrenal cortex

Renin responds to a reduced blood supply experienced by the kidney, and acts in several ways. Encountering the inactive form of angiotensin in the bloodstream, it converts this molecule to active angiotensin I and then to the very active angiotensin II. The angiotensins constrict the blood vessels, thus raising the blood pressure. They also stimulate thirst, leading to increased water intake, another way of raising the blood pressure. The angiotensins also cause the kidneys to retain water and salt. Thus the angiotensins increase blood pressure by several means at once.

Renin and angiotensin also stimulate the adrenal cortex to secrete the hormone aldosterone. This hormone's target organ is also the kidney, which responds by excreting less sodium and, with it, less water. The effect is to retain more water in the bloodstream — thus, again, raising the blood pressure.

In most instances, hormones work to improve the body's functioning. The example just given illustrates this point. You *need* your blood pressure to rise whenever the blood volume falls, because blood must continue to be delivered to every body organ at all times.

The body's pressure-raising response to lowered blood volume is an adaptive response that takes care of accidental injuries and all situations in which there is blood loss. Water substitutes for blood in the circulatory system, enabling the heart to keep pumping this precious fluid to all the organs that depend on it for their life.

However, hormones can be led astray by circumstances the body is not accustomed to dealing with. Take raised sodium, for example. In nature the human animal (our cave-dwelling ancestor) would seldom run across a dose of salt large enough to raise body sodium, but loss of water, causing raised sodium, would often be experienced. The adaptive response would be to retain water and decrease sodium excretion, and this is what the renin-angiotensin mechanism accomplishes. The body has evolved slowly, over time, to deal with the variety of circumstances it has experienced.

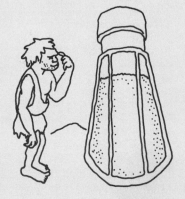

Salt in abundance in foods is a relatively new factor in the human environment. Not everyone's kidneys can excrete the sodium of salt as fast as we can consume it, and when the kidneys can't keep up, blood pressure rises undesirably high. This would benefit the person who had high blood sodium caused by loss of blood and body fluids, because it would keep blood flowing to the body parts that need it. But in the person who has high blood sodium from overeating salt, raised blood pressure confers no benefit. In fact, it causes wear and tear on the heart and can shorten life.

The subject of sodium and heart disease is treated extensively in Part Five; this digression is intended to make the point that sometimes the hormones can be fooled. The "new" substances, like pure salt and pure sugar, which have only been widely consumed for a hundred years or so, may disturb the body's balances. If a person already has a disorder, such as an underlying tendency towards high blood pressure, then salt restriction may be advisable. Sugar, too, may be hard for some people's hormone systems to handle. Some authorities believe that large quantities of sugar play a causal role in the disorders of glucose metabolism: hypoglycemia and diabetes.

There remain three sets of hormones and hormone-like substances to be discussed. These are the gastrointestinal hormones, the sex hormones, and the prostaglandins.

The Gastrointestinal Hormones   Three hormones are known to be produced in the stomach and intestines in response to the presence of food or the components of food:

- gastrin, from the stomach and duodenum
- cholecystokinin, from the duodenum
- secretin (enterogastrone), from the duodenum

gastrointestinal (GI): having to do with the stomach and intestines.

gastro = stomach

For more about the GI hormones, see Chapter 5.

Gastrin stimulates the stomach to make and release its acid and digestive juices and to move and churn its contents actively. Cholecystokinin signals the gall bladder and pancreas to release their contents into the intestine to aid in digestion. Secretin calls forth acid-neutralizing bicarbonate from the pancreas into the intestine, and slows the action of the stomach and its secretion of acid and digestive juices. These hormones are dealt with in more detail in Chapter 5.

The Sex Hormones   The three major sex hormones are:

- testosterone, from the testes
- estrogens, from the ovary
- progesterone, from the ovary's corpus luteum in preparation for, and during, pregnancy

Testosterone, in the male, in response to LH (remember LH?) acts on all the tissues that are involved in male sexuality and promotes their sexual development and maintenance. Estrogens, in response to both FSH and LH, do the same thing in the female. Progesterone, in response to raised LH and prolactin, acts on the uterus and mammary glands, stimulating them to grow and develop.

The Prostaglandins   The prostaglandins are a group of hormones produced by many different body organs with a multitude of diverse effects. More recently discovered than the other hormones, they don't have descriptive names but are designated by letters and numbers: E_1, E_2, and so forth. One, produced in the kidney in response to angiotensin

testosterone: a steroid hormone from the testes. The steroids, as explained in Chapter 2, are chemically related to, and some are derived from, the lipid cholesterol.

sterone = a steroid hormone

estrogens: hormones responsible for the menstrual cycle and other female characteristics.

oestrus = the egg-making cycle
gen = gives rise to

progesterone: the hormone of gestation (pregnancy).

pro = promoting
gest = gestation (pregnancy)
sterone = a steroid hormone

prostaglandin: so named because the first of those hormones to be discovered was found in association with the prostate gland.

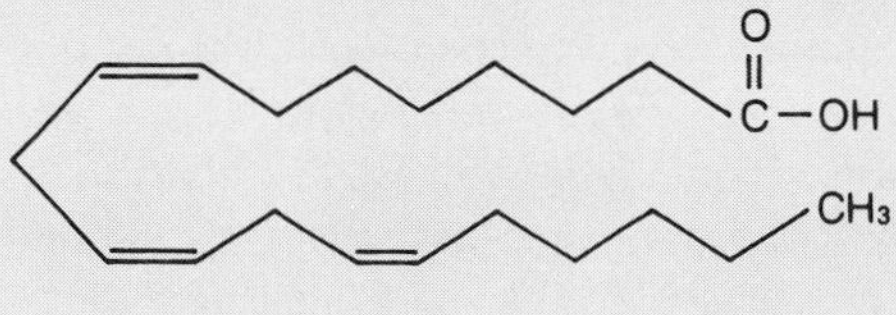

A 20-carbon essential fatty acid related to linolenic acid, from which some of the prostaglandins are made. Notice the similarity of structures:

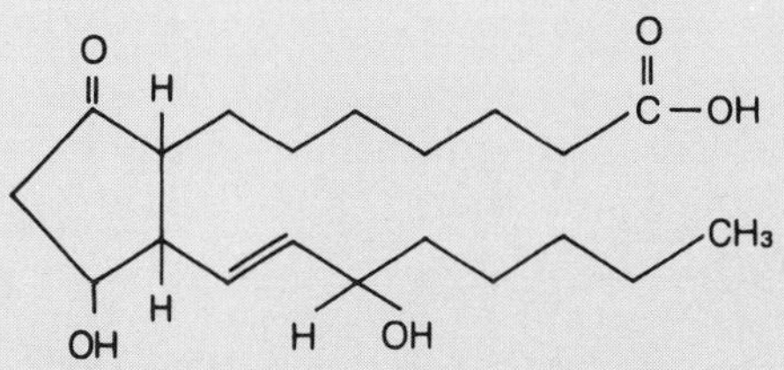

Prostaglandin E_1.

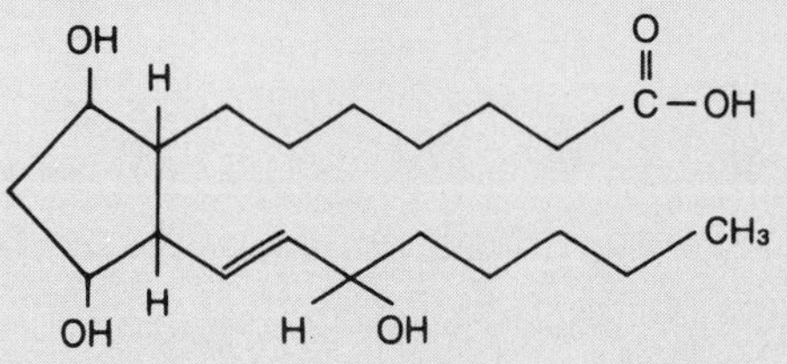

Prostaglandin F_{1a}

and increased epinephrine, dilates and/or constricts blood vessels, working especially on those of the kidney itself. The lung and liver rapidly inactivate this hormone so that it will not work in these organs. Another prostaglandin, produced in the neural tissue in response to certain nerve activity, alters transmission of nerve impulses. Still another, produced by many of the body's cells, alters their response to hormones. The prostaglandins are all derived from the polyunsaturated fatty acids, and account in part for the essentiality of these fatty acids in the diet.

The description of the hormones just given names the major ones and lists a function or two for each. If you are new to the subject, this should be more than enough to provide an awareness of the enormous impact these compounds have on body processes. The other overall regulating agency, the nervous system, will receive even briefer treatment. The reminder is offered once more: The point is not to learn the details but to know that they are there.

The Nerves

Like the hormones, the nerves coordinate the actions of all the body systems. Unlike the hormones, however, their actions are specific, point-to-point. Nerves generally control the action of specific muscles and glands, whereas hormones tend to regulate overall metabolic processes.

The most familiar example of nerve action is the working of the reflex arc. In response to a stimulus at one part of the body — such as pain — nerves will activate muscles that will adjust that part — for example, pull the limb away from the source of the pain.

A major difference, then, between the hormonal and the nervous system is that the hormones are released into the bloodstream and travel indiscriminately to all parts of the body. The characteristics of the target organs determine whether they respond. Nerve messages, however, are transmitted selectively down specific channels to specific end organs. Another difference is that a nerve message travels extremely fast, eliciting a muscular response in a fraction of a second; hormonal messages occur over a broader range of time intervals, taking anywhere from a few seconds (the stress response) to several days (the ovulatory cycle) or years (sexual maturation).

The two systems, hormonal and nervous, have major features in common, however. Both act to promote homeostasis, the returning of the body's internal environment to the normal or optimal state whenever a disturbance is imposed from outside. Both have systems to detect these disturbances, chains of reactions to correct them, ways of detecting when the corrections have been made, and ways of stopping the reactions from going too far. The two systems work harmoniously together, cooperating to bring about health in response to the same stimuli. Stress, for example, elicits both hormonal and nerve responses; milk production responds to both hormonal and nerve messages.

The hormonal and nervous systems share a common chemistry, too; some of the hormones that have generalized whole-body effects can also be secreted at specific nerve endings where they act as the transmitters of nerve impulses along selected channels. The two systems are tied together by the brain, where the major controlling gland, the pituitary, lies. The brain's hypothalamus — which produces and releases the hormones that control the pituitary and other master glands — is itself made of nerve cells, and it has both nerve and endocrine functions. Some additional details about the way nerves function appear in Highlight 5: Nutrition and the Brain.

The hormonal and nervous systems coordinate the body's overall responses to disturbances, but they are not the only homeostatic systems operating. Each individual cell also has the capacity to respond to changes in local conditions. Some of the cells' strategies for maintaining homeostasis within their boundaries are described in Highlight 7B.

Hormones, Nerves, and Nutrients

A definition and description of homeostasis appeared in Highlight 1.

Up to now, the message has been repeated that nutrients often fail to affect body systems, because the hormones and nerves are in control. With the introduction just presented, however, you are in a position to see that some nutrients *do* affect the systems that control the body. The examples that follow show some of the major relationships that are known between nutrients and the body's hormonal and nervous systems. The order of presentation has no special significance but is merely the order in which the nutrients are presented in this book: carbohydrate, fat, protein, vitamins, minerals, water.

As you already know, when you eat *carbohydrate* your pancreas secretes insulin as soon as it detects a rise in blood glucose concentration. The insulin brings the glucose level down. You may know, too, that in most diabetics the major problem seems to be that they don't secrete enough insulin, or soon enough, or insulin that is effective enough, to bring the glucose level down to normal. The naive approach to solving this problem would be to ask, "What can we feed that will not raise the glucose level so high?" and the diet that results from this approach is a low-carbohydrate diet, high in fat and protein. Such a diet has been used for years in the treatment of diabetes.

When you appreciate the role the hormones play in the regulation of blood glucose, however, you can ask a more sophisticated question: "What can we feed that will stimulate a more adequate, effective insulin response?" Recent research has revealed that diets that contain carbohydrate stimulate the body (even in a diabetic) to regulate its glucose level more appropriately after a meal, so that the body can handle a greater glucose load. The new diet therapy for diabetes emphasizes diets that are *high*, not low, in complex carbohydrate.[1]

(Diabetics still have to avoid eating concentrated sweets, though.)

When you eat *fat*, as you already know, one of the body's hormonal responses is to slow the action of the GI tract. This gives the intestines a longer time to digest and absorb the fat, and also lengthens the time it takes to digest a meal containing fat. The result: you feel satisfied longer. The knowledgeable diet therapist uses this information to help the weight-loss dieter. Even though fat is higher in kcalories-per-gram than carbohydrate and protein, it can make you feel full, so that a person using it judiciously can end up eating fewer kcalories and spacing meals further apart than if fat were omitted altogether.

As for *protein*, you may remember from Chapter 1 that this nutrient elicits a response not only from insulin but also from insulin's opposing hormone, glucagon, as well (and other hormones too). This is why it helps to eat protein frequently to stabilize blood glucose level, especially for a person who tends to be hypoglycemic.

Protein *lack* has far-reaching effects on every body organ. It isn't just that they lack amino acids with which to synthesize new tissues. The body's hormone balance changes one way in protein deficiency, when kcalories are fed, and changes another way in straight starvation, so the effects of the two kinds of malnutrition (kwashiorkor and marasmus) are different. The edema of kwashiorkor, the fatty liver, the apathy, and other symptoms are due to the different hormonal climate produced by the lack of protein (see Chapter 4).

The interactions of *vitamins* and *minerals* with hormones are numerous. For example, vitamin B_6 interacts with the cellular receptors that normally respond to the glucocorticoids and helps to modulate the action of the steroid hormones. Iodine is a part of the hormone thyroxine; zinc is a part of insulin. Other examples abound in Chapters 9 to 13, and some special relationships are also described in Highlight 5. But the point has been made. A person's nutritional state may affect the body by way of its hormonal system and so may have more far-reaching effects than anyone might at first presume. The hormonal state (it's been called "endocrine resiliency") in turn affects the body's ability to use nutrients. The health worker who wishes to have a maximum beneficial effect must have a keen interest in and appreciation for both.

Most adult diabetics secrete insulin, but its action is ineffective or delayed. This type of diabetes has recently been renamed **non-insulin-dependent diabetes** (see Chapter 25).

Summing Up

This Highlight has introduced the body's major regulatory systems and presented considerable terminology. Hopefully it will enable someone without a background of physiology to appreciate the stability of the body's self-regulatory systems. Blood pressure, temperature, growth,

[1]E. L. Bierman, guest ed., Dietetic management of diabetes mellitus, *Dietetic Currents*, *Ross Timesaver*, March-April 1980.

glucose levels, calcium, and every condition that may vary and that affects well-being is constantly monitored and adjusted to achieve the optimum balance. It would be appropriate, now, to stop for a moment and remember the questions raised at the start of Highlight 1. If I have low blood glucose, how can I change that ("fix" it)? How can I prevent the loss of calcium from my bones, so common, especially, in older women? It should now be apparent why the conclusion was reached at the end of Highlight 1 that we cannot change body conditions by naively pushing nutrients in (glucose, calcium) or by withholding them (cholesterol). Rather, we must understand how the body's controls work, so that we can cooperate with them to correct undesirable conditions. The rest of this book will illustrate this principle over and over again.

To Explore Further

In 1932, in the early days of study of physiology, a physiologist, who was wonderstruck at the ways the body achieves homeostasis, wrote a book to tell the world about it:

● Cannon, W. B. *The Wisdom of the Body.* New York. Norton, 1932.

The title of this Highlight is taken from Cannon's book.

The information in this Highlight can be studied in greater detail in any physiology text. The one we've used and recommend highly is:

● Eckert, R. O. *Animal Physiology,* with Chapters 13 and 14 by D. Randall. San Francisco: Freeman, 1978.

Some thought-provoking and, we think, wise comments on the interactions of nutrition with the hormonal system were made by a professor of biological chemistry twenty years ago:

● Griffith, W. H. Food as a regulator of metabolism. *American Journal of Clinical Nutrition* 17 (1965):391-398.

More recently, another biochemist-physician made clear some of the intricacies of the interacting systems:

● Olson, R. E. Introductory remarks: nutrient, hormone, enzyme interactions. *American Journal of Clinical Nutrition* 28 (1975):626-637.

The ultimate authority on physiology for the advanced student is a text whose users refer to it familiarly as "Guyton." Its 6th edition is the best yet:

● Guyton, A. C. *Textbook of Medical Physiology,* 6th ed. Philadelphia: Saunders, 1981.

Fat

From your Self-Study at the end of the Introduction, answer the following questions:

1. How many grams of fat do you consume in a day?

2. How many kcalories does this represent? (Remember, a gram of fat contributes 9 kcalories.)

3. What percentage of your total kcalories is contributed by fat (fat kcalories ÷ total kcalories × 100)?

4. How does this figure compare with the dietary goal that fat should represent 30 percent of total kcalories?

Optional Extras

5. Figure out your P:S ratio. Within total fat consumption, a 1 to 1 ratio of polyunsaturated to saturated fat items is sometimes recommended. Using Appendix H, you can calculate your intake of linoleic acid to represent polyunsaturated fat. The appendix provides a direct estimate of your saturated fat intake. What is your P:S ratio? (See Appendix D for help with calculating ratios and proportions.) If it isn't at least 1 to 1, what specific foods would you cut down on and what foods could you add to bring the ratio closer to 1 to 1?

6. Study your cholesterol consumption. How does your cholesterol consumption compare with the recommendation that it be not more than 300 mg/day (see Appendix G)?

7. Notice your linoleic acid intake. It is recommended that 3 percent of your kcalories come from linoleic acid.[1] Is your diet in accord with this recommendation?

8. Adjust your diet. If any of your findings from the above calculations do not square with your own goals, think through and outline changes in terms of foods that would bring them more closely into line. For example, how would exchanging 6 oz fish for 6 oz beef alter your P:S ratio?

9. Visualize how much fat you eat. You may not be clearly aware of how large your meat portions are. Weigh them for a day or so to see. Then calculate how much fat you derive from meat in a day. To visualize this amount of fat, measure it from your butter or margarine dish onto a plate.

[1]*Recommended Dietary Allowances*, 9th ed. (Washington, D.C.: National Academy of Sciences, 1980): pp. 33-35.

CHAPTER 3

CONTENTS

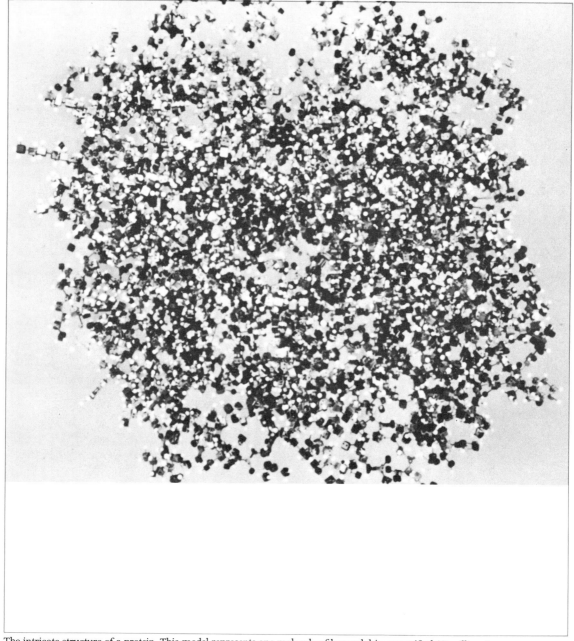

The intricate structure of a protein. This model represents one molecule of hemoglobin, magnified 27 million times.

PROTEIN: Amino Acids

To make an organism demands the right substances in the right proportions and in the right arrangement. We do not think that anything more is needed —but that is problem enough.

GEORGE WALD

Everybody knows that protein is important. It is advertised on every cereal box; it is said to "build strong bodies" and to provide "super go power." In fact, as you will see, protein has been so overemphasized that many people eat more than enough, sometimes at the expense of other nutrients that are equally important. An understanding of the quantity and quality of protein will help put it in its proper place—as only one of the many essential nutrients needed in correct proportions to achieve a balanced diet.

The preceding two chapters, on carbohydrates and lipids, began with sections describing the roles of these nutrients in the body, then moved on to a consideration of their structure. This chapter, on the contrary, describes the structure of protein first, because protein's structure enables it to play many more roles than carbohydrate or lipid. All three nutrients are important, and all three share the common function of providing energy, but protein is far more versatile.

Protein structure is also far more interesting than that of carbohydrate or lipid. The regularity and simplicity of protein structure have yielded only recently to human investigation. Those who have worked on elucidating the structure of protein have been rewarded with a rare insight into the elegance of nature's designs.

The Chemist's View of Protein

A protein is a chemical compound composed of the same atoms as carbohydrate and lipid—carbon, hydrogen, and oxygen—but protein also contains nitrogen atoms. These C, H, O, and N atoms are arranged into amino acids, which are linked into chains to form proteins. It is easy to construct a protein once we know what an amino acid looks

protein: a compound composed of C, H, O, and N, arranged into amino acids linked in a chain. Proteins also contain some S (sulfur).

like, and the unit structure of an amino acid is simpler than that of either carbohydrates (monosaccharides) or lipids (glycerol and fatty acids).

Amino Acid Structure An amino acid has a backbone of one nitrogen and two carbon atoms linked together. Recall that carbons must form four bonds with other atoms, oxygens two, and hydrogens one. In amino acids, nitrogens form three bonds with other atoms. The structure that all amino acids have in common fulfills these requirements:

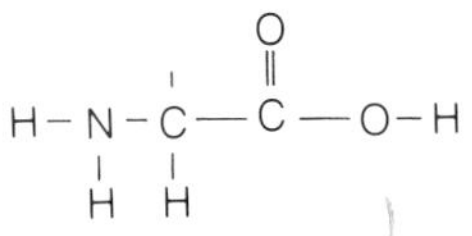

amino (a-MEEN-oh) **acid:** a building block of protein; a compound containing an amino group and an acid group attached to a central carbon, which also carries a distinctive side chain.

amino = containing nitrogen

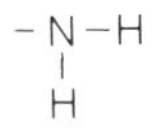

Amino group 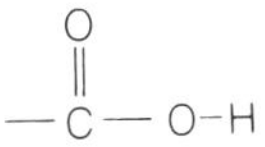   Acid group

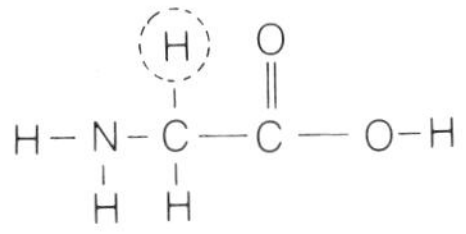

Glycine

At one end is an amino group (NH_2); at the other is an acid group (COOH). Both are attached to a central carbon that also carries a hydrogen (H). As you can see, on this drawing one position is left unfilled: The central carbon atom must have another atom or group of atoms attached to it to make a complete structure.

This central carbon atom and the attached structures are what make proteins so different from either carbohydrates or lipids. A polysaccharide (starch, for example) is composed of glucose units one after the other. It may be 100 or 200 units long, but every unit in the chain is a glucose molecule just like all the others. In a protein, on the other hand, 22 different amino acids may appear. Each differs from the others in the nature of the side group that it carries on the central carbon. The simplest amino acid, glycine, has a hydrogen atom in that position. A slightly more complex amino acid, alanine, has an extra carbon with three attached hydrogen atoms. Other amino acids have still more complex side groups. For example, one amino acid may have an acid group, another may have an amino group. Still others may have aromatic ring structures. Thus although the basic structure of an amino acid is simple, the side groups may be quite elaborate.

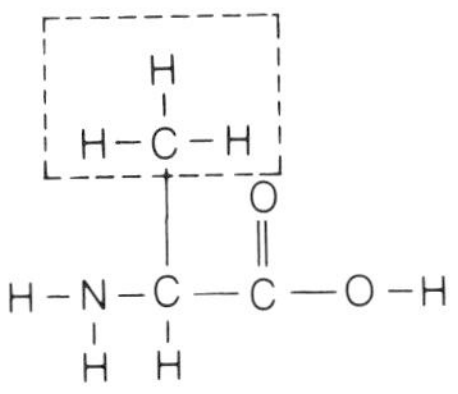

Examples of amino acids.

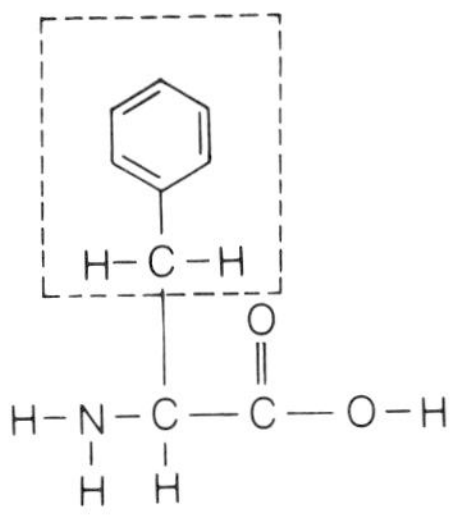

Alanine   Aspartic acid   Phenylalanine

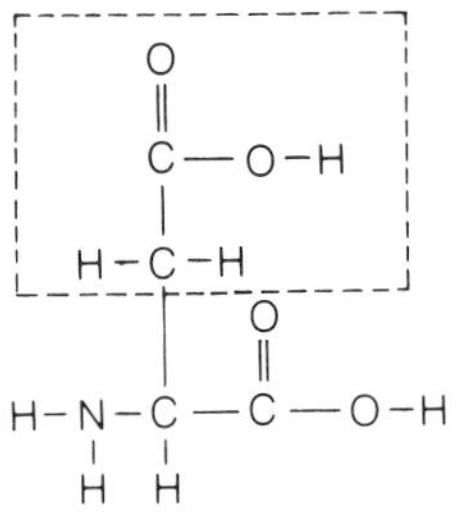

Amino Acid Sequence The 22 different common amino acids may be linked together in a great variety of ways to form proteins. They connect by means of a condensation reaction similar to those you have seen before. An OH is removed from the acid end of one and an H from the amino group of another amino acid. A bond forms between the two amino acids, and the H and OH join to form a molecule of water. The resulting structure is called a dipeptide:

Condensation reactions: see pp. 25, 60.

dipeptide: two amino acids bonded together. The bond between two amino acids is a **peptide bond**.

di = two
peptide = amino acid

Formation of a dipeptide by condensation of two amino acids.

By the same reaction, the OH can be removed from the acid end of the second amino acid and an H from the amino group of a third to form a tripeptide. As additional amino acids are added to the chain, a polypeptide is formed. Most proteins are polypeptides, 100 to 300 amino acids long.

It would be misleading, however, to end the description here, because in showing the structures on paper we have drawn a straight, flat chain. Actually, polypeptide chains fold and tangle so that they look not like rods but like crazy jungle gyms or tangled balls of yarn. The sequence of amino acids in a protein determines which specific way the chain will fold.

tripeptide: three amino acids bonded together by peptide bonds.

tri = three

polypeptide: many amino acids bonded together by peptide bonds. *Many* refers to 10 or more. An intermediate string of between 4 and 10 amino acids is an **oligopeptide**.

poly = many
oligo = few

Folding of the Chain The chain structure can best be visualized by keeping in mind that each side group on the amino acids has special characteristics that attract it to other groups. Some side groups are negatively charged, others are positively charged, and the aromatic rings are attracted to other aromatic rings. As amino acids are added to a polypeptide chain and the chain lengthens, the acids that are negatively charged move as close as possible to those that are positively charged. Since the molecule is in a watery solution, these charged groups, being hydrophilic (see p. 67), tend to expose themselves on the outer surface of the completed protein; the aromatic groups, being hydrophobic (see p. 67), tend to tuck themselves inside. The shape the polypeptide finally assumes is usually globular, giving it the maximum stability possible in water solution. Finally, two or more of these giant molecules may associate to form a still larger working aggregate. Thus

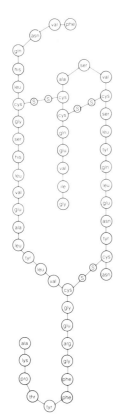

The change in a protein's shape brought about by heat, acid, or other conditions is known as **denaturation**. Past a certain point, denaturation is irreversible.

tryptophan (TRIP-toe-fane) and **serine** (SEAR-een): amino acids.

maltase: the enzyme that hydrolyzes maltose to two glucose units.

maltose: the disaccharide composed of 2 glucose units (see p. 30).

ase: a suffix denoting an enzyme, usually identifying the compound that the enzyme works on. Thus maltase is the enzyme that works on maltose.

(Figure at left)
The complete amino acid sequence of insulin, a small protein. S-S represents the cross-links between cystine molecules, known as disulfide bridges.

the completed protein is one or more very complex tangled chains of amino acids, bristling on the surface with positive and negative charges.

When a protein molecule is subjected to heat, acid, or other conditions that disturb its stability, it uncoils or changes its shape, thus losing its function to some extent. That is what happens to an egg when it is cooked; alterations of the egg proteins during cooking largely account for the observable changes in the egg white and yolk.

The Completed Protein If you could step onto a carbohydrate molecule like starch and walk along it, the first stepping stone would be a glucose. Your next stepping stone would be glucose again, and then glucose, and then glucose, and then glucose. But if you were to step onto one end of a polypeptide chain, your first stepping stone might be a glycine. Your second might be an alanine. The third might be a glycine again, and the fourth a tryptophan, then a serine, and so on. In other words, the variety of units in a protein, in both their nature and their sequence, is far greater than it is in a carbohydrate molecule.

By way of another analogy, if you were to try to make a sentence using only the letter G, you could only speak gibberish: G-G-G-G-G-G-G. But with 26 different letters available, you can say, "To be or not to be, that is the question"—or on a different plane, "The way to a man's heart is through his stomach." The Greek alphabet contains only 24 letters, and all of Homer was written with it.

The variety of sequences in which the 22 amino acids can be linked together is even greater than that possible for letters in a sentence, because proteins do not have to be pronounced. This gives them a tremendous range of possible surface structures, which in turn enable them to perform very distinct, individual, and specialized functions.

Enzymes: A Function of Protein

In Chapter 1 we mentioned enzymes for the first time, and we promised that we would look at these magnificent molecules more closely when protein structure had been explained. Let's start by looking at the enzyme maltase.

A typical protein, maltase is a tangled ball-shaped polypeptide chain, 100 or so amino acids long. The little molecule maltose, on the other hand, is a disaccharide perhaps 100 times smaller. If you were one of the glucoses in maltose, you would be joined to the other glucose like a Siamese twin, incomplete and unable to stand alone for lack of an H or an OH. Suppose you were swallowed by a person: You would travel down her esophagus, and after spending some time in her stomach, you would find yourself floating around in the watery medium of her small intestine. Looking about, you would see many giant enzymes working on, breaking down, and putting together a variety of other compounds like yourself. Sooner or later you would find yourself snapping into position on the surface of a maltase, an enzyme custom-designed to fit your contours. On this surface you would encounter a molecule of water, and as you split away from your glucose twin, the water would also split apart, its H being added to one of you and its OH to the other. Released as a free glucose, you might turn around to see other pairs being attracted into that same position and being hydrolyzed just as you had been.

Enzymes and what they do are so fundamental to all life processes that it may be worthwhile to introduce a somewhat fanciful analogy in order to clarify two important characteristics they all share. Enzymes could be compared to the ministers and judges who respectively make and dissolve human matrimonial bonds. When two individuals come to a minister to be married, the couple leaves with a new bond between them. They are joined together. But the minister is only momentarily involved in this process and remains unchanged and available to perform other ceremonies between other pairs of people. One minister can perform thousands of marriage ceremonies. In a divorce court, the judge plays a similar but opposite role. A couple enters the court, the judge performs the dissolution, and the couple leaves as two separate individuals. Like the minister, the judge may decree many divorces before he dies or retires.

The minister represents enzymes that synthesize larger compounds from smaller ones—the synthetases, which build body structures. The judge represents enzymes that hydrolyze larger compounds to smaller ones—the proteases, lipases, carbohydrases, disaccharidases, and others. Maltase is a disaccharidase.

The first point to be learned is that some enzymes put compounds together and others take them apart. Since you yourself are a very "put-together" kind of organism, superbly organized out of billions of molecules that have been bonded together to make muscle, bone, skin, eyes, and blood cells, you can imagine how numerous and very active in your body are the enzymes that put things together.

The second point to be learned is that the enzymes are not themselves affected in the process of facilitating chemical reactions: They are catalysts. The technical definition of an enzyme, which biologists and chemists use, is a protein catalyst.

What makes you unique and distinct from any other human being is minute differences in your body proteins (enzymes, antibodies, and others). These differences are determined by the amino acid sequences of your proteins, which are written into the genetic code of the DNA you inherited from your parents and ancestors. Each person receives at conception a unique combination of DNA codes for these sequences. The DNA code directs the making of all the body's proteins, as shown in Figure 1.

An apology for the use of fanciful descriptions appears in the Note to the Student.

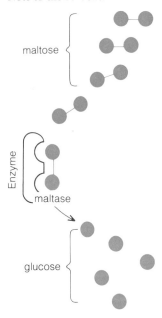

Model of enzyme action.

synthetase (SIN-the-tase): an enzyme that synthesizes compounds.

protease (PRO-tee-ase): an enzyme that hydrolyzes proteins.

lipase (LYE-pase): an enzyme that hydrolyzes lipids.

The definitions of **carbohydrase, disaccharidase, sucrase, lactase,** and **phospholipase** are self-evident.

catalyst (CAT-uh-list): a compound that facilitates chemical reactions without itself being destroyed in the process.

enzyme: a protein catalyst.

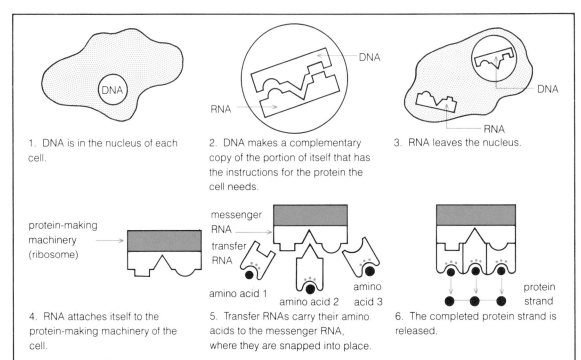

1. DNA is in the nucleus of each cell.

2. DNA makes a complementary copy of the portion of itself that has the instructions for the protein the cell needs.

3. RNA leaves the nucleus.

4. RNA attaches itself to the protein-making machinery of the cell.

5. Transfer RNAs carry their amino acids to the messenger RNA, where they are snapped into place.

6. The completed protein strand is released.

Figure 1 Protein synthesis. The instructions for making every protein in a person's body are transmitted in the genetic information he or she receives at conception. This body of knowledge is filed away in the nucleus of every cell. The master file is the DNA (deoxyribonucleic acid), which never leaves the nucleus. The DNA is identical in every cell and is specific for each individual. Each specialized cell has access to the total inherited information but calls on only the instructions needed for its own functions.

In order to inform the cell of the proper sequence of amino acids for a needed protein, a "photocopy" of the appropriate portion of DNA is made. This copy is messenger RNA (ribonucleic acid), which is able to escape through the nuclear membrane. In the cell fluid it seeks out and attaches itself to one of the ribosomes (a protein-making machine, itself composed of RNA and protein). Thus situated, the messenger RNA presents the specifications for the amino acids to be linked into a protein strand.

Meanwhile, another form of RNA, called transfer RNA, collects amino acids from the cell fluid and brings them to the messenger. For each of the 22 amino acids there is a specific kind of transfer RNA. Thousands of these trans-fer RNAs, with their loads of amino acids, cluster around the ribosomes, like vegetable-laden trucks around a farmer's market awaiting their turn to un-load. When an amino acid is called for by the messenger, the transfer RNA carrying it snaps into position. Then the next and the next and the next loaded transfer RNAs move into place. Thus the amino acids are lined up in the right sequence. Then an enzyme bonds them together.

Finally, the completed protein strand is released, the messenger is degraded, and the transfer RNAs are freed to return for another load. It takes many words to describe these events, but in the cell, 40 to 100 amino acids can be added to a growing protein strand in only a second.

Perhaps you have realized by now that the protein story moves in a circle. All enzymes are proteins. All proteins are made of amino acids. Amino acids have to be put together to make proteins. Enzymes put together the amino acids. Only living systems work with such self-renewal. A broken toaster cannot be fixed by another toaster. A car cannot make another car. Only living creatures and those parts that they are composed of—the cells—can duplicate themselves and make the parts of which they are made. To follow the circle in nutrition, start with a person eating proteins. The proteins are broken down by proteins (enzymes) into amino acids. The amino acids enter the cells of the body, where proteins (enzymes) put them together in long chains with sequences specified by DNA. The chains fold and become enzymes themselves. These enzymes may then be used to break apart other compounds or to put other compounds together. Day by day, billion reactions by billion reactions, these processes repeat themselves and life goes on.

A Closer Look at Enzyme Action

If you look closely at the details of the reaction sequences governed by enzymes, some additional important facts emerge. The following description is an example of the way enzymes work to alter the structure of a compound. It is the only example in this book of biochemistry at the level biochemists actually think about it. The object is to give you an insight into the kinds of processes that account for human nutritional needs.

Let's look at a biochemical pathway partway along its length and see how each enzyme alters the structure of a compound until one thing has been converted into another quite different thing. Beginning with glucose, a six-carbon compound, enzymes add a phosphate group, altering and breaking this structure until a three-carbon compound results—which looks like compound A.

An intermediate in glucose metabolism (compound A).

Compound A floats around until it encounters an enzyme with the specialized function of removing hydrogen atoms (from these compounds). The encounter results in the altered compound, compound B.

Removal of hydrogen from the intermediate by a dehydrogenase (compound B).

Compound B is released from the enzyme and later encounters another enzyme, which removes oxygens and substitutes amino groups. What results is compound C.

$$H-O-\overset{\displaystyle \underset{||}{O}}{\underset{|}{P}}-O-\overset{\displaystyle \underset{|}{H}}{\underset{|}{C}}-\overset{\displaystyle \underset{|}{\overset{N-H}{|}}}{\underset{|}{C}}-\overset{\displaystyle \underset{||}{O}}{C}-O-H$$

Removal of oxygen and substitution of H and NH_2 by a transaminase (compound C).

$$H-O-\overset{\displaystyle \underset{|}{H}}{\underset{|}{C}}-\overset{\displaystyle \underset{|}{\overset{N-H}{|}}}{\underset{|}{C}}-\overset{\displaystyle \underset{||}{O}}{C}-O-H$$

Removal of phosphate by a phosphatase (compound D).

$$H-\overset{\displaystyle \underset{|}{H}}{\underset{|}{C}}-\overset{\displaystyle \underset{||}{O}}{C}-O-H$$

What is it (compound E)?

essential amino acid: an amino acid that the body cannot synthesize in amounts sufficient to meet physiological need. The eight amino acids known to be essential for human adults:

methionine (meh-THIGH-o-neen)
threonine (THREE-o-neen)
tryptophan (TRIP-toe-fane)
isoleucine (eye-so-LOO-seen)
leucine (LOO-seen)
lysine (LYE-seen)
valine (VAY-leen)
phenylalanine (fee-nul-AL-uh-neen)

Infants also require **histidine** (HISS-tuh-deen).[1]

Students attempting to learn these by heart often use the device "TV TILL PM" to recall their first letters.

The next enzyme removes the phosphate group from the end carbon and replaces it with a hydrogen, leaving compound D.

If you look closely at the picture of compound D, you may recognize its characteristics and not be surprised by the statements that follow. But first let us take the process one more step. Another enzyme, whose function is to remove CH_2OH groups from these molecules, forms compound E. Look at this product closely. It is one that you may recognize because you have seen it before. It has an amino group at one end, an acid group at the other, and a central carbon carrying two Hs. It is the amino acid glycine (p. 96).

Well, how about that! We started with a molecule of glucose, a derivative of dietary carbohydrate, and by making one minute change after another, we transformed it into an amino acid, a member of the protein family.

The lesson to be learned from this sequence of events is that the body can make, from glucose and nitrogen-containing compounds, many of the amino acids needed to build body proteins. Glycine is one of those. Compound D, which precedes glycine, is the amino acid serine (which has a CH_2OH on its central carbon). This too is an amino acid the body can make.

The Essential Amino Acids

It should now be clear that the role of protein in food is not to provide body proteins directly but to supply the amino acids from which the body can make its own proteins. Since the body can make glycine and serine for itself, the proteins in the diet need not contain these two amino acids. But there are some amino acids that the body cannot make at all, and some that it cannot make fast enough to meet its need. (This is because the body does not possess the genetic code for making the enzymes necessary to synthesize these amino acids, or because the enzymes it does make work too slowly.) These amino acids are referred to as essential amino acids; it is essential that they be included in the diet.

[1] R. E. Olson, Clinical nutrition: An interface between human ecology and internal medicine, *Nutrition Reviews* 36 (June 1978): 161-178.

In Chapter 2, one fatty acid was singled out as a dietary essential for the same reason: because it cannot be synthesized in the body. All compounds in your body are needed for your health, but those that you cannot make for yourself are needed in your diet, and these are called essential nutrients. With the addition of the eight essential amino acids, your list of essential nutrients has now expanded to nine.

To make body protein, a cell must have all 22 amino acids available simultaneously. The first important characteristic of dietary protein is therefore that it should supply at least the eight essential amino acids plus enough additional nitrogen for the synthesis of the others.

Protein Quality

A complete protein is a protein that contains all of the essential amino acids; it may or may not contain all of the others. A high-quality protein is one that is not only complete but also contains the essential amino acids in amounts proportional to the body's need for them.

Ideally, dietary protein would supply each amino acid in the amount needed for protein synthesis in the body. If one amino acid is supplied in an amount smaller than is needed, the total amount of protein that can be synthesized from the others will be limited. By analogy, suppose that a signmaker plans to make 100 identical signs, each saying LEFT TURN ONLY. He needs 200 Ls, 200 Ns, 200 Ts, and 100 of each of the other letters. If he has only 20 Ls, he can make only 10 signs, even if all the other letters are available in unlimited quantities. The Ls limit the number of signs that can be made. If he doesn't get some more Ls, he will have to throw away all his other letters.

When the body uses a protein of poor quality, it wastes many of the amino acids. What happens is that enzymes strip off the nitrogen-containing amino groups and fix them into the compound urea, and the urea is excreted in the urine. The carbon skeletons that remain can be used to make glucose or fat, but the nitrogen from amino acids cannot be stored in the body. The amount of urea excreted is thus a measure of the number of wasted amino acids.

The quality of dietary protein thus depends partly on whether the protein supplies all the essential amino acids and, more importantly, on the extent to which it supplies them in the needed proportions. An excellent protein by these standards is egg protein, whose nitrogen tends to be retained in the body. Egg protein has been designated the reference protein and has been assigned a biological value of 100 by the Food and Agriculture Organization of the United Nations and the World Health Organization, which set world standards.

The amino acid composition of a test protein can be compared with the composition of egg protein, and a chemical score can be derived to express the theoretical value of the test protein. A test protein with a chemical score of 70, for example, contains a limiting amino acid, and

complete protein: a protein containing all of the amino acids essential for humans.

high-quality protein: a complete protein whose amino acids fit the pattern needed by humans. (A true high-quality protein is also easily digestible.)

EFT TURN ON Y

limiting amino acid: the amino acid found in the shortest supply relative to the amounts needed for protein synthesis in the body.

How urea is made: see Chapter 7.

reference protein: egg protein; used by FAO/WHO as a standard against which to measure the quality of other proteins.

chemical score: a rating of the quality of a test protein arrived at by comparing its amino acid pattern with that of a reference protein.

digestibility: the amount of protein absorbed from a given intake. To learn why liquid protein is less digestible than whole protein, even though it is delivered in small fragments, turn to p. 157.

biological value (BV): the amount of protein retained from a given amount absorbed.

that amino acid is present in only 70 percent of the amount found in the ideal amino acid pattern. If you fed that test protein to a human being, you could expect 30 percent of its amino acids to be wasted (30 percent of its nitrogen to be excreted in the urine).

In a world where food is scarce and where many people's diets contain marginal or inadequate amounts of protein, it is important to know which foods contain the highest-quality protein. It is now possible to determine the amino acid composition of any protein relatively inexpensively, but unfortunately chemical scoring does not always give an accurate reflection of the way a protein will be used by the body. One reason is that proteins also differ in digestibility. If a protein can't be digested to small fragments—amino acids, dipeptides, and tripeptides—then its amino acids will not pass across the intestinal wall into the blood but will be lost in the feces.

To determine the actual value of a protein as it is used by the body, it is therefore necessary to measure not only urinary but also fecal losses of nitrogen when that protein is actually fed to human beings under test conditions. (Even then, small additional losses from sweat, shed skin, and the like will be missed.) This kind of experiment provides the determinations of biological value (BV) of protein that are used internationally. (The mathematics of chemical scoring and biological value determinations are presented in Appendix E for those who are interested.) The biological values of the protein in some sample foods are shown below. Generally, a biological value of 70 or above indicates acceptable quality.

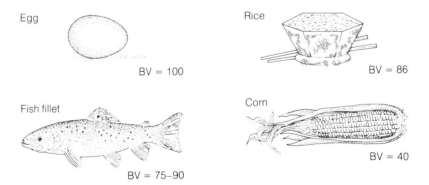

Egg   BV = 100

Rice   BV = 86

Fish fillet   BV = 75–90

Corn   BV = 40

protein efficiency ratio (PER): a measure of protein quality derived by feeding a test protein to growing animals and determining their weight gain.

As you may well imagine, determining the biological value of a protein is a cumbersome and expensive procedure. A different laboratory test involves feeding a test protein to young animals (usually rats) and measuring their growth rate. This measure, the protein efficiency ratio (PER), is used to qualify statements about daily protein requirements in the United States. You are assumed to eat protein with a PER of 70 or above; if the PER is lower, you need more protein.

For those who choose not to tangle with the formulas for BV and PER, a convenient way to distinguish among proteins is to think of animal proteins as being generally of higher quality than plant proteins. However, the educated vegetarian can design a perfectly acceptable diet around plant foods alone.

Diet planning for the vegetarian: see Highlight 4.

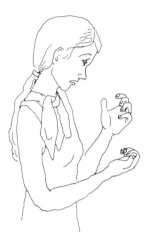

"Animal proteins are generally of higher quality than plant proteins." This statement, like all generalizations, does not quite stand up to close inspection. One animal protein that is not complete is gelatin (it lacks tryptophan). Ironically, this is the protein often recommended for correcting cracked nails and dull or brittle hair. The logic is that, because these tissues are made of protein, a drink of protein will improve their texture. Even if this were the case, however — and a symptom, you remember, is not a deficiency disease — gelatin supplements would help only if protein containing tryptophan had already been supplied. And if that protein were complete, then the gelatin would not be needed!

There is a place for low-quality proteins in the diet, however. An excellent way to support the efficient use of high-quality animal protein is to eat plenty of plant protein along with it. Research has shown that expensive meat protein is far more efficiently used when ample bread, cereal, and vegetable protein accompanies it. An adult needs only 20 percent of his total protein as essential amino acids.[2]

There is one circumstance in which dietary protein—no matter how high the quality—will not be used efficiently by the body and will not support growth: when energy from other energy nutrients is lacking. The body assigns top priority to meeting its energy needs, and when kcalories from other sources are not available, it will break down protein to meet this need. Stripping off and excreting the nitrogen from the amino acids, it will use their carbon skeletons in much the same way it uses those from glucose or from fat.

Carbohydrate and fat allow amino acids to be used to build body proteins. This is known as the **protein-sparing action** of carbohydrate and fat.

Energy value of protein: 1 g provides 4 kcal.

Other conditions may also affect the body's use of protein. The presence of other nutrients—vitamins, minerals, and water—is needed to process the protein, and the body itself must be in a healthy state in order to absorb and assimilate it. Cooking methods affect digestibility: Moist heat enhances it, and dry heat may reduce it.

In summary, to be used with maximum efficiency a protein must contain an amino acid pattern tailored to meet the body's needs; it must be digestible; it must be consumed with sufficient kcalories from other sources so that it will not be used for energy; it must be accompanied by the needed vitamins, minerals, and water; and it must be received by a body that is healthy and equipped to use it.

[2]M. C. Crim and H. N. Munro, Protein, in *Nutrition Reviews' Present Knowledge in Nutrition*, 4th ed. (Washington, D. C.: Nutrition Foundation, 1976), pp. 43-54.

Recommended Protein Intakes

nitrogen balance: the amount of nitrogen consumed (N-in) as compared with the amount of nitrogen excreted (N-out) in a given period of time. To learn about nitrogen balance and the athlete, turn to Chapter 16.

The average amino acid weighs about 6.25 times as much as the nitrogen it contains, so the laboratory scientist can estimate the protein in food by multiplying the weight of the food nitrogen by 6.25.

nitrogen equilibrium (zero nitrogen balance): N-in = N-out.

positive nitrogen balance: N-in > N-out.

negative nitrogen balance: N-in < N-out.

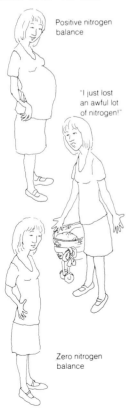

Positive nitrogen balance

"I just lost an awful lot of nitrogen!"

Zero nitrogen balance

Quality and total kcalories are not the only important factors in selecting protein for your diet. The quantity of protein that you need depends on the amount of lean tissue in your body. Fat tissue requires relatively little protein to maintain itself, but the muscles and blood and other metabolically active tissues must be maintained by a continuous supply of essential amino acids. To determine how much protein a person needs, the laboratory scientist can perform a nitrogen balance study.

Protein is the only one of the three energy nutrients that contains nitrogen, so it is possible to follow its path through the body simply by following the nitrogen. Furthermore, the amount of nitrogen in a mixture of substances can easily be measured. When we measure the amount of nitrogen in a meal, we are also measuring indirectly the amount of protein in the meal. When we measure the nitrogen excreted by a person in feces and urine (and to a lesser extent in hair, fingernails, and perspiration), we are indirectly measuring the amount of protein that is being lost from the body.

Under normal circumstances healthy adults are in nitrogen equilibrium or zero nitrogen balance—they have at all times the same amount of total protein in their bodies. When nitrogen-in exceeds nitrogen-out, they are said to be in positive nitrogen balance; this means that somewhere in their bodies more proteins are being built than are being broken down and lost. When nitrogen-in is less than nitrogen-out, they are said to be in negative nitrogen balance. Let's consider some of the circumstances in which these non-zero balances occur.

Growing children add to their bodies every day new blood, bone, and muscle cells. Since these cells contain protein, children must have in their bodies more protein (and therefore more nitrogen) at the end of each day than they had at the beginning. A growing child is therefore in positive nitrogen balance. Similarly, when a woman is pregnant she is in essence growing a new organism; she too must be in positive nitrogen balance (although on the day she gives birth she loses at one fell swoop a tremendous amount of the protein she has accumulated). When she is lactating, she may be in equilibrium again, but it is a sort of enhanced equilibrium. She is eating more protein than before to make her milk and is excreting it whenever the baby nurses.

Negative nitrogen balance occurs when muscle or other protein tissue is broken down and lost. When people have to rest in bed for a period of time, their muscles atrophy, and they suffer a net loss of protein. One of several problems faced by nutritionists responsible for the welfare of the astronauts was that of the negative nitrogen balance that occurred when they were confined for days in the space capsule; their muscles failed to receive enough exercise to maintain themselves.

On the basis of nitrogen balance studies and other experiments, governments attempt to set recommendations for people's protein intakes. Some of these recommendations are described in the following sections.

U.S. Recommendations One recommendation for protein intake has already been mentioned in the preceding chapters. The Senate committee that published the *Dietary Goals for the United States* observed that protein intake has been relatively constant in U.S. diets for many decades, representing about 12 percent of the total kcalories consumed. In setting the Dietary Goals for protein, fat, and carbohydrate, the committee recommended that you continue to consume about 12 percent of your kcalories from protein. They reasoned that your intakes need not be higher in protein than they already are and that a reduction in protein intake, which might require drastic alterations in your lifestyle, would not pay off in any predictable benefits. The Dietary Goals for the three energy nutrients, then, were:

- *Protein.* 12 percent of kcalories (more loosely, 10 to 15 percent is fine).
- *Carbohydrate.* 58 percent of kcalories (or more).
- *Fat.* 30 percent of kcalories (or less).

A much more formal recommendation for protein intake is the Recommended Dietary Allowance (RDA). (Don't confuse the RDA with the U.S. RDA used on labels: see pp. 428-429.) Protein is the first nutrient discussed in this book for which there is an RDA, so some discussion of the RDA is in order here. The agency that has responsibility for setting formal recommendations for nutrient intake for U.S. citizens is the Committee on RDA of the Food and Nutrition Board. Its most recent recommendations for protein intakes were published in 1979-1980. The Committee on RDA stated that a generous protein allowance for a healthy adult would be 0.8 g of high-quality protein per kilogram of ideal body weight per day. Suppose that your ideal weight is 50 kilograms; your protein RDA would then be 0.8 times 50, or 40 g of protein each day.

The Committee uses the ideal, not the actual, weight for this calculation because that weight is proportional to the lean body mass of the average person. If you gain weight, your fat tissue increases in mass; but fat tissue is composed largely of fat—C, H, and O—and does not require much protein for maintenance.

The RDAs have been much misunderstood. One young woman, on first learning of their existence, was outraged: "You mean Uncle Sam tells me that I must eat exactly 40 g of protein every day?" This is not the government's intention, and the RDAs are not commandments. The following facts will help put the RDAs in perspective:

- They are published by the government, but the study group that recommends them is composed of nutritionists and other scientists, not politicians.

Recommended Dietary Allowances (RDA): published by the Food and Nutrition Board (FNB) of the National Academy of Sciences/National Research Council (NAS/NRC).

To figure your protein RDA, follow the directions in the Self-Study at the end of Highlight 3.

- They are based on available scientific evidence to the greatest extent possible and are revised about every five years for this reason.

- They are recommendations, not requirements, and certainly not minimum requirements. They are thought by the Food and Nutrition Board to include a margin of safety for most people, being perhaps about 30 percent higher than the average requirement.

- They are based on the understanding that people's nutrient needs are not identical but fall within a range. They recommend an intake thought to be near the upper end of that range.

- They are for healthy persons only; medical problems alter nutrient needs.

RDA tables: see the inside front cover.

RDAs are published for protein and several vitamins and minerals as well as for kcalories. Separate recommendations are made for different groupings of people. Children 4 to 6 years old are distinguished from men 19 to 22, for example. Each individual can look up the recommendations for his or her own age-sex group. No RDA is set for carbohydrate or fat. The assumption is that you will use a certain number of kcalories meeting your protein needs and then will distribute the remaining kcalories among carbohydrate and fat and possibly alcohol, according to your personal preference, to meet your energy RDA.

The RDA for Protein   The most important thing to understand about the RDA at first is the way the numbers were chosen, and a theoretical discussion will illustrate this.

Suppose we were the Committee on RDA and we had the task of setting an RDA for nutrient X. Ideally, our first step would be to try to find out how much of that nutrient individual people need. We might review and select the most valid balance studies. We would note the subjects' losses of the nutrient and determine exactly what intake they needed to stay in balance. For each individual subject, we could determine a *requirement* for nutrient X. Below the requirement, that person would slip into negative balance and begin to develop a deficiency.

requirement: the amount of a nutrient that will just prevent the development of specific deficiency signs.

We would find that different individuals have different requirements. Mr. A might need 40 units of the nutrient each day to maintain balance, Ms. B might need 35, and Mr. C, 65. If we looked at enough individuals, we might find that their requirements fell into a normal distribution, that most were somewhere close to the mean and only a few were at the extremes. Figure 2 depicts this situation.

normal distribution: a distribution in which the majority of points cluster near the mean. The graph of this distribution is symmetrical and bell-shaped.

Then we would have to decide what intake to recommend for everybody: We would have to set the RDA. Should we set it at the mean (shown in Figure 2 at 45 units)? This is the average requirement for nutrient X; it is the closest to everyone's need. But if people took us literally and consumed exactly this amount of nutrient X each day, half of the population would develop deficiencies, Mr. C among them.

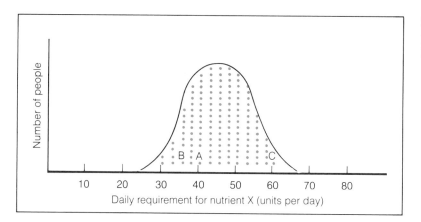

Figure 2   Each dot represents a person. A, B, and C are Mr. A, Ms. B, and Mr. C.

Perhaps we should set the RDA for nutrient X at or above the extreme—say, at 70 units a day—so that everyone would be covered. (Actually, we didn't study everyone, so we would have to worry that some individual we didn't happen to test would have a still-higher requirement.) This might be a good idea in theory, but what if nutrient X is expensive or scarce? A person like Ms. B, who needs only 35 units a day, would then try to consume twice that, an unnecessary strain on her resources. Or she might overeat as a consequence or overemphasize foods containing nutrient X to the exclusion of foods containing other valuable nutrients.

The choice we would finally make, with some reservations, would be to set the RDA at a reasonably high point so that the bulk of the population would be covered. In this example, a reasonable choice might be to set it at 63 units a day. By moving the RDA further toward the extreme, we would pick up very few additional people but inflate the recommendation as it applies to most people (like Mr. A and Ms. B).

It was this kind of choice that the Committee made with respect to protein. They set the RDA two standard deviations above the mean requirement, as best they could determine it from the available data. (Actually, they didn't even have enough data to be sure that the population's requirements fit the normal distribution.) Assuming a normal distribution of requirements, this choice would theoretically meet the needs of 97.5 percent of the population.[3]

The RDA for protein, then, is 0.8 g per kilogram of ideal body weight, but this number cannot be taken literally by any individual. Remember, no individual knows exactly what his or her personal requirement may be. Remember, too, that the Committee on RDA made several assumptions that would not apply to all real situations: They assumed,

standard deviation: describes the spread of a distribution. If the standard deviation is small, the curve is narrow; if large, the curve is broad. One standard deviation each side of the mean includes 68 percent of the sample; two include 95 percent. To determine the standard deviation of a particular distribution, the statistician adds up the squares of all the deviations from the mean, divides that total by the number of cases minus one, and finds the square root of the resulting number. The square root figure equals the standard deviation.

[3]A. E. Harper, Those pesky RDAs, *Nutrition Today,* March/April 1974, pp. 15-16, 19-22, 27-28.

among other things, that the protein would be of high quality (a PER of 70 or above), that it would be consumed with adequate kcalories from carbohydrate and fat, and that other nutrients in the diet would be adequate.

The RDAs have many uses. One use is to provide a yardstick against which the nutrient intakes of segments of the population can be measured. If, for example, all the children in a community are healthy and all are consuming over 100 percent of the RDA for protein, we can assume that we have no need to worry about their diets with respect to this nutrient. But if half the children are consuming less than 75 percent of the RDA for protein, we have cause for alarm because as many as half of these children may not be meeting their needs fully.

Another use of the RDAs is to set a standard for diet planning. In feeding large groups of people, a planner is well advised to aim at providing 100 percent of the recommended intakes for each nutrient to each person each day.

Before applying these numbers to individuals, however, it is important to understand that any application of statistical norms to individuals has inherent limitations. The RDAs have been so widely misinterpreted, misunderstood, and misused that the American Dietetic Association has published a paper titled "The RDAs Are Not for Amateurs."[4]

Note: The RDA is not the same as the U.S. RDA. To use the U.S. RDA for interpreting labels, see Highlight 12.

The Minimum Daily Requirements (MDR), formerly used for purposes similar to the RDA, have been discontinued.

There are two important cautions to apply when the RDAs are used as a yardstick to measure individual intakes:

● The RDAs are not minimum daily requirements. Most people do not have to consume 100 percent of their RDAs for all nutrients in order to be adequately nourished.

CAUTION WHEN YOU READ!

A margin of safety is built into the RDAs. R stands for Recommended—not for Required.

● The RDAs apply only to healthy persons. Illness, malnutrition, or other stress may greatly increase an individual's needs for certain nutrients.

[4]R. M. Leverton, The RDAs are not for amateurs, *Journal of the American Dietetic Association* 66 (1975): 9-11.

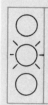

CAUTION WHEN YOU READ!

The RDAs apply to healthy persons only.

Additional cautions regarding interpretation of the RDAs are offered in later chapters.

Canadian Recommendations   The Canadian equivalent to the RDAs is the Dietary Standard for Canada, a table of Recommended Daily Nutrient Intakes (shown in Appendix O). The Canadian recommendations differ from the RDAs in several important respects, because conditions in Canada differ somewhat from those in the United States. The protein recommendation, however, is similar to the RDA.

FAO/WHO Recommendations   The protein recommendation of the Food and Agriculture Organization and the World Health Organization is considerably lower than the RDA for protein: 0.57 g per kilogram for the adult male and 0.52 for the adult female. These figures are much closer to the average *requirement* for protein and are not a generous *allowance* like the RDA. FAO/WHO has a somewhat different task from that of the Committee on RDA, however. It must find acceptable levels of nutrient intakes for a world in which poverty makes generous intakes a luxury. FAO/WHO carefully defines its protein recommendation in terms of egg or milk protein and also publishes a set of graded recommendations for proteins of lower quality. There is some concern that the FAO/WHO recommendation is too low to support health, and this matter is still under study.[5]

The FAO/WHO tables are shown in Appendix O. What may interest you the most about them is the way they differ from the U.S. and Canadian standards, a difference that reflects realities in the societies they are designed for.

Protein in Foods

In the exchange system, the foods that supply protein in abundance are those in the milk and meat lists. One milk exchange provides 8 g of protein; one meat exchange provides 7 g, as shown in Table 1.

[5]N. S. Scrimshaw, Strengths and weaknesses of the committee approach: An analysis of past and present Recommended Dietary Allowances for protein in health and disease, *New England Journal of Medicine* 294 (1976): 136-142.

Table 1. Protein Content of the Six Exchange Groups

Exchange group	Serving size	Carbohydrate (g)	Protein (g)	Fat (g)	Energy (kcal)
(1) **Skim milk**	1 c	12	8	0	80
(2) Vegetables	1/2 c	5	2	0	25
(3) Fruit	varies	10	0	0	40
(4) Bread	1 slice	15	2	0	70
(5) **Lean meat**	1 oz	0	7	3	55
(6) Fat	1 tsp	0	0	5	45

Foods containing protein:

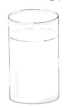

8 g in 1c milk

7 g in 1 oz meat

2 g in 1/2 c vegetables

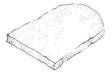

2 g in a slice of bread

As the table also shows, the foods in the vegetable and bread lists contribute small but significant amounts of protein to the diet.

The exchange system provides an easy way to estimate the amount of protein a person consumes in a day. For example, the day's meals described on p. 43 supplied the following amounts.

Breakfast	*Exchanges*	*Grams Protein*
1 egg	1 meat	7
1 slice toast	1 bread	2
Lunch		
2 slices bread	2 bread	4
2 tbsp peanut butter	1 meat	7
1 c milk	1 milk	8
Dinner		
6-oz steak	6 meat	42
1/2 c beans	1 vegetable	2
1 c mashed potato	2 bread	4
Dessert		
shortcake	1 bread	2
	Total	78 g protein

This menu provides more than enough protein for the day.

Recall from the discussion of the RDAs that the protein recommendation is a generous intake for most people. If your recommended intake is 40 g, then you will need only about 14 g of protein at each meal—provided, of course, that the protein is of high quality. From the exchange lists it is clear that 1 c milk or 1 oz meat along with the incidental additional protein provided by a few servings of vegetables, bread, or cereal will provide this amount. This means that 2 c milk and a very small serving of meat would suffice for a day. Needless to say, most people in the developed countries consume a great deal more high-quality protein than they need. Further considerations relating to the consumption of protein and to the special needs and problems of vegetarians are offered in Highlight 4.

Too Much Protein?

As the essential nutrients were discovered early in the history of nutrition, great emphasis was placed on the concept of minimum intakes. It was important to get enough. More recently the notion has arisen that it is possible to get too much, even of a valuable nutrient such as protein. One authority puts it this way:

> As the amount of any nutrient in the diet is increased from zero, a level is approached that prevents clinical symptoms and is considered the minimal requirement. With further additions of the nutrient, when body stores are saturated, the optimal requirement is reached. Still further nutrient additions may result in toxic or adverse effects.[6]

Is it possible to consume too much protein? Research designed to answer this question is now under way, and several facts are already known. Infants and children do not adjust well to diets containing large amounts of protein.[7] Animals fed high-protein diets experience a "protein overload effect," seen in the hypertrophy of their livers and kidneys. There are evidently no benefits to be gained by consuming a diet that derives more than 15 percent of its kcalories from protein, and there are possible risks.[8] The higher a person's intake of such protein-rich foods as meat and milk, the more likely it is that fruits, vegetables, and grains will be crowded out of the diet, making it inadequate in other nutrients. And diets high in protein necessitate higher intakes of calcium as well because such diets promote calcium excretion.

hypertrophy (high-PURR-tro-fee): growing too large.

hyper = too much
trophy = growth

This discussion illustrates a point to remember about nutrient needs. It is naive to think only in terms of minimum intakes. A more accurate view is to see one's nutrient needs as falling within a range, with danger zones below and above it.[9] The figure in the margin illustrates this point.

At the end of Chapter 2 we recommended that the diet be designed around the principles of dilution and variety. To these should now be added two more watchwords for diet planning: moderation and balance.

Nutrient needs:

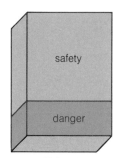

Naive view

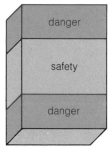

Accurate view[7]

[6]M. E. Swendseid, Nutritional implications of renal disease: 3. Nutritional needs of patients with renal disease, *Journal of the American Dietetic Association* 70 (1977): 488-492.

[7]A. A. Albanese and L. A. Orto, The proteins and amino acids, in *Modern Nutrition in Health and Disease*, 5th ed., eds. R. S. Goodhart and M. E. Shils (Philadelphia: Lea and Febiger, 1973), pp. 28-88; and L. E. Holt, Jr., Protein economy in the growing child, *Postgraduate Medicine* 27 (1960): 783-798.

[8]J. G. Chopra, A. L. Forbes, and J. P. Habicht, Protein in the U.S. diet, *Journal of the American Dietetic Association* 72 (1978):253-258.

[9]Holt, 1960.

Summing Up

Proteins are composed of carbon, hydrogen, oxygen, and nitrogen atoms arranged as amino acids, which are linked in chains some 100 to 300 amino acids long. The sequence of a protein's amino acids determines how it folds. The final configuration establishes the surface characteristics that enable the protein to act in specific ways—for example, as an enzyme that catalyzes a particular chemical reaction. (Other roles of protein are described in Chapter 4.)

Many amino acids can be synthesized in the body from other energy nutrients and a nitrogen source. Eight (listed on p. 102) cannot; these are the essential amino acids. An additional amino acid, histidine, is required by infants. The major role of dietary protein in human nutrition is therefore to supply amino acids for the synthesis of proteins needed in the body, although dietary protein can also serve as an energy source, providing 4 kcal per gram.

A complete protein is defined as one that supplies all of the essential amino acids; a high-quality protein is one that not only supplies them but also provides them in the appropriate amounts relative to human physiological need. When one essential amino acid is in short supply relative to the others in a protein source, it is said to be a limiting amino acid; that is, it limits the total amount of protein that can be synthesized from that source. Egg protein is the World Health Organization's reference protein; it is a high-quality protein used as a standard for measuring the quality of other proteins.

Ways of measuring protein quality include chemical scoring; measuring the extent to which protein supports growth in a young animal (protein efficiency ratio, or PER); or measuring nitrogen intake and losses under test conditions (biological value, or BV). Animal protein sources are generally of higher quality than vegetable protein sources, but a vegetarian can design a diet that is adequate in protein by exercising some care.

The amount of protein needed by humans can be determined by nitrogen balance studies. The RDA for protein for the healthy adult is 0.8 g of protein per kilogram of ideal body weight (determined by the Committee on RDA of the Food and Nutrition Board). This is a generous allowance, set high enough to cover even people whose individual needs for protein (as determined by nitrogen balance and other studies) reach as high as two standard deviations above the mean. The Canadian recommendation for protein is similar; the FAO/WHO recommendation is lower and is heavily qualified to ensure consumption of proteins of acceptable quality.

In the exchange system, the exchange groups that supply protein in abundance are the milk list (8 g per exchange, or per cup) and the meat list (7 g per ounce and therefore 28 g per 4-oz serving). Vegetable and bread exchanges contribute 2 g protein per exchange. Most people's average consumption of protein is considerably higher than the RDA and is largely from high-quality sources. Diets that are especially high in protein might actually be hazardous.

To Explore Further

A paperback that offers a clear picture of our new and profound understanding of how genes code for enzymes, which in turn determine the structure and function of cells, tissues, and whole organisms:

- Watson, J. D. *Molecular Biology of the Gene*, 3d ed. Menlo Park, Calif.: W. A. Benjamin, 1976.

An amusing autobiographical account (paperback) of Watson and Crick's discovery of the structure of DNA:

- Watson, J. D. *The Double Helix.* New York: Atheneum, 1968.

The 1980 RDA book provides readable and interesting accounts of the reasoning behind the latest recommendations:

- *Recommended Dietary Allowances*, 9th ed. Washington, D.C.: National Academy of Sciences, 1980.

Inborn Errors

Knowing how proteins are put together (Chapter 3) has made possible insight into and control over some diseases that once were utterly mysterious and unconquerable. The so-called inborn errors of metabolism provide a dramatic example of these victories.

Imagine a happy pair of parents proudly viewing their beautiful baby in the hospital nursery. She looks flawless, and they are thrilled, after waiting so long, to welcome her into the world. But unknown to them she has a hidden disease — phenylketonuria (PKU) — whose symptoms have not yet emerged.

Before screening for PKU became routine, this story would have become a tragedy. The parents would take their child home, and she would behave like any other baby — for a while. But gradually, signs of retardation would begin to appear. By half a year of age the baby would be more irritable and active than other babies. By a year, she would be noticeably abnormal; she would wave her arms, grind her teeth, and might even have convulsions. She would become overdependent and immature. Already, irreversible brain damage would have occurred. By two years, more symptoms would appear: She might be unable to walk, she would never learn to talk, and her IQ would

Fundamentally, genes control enzymes, and enzymes control the chemistry of life. If any mutation or change takes place in the structure of a gene, there will be a functional disturbance somewhere in the body. . . . In a delicately balanced system like the gene complex, as in the engine of a motorcar or a television set, almost any change is likely to be for the worse.

WILLIAM BOYD

probably be below 30, maybe as low as 20. It is hard to believe that a simple change in diet, early in the child's life, could have prevented this, but in the case of PKU and many diseases like it, it is true.

Cause of PKU PKU results from an enzyme defect. The enzyme that should act on the amino acid, phenylalanine, to convert it to tyrosine is malfunctioning (see Figure 1). The result: Abnormally high concentrations of phenylalanine and other compounds derived from it accumulate and damage the developing nervous system. Simultaneously, the needed amino acid tyrosine is lacking, and the lack causes further damage. In effect, tyrosine has become an *es-*

sential amino acid. Needed compounds derived from tyrosine are also lacking. One of these is the hormone epinephrine.

Nutritional Therapy The effect of nutrition intervention in PKU is like magic. In almost every case, the devastating array of symptoms just described can be greatly modified or almost completely prevented. How? By controlling the amount of phenylalanine given in the diet so that tissue levels do not rise to the point where they can cause damage. To achieve this, special formulas and foods have been developed that contain normal amounts of *all of the amino acids except phenylalanine.* (Sometimes, extra tyrosine has to be added to the diet too.) Phenylalanine is an essential amino acid; that is, the body can't make it and it is needed to build protein, so it can't be completely excluded from the diet. The goal of treatment is to feed just that amount that will be locked up by the child's body into proteins where it will do good, not harm. To be sure of doing this, the dietitian, nutritionist, or clinician responsible for diet reviews periodic tests to monitor the concentration of phenylalanine in the blood, and alters the diet when necessary. If phenylalanine intake is controlled, the child can lead a much more normal life.

Figure 1   The biochemical defect in PKU.

Normal:

phenylalanine

major route

minor route

tyrosine

phenylpyruvic acid

Tyrosine then goes on to form other compounds. Among them are the very important hormone epinephrine, and the pigment melanin.

other compounds (phenyl acetic acid and phenyl acetyl glutamine)

A. Normally, the amino acid phenylalanine encounters two enzymes that convert it to other compounds. One (the major one) adds an OH group to it to form the very similar but distinct amino acid, tyrosine. The other enzyme (which can't handle much phenylalanine at a time) removes its amino group to make the compound phenylpyruvic acid. Other enzymes act on this compound to make other phenyl acids. (Do you see the subtle differences in structure among these three compounds?)

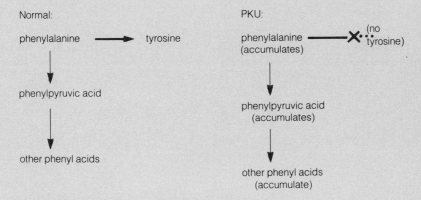

B. In PKU, the major enzyme is malfunctioning, so that little or no conversion of phenylalanine to tyrosine can take place. The minor enzyme works to capacity, producing abnormal amounts of the phenyl acid products. Phenylalanine itself also accumulates (not all is processed). Abnormally high concentrations of these substances accumulate all over the body and, together with the relative lack of tyrosine, cause irreversible damage to the developing brain.

Screening for PKU   In nearly every state, all hospitals are required to screen all their newborns to detect PKU before it can damage development. Any of several tests, administered after the baby has first been fed protein, can pick up on high phenylketone concentration in the blood or urine. When the abnormality is found, further testing is undertaken to pin down the diagnosis. About one in every 14,000 babies has PKU — not many, but before they were identified and treated they may have accounted for one out of every 100 or 200 institutionalized mentally retarded. Today, fifty years after the disease was first recognized, there are clinics, teaching programs for parents, commercial products, cookbooks, and ongoing research programs devoted to PKU.

The Carrier of PKU   PKU is a recessive trait; that is, it normally does not appear in a person who carries just one gene for it. Like all genes, the gene for the enzyme that is defective in PKU comes in two copies: one from the mother, the other from the father. The baby who inherits a defect-free gene from one parent will be able to make a functioning enzyme; that is, the normal type is dominant. Only if defective genes from both parents turn up in the child does the defect become

apparent. Another way to say this is that only if both parents are carriers can they have a PKU child; and even then, they may not, because either one or both may pass on a defect-free gene to each child (see Figure 2). A person may not even know that he/she is a carrier; hence the importance of testing all members of a family in which PKU has appeared, and of genetic counseling for carriers who consider having children.

The PKU Adult: Special Diet During Pregnancy
It is not known for how long the nervous system is vulnerable to the PKU defect. When the critical events have taken place, it may be that the diet can be discontinued. If the person eats the same foods as everyone else, however, the tissue levels of phenylalanine and associated products will again rise. If a female with PKU becomes pregnant, she must go back on the phenylalanine-restricted, tyrosine-

Figure 2   Inheritance of PKU.

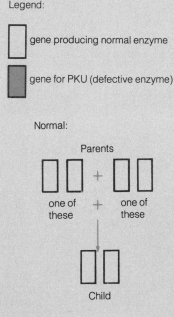

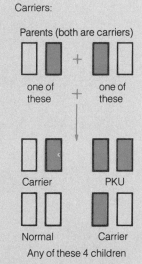

Any of these 4 children

Figure 2a   If both parents possess two copies of the normal enzyme for processing phenylalanine, their children will of course inherit defect-free genes from both.

Figure 2b   If both parents are carriers (possess one gene for PKU), then they can both pass on the PKU gene to any of their children. For each birth, there is one chance in four that the child will have PKU, two chances that the child will be a carrier, and one chance that it will be PKU-free.

supplemented diet for the term of her pregnancy, so as to avoid damaging her baby's developing nervous system.

The account of PKU just given is necessarily brief. It does not give insight into the variations on PKU, the differences of opinion regarding appropriate times to discontinue the diet, or the challenge a family faces in actually coping with the problems of a PKU child (but see To Explore Further). This Highlight's purpose has been served, however. From this one example, you can see how devastating the consequences can be when a single enzyme is missing or cannot do its job. You can see the dramatic benefits gained from our new understanding of protein nutrition and of each amino acid's role in metabolism. And you are in a position to appreciate the importance of fitting the appropriate nutrition therapy to a disease that can respond to it.

Galactosemia   To give you some idea of the variety of inborn errors like PKU, now known, another can be used for contrast. Galactosemia is a disorder in which the monosaccharide galactose

can't be normally utilized by the body. *Three* enzymes are involved in handling galactose, and any one may be missing or defective. In the more severe case, an infant given milk, which contains a

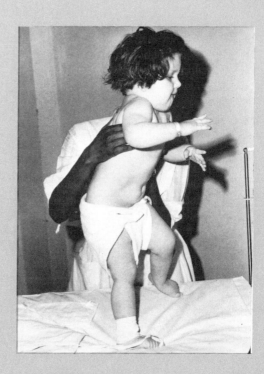

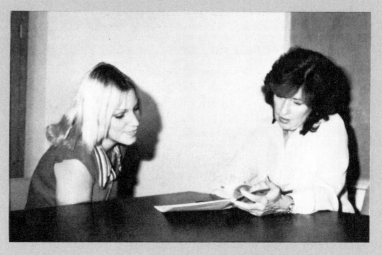

galactose unit in each molecule of lactose, vomits and has diarrhea after the very first milk feeding. Growth begins to fail within days after birth and liver damage is apparent within a week. Death may follow soon after. If the child lives, the unmetabolized galactose is shunted along an alternative pathway to form an abnormal product that causes cataracts, damage to the sexual organs, and brain damage to the point of mental retardation. A diet restricted in galactose can prevent or minimize these symptoms.

Galactosemia differs from PKU in several ways. First, galactose is not an essential nutrient (as phenylalanine is), so dietary adjustment is simpler. The PKU diet is a balancing act of providing just enough for normal protein synthesis, without enough left over to be toxic; the galactosemia diet involves simply excluding galactose. Since galactose occurs only in lactose (the sugar in milk), milk and milk products must be avoided. Secondly, the problem of phenylalanine toxicity may be time-limited, so that perhaps the diet can be discontinued after a while; galactosemia, in contrast, is known to require lifelong adherence to a galactose-free diet. Thirdly, *carriers* of galactosemia (carrying one gene for the trait) are not symptom-free. Their bodies

can't manage galactose quite as well as those who have three perfect genes; reduced enzyme activity can be detected. Even though they can eat a normal diet, it is thought that during pregnancy they should eliminate galactose to avoid damage to the fetus.

Galactosemia is perhaps two or three times more rare than PKU, but must be treated immediately if its consequences are to be averted. It can be detected even before a baby is born, by measuring the enzyme level in blood taken from the umbilical cord.

Other Inborn Errors

Phenylalanine is an amino acid. Galactose is a monosaccharide. When the enzyme that metabolizes phenylalanine is defective, PKU results. When any of the enzymes that metabolize galactose is defective, galactosemia results. What other enzymes are subject to defects that can cause diseases? How many inborn errors are possible?

Every enzyme the body makes has its code carried by a gene (Chapter 3, Figure 1). Any gene can mutate, so that the protein it makes differs from the normal protein in some way. In 999 cases out of 1,000, the result of a mutation is a disadvantage or disaster for the organism.

One of the smallest types of cells ever studied, a bacte-

rial cell, bears genes for at least 1,000 different enzymes. Mutations are possible in all of these genes. Human cells probably have at least 100 to 1,000 times as many proteins of major importance and, in theory, any of them can appear in many different mutant forms. Not only the genes for enzymes but also those for other proteins such as the "pumps" that move nutrients into and out of cells, the carriers that transport them in the blood, and the structural proteins of cell membranes, connective tissue, and the like can be affected by alterations in genes.

In many cases, a mutation in a gene will produce such catastrophic effects that the organism inheriting that gene will not survive; it will die before birth (a lethal mutation) or before reaching reproductive age. In such a case, the mutation will not be passed on to any offspring; it is "selected out" of the gene pool. But in other cases a mutant gene can be carried by an individual so long as it is paired with a normal gene that permits production of the needed protein. Only when two mutant genes from two different carriers segregate into the same individual do the effects of the protein's malfunction appear. Such is the case with PKU and most of the other inborn errors of metabolism. They are rare, recessive traits.

PKU has been known for fewer than 50 years. Following its discovery, a multitude of other inborn errors have been recognized. A familiar one is sickle-cell anemia, in which one of the amino acids of the hemoglobin molecule is replaced by a different amino acid at one of the molecule's dozens of sites. Some 150-odd other mutant forms of hemoglobin are known (most have no observable effects), and about one of every 600 people probably carries one.[1] Another is familial hypercholesterolemia, which may account for about 20 percent of all heart attacks that occur before 60 years of age. The defective protein is one in the liver cell membranes that removes cholesterol from the blood. About one in every 500 persons carries one copy of the mutant gene.[2]

These examples could be multiplied many times, but they are enough to convey the intended message. Understanding protein structure and function makes it possi-

---

Miniglossary

carrier: an individual who possesses one dominant and one recessive gene for a recessive trait such as an inborn error. Such a person may show no signs of the trait but can pass it on.

dominant: see *recessive.*

familial hypercholesterolemia: a hereditary disease characterized by inability of the liver cells to remove cholesterol from the blood.

hyper = too much
emia = in the blood

galactosemia: an inborn error of metabolism in which galactose cannot be metabolized normally to compounds the body can handle. An alternative metabolite accumulates in the tissues, causing damage.

mutant: an organism carrying a mutation that shows up. Often a mutant must carry two copies of the mutation, one in each gene, before the effects are seen.

muta = change

mutation: an alteration in a gene, such that an altered protein is produced.

phenylketonuria (PKU): an inborn error of metabolism in which phenylalanine cannot be converted to tyrosine. Alternative metabolites of phenylalanine (phenylketones) accumulate in the tissues causing damage, and overflow into the urine.

phenyl = a ring structure found in many important molecules
ketone (see Chapter 2)
uria = in the urine

recessive: of a mutated gene, one that has no observable effect on an organism as long as it is paired with a normal gene that can produce a normal product. The normal gene is said to be *dominant.*

sickle-cell anemia: a hereditary disease caused by an alteration in the hemoglobin molecule. The altered hemoglobin carries oxygen less efficiently and also causes a change in the red blood cells so that they become sickle-shaped.

---

[1]N. A. Holtzman, M. L. Batshaw, and D. L. Valle, Genetic aspects of human nutrition, in R. S. Goodhart and M. E. Shils, eds., *Modern Nutrition in Health and Disease,* 6th ed. (Philadelphia: Lea and Febiger, 1980), pp. 1193-1219.

[2]J. M. Osten and O. W. Neuhaus, *Human Biochemistry,* 9th ed. (St. Louis: Mosby, 1975), p. 778.

ble to compensate for inborn errors of metabolism that otherwise would destroy the quality of life. Diet can not always be tailored to prevent completely the defects of inborn errors, but a 1980 authority lists 90 such diseases that are diet-responsive.[3] The diet therapist can be rewarded with the chance to make a great difference in people's lives.

[3]Holtzman, Batshaw, and Valle, 1980.

To Explore Further

A nurse whose child was diagnosed as having PKU describes the resulting disruption of her family's life and how they rose to the challenge, in:

● Reyzer, N. Diagnosis: PKU. *American Journal of Nursing* 78 (1978):1895-1898.

A physician expresses his concerns about the risks of discontinuing the PKU diet too early in childhood:

● Diet termination for PKU: Yes or No? (Medical News). *Journal of the American Medical Association* 240 (1978):1471.

A group of clinicians explain how to get infants started on the PKU diet:

● Acosta, P.B., Wenz, E., Williamson, M., and Writing Committee, Collaborative Study of Children Treated for Phenylketonuria. Methods of dietary inception in infants with phenylketonuria. *Journal of the American Dietetic Association* 72 (1978):164-169.

Techniques for managing the pregnant woman's diet are outlined in:

● Pueschel, S. M., Hum, C., and Andrews, M. Nutritional management of the female with phenylketonuria during pregnancy. *American Journal of Clinical Nutrition* 30 (1977):1153-1161.

A thoughtful review, for the advanced student, of the relationship of PKU to mental retardation suggests that some of the PKU defects are due to tyrosine deficiency and can even be caused in the fetus of a carrier mother if she doesn't eat ample protein:

● Bessman, S. P. The justification theory: The essential nature of the non-essential amino acids. *Nutrition Reviews* 37 (1979):209-220.

A major technical reference on the diet-responsive inborn errors is:

● Winick, M., ed. Nutritional Management of Genetic Disorders. Current Concepts in Nutrition, Vol. 8. New York: Wiley, 1979.

Another is:

● Stanbury, J. B. and Wyngaarden, J. B. The Metabolic Basis of Inherited Disease, text ed. New York: McGraw-Hill, 1977.

A clear exposition of the genetics underlying inborn errors and of the principles of dietary management is available in:

● Holtzman, N. A., Batshaw, M. L., and Valle, D. L. Genetic aspects of human nutrition, in Goodhart, R. S., and Shils, M. E., eds., *Modern Nutrition in Health and Disease*, 6th ed. Philadelphia: Lea and Febiger, 1980, pp. 1193-1219.

Protein

1. Calculate your protein RDA as suggested in this chapter. Compare your protein intake from the Introduction Self-Study with the RDA. If you are "average," two-thirds of the RDA is probably sufficient for you. How much more (or less) do you consume? Are you spending protein prices for an energy nutrient?

2. How many kcalories a day do you consume from protein? (Remember, protein contributes 4 kcal/g.) What percentage of your total daily kcalories does protein contribute? How does this figure compare with the suggested goal of 10 to 12 percent of kcalories from protein?

3. How many of your protein grams are from animal, and how many from plant, sources? It is desirable to get about half or more from plant sources. Should the proportion be changed? If you decreased your intake of animal protein and increased your plant protein, what effect would this have on the relative amounts of polyunsaturated and saturated *fat* in your diet?

Optional Extras

4. Notice the timing of your protein intake. How is your protein intake distributed throughout the day? (Study the twenty-four-hour record you made for the Introduction Self-Study.) Do you have amino acids at breakfast time to stabilize your blood glucose supply from carbohydrate? At lunchtime, to steady you for the afternoon? At dinnertime, to sustain you through the evening?

5. Be aware of the units in which protein is measured. A "high-protein supplement" advertises that it supplies "an unbelievable 690 milligrams of purified high-quality protein in every tablet!" Using the RDA as a yardstick, what percentage of a person's daily need for protein does a tablet supply? (Check the Introduction Self-Study to compare milligrams with grams.)

CHAPTER 4

CONTENTS

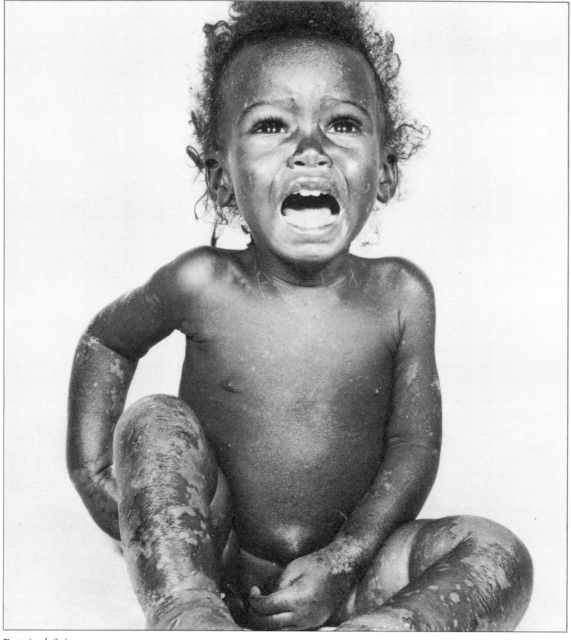

Protein deficiency.

PROTEIN IN THE BODY

There is present in plants and in animals a substance which . . . is without doubt the most important of all the known substances in living matter, and, without it, life would be impossible on our planet. This material has been named Protein.

GERARD JOHANNES MULDER, 1838

The elaborately coiled configuration of the body's gigantic protein molecules enables them to do the thousands of tasks that maintain life. This chapter describes a few of those tasks so that you may understand the tremendous importance of obtaining the amino acids you need. The following discussion focuses on the tasks performed by protein in which other nutrients (vitamins and minerals) cooperate. The minerals sodium and potassium, for example, help proteins maintain the water balance; vitamin C helps make the protein collagen which is involved in scar formation. For the present, we suggest that you read the following with the thought in mind that "proteins do all these things." Then you will have the background to appreciate the roles of the helper nutrients, details of which are given in Chapters 9 through 14. When you read those chapters, you can recall that "these other nutrients help the proteins do all these things." Margin references in this chapter show where each of the helper nutrients is described.

Some proteins act as enzymes. Our earlier description of enzyme molecules depicted them as giant tangled chains of amino acids, bristling with positive and negative charges, and bouncing about in the fluids of the body. Because of their differing surface characteristics, each enzyme is able to perform a different role. Each can work on a different compound—to break it apart into smaller compounds, to add something to it and make it larger, or to change some part of it in order to change its chemical identity.

There are many other proteins besides enzymes in the body. The roles of some of these are understandable at the molecular level if you keep this "bristling ball" picture in mind.

Enzyme: see pp. 98-102.

Helper nutrients: coenzymes (like the B vitamins) and cofactors (minerals). See Chapters 9, 12, and 13.

water balance: distribution of body water among the body compartments.

intravascular space: the continuous space inside the circulatory system (heart, arteries, capillaries, and veins).

intra = inside (within)
vascular = vein

intracellular space: the spaces inside the cells.

Fluid Balances

Proteins help maintain the water balance. To understand how this extremely important function is managed, you must know that there are three principal compartments for fluids in the body: the intravascular space, the intracellular space, and the interstitial space. In normal, healthy people, each of these compartments contains the

125

interstitial (in-ter-STISH-ul) **space:** the spaces between the cells and outside the vascular system.

interstice = space between

Minerals are helper nutrients (see pp. 482-496).

The flow of water across a membrane in the direction of a solute, such as protein or minerals, is due to osmotic pressure (see Chapter 14).

edema (uh-DEE-muh): accumulation of fluid in the interstitial spaces. In the special case where edema occurs in the abdomen, it is known as **ascites** (uh-SITE-eez).

diuretic (dye-yoo-RET-ic): a drug that stimulates increased renal water excretion.

renal = kidney

Kidneys: see the illustration on p. 179.

proper amount of fluid. Fluid can flow back and forth across the boundaries between them, but whenever the volume of fluid deviates, it is rapidly brought back to normal. Protein (with certain minerals) helps to maintain the amount of water at the proper volume in each compartment.

The way this works is neat and simple. Proteins are so large that they cannot pass freely across the walls or membranes that separate the compartments. They are trapped where they are. They are also hydrophilic, or attractive to water molecules, so the water molecules stay with or near the proteins. By regulating the amount of protein (and minerals) in each compartment, the body indirectly regulates the amount of water.

When something goes wrong with this system—when a person is suffering from a condition in which the blood protein concentration falls, for example—fluid may leak out of the vascular system and accumulate in the interstitial tissues. The result is a symptom known as edema, a visible swelling or puffiness in the tissues. It is not uncommon for pregnant women to suffer a swelling of the ankles, which reflects fluid leakage from the leg veins. In other people fluid may leak out of the veins into the abdominal cavity, resulting in a swollen "pot belly." In others the hands may swell or the face may become puffy.

The uninformed person may believe that the way to prevent this swelling is to drink less water or to increase excretion by taking a diuretic. If edema has become extreme, these measures, as well as salt restriction, may indeed be a necessary part of treatment. Yet you can never cause edema by drinking too much water. The more you drink, the more you carry in your vascular system, and (because the vascular fluid is circulated through your kidneys) the more you automatically excrete.

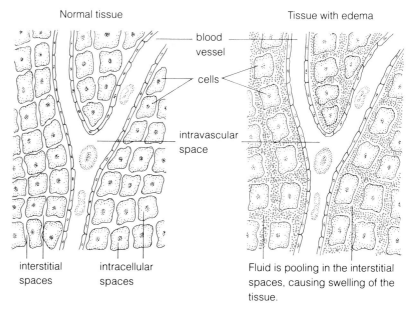

Normal tissue   Tissue with edema

blood vessel

cells

intravascular space

interstitial spaces   intracellular spaces   Fluid is pooling in the interstitial spaces, causing swelling of the tissue.

This discussion illustrates a principle that pervades the study of health. Provided that you are healthy, your body will maintain its own health. No known drug renders the healthy body more capable of regulating its own functions than it is already. Drugs are needed only to remedy situations in which body functions have become impaired. Diuretics may be needed only when excess fluid has already accumulated. They are not useful as preventive medicine.

Since the taking of a diuretic increases water excretion, it causes a sudden weight loss. A healthy person who fails to distinguish between loss of body fat and loss of water may see this as a desirable effect and start using diuretics for this purpose. But because the only loss induced is water loss, the only achievement gained is dehydration.

So what does cause edema? One thing is a protein-deficient diet. When protein intake falls below a certain limit, blood proteins become depleted and the body's hormonal balance becomes upset. The water that should be held within the bloodstream then leaks into the interstitial space causing swelling. This water is not available to the kidneys to excrete; the kidneys do not "know" it is there. (Remember, the kidneys can only "see" what is in the bloodstream that travels through them.) Hence the remedy may not be less water but more protein.

Another fluid balance that proteins help maintain is that between acids and bases. An acid solution is one in which there are hydrogen ions floating around. The more hydrogen ions, the more concentrated the acid. Proteins (and minerals), which have negative charges on their surfaces, attract hydrogen ions, and hydrogen ions in turn attract proteins. As long as the concentration of hydrogen ions—that is, the strength of the acid—stays within certain limits, the proteins maintain their integrity. If the acid becomes too strong, however, the extra positive charges surrounding the protein molecules deform them and, so to speak, pull them out of shape. When this happens the proteins can no longer function.

Of all the consequences that stem from exceeding the normal limits of acid-base balance in the body, the most direct and serious is a disturbance of the shapes of the proteins that carry out so many of the vital body functions. Acidosis and alkalosis both are lethal if unchecked. The proteins in the plasma, such as albumin, help to prevent these conditions from arising. In a sense the proteins protect one another by binding or sequestering extra hydrogen ions when there are too many in the surrounding medium and by releasing them when there are too few. This ability to regulate the acidity of the medium is known as the buffering action of proteins.

acid-base balance: the balance maintained in the body between too much and too little acid. Blood pH, for example, is regulated normally between 7.38 and 7.42 (pH: see below).

Minerals are helper nutrients (see pp. 482-496).

Ion: see p. 67, Appendix B.

pH: the concentration of H^+ ions (see Appendix B). The lower the pH, the stronger the acid. Thus pH 2 is a strong acid, pH 6 a weak acid (pH 7 is neutral). A pH above 7 is alkaline, or basic (a solution in which acid-accepting ions such as OH^- predominate).

acidosis: too much acid in the blood and body fluids.

alkalosis: too much base in the blood and body fluids.

lethal: causing death.

sequester (see-KWES-ter): to hide away or take out of circulation.

buffer: a compound that can reversibly combine with H^+ ions to help maintain a constant pH. Figure 1 in Chapter 14 shows how a buffer works.

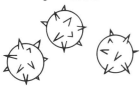

1. Body is challenged with foreign invaders.

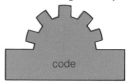

2. Body makes code for manufacturing antibody.

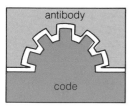

3. Code makes antibody.

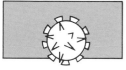

4. Antibody inactivates foreign invader.

Crunch!

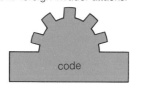

5. Code remains to make antibodies faster the next time this foreign invader attacks.

Development of immunity. The relationships of nutrients to the immune system are the subject of Highlight 22.

Antibodies and Hormones

Other major proteins found in the blood—the antibodies—act against disease agents. When a body is invaded by a virus—whether it is a flu virus, smallpox virus, measles virus, or virus that causes the common cold—the virus enters the cells and multiplies there. One virus may produce a hundred replicas of itself within an hour or so. These burst out and invade a hundred different cells, soon yielding ten thousand virus particles, which invade ten thousand cells. After several hours there may be a million viruses and then a hundred million and so on. If they were left free to do their worst, they would soon overwhelm the body with the disease they cause.

The antibodies, giant protein molecules circulating in the blood, are a defense against viruses, bacteria, and other "foreign agents." The surface of each antibody molecule has characteristics that enable it to combine with and inactivate a specific foreign protein, like that in a virus coat or bacterial cell membrane. The antibodies work so efficiently that in a normal healthy individual the many disease agents that attempt to attack never have a chance to get started. If a million bacterial cells are injected into the skin of a healthy person, fewer than ten are likely to survive for five hours.[1]

Once the body has manufactured antibodies against a particular disease agent (such as the measles virus), the cells never forget how to produce them. The next time the antibodies will respond even more quickly. The immunological response of the antibody-producing cells and the way they achieve their molecular memory of the body's enemies is beyond the scope of this book, but Highlight 22 offers some further details.

Hormones are also carried by the blood, and some are pure protein. Among them are the familiar thyroid hormone and insulin. The thyroid hormone regulates the body's metabolic rate—the rate of the chemical reactions that yield energy. Insulin regulates the concentration of the blood glucose and its transportation into cells, upon which the functioning of the brain and the nervous system depend. Hormones have many other profound effects on the body, as discussed in Highlight 2.

Transport Proteins

Some proteins move nutrients into and out of cells. There are proteins in the membrane of every cell of the body, each one specific for a certain compound (or group of related compounds). Each of these proteins is confined to the membrane but can rotate or shuttle from one side to the other. These protein "pumps" can pick up a compound on one side of the membrane and release it on the other, thus enabling the cells to

[1] R. Y. Stanier, M. Doudoroff, and E. A. Adelberg, *The Microbial World*, 3rd ed. (Englewood Cliffs, N.J.: Prentice-Hall, 1970), p. 784.

choose what substances to take up and what to release. For example, the glucose pump and the potassium pump transport glucose and potassium into cells faster than they can leak out, and the sodium pump transports sodium out of cells. Thanks to these pumps, a higher concentration of glucose and potassium is maintained inside than outside the cells, and the reverse is true of sodium. It may not be obvious why the cells go to so much trouble to maintain these concentration gradients, but many reasons will become apparent in later chapters. To anticipate one of them very simplistically: The sodium-potassium distribution across the membranes of nerve cells is what makes it possible for nerve impulses to travel—and so for you to think.

The mineral calcium enters the body with the help of a protein too, the calcium-binding protein in the intestinal tract. In fact, almost every water-soluble nutrient seems to have its own pump in cell membranes. (By contrast, lipids can cross membranes without the help of pumps if they are small and simple enough. Cells seem to regulate lipid transport by taking them apart so they can move across the membranes, then putting them back together again to keep them from escaping.)

Many of the cell membrane pumps can be switched on or off according to the body's needs. Often hormones do the switching, with a marvelous precision. Suppose, for example, there is too much glucose in the blood. High blood glucose causes the pancreas to step up its output of the hormone insulin; the insulin stimulates glucose uptake in the membranes of the liver and fat cells (and is destroyed in the process); these cells pick up the excess glucose; then when the blood glucose concentration is normal, the pancreas reduces its insulin output. The absorption of calcium is regulated by the hormones calcitonin and parathormone in a similar manner. These examples illustrate how hundreds of different body proteins maintain the distribution of substances into the various body spaces.

Another type of transport protein is the carriers in the body fluids. Many nutrients travel freely in the vascular system, but others have to be carried. The lipids are an example. You have already read about the problem these cumbersome molecules pose for the digestive system: They have to be emulsified in order to be made accessible to the enzymes that hydrolyze them. Even after absorption they require special handling. Each major lipid has to be wrapped in protein before it can be transported in the blood. These complexes are called lipoproteins. They are giant aggregates, much larger than lipids by themselves, but they travel easily in water because their protein coats are hydrophilic. (Only the smaller lipids—monoglycerides, glycerol, and fatty acids—can travel freely without carriers.) The fat-soluble vitamins are also carried by special proteins.

The mineral iron is a nutrient whose handling in the body illustrates especially well how precisely proteins operate. On leaving the intestine, iron is picked up by an iron-carrying protein in the bloodstream known as transferrin. Transferrin may transfer the iron to a storage protein in

antibody: a large protein of the blood, produced in response to invasion of the body by foreign protein; inactivates the foreign protein.

immunology (im-yoo-NOLL-uh-gee): the study of immunity and the way in which it is achieved by antibodies and other agents of disease resistance.

Hormone: see p. 82.

Iodine (part of the thyroid hormone) and zinc (part of insulin) are helper nutrients (see pp. 451-456).

These membrane-associated proteins are variously called **permeases, vectorial enzymes,** and **transferases.**

concentration gradient: a difference in concentration of a **solute** (SOLL-yoot), a dissolved substance, on two sides of a semipermeable membrane.

Regulation of calcium absorption: see p. 417.

Emulsify: see pp. 67-68.

Lipoprotein: see p. 182.

hydrophilic (high-dro-FILL-ic): water-loving (see also p. 67).

the bone marrow known as ferritin. This protein finally releases the iron to become part of the protein hemoglobin, which is synthesized in new red blood cells as they are formed.

The protein hemoglobin is a giant molecule that contains four atoms of iron. The iron can combine with oxygen and then release it. As the red cells flow through the lungs, the hemoglobin iron picks up oxygen. Then as the red cells flow through the tissues, the iron releases the oxygen into the body cells, where it can oxidize other nutrients to provide energy. (As a carbon-hydrogen-oxygen compound such as carbohydrate or fat is oxidized, the H combines with O to form water—H_2O—and the C combines with O to form carbon dioxide—CO_2.) The blood plasma then dissolves the carbon dioxide released by the cells. When the blood returns to the lungs, this carbon dioxide is released into the air spaces in the lungs and exhaled. The oxygen carrier of muscle, myoglobin, is also a protein.

Other Proteins

Proteins perform many other roles in the body. Only a few more examples will serve to illustrate their diversity.

thrombin: a protein carried in the blood, involved in blood clotting.

thrombo = clot

The other protein circulating in the blood, ready to react with thrombin, is **fibrinogen** (fye-BRIN-o-gen). The reaction between these two and other protein factors produces **fibrin** (FYE-brin), the protein material of the clot.

fibr = fibers
ogen = gives rise to

Vitamin K (involved in the production of thrombin) and calcium (needed for blood to clot) are helper nutrients (see p. 397).

Collagen: see also p. 353.

Vitamin C (needed to form collagen) and minerals (to calcify bones and teeth) are helper nutrients (see pp. 353, 413).

Blood Clotting   Blood is unique and wonderful in its ability to remain a liquid tissue even though it carries so many large molecules and cells through the circulatory system. But blood can also turn solid within seconds when the integrity of that system is disturbed. If it did not clot, a single pinprick could drain your entire body of all its blood, just as a tiny hole in a bucket makes the bucket forever useless for holding water. When you cut yourself, the injured blood cells react immediately by releasing a protein called thrombin. The thrombin encounters another protein already circulating in the fluid part of the blood and converts it to fibrin, a stringy, insoluble mass of fibers that plugs the cut and stops the leak. Later, more slowly, a scar forms to replace the clot and permanently heal the cut.

Connective Tissue   Proteins help make scar tissue, bones, and teeth. When the construction of a bone or a tooth begins, the shape is first roughed out by laying down a protein matrix known as collagen, which forms a cartilage. Later, crystals of calcium, phosphorus, fluoride, and other minerals are laid down on this matrix, and the hardened bone begins to form. When a bone breaks, again the protein collagen precedes the bony material in the mending process. Collagen is also the mending material in torn tissue, forming scars to hold the separated parts together. It forms the material of ligaments and tendons and is a strengthening constituent between the cells of the artery walls, which must be able to withstand the pressure of surging heartbeats.

Visual Pigments   The light-sensitive pigments in the cells of the retina are molecules of the protein opsin. Opsin responds to light by changing its shape, thus initiating the nerve impulses that convey the sense of sight to the higher centers of the brain.

Opsin: see p. 379.

Vitamin A is a helper nutrient (see pp. 377-380).

Growth and Maintenance

Proteins are needed for growth and maintenance of all body tissues. Whenever you take a bath, you wash off whole cells from the surface layers of your skin, losing protein. Your hair and fingernails are growing constantly; since you ultimately cut them off (or break or chew them), these processes also result in a net loss of body protein. Similar processes occur inside your body. When you swallow food, it passes down your intestinal tract. Ultimately the undigested materials—fiber, water, and waste—leave your body, carrying with them cells that have been shed from the intestinal lining. Both inside and outside you must constantly build new cells to replace those lost from the exposed surfaces. In fact, it is said that a person's skin is replaced totally every seven years.

Given either fat or carbohydrate (composed of C, H, and O) as an energy source, the body can construct many of the materials (also composed of C, H, and O) needed to replace these lost cells. But to replace the protein, it must have protein from food, because food protein is virtually its only available source of nitrogen.

If the body is growing, it must manufacture more cells than are lost. Children end each day with more blood cells, more muscle cells, more skin cells than they had at the beginning of the day. So protein is needed both for routine maintenance (replacement) and growth (addition) of body tissue.

The above list of protein functions is by no means exhaustive, but it does give some sense of the immense variety and importance of proteins in the body. With this information as background, you are in a position to appreciate the significance of the world's most serious malnutrition problem: protein-kcalorie deficiency.

Protein-kCalorie Deficiency

The most ominous specter haunting the populations of the world's underdeveloped countries is protein-kcalorie malnutrition. Protein and kcalories (energy) are all-pervasive in human nutrition; they are involved in every body function. When children are deprived of food and suffer a kcalorie deficit, they degrade their own body protein for

protein-kcalorie malnutrition: a deficiency of protein or kcalories or both.

PCM: protein-calorie malnutrition.

Marasmus: see also p. 213.

kwashiorkor (kwash-ee-OR-core, kwash-ee-or-CORE): the protein-deficiency disease.

energy and thus indirectly suffer a protein deficiency as well as a kcalorie deficiency.

Protein and kcalorie deprivation go hand in hand so often that public health officials have adopted an abbreviation for the overlapping deficiency: PCM (protein-calorie malnutrition). Cases are observed at both ends of the spectrum, however. The classic kcalorie deficiency disease is marasmus, and the protein deficiency disease is kwashiorkor.

Classical marasmus is discussed in the chapter on energy balance (Chapter 7), because it can more easily be understood after some facts about energy metabolism have been presented. Kwashiorkor, however, is understandable on the basis of what we have already said about protein. These two diseases have a tremendous impact on the world's people and serious implications for the future of humankind. The problem is so complex that it requires separate emphasis; it is the subject of Highlight 18.

Kwashiorkor The word *kwashiorkor* originally meant "the evil spirit which infects the first child when the second child is born." It is easy to see how this superstitious belief arose among the Ghanaians who named the disease. When a mother who has been nursing her first child bears a second child, she weans the first and puts the second on the breast. The first child soon begins to sicken and die, just as if an evil spirit had accompanied the new baby into the world and set out to destroy the older child. What actually happens, of course, is that protein deficiency follows soon after weaning. Breast milk provides a child with sufficient protein, but these children are generally weaned to a starchy, protein-poor gruel. The gruel does not supply enough amino acids even to maintain a child's body, much less enough to enable it to grow.

Kwashiorkor occurs not only in Africa but also in Central America, South America, the Near East, the Far East—and in some wealthier countries as well. In all these regions, mother's milk is the only reliable and readily available source of protein for infants. Thus kwashiorkor typically sets in around the age of two. By the time the child is four, his growth is stunted; he is no taller than he was at two. His hair has lost its color; his skin is patchy and scaly, sometimes with ulcers or open sores that fail to heal. His belly, limbs, and face become swollen with edema; he sickens easily and is weak, fretful, and apathetic. Figure 1 is a picture of such a child.

The body follows a priority system when there is not enough protein to meet all its needs. It abandons its less vital systems first. When it cannot obtain enough amino acids from dietary sources, the body switches to a "metabolism of wasting": It begins to digest its own protein tissues in order to supply the amino acids needed to build the most vital internal proteins and thus to keep itself alive. Hair and skin pigments (which are made from amino acids) are dispensable and are not manufactured. The skin needs less integrity in a life-or-death situation than the heart does, so its maintenance ceases and skin sores

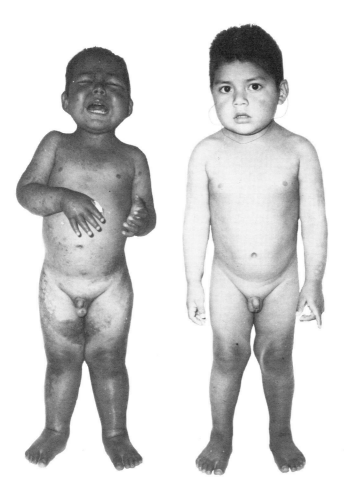

Figure 1 Kwashiorkor. The child at left has the characteristic "moon face" (edema) and the edematous swelling, which stretches the skin of his hands, belly, legs, and feet. His skin shows the typical patchy dermatitis of kwashiorkor. Without the swelling of edema, he would appear emaciated. At right, the same child after nutritional therapy.

Courtesy of Dr. Robert S. Goodhart, M.D.

fail to heal. Many of the antibodies are also degraded so that their amino acids may be used as building blocks for heart and lung and brain tissue. A child with a lowered supply of antibodies cannot resist infection and readily contracts dysentery, a disease of the digestive tract. Dysentery causes diarrhea, leading to rapid loss of nutrients—including amino acids—that the child may be receiving in food. Thus dysentery worsens the protein deficiency, and the protein deficiency in turn increases the likelihood of a second or third or tenth attack of dysentery.

The water loss in diarrhea increases losses of the water-soluble B vitamins and vitamin C. The child's inability to manufacture protein carriers for the fat-soluble vitamins creates a deficiency in vitamins A and D as well. The child's inability to manufacture protein carriers for fat often leaves him with fat accumulated in the liver tissue, from which it would normally be carried away. As the liver clogs with fat, its cells lose their ability to carry out their other normal functions, and gradually they atrophy and die.

dysentery (DIS-en-terry): an infection of the gastrointestinal tract caused by an amoeba or bacterium and giving rise to severe diarrhea.

When two variables interact so that each increases the other, they are said to be acting synergistically. Malnutrition and infection are a deadly combination because they work this way.

synergism (SIN-er-jism): the effect of two factors operating together in such a way that the sum of their actions is greater than the actions of the two considered separately.

Edema: see pp. 126-127.

A malnourished child who contracts measles cannot fight it off. In our country, where protein deficiency is not a problem, the child with measles may expect to recover within five to seven days; the kwashiorkor child dies within the first two days. Other diseases also take their toll.

The swollen belly of the kwashiorkor child is due to edema; blood protein is low and hormonal balance is disturbed so that fluid leaks out of the blood vessels into the body tissues and spaces. The child is too weak to stand much of the time, so the fluid settles in the belly—the lowest available space. Thus a child with this problem often has skinny arms and legs and a greatly swollen belly. On first glance you might think the child is fat, but if the fluid could be drawn off, his true condition would be revealed: He is actually a wasted skeleton, just skin and bones.

Adult Protein Deficiencies   Kwashiorkor is only one of several diseases associated with protein deficiency. Another that is closer to home for most of us is the nutritional liver disease associated with alcoholism. The alcoholic person, like the kwashiorkor child, consumes abundant kcalories, but up to three-fourths of his kcalories may come from alcohol, a nonprotein substance. Like the kwashiorkor child, the malnourished alcoholic may have a swollen belly; puffy hands, feet, and face; skin sores; and a reduced ability to withstand infection. Also like the kwashiorkor child, the chronic alcoholic develops a fatty liver. If the situation goes unremedied for too long, the liver cells ultimately die and are replaced by inert scar tissue. This is the progression to cirrhosis, which is so often caused by alcoholism.

The "beer belly" of the alcoholic sometimes reflects ascites (edema in the abdomen), although it is usually rightly attributed to an excess of kcalories.

cirrhosis (seer-OH-sis): irreversible liver damage involving death of liver cells and their replacement by scar tissue.

For the effects of alcohol on the liver, see Chapter 24.

Adult kwashiorkor and marasmus also occur in hospital patients whose diets have been inadequate. A person undergoing surgery or fighting an infection has a greatly increased need of protein and kcalories. At the same time, she may feel too sick to eat or may be fed only liquids or intravenous fluids, which are not nearly nutritious enough even to maintain a healthy body. Hospital malnutrition occurs in up to 50 percent of the patients in some hospitals and increases the risks associated with surgery and infection. Physicians, whose medical school training has until recently almost totally neglected nutrition, are now becoming increasingly aware of its importance in the treatment of the sick. Some hospitals now maintain staffs to assess the nutrition status of the patients and to provide nutrition support.[2]

Highlight 20B describes a nutrition support team in action.

It must by now be abundantly clear that protein is more than just an energy source. It is the body's molecular machinery; it does the body's work. Understanding what proteins are and what they do permits perspective on the roles of nutrients in health and disease.

[2]G. L. Blackburn and B. R. Bistrian, Nutritional support resources in hospital practice, in *Nutritional Support of Medical Practice*, eds. H. A. Schneider, C. E. Anderson, and D. B. Coursin (Hagerstown, Md.: Harper & Row, 1977), chap. 10.

Summing Up

In addition to acting as enzymes, as described in Chapter 3, proteins perform many other functions in the body. They provide osmotic pressure, which regulates the distribution of water in the various body compartments (the water balance). They provide a buffering action in the body fluids, which helps to maintain the acid-base balance. Antibodies, which convey immunity, and some hormones, such as thyroid hormone and insulin, are made of protein. In the cell membrane, protein "pumps" confer on the cell the ability to select and take up specific compounds while excluding others, thus establishing concentration gradients. The absorption of many nutrients from the gastrointestinal tract depends on this function. Protein carriers are necessary to transport fats and fat-soluble vitamins in the circulatory system. Proteins are hydrophilic and so can carry these compounds in the watery fluid of the blood. The body's oxygen carriers, the hemoglobin of red blood cells and the myoglobin of muscles, are also proteins. Other important body proteins include collagen—the building material of scar tissue, cartilage, ligaments, bones, and teeth—and the light-sensitive pigments of the retina.

Since all body cells contain protein, routine maintenance and repair of body tissues requires a continual supply of amino acids to synthesize proteins. Growth of new tissue requires additional protein.

Kwashiorkor is the name for the disease in which protein is lacking but kcalories are adequate. (kCalorie deficiency, known as marasmus, is treated in Chapter 7.) Kwashiorkor typically occurs in children after weaning, with severest symptoms being observed after the age of two. Symptoms include stunted growth, loss of pigment in the hair and skin, ulceration of the skin, edema, weakness, and apathy. The kwashiorkor victim often develops a fatty liver caused by a lack of the protein carriers that transport fat out of the liver. Reduced antibody formation makes the child extremely vulnerable to such diseases as dysentery and measles. These diseases work synergistically with the malnutrition, leaching nutrients from the body. Similar symptoms are seen in the alcoholic with nutritional liver disease and in the undernourished hospital patient.

Protein deficiency occurs whenever protein itself is lacking in the diet or when kcalories are inadequate. In the latter case, amino acids are degraded for energy, causing protein deficiency indirectly. The two deficiencies of protein and kcalories, which often go hand in hand, are together called PCM (protein-calorie malnutrition); this is the world's most serious malnutrition problem. PCM afflicts millions of people, especially children.

To Explore Further

A chapter on immunology provides a clear and understandable explanation of the way antibodies are constructed and how they work:

- Stanier, R. Y., Doudoroff, M., and Adelberg, E. A. *The Microbial World*, 3rd ed. Englewood Cliffs, N.J.: Prentice-Hall, 1970.

A detailed treatment of antibodies written for the general reader is:

- Nossal, G. J. V. *Antibodies and Immunity.* New York: Basic Books, 1969.

Meat Eaters versus Vegetarians

"Boy!" said the cave lady, as we stood with them before the solemn, clergyman-like head of an enormous moose. "Would he be good with onions!"

ALDOUS HUXLEY

The middle-aged man who says with braggadocio that he is a "meat and potatoes man" and the college-aged person who almost defiantly disdains any restaurant that will not serve a meal of vegetables, fruit, and nuts have a lot more in common than either would like to believe. Both are extremists in their use of a valuable class of food — protein — and both could be suffering from malnutrition due to the rigidity of their ideas about what constitutes a "good" food plan. In today's world, where overconsumption in affluent nations contrasts with famines in poorer nations, there is a need for better understanding of protein nutrition by everyone, from policy makers to consumers.

In earlier times, recommendations on proper diet were made on the basis of observation only. A doctor might have noted, for instance, that people who ate meat and eggs and drank milk were healthier, stronger, taller, or more resistant to infections. Therefore, he might have recommended to all his patients that they needed more protein and should include animal and dairy products in their diets. Later, when more sophisticated laboratory tests had been developed, it became clear that it was necessary to include certain amino acids in the diet and that animal and dairy products contained all of these essential amino acids. Vegetables, it was found, lacked one or more of these. Another observation was that populations subsisting on cereal diets, for reasons either of meat taboos or of economic necessity, were malnourished. The evidence was their relatively short stature, low resistance to diseases, short life span, and high infant mortality. All these observations and supporting laboratory work underscored a common belief that animal and dairy products were "good" protein foods and that plants were "poor" protein foods. Present-day investigations have shown that this notion was not entirely justified.

It is true that animal and dairy foods contain complete proteins; it does seem to be true that populations that consume milk and meat are generally healthier than grain-eating populations. But it has been shown by clinical tests that if the vegetables, legumes, fruits, and grains are wisely chosen, children grow as well on a diet devoid of animal protein as on one that includes milk and other animal proteins.[1]

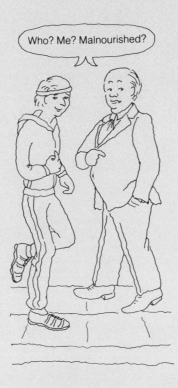

Who? Me? Malnourished?

[1]U. D. Register and L. M. Sonnenberg, The vegetarian diet, *Journal of the American Dietetic Association* 62 (1973):253-261.

137

In the United States and Canada, a love affair with meat has been flourishing for a century or more. No doubt the wide expanses of grazing land and the easy availability of wild animals to be had for the hunting (especially in earlier times) contributed to the acquisition of a taste for meat three times a day. In this century in the United States, the percentage of total protein consumed from animal sources has increased from half to two thirds of the total while protein consumed from plant sources has decreased from half to only one third of the total.[2]

However, a countertrend has been developing among many people, who are turning from the meals made up of eggs and bacon, hamburger and french fries, and steak and potatoes toward vegetarian diets. There is a wide variation in the reasons for this change given by the "new" vegetarians:[3] Some have been influenced by Eastern religions; some choose vegetarianism for reasons of health; some exclude meat on humanitarian grounds; some believe meat is too costly in money or in terms of land use; some are expressing antiestablishment feelings; and some are merely caught up in a new fad. There is also a wide variation in the extent to which meat and dairy products are excluded from these diets, ranging from the highest "Zen" macrobiotic diet, made up exclusively of rice, to those that eliminate animal meat but include fish or animal products such as eggs, milk, and cheese.

In order to help us gain an understanding of the nutritional problems of these two groups, let's examine the kcalorie, protein, and fat content of a "meat-and-potatoes" diet and a "vegetables, fruits, and nuts" diet to see why anyone who relies on either may be malnourished.

To make a valid comparison, we must use people of the same age and sex. If both are men under 35 and their ideal weight is 70 kilograms (154 pounds), their daily kcalorie allowance would be 2,700 kcal (see Appendix O). The RDA for protein is 0.8 g for each kilogram of ideal body weight, or 56 g protein for our subjects. If we assume that each eats a third of his kcalorie and protein allowance at each meal, then dinner should provide 900 kcal, and 19 g of protein.

[2]B. Friend and R. Marston, *Nutritional Review,* 1975 (bulletin of the Consumer and Food Economics Institute, U.S. Department of Agriculture, 1976).

[3]J. T. Dwyer, R. F. Kandel, L. D. V. H. Mayer, and J. Mayer, The new vegetarians, *Journal of the American Dietetic Association* 64 (1974):376-381.

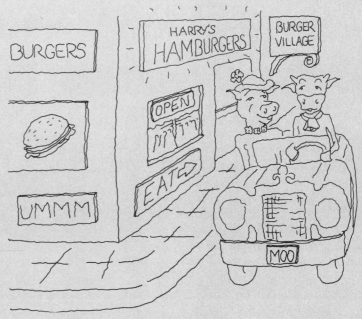

"This neighborhood always makes me nervous."

The Meat-and-Potatoes Diet What health implications can we see in the diet of the meat-and-potatoes man? The first observation must concern his excess *kcalories*. It is relatively easy to exceed the energy allowance when a large portion of the kcalories comes from animal meat. Some fat can be trimmed from the meat, but much of it is in the marbling. In addition to fat visible in the marbling, there may also be considerable invisible fat. The fat tastes delicious, so the eater eats more of the meat.

The *protein* needs for the entire day have almost been met in this one meal alone — 49 g of the 56 g required. Protein is important, of course, but only up to a point. If after ingestion more amino acids are present for several hours than are needed by the body, these amino acids will be degraded to carbon fragments that will be used for energy. If the carbon fragments are not needed for energy, they will be used to build body fat. Thus, overconsumption of essential amino acids, even though they are valuable in the proper quantity, can lead to obesity.

Beef used for *kcalories* is costly. If a cut of beef costs $5.50 a pound, its cost is 46 cents for 100 kcal; if an 18-oz box of rolled oats costs $1.50, its cost is only 6 cents for 100 kcal. If it is energy rather

than amino acids you are buying, it is obvious which of these is the better buy.

Plant kcalories also cost less land. A million kcalories in wheat can be produced on less than an acre of land; a million kcalories in beef require 17 acres.[4] (These figures have some striking implications for groups interested in solving the nutrition problems in developing countries; introducing meat into a vegetarian economy may worsen the food balance. Even in the United States we may soon find that we cannot afford the luxury of using 17 times as much land to produce the same amount of energy food.)

[4]F. J. Stare, Sugar in the diet of man, in *World Review of Nutrition and Dietetics* 22, ed. G. F. Bourne (Basel: S. Karger, 1975), pp. 239-247.

As for *fat*, 83 g were consumed in this meal. Each gram of fat produces 9 kcal, so about 750 out of 1,270 kcal in this meal came from fat — more than 55 percent. It is recommended that fat contribute no more than 30 to 35 percent of the total kcalories and, furthermore, that saturated fat consumption be reduced. A diet high in fat has serious implications for the development of atherosclerosis (see Chapter 26) and perhaps some forms of cancer (Highlight 28). Fat also has a high satiety value, but this is not desirable when the appetite is satisfied before enough vegetables, fruits, and grains have been consumed to ensure that all the needed vitamins and minerals have been included.

Finally, this is a low *fiber* meal. Fiber aids in digestion and may be important for

Table 1. The Meat-and-Potato Dinner

Food	Exchanges*	Energy (kcal)	Protein (g)	Fat (g)
6 oz boneless	6 lean meat	330	42	18
beefsteak	6 fat	270	—	30
1 large baked potato	2 bread	140	4	—
2 tsp margarine	2 fat	90	—	10
1 lettuce salad	vegetable (free)	—	—	—
2 tbsp French dressing	2 fat	90	—	10
1 slice (1/7) apple pie†		350	3	15
TOTAL		1,270	49	83

*Food composition values are from the exchange lists in Appendix L.
†Calculated by using the Table of Food Composition (Appendix H).

the prevention of diverticulosis (Chapter 23) and cancer of the colon,[5] as well as atherosclerosis[6] (Chapter 26). People who are interested in prevention of these diseases would be wise to increase their consumption of vegetables, fruits, and grains.

In summary, this meal contains more than enough protein and an excess of kcalories, largely from fat. At the same time, it offers too few vegetables and fruits to ensure that all essential nutrients and adequate fiber are present. It is an unbalanced diet.

[5] D. P. Burkitt, Relationships between diseases and their etiological significance, *American Journal of Clinical Nutrition* 30 (1977):262-267.

[6] D. Kritchevsky and J. A. Story, Binding of bile salts in vitro by nonnutritive fiber, *Journal of Nutrition* 104 (1974):458-462.

Miniglossary

extrapolation (ex-trap-ah-LAY-shun): an educated guess, from a known series of numbers, as to what others may be. For example, knowing that the world population was 2 billion in 1930, 3 billion in 1960, and 4 billion in 1977, we can extrapolate that it will be 6 billion in 2000.

lacto-ovo-vegetarian: a vegetarian who excludes animal flesh but eats such animal products as milk and eggs.

  lacto = milk
  ovo = eggs

lacto-vegetarian: a vegetarian who excludes animal flesh and all animal products except milk.

marbling: a lacy network of fat embedded in meat, sometimes so fine as to be invisible. Sometimes called invisible fat, in contrast to the visible fats — butter, margarine, oil, and the fats removable from meat.

mutual supplementation: the strategy, used by vegetarians, of combining two incomplete protein foods in a meal so that each food provides the essential amino acid(s) lacking in the other. The resulting protein mixture is called complementary protein.

ovo-vegetarian: a vegetarian who excludes animal flesh and all animal products except eggs.

satiety (suh-TIE-uh-tee): the feeling of fullness or satisfaction after a meal. Fat provides satiety more than carbohydrate or protein because it slows gastric motility.

vegan (VAY-gun, VEJ-an): a strict vegetarian; one who excludes all animal flesh and animal products, eating only plant foods.

In the introduction to Part One we stated that the only unequivocal statement about the nutritive quality of a food is a statement of the specific nutrients it contains and the amount of each. In this Highlight the nutritive quality of two diets is being examined, and the above statement can be amplified. In assessing these diets it is useful (1) to note the specific nutrients they contain and (2) to state the amount of each. We also undertake two additional means of evaluation: (3) to examine the quality of the nutrients (complete or incomplete protein, saturated or polyunsaturated fat) and (4) to compare the amounts of the nutrients with the recommended intakes. Each of these two additional judgments deserves a comment.

Notice that in assessing the quality of the nutrients we are not concerned about their source but about their molecular characteristics. The food sources of amino acids need not be "organically grown," but they do need to contribute a complete and balanced spectrum of essential amino acids. The fat need not be "natural," but it does need to have a high percentage of polyunsaturated fatty acids. These observations reinforce the points made in the first Digression of Chapter 2.

In comparing the amounts of the nutrients with the RDAs, we can make a meaningful statement about their contribution to a person's needs. Failing to use such a yardstick can cause serious misunderstanding on the part of a careless reader/consumer. For example, when you read that a diet pill contains "570 mg of solid natural protein," you may believe that you are taking a pill that contains significant protein. Only when you measure this amount against the RDA for protein (56,000 mg for each of our subjects) do you realize that you would have to take nearly a hundred diet pills a day to meet the protein recommendation.

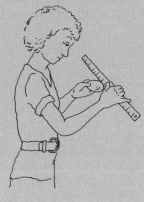

CAUTION WHEN YOU READ!

Make a habit of using a yardstick to measure quantities.

Many food companies make statements about their products that can be critically analyzed this way. A "high-protein cereal" may sound like a cereal that provides a lot of protein for human needs, but on closer examination it turns out to be high in protein only when compared with other cereals. In small lettering on the side panel, the label of such a cereal may reveal that one serving, even including the milk added to it, supplies only 10 percent of the RDA for protein!

If there is no statement of quantity on the label or in the advertisement, beware. The statement that a food contains a nutrient, without specifying how much, may be intended to mislead.

A FLAG SIGN OF A SUSPECT CLAIM IS THE STATEMENT THAT: This product contains X (with no amount specified).

Now let's look at the "vegetables, fruits, and nuts" diet.

The Vegetables, Fruits, and Nuts Diet   This one meal is not typical of a knowledgeable vegetarian's diet, but it illustrates several of the difficulties an amateur vegan may encounter. There is a very large quantity of food in this meal, yet the energy is deficient by about 250 kcal. This deficiency, amounting to about 750 kcal per day, could result in a loss of about a pound every four to five days — unless, of course, it is corrected at the other meals. As a matter of fact, a common observation about vegans is that they are usually underweight and must eat huge amounts of food if they are to maintain their weight.

Another obstacle the vegan faces in planning meals is obtaining sufficient protein. This vegetarian dinner provides about half the recommended amount of protein. Furthermore, the protein that is present has a poor combination of essential amino acids. Vegetables must be chosen carefully if they are to be the only source of protein. Potatoes and carrots provide many important nutrients as well as adding to the fiber content of the diet, but a

Table 2.   The Vegetables, Fruits, and Nuts Dinner

Food	Exchanges*	Energy (kcal)	Protein (g)	Fat (g)
1 c cooked cabbage	2 vegetable	50	4	—
1 tsp safflower oil	1 fat	45	—	5
1/2 c cooked carrots	1 vegetable	25	2	—
1 large baked potato	2 bread	140	4	—
1 tbsp margarine	3 fat	135	—	15
fruit salad:				
1 small banana	2 fruit	80	—	—
1 small apple	1 fruit	40	—	—
1/2 c pineapple	1 fruit	40	—	—
2 tbsp raisins	1 fruit	40	—	—
6 nuts	1 fat	45	—	5
TOTAL		640	10	25

*See the exchange lists in Appendix L.

child would not grow properly on a diet in which the only sources of protein were potatoes and carrots.

In selecting *protein* sources for the diet, you must not only know the amount of protein in the source but also be certain that the essential amino acids are present. Most of the vegetables and grains are low in such essential amino acids as lysine, methionine, threonine, or tryptophan; however, by eating specific combinations at the same meal, you can obtain the equivalent of a complete protein. Use of two protein sources in such a way that each lacks a different amino acid, but provides the amino acid missing from the other, is called mutual supplementation. A rule of thumb: Mixtures of grains and legumes eaten *at the same meal* provide a fairly good proportion of the essential amino acids.

Some sincere vegetarians, when they first learn how important it is to eat complementary proteins at the same meal, are eager to know how much of each essential amino acid is required daily. They also want to know exactly how much of each is contained in their favorite plant foods.

This information is available. The laboratory work has been done, and the results are contained in advanced nutrition references.[7] However, much time can be squandered calculating the amino acid content of a meal. The calculations won't be useful because they tell you only how much amino acid is present, not how much your body will derive from it. The way the digestive system handles proteins is highly complex. For example, on some plant proteins the exposed bonds may resist early digestive steps, so that the entire protein remains intact. In this instance, even if the amino acids were present in the diet, they would not be available to the body; they would simply be excreted in the feces.

To avoid the hassle of computing specific amino acid quantities from tables only to come up with meaningless numbers, the vegetarian can adopt the strategy of eating a wide variety of protein sources

[7] H. N. Munro and M. C. Crim, The proteins and amino acids, in *Modern Nutrition in Health and Disease*, 6th ed., eds. R. S. Goodhart and M. E. Shils (Philadelphia: Lea and Febiger, 1980), pp. 82-95.

in generous servings. It is then practical to ask the question: What mixtures of plant foods contain a complete spectrum of essential amino acids? Armed with these strategies, the vegetarian can plan a menu that provides for his body's protein needs. Here is an answer[8] to that question:

Peanut protein	+	Wheat, oats, corn, rice, or coconut
Soy protein	+	Corn, wheat, rye, or sesame
Legumes	+	Cereals
Leafy vegetables	+	Cereals

[8]Register and Sonnenberg, 1973.

Mutual supplementation.

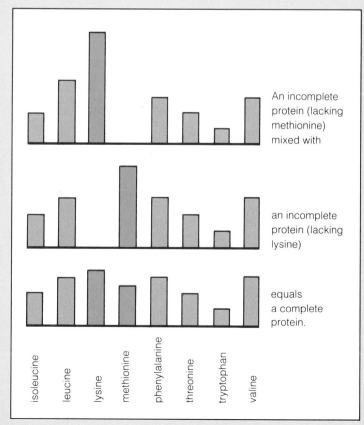

An incomplete protein (lacking methionine) mixed with

an incomplete protein (lacking lysine)

equals a complete protein.

isoleucine   leucine   lysine   methionine   phenylalanine   threonine   tryptophan   valine

Another point to consider in planning the protein for a meal is that there must be sufficient *kcalories* so that the amino acids will not be degraded for energy (that is, sufficient to "spare" the protein). With a 250-kcal deficit, the 10 g protein in this vegetarian's meal will most likely be used for energy rather than for building and maintaining his body tissues.

When we examine the *fat* content of the vegetarian's meal, we find only 25 g; this amount supplies 225 kcal, or about 35 percent of the total kcalories for the meal. This approaches the optimum fat consumption. In addition, about a third of the fat is the essential fatty acid, linoleic acid, whereas only a sixth of the fat in the meat-and-potatoes diet is linoleic acid. Also, there is no cholesterol in this meal. These are among the advantages of the vegetarian diet as compared to the meat-and-potatoes diet. Plant sources are high in polyunsaturated fat and, except for coconut, palm, and cocoa fat, contain very little saturated fat.

You have seen that this one meal of vegetables, fruits, and nuts contains a large quantity of food but a deficit of kcalories. This deficit could lead not only to loss of weight but also to poor utilization of the protein that·is present. The minimal amount of protein has a poor amino acid spectrum, since the two protein sources are not mutually supplemental. The meal does, however, contain a wide variety of fruits and vegetables, which would ensure an ample supply of vitamins and minerals and a good *fiber* content.

Diet Planning for the Vegetarian The discussion just concluded has shown that the vegetarian has some problems, albeit different ones from the meat-eater, with diet planning. Getting enough kcalories can be one. Getting enough protein, and protein of sufficiently high quality, can be another. The vegetarian who uses milk, dairy products, and eggs

Four Food Group Plan for the Vegetarian[9]

2 servings milk or milk products (or soy milk fortified with vitamin B_{12})

2 servings protein-rich foods (include 2 c legumes daily to help meet women's iron requirements; count 4 tbsp peanut butter as a serving)

4 servings whole-grain foods

4 servings fruits and vegetables (include 1 c dark greens to help meet women's iron requirements)

[9]Register and Sonnenberg, 1973.

(lacto-ovo) solves these problems rather easily. The vegan (no animal products) has to work harder at it.

The vegan also faces problems with other nutrients; these will be discussed later but should be recognized here. With the absence of milk and milk products, calcium, riboflavin, vitamin B_{12}, and vitamin D must be obtained in other ways. Occasional use of dark green leafy vegetables, legumes, and nuts will not supply enough calcium and riboflavin, but the daily use of 2 c soybean milk will protect against deficiencies of these two nutrients.[10] Soybean milk has been on the market for many years as a milk substitute for infants who are allergic to cow's milk. Soybean milk contains no vitamin B_{12}, however, so all vegans should supplement their diets with this vitamin or make a point of getting specially fortified soy milk.[11] Vitamin D can normally be obtained by exposure to the sun, but supplements are necessary otherwise, especially for growing children. The minerals iron and zinc may also be a problem: iron, because meat is omitted from the diet; and zinc, because it is

[10]Shands Teaching Hospital and Clinics, Food and Nutrition Service, *Vegetarian Food Choices* (Gainesville: University of Florida, 1976).

[11]Register and Sonnenberg, 1973.

not well absorbed from most plant foods. All this adds up to the fact that a vegetarian must be well informed about foods and diet planning.[12]

The vegan should take one other precaution in menu planning: Avoid the use of empty-kcalorie foods. Vegans must eat large quantities of food to meet their protein needs. They are dependent on the accumulation of small amounts of amino acids from each of many items. Empty-kcalorie foods would contribute no protein, vitamins, or minerals. The table in the corner shows a food group plan specifically designed for the vegetarian.

Which is the Better Diet? This comparison of the meat-eater's and the vegetarian's diet has turned up some flaws in each. The ideal diet lies somewhere between the two examples we've just studied. The person on a diet of meat and potatoes should select smaller servings of leaner meat and include a variety of vegetables, fruits, and cereals. Substituting meats that are lower in saturated fats (such as fish, chicken, and veal) for beef and pork would lower the fat and cholesterol con-

[12]J. H. Freeland-Graves, P. W. Bodzy, and M. A. Eppwright, Zinc status of vegetarians, *Journal of the American Dietetic Association* 77 (1980):655-661.

tent of this diet as well as the total kcalorie content. Conversely, the pure vegetarian would do well to shift *toward* the use of animal products. If vegans would decide to become lacto-ovo-vegetarians, they could easily correct most of the deficiencies noted in their diet. One egg and 2 c milk (2% fat) would provide 23 g of complete protein and 305 kcal as well as other valuable nutrients.

If vegetarians insist on omitting all animal and dairy products, they should be especially careful to meet their protein needs, should use a vitamin B_{12} supplement, and should meet their energy needs without resorting to empty-kcalorie foods. They must also be willing to become very well informed on nutrition and strict about including, at every meal, plant proteins that complement one another.

The lesson from these two examples seems to be that people can get into trouble nutritionally when they emphasize foods from just one or two categories, even if these are high-quality, important foods. By the same token, if they avoid one entire group of foods, as some vegetarians do, they are likely to develop deficiencies. The old maxim among nutritionists appears to be true: Good nutrition depends mostly on including a wide variety of foods in the diet.

To Explore Further

The American Dietetic Association has published a position paper on vegetarianism, defining terms and types of vegetarians, describing nutritional risks, and making recommendations:

- Position paper on the vegetarian approach to eating. *Journal of the American Dietetic Association* 77 (1980):61-69.

An easy book for the vegetarian, with an especially good discussion of complementary amino acids, is the paperback:

- Lappe, F. M. *Diet for a Small Planet.* New York: Ballantine Books, 1971.

Lappe's ideas are translated into attractive recipes in the paperback:

- Ewald, E. B. *Recipes for a Small Planet.* New York: Ballantine Books, 1973.

Two other cookbooks that we like are:

- Robertson, L. Flinders, C., and Godfrey, B. *Laurel's Kitchen: A Handbook for Vegetarian Cookery and Nutrition.* Berkeley, Calif.: Nilgiri Press, 1976.

- Thomas, A. *The Vegetarian Epicure.* New York: Knopf, 1972 paperback.

An excellent alternative to the two extreme diets described in this Highlight is presented by Chinese cookery, which uses small amounts of meat in dishes with great varieties of vegetables. The advantages of Chinese cookery are well described in the article:

- Newman, J. M. Chinese-American food: The diet of the future? *Journal of Home Economics* 68 (November 1976):39-43.

CHAPTER 5

CONTENTS

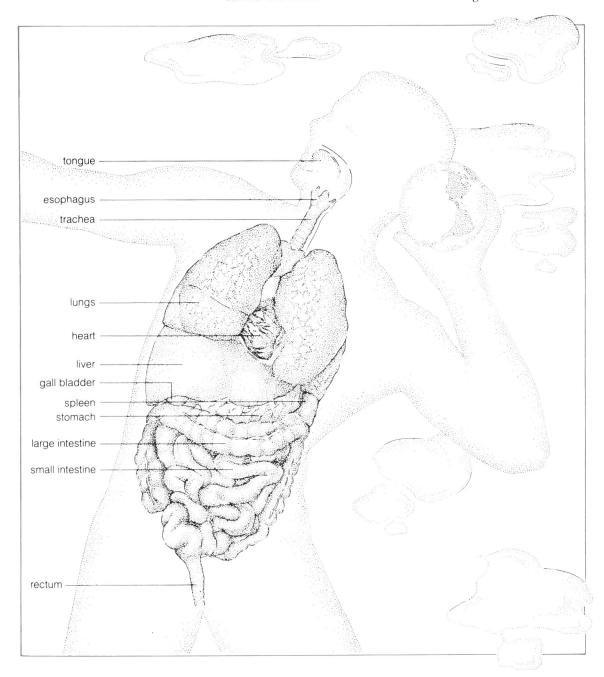

tongue

esophagus

trachea

lungs

heart

liver

gall bladder

spleen

stomach

large intestine

small intestine

rectum

DIGESTION

Food does not become nutrition until it passes the lips.

RONALD M. DEUTSCH

Lynn, age one, is playing with her mother's necklace. As one-year-olds do, she puts it in her mouth and chews on it. The necklace breaks. Lynn puts the beads into her mouth one by one and swallows them. An hour later her mother finds her with only a few of the hundred beads left on the table. In a panic, her mother calls the doctor. "Doctor," she says, "my daughter has just swallowed a necklace!" "Don't panic," says the doctor. "What was the necklace made of?" "Glass beads," says the mother. "And how big were the beads?" "About the size of a pea," says the mother. "That's all right then," says the doctor. "You'll get them back. Just watch her diapers for a day or so."

One of the beauties of the digestive tract is that it is selective. Materials that are nutritive for the body are broken down into particles that can be assimilated into the bloodstream. Those that are not are left undigested and pass out the other end of the digestive tract. In a sense, the human body is doughnut-shaped, and the digestive tract is the hole through the doughnut. You can drop beads through the hole indefinitely, and none of them will ever enter the doughnut proper. Two days after Lynn has swallowed them, her mother has recovered and restrung all the beads—and is again wearing the necklace!

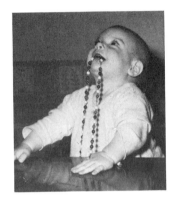

The problems associated with the nonnutritive dietary contaminants that can be absorbed are treated in Highlight 14.

The Problems of Digestion

Should you ever accidently swallow a necklace, you would be protected from any serious consequences by the design of your digestive tract. The system solves many other problems for you without your having to make any conscious effort. In fact, the digestive tract is the body's ingenious way of getting the nutrients ready for absorption. Let's consider the problems that are involved:

1. Human beings breathe as well as eat and drink through their mouths. Air taken in through the mouth must go to the lungs; food and liquid must go to the stomach. The throat must be arranged so that food and liquid do not travel to the lungs.

2. Below the lungs lies the diaphragm, a dome of muscle that separates the upper half of the major body cavity from the lower half. Food must be conducted through this wall to reach the abdomen.

3. To pass smoothly through the system, the food must be ground to a paste and must be lubricated with water. Too much water would cause the paste to flow too rapidly; too little would compact it too much, which could cause it to stop moving. The amount of water should be regulated to keep the intestinal contents at the right consistency.

4. When digestive enzymes are working on food, it should be very finely divided and suspended in a watery solution so that every particle will be accessible. Once digestion is complete and all the needed nutrients have been absorbed out of the tract into the body, only a residue remains, which is excreted. It would be both wasteful and messy to excrete large quantities of water with this residue, so some water should be withdrawn, leaving a paste just solid enough to be smooth and easy to pass.

5. The materials within the tract should be kept moving, slowly but steadily, at a pace that permits all reactions to reach completion. The materials should not be allowed to back up, except when a poison or like substance has been swallowed. At such a time the flow should reverse, to get rid of the poison by the shortest possible route (upward). If infection sets in farther down the tract, the flow should be accelerated, to speed its passage out of the body (downward).

6. The enzymes of the digestive tract are designed to digest carbohydrate, fat, and protein. The walls of the tract, being composed of living cells, are made of the same materials. These cells need protection against the action of the powerful juices that they secrete.

7. Once waste matter has reached the end of the tract, it must be excreted, but it would be inconvenient and embarrassing if this function occurred continuously. Provision must be made for periodic evacuation.

The following sections show how the body solves these problems, with elegance and efficiency.

GI tract: the gastrointestinal tract or alimentary canal; the principal organs are the stomach and intestines.

gastro = stomach
aliment = food

Anatomy of the Digestive Tract

The gastrointestinal (GI) tract is a flexible muscular tube measuring about 26 feet in length from the mouth to the anus. The voyage of the blue glass beads traces the path followed by food from one end to the other (see Figure 1).

When Lynn swallowed the beads, they first slid across her epiglottis, bypassing the entrance to her lungs. This is the body's solution to problem 1: Whenever you swallow, the epiglottis closes off your air passages so you do not choke. (You may wonder, however, what happens when a person does choke; that question is answered later in this chapter.)

Next the beads slid down the esophagus, which conducted them through the diaphragm (problem 2) to the stomach. There they were retained for a while. The cardiac sphincter at the entrance to the stomach closed behind them so that they could not slip back (problem 5). Then one by one they popped through the pylorus into the small intestine, and the pylorus too closed behind them. At the top of the small intestine they bypassed an opening (entrance only, no exit) from a duct (the common bile duct), which was dripping fluids (problem 3) into the small intestine from two organs outside the GI tract—the gallbladder and the pancreas. They traveled on down the small intestine through its three segments—the duodenum, the jejunum, and the ileum—a total of 20 feet of tubing coiled within the abdomen.

Having traveled through these segments of the small intestine, the beads arrived at another sphincter (problem 5 again)—the ileocecal valve—at the beginning of the large intestine (colon) in the lower right-hand side of the abdomen. As the beads entered the colon they passed another opening. Had they slipped into this opening they would have ended up in the appendix, a blind sac about the size of your little finger. They bypassed this opening, however, and traveled along the large intestine up the right-hand side of the abdomen, across the front to the left-hand side, down to the lower left-hand side, and finally below the other folds of the intestines to the back side of the body, above the rectum.

During passage through the colon, water was withdrawn, leaving semisolid waste (problem 4). The beads were held back by the strong muscles of the rectum. When the child chose to defecate, this muscle relaxed (problem 7), and the last sphincter in the system, the anus, opened to allow their passage.

To sum up, the path followed by the beads was

Epiglottis
Esophagus
Cardiac sphincter
Stomach
Pylorus
Common bile duct
Gallbladder
Pancreas
Duodenum
Jejunum
Ileum
Ileocecal valve
Colon
Appendix
Rectum
Anus

see Figure 1.

Mouth (epiglottis) → esophagus (cardiac sphincter) → stomach (pylorus) → small intestine (duodenum, with entrance from gallbladder and pancreas → jejunum → ileum) → large intestine (appendix) → rectum (anus)

This is not a very complex route, considering all that happens on the way. If you understand the anatomy of the system and the way the parts are connected, you can understand a number of common experiences: what happens when you choke on food (and what to do about it), when you vomit, when you get constipated, or when you have an ulcer. These experiences are explained in a section of Chapter 23.

epiglottis (epp-ee-GLOT-is): cartilage in the throat that guards the entrance to the trachea and prevents fluid or food from entering it when a person swallows.

epi = upon (over)
glottis = back of tongue

trachea (TRAKE-ee-uh): windpipe.

esophagus (e-SOFF-uh-gus): food pipe.

cardiac sphincter (CARD-ee-ack SFINK-ter): sphincter muscle separating the esophagus from the stomach.

cardiac = near the heart

sphincter: circular muscle surrounding and able to close a body opening.

sphincter = band (a binder)

pylorus (pie-LORE-us): sphincter muscle separating the stomach from the small intestine.

pylorus = gatekeeper

gallbladder and pancreas: see pp. 155-156.

duodenum (doo-oh-DEEN-um, doo-ODD-num): the top portion of the small intestine (about "12 fingers' breadth" long).

duodecim = twelve

jejunum (je-JOON-um): the first two-fifths of the small intestine beyond the duodenum.

ileum (ILL-ee-um): the last segment of the small intestine.

ileocecal (ill-ee-oh-SEEK-ul) **valve:** sphincter muscle separating the small and large intestines.

colon (COAL-un): the large intestine. Its segments are the ascending colon, the transverse colon, the descending colon, and the sigmoid colon.

sigmoid = shaped like the letter S (sigma)

appendix: a narrow blind sac extending from the beginning of the colon; a vestigial organ with no function.

rectum: the muscular terminal part of the intestine, from the sigmoid colon to the anus.

anus (AY-nus): terminal sphincter muscle of the GI tract.

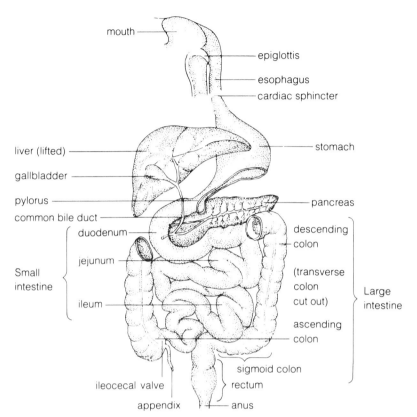

mouth

epiglottis

esophagus

cardiac sphincter

stomach

liver (lifted)

gallbladder

pylorus

common bile duct

pancreas

duodenum

descending colon

jejunum

(transverse colon cut out)

Small intestine

ileum

Large intestine

ascending colon

sigmoid colon

ileocecal valve

rectum

appendix

anus

The Involuntary Muscles and the Glands

You are usually unaware of all the activity that goes on between the time you swallow and the time you defecate. Like so much else that goes on in the body, the muscles and glands of the digestive tract meet internal needs without your having to exert any conscious effort to get the work done.

Chewing and swallowing are under conscious control, but even in the mouth there are some automatic processes that you have no control over. The salivary glands squirt just enough saliva into each mouthful of food so that it can pass easily down your esophagus (problem 3). (Occasionally, as you have noticed, they will squirt when you definitely do not want them to—when your mouth is open.) After a mouthful of food has been swallowed, it is called a bolus.

At the top of the esophagus peristalsis begins. The entire GI tract is ringed with muscles that can squeeze it tightly. Within these rings of muscle lie longitudinal muscles. When the rings tighten and the long muscles relax, the tube is constricted. When the rings relax and the long muscles tighten, the tube bulges. These actions follow each other so

gland: a cell or group of cells that secretes materials for special uses in the body. The salivary glands are **exocrine** (EX-o-crin) glands, secreting saliva "out" (not into the blood) into the mouth.

exo = outside

endocrine: secreting into the blood.

endo = within

bolus (BOH-lus): the portion of food swallowed at one time.

peristalsis (peri-STALL-sis): successive waves of involuntary contraction passing along the walls of the intestine.

peri = around
stellein = to wrap

Peristalsis.

Tube with longitudinal (L) and circular (C) muscles

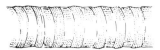

that the intestinal contents are continuously pushed along (problem 5). (If you have ever watched a lump of food pass along the body of a snake, you have a good picture of how these muscles work.) The waves of contraction ripple through the GI tract all the time, at the rate of about three a minute, whether or not you have just eaten a meal. Peristalsis—along with the sphincter muscles that surround the tract at key places—prevents anything from backing up.

Tube with longitudinal (L) and circular (C) muscles

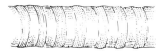

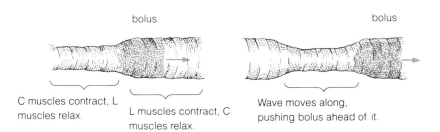

C muscles contract, L muscles relax.

L muscles contract, C muscles relax.

Wave moves along, pushing bolus ahead of it.

segmentation: a periodic squeezing or partitioning of the intestine by its circular muscles.

During the pushing motion, the intestines also periodically squeeze in short bands—as if you had put a string around them and pulled it tight. This motion, called segmentation, forces their contents backward a few inches at intervals, mixing them and allowing the digestive juices and the absorbing cells of the walls to make better contact with them.

Four major sphincter muscles work along the tract. The cardiac sphincter prevents reflux of the stomach contents into the esophagus. The pyloric sphincter, which stays closed most of the time, also prevents backup of the intestinal contents into the stomach and holds the bolus in the stomach long enough so that it can be thoroughly mixed with gastric juice and liquefied. At the end of the small intestine, the ileocecal valve performs a similar function. Finally, the tightness of the rectal muscle is a kind of safety device; together with the anus, it prevents elimination until you choose to perform it voluntarily (problem 7).

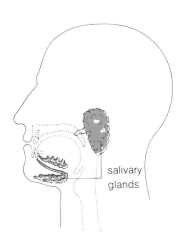

salivary glands

Smaller and Smaller

Besides forcing the bolus along, the muscles of the GI tract help to liquefy it so that the digestive enzymes will have access to all the nutrients. The first step in this process takes place in the mouth, where chewing, the addition of saliva, and the action of the tongue reduce the food to a coarse mash suitable for swallowing. A further mixing and kneading action then takes place in the stomach.

Of all parts of the GI tract, the stomach has the thickest walls and strongest muscles; in addition to the circular and longitudinal muscles, it has a third layer of transverse muscles that also alternately contract and relax.

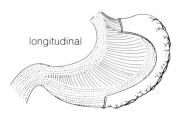 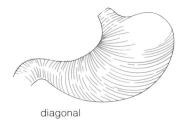 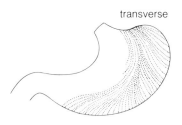

longitudinal

diagonal

transverse

Stomach muscles.

While these three sets of muscles are all at work forcing the bolus downward, the pyloric sphincter usually remains tightly closed, preventing the bolus from passing into the duodenum. Meanwhile, the gastric glands release juices that mix with the bolus. As a result, the bolus is churned and forced down, hits the pylorus, and bounces back. When the bolus is thoroughly liquefied, the pylorus opens briefly, about three times a minute, to allow small portions through. From this point on the intestinal contents are called chyme. They no longer resemble food in the least.

How Food Becomes You

One person may be a vegetarian, eating only fruits, vegetables, legumes, and nuts; another may have a meat-and-potatoes diet, eating very few fruits and vegetables. Whatever the diet—as long as it provides the needed nutrients in one form or another—people's body composition remains very much the same. It is impossible to tell from looking at a person whether he has just eaten a bowl of spaghetti and meatballs or a mixed green salad; in either case he has converted the materials in his food into the flesh, skin, and bones he is made of. How does he do it? It all comes down to the fact, of course, that the body renders food—whatever it was to start with—into the basic units that carbohydrate, fat, and protein are composed of. The body absorbs these units and builds its tissues from them. The final problem of the GI tract is to digest the food.

For this purpose there are five body components that contribute digestive juices: the salivary glands, the gastric glands, the intestinal glands, the liver, and the pancreas.

In addition to water and salts, saliva contains amylase, an enzyme that hydrolyzes starch to maltose. The digestion of starch thus begins in your mouth. In fact, you can taste the change if you choose. Starch has very little taste, but maltose has a subtly sweet flavor that you may associate with malted milk. If you hold a piece of starchy food like white bread in your mouth without swallowing it, you can taste it getting sweeter as the enzyme acts on it.

gastric glands: exocrine glands in the stomach wall that secrete gastric juice into the stomach.

gastro = stomach

chyme (KIME): the semiliquid mass of partly digested food expelled by the stomach into the duodenum.

chymos = juice

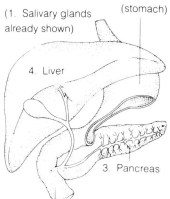

(1. Salivary glands already shown)

2. Gastric glands (stomach)

4. Liver

3. Pancreas

5. Intestinal glands

Organs that secrete digestive juices.

saliva: the secretion of the salivary glands; the principal enzyme is salivary amylase.

amylase (AM-uh-lase): an enzyme that hydrolyzes amylose (a form of starch). An older name for salivary amylase is **ptyalin** (TY-uh-lin).

hydrolyze (HIGH-dro-lies): to split by hydrolysis (see p. 25).

Mouth:		
Carbohydrate	Starch $\xrightarrow{\text{amylase}}$ maltose	
Fat	No chemical action	
Protein	No chemical action	
Vitamins	No chemical action	
Minerals	No chemical action	
Water	Added	
Fiber	Remains	

gastric juice: the secretion of the gastric glands. The principal enzymes are rennin (curdles milk protein, casein, and prepares it for pepsin action), pepsin (acts on proteins), and lipase (acts on emulsified fats).

pH: see p. 127.

mucus (MYOO-cuss): a mucopolysaccharide secreted by cells of the stomach wall. The cellular lining of the stomach with its coat of mucus is known as the mucous membrane.

Gastric juice is composed of water, enzymes, and hydrochloric acid. The acid is so strong (at or below pH 2) that if it chances to reflux into the mouth, it burns the throat. To protect themselves from gastric juice, the cells of the stomach wall secrete mucus, a thick, slimy, white polysaccharide that coats the cells, protecting them from the acid and enzymes that would otherwise digest them (problem 6).

It should be noted here that the strong acidity of the stomach is a desirable condition—television commercials for antacids notwithstanding. A person who overeats or who bolts her food is likely to suffer from indigestion. The muscular reaction of the stomach to unchewed lumps or to being overfilled may be so violent as to cause regurgitation (reverse peristalsis, another solution to problem 5). When this happens, the overeater may taste the stomach acid in her mouth and think she is suffering from "acid indigestion." Responding to TV commercials, she may take antacids to neutralize the stomach acid. The consequence of this action is a demand on the stomach to secrete more acid to counteract the neutralizer and enable the digestive enzymes to do their work. So the consumer ends up with the same amount of acid in her stomach but has had to work against the antacid to produce it.

Antacids are not designed to relieve the digestive discomfort of the hasty eater. Their proper use is to correct an abnormal condition, such as that of the ulcer patient whose stomach or duodenal lining has been attacked by acid. Antacid misuse is similar to the misuse of diuretics already described.

> A FLAG SIGN OF A SPURIOUS CLAIM IS THE IMPLICATION THAT:
>
> Medication designed to correct an abnormal condition is needed for the normal, healthy person.

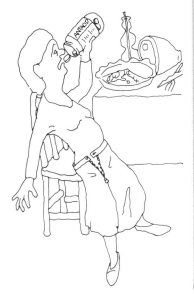

What our misguided consumer actually needs to do is to chew her food more thoroughly, eat it more slowly, and possibly eat less at a sitting.

All proteins are responsive to acidity; the stomach enzymes work most efficiently in a fluid of pH 2 or lower. However, salivary amylase—which is swallowed with the food—does not work in acid this strong, so the digestion of starch gradually ceases as the acid penetrates the bolus. In fact, salivary amylase becomes just another protein to be digested; its amino acids end up being recycled into other body proteins.

The major digestive event in the stomach is the hydrolysis of proteins. Both the enzyme pepsin and the stomach acid itself act as catalysts for this reaction. Minor events are the hydrolysis of some fat by a gastric lipase, the hydrolysis of sucrose (to a very small extent) by the stomach acid, and the attachment of a protein carrier to vitamin B_{12}.

pepsin: a gastric protease. It circulates as a precursor, pepsinogen, and is converted to pepsin by the action of stomach acid.

Vitamin B_{12} and the intrinsic factor: see Chapter 9.

Stomach:	
Carbohydrate	Minor action
Fat	Minor action
Protein	Protein $\xrightarrow[\text{HCl}]{\text{pepsin}}$ smaller polypeptides
Vitamins	Minor action
Minerals	No chemical action
Water	Added
Fiber	Remains

intestinal juice: the secretion of the intestinal glands; contains enzymes for the digestion of carbohydrate and protein and a minor enzyme for fat digestion.

pancreatic (pank-ree-AT-ic) **juice:** the exocrine secretion of the **pancreas**, containing enzymes for the digestion of carbohydrate, fat, and protein. (The pancreas also has an endocrine function, the secretion of insulin and other hormones; see p. 19). Juice flows from the pancreas into the small intestine through the pancreatic duct. When the pancreas fails, fat digestion is seriously impaired, since the intestine has no major lipase.

By the time food has left the stomach, digestion of all three energy nutrients has begun. But the action really gets going in the small intestine, where three more digestive juices are contributed. Glands situated in the intestinal wall secrete a watery juice containing all three kinds of enzymes—carbohydrases, lipases, and proteases—and others as well. In addition, both the pancreas and the liver make contributions by way of ducts leading into the duodenum. The pancreatic juice also contains enzymes of all three kinds, plus others.

Food evidently needs to be digested completely. The presence of two sets of enzymes for this purpose at this point underscores the body's determination to get the job done. If the pancreas fails, the intestine can largely carry on; if the intestine fails, the pancreas can substitute at least in part. Such duplication of effort is never seen in nature unless the job is absolutely vital, as it is in this case.

In addition to enzymes, the pancreas secretes sodium bicarbonate, which neutralizes the acidic chyme leaving the stomach. From this point on the contents of the digestive tract are at a neutral or slightly alkaline pH. The enzymes of both the intestine and the pancreas work best at this pH.

Bile, a secretion from the liver, also flows into the duodenum. The liver secretes this material continually, but it is needed only when fat is present in the intestine. The bile is concentrated and stored nearby, in the gallbladder, which squirts it into the duodenum on request. As explained in Chapter 2, bile is not an enzyme but an emulsifier; it brings fats into suspension in water so the enzymes can work on them.

bicarbonate: an alkaline secretion of the pancreas, part of the pancreatic juice. Bicarbonate also occurs widely in all cell fluids.

bile: an exocrine secretion of the liver (the liver also performs a multitude of metabolic functions). Bile flows from the liver into the gallbladder, where it is stored.

gallbladder: an organ that stores and concentrates bile. The gallbladder has no secretory function. Bile flows from the gallbladder into the small intestine through the bile duct.

The pancreatic and bile ducts conduct pancreas and liver secretions into the duodenum.

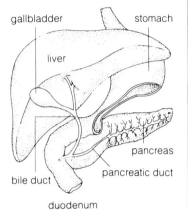

Details of pancreas, liver, gallbladder, and ducts.

Thanks to all these secretions, all the energy nutrients are digested in the small intestine.

Small intestine:

Carbohydrate	All carbohydrates ——→ monosaccharides	
Fat	All fats ——bile——→ emulsified fats	
	Emulsified fats ——→ monoglycerides or glycerol and fatty acids	
Protein	All proteins ——→ di- and tripeptides and amino acids	
Vitamins	No chemical action	
Minerals	No chemical action	
Water	Added	
Fiber	Remains	

Denaturation: see p. 98.

Most proteins are broken down to di- and tripeptides and amino acids before they are absorbed. With this in mind, you will be in a position to refute certain untrue claims made about foods. For instance:

"Don't eat store-bought beef. They injected a tenderizer into the blood of the steer before they killed it. When it gets into your blood, this enzyme will digest and destroy your tissues."

Just before slaughtering, pancreatic enzymes are sometimes injected into the steer's circulatory system; they do digest tough connective tissue in the vessel walls and make the meat easier to chew. But when you eat the meat, these enzymes have been denatured by cooking and cannot function as enzymes. They are but a few among thousands of different proteins in your digestive tract; they are broken down to amino acids identical to those from the other proteins you eat. Your body cannot tell the source of a particular amino acid any more than it can tell where its vitamin C comes from (Introduction).

"Eat brains. The materials they are made of will nourish your brain."

Like any other nutrients, the proteins, fats, and carbohydrates in brain tissue will be digested and absorbed and will nourish the body. But they are no better than hamburger, in the sense that both are digested to basic units before absorption. Each body builds its own brain tissue from basic units that can be obtained as well from hamburger as from brains.

"Eat predigested protein as amino acid mixtures so your digestive tract won't have to work so hard to digest protein."

It used to be believed that protein was digested all the way to amino acids before it was absorbed. Now we know that protein digestion in the fluid of the intestinal tract proceeds only as far as small peptides in many cases. These then enter the cells of the intestinal lining, and there they are digested further to amino acids. As a matter of fact, whole proteins are better absorbed and utilized, even by the body of a very sick, malnourished person, than are hydrolyzed amino acid mixtures.[1] This surprising finding has come to light through actual experiments, not through the exercise of reasoning from what was known before. It has given the lie to advertisers who try to sell protein supplements to athletes, sick people, dieters, and others. The "best" protein is food protein. The reasons why will be made clearer in Chapter 6, where a closer look at the intestinal cells shows how they handle protein.

This discussion stresses a point that is important for the informed consumer to remember. The argument that a food (tenderized beef) is harmful or that a food (brains) is beneficial can be identified as spurious by the flag sign mentioned before (p. 64). In addition, although these arguments are logical, they are not based on evidence. They sound convincing, as logical statements do, but if you know the facts of nutrition you can see through them.

In the hospital, there is a proper use for partially digested proteins. See Chapter 20.

A FLAG SIGN OF A SPURIOUS CLAIM IS:

The use of logic rather than evidence.

Such mistaken notions are as old as humankind. Will eating beets build good red blood? Will eating polished rice rather than brown rice give you a clear white complexion? Will you get pregnant from drinking cow's milk? You know these statements are preposterous, but all of them are still believed by thousands of people less well informed than yourself. The level of misleading statements now being circulated to our better-educated public has also been raised.

On the other hand, once logical statements are tested, they often prove true. In a susceptible or upset system, especially in that of a young infant, whole proteins from an uncooked food such as milk may be absorbed. They may be beneficial, as when antibodies from the mother's milk confer immunity on the infant. But they may cause allergy; in fact, the most common cause of food allergy is milk

Milk allergy: see p. 417.

[1]E. M. N. Hamilton and E. N. Whitney, Controversy 6: Liquid Protein, in *Nutrition: Concepts and Controversies*, 2d ed. (St. Paul: West, 1982), pp. 176-179.

protein "leaking" into the system through a defect in the wall. When a question like this is raised, experimental research must be undertaken to ascertain what really happens.

This Digression is not intended to review the evidence on protein absorption but to remind you that questions regarding whether or not a constituent of food is harmful can be answered only by experimentation.

The story of how food is broken down into nutrients that can be absorbed is now nearly complete. All that remains is to recall what is left in the GI tract. The three energy nutrients—carbohydrate, fat, and protein—are the only ones that must be disassembled to basic building blocks before they are absorbed. The other nutrients—vitamins, minerals, and water—are mostly absorbable as is. The function of the indigestible residues, such as fiber, is not to be absorbed but rather to remain in the digestive tract—mainly to provide a semisolid residue that can stimulate the muscles of the tract so that they will stay in tone and perform peristalsis. Fiber also retains water, keeping the stools soft. Furthermore, it carries bile acids, sterols, and fat with it out of the body.[2]

However there are some alterations made in the form of some minerals and vitamins. For oxidative changes of iron, see p. 440; for the binding of iron, p. 442. For the B_{12} carrier, or intrinsic factor, see pp. 332-333.

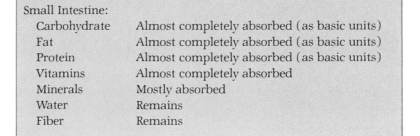

Small Intestine:

Carbohydrate	Almost completely absorbed (as basic units)
Fat	Almost completely absorbed (as basic units)
Protein	Almost completely absorbed (as basic units)
Vitamins	Almost completely absorbed
Minerals	Mostly absorbed
Water	Remains
Fiber	Remains

The process of absorbing the nutrients presents its own problems, which are taken up in Chapter 6. For the moment, let us assume that the digested nutrients simply disappear from the GI tract as soon as they are ready. Virtually all are gone by the time the contents of the GI tract reach the end of the small intestine. Little remains but water, a few dissolved salts and body secretions, indigestible materials such as fiber, and an occasional blue glass bead. These enter the colon, where intestinal bacteria degrade some of the fiber to simpler compounds.

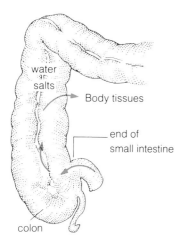

water salts
Body tissues
end of small intestine
colon

Detail of the large intestine.

[2]J. Scala, Fiber, the forgotten nutrient, *Food Technology* 28 (1974): 34-36.

The colon retrieves from its contents the materials that the conservative body is designed to recycle—much of the water and the dissolved salts (problem 4).

Large Intestine (Colon):
   Minerals   Reabsorbed
   Water   Some reabsorbed
   Fiber   Some digested by bacteria; some remains

At the end of the colon what is left is a semisolid waste of a consistency suitable for excretion.

The Regulation of GI Function

This is the first chapter of the book that takes you inside the body. While you are there, watching the motions of the muscles and the secretion of the digestive juices responding to the presence of food, it is only fair to give you a glimpse of the puppeteers who pull the strings. The story of digestion told above, although complete in outline and fair in emphasis, fails to give credit to the two marvelous systems that coordinate all the digestive processes and ensure that nothing goes wrong: the hormonal (or endocrine) system and the nervous system. This is not the place for a detailed description of advanced physiology; accordingly, the five examples given below are intended only as vignettes to illustrate the principles of the body's regulation of its internal environment.

The stomach normally remains at pH 1.5 to 1.7. How does it stay that way? One of the regulators of the stomach pH is a hormone, gastrin, produced by cells in the stomach wall. The entrance of food into the stomach stimulates these glands to release the hormone. The hormone in turn stimulates other stomach glands to secrete the components of hydrochloric acid. When pH 1.5 is reached, the gastrin-producing cells cannot release the hormone, so they stop. (The acid itself turns them off.) The acid-producing glands, lacking the hormonal stimulus, then stop secreting hydrochloric acid. Thus the system adjusts itself automatically.

Another regulator consists of nerve receptors in the stomach wall. These receptors respond to the presence of food and stimulate activity by both the gastric glands and muscles. As the stomach empties, the receptors are no longer stimulated, the flow of juices slows, and the stomach quiets down.

Highlight 2 is an optional chapter devoted to all the major hormones. The only ones mentioned here are a few of the GI tract hormones.

Hormone: see p. 82.

gastrin: a hormone produced by cells in the stomach wall. Target organ: the stomach. Response: secretion of gastric juice.

Gastrin regulation of stomach pH.

1. Food enters stomach.

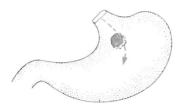

2. Stomach wall secretes gastrin into blood.

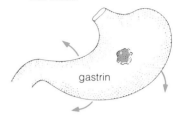

gastrin

3. Stomach glands respond by secreting acid.

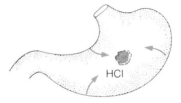

HCl

4. Acid stops gastrin secretion. Digestion proceeds at pH 1.5.

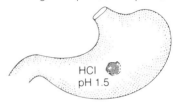

HCl
pH 1.5

The pylorus opens to let out a little chyme. How does it know when to close? When the pylorus relaxes, acidic chyme slips through. The acid itself touching that muscle on the far side causes the pylorus to close tightly. Only after the chyme has been neutralized by pancreatic bicarbonate and the medium surrounding the pylorus has become alkaline can the muscle relax again. This process ensures that the chyme will be released slowly enough to be neutralized as it flows through the small intestine. This is important because the small intestine has less of a mucous coating than the stomach does and therefore is not so well protected from acid.

Acid regulation of pylorus opening.

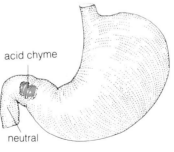

acid chyme

neutral

1. Pylorus opens.

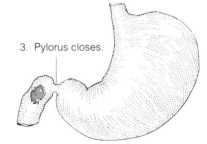

3. Pylorus closes.

2. Acid chyme passes through, touches far side of pyloric muscle.

secretin (see-CREET-in): a hormone produced by cells in the duodenum wall. Target organ: the pancreas. Response: secretion of pancreatic juice. Secretin has another name and function; see *enterogastrone*, p. 162.

As the chyme enters the intestine, the pancreas adds bicarbonate to it, so that the intestinal contents always remain at a slightly alkaline pH. How does the pancreas know how much to add? The duodenal contents stimulate cells of the duodenum wall to release the hormone secretin into the blood. As this hormone circulates through the pancreas, it stimulates the pancreas to release its juices. Thus whenever there is an acid in the duodenum, the pancreas responds by sending bicarbonate to neutralize it. When the need has been met, the secretin cells of the duodenal wall are no longer stimulated to release the hormone, the hormone no longer flows through the blood, the pancreas no longer receives the message, and it stops sending pancreatic juice. Nerves also regulate pancreatic secretions.

acid chyme in duodenum

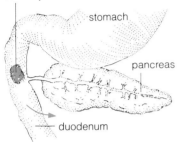

stomach

pancreas

duodenum

1. Duodenal wall releases secretin into blood.

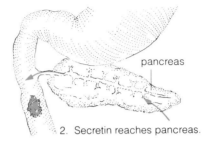

pancreas

2. Secretin reaches pancreas.

3. Pancreas secretes juice into duodenum.

4. Acid chyme is neutralized. Secretin release (1) stops.

Secretin regulation of pancreatic secretion.

When fat is present in the intestine, the gallbladder contracts to squirt bile into the intestine, to emulsify the fat. How does the gallbladder get the message that fat is present? Fat in the intestine stimulates cells of the intestinal wall to release the hormone cholecystokinin. This hormone, reaching the gallbladder by way of the blood, stimulates it to contract, releasing bile into the small intestine. Once the fat in the intestine is emulsified and enzymes have begun to work on it, it no longer provokes release of the hormone, and the message to contract is canceled.

cholecystokinin (coal-ee-sis-toe-KINE-in): a hormone produced by cells of the intestinal wall. Target organ: the gallbladder. Response: release of bile.

Cholecystokinin regulation of bile secretion.

stomach

gallbladder

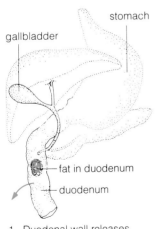

fat in duodenum

duodenum

1. Duodenal wall releases cholecystokinin into blood.

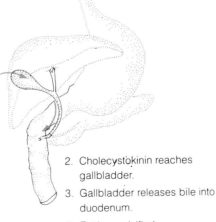

2. Cholecystokinin reaches gallbladder.

3. Gallbladder releases bile into duodenum.

4. Fat is emulsified. Cholecystokinin release (1) stops.

enterogastrone (enter-oh-GAS-trone): actually secretin by another name (once thought to be a different hormone). Enterogastrone is produced in the intestine in response to the presence of fat. Target organ: the stomach. Response: slowing of peristalsis.

The digestion of fat takes longer than that of carbohydrate. When fat is present, intestinal motility slows to allow time for its digestion. How does the intestine know when to slow down? Fat stimulates the release of the hormone enterogastrone, which suppresses the nerves that stimulate gastrointestinal motility, thus keeping food in the stomach longer. You may recall that a mixed breakfast of carbohydrate, fat, and protein was recommended in Chapter 1, partly because fat slows the digestion of carbohydrate, helping to keep the blood glucose level steady. Hormonal and nervous mechanisms like these account for much of the body's ability to adapt to changing conditions.

Once you have begun asking questions like these, you may not want to stop until you have become a full-fledged physiologist. For now, however, these few will be enough to make the point. Throughout the digestive system and all other body systems, all processes are precisely and automatically regulated, without your conscious efforts. This leaves you free to compose a symphony or to gaze at the stars instead of tying up your energy in worrying about how much acid to secrete or when to close your pylorus. This remarkable arrangement once prompted the physiologist Claude Bernard to remark, "Stability of the internal environment is the condition of free life." Walter Cannon, another physiologist, wrote a whole book about these processes, aptly titled *The Wisdom of the Body.* We took his title for the second Highlight of this book.

The kinds of regulation described are all examples of **feedback** mechanisms: a certain condition demands a response to change that condition. The change produced becomes itself the signal to cut off the response. Thus the system is self-corrective.

Summing Up

Let's follow some food through the digestive tract to the point where all needed nutrients have been absorbed. Whether it be a hamburger or a piece of chocolate cake, the same processes occur. The food is lubricated by saliva and broken up into particles by chewing. Starch digestion proceeds no farther than maltose in the mouth.

The food is swallowed and carried down the esophagus and through the cardiac sphincter by peristalsis, a muscular squeezing action that continues throughout the length of the tract. In the stomach further liquefication occurs, and the digestion of proteins begins through the action of pepsin and hydrochloric acid. The pylorus releases small portions of the liquefied acidic contents into the duodenum.

In the duodenum the emulsification of fats occurs—thanks to bile, a secretion of the liver that is concentrated and stored in the gallbladder until needed. Pancreatic bicarbonate neutralizes the intestinal contents to allow the enzymes of the intestinal and pancreatic juices to work, and fat, protein, and carbohydrate digestion all proceed further.

As the liquefied mixture of nutrients passes along the small intestine, the three energy nutrients continue being digested. By the time the mixture reaches the ileocecal valve, these nutrients have been almost completely rendered into the simpler compounds—the carbohydrates to monosaccharides; the lipids to monoglycerides, glycerol, and fatty acids; the proteins to di- and tripeptides and amino acids—and have been absorbed. The vitamins and minerals have also largely been absorbed by this time. For the most part, only water, fiber, and some dissolved salts remain.

In the large intestine, water and salts are reabsorbed, leaving a semisolid waste that is excreted from the rectum when the anus opens. The regulation of GI functions is accomplished by various hormonal and nerve-mediated messages that coordinate the supply of digestive juices and the action of the tract's muscles with demand.

To Explore Further

The early classic in physiology is:

● Cannon, W. B. *The Wisdom of the Body.* New York: Norton, 1932.

Cannon reveals and marvels at the ways the body maintains homeostasis.

One of many excellent recent physiology textbooks is:

● Eckert, R. *Animal Physiology.* San Francisco: Freeman, 1978.

An excellent, readable text about hormones, intended for college undergraduate chemistry students, is:

● Frieden, E., and Lippner, J. *Biochemical Endocrinology of the Vertebrates.* Foundations of Modern Biochemistry Series, Englewood Cliffs, N. J.: Prentice-Hall, 1971.

A teaching aid, *GI Function and Dysfunction,* includes four different slide presentations, each with an annotated syllabus. These can be purchased from the Nutrition Today Society (address in Appendix J).

Nutrition and the Brain

We ... have the fascinating prospect that the normal function of the central nervous system may depend on several transmitter substances, some stimulatory and others inhibitory.

KNUT SCHMIDT-NIELSEN

Have you ever wondered if what you eat affects how you think? Do certain foods calm you down? Does any food or nutrient help to put you to sleep? Could a food help to relieve depression or pain? Do people only imagine these things — is it all psychological — or is there a basis of reality beneath the imaginings?

Not long ago, most serious-minded scientists would have pooh-poohed the idea that food could affect mood, behavior, or wakefulness. But recent research has shown not only that it does have such effects but is beginning to show how the effects are brought about, at the molecular level. Two of the foremost researchers working in this area are R. J. Wurtman and J. J. Wurtman, who have been assembling their own and other workers' research into a massive work, *Nutrition and the Brain*, that has been appearing in published form, volume by volume, since 1977.[1] This Highlight focuses on a few of the areas their work has revealed.

How Nutrients Reach the Brain As the body's master controller, the brain is more carefully protected from harmful influences than any other organ in the body.

Three barriers separate the brain from direct exposure to what you eat. First, the GI tract cells themselves are selective; they refuse to absorb materials they don't recognize as foodstuffs (although they can be fooled sometimes). Second, all the materials absorbed into the blood circulate through the liver, which selectively removes toxins, drugs, and excess quantities of nutrients before allowing the blood to reach other parts of the body (Chapter 6). Thus the blood contents arriving at the brain have already been twice adjusted and cleansed; but the brain has its own molecular sieve to safeguard it further. Called the blood-brain barrier, this protective device normally keeps out all substances except those the

brain cells particularly need: glucose (or ketones), oxygen, amino acids (the ones not needed), nutrients (but not excessively large amounts).[2] As for the complex molecules that the brain cells themselves are made of, they make these for themselves out of the simple building blocks that they accept from the passing supply. If there is a *deficiency* of an essential nutrient, the brain's supply falls short, of course. The chapters on vitamins and minerals provide many examples of severe effects of deficiencies on brain function. But in general, the internal contents of brain cells do not reflect fluctuations in the supply from the diet.

An exception to these statements is the neurotransmitters, the substances that transmit impulses from one nerve cell to the next (Figure 1). These compounds, or at least some of them, are unusual in being subject to precursor control; that is, the nerve cells respond to the available supply of building blocks by making larger amounts of neurotransmitters. Furthermore, the building blocks (precursors) are able to penetrate the blood-brain barrier; and they are nutrients derived from food. Thus the food you eat can influence your brain chemis-

[1] R. J. Wurtman and J. J. Wurtman, eds., *Nutrition and the Brain*, vol. 4 (New York: Raven Press, 1979).

[2] The blood-brain barrier is not anatomic but physiological.

try, to the extent that it produces high concentrations of the neurotransmitter-precursor nutrients in an available form. These facts link nutrition to brain activity in some intriguing ways. A few examples will illustrate, but first it is necessary to know how neurotransmitters work.

How Neurotransmitters Work

Nerve cells are elongated structures, analogous to the wires or cables in electrical communications equipment. Each nerve cell has a receiving end, where a stimulus may initiate an electrical impulse, and a transmitting end, where the impulse may be passed on to another nerve cell or to a muscle cell (see Figure 1). The electrical impulse can in some cases jump unaided from one cell to the next, but in most cases the gap between cells prevents electrical transmission. This gap is the synapse.

Communication across synapses usually involves neurotransmitters. The first neuron (the one sending the impulse) releases a quantity of these molecules and they diffuse across the synapse and reach the second (receiving) neuron. On arrival, they may make the receiving neuron either *more* or *less* likely to fire. Thus a neurotransmitter can either *stimulate* or *inhibit* the postsynaptic neuron. If it stimu-

lates it, and the neuron fires, then an electrical impulse starts up which travels along the nerve to the other end, the next synapse. Thus messages are carried along nerves by electrical impulses and from one nerve to the next by chemical compounds, until they result in action (storage, integration of information, contraction of a muscle) or die away.

A nerve cell "decides" to fire based on inputs from all the other neurons that are in contact with it. If the amount of stimulation relative to the amount of inhibition is great enough to initiate an impulse, then the nerve cell will fire. Figure 1 shows a nerve cell causing another to fire by dispatching a neurotransmitter to stimulate it.

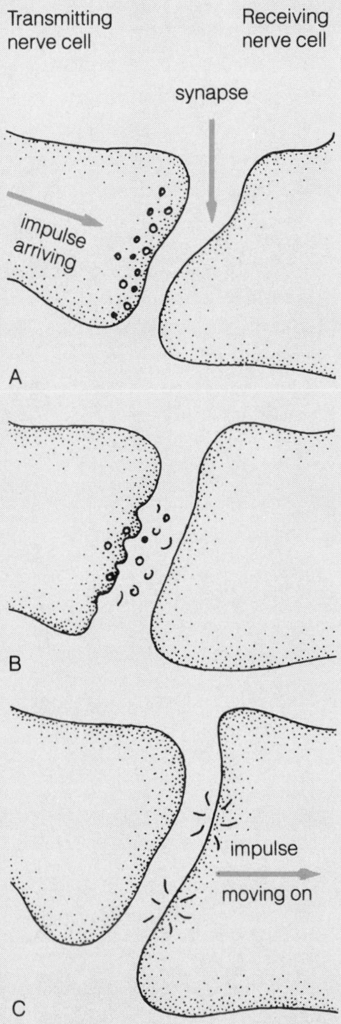

Transmitting nerve cell   Receiving nerve cell

synapse

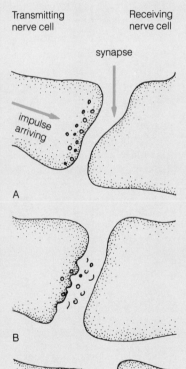

A

B

C

Figure 1   How nerve cells transmit messages.

Figure 1a   The impulse arrives at the end of the first nerve cell. Clustered just inside the nerve cell ending are a multitude of little sacs (vesicles) filled with the neurotransmitter.

Figure 1b   The vesicles fuse with the nerve cell membrane, releasing the neurotransmitter into the synaptic cleft.

Figure 1c   The neurotransmitter arrives at the receiver cell and (in this instance) stimulates it to generate an impulse that will travel along its length. Simultaneously, the receiver cell destroys the molecules of neurotransmitter at its membrane or the transmitter cell takes them up again to re-use them. Total elapsed time: a fraction of a second.

Nerve cells manufacture and release amounts of neurotransmitters that vary in response to diet. Thus dietary factors affect the overall chemical climate of the brain. If a transmitter's action within a cluster of cells is primarily inhibitory, then an increase in the supply of that transmitter will inhibit the cells further. If the same transmitter has an excitatory effect on another group of cells, then an increase will excite them. A change in the supply of a single neurotransmitter could increase some kinds of activity and decrease others, thus altering the balance of activities in the brain. Among the diet-responsive neurotransmitters are serotonin, norepinephrine, and acetylcholine. We'll use serotonin as an example of how they all work.

Serotonin The neurotransmitter serotonin is made in the brain from the essential amino acid tryptophan (Figure 2). The amount of serotonin made normally varies with the amount of tryptophan that is available. Tryptophan availability, in turn, depends on what is eaten (remember, an essential amino acid can't be made in the body). And a lack of tryptophan flowing into the brain can manifest itself in wakefulness, enhanced sensitivity to pain, and possibly depression.[3] In the presence of these symptoms, we have reason to believe that it is indeed seroto-

[3]J. D. Fernstrom, Effects of the diet on brain neurotransmitters, *Metabolism* 26 (1977):207-223; S. H. Zeisel and J. H. Growdon, Diet and brain neurotransmitters, *Nutrition and the MD*, April 1980.

nin that is being affected by a lack of dietary tryptophan, because sleep, pain sensitivity, and some forms of depression involve nerve cells that use serotonin as their neurotransmitter. And in the case of pain, animals that have been made tryptophan-deficient have a lowered threshold for pain; when they are given a single injection of tryptophan they manifest simultaneous restoration of their brain serotonin levels and a normalized pain threshold.[4]

Findings like these are of great interest to researchers who seek insight into brain function because they suggest ways of altering it when there is a need. Both sleep and the experience of pain are of great importance in

[4]Fernstrom, 1977.

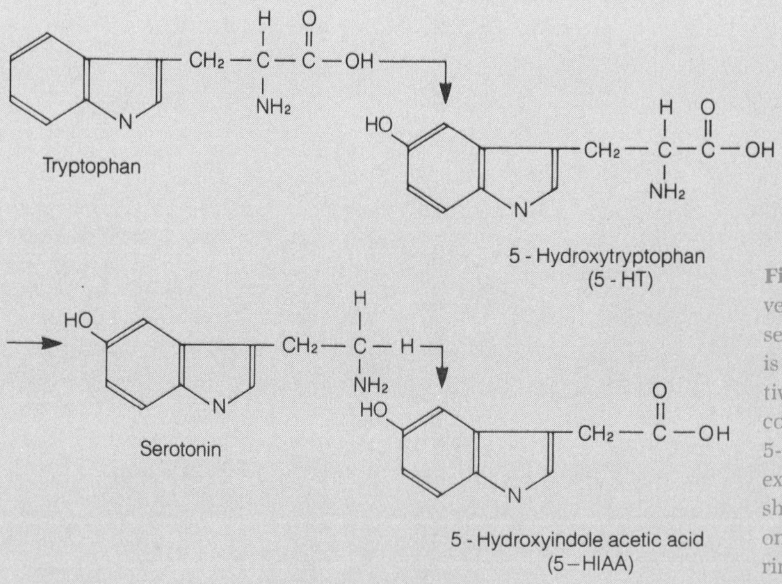

Figure 2 Tryptophan is converted to the neurotransmitter serotonin in two steps. Serotonin is then broken down to the inactive product 5-HIAA when its concentration rises too high, and 5-HIAA leaves the brain to be excreted. The chemical drawings shown here are simplified by omitting the Cs and Hs in the ring structures.

health and in illness. So the question has been asked — and answered — exactly how the diet can be adjusted to alter the amount of tryptophan flowing into the brain. It isn't as simple as you might think at first but experiments with animals have shown what the key factors are.

If tryptophan is fed or injected by itself, as a single amino acid, its concentration in the blood rises, it flows into the brain, and brain serotonin increases proportionately. If protein containing tryptophan is fed, blood tryptophan also rises, but it does *not* flow into the brain. It turns out that some of the other large amino acids in the protein compete with tryptophan for entry into the brain; they use the same carrier.[5] So protein, even though it contains the amino acid tryptophan, does not effectively enhance brain serotonin synthesis.

On the other hand, if insulin is injected, or if a diet high in carbohydrate is fed (which raises blood insulin), blood tryptophan rises and enters the brain. It seems that insulin drives the other amino acids, but not tryptophan, into cells, thus leaving the tryptophan free to enter the brain without competition. Thus, paradoxically,

[5]The amino acids that share this carrier are tyrosine, phenylalanine, leucine, isoleucine, and valine.

Miniglossary

acetylcholine: a compound that is related in structure to (and made from) the B vitamin choline and that serves as one of the brain's principal neurotransmitters.

blood-brain barrier: a physiological barrier, nature unknown, that prevents most of the substances in the bloodstream from entering the nerve cells.

neurotransmitter: a substance that is released at the end of one nerve cell when a nerve impulse arrives there, diffuses across the synapse, and alters the membranes of the next nerve cell in such a way that it is either less or more likely to fire (or does fire).

norepinephrine: a compound related in structure to (and made from) the amino acid tyrosine. When secreted by the adrenal medulla, it acts as a hormone; when secreted at the ends of nerve cells, it acts as a neurotransmitter.

precursor: a substance that is converted into another substance.

precursor control: control of a compound's synthesis by the availability of that compound's precursor. (The more precursor there is, the more of the compound is made.)

serotonin: A compound that is related in structure to (and made from) the amino acid tryptophan and that serves as one of the brain's principal neurotransmitters.

synapse: The gap between one nerve cell and the next cell with which it communicates; or between a nerve cell and the muscle cell it stimulates.

a meal that is high in carbohydrate, but not one high in protein, causes a rise in tryptophan in both the blood and the brain and promotes serotonin synthesis. It's not the total amount of tryptophan, then, but the amount relative to the competing amino acids, that affects brain serotonin level.[6]

With this knowledge, researchers have some fascinating avenues open to them. Experimentation is active in all the relevant areas. The objective is to learn how diet modification can benefit people with sleep disturbances, pain, and depression.

[6]Fernstrom, 1977. The reader acquainted with this research may recall that it was at one time thought that *free* tryptophan (i.e., that not bound to albumin) was the key variable and that therefore other substances that bind albumin such as fatty acids might affect tryptophan availability to the brain. The paper cited here presents evidence that the binding of tryptophan to albumin is loose and has little or no effect on its availability to the brain.

An emphatic cautionary word is in order. *None* of the information being presented here is in a form to be used, yet, by the man on the street or even by the very knowledgeable student of nutrition, nursing, or medicine. Much of this information has reached the popular media, and health food stores make available preparations labeled "tryptophan . . . take two . . . for sleep" and the like as if it were possible to diagnose and treat sleep or other disorders with them as we self-medicate ourselves for simple cold symptoms. Research into the therapeutic effects of any of the nutrients in such disorders is still very much in the exploratory stage. Anyone who tried to apply what is known in a real-life situation would be opening him/herself to the double hazard of upsetting the body's balance with unpredictable consequences and of failing to obtain knowledgeable medical attention for what could be a serious — and treatable — condition.

Because this book is intended for an audience of responsible readers, it is expected that this information will not be misused. At this point in time

its only proper use, outside of strictly controlled, clinical investigation, is to shed light on the fascinating interrelationships of nutrients, the brain, and the mind; to enhance your appreciation of the complexity of those interrelationships; and to motivate you to want to learn more.

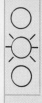

CAUTION WHEN YOU READ!

Before "prescribing" any nutrient you read about to alter brain function or behavior, think twice. And your second thought should be: DON'T.

Applications   While the research on diet and neurotransmitters progresses, and before its applications and limitations are satisfactorily defined, is there any way in which we can safely use what we know? Popular magazines have published some suggestions; are they OK to follow? The Rodale Press' *Executive Fitness Newsletter*, for example, says that if you want to go to sleep easily at night, you'd better have a turkey sandwich — turkey for the tryptophan, bread for the carbohydrate to "liber-

ate" it.[7] Is this good advice? The turkey may be superfluous in a body where plenty of tryptophan is already circulating, but the carbohydrate may help to facilitate its entry into the brain. *Health* magazine recommends a cup of warm milk as a nightcap.[8]

There may or may not be a basis in fact for these or other choices, but at least one feature stands out in their favor: They probably will do no harm. Many people feel that they can't sleep well on an empty stomach. Babies and animals slumber after eating. The next Highlight will touch on another effect of food on brain chemistry, the production of natural tranquilizers that help to relieve both pain and stress. And the increased synthesis of serotonin after a carbohydrate feeding provides a possible explanation for at least part of the soothing effect such a feeding may have. Research presently under way is investigating the possibility that the serotonin-using nerves may even provide feedback control of their own tryptophan supply. When they have enough serotonin neurotransmission going on, they

[7]What to eat if you're going to eat before going to bed, *Executive Fitness Newsletter* 12 (January 10, 1981).

[8]News about nightcaps, *Health*, November/December 1981, p. 6.

suppress carbohydrate consumption.[9] When they lack serotonin, perhaps they signal a need for carbohydrate.

All of these and many other observations hint at answers to the questions raised at the start. Perhaps what you eat does affect how you think and feel. Perhaps carbohydrate plays a special role in modulating these effects. The research reviewed in this Highlight has answered one or two questions but has raised a dozen more.

Highlight 16 returns to the subject of carbohydrate once again — specifically, to the fascinating question of sugar addiction. After reading that Highlight, you will probably find you have still more questions. If so, then you are thinking like a research scientist who is willing to live in a world where the questions are many and the answers are scarce. The scientist's task is to make educated guesses (hypotheses), and then to design and execute experiments that will confirm or deny those guesses.

Research into the roles of nutrients in the brain is relatively new, but has branched out into many lines of investigation. Investigators are studying relationships of several other substances besides tryptophan to neurotransmission: the mineral iron, the B vitamin choline, and the amino acid tyrosine. The more they learn, the more they want to find out, because so much territory remains to be explored. Hopefully, research into these areas will continue to be supported, because they are of great interest, and also because they have great potential for enhancing human life.

9Zeisel and Growdon, April 1980.

To Explore Further

The two principal sources from which much of this information was taken are technical papers intended for the advanced student but written very clearly. The first is especially helpful about general principles and about acetylcholine; the second is a thorough review of all three systems — those involving acetylcholine, norepinephrine, and serotonin:

- Growdon, J. L., and Wurtman, R. J. Dietary influences on the synthesis of neurotransmitters in the brain. *Nutrition Reviews* 37 (1979):129-136.

- Fernstrom, J. D. Effects of the diet on brain neurotransmitters. *Metabolism* 26 (1977):207-223.

A brief (two-page), less technical review of the same subject is provided in:

- Growdon, J. L., and Wurtman, R. J. Nutrients and neurotransmitters. *Contemporary Nutrition*, December 1979.

CHAPTER 6

CONTENTS

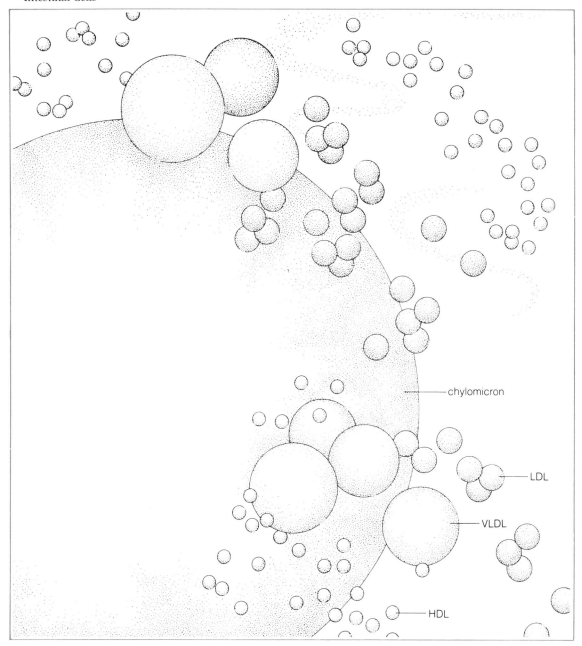

chylomicron

LDL

VLDL

HDL

The lipoproteins.

ABSORPTION AND TRANSPORT

I know there have been certain philosophers, and they learned men, who have held that all bodies are endowed with sense; nor do I see, if the nature of sense be set alongside reaction solely, how they can be refuted.

THOMAS HOBBES

Problem: Given an elaborate production in which 1,000 actors are on stage at once, provide a means by which all can exit simultaneously! This is the problem of absorption. Within three or four hours after you have eaten a steak dinner with potato, vegetable, salad, and dessert, your body must find a way to absorb some two hundred thousand million, million, million amino acid molecules one by one, to say nothing of the other nutrient molecules. For the stage production, the manager might design multiple wings that all of the actors could crowd into, 20 at a time. If the manager were a mechanical genius, he might somehow design moving wings that would actively engulf the actors as they approached. The absorptive system is no such fantasy; in 20 feet of small intestine it provides over a quarter-acre of surfaces where the nutrient molecules can make contact and be absorbed. To remove them rapidly and provide room for more to be absorbed, a rush of circulation continuously bathes the underside of these surfaces, washing away the absorbed nutrients and carrying them to the liver and other parts of the body.

Anatomy of the Absorptive System

The inner surface of the small intestine looks smooth to the naked eye, but through a microscope it appears to be wrinkled into hundreds of folds. Each of these folds is covered with thousands of nipplelike projections, as numerous as the nap hairs on velvet fabric. Each of these small intestinal projections is a villus. If you could look still closer, you would see that each villus is covered with minute hairs, the microvilli.

villi (VILL-ee), singular **villus:** fingerlike projections from the folds of the small intestine.

microvilli (MY-cro-VILL-ee), singular **microvillus:** projections from the membranes of the cells of the villi.

Figure 1a Five folds in the wall of the small intestine. Each is covered with villi.

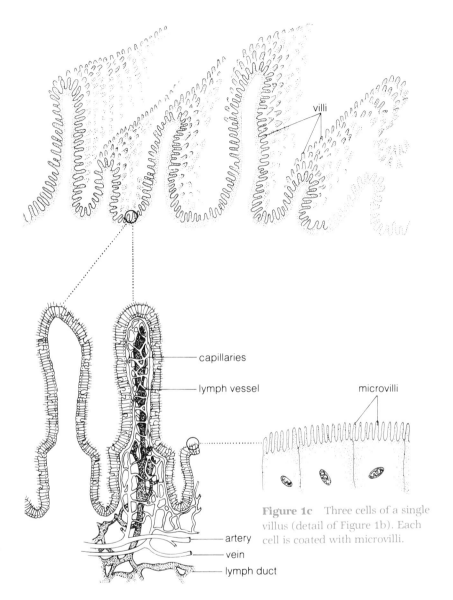

villi

capillaries

lymph vessel

microvilli

Figure 1c Three cells of a single villus (detail of Figure 1b). Each cell is coated with microvilli.

artery

vein

lymph duct

Figure 1b Two villi (detail of Figure 1a). Each villus is composed of several hundred cells.

A nutrient molecule, such as an amino acid, that encounters any part of this surface, is drawn into the cells that compose it.

The villi are in constant motion, waving, squirming, and wriggling like the tentacles of a sea anemone. They actively reach for and engulf nutrient molecules, aided by a thin sheet of muscle that lines each of them.

Once a molecule has entered a cell in a villus, the next problem is to transport it to its destination elsewhere in the body. Everyone knows that the bloodstream performs this function, but you may be surprised to learn that there is a second transport system—the lymphatic system. Both of these systems supply vessels to each villus, as shown in Figure

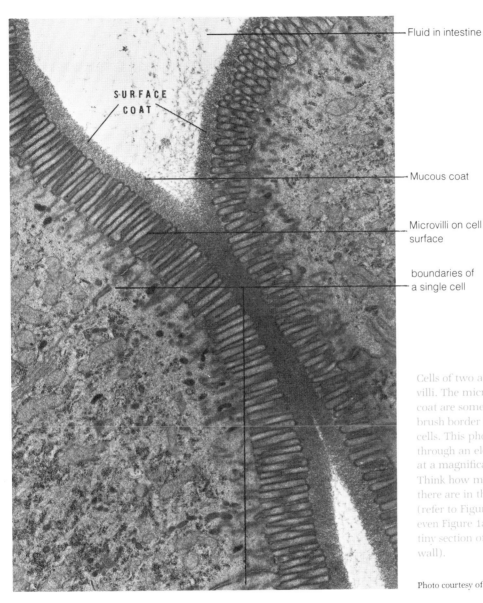

Fluid in intestine

SURFACE COAT

Mucous coat

Microvilli on cell surface

boundaries of a single cell

Cells of two adjacent intestinal villi. The microvilli and mucous coat are sometimes called the brush border of the intestinal cells. This photograph was taken through an electron microscope at a magnification of 51,000X. Think how many of these cells there are in the small intestine (refer to Figure 1 and notice that even Figure 1a represents but a tiny section of the intestinal wall).

Photo courtesy of Dr. Susumu Ito.

1b. When a nutrient molecule has crossed the cell of a villus, it may enter either the lymph or the blood. In either case the nutrients end up in the blood, at least for a while.

A Closer Look at the Intestinal Cells

The cells of the villi are among the most amazing in the body, for they recognize, select, and regulate the absorption of the nutrients the body needs. It is thanks to these cells that blue glass beads (see Chapter 5)

lymph (LIMF): the body's interstitial fluid, between the cells and outside the vascular system. Lymph consists of all the constituents of blood that can escape from the vascular system; it circulates in a loosely organized system of vessels and ducts known as the **lymphatic system.**

never enter the body proper to lodge in inconvenient places. But they are far more sophisticated in the distinctions they can make, and they not only absorb but also process many of the nutrients you consume in food. A closer look at them is worthwhile, because it will help to explode a number of common misconceptions about nutrition.

Some people believe, for example, that eating predigested protein—amino acid preparations such as the "liquid protein" products sold to dieters—saves the body the work of having to digest protein, so that the digestive system won't "wear out" so easily. Nothing could be further from the truth. Others believe that people shouldn't eat certain food combinations (for example, fruit and meat) at the same meal, because the digestive system can't handle more than one task at a time. The art of "food combining" is based on this gross underestimation of the body's capabilities.

Each cell of a villus is coated with thousands of microvilli (Figure 1c), which project from its membrane. In these microvilli and in the membrane lie hundreds of different kinds of enzymes and "pumps," which recognize and act on different nutrients. For example, one of the enzymes is lactase, which breaks apart the disaccharide lactose, or milk sugar. The presence of lactase at the cell surface ensures the efficient absorption of this sugar, because as soon as it is broken into its component parts (glucose and galactose), those parts are easily contacted by the nearby pumps, which move them into the interior of the cell.[1] This arrangement makes it easy for a newborn infant to absorb and use milk sugar, even though his gastrointestinal tract may in some ways still be immature.

Enzymes for cleaving di- and tripeptides also lie in the surface structures of the intestinal cells. Whole proteins—long polypeptides—are digested to shorter chains out in the fluid of the intestine, but once they have been rendered into short fragments, these fragments are contacted and trapped by the microvilli, where the final stages of digestion occur.[2] The cells' enzymes then can deliver the final products—amino acids—directly to the pumps, which carry them into the cells.

There is nothing random about this process. The anatomical arrangement guarantees not only digestion but also delivery of its products into the body. Digestion and absorption are coordinated.

When hydrolyzed proteins (that is, mixtures of amino acids) are consumed, there can be no such coordination. They arrive en masse in the intestine, presenting it with the problem of trying to absorb them all at once. At first, floating free in the fluid, they exert an

[1] R. Levine and D. E. Haft, Carbohydrate homeostasis (first of two parts), *New England Journal of Medicine* 283 (1970): 175-183.

[2] D. M. Matthews and S. A. Adibi, Peptide absorption, *Gastroenterology* 71 (1976): 151-161.

attractive force (remember that charged molecules attract water). As a result, excess water is drawn into the GI tract, causing at the least discomfort and at the worst cramping, nausea, and diarrhea.

Chapter 3 showed that most people (in the developed countries) eat more protein than they need. Chapter 4, in describing the remarkable roles of protein, explained perhaps why they do: Protein is an impressively important nutrient, and the more we learn about it the more its importance staggers the imagination. Still, excess protein in any form does no good and may do harm; and protein in the form of completely predigested supplements is dangerous. Even in the hospital, in the treatment of very sick, starving people, it is now recognized that the well-meaning attempt to provide amino acids when whole protein can be used is misguided. It is based on "a misconception concerning the digestive capacities of the human gastrointestinal tract in emaciation, disease, and after surgery. Actual feeding experiments have proven . . . that even in extreme starvation proteins can still be digested as long as food can be swallowed."[3]

It is unwise to try to second-guess the body. It has evolved over millions of years to derive its nutrients efficiently from foods. How could we presume, after five minutes of listening to a health food salesman or fad diet promoter, to improve on this natural capacity by feeding the body "liquid protein" or any other such nostrum?

This attractive force is osmotic pressure (see pp. 488-489).

The clinical nutritionist finds some legitimate uses for *partially* hydrolyzed protein in formulas. In some hospital situations, amino acids are also appropriate, but only in the hospital. See Chapter 20.

An additional refinement of the system for digesting and absorbing protein gives a further reason for not tampering with it. The amino acid pumps are not specific for individual amino acids but for groups of them. For example, there is one pump for the basic amino acids and another for the neutral ones. Each group of amino acids with similar structures shares a carrier. This means that competition can occur: The amino acids within a group can interfere with each other's absorption.

Normally, no problems arise with this arrangement. Food proteins deliver balanced assortments of amino acids to the GI tract, digestion occurs slowly, fragments are delivered in leisurely fashion to the microvilli, and the final steps of digestion-absorption occur without much mutual interference.

If, however, a person takes pure amino acids rather than protein, the competition for carriers is more severe and some amino acids are lost. If the person still more foolishly presumes to decide that she needs certain specific amino acids and takes an overdose of one, she may well precipitate a deficiency of the others that share its carrier. If the lost amino acids are essential ones, the net effect will be to reduce her total supply of usable protein.

Essential amino acids:
see p. 102.

[3]A. A. Albanese and L. A. Orto, The proteins and amino acids, in *Modern Nutrition in Health and Disease*, 5th ed., eds. R. S. Goodhart and M. E. Shils (Philadelphia: Lea and Febiger, 1973), p. 37.

This is not to say that some food proteins can't be improved by amino acid supplementation. A plant protein of very poor quality may be better utilized by the body if the limiting amino acid(s) are added to it. In this instance, adding amino acids provides a balance closer to what the body needs. This theory has been scientifically tested and confirmed—for example, in growth experiments on children.[4]

"Very well, then, it is best to eat food proteins rather than artificial amino acid mixtures. But surely, if you ask the GI tract to perform all the fancy maneuvers of digesting and absorbing protein, it would be best not to ask it to handle other nutrients at the same time. Surely there is a limit to how much those little cells can do at once." (This is logic speaking.)

On the contrary, there seems to be no interference—other than the specific kind of competition just mentioned—between the absorption and utilization of one kind of nutrient and that of another. In fact they often seem to enhance each other. For example, sugars taken at the same time as protein (within four hours) seem to promote better retention of the protein.[5] The sugars may slow the digestive process so that it is more complete, or they may provide precursors for some nonessential amino acids so that whole proteins can be produced more readily and retained in the body. Whatever the mechanism, the facts support the practice of taking mixed meals composed of a wide variety of foods to supply nutrients together so that they can act cooperatively wherever possible. There is no basis in any known facts about the digestive system for thinking that combining foods (for example, fruit and meat) in a meal taxes the ability of the GI tract to handle them. More likely, the combination enhances its most efficient functioning.

Not only is there a beneficial interaction between the energy nutrients in these two foods (protein in meat and carbohydrate in fruit); there are others that have to do with the vitamins and minerals. For example, the vitamin C in one food enhances the absorption of the iron in another food. This phenomenon and many others like it are described in Part Two.

A FLAG SIGN OF A SPURIOUS CLAIM
IS THE IMPLICATION THAT:

We can second-guess the body and make its work easier.

[4]Albanese and Orto, 1973, p. 51.

[5]Albanese and Orto, 1973, p. 57.

The preceding discussion has illuminated some aspects of the absorption of carbohydrate and protein but has said nothing about lipids. The absorption of lipids differs in that pumps are not involved. Cell membranes dissolve lipids easily because they are made largely of lipid themselves. After the digestion of triglycerides to monoglycerides or to glycerol and fatty acids, for example, they simply diffuse across the cell membrane. The cell retains them by reassembling them.

As you can see, the cells of the intestinal tract wall are beautifully designed to perform their functions. A further refinement of the system is that the cells of successive portions of the tract are specialized for different absorptive functions. The nutrients that are ready for absorption early are absorbed near the top of the tract; those that take longer to be digested are absorbed farther down. Thus the top portion of the duodenum is specialized for the absorption of calcium and several B vitamins, such as thiamin and riboflavin; the jejunum absorbs most of the products of triglyceride digestion; and vitamin B_{12}, which requires extensive preparation, is absorbed at the end of the ileum. The rate at which these nutrients travel is finely adjusted to maximize their availability to the appropriate absorptive segment of the tract when they are ready. The lowly "gut" turns out to be one of the most elegantly designed organ systems in your body.

Vitamin B_{12} is first attached to a special carrier in the stomach. For further details about the absorption of vitamins and minerals, see Part Two.

Release of Absorbed Nutrients

Once inside the intestinal cells, the products of digestion must be released for transport to the rest of the body. The water-soluble nutrients—monosaccharides (from carbohydrate), amino acids (from protein), and small lipid components such as short-chain fatty acids and glycerol—are released directly into the bloodstream. The water-soluble vitamins and minerals also follow this route.

WATER-SOLUBLE NUTRIENTS

Carbohydrates
   monosaccharides ————————————————→blood

Lipids
   glycerol
   medium- and short-chain fatty acids ——————→blood

Proteins
   amino acids—————————————————→blood
Vitamins
   B vitamins ⎤
   vitamin C ⎦————————————————→blood

Minerals ————————————————————→blood

Things get into cells in several ways:

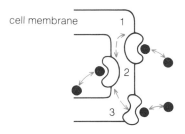

Diffusion.   Some substances cross membranes freely. Water is an example. The concentration of water tends to equalize on the two sides of a membrane: as long as it is higher outside the cell, it flows in; if it is higher inside the cell, it flows out. The cell cannot regulate the entrance and exit of water directly but can control it indirectly by concentrating some other substance to which water is attracted, such as protein or sodium. Thus the cell can pump in sodium, and water will follow passively. This is the way the cells of the wall of the large intestine act to retrieve water for the body. Since nearly all the sodium is taken into these cells before waste is excreted, nearly all the water is absorbed too. Small lipids also cross cell membranes by diffusion.

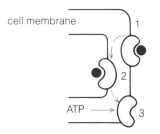

Facilitated diffusion.   Other compounds cannot cross the membranes of the intestinal wall cells unless there is a specific carrier or facilitator in the membrane. The carrier may shuttle back and forth from one side of the membrane to the other, carrying its passengers either way, or it may affect the permeability of the membrane in such a way that the compound is admitted. Insulin probably works the latter way to facilitate the entrance of glucose into liver and other cells. The end result is the same as for diffusion: Equal concentrations are reached on both sides. By providing carriers only for the desired compounds, the cell effectively bars all others (except those to which it is freely permeable). Facilitated diffusion is also termed carrier-mediated diffusion or passive transport.

1. Carrier loads particle on outside of cell.

2. Carrier releases particle on inside of cell.

3. Or the reverse.

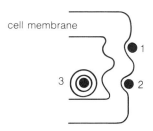

Active transport.   For compounds that must be absorbed actively, the two types of diffusion systems mentioned above will not suffice. The best a cell can do using only diffusion is to take up a compound until the concentration inside the cell is equal to that outside. An effective means of concentrating a substance inside the cell is to pump it in, consuming energy in the process. The monosaccharides, amino acids, and other nutrients are absorbed by intestinal wall cells in this manner.

1. Carrier loads particle on outside of cell.

2. Carrier releases particle on inside of cell.

3. Carrier returns to outside to pick up another, powered by the energy carrier, ATP (see p. 230).

Pinocytosis.   This process involves a large area of the cell membrane, which actively engulfs whole particles and "swallows" them into the cell. Although it is not of great importance in the GI tract, this process is one way that the white blood cells are able to engulf invading viruses and bacteria in order to dispose of them.

1. Particle touches cell membrane.

2. Membrane wraps around particle.

3. Portion of membrane surrounding particle separates into cell.

The selective cell membranes.

As for the larger lipids and the fat-soluble vitamins, access directly into the bloodstream is impossible. They are apparently too insoluble and cumbersome to cross the walls of the blood vessels. Monoglycerides and long-chain fatty acids are assembled into larger molecules—triglycerides—the form in which the cells can best handle them. These and the other large lipids, cholesterol and the phospholipids, are wrapped in protein by a special arrangement (to be described beginning on p. 182) and are released into the lymphatic system. They can then "squish" through the lymph spaces until they move to a point of entry into the bloodstream near the heart.

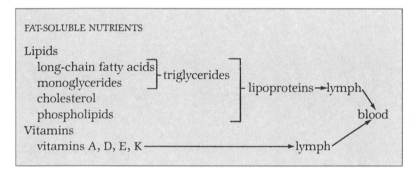

FAT-SOLUBLE NUTRIENTS

Lipids
  long-chain fatty acids
  monoglycerides   } triglycerides
  cholesterol   } lipoproteins → lymph
  phospholipids   blood
Vitamins
  vitamins A, D, E, K ──────────────→ lymph

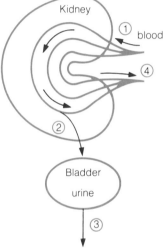

1. Blood enters the kidney by way of the arteries.
2. Waste is removed and sent as urine to the bladder.
3. Urine is periodically eliminated.
4. Cleansed blood is returned to the general circulation.

Anatomy of the Circulatory Systems

Once a nutrient has entered the bloodstream or the lymph circulatory system, it may be transported to any part of the body and thus become available to all the body cells, from the tips of the toes to the roots of the hair. To understand the way nutrients arrive at the toes or the hair roots, you must understand the anatomy of the circulatory systems.

The Vascular System   The vascular or blood circulatory system is a closed system of vessels through which blood flows continuously in a figure eight, with the heart serving as a pump at the crossover point. The system is diagramed in Figure 2. As the blood circulates through this system it picks up and delivers materials as needed.

All the body tissues derive oxygen and nutrients from the blood and deposit carbon dioxide and other wastes into it. The lungs are the place for exchange of carbon dioxide (which leaves the blood to be breathed out) and oxygen (which enters the blood to be delivered to all cells). The digestive system is the place for nutrients to be picked up. The kidneys are the place where wastes other than carbon dioxide are filtered out of the blood to be excreted in the urine. There is something special about the routing of the blood past the digestive system that requires a little explanation.

Blood leaving the right side of the heart circulates by way of arteries into the lung capillaries and then back through veins to the left side of

artery: a vessel carrying blood away from the heart.

capillary (CAP-ill-ary): a small vessel that branches from an artery. Capillaries connect arteries to veins. Exchange of blood and tissue components takes place across capillary walls.

vein: a vessel carrying blood back to the heart.

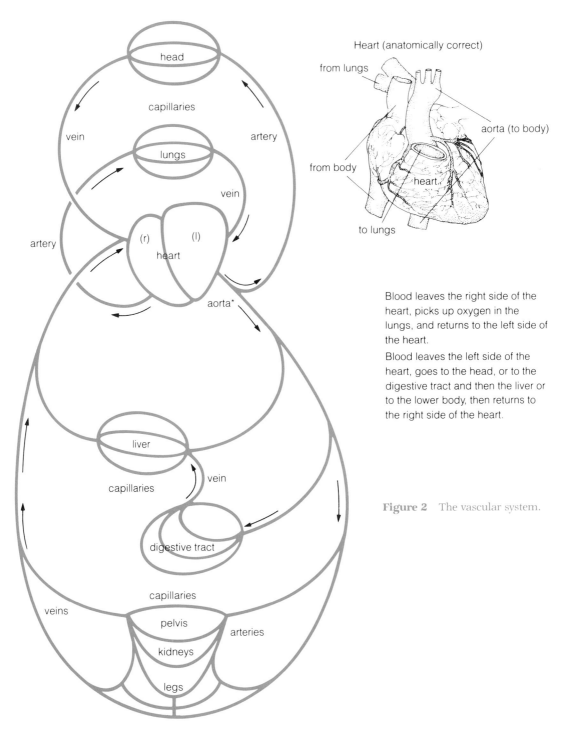

Heart (anatomically correct)

from lungs

aorta (to body)

from body

heart

to lungs

Blood leaves the right side of the heart, picks up oxygen in the lungs, and returns to the left side of the heart.

Blood leaves the left side of the heart, goes to the head, or to the digestive tract and then the liver or to the lower body, then returns to the right side of the heart.

Figure 2   The vascular system.

*The aorta is the main artery that launches blood on its course through the body. The picture is not anatomically correct but is drawn this way for clarity. The aorta arises behind the left side of the heart and arcs upward, then divides.

the heart. The left side of the heart then pumps the blood out through arteries to all systems of the body. The blood circulates in the capillaries and then collects into veins, which return the blood again to the right side of the heart (see Figure 2). In all cases but one, blood leaving the heart travels this simple route:

$$\text{Heart} \rightarrow \text{arteries} \rightarrow \text{capillaries} \rightarrow \text{veins} \rightarrow \text{heart}$$

Only in the case of the digestive system does the blood flow twice through a capillary bed before returning to the heart. Surrounding and supporting the stomach and intestines is the strong, flexible mesenteric membrane. A major artery from the heart leads into this membrane and branches into smaller arteries and then into tiny capillaries, which penetrate every villus of the intestine. These capillaries rejoin to form veins, which return to the mesenteric membrane and merge into a single large vein, the portal vein. This vein connects directly to the liver, where it again branches into capillaries. Thus all the blood leaving the digestive system must go through a second capillary bed in the liver:

$$\text{Heart} \rightarrow \text{arteries} \rightarrow \text{capillaries (in intestines)} \rightarrow \text{vein} \rightarrow$$
$$\text{capillaries (in liver)} \rightarrow \text{veins} \rightarrow \text{heart}$$

An anatomist studying this system knows there must be a reason for it. He concludes that the liver is placed in the circulation at this point in order to have the first chance at the materials absorbed from the GI tract. In fact the liver has many jobs to do preparing the absorbed nutrients for use by the body. It is the body's major metabolic organ.

You might guess that in addition the liver may stand as a gatekeeper to waylay intruders that might otherwise harm the heart. Perhaps this is why, when people ingest poisons that succeed in passing the first barrier (the intestinal cells) and enter the blood, it is the liver that suffers the damage—from hepatitis virus, from drugs such as barbiturates, from alcohol, from poisons such as DDT, from toxic metals such as mercury. Perhaps, in fact, you have been undervaluing your liver, not knowing what quiet and heroic tasks it performs for you. (Chapter 24 focuses on the liver, in case you are interested in more information about this noble organ.)

The Lymphatic System   The lymphatic system is an open system that can be pictured simply as being similar to the spaces in a sponge. If you wet a sponge, its spaces fill with water. If you squeeze it, you can force the water from one end of the sponge to the other. Between the cells of the body there are spaces similar to those in the sponge; the fluid circulating in them is the lymph. This fluid is almost identical to the fluid of the blood except that it contains no red blood cells, because they cannot escape through the blood vessel walls. The spaces between the cells are somewhat imprecisely called lymphatic "vessels."

The lymphatic system has no pump; like the water in a sponge, lymph "squishes" from one portion of the body to another as muscles contract and create pressure here and there. Ultimately much of the

mesenteric (mez-en-TERR-ic) **membrane,** or **mesentery** (MEZ-en-terr-ee): the strong, flexible membrane that surrounds and supports the abdominal organs.

The vein that collects blood from the mesentery and conducts it to capillaries in the liver is the **portal vein.**

portal = gateway

The vein that collects blood from the liver capillaries and returns it to the heart is the **hepatic vein.**

hepat = liver

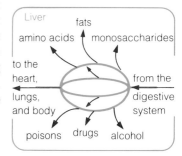

The liver removes many materials from the blood.

thoracic (thor-ASS-ic) **duct:** a duct of the lymphatic system that collects lymph that has circulated to the upper portion of the body. The **subclavian vein** connects this duct with the right upper chamber of the heart, providing a passageway by which lymph can be returned to the vascular system.

lipoprotein (lip-oh-PRO-tee-in): a complex of lipids with proteins. The lipids apparently orient with their hydrophobic ends in; the proteins associate with the outside of the cluster, rendering the entire complex water-soluble.

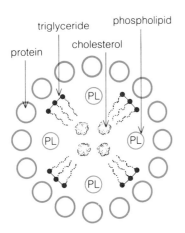

A lipoprotein.

chylomicron (kye-lo-MY-cron): the lipoprotein formed in intestinal wall cells following digestion and absorption of fat. Released from these cells, chylomicrons transport ingested fats to liver cells. The liver cells dismantle the chylomicrons and construct other lipoproteins for further transport.

lymph collects in a large duct behind the heart called the thoracic duct. This duct terminates in a vein that conducts the lymph into the heart. Thus materials from the GI tract that enter lymphatic vessels in the villi ultimately enter the blood circulatory system and then circulate through arteries, capillaries, and veins like the other nutrients. In other words, nutrients that are first absorbed into lymph soon get into the blood.

Transport of Lipids: A Special Arrangement

Once inside the body, the nutrients can travel freely to any destination and can be taken into cells and used as needed. What becomes of them is the subject of Chapter 7. Before leaving the transport system, however, you might be interested in looking more closely at the forms in which lipids travel.

Within the circulatory systems, lipids always travel from place to place wrapped in protein coats—that is, as lipoproteins. Lipoproteins are very much in the news these days. In fact, when the doctor measures a person's blood lipid profile, she is interested not only in the types of fat she finds (triglycerides and cholesterol) but also in the types of protein coats they are wrapped in. Newly absorbed lipids leaving the intestinal cells are mostly packaged in the lipoproteins known as chylomicrons. Lipids that have been processed or made in the liver are released in lipoproteins known as VLDL and LDL. Lipids returning to the liver from other parts of the body are packaged in lipoproteins known as HDL. The distinction of interest, because it has implications for the health of the heart and blood vessels, is the distinction between HDL and the other lipoproteins. Raised HDL concentrations are associated with a low risk of heart attack.[6]

A brief look at each of these types of particles will help you to interpret the news about them as new findings continue to emerge—and to understand the significance of tests the doctor may run to determine your own lipid profile. (An artist's conception of what they look like appears at the start of this chapter.)

Chylomicrons: From the Intestinal Cells   The lipids you eat are in the form of water-insoluble triglycerides, cholesterol, and phospholipids, with the triglycerides predominating (composing about 95 percent of dietary fat). Both of the body's transport systems—lymph and blood—are watery fluids. Clearly, if the lipids were dumped "as is" into the bloodstream, they would clump together to form globs of fat that would clog the arteries. You are familiar with this effect if you have ever carelessly dumped greasy foods down the kitchen sink: The drain became clogged and the grease had to be removed, at great expense to you. The body is smarter with lipids than you may be with your kitchen

[6]High blood lipid levels can be good or bad—depending on the lipid. *Journal of the American Medical Association* 237 (1977):1066-1070.

grease. Although arteries sometimes clog (see Chapter 26), it is not because pure, unadulterated grease ever travels through them.

An intestinal cell allows a cluster of triglycerides to form, then wraps the cluster with a protein coat to form a chylomicron. The fat-loving tails of the fatty acids position themselves as far away from the water as they can get, some phospholipids and cholesterol arrange themselves nearby, and the small skin of protein forms around the entire aggregate. In this ingenious configuration, the fat can be released from the intestinal cell and can travel through the lymph to the blood.

The protein of the chylomicrons is recognized by the liver cells, which make it their business to remove these lipoproteins from the blood, to dismantle them, and to custom-design new lipids for use by other body cells. Chylomicrons are large, fluffy particles that float at the top of a blood sample in a test tube. This floating layer of fat does not appear if blood is drawn 14 hours after a meal, for in this period of time the liver has completely disposed of all of it.

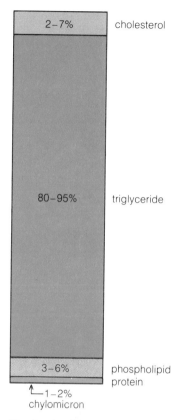

From the intestine:

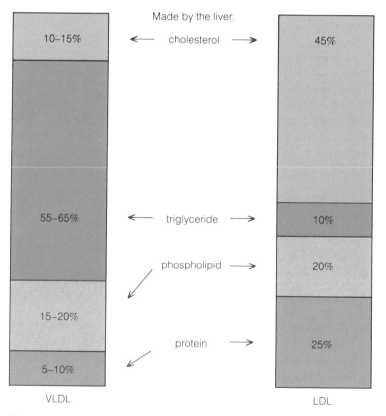

Made by the liver:

Compare these particles with the chylomicrons and HDL. Note that "high blood cholesterol" might easily reflect a high LDL concentration.

The density of these particles is very, very low because they contain so little protein and so much triglyceride. You can see how the laboratory report that a person has "high blood triglycerides" might easily reflect a high concentration of chylomicrons in his blood.

VLDL: very low density lipoprotein. This type of lipoprotein is made by liver cells (and to some extent by intestinal cells[7]). An alternative name is "pre-beta" lipoprotein.

LDL: low-density lipoprotein. This type of lipoprotein may be made by liver cells or derived from VLDL as cells remove triglycerides from them.[8] An alternative name is "beta" lipoprotein.

[7]H. B. Brown and M. Farrand, What a dietitian should know about hyperlipidemia, *Journal of the American Dietetic Association* 63 (1973): 169-170.

[8]An intermediate form, IDL, is now recognized by some authorities. A. K. Khachadurian, guest editor, Hyperlipoproteinemia, *Dietetic Currents, Ross Timesaver* 4 (July/August 1977).

Returned to the liver:

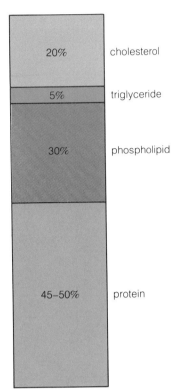

20%	cholesterol
5%	triglyceride
30%	phospholipid
45–50%	protein

HDL

These particles are denser than the others because they contain such a high percentage of protein.

HDL: high-density lipoprotein. These lipoproteins seem to transport lipids back to the liver from peripheral cells. An alternative name is "alpha" lipoprotein.

VLDL and LDL: From the Liver The liver cells rearrange most of the triglycerides from the chylomicrons. They break the fatty acids down to fragments and use them to make other fatty acids, cholesterol, and other compounds. (At the same time, if they are metabolizing carbohydrates, they may be making lipids from some of these.) Ultimately, some of the lipids they manufacture will need to be used or stored in other parts of the body. To send them there, the liver once again wraps them in proteins, this time as VLDL and LDL.

The VLDL and LDL made by the liver contain relatively more cholesterol and phospholipid than the chylomicrons do. Released from the liver into the blood, they circulate throughout the body, making their fat available to all the body cells—muscle, including the heart muscle, adipose tissue, the mammary glands, and others. The body cells can select fat from these particles to build new membranes, to make hormones or other compounds, or to store for later use. Both VLDL and LDL are much smaller and denser than the chylomicrons, but the VLDL are still large enough to give the blood a milky appearance if there are enough of them.

HDL: From the Body Cells When energy is in short supply, the cells may have only their own stored fat to rely on. At such a time they mobilize fat; that is, they take it out of storage. Most of the triglycerides are used for energy, and the cells return the unused fat—mostly cholesterol and phospholipid—to the blood. The packages in which unused fats are returned are the HDL, and it is believed that these are returned to the liver for recycling or disposal.

Atherosclerosis and the Lipoproteins The lipoproteins have become headline news in recent years, as researchers have discovered that they may be an important clue to the risks of heart and artery disease. In the early years, scientists spoke of "hyperlipidemia"—too much lipid in the blood. Now they refer to "hyperlipoproteinemia," recognizing the carrier in which the lipid appears.

The formation of plaques in the artery walls is described in Chapter 2. The cholesterol deposited in these plaques is available to them from the lipoproteins that carry it in the bloodstream. Those that carry the most cholesterol are the LDL, and the LDL correlate most closely with atherosclerosis.[9] LDL have an affinity for the artery walls, perhaps because of the character of their protein.[10] Generally speaking, *high serum cholesterol* reflects a high LDL concentration.

But the HDL also carry cholesterol, and raised HDL concentrations represent lower total body cholesterol, a lower risk of developing atherosclerosis, and a lower risk of heart attack. It is clearly not useful

[9]Interdisciplinary Cluster on Nutrition, President's Biomedical Research Panel, Assessment of the state of nutrition science, part 2, *Nutrition Today*, January/February 1977, pp. 24-27.

[10]D. M. Small, Cellular mechanisms for lipid deposition in atherosclerosis (first of two parts), *New England Journal of Medicine* 297 (1977):873-877.

simply to measure the amount of cholesterol in the blood; it is necessary to know whether it is LDL or HDL cholesterol.

Some people have abnormal lipid profiles (high in chylomicrons, VLDL, or LDL) for genetic reasons, but apparently some may have them due to such poor health habits as overeating, overconsumption of fat, or underactivity. To normalize their blood lipid profiles, such people may need to eat less fat and lose weight. Activities that raise HDL concentrations—such as frequent, intensive, and sustained exercise—may help to reverse degenerative disease processes such as atherosclerosis. (For more about HDL and atherosclerosis, see Chapter 26.)

Excretion of Cholesterol with Fiber   Knowing how the digestive and circulatory systems are arranged, you can better appreciate the relationship of dietary fiber to the body's cholesterol content. Cholesterol is used by the liver largely to manufacture bile. The bile collects in the gallbladder and stays there until fat arrives in the intestine; then the bile is squirted into the intestine to emulsify the fat.

When emulsified fat is absorbed, some of the bile accompanies it into the intestinal cells. The cells can't use this bile, and they excrete some of it back into the GI tract and return the rest to the bloodstream, where it travels by way of the portal vein back to the liver. There it may either be degraded or returned once again to the gallbladder for further recycling to the intestine.

The bile that is left in the intestine travels down the GI tract with the waste materials and is excreted from the body with them. Certain kinds of fiber have an affinity for bile, and when the diet is rich in those fibers, more bile is excreted. This effectively reduces the total body cholesterol content and is one reason for interest in dietary fiber as a possible means of retarding the development of atherosclerosis.

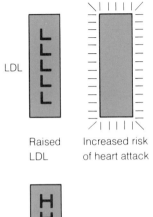

LDL

Raised LDL

Increased risk of heart attack

HDL

Raised HDL

Decreased risk of heart attack

The circulation of bile from the liver to the gallbladder to the intestine and back to the liver is known as the **enterohepatic circulation** of bile.

enteron = intestines

People who have learned that "fiber lowers blood cholesterol" have not learned quite enough to take advantage of this knowledge. If you accept oversimplified statements like this one, you may find yourself on a bandwagon like the fiber fad. Faddists have for some years been buying purified fiber to sprinkle into their foods, in the hope of improving their health. But it happens that the purified fiber they buy is most often wheat bran, the only type known to have no such effect.[11] (Bran is, however, an excellent stimulator of peristalsis and promotes the maintenance of healthy muscle tone in the GI tract.) Fibers that do lower blood cholesterol levels include pectin (the fiber of apples and other fruits) and hemicellulose (a fiber found in cereal

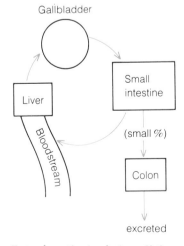

Enterohepatic circulation of bile.

[11]A. M. Connell, C. L. Smith, and M. Somsel, Absence of effect of bran on blood-lipids, *Lancet* I (March 1975), pp. 496-497.

grains). Most effective is an as-yet-unidentified fiber found in legumes such as chickpeas.[12]

Once again, the lesson seems to be that foods, not purified nutrients or other food components, are most likely to offer the greatest benefits to those who seek good health—and not so much any particular foods as a variety of foods. You may recall that other nutrition knowledge points in the same direction (see pp. 6, 157, 164).

Practical Applications

We have described the anatomy of the digestive tract on several levels: the sequence of digestive organs, the structures of the villi and of the cells that compose them, and the selective machinery of the cell membranes. The intricate architecture of the GI tract makes it sensitive and responsive to conditions in its environment. Knowing what the optimal conditions are will help you to promote the best functioning of your system.

One indispensable condition is good health of the digestive tract itself. This health is affected by such factors of lifestyle as sleep, exercise, and state of mind. Adequate sleep allows for repair, maintenance of tissue, and removal of wastes that might impair efficient functioning. Exercise promotes healthy muscle tone. As for mental state: When you read Highlight 6, you will see that stress profoundly affects digestion and absorption. In a person under stress digestive secretions are reduced and the blood is routed to the skeletal muscles more than to the digestive tract, so that efficient absorption of nutrients is impaired. To digest and absorb food best, you should be relaxed and tranquil at mealtimes.

Another factor is the kind of diet you eat. Three characteristics of the diet promote optimal absorption of nutrients: balance, variety, and adequacy. Balance means having neither too much nor too little of any dietary component. For example, some fat is needed to stimulate the release of bile from the gallbladder, not only for its own emulsification but also to help absorb the fat-soluble vitamins. Fat also slows down intestinal motility, permitting time for some of the slower nutrients to be absorbed. Too much fat, however, can form an insoluble, soapy scum with calcium and so rob the body of this mineral. A well-planned meal presents you with perhaps 20 to 30 percent of its kcalories as fat.

Another example of diet balance is already familiar to you: Fiber stimulates intestinal motility. With too little fiber the intestines are

[12]E. M. N. Hamilton and E. N. Whitney, Controversy 5: Cholesterol, in *Nutrition: Concepts and Controversies* (St. Paul: West, 1979), pp. 109-114.

likely to be sluggish; they may then fail to mix their contents or fail to bring materials into contact with the sites on the walls where they can be absorbed. Too much fiber, however, causes the contents of the intestines to move so fast through the tract that they are not in contact with the walls long enough to be absorbed. A well-planned meal delivers a moderate amount of fiber along with a generous assortment of nutrients.

Variety is important for many reasons but partly because a peculiar interaction takes place between some food constituents and certain nutrients. Compounds known as binders combine chemically with certain nutrients so that the nutrients cannot be absorbed. For example, phytic acid and oxalic acid combine with iron and calcium to prevent their absorption. Phytic acid is found in oatmeal and other whole-grain cereals, and oxalic acid in rhubarb and spinach, rendering some of the calcium and iron in these foods "unavailable." This does not mean that oatmeal or spinach is an undesirable food; both are rightly praised for their nutrient contributions. But it does mean that a person who consumes oatmeal as his only grain food or spinach as his only dark-green vegetable may be deriving less calcium and iron from his diet than he would if he were to vary his choices.

As for adequacy—in a sense this entire book is about dietary adequacy. But here, at the end of this chapter, is a good place to underline the interdependence of the nutrients, which makes it necessary to supply them all in the amounts needed in order to achieve optimum health. It could almost be said that every nutrient depends on every other. Whimsically, we might attempt to sum up this notion in one overlong, oversimplified sentence. (Don't take this seriously; it is not for memorizing. Details we think you should learn are presented more systematically.) The sentence shows the needed nutrients in capital letters and those they interact with in italics.

You need PROTEIN to attract *water* into cells; to provide pumps and diffusion-mediators for *amino acids, monosaccharides, minerals,* and the *water-soluble vitamins;* to provide carriers for *iron,* the *lipids,* and the *fat-soluble vitamins;* and to provide hormone regulators for many of these; you need LIPID to stimulate the release of bile to emulsify *lipids* and *fat-soluble vitamins* and to slow down intestinal motility to allow time for absorption of certain *minerals;* you need CARBOHYDRATE as *glucose* to provide energy for the active transport of many nutrients into cells; as *lactose* to help calcium absorption (after being converted to an acid by bacteria in the intestines) and as *cellulose (fiber)* to stimulate the mixing and moving-along of *all* the nutrients; you need VITAMIN D for *calcium* absorption, VITAMIN C to help provide the acid environment needed for absorption of *iron* and *calcium,* and VITAMIN B_6 to help the

One long sentence

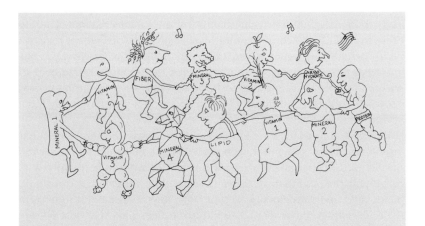

transport systems for *amino acids*; you need MINERALS such as *chlorine*, to make the hydrochloric acid that provides the stomach acidity that facilitates the digestion of *protein* and the absorption of *iron* and *calcium*; *sodium*, to provide the sodium bicarbonate secreted by the pancreas to neutralize stomach acid when it reaches the duodenum, to help with the withdrawal of *water* into cells, and to assist the transport system for *glucose*; and *phosphorus*, to assist *vitamin B₆*, which in turn assists the transport systems for *amino acids*; and you need WATER to suspend *all* of the above nutrients in a finely divided state so that they are accessible to the absorptive machinery.

You need not eat all of these nutrients at the same time in every meal, but they all work together and are all present in the cells of a healthy digestive tract. The point of all of this must be abundantly clear: To maintain health and promote the functions of the GI tract, adequacy, balance, and variety should be features of every day's menus.

Summing Up

Chapter 5 ended at the point where a hamburger or a piece of chocolate cake had been completely digested and the nutrients were ready for absorption. This chapter sums up the next part of the story. From carbohydrates, the monosaccharides — glucose, fructose, and galactose — are absorbed mostly from the small intestinal villi into the capillaries of the mesenteric membrane; the capillaries converge into veins, which in turn converge into the single large portal vein. The next stop is the liver.

From lipids, the medium- and short-chain fatty acids a
follow the same route. The long-chain fatty acids and mor
are reassembled into triglycerides and packaged, tog
cholesterol and phospholipids, in protein to form chylomic
leave the intestinal cells by way of the lymphatic sys
lipoproteins later join the general circulation through a ve
lymphatic system into the heart, and ultimately most
cleared by the liver.

From proteins, the amino acids follow the same r
monosaccharides, traveling through the mesenteric ca
veins and finally through the portal vein to the liver. The
B vitamins, vitamin C, and the minerals accompany the monosaccharides and amino acids; the fat-soluble vitamins (A, D, E, and K) are
attached to carriers and follow the path of the larger fats. Some water
moves with all of these nutrients; the water that remains is retrieved in
the large intestine. Undigested fiber remains in the GI tract until it is
excreted from the body.

The lipoproteins made in intestinal cells are mostly chylomicrons,
and these are composed predominantly of triglycerides. These travel by
way of the lymph and blood to the liver, which clears them and makes
other lipoproteins—the VLDL and LDL. The VLDL and LDL transport
lipids from the liver to the peripheral cells. The LDL may also deposit
cholesterol in arterial plaques, contributing to atherosclerosis. Fats
returning to the liver for dismantling and disposal are packaged in
HDL; a raised HDL level correlates with a reduced risk of atherosclerosis.

In the process of absorption many compounds are interdependent.
The absorption of many nutrients depends on protein; the absorption of
many others, on minerals and vitamins. The whole picture is one of
complex interrelationships, suggesting that for optimal functioning a
mixture of nutrients should be taken together at each meal.

"When I'm under st
can't eat a thing,"
says. Another
"When I'm
like a hor
notice
und

Stress and Nutrition

Stress is not even necessarily bad for you; it is also the spice of life, for any emotion, any activity causes stress. But, of course, your system must be prepared to take it.

HANS SELYE, M.D.

...ess, I ...one person ...esponds, ...nder stress, I eat ...se." And a third ..., "My friend was ...r severe stress for a ...hile and it took so much out of her. . . . She looks years older."

You may suffer from stress, or you may thrive on it. Whatever your reaction may be, it is virtually certain that your eating behavior is one of the many things affected. And because stress can "take a lot out of you," literally, it is important to know what happens to your body during periods of stress and what you can do before, during, and after, to protect yourself from the most severe effects.

To begin by defining terms, *stress* can be loosely described as anything that you experience as a threat to your stability or equilibrium; Table 1 gives examples. The *stress response* is the body's way of responding to such a perceived threat. As you are already aware, it involves hormones that affect all body tissues.

The Stress Response The stress response readies the body to deal with danger efficiently and effectively. In today's world, it stimulates people to solve problems and achieve great objectives. Yet it can wreak havoc with your health. Stress in the extreme is known to destroy mental

and physical health, and to shorten life. To understand why, you have to realize that the stress response is designed to enable the body to cope with *physical* danger, while many of the threats we experience today are psychological. The stress response readies the body for the vigorous muscular activity of fight or flight, not for the uptight, anxious posture of a person holding it all in.

The reaction begins when a threat to your equilibrium is perceived by the brain. The sight of a car hurtling toward you; the terror that an enemy is concealed around a nearby corner; the excitement of planning for a party, a move, or a wedding; the feeling of pain; or any other such disturbance perceived by the

brain serves as an *alarm signal*. There follows the chain of events depicted in Figure 1, which acts via both nerves and hormones to bring about a state of readiness in every body part. The effects all favor physical action (fight or flight). Notice the tremendous array of target organs in the paragraph that follows.

The pupils of the *eyes* widen so that you can see better; the *muscles* tense up so that you can jump, run, or struggle with maximum strength; breathing quickens to bring more oxygen into the *lungs*, and the *heart* races to rush this oxygen to the muscles so that they can burn the fuel they need for energy. The *liver* pours forth the needed fuel — glucose — from its stored supply, and the *fat cells* release fatty acids and ketones as alternative fuels. Body *protein tissues* break down to supply amino acids to back up the glucose supply and to be ready to heal wounds if necessary. The *blood vessels* of the muscles expand to feed them better while those of the *GI tract* constrict; and GI tract glands shut down (digestion is a low-priority process in time of danger). Less blood flows to the *kidney*, thus fluid is conserved; and less flows to the *skin*, so that blood loss will be minimized at any wound site. More *platelets* form, so the blood will clot faster if need be. *Hearing*

Table 1.   Events People Perceive as Stressful

People ranked these events, according to how stressful they perceived them to be, on a scale from 1 to 100. Note that some "happy" events are included here. Individual people score these events higher or lower than they are here.

Life event	"Stress points"
Death of spouse	100
Divorce	73
Marital separation	65
Jail term	63
Death of close family member	63
Personal injury or illness	53
Marriage	50
Being fired at work	47
Marital reconciliation	45
Retirement	45
Change in health of a family member	44
Pregnancy	40
Sex difficulties	39
Gain of new family member	39
Business readjustment	39
Change in financial state	38
Death of close friend	37
Change to different line of work	36
Change in number of arguments with spouse	35
Mortgage over $10,000	31
Foreclosure of mortgage or loan	30
Change in responsibilities at work	29
Son or daughter leaving home	29
Trouble with in-laws	29
Outstanding personal achievement	28
Wife beginning or stopping work	26
School beginning or ending	26
Change in living conditions	25
Revision of personal habits	24
Trouble with boss	23
Change in work hours or conditions	20
Change in residence	20
Change in schools	20
Change in recreation	19
Change in church activities	19
Change in social activities	18
Mortgage or loan less than $10,000	17
Change in sleeping habits	16
Change in number of family get-togethers	15
Change in eating habits	15
Vacation	13
Christmas	12
Minor violations of the law	11

sharpens, and the *brain* produces local opium-like substances, dulling its sensation of pain which during an emergency might distract you from taking the needed action. And your *hair* may even stand on end — a reminder that there was a time when our ancestors had enough hair to bristle, look bigger, and frighten off their enemies.

This tightly synchronized, adaptive reaction to threat provides superb support for emergency physical action. You probably remember having had to take such action; you may have performed an amazing feat of strength or speed for a few minutes, and only after it was over did you notice your heart was hammering, your breathing was fast, your fingers cold, your skin tingling, your mouth dry, and the sensation of pain or exhaustion just beginning to come through as the adrenaline drained away.

Anyone can respond in this magnificent fashion to sudden physical stress for a short interval of time. But if the stress is prolonged, and especially if physical action is not a permitted response to it, then it can drain the body of its reserves and leave it weakened, aged, and susceptible to illness. How can we best prepare to deal with periods of stress? How can we best get through them? And how can we recover most rapidly and completely afterwards?

Figure 1 The stress response. Effects with nutritional implications are shaded.

Adapted from M. B. Marcinek, Stress in the surgical patient, *American Journal of Nursing* 77, November 1977, 1809-1811, and from M. V. Kaminski, Jr., R. P. Ruggiero, and C. B. Mills, Nutritional assessment, a guide to diagnosis and treatment of the hypermetabolic patient, *Journal of the Florida Medical Association* 66 (1979):390-395.

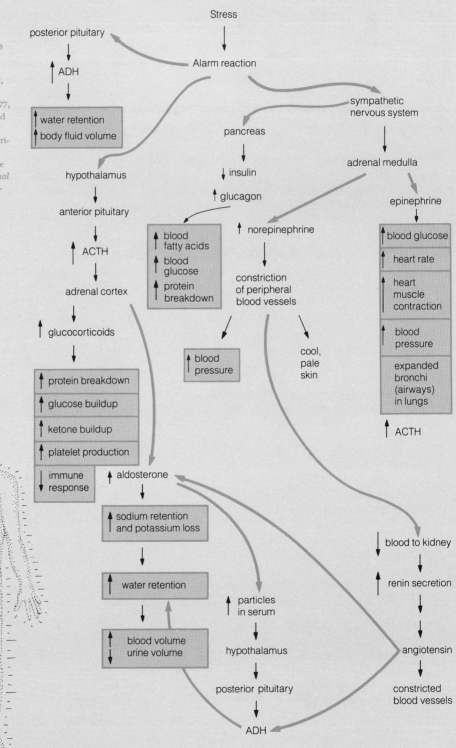

Body Reserves Drawn on During Stress   All three energy fuels — carbohydrate, fat, and protein — are drawn from body stores in increased quantities during stress. If the stress requires vigorous physical action, and if there is injury, all three are used. While the body is busy responding, eating is impossible, so the fuels must be drawn from body stores.

The conservation of *water* at such a time is of utmost importance, as you can deduce from a look at Figure 1. The body takes several measures to conserve water; one is to retain sodium — but to retain sodium the kidney exchanges, and loses, potassium. Thus you need to have ample stores of potassium to be able to afford this loss.

As for the energy nutrients: *Glucose* is taken from stored glycogen in the liver for as long as the supply lasts, but the supply is exhausted within 24 hours. Thereafter, body *protein* provides the only significant continuing glucose supply, and this is drawn primarily from muscle. Amino acids from muscle also have to be used to make scar tissue to heal wounds. Tissues that can use *fat* for energy do so, and in a normally nourished person, fat stores are adequate to meet the need for many days. Chapter 7 displays these processes as they occur during the stress of fasting; for now what is im-

portant to notice is that the body uses not only *dispensable* supplies (those that are there to be used up, so to speak, like stored fat) but also functional tissue that one doesn't want to lose, like muscle tissue. Two thoughts come to mind. First, in preparation for prolonged periods of stress, one would want to have stored as much protein in the muscle as possible. Second, one would want to take measures to minimize the wasting of muscle during stress.

Another nutrient lost from the body during stress is *calcium* from the bones. The evidence is not completely clear on this, but it has been observed that people lose widely varying amounts of this important bone mineral, depending partly on their hormonal state.[1] Adult bone loss is a common occurrence anyway, especially among women, so the same considerations apply here: one wants to know, first, how to be prepared to sustain these losses and second, how to minimize them.

Nutrition Prior to Periods of Stress   The body that is healthy, with filled stores of the needed nutrients, is best prepared for stress. Protein and calcium are among the nutrients just mentioned;

[1]W. H. Griffith, Food as a regulator of metabolism, *American Journal of Clinical Nutrition* 17 (1965):391-398.

how do you fill your stores with these nutrients? In both cases the answer is the same: by eating foods that provide ample amounts of these nutrients (easy), and, equally important, by exercising so as to make them "stick" (takes work). Muscles don't grow and retain protein without activity, even if they are bathed in an amino-acid rich fluid. They don't respond passively to what's in their environment, but actively to the demands that are put upon them. Only when they are called upon to *work*, do they grow and store protein. So being healthy, in this sense, means more than just nutrition; it means nutrition-and-exercise. It means daily or every-other-day workouts, prolonged and demanding enough to bring about a training effect, the building of muscle. (Don't get scared, though. This means only 20 or so minutes of pleasantly vigorous exercise every other day at first. See To Explore Further.) Then when stress hits, even if eating is altogether impossible for a while, the wasting that may inevitably occur will have less severe impact. (And incidentally, in having increased your muscle mass, you will have added significantly to your potassium supplies.)

Bones, like muscles, do not store their component nutrients (calcium, in this case) passively. No matter how many glasses of milk you drink a day, the extra calcium will not be deposited in bone but will be excreted as fast as you take it in — unless you work your bones. In response to stress (the "good" stress of physical work), bones store calcium and become denser, stronger, and able to carry more weight. Like the muscles, then, when they respond to the weakening effects of the "bad" stress of anxiety, illness, or the like, they can better afford to give up their calcium without becoming dangerously weak.

In short, the best nutritional preparation for stress is a balanced and varied diet as part of a lifestyle in which exercise plays a constant part. Notice that nothing is said here about supplements or gimmicks. Just eat well and work out regularly, and your body will be as well prepared as it can be to withstand the impact of periods of unavoidable stress.

Nutrition During Stress
The appetite is suppressed during severe stress. We've already said why. It's an adaptive reaction to a *physical* threat, the kind of threat that our ancestors experienced during their evolution. Energy at such a time is needed for fight or flight; it would be wasteful and risky to spend it looking for or eating food. The blood supply has been diverted to the muscles to maximize

strength and speed; so even if you swallow food you may not be able to digest or absorb it efficiently. (In a severe upset, the stomach and intestines will even reject solid food; vomiting and/or diarrhea are their way of disposing of a burden they can't handle.) All of this means that it is poor advice to someone under severe stress to tell them to eat. They can't; or if they can, they can't assimilate what they've eaten.

On the other hand, fasting is itself a stress on the body and the longer you go without eating, the harder it can be to get started again. So it can be a no-win situation. It is frightening to see the downward spiral that people can get into once they have let stress affect them to the point where they can't eat, and not eating makes it harder for them to handle the stress.

It is therefore desirable not to let stress become so overwhelming that eating becomes impossible. Managing stress, so that it does not overwhelm, is not only a nutritional but also a psychological task.

If you can eat, do so, of course. Take only a little if that's all you can handle, and eat more often to keep meeting your nutrient and kcalorie needs. Choose a variety of foods from all food groups to meet all needs. Listen to your body, remember

what you know about nutrition, and try to keep in tune with what you need and can handle. Drink fluids, too. Although the body conserves fluids during stress, it will excrete what it does not need, and by taking in water you enable your kidneys to excrete the sodium they might otherwise have to retain.

Whenever someone can't eat, there will inevitably be depletion of nutrients. Aside from the protein, calcium, and potassium already mentioned, the nutrients most susceptible to this depletion are the vitamins and minerals that are not stored in substantial quantities. People are aware that the water-soluble vitamins (B vitamins and vitamin C) fall into this category; they are less likely to know that some two dozen minerals do, too. When the question arises whether one should take vitamin supplements during periods of stress, the answer should probably be: "Yes, if you can't eat — but not just vitamin supplements. Take a multivitamin-mineral preparation that supplies a balanced assortment of all the nutrients that might be needed, not in 'mega' doses, but in amounts comparable to the RDA."

The vitamins and minerals occupy five chapters later in the book, but it seems important to say this much about them here. Generally, people consuming less than 1,200 to 1,500 kcal/day of food need such supplements; the RDA table on the inside front cover shows the amounts to look for.

Stress Eating   All that has been said so far has been directed at the person who loses appetite during stress. What about the one who eats more than usual? It is not clear why stress drives some people to eat more, but it certainly does happen.[2] One possible explanation is this sequence of events: glucose is drawn from stores, the body fails to use it up by way of physical exertion, and instead stores it as fat, then the person feels hungry because blood glucose has fallen. Another possibility is that the *behavior* of eating helps to relieve stress by occupying the nervous system with a familiar activity that discharges its nerves without doing harm as fighting might do. (This is a phenomenon that biologists call displacement activity.[3]) It may be that eating, or the food eaten, leads to release of

substances in the brain that you experience as soothing. Highlight 5 showed that neurotransmitter levels change when carbohydrate-containing food is eaten. Something else happens, too, that is worth a paragraph of explanation.

It seems that eating leads to the production of substances in the brain that act in the same way as opiates like morphine do. Stress uses up these opiates in the emotion-governing brain centers, and eating helps to restore them to levels that relieve the stress.[4] Much remains to be learned about these endogenous opiates, but it already seems likely that they help to explain stress-induced eating. The person who is subject to this behavior and who is threatened with obesity on account of it, would be well-advised to find an alternative way of raising the level of internal tranquilizers — exercise, meditation, listening to music, or the like.

The phenomenon of stress eating shows why exercise is important during stress as

well as before. In fact it may be positively harmful *not* to exercise in response to acute stress. As just described, in the stress response, muscle fuel floods the bloodstream; it needs to be used, or else it will be stored as fat. For psychological reasons, too, it is desirable if you are upset, angry, anxious, or even happy, to express those feelings through physical action: Cry, scream, laugh, punch a pillow, pace, run, lift weights, dance, or whatever else you choose. Actions like these release tensions that otherwise build up and increase stress.

Exercise during stress has at least two other beneficial effects. It builds muscle and bone as already explained, promoting the storage of needed nutrients. And it may release the same pain-killing chemicals (endorphins) that stress does, helping to heighten mood.

Nutrition in the Recovery Period   When the stressful time is over and the body can recover, comes the opportunity to replenish depleted stores. If you have lost weight you need to gain it back — not just by eating and putting on fat, but by eating-and-exercising to restore both lean and fat tissue. If you have gained weight, it is time to get back in trim with a combination of diet and exercise. But perhaps more important than nutrition

[2]A. S. Levine and J. E. Morley, Stress-induced eating, in *Food in Contemporary Society,* a symposium sponsored by Stokely-Van Camp and conducted at The University of Tennessee, Knoxville, May 27-29, 1981, pp. 126-135; J. Slochower and S. P. Kaplan, Anxiety, perceived control, and eating in obese and normal weight persons, *Appetite* 1 (1980):75-83.

[3]Levine and Morley, 1981.

[4]This has been demonstrated in experiments using rats and is believed to account for what is seen with humans as well. Levine and Morley, 1981; also Morley and Levine, The endorphins and enkephalins as regulators of appetite, in *Food and Contemporary Society* (already cited), pp. 136-148; also J. E. Morley and A. S. Levine, Stress-induced eating is mediated through endogenous opiates, *Science* 209 (1980):1259-1261.

Miniglossary

endogenous opiates: morphine-like compounds produced in the brain in response to a variety of events and activities including stress, eating, and exercise.

endo = within (the body)
gen = arising

endorphins: See *endogenous opiates.*

general adaptation syndrome: see *stress response.*

stress: Any threat to a person's well-being. The threat may be physical or psychological, desired or feared, but the reaction is always the same. See *stress response.*

stress eating: The behavior of eating in response to stress; causes unknown as yet.

stress response: The body's response to stress, mediated by both nerves and hormones initially; begins with an *alarm reaction*, proceeds through a stage of *resistance*, and then to recovery or, if prolonged, to *exhaustion.* This three-stage response has also been termed the *general adaptation syndrome.*

techniques would be the learning of mind-control techniques to prevent the next stressful event from being so overwhelming and debilitating.

Stress Management A clue to the management of stress comes from the fact that it is not the event itself but the individual's reaction to it that determines how much it will strain the body's resources. Remember, stress is defined as anything you *perceive* as a threat to your equilibrium. Divorce is considered extremely stressful by most people (it receives an average score of 73 in Table 1), but it may threaten one person much more than another. Psychological counselors urge that you learn stress management techniques to ride through the disruptive changes in your life. They suggest that you:

● Change how you perceive the event so you will react less violently to it (learn to see it not as a disaster that may destroy you but as a change you can handle).

● Learn to express yourself (ventilate), so that you will not be so uptight. This involves muscular action and deep breathing with vigorous and dramatic demonstration of your feelings (when and where appropriate).

● Take time out. Meet your need for relief from pain, anxiety, or anger by way of meditation, relaxation techniques, exercise, or the like.

● Expand your social support system. Much that is exhausting and painful to handle alone is easier to manage when you have understanding from a circle of supportive friends and/or helpers.

This Highlight necessarily ends by putting nutrition in perspective as part of a much larger picture in which many nonnutritional factors are of great importance. But it has also shown that nutrition *is* important, and has given some practical pointers for everyone to apply. Chapter 22 expands on this theme by describing the severe stress hospital patients experience, and the special considerations involved in providing them with nutrition support.

To Explore Further

The "father of stress," who coined the term and spent his life studying it, is Hans Selye. A popular paperback of his, written in nontechnical language, is:
● Selye, H. *The Stress of Life*, revised ed. New York: McGraw-Hill, 1976.

A series of four excellent articles on stress appeared in the *American Journal of Nursing*. They show how the nurse can recognize and cope with stress in her very demanding job, and also how she can recognize it in patients or clients and help them to cope with it:

● Smith, M. J. T., and Selye, H. Reducing the negative effects of stress. *American Journal of Nursing* 79 (November 1979):1953-1955.

● O'Flynn-Corniskey, A. J. The type A individual. *American Journal of Nursing* 79 (November 1979):1956-1958.

● Morris, C. L. Relaxation therapy in a clinic. *American*

Journal of Nursing 79 (November 1979):1958.

- Richter, J. M., and Sloan, A. A relaxation technique. *American Journal of Nursing* 79 (November 1979):1960-1964.

The article by Smith and Selye also lists the "diseases of adaptation," showing how each person has a different body system or part that may be the first to succumb to excessive stress, so that one person gets heart disease, another ulcers, another allergies, and so forth.

The standard-bearer for accuracy in vitamin claims, Victor Herbert, shows how the notion of "stress vitamins" arose and why we should not take it seriously:

- Herbert, V. The vitamin craze. *Archives of Internal Medicine* 140 (1980):173-176.

The psychological means of managing stress are nicely described in Chapter 4 of the delightful book:

- Farquhar, J. W. *The American Way of Life Need Not Be Hazardous to Your Health.* New York: Norton, 1978.

Farquhar's bibliography for that chapter suggests other good references.

To get in shape physically, we suggest you use one of the following books as a guide. The first is the easiest and most fun to read; the last is the most technically accurate and deals only with running.

- Bailey, C. *Fit or Fat?* Boston: Houghton Mifflin, 1977.
- Katch, F. I., McArdle, W. D., and Boylan, B. R. *Getting in Shape.* Boston: Houghton Mifflin, 1979.
- Costill, D. L. *A Scientific Approach to Distance Running.* Los Altos, Calif: Track and Field News, 1979.

The first study in which severe psychological stress has been shown to produce a measurable abnormality in immune function is:

- Bartrop, R. W., Lazarus, L., Luckhurst, E., Kiloh, L. G., and Penny, R. Depressed lymphocyte function after bereavement. *Lancet* 1 (1977):834-836.

This book is written for doctors by a doctor:

- Altschule, M. D. *Nutritional Factors in General Medicine: Effects of Stress and Distorted Diets.* Springfield, Ill.: Charles C. Thomas, 1978.

A teaching aid, *Stress: On Just Being Sick*, by H. Selye, is a set of 13 slides designed to depict the consequences of stress. The set can be ordered from the Nutrition Today Society (address in Appendix J).

CHAPTER 7

CONTENTS

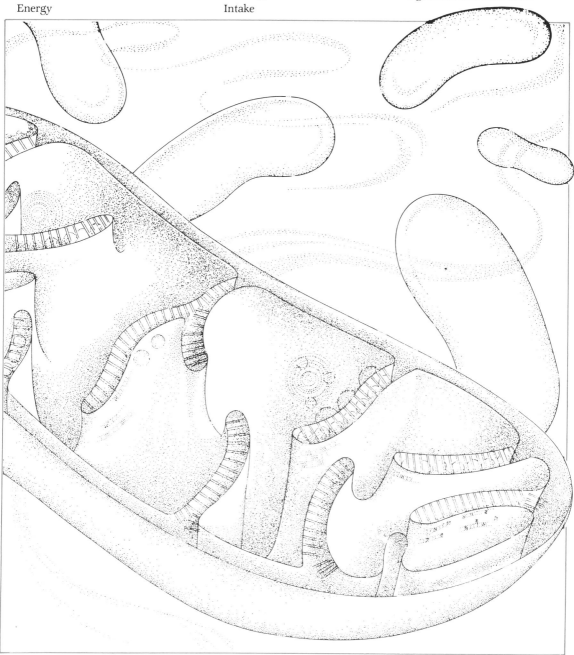

Much of the cell's metabolic activity takes place in structures like this one (a mitochondrion). A million enzyme-complexes are mounted on the membranes inside this particle, and there may be hundreds of such particles inside an active cell. Within each complex the enzymes are mounted in the order in which they perform their reactions.

METABOLISM:
Feasting, Fasting, and Energy Balance

The course of nature ... seems delighted with transmutations ...

SIR ISAAC NEWTON

When you eat too much you get fat; when you eat too little you get thin. Everybody knows these simple facts, but nobody knows exactly how to account for them. The mission of this chapter is to shed some light on what we do know and to provide answers to some of the questions people often ask about diets. What makes a person gain weight? Are carbohydrate-rich foods more fattening than other foods? What's the best way to lose weight: Is fasting dangerous? Are low-carbohydrate diets dangerous? The answers to these and many other questions lie in an understanding of metabolism.

Metabolism could be defined as the way the body handles the energy nutrients; a more precise definition appears in the margin. But before getting into the body cells to see metabolism in progress, a brief review of the energy nutrients themselves may be helpful.

metabolism: the sum total of all the chemical reactions that go on in living cells.

meta = among
bole = change

Starting Points

The first four chapters introduced the energy nutrients—carbohydrate, fat, and protein—as they are found in foods and in the human body. Chapters 5 and 6 followed the nutrients through digestion to the simpler units they are composed of and showed these units disappearing into the blood. Four of these units will be followed here.

(1) *Carbohydrates* come in several varieties in the diet: principally as the polysaccharide starch, the disaccharides, and the monosaccharides. During digestion, these units are all broken down to monosaccharides — glucose, fructose, and galactose — and are absorbed into the blood. The latter two are then taken into liver cells and converted to glucose or to very similar compounds. Thus to continue the story of what happens to carbohydrate thereafter, we will simply follow glucose.

(2 & 3) *Lipids* also come in several varieties, but 95 percent of those found in foods are *triglycerides*. The triglycerides undergo several transformations during digestion and absorption, but many of them end up once again as triglycerides in body cells. There they can be

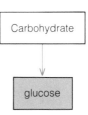

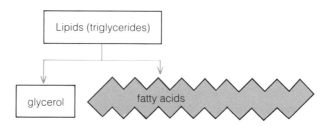

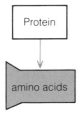

dismantled to glycerol and fatty acids. Following the further transformations of glycerol and fatty acids will show the principal fates of dietary fat.

(4) *Protein* is digested to amino acids, absorbed into blood, and carried to the liver, where further transformations occur. Thus to follow protein through metabolism, we will trace the steps by which amino acids are further transformed.

Building Body Compounds

You already know what may happen to some of these basic units when their energy is not needed by the cells: They may be stored "as is," being used to build body compounds. Glucose units may be strung together to make glycogen chains. Glycerol and fatty acids may be assembled into triglycerides. Amino acids may be used to make proteins. These building reactions, in which simple compounds are put together to form larger, more complex structures, involve doing work—and so require energy. They are called anabolic reactions.

anabolism: those reactions in which small molecules are put together to form larger ones. Anabolic reactions involve reduction and require energy.

ana = up

Arrows pointing up represent anabolic reactions. These reactions take place in many of the body's cells.

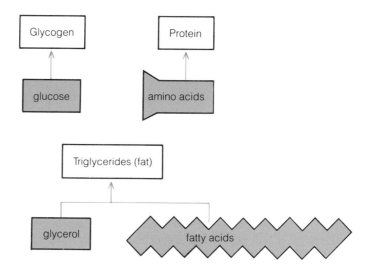

Breaking Down Nutrients for Energy

If the body does need energy, however, it may break apart any or all of these units into fragments. The breakdown reactions, which release energy, are called catabolic reactions.

At this point you must stop thinking about these compounds as the basic units of the nutrients and remember that they are composed of still more basic units, the atoms. During metabolism, the body goes to work with an "electron saw" and actually separates the atoms from one another. It will help if you recall the structures of these compounds (introduced in the first four chapters). There is no need to remember exactly how they are put together; it is enough to remember how many carbons are in their "backbones":

catabolism: reactions in which large molecules are broken down to smaller ones. Catabolic reactions involve oxidation and release energy.

kata = down

Arrows pointing down represent catabolic reactions. Much of the body's catabolic work is done in the liver cells, and all of the reactions described in this chapter can take place there.

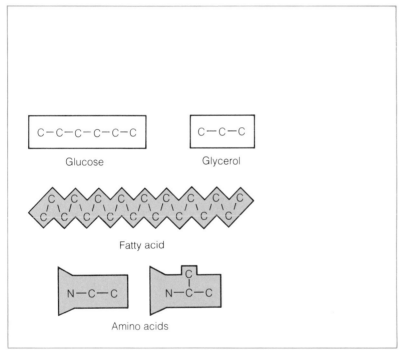

The main point to notice in the following discussion is that compounds that have a three-carbon skeleton can be used to make the vital nutrient glucose, but those that have two-carbon skeletons cannot.

The story of what happens to these compounds inside of cells can be told most simply by starting with glucose. Two new names appear — pyruvate (three carbons) and acetyl CoA (two carbons) — and once you have learned these, the rest of the story falls into place around them.

Glucose   In breaking down, glucose first splits in half releasing energy. One product is the three-carbon compound pyruvate, and the other is converted into pyruvate, so that two identical halves result from this step.

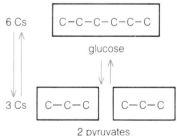

pyruvate (PIE-roo-vate): a salt of pyruvic acid. (Throughout this book the ending *ate* is used interchangeably with *ic acid*. Thus acetate is the same as acetic acid.)

Should a cell "change its mind" after splitting glucose to pyruvate, it could reverse this step. It could put the two halves back together to make glucose again.

If the cell still needs energy, however, it breaks the pyruvate molecules apart further, cleaving a carbon from each. The lone carbon is combined with oxygen to make carbon dioxide, which is released into the blood, circulated to the lungs, and excreted (breathed out). The two-carbon compound that remains is acetyl CoA. Should the cell "change its mind" at this point and want to retrieve the carbons and make glucose, it could not do so. The step from pyruvate to acetyl CoA is metabolically irreversible: It is a one-way step.

CoA (coh-AY): nickname for a compound described further in Chapter 9. As pyruvate loses a carbon and becomes a 2-carbon compound (acetate), a molecule of CoA is attached to it, making **acetyl CoA** (ASS-uh-teel co-AY).

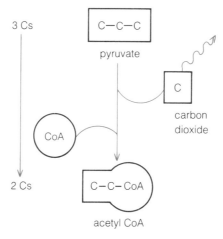

Finally acetyl CoA may be split, yielding two more carbon dioxide molecules. The energy released in this step powers most of the cell's activities. The process by which acetyl CoA splits and releases its energy is known as the TCA cycle; its details are not necessary to a basic understanding of nutrition but are given in Highlight 7A for those who are interested.

The reactions by which the complete oxidation of acetyl CoA is accomplished are those of the **TCA** (tricarboxylic acid) or **Krebs cycle** (named for the biochemist who elucidated them) and **oxidative phosphorylation.** Details are given in Highlight 7A.

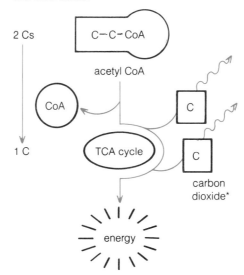

To sum up, then, the steps in the complete breakdown of glucose are:

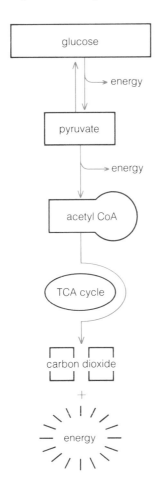

Only the first step is reversible. Energy is released at every step, but the breakdown of acetyl CoA provides most of the energy that powers the cell.

Why should you bother to learn about the intermediate compounds, pyruvate and acetyl CoA? What happens to these two compounds explains the most interesting and important aspects of nutrition and makes it possible to answer questions like those asked at the outset. The breakdown of protein and fat, as well as glucose, yields pyruvate and acetyl CoA. The parts of protein and fat that can be converted to pyruvate (3 carbons) *can* provide glucose for the body; those that are converted to acetyl CoA can *not* do so. And glucose is all-important to survival.

Glycerol and Fatty Acids   The typical triglyceride consists of a molecule of glycerol (3 carbons long) and three fatty acids (about 18 carbons each, or 54 carbons in all). When such a molecule is broken

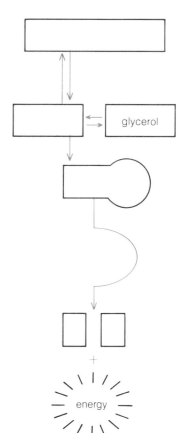

down inside a cell, these parts are first separated. The glycerol is easily converted to pyruvate (also three carbons long) and then may go either "up" to form glucose or "down" to form acetyl CoA and finally carbon dioxide. Thus one tiny piece of each fat molecule—about 5 percent of the total weight—can be used to meet the body's need for glucose.

But the three fatty acids are taken apart two carbons at a time to make acetyl CoA, and this cannot be used to make glucose. It is either broken down further, yielding energy, or put together to make compounds such as other fatty acids, cholesterol, or ketones. So fat is a very poor, inefficient source of glucose. About 95 percent of it cannot be converted to glucose at all.

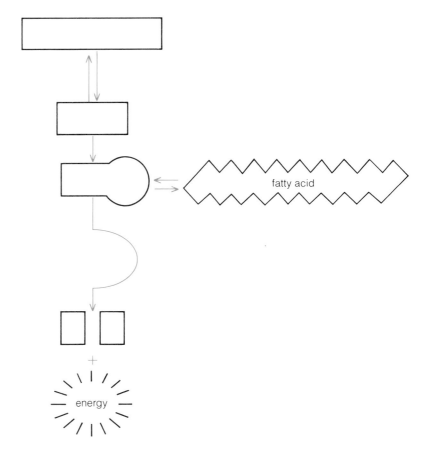

Amino Acids   Protein enters the body as an array of different amino acids. Ideally they will be used to build needed body proteins. But if energy needs are not met by carbohydrate and fat, then the amino acids will be sacrificed to provide energy. When this occurs, they are stripped of their nitrogen (see the next section) and then treated in a variety of

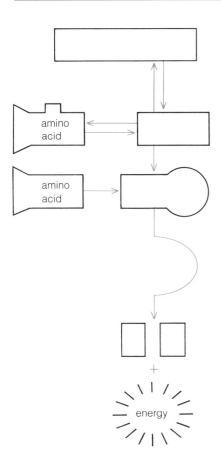

ways.[1] The net effect is that about half of amino acids can be converted to pyruvate; the other half go either to acetyl CoA or directly into the TCA cycle. Those that can be used to make pyruvate can provide glucose for the body. Thus protein, unlike fat, is a fairly good source of glucose when carbohydrate is not available.

Amino acids break down when energy needs are not met by carbohydrate and fat, as just described, but they also break down in the same way under another set of conditions: when surplus kcalories and protein are consumed. Surplus protein cannot be stored in the body as such; it has to be degraded. If you eat more protein than you can use at a given time, the excess amino acids quickly lose their nitrogens and most are converted to acetyl CoA either directly or indirectly (through pyruvate). But this acetyl CoA is not broken down further, because energy is not needed. Instead it is strung together into chains—fatty

The making of glucose from protein or fat is **gluconeogenesis** (gloo-co-nee-o-GEN-uh-sis). About 5 percent of fat (the glycerol portion of triglycerides) and about half of the amino acids (those that are glucogenic) can be converted to glucose.

gluco = glucose
neo = new
genesis = making

[1] Some are rearranged to form pyruvate. Others are four-carbon compounds that split into two acetyl CoA. One, which contains only two carbons after the nitrogen is removed, is rearranged directly to become acetyl CoA. Still others become compounds that enter the TCA cycle (see Highlight 7A).

acids—and stored in body fat. Thus even the so-called "lean" nutrient, protein, can make you fat if you eat too much of it.

What Happens to the Nitrogen? When amino acids are degraded for energy or to make fat, the first step is removal of their nitrogen-containing amino groups, a reaction called deamination. The product is ammonia, chemically identical to the ammonia in the bottled cleaning solutions used in hospitals and in industry. It is a strong-smelling and extremely potent poison.

deamination: removal of the amino (NH_2) group from a compound such as an amino acid.

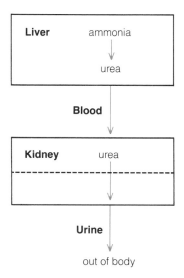

A small amount of ammonia is always being produced by liver deamination reactions. Some of this ammonia is captured by liver enzymes and used to synthesize other amino acids, but what cannot be used is quickly combined with a carbon-oxygen fragment to make urea, an inert and less toxic compound.

Urea is released from the liver cells into the blood, where it circulates until it passes through the kidneys. One of the functions of the kidneys is to remove urea from the blood for excretion in the urine. Urea is the body's principal vehicle for excreting unused nitrogen; water is required to keep it in solution and excrete it. This explains why people who consume a high-protein diet must drink more water than usual.

(After excretion, urea may be converted spontaneously or by

urea (yoo-REE-uh): the principal nitrogen-excretion product of metabolism. Two ammonia fragments are combined with a carbon-oxygen group to form urea. The diagram greatly over-simplifies the reactions.

bacterial action back to ammonia. This accounts for the ammonia odor of the diaper pail.)

Putting It All Together   After a normal mixed meal, if you do not overeat, the body handles the nutrients in all of the ways just described (see Figure 1).

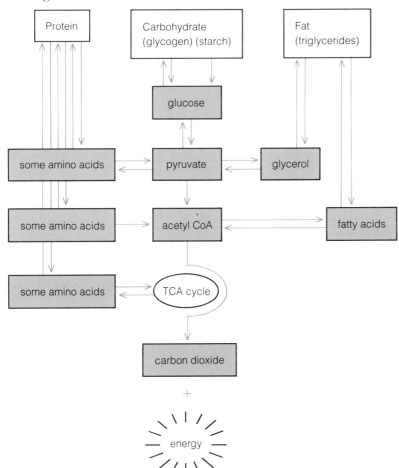

Figure 1   The central pathways of metabolism. This diagram is repeated five times on the next few pages, highlighting a different part each time.

The carbohydrate yields glucose: Some is stored as glycogen, and some is taken into brain and other cells and broken down through pyruvate and acetyl CoA to provide energy. The protein yields amino acids: Some are used to build body protein, and (if there is a surplus) some are broken down through the same pathways as glucose to provide energy. The fat yields glycerol and fatty acids: Some are put together and stored as fat, and others are broken down through the same pathways as glucose to provide energy.

A few hours after the meal, the stored glycogen and fat begin to be released from storage to provide more glucose, glycerol, and fatty acids to keep the energy flow going. When all of the energy supplied from the last meal has been used up and reserves of these compounds are running low, it is time to eat again.

The average person consumes more than a million kcalories a year and expends more than 99 percent of them, maintaining a stable weight for years on end.[2] This remarkable achievement, which most people manage without even thinking about it, could be called the economy of maintenance: The body's energy budget is balanced. Some people, however, eat too little and get thin; others eat too much and get fat. The possible reasons for this are explored in Chapter 8; the metabolic consequences will be discussed here.

The Economy of Feasting

The pathways of metabolism just described make it clear why consuming too much of any energy nutrient can make you fat. Surplus carbohydrate (glucose) can be stored as glycogen, but there is a limit to

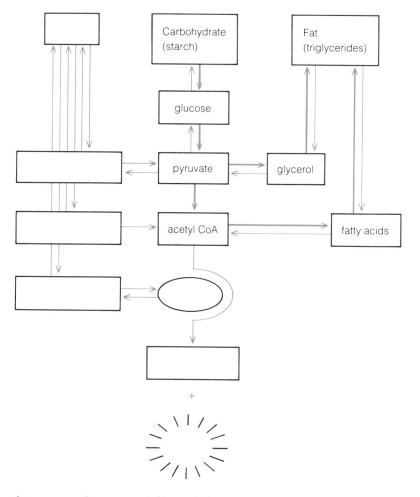

the capacity of the glycogen-storing cells. Once glycogen stores are filled, the overflow is routed to fat (note the heavy arrows in the diagram above). Fat cells expand as they fill with fat, and they seem to be able to expand indefinitely. Thus excess carbohydrate, above and beyond the kcalorie need, can contribute to obesity.

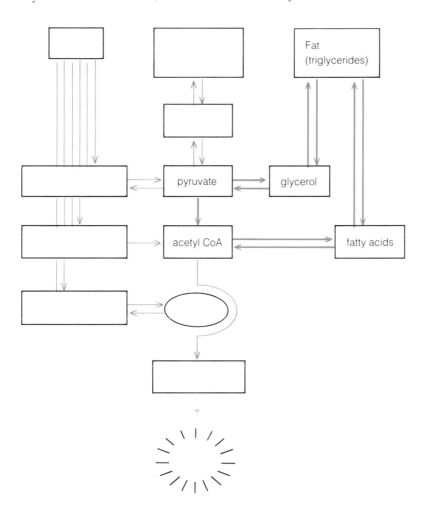

Of course, surplus fat in the diet can also contribute to the body's fat stores (note the heavy arrows in the diagram above). It may break down to fragments such as acetyl CoA, but if energy flow is already rapid enough to meet the demand, these fragments will not enter the energy-yielding pathway. They will be diverted back again to the assembly of triglycerides and stored in the fat cells.

Finally, surplus protein may encounter the same fate (note the heavy arrows on the next page). If not needed to build body protein or to meet present energy needs, amino acids will lose their nitrogens and be converted through the intermediates, pyruvate and acetyl CoA, to triglycerides. These, too, swell the fat cells and increase body weight.

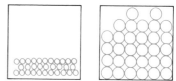

Fat cells enlarge.

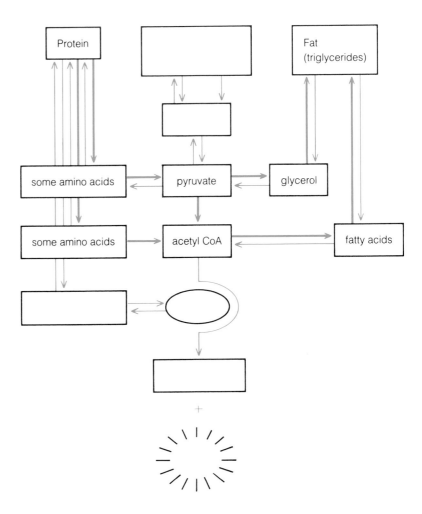

The Economy of Fasting

Even when you are asleep and totally relaxed, the cells of many organs are hard at work spending energy. In fact, the work that you are aware of, that you do with your muscles during waking hours, represents only about a third of the total energy you spend in a day. The rest is the metabolic work of the cells, for which they constantly require fuel.

The body's top priority is to meet these energy needs, and its normal way of doing so is by periodic refueling—that is, by eating. When food is withdrawn, the body must find other fuel sources in its own tissues. If people choose not to eat, we say they are fasting; if they have no choice (as in a famine), we say they are starving; but there is no metabolic difference between the two. In either case the body is forced to switch to a wasting metabolism, drawing on its stored reserves of carbohydrate and fat and within a day or so on its protein tissues as well.

Fuel must be delivered to every cell. As the fast begins, glucose and fatty acids are both flowing into cells, breaking down to yield acetyl CoA, and delivering energy to power the cells' work. Several hours later, however, most of the glucose is used up, the available glycogen has been withdrawn from storage to replenish it, and this source in turn is being exhausted.

At this point, most of the cells are depending on fatty acids to continue providing their fuel. But the brain cells cannot; they still need glucose. (The problem is that the only nutrient that can get through their membranes is glucose. Once inside, this glucose breaks down to acetyl CoA and is processed the same way as in other cells.) Normally the brain consumes about two-thirds of the total glucose used each day.

The brain's special requirement for glucose poses a problem for the fasting body. It can use its stores of fat, which may be quite generous, to furnish most of its cells with energy, but for the brain it must supply energy in the form of glucose. This is why body protein tissues, such as

The liver releases both fat and glucose to be used as fuel by the body's cells, but the brain can accept and use only the glucose.

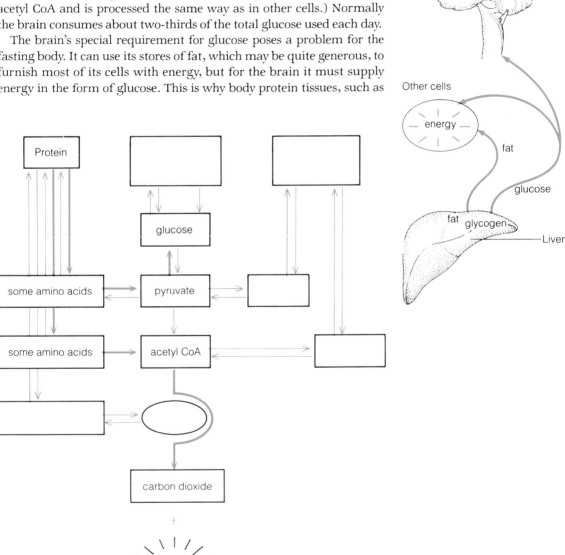

ketone (KEE-tone): a compound formed during the incomplete oxidation of fatty acids. Ketones contain a C=O group between other carbons; when they also contain a COOH, or acid group, they are called keto-acids. Small amounts of ketones are a normal part of the blood chemistry, but when their concentration rises, they spill into the urine. The combination of high blood ketones (ketonemia) and ketones in the urine (ketonuria) is termed **ketosis.**

muscle, always break down to some extent during fasting. Only those amino acids that yield three-carbon pyruvate can be used to make glucose, and to obtain them, whole proteins must be broken down and the other amino acids have to be disposed of. This is an expensive way to gain glucose. But to extract glycerol from fat is even more expensive: Every little three-carbon glycerol taken from fat obligates the body to dispose of some 50 or 60 carbons' worth of fatty acids. In the first few days of a fast, body protein provides about 90 percent of the needed glucose, and glycerol about 10 percent. If body protein loss were to continue at this rate, death would ensue within three weeks.

As the fast continues, the body adapts by producing an alternate energy source—ketones—by condensing together fragments derived from fatty acids. Normally produced and used in only small quantities, ketones can enter some brain cells and serve there as a fuel. Ketone production rises until, at the end of several weeks, it is meeting about half or more of the brain's energy needs. Still, many areas of the brain rely exclusively on glucose, and body protein continues to be sacrificed to produce it.[3]

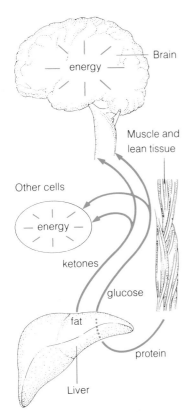

In fasting, muscle and lean tissue atrophy to supply protein for conversion to glucose. This glucose and the ketones produced from fat fuel the brain's activities.

Acetone (ASS-uh-tone) is familiar to some as the solvent used in nail polish remover. "Acetone breath" indicates that a person is in ketosis.

2 acetyl CoA   (−2 CoA)⟶   A ketone (keto-acid)

This ketone may lose a molecule of carbon dioxide to become another ketone:

Acetone

Simultaneously, the body drastically reduces its energy output in order to conserve both its fat and lean tissue. As the lean (protein-containing) organ tissue shrinks in mass, it performs less metabolic work, reducing energy needs. As the muscles waste, they do less work, enhancing this effect. Because of the slowed metabolism, the loss of fat falls to a bare minimum—less, in fact, than the fat that would be lost on a low-kcalorie diet.[4] Thus although weight loss during fasting may be quite dramatic, fat loss may be less than when at least some food is supplied.

[3]R. A. Hawkins and J. F. Biebuyck, Ketone bodies are selectively used by individual brain regions, *Science* 205 (1979):325-327.

[4]M. F. Ball, J. J. Canary, and L. H. Kyle, Comparative effects of calorie restriction and total starvation on body composition in obesity, *Annals of Internal Medicine* 67 (1967):60-67.

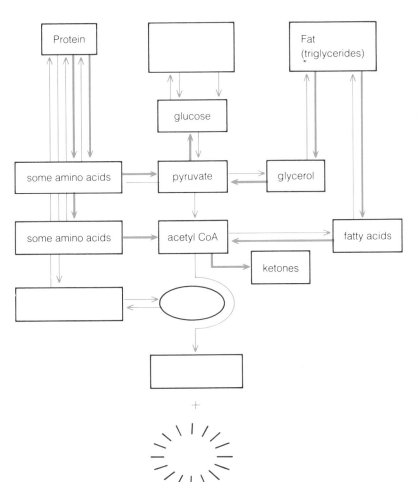

Figure 2 Metabolism during fasting. Protein breakdown supplies some glucose for the brain. Ketone production helps to support brain function. Heavy arrows show which pathways are speeded up during ketosis.

Marasmus These adaptations also occur in the starving child and help to prolong its life. The severe malnutritional state resulting from starvation is termed marasmus. Together with protein deficiency, it is the most widespread malnutrition problem in the world. Children with marasmus suffer symptoms similar to those of children with the protein-deficiency disease kwashiorkor, due to the loss of body protein tissue; differences are that kwashiorkor children retain some of their stores of body fat, accumulate fat in their livers, and develop edema.

A marasmic child looks like a wizened little old person—just skin and bones. He is often sick, because his resistance to disease is low. All his muscles are wasted, including his heart muscle, and his heart is weak. His metabolism is so slow that his body temperature is subnormal. He has little or no fat under his skin to insulate against cold. The experience of hospital workers with victims of this disease is that their primary need is to be wrapped up and kept warm. They also need love, because they have often been deprived of maternal attention as well as food.

marasmus (ma-RAZ-mus): overt starvation due to a deficiency of kcalories from any source.

Kwashiorkor: see p. 132.

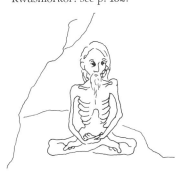

Unlike the kwashiorkor child, who is fed milk until weaning, the marasmic child may have been neglected from early infancy. The disease occurs most commonly in children from 6 to 18 months of age in all the overpopulated city slums of the world. Since the brain normally grows to almost its full adult size within the first two years of life, marasmus impairs brain development and so may have a permanent effect on learning ability.

For the effect of early malnutrition on brain development, see Highlight 18.

Marasmus also occurs in adults in countries where kcalorie deficiency is prevalent. The causes are manifold; Highlight 18 attempts to sort them out and put them in perspective. In recent years marasmus has also been seen to occur in many undernourished hospital patients.

The Low-Carbohydrate Diet A similar economy prevails if a low-carbohydrate diet is consumed. Advocates of the low-carbohydrate diet would have you believe that there is something magical about ketosis, which promotes faster weight loss than a regular low-kcalorie diet. In fact, the low-carbohydrate diet presents the same problem as a fast. Once the body's available glycogen reserves are spent, the only remaining source of energy in the form of glucose is protein. The low-carbohydrate diet provides a little protein from food, but some must still be taken from body tissue. The onset of ketosis is the signal that this wasting process has begun.

Low-carbohydrate diet = eating protein and fat almost exclusively.

In a diet that provides fewer than about 900 kcal (for the average-size adult), it is pointless to supply any protein at all, because the protein will only be wasted to provide energy. Body protein is lost at the same rate in adults on such a diet whether or not they are given any food protein.[5]

One conclusion to draw from this is that a person who diets at the level of 900 kcal a day might as well eat carbohydrate and fat alone, without protein. This conclusion is valid: Carbohydrate-containing foods are less expensive than protein-rich foods, and both will serve the same purpose—supplying glucose. This is the choice made by the person on a juice fast, for juices contain only carbohydrate. But a wiser conclusion is that such a diet is unnecessarily low in kcalories, even dangerously so. The person who wishes to lose body *fat* will select a balanced diet of 1,200 or more kcalories, one containing carbohydrate, fat, *and* protein. At this level, body protein will be spared, ketosis need not occur, vital lean tissues (including both muscle and brain) will not starve, and only the unwanted *fat* will be lost.

Juice fast = eating only carbohydrate.

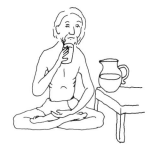

People are attracted to the low-carbohydrate diet because of the

[5]A. A. Albanese and L. A. Orto, The proteins and amino acids, in *Modern Nutrition in Health and Disease*, 5th ed., eds. R. S. Goodhart and M. E. Shils (Philadelphia: Lea and Febiger, 1973), p. 56.

dramatic weight loss it brings about within the first few days. They would be disillusioned if they realized that much of this weight loss is a loss of protein, and with it, quantities of water and important minerals. A woman who boasts of losing seven pounds in two days on her diet may be unaware that at best, she has lost a pound or two of fat and five or six of lean tissue, water, and minerals. When she goes "off" her diet, her body will avidly devour and retain these needed materials, and her weight will zoom back to within two pounds of where she started.

CAUTION:

Beware of those who promote quick-weight-loss schemes. Learn to distinguish between loss of *fat* and loss of *weight*.

The Protein-Sparing Fast   A variant on fasting is the technique of feeding the patient only protein. The hope is that the protein will spare lean tissue and that the patient will break down his own body fat at a maximal rate to meet his other energy needs. You may suspect that this is not so different from the low-kcalorie diet and will guess that this protein—together with the body's lean tissues—will be used to provide glucose. You are probably right. The idea sounded good when it was first advanced, but it has met with mixed results. It seems effective only after considerable lean tissue has already been lost, at which time the body may be conserving itself quite efficiently anyway, and the fast has not been shown more effective than a mixture of protein and carbohydrate.[6] Furthermore, it doesn't seem to "stick" very well; most patients regain the lost weight.[7] Thus the protein-sparing fast has to be judged at best a very moderate success and at worst a failure, for the ultimate criterion of success in any weight-loss program is maintenance of the new low weight.

The idea of a protein-sparing fast originated with some responsible physicians who experimented carefully with it, using whole natural protein foods such as fish and lean beef. Unfortunately, the idea was then seized upon and began to be misused by the public with the publication of a popular book, *The Last Chance Diet*, in 1977.[8] Fad dieters, usually without any medical supervision, drank liquid protein potions prepared in questionable ways, and lost dramatic amounts of weight (including, of course, body lean tissue, water, and vital minerals). Within the year, 11 deaths had been ascribed to the fad and

Protein-sparing fast = eating only protein.

[6]T. B. Van Itallie and M. U. Yang, Current concepts in nutrition: Diet and weight loss, *New England Journal of Medicine* 297 (1977):1158-1161.

[7]Morbid obesity: Long-term results of therapeutic fasting, *Nutrition Reviews* 36 (January 1978):6-7.

[8]R. Linn and S. L. Stuart, *The Last Chance Diet* (New York: Bantam Books, 1977).

the FDA had issued a stringent warning about liquid protein preparations.[9] Since then, many more have died on the fast, due to sudden stopping of the heart caused probably by mineral losses.[10]

The term *protein-sparing* has also been used in another connection. Malnourished hospital patients also lose body protein, and this is especially likely—and especially dangerous—if they are simultaneously fighting infection. The knowledgeable physician makes every effort to prevent the loss of vital lean tissue and supplies amino acids as well as glucose in some form—through a vein if the patient can't eat. The effort to provide protein-sparing *therapy* in these circumstances has met with notable success and has significantly reduced the death and disease rate in cases of severe hospital malnutrition. These praiseworthy efforts should not be confused with the profiteering efforts of faddists to sell the protein-sparing *fast*.

Moderate Weight Loss The body's cells and the enzymes within them make it their task to convert the energy nutrients you eat into those you need. They are extraordinarily versatile and relieve you of having to compute exactly how much carbohydrate, fat, and protein to eat at each meal. As you have seen, they can convert either carbohydrate (glucose) or protein to fat. To some extent, they can convert protein to glucose. To a very limited extent, they can even convert fat (the glycerol portion) to glucose. But a grossly unbalanced diet or one that is severely limited in kcalories imposes hardships on the body. If kcalories are too low or if carbohydrate and protein kcalories are undersupplied, the body is forced to degrade its own lean tissue to meet its glucose need.

Someone who wants to lose body fat must reconcile himself to a hard fact: There is a limit to the rate at which this tissue will break down. The maximum rate, except for a very large person, is one to two pounds a week. To achieve this kind of weight loss, the sensible course is to adopt a balanced low-kcalorie diet supplying all three energy nutrients in reasonable amounts and possibly to increase energy expenditure by getting more exercise. In effect, this means adjusting the energy budget so that intake is 500 to 1,000 kcal per day less than output. A person who wants to gain weight needs to make the opposite adjustment. It might seem that both efforts would require tedious counting of kcalories, but the following sections show that shortcuts are possible.

[9]"These liquid protein diets are made from hydrolyzed (predigested) collagen or gelatin obtained from animal hides, tendons, and bones. . . . None is nutritionally complete. . . . Liquid protein diets are neither registered nor approved by FDA. FDA is responsible for the labeling of such products, but generally the labeling does not give directions for weight-loss regimens. Such claims are made in books, by word of mouth, or in the media, which are beyond FDA's control. FDA can take action, such as seeking recall or seizing the product, only if the product has become adulterated." Predigested protein drinks and "modified fasting" diets, *Journal of the American Dietetic Association* 71 (1977): 609.

[10]T. B. Van Itallie, Liquid protein mayhem, *Journal of the American Medical Association* 240 (1978): 144-146.

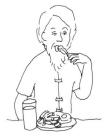

1 lb = 3,500 kcal A pound of body fat (adipose tissue) is actually composed of a mixture of fat, protein, and water and yields 3,500 kcal on oxidation. A pound of pure fat (454 g) would yield 4,086 kcal (at 9 kcal per gram).

The Energy in Food: kCalorie Intake

A bomb calorimeter is a device for measuring food energy by the heat given off when food is burned. The number of potential kcalories can be determined in a portion of any food. Researchers have found that the values produced by this method are higher than the number of kcalories the same food would give to an animal. This apparent discrepancy is explained by the fact that not all the food is metabolized by an animal all the way to carbon dioxide, as it is in a bomb calorimeter. Adjustments of bomb calorimeter values have resulted in tables showing the kcalorie content of foods and the values for kcalories in carbohydrate, protein, fat, and alcohol. If you want to balance your energy budget, you can rely on the kcalorie values given in Appendix H for the highest degree of accuracy available.

But looking up every food in kcalorie charts is boring and inconvenient, and only the most motivated will persist at it for a prolonged period of time. For the rest of us who may want to keep track of kcalories, some acquaintance with groups of foods, such as those described at the end of Chapter 1, provides a simpler method. The foods depicted below here could be found one by one in Appendix H, but it's quicker to translate them into exchanges and add up the kcalorie values to get a rough idea of the number. With some practice, you can look at any plate of food and "sense" the number of kcalories it represents. Some kcalorie amounts to remember are:

1 c skim milk (a milk exchange) (for whole milk, add 2 fat exchanges)	80 kcal
1 serving vegetable (a vegetable exchange)	25 kcal
1 serving fruit (a fruit exchange)	40 kcal
1 slice bread (a bread exchange)	70 kcal
1 oz lean meat (a meat exchange) (for medium-fat meat, add 1/2 fat exchange; for high-fat meat, add 1 fat exchange)	55 kcal
1 tsp fat or oil (a fat exchange)	45 kcal

In case you'd like to try guessing how many kcalories are in the meal depicted below, the answer is provided at the bottom of the next page.

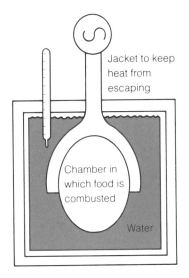

Bomb calorimeter.

When an organic substance such as food is burned, the energy in the chemical bonds that held its carbons and hydrogens together is released in the form of heat. The amount of heat that is released can be measured; this direct measure of the amount of energy that was stored in the chemical bonds in the food is termed **direct calorimetry.**

As the chemical bonds in food are broken, the carbons (C) and hydrogens (H) combine with oxygen (O) to form carbon dioxide (CO_2) and water (H_2O). Measuring the amount of oxygen consumed in the process gives an indirect measure of the amount of energy released, termed **indirect calorimetry.**

calorimetry (cal-o-RIM-uh-tree): the measurement of energy.

  calor = heat
  metron = measure

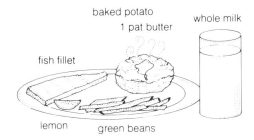

baked potato
1 pat butter
whole milk
fish fillet
lemon   green beans

The Body's Energy Needs: kCalorie Output

Counting the kcalories in your food tells you your energy income, but to balance your budget you also need to know your expenditure. How can you count the kcalories you expend in a day?

Government Recommendations   Government authorities such as the U.S. Committee on RDA and the Canadian Ministry of Health and Welfare have published recommended energy intakes for various age-sex groups in their populations. These are useful for population studies, but the range of energy needs for any one group is so broad that it would be impossible to guess an individual's needs without knowing more about his lifestyle. The U.S. recommendations shown in the accompanying material on pages 219-220 make this obvious: a 20-year-old woman, for example, may need about 2,100 kcal per day—if she is 5 feet 4 inches tall, if she weighs about 120 pounds, and if she typically engages in light activity. But very few 20-year-old women fit this description exactly.

We figure about 530 kcal for the meal below:

1 c milk (milk exchange plus 2 fat exchanges)	170 kcal
1/2 c beans (vegetable exchange)	25 kcal
1 small potato (bread exchange)	70 kcal
1 pat butter (fat exchange)	45 kcal
4 oz fish (4 lean-meat exchanges, assuming no fat is added)	220 kcal
1 lemon wedge	0 kcal
	530 kcal

Appendix H values yield a total of about 500 kcalories, lower because these foods are low-kcalorie choices within the exchange groups. Any answer within about 50 to 100 kcalories of this is a good estimate.

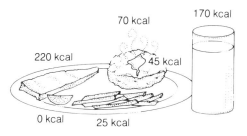

The Energy RDA for Adults (kcal)

Table 1. Recommended Daily Energy Intakes for Adults (kcal)

Age	Men	Women
19-22	2,900 (2,500-3,300)	2,100 (1,700-2,500)
23-50	2,700 (2,300-3,100)	2,000 (1,600-2,400)
51-75	2,400 (2,000-2,800)	1,800 (1,400-2,200)
76+	2,050 (1,650-2,450)	1,600 (1,200-2,000)

The recommendations in Table 1 are useful for population studies, but they are made for the "average person"—and no one, of course, is exactly average. The man used as a reference figure is 5 feet 10 inches tall and weighs 154 pounds (178 centimeters, 70 kilograms). The woman is 5 feet 4 inches tall and weighs 120 pounds (163 centimeters, 55 kilograms). Both engage in light activity: They sleep or lie down for eight hours a day, sit for seven hours, stand for five, walk for two, and spend two hours a day in light physical activity.

Very few people fit these descriptions exactly, although most fall close to the mean. The total span of needs is broad: For adults, it is believed that an 800-kcal range covers most individuals, but some are no doubt excluded at both the lower and upper ends of the range.

In setting the RDA for *protein*, the authorities considered two important facts: First, that the protein needs of individuals vary over a wide range; second, that the consequences of a protein deficiency are severe but that those of an excess of protein are not. In deciding what amount of protein to recommend for an individual of a given age-sex group, the Committee on RDA chose to set the recommendation rather high, so that it would cover the majority of the population. For an average person, whose protein needs fall near the mean, the RDA provides half again as much protein in a day as actually needed. For a vital nutrient such as protein, this recommendation makes sense, and it will do no harm to consume somewhat more than the actual need. kCalories, on the other hand, are harmful in excess, because they lead to obesity; a deficit (within reason) is not harmful.

Like protein needs, the energy needs of individuals vary, with most people needing some amount of energy near the middle of the range. In setting the RDA for energy, the Committee on RDA elected to draw the line right at the mean. This ensured (if all members of our population were to consume exactly the recommended intake) that half would be consuming somewhat less than they actually needed as individuals, and that half would be consuming somewhat more.

The nutrient RDAs are set so that only a few people's requirements will not be met by them. The energy RDAs are set so that half of the population's requirements will fall below and half above them.

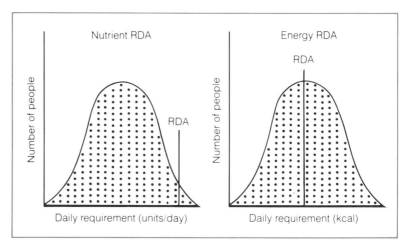

This choice minimizes the risk of encouraging excessive obesity or excessive thinness.

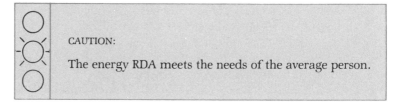

CAUTION:

The energy RDA meets the needs of the average person.

The Committee on RDA has made no recommendation for daily consumption of the energy nutrients (carbohydrate or fat)—only for total energy and protein. To understand the reason for this, recall that all three energy nutrients contribute kcalories, protein being unique among them because it also contributes nitrogen. You must therefore meet the RDA for protein to obtain the nitrogen you need. When you have consumed that amount of protein, you will have simultaneously consumed a certain number of kcalories. The remaining kcalories you need can come from carbohydrate and fat. It is left to you to choose how to balance these two nutrients in meeting your energy allowance.

The complete tables of heights and weights and recommended energy intakes for all age-sex groups are shown in Appendix O. The Canadian and FAO/WHO recommendations are also in Appendix O.

Diet Record Method   For an individualized estimate of your energy needs, the best indicator is the stability of your body weight over a period of time in which your activities are typical of your lifestyle. If you keep a strictly accurate record of all the food and beverages you consume for a week or two and if your weight does not change during that time, you can assume that your energy budget is balanced: kCalories-in equal kcalories-out. Records have to be kept for at least a week, however, because intakes fluctuate from day to day. (On about half the days you eat less, on the other half more kcalories than the average.) If during the week you gain a pound, you can assume that you expended 3,500 kcal less than you consumed, or an average of 500 kcal per day for seven days.

Laboratory Methods   Energy expenditures can also be accurately measured using laboratory equipment designed for this purpose. Two principles underlie the design of such machines. First, because heat is always a byproduct of energy expenditure, a device that measures escaping heat gives a direct measure of the kcalories being spent. Early efforts to accomplish this involved putting a person inside a large insulated, tightly sealed room with water circulating about it. The rise in the water's temperature indicated the number of kcalories being generated by the person's body. Inside the room, the person could be at rest or engaged in an activity such as studying or bicycle riding.

This clumsy and expensive method was replaced by a portable and much less expensive machine using the principle that the amount of oxygen consumed and carbon dioxide expelled is in direct proportion to the heat released. If twice as much heat is generated in one instance as in another, then twice as much oxygen will also be used. This advance made it possible to measure the kcalories expended during a wider range of physical activities. Laboratory studies of energy output by humans have been so extensive that tables are now available giving averages from which most people can estimate their own needs quite accurately. (An example appears in the Self-Study on Energy Output that follows Highlight 7B).

Estimating from Basal Metabolism and Activities   Human energy is spent in two major ways—on the basal metabolic processes and on voluntary activities. In order to calculate how much energy you spend in a day, you must obtain an estimate for the energy spent in each of these categories. A third way of spending energy, much smaller but still significant, is on digesting, absorbing, and metabolizing food. Let's take these up one by one.

● *Energy for basal metabolism.* Certain processes necessary for the maintenance of life proceed without your conscious awareness. The beating of the heart, the inhaling of oxygen and the exhaling of carbon dioxide, the ongoing metabolic activities of each cell, the maintenance of body temperature, and the sending of nerve impulses from the brain to direct these automatic activities are the basal metabolic processes that maintain life. Their minimum energy needs must be met before any kcalories can be used for physical activity or for the digestion of food.

The basal metabolic rate (BMR) is the rate at which kcalories are

basal metabolism: the total energy output of a body at rest after a 12-hour fast. Also called **basal metabolic rate** or **BMR.**

Shortcut for Estimating Energy Output

1. *Basal metabolism (BMR).* To get a rough approximation of the energy spent on BMR, use the factor 1.0 kcal per kilogram per hour (for men) or 0.9 kcal per kilogram per hour (for women). Example: for a 150-pound woman,

a. Change pounds to kilograms:

$$150 \, \text{lb} \times \frac{1 \, \text{kg}}{2.2 \, \text{lb}} = 68 \, \text{kg}$$

b. Multiply weight in kilograms by the BMR factor for women:

$$68 \, \text{kg} \times \frac{0.9 \, \text{kcal}}{\text{kg per hr}}$$
$$= 61 \, \text{kcal per hr}$$

c. Multiply the kcalories used in one hour by the hours in a day:

$$61 \, \text{kcal per hr} \times \frac{24 \, \text{hr}}{1 \, \text{day}}$$
$$= 1,464 \, \text{kcal per day for BMR}$$

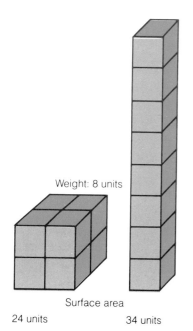

Weight: 8 units

Surface area

24 units   34 units

Both weigh the same, but the tall, thin structure will lose more heat to its surroundings.

spent for these maintenance activities, usually expressed as kcal per hour. The BMR varies from one person to another and may vary for one individual with a change in circumstance, physical condition, or age. The BMR is lowest when you are lying down in a room with a comfortable temperature and not digesting or metabolizing any food. In this relaxed state, few digestive juices are flowing, intestinal muscles are quiet, and other body muscles are just tense enough to keep them in good tone. At this time you need the least amount of oxygen and your cells are generating the least amount of heat. During sleep, you are probably more relaxed, but there is more muscular activity. That's why the basal metabolic rate is usually measured when the person is awake and can cooperate. She must be comfortable and relaxed and must have been without food or heavy exercise for at least 12 hours.

The BMR is surprisingly large. A woman whose total energy needs are 2,000 kcal a day may spend more than half of these, as much as 1,200 to 1,400 kcal, maintaining her basal metabolic processes. People often do not realize that so much of their energy is going to support the basic work of their bodies' cells, because they are unaware of all the work these cells do to maintain life.

The BMR is influenced by a number of factors. In general, the younger a person is, the higher the basal metabolic rate. This seems to be due to the increased activity of cells undergoing division, because it is most pronounced during the growth spurts that take place in infancy, puberty, and pregnancy. After growth stops, the BMR decreases by about 2 percent per decade throughout life.[11]

Body surface area also influences the BMR. Research has shown that it is indeed surface area, not weight, that is crucial. The greater the amount of body surface area, the higher the BMR. Thus of two people with different shapes who weigh the same amount, the short fat person will have a slower BMR than the tall thin person. The tall thin person has a greater skin surface from which heat is lost by radiation and so must run her metabolism faster to generate heat to replace it.

A third factor that influences BMR is gender. Males generally have a faster metabolic rate than females. It is thought that this may be due to the greater percentage of lean tissue in the male body. Muscle tissue is highly active even when it is resting, whereas fat tissue is comparatively inactive.

Fever also increases the energy needs of cells. Their increased activities to fight off infection require more energy and generate more heat than normal.

Fasting and constant malnutrition lower the BMR, in part because of the loss of lean tissues as well as the shutdown of functions the body can't afford to support. This lowering of BMR seems to be a protective mechanism to conserve energy when there is a shortage.

[11]Food and Nutrition Board, Committee on Recommended Allowances, *Recommended Dietary Allowances*, 8th ed. (Washington, D. C.: National Academy of Sciences, 1974).

Some glandular secretions influence the BMR. The adrenal glands secrete the hormone epinephrine into the blood in response to stress. The stress may be caused by as simple a situation as the command "Hurry, or you'll be late to work" or by as threatening a dilemma as the discovery of an intruder in the house. Whatever the cause, the body reacts by marshaling all its forces to meet the emergency. The increase in epinephrine increases the energy demands of every cell and thus temporarily raises the BMR.

The activity of the thyroid gland has a direct influence on basal metabolic rate. The less thyroxin secreted, the lower the energy requirement for maintenance of basal functions. Some people move about their tasks in a slow, deliberate fashion, due in part to the lower activity of their thyroid glands. Others race through the day, breaking dishes and becoming irritable, due to thyroid oversecretion. The difference in the two personalities may reflect a difference in their basal metabolic rates.

Contrary to what you might expect, physical training seems not to influence BMR. It might seem logical that athletes, with their greatly developed muscle tissue, would have a higher BMR than nonathletes of the same sex. Heavy exercise like jogging does speed up the basal metabolic rate, and it remains raised for several hours afterwards. However, research has revealed only a negligible difference in BMR between athletes and nonathletes under conditions of the BMR test—that is, after 12 hours of rest, when epinephrine secretion has returned to normal.

To sum up, basal metabolic rate is higher in the young, in people with a large surface area, in males, in people with fever or under stress, and in people with high thyroid gland activity. It is lowered by increasing age, fasting, and malnutrition, and it is unaffected by physical conditioning.

- *Energy for muscular activity.* The second of the three components of energy output is physical activity voluntarily undertaken and achieved by use of the skeletal muscles. The amount of energy needed for an activity like playing tennis or studying for an exam depends on the involvement of the muscles, on the amount of weight being moved, and on the length of time the activity is engaged in.

As disheartening as it may be for you to discover, mental activity requires very little energy, although it may make you very tired. Contraction of muscles, on the other hand, uses up a great many kcalories. In addition to the muscles involved in moving the body, the heart must beat faster to send nutrients and oxygen to the muscles, and the lungs must move faster to get rid of the carbon dioxide and bring in additional oxygen. The heavier person obviously needs more kcalories when performing the same task in the same time as a lighter person, because it takes extra effort to move her additional body weight. The longer the activity continues, the more kcalories will be used. The measurement of energy needed for a particular

thyroxin (thigh-ROX-in): a hormone secreted by the thyroid gland; regulates the basal metabolic rate.

2. *Activities.* To estimate the energy spent on muscular activities, classify the person's lifestyle as either sedentary, lightly active, moderately active, or very active and add the appropriate percentage to the BMR. The figures below are crude approximations based on the amount of muscular work performed. To select the one appropriate for you, remember to think in terms of the amount of *muscular* work you perform; don't confuse being busy with being active.

- For sedentary (mostly sitting) activity (a typist), add 20 percent of the BMR.
- For light activity (a teacher), add 30 percent.
- For moderate activity (a nurse), add 40 percent.
- For heavy work (a roofer), add 50 percent.

If the woman we're using as an example were a typist, we would estimate the energy she needs for physical activities by multiplying the BMR kcalories per day by 20 percent:

1,464 kcal per day × .20
= 293 kcal per day for physical activities

Energy for metabolizing food is called the **specific dynamic effect** (SDE), the specific dynamic energy, or the specific dynamic activity (SDA).

3. *SDE.* Energy spent by the body to deal with the food it receives represents a "tax" of about 10 percent of the kcalories in that food. If our woman ate 2,000 kcal in a day, the SDE "tax" would amount to

2,000 kcal × .10 = 200 kcal per day for the effect of food

4. *Total energy spent.* Now add items 1, 2, and 3 to obtain an estimate of the total energy spent in a day:

1,464 kcal + 293 kcal + 200 kcal = 1,957 kcal total per day (ANS.)

[If we didn't know how much she ate, we could guess. Assuming that her energy budget was balanced, we could reason that she ate about enough to meet her needs for items 1 and 2, and we could take 10 percent of that total to derive item 3:

1,464 kcal (BMR) + 293 kcal (activities) = 1,757 kcal

1,757 kcal × .10 = 176 kcal per day for the effect of food (SDE)

1,464 + 293 + 176 = 1,933 kcal per day (ANS.)]

Thus this woman's total energy needs for a day might be about 1,925 to 1,975 kcal. The exact figure is based on several estimates, so it's probably best to express her needs as falling within a 50-kcal range.

physical activity, then, is expressed in three units: kcalories per weight per unit of time.

As people age, their activities taper off somewhat. This slowing down varies greatly from one person to the next but averages out in such a way that people's total energy needs (including BMR) probably decrease by about 5 percent per decade after the age of 20.

● *Energy for metabolizing food.* The third component of energy expenditure has to do with processing food. When food is taken into the body, many cells that have been dormant begin to be active. The muscles that move the food through the intestinal tract speed up their rhythmic contractions; the cells that manufacture and secrete digestive juices begin their tasks. All these cells and others need extra energy as they "come alive" to participate in the digestion, absorption, and metabolism of food. In addition, the presence of food stimulates the general metabolism. This stimulation is the specific dynamic effect (SDE) of food, or the specific dynamic activity (SDA), and is generally thought to represent about 6 to 10 percent of the total food energy taken in. Because food energy taken in normally equals energy expended, the SDE is usually calculated by taking 10 percent of the total kcalories used for BMR and physical activity.

Food faddists make a big thing out of the specific dynamic effect, suggesting that a high-protein diet stimulates such tremendous energy losses that it will increase the rate of weight loss. Actually, high-protein and low-protein diets have the same effect.[12]

Weight Loss and Gain Rates

A deficit of 500 kcal a day brings about loss of body fat at the rate of a pound a week; of 1,000 kcal, two pounds a week. Extraordinarily active people, by virtue of their activities, or extremely obese persons, by virtue of the metabolic demands made by the sheer bulk of their body cells, can lose more. For those who are only moderately obese, the maximum possible rate of fat loss is one to two pounds a week, which for most people means an intake of about 1,000 to 1,500 kcal a day. Below 1,200, the dieter will be losing lean tissue, and at this restricted kcalorie level, the diet planner is hard put to achieve adequacy for all the vitamins and minerals.

The principles outlined in this chapter are simple, but putting them into practice is more difficult than you might imagine. Obesity and underweight are complex problems with social and psychological ramifications, as well as the metabolic ones just described. Chapter 8 provides some practical pointers for the dieter but deals first with all the factors that contribute to the problems of underweight and obesity.

[12]R. L. Pike and M. L. Brown, *Nutrition: An Integrated Approach*, 2nd ed. (New York: Wiley, 1975), p. 835.

Summing Up

Figure 1 summarizes the central pathways of metabolism. The principal compounds derived from carbohydrate, fat, and protein in the diet are glucose, glycerol and fatty acids, and amino acids. Glucose may be anabolized to glycogen or catabolized to pyruvate, which in turn yields acetyl CoA. Glycerol and fatty acids may be anabolized to triglycerides or catabolized (glycerol to pyruvate, fatty acids to acetyl CoA). Amino acids may be anabolized to protein or catabolized (after deamination) to pyruvate, acetyl CoA, or TCA cycle intermediates.

Pyruvate is reconvertible to glucose, but the reaction yielding acetyl CoA from pyruvate is irreversible. Hence fatty acids cannot serve as a source of glucose in the body. All three energy nutrients are convertible to acetyl CoA, however, and hence can be used to manufacture body fat.

If a person fasts or if carbohydrate is undersupplied, lean body tissue is catabolized to meet the brain's need for glucose. Within a day or so ketosis sets in: Fatty acids are metabolized to ketones, which can meet some of the brain's energy need. The nitrogen removed from protein is combined with carbon and oxygen in urea and excreted. Below about 900 kcal a day, a diet imposes lean tissue loss and ketosis, and the protein kcalories in such a diet are equivalent to carbohydrate kcalories in their protein-sparing effect. Weight loss may be dramatic, but fat loss may be slower than on a moderate, balanced low-kcalorie diet. To design such a diet requires adjusting energy balance so that the intake is reduced, the output is increased, or both.

Energy intake can be computed by adding up the kcalorie values of the foods consumed or can be estimated by using the averaged exchange system values for many foods. The energy available from food was originally determined by measuring the heat lost when the food was completely burned. Before tables of the kcaloric values of foods were published, adjustments were made for the incomplete breakdown of food in the body.

Energy outputs for various age-sex groups are provided by recommendations such as the RDA, but lifestyle has to be taken into account when estimating an individual's energy needs. Machines designed to measure energy expenditure work by measuring heat lost from the body or oxygen used. Data collected in this way have yielded tables from which you can estimate your energy needs quite accurately.

The body's total energy output falls into three categories: energy to support the basal metabolism, energy for muscular activity, and energy to digest, absorb, and metabolize food (SDE, the specific dynamic effect of food). Basal metabolic activities are estimated to require about 1.0 kcalorie per kilogram of body weight per hour (0.9 for women). Muscular activity requires an additional 20 to 50 percent above the basal metabolism. The effect of food adds another 10 percent to the total energy expenditure.

The basal metabolic rate is influenced primarily by age and growth rate, body shape, and sex (males have a higher BMR). It is also affected by fever, fasting, and hormonal secretions (especially epinephrine and thyroxin) but not by body conditioning.

An energy deficit of 3,500 kcal is necessary for the loss of a pound of body fat. Loss of body fat in excess of two pounds a week can rarely be sustained. A diet supplying fewer than 1,200 kcal per day can be made adequate in vitamins and minerals only with great difficulty.

To Explore Further

What happens during fasting is clearly and completely explained in an article for the general reader:

● Young, V. R., and Scrimshaw, N. S. The physiology of starvation. *Scientific American* 225 (1971):14-21.

The Healthy Way to Weigh Less and *Critique of Low Carbohydrate Ketogenic Weight Reduction Regimens*, a pamphlet and a reprint, can be ordered from the American Medical Association (address in Appendix J).

HIGHLIGHT 7A

AN OPTIONAL CHAPTER
Extracting Energy from
Carbohydrate, Fat, and Protein

It is through this structure, in the process of metabolism, that matter and energy flow. Entering in various forms and quantities, they are temporarily shaped exactly to the form and condition of the organism; they conform to the characteristics of the kingdom, class, order, family, genus, species, and variety to which it belongs, and they assume even the characteristics of the individual itself. Then they depart through the various channels of excretion.

LAWRENCE J. HENDERSON

When you were a student in the elementary grades, your teacher probably taught you that you ate food because it gave you energy to run and play. That is one level of understanding metabolism. Later you enlarged your knowledge to include the fact that when you ate meat you were receiving the energy of the sun, which had fallen on green plants to make glucose that was consumed by the grazing animal. Today you can embellish this fact with many chemical and biological details.

You do not need a deeper level of understanding of metabolism than the preceding chapters have given to master the remaining concepts in this book; however, metabolism is such a fascinating subject that we want to make the next level available to you. This optional chapter provides no more than a glimpse at the wonders of metabolism as seen by scientists, but we warn you that it may encourage you to pursue the subject further.

Energy

One of the strangest notions that human beings who study the nature of things have ever come up with is the idea of energy. Energy has no concrete existence; it weighs nothing. And yet it can move mountains and make itself felt over great distances. Energy is apparent to us sometimes as light, at other times as heat; one seems to turn into the other. Energy has no mass, and yet it possesses a characteristic that

energy: the capacity to do work.

Forms of energy: heat, light, electrical, mechanical, chemical.

Sunlight provides the energy for life on earth. This photo, taken from an Apollo spacecraft, shows the Florida peninsula, with the Gulf of Mexico in the foreground.
Courtesy of NASA.

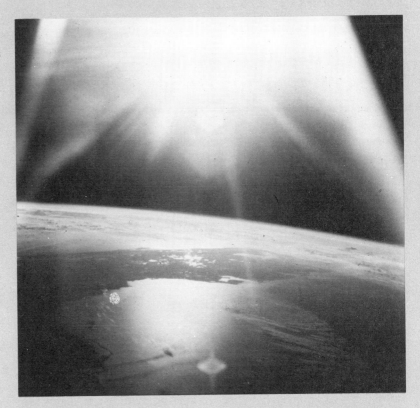

work: the moving of a mass through a distance.

First Law of Thermodynamics: Energy is neither created nor destroyed during chemical or physical processes, but it may be transformed from one form to another.

physicists call charge—and so it can do the work of electricity. Physicists have measured energy and have satisfied themselves that energy is never created or destroyed. Instead, as it is converted from one form to another, energy is conserved. Wherever there is motion there is energy, and yet energy may seem to stand still, like the energy stored in a boulder at the edge of a mountain precipice. Wherever there is the power to move things there is also energy—like the energy in the storage battery of your car. If you like to ponder the mysteries of the universe, one of the most wonderful (wonder-full) is that energy is real. It exists; it has been measured; it works.

The energy in food, or more properly in the nutrients of which food is composed, is found in what we have somewhat imprecisely called the bonds that hold the atoms of those nutrients together. The glucose molecule, with which you are by now thoroughly familiar, possesses 24 atoms held together by 23 such bonds, each composed of a pair of electrons. As glucose is taken apart during catabolism, some of the electron energy that constitutes those bonds becomes available to form bonds between other atoms. As a glucose molecule is broken down from a six-carbon compound to two three-carbon compounds, your system can capture the energy that held the two three-carbon chains together and use that energy to combine two other molecules. Let's call the two molecules B and C and the new, larger compound B-C. Later, by breaking B-C, you can retrieve the energy and use it to put together two amino acids and begin forming a protein. The proteins of hair, for example, are formed by the addition of amino acids to a chain in a process fueled by energy released in the breaking of bonds like those in glucose.

Only living systems can perform this remarkable feat of transferring the energy from the breaking of bonds (catabolism) in one molecule to the synthesis of bonds (anabolism) between two other molecules without a significant rise in temperature or a shift in the acidity of the environment. Breaking of molecules also occurs in dead organic systems, but when such a breakdown occurs (for example, when firewood burns), the released energy is not captured in a usable form but is converted to heat and light energy, which radiate away from the object. The process by which the body breaks down glucose is ultimately similar to that by which the glucose (cellulose) in firewood is broken down when it burns: Oxygen is consumed and energy is released (along with carbon dioxide and water). But unlike burning firewood, the body doesn't go up in flames. Instead, it retains most of the energy in the chemical bonds of body compounds and releases only a little as heat.

In some ways, the metabolism of the nutrients is analogous to the transformations that can be performed with Tinker Toys. The wheels are atoms, the sticks electrons. A toy jungle gym built with these pieces, like a nutrient molecule, can be taken apart, and the same wheels and sticks can be used to build a toy crane (analogously, a body structure like hair). There are two important differences, however: A dismantled Tinker Toy can lie around for days before the pieces are used to build another one, but in chemical reactions, the electrons never stay still. They either escape or immediately become associated with atoms, holding them together. So in the body, electron energy removed from glucose and other nutrients is immediately used to form bonds in other compounds.

The other difference is that the sticks may be used over and over again without losing their binding ability, but in chemical reactions a little energy is lost (as heat) in each transfer. The loss of energy from your metabolic system literally heats you up; your body is maintained at 98.6° F by the rate of the metabolic reactions it performs. This continual loss of heat energy from the body makes it necessary for people to refuel periodically—that is, to obtain a new energy supply from food to continue their metabolic work.

Second Law of Thermodynamics: The natural tendency of any physical system consisting of a large number of individual units is to go from a state of order to a state of disorder, thus decreasing the usable energy.

Where does this heat energy go? The total amount of energy in the universe remains constant; in that sense this energy is not lost. But it is lost to you: You can only use energy in forms—such as chemical bonds—that can do your metabolic or mechanical work. Pondering this question has brought physicists to the brink of metaphysics and philosophy, areas outside our province as nutritionists. References at the end of this Highlight will carry you further in these directions should you choose to follow them.

As you try to put together your own mental picture of what happens to energy during metabolism, you may anticipate that a molecule B and a molecule C are available somewhere nearby while nutrients are being broken down. These molecules can be put together whenever energy becomes available. This is indeed the way the system works. Molecules B and C are floating around in all your body cells; wherever energy is made available to put them together, the compound B-C is formed. The energy is captured between them. B and C are brought together on the surface of an enzyme-complex that takes apart some other molecule, releasing energy.

The enzymes that can perform this energy transfer are those that catalyze coupled reactions. An example will illustrate. Picture an enzyme-complex (a cluster of giant molecules whose surfaces are bristling with positive and negative charges) that has on its surface a place for splitting glucose and elsewhere on its surface a place where B and C can be put together. A molecule of glucose approaches this enzyme-complex and begins to split in half. For the coupled reaction to occur, B and C must also be present at the other site. As the glucose splits, the electron energy that bonded it together is transferred to the bond between B and C (losing only a little energy as heat). At no time can the energy that bonded the glucose be freed or lost altogether as heat or light.

Loading Energy into Carriers

It is a strange paradox that even though energy weighs nothing, it still must be carried. When it is being held in the cells of animals for future use, it is carried in a compound like adenosine triphosphate (ATP). ATP is the compound B-C we have been using in our example of coupled reactions. Molecule B is adenosine diphosphate (ADP, containing two phosphates) and molecule C is another phosphate. When a molecule of any of the energy nutrients gives up some of its energy, ADP and P use that energy to combine into ATP, which has three phosphates.

coupled reaction: a chemical event in which an enzyme-complex catalyzes two reactions simultaneously; often involves the breakdown of one compound to two and the synthesis of another from two.

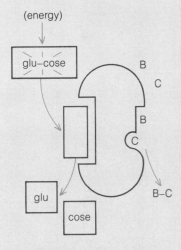

ATP or adenosine triphosphate (ad-DEN-o-sin try-FOS-fate): the commonest energy carrier in cells.

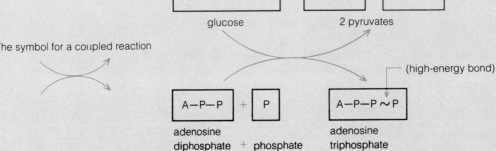

The symbol for a coupled reaction

(It is not important to learn the structures of these compounds. ADP is merely another molecule like others you are familiar with, composed of C, H, O, and N and containing two phosphorus—P—atoms derived from the mineral phosphorus in the diet. Free phosphate, also derived from dietary phosphorus, abounds in cells too.)

Not all bonds in the nutrients possess enough energy to bind phosphate to ADP; there are high-energy bonds and low-energy bonds. Hence not every reaction in which a large molecule is broken down yields energy that can be captured in this way; many yield heat only. Then, too, some high-energy bonds cannot be used in the body because humans do not possess the necessary enzymes to make the transfer. This is why protein, fat, and carbohydrate (and alcohol) are the only molecules that serve as energy nutrients: During their breakdown your body cells can extract the energy from them in a usable form—high-energy compounds like ATP.

The metabolism of alcohol is described in Highlight 9.

There are billions and billions of molecules of ATP in your cells. When you use or spend this energy, the above reaction is reversed. ATP breaks down to ADP and P in a coupled reaction, using the energy to power the chemical work of the cell—whether that is the building of a protein or the contraction of a muscle. (The symbol for a coupled reaction is two arrows that first converge and then diverge, as illustrated in the margin.)

The reversible reaction between ADP + P and ATP provides an energy-carrying system that is universal in animal organisms. Any other two molecules could be used in theory, and some are to a limited extent; the only requirement is that a high-energy bond be formed when they are put together. As it happens, animals have evolved to use the ATP system as a most convenient way of carrying and exchanging energy between molecules in their cells.

Other energy carriers in animal systems:

Guanosine (GWON-o-sine) diphosphate (GDP) + phosphate (P) → guanosine triphosphate (GTP) (used in protein synthesis).

Creatine (CREE-uh-tin) + P → creatine phosphate (used in muscle contraction).

Generating ATP: A Closer Look

Throughout this book we refer to glucose as a six-carbon compound that breaks apart into two molecules of pyruvate, yielding energy. This is true but not true enough for you who are studying this optional chapter. If you are to understand how the energy in nutrients is parceled out into ATPs, we must fill in the missing details. What happens between the time a molecule of glucose arrives in the cell and the time it is converted to pyruvate and then to acetyl CoA?

The conversion of a molecule of glucose to carbon dioxide and water yields a great deal of energy—far more than could be picked up by ADP all at once. Therefore, the release of this energy is accomplished by many small steps. This conversion takes place in two sets of reactions. The first of these, leading from glucose to pyruvate, is anaerobic (without oxygen) and is called glycolysis. The next set, leading from acetyl CoA to carbon dioxide, is aerobic (with oxygen) and involves the tricarboxylic acid (TCA) cycle.

anaerobic: taking place in the absence of oxygen.

an = without
aero = air (oxygen)

glycolysis (gligh-KOLL-ih-sis): the breakdown of glucose to pyruvate; an anaerobic process.

aerobic: taking place in the presence of oxygen.

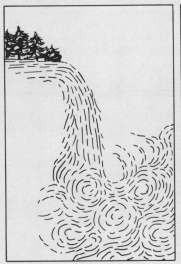

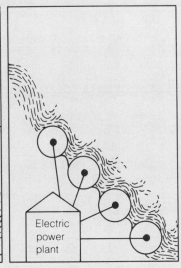

Energy of falling water too great to capture

Energy of falling water captured by a series of water wheels

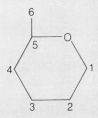

This is the way chemists number the carbons in a glucose molecule

NAD⁺: an organic ion. For a discussion of ions, see Appendix B. NAD^+ is further defined as a coenzyme in Chapter 9.

Glycolysis Glucose must be given some activation energy before it can proceed toward the release of its own energy, just as a log must be given some heat from twigs and paper before it will burn spontaneously. This activation of glucose is accomplished in a coupled reaction with ATP.

In the process of activation, a phosphate is attached to the carbon that chemists call number 6. The product is called, logically enough, glucose-6-phosphate. In the next step, glucose-6-phosphate is rearranged by an enzyme, and a phosphate is added in another coupled reaction with ATP. The product this time is fructose-1,6-diphosphate. At this point the six-carbon sugar has been activated. It has a phosphate group on its first and sixth carbons and enough energy to break apart. Two ATPs have been used to accomplish this.

(From this point to the production of pyruvate we will use letters in place of compound names. The names are in the drawing of the reactions on the next page, for those who wish to know them.)

When fructose-1,6-diphosphate breaks in half, the two three-carbon compounds (A and A′) are not identical. Each has a phosphate group attached, but only one converts directly to pyruvate. The other compound converts easily to the first. (Compound A′ is usually ignored, except for its role as the point of entry for glycerol; we say that two molecules of compound A are derived from one glucose.)

In the step from compound A to compound B, enough energy is released to convert NAD^+ to $NADH + H^+$. Also, in the steps from B to C and from E to pyruvate, ATP is regenerated. Remember that there are effectively two molecules of compound A coming from glucose;

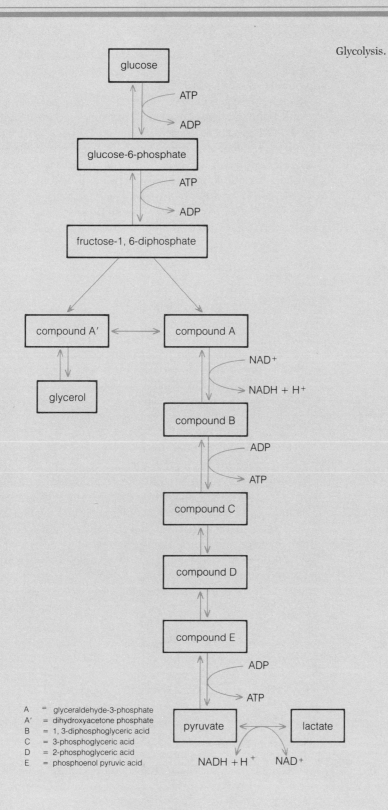

Glycolysis.

therefore, four ATP molecules are generated. Two ATPs were needed to get the sequence started, so the net gain at this point is two ATPs and two molecules of NADH + H$^+$.

So far, no oxygen has been used; the process has been anaerobic. But at this point, oxygen is needed. If oxygen is not immediately available, pyruvate converts to lactic acid, to soak up the hydrogens from the NADH + H$^+$ that was generated. Lactic acid accumulates until oxygen becomes available. However, in the energy path from glucose to carbon dioxide, this side step usually is not necessary. As you will see later, each NADH + H$^+$ moves to the electron transport chain to unload its hydrogens onto oxygen. The associated energy produces 2 ATPs, making the total yield 8 ATPs for the process from glucose to pyruvate.

The body's disposal of lactic acid is of great interest to the athlete who knows that its accumulation in his muscles will cause fatigue. The muscle cells draw their energy in the first burst of activity from the available high-energy compounds (similar to ATP) but soon exhaust this source. To replenish it, they then start breaking down their stored glycogen. So far, so good, but if the exertion is very severe, the heart cannot pump oxygen to them fast enough to permit aerobic metabolism to proceed at full speed. So lactic acid accumulates. At the end of the activity, the oxygen debt is repaid, and lactic acid is shunted back into the main stream of metabolism by being reconverted to pyruvate.

The muscles would be completely debilitated by the accumulation of lactic acid after a while, because they can't dispose of it. But they do have an alternative: They can release it into the bloodstream, and the liver can pick it up and reconvert it to glucose. To be well prepared for an endurance event, the athlete takes two steps based on these facts: He ensures that his muscles are well supplied with glycogen at the start (see page 20), and he warms up so that the cycling of lactate to the liver will already be underway when he enters the competition.

The Tricarboxylic Acid Cycle (TCA Cycle)   The TCA cycle is the name given to the set of reactions involving oxygen and leading from acetyl CoA to carbon dioxide (and water). To link glycolysis to the TCA cycle, pyruvate is converted to acetyl CoA. This set of aerobic reactions is not restricted to the metabolism of carbohydrate. It also includes fat and protein, as shown in the diagram that follows. Any substance that can be converted to acetyl CoA directly, or indirectly through pyruvate, may enter the cycle.

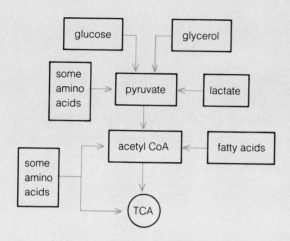

The step from pyruvate to acetyl CoA is an exceedingly complex one. We have included only those substances that will help you understand the transfer of energy from the nutrients. When pyruvate is in the presence of oxygen, it loses a carbon in the form of carbon dioxide, and CoA is attached. In the process NAD^+ picks up two hydrogens with their associated energy, becoming $NADH + H^+$.

As the acetyl CoA breaks down to carbon dioxide and water, its energy is captured in ATP. Let's follow the steps by which this occurs (see Figure 1):

1. Acetyl CoA combines with a four-carbon compound, oxaloacetate. The CoA comes off, and the product is a six-carbon compound, citrate.

2. The atoms of citrate are rearranged to form isocitrate.

3. Now NAD^+ reacts with isocitrate. Two Hs and two electrons are removed from the isocitrate. One H becomes attached to the NAD^+ with the two electrons; the other H is released as a free proton. Thus NAD^+ becomes $NADH + H^+$.

> Remember this $NADH + H^+$. It is carrying the Hs and the energy from the last reaction. But let's follow the carbons first.

A carbon is removed and combined with oxygen, forming carbon dioxide (which diffuses away in the blood and is exhaled). What is left is the five-carbon compound alpha-ketoglutarate.

4. Now two compounds interact with alpha-ketoglutarate—a molecule of CoA and a molecule of NAD^+. In this complex reaction a carbon is removed and combined with oxygen (forming carbon dioxide); two Hs are removed and go to NAD^+ (forming $NADH + H^+$); and the CoA is attached to the remaining four-carbon compound, forming succinyl CoA.

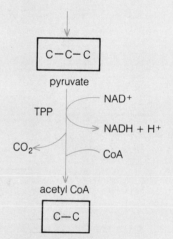

(TPP is a helper compound containing the B vitamin thiamin; see Chapter 9.)

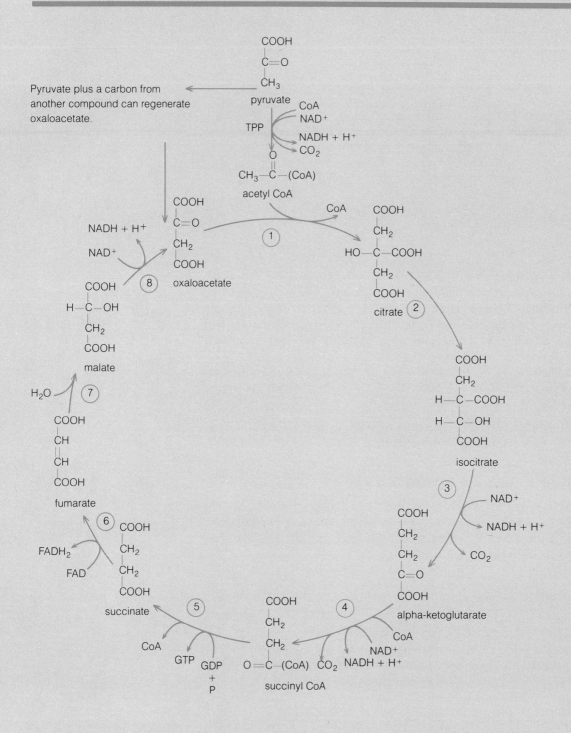

Figure 1 The TCA cycle.

> Remember this NADH + H$^+$ also.
> You will see later what happens to it.

5. Now two molecules react with succinyl CoA—a molecule called GDP and one of phosphate (P). The CoA comes off, the GDP and P combine to form the high-energy compound GTP, and succinate remains.

> Remember this GTP.

6. In the next reaction two Hs with their energy are removed from succinate and are transferred to a molecule called FAD (an electron-hydrogen receiver like NAD$^+$) to form FADH$_2$. The product that remains is fumarate.

> Remember this FADH$_2$.

7. Next a molecule of water is added to fumarate, forming malate.

8. A molecule of NAD$^+$ reacts with the malate; two Hs with their associated energy are removed from the malate and form NADH + H$^+$. The product that remains is the four-carbon compound oxaloacetate.

> Remember this NADH + H$^+$.

We are back where we started. The oxaloacetate formed in this process can combine with another molecule of acetyl CoA (step 1), and the cycle can begin again. (The whole scheme is shown in Figure 1.)

So far, what you have seen is that two carbons are brought in with acetyl CoA and that two carbons end up in carbon dioxide. But where is the energy and the ATP we promised you?

Each time a pair of hydrogen atoms is removed from one of the compounds in the cycle, it carries a pair of electrons with it. This chemical bond energy is thus captured into the compound to which the Hs become attached. A review of the eight steps of the cycle shows that energy is thus transferred into other compounds in steps 3, 4, 6, and 8. In step 5, energy is harnessed to bind GDP and P together to form GTP. Thus the compounds NADH + H$^+$ (three molecules), FADH$_2$, and GTP are built with energy originally found in acetyl CoA. To see how this energy ends up in ATP, we must follow the electrons further. Let us take those attached to NAD$^+$ as an example.

The six reactions described here are those of the **electron transport chain.** Since oxygen is required for these reactions and ADP and P are combined to form ATP in several of them (ADP is phosphorylated), they are also called **oxidative phosphorylation.**

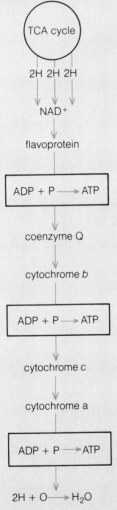

Electron transport. The electrons associated with the Hs move from compound to compound.

The Electron Transport Chain An important concept to remember at this point is that an electron is not a fixed amount of energy. The electrons that bond the H to NAD$^+$ in NADH have a relatively large amount of energy. In the series of reactions that follow, they lose this energy in small amounts, until at the end they are attached (with Hs) to oxygen (O) to make water (H_2O). In some of the steps, the energy they lose is captured into ATP in coupled reactions.

In the first step of the electron transport chain, NADH reacts with a molecule called a flavoprotein, losing its electrons (and their Hs). The products are NAD$^+$ and reduced flavoprotein. A little energy is lost as heat in this reaction.

The flavoprotein passes on the electrons to a molecule called coenzyme Q. Again they lose some energy as heat, but ADP and P participate in this reaction and gain much of the energy to bond together and form ATP. This is a coupled reaction.

$$ADP + P \rightarrow ATP$$

Coenzyme Q passes the electrons to cytochrome b. Again the electrons lose energy.

Cytochrome b passes the electrons to cytochrome c in a coupled reaction in which ATP is formed.

$$ADP + P \rightarrow ATP$$

Cytochrome c passes the electrons to cytochrome a.

Cytochrome a passes them (with their Hs) to an atom of oxygen (O), forming water (H_2O). This is a coupled reaction in which ATP is formed.

$$ADP + P \rightarrow ATP$$

The entire electron transport chain is diagrammed in Figure 2. As you can see, each time NADH is oxidized (loses its electrons) by this means, the energy it loses is parceled out into three ATP molecules. When the electrons are passed on to water at the end, they have much less energy than they had to begin with. This completes the story of the electrons from NADH.

As for FADH$_2$, its electrons enter the electron transport chain at coenzyme Q. From coenzyme Q to water there are only two steps in which ATP is generated. Therefore, FADH$_2$ coming out of the TCA cycle yields just two ATP molecules.

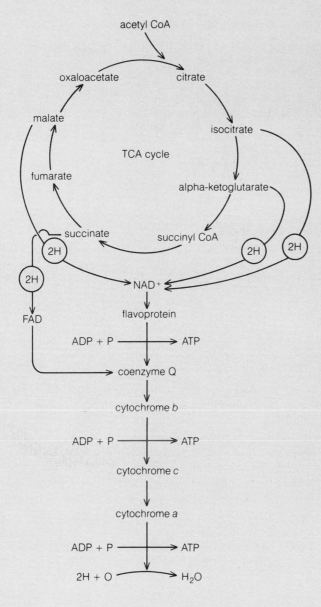

Figure 2 The electron transport chain.

One energy-receiving compound of the TCA cycle (GTP) does not enter the electron transport chain but gives its energy directly to ADP in a simple phosphorylation reaction.

You are now ready to look at the balance sheet of glucose metabolism (see table on p. 240). Glycolysis has yielded 4 NADH + H$^+$ and 4 ATP molecules and has spent 2 ATP. The 2 acetyl CoAs going through the TCA cycle have yielded 6 NADH + H$^+$, 2 FADH$_2$, and 2 GTP molecules. After the NADH + H$^+$ and FADH$_2$ have gone through the electron transport chain, there are 34 ATP. Added to these are the 4 ATP from

Table 1. Balance Sheet for Glucose Metabolism

	Expenditures	Income
Glycolysis:		
1 glucose	2 ATP	4 ATP
1 fructose-1,6-diphosphate		2 NADH + H$^+$
2 pyruvate		2 NADH + H$^+$
TCA cycle:		
2 isocitrate		2 NADH + H$^+$
2 alpha-ketoglutarate		2 NADH + H$^+$
2 succinyl CoA		2 GTP
2 succinate		2 FADH$_2$
2 malate		2 NADH + H$^+$
Total ATPs collected:		
From glycolysis	2 ATP	4 ATP
From 10 NADH + H$^+$		30 ATP
From 2 GTP		2 ATP
From 2 FADH$_2$		4 ATP
Totals:	2 ATP	40 ATP
Balance on hand from 1 molecule glucose:		38 ATP

glycolysis and the 2 ATP from GTP, making the total 40 ATP generated from one molecule of glucose. After the expense of 2 ATP is subtracted, there is a net gain of 38 ATP.

The TCA cycle and the electron transport chain are the body's major means of capturing the energy from nutrients in ATP molecules. There are other means that contribute (glycolysis is one), but these are the most efficient. Biologists and chemists understand much more about these processes than has been presented here. To Explore Further at the end of this Highlight suggests some readings that were selected for the clarity with which they present further details. Some considerations relating to the release of energy from ATP will complete this overview of the way in which energy from food does the body's work.

Unloading Energy from Carriers

Okay—so now you are full of energy. You have just eaten a meal and catabolized the carbohydrate, fat, and protein in it, making billions of molecules of ATP. What do you do with it? Fortunately, you don't have to make all of these decisions consciously. About two-thirds of your energy is spent automatically to maintain your vital functions, using a priority system that guarantees that the most important work is done first. The other third you are free to spend as you wish—contemplating the mysteries of nature, playing tennis, or doing whatever else you choose to do.

Two major classes of activities consume human energy each day. The first are the basal metabolic processes, which go on all the time, even during sleep. These are vital processes: the maintenance of the heartbeat, respiration, nerve function, glandular activity, generation of heat, and the like, without which you could not be said to be alive. The second are the voluntary activities, over which you have conscious control: sitting, standing, running, eating, playing the piano, and the like. The amount of energy spent on each of these types of activity can be measured, and their total (plus a little energy needed to metabolize food) represents the total amount of energy you must consume each day to stay in balance. These measurements and the concept of energy balance were the subjects of Chapter 7. But it seems worthwhile to give a few examples here of the way the energy taken from nutrients and transferred into ATP is used to power these activities.

Basal metabolism is defined and discussed further in Chapter 7.

• *ATP provides energy for catabolism.* A most vital need is to ensure that you have a continuous influx of energy to replace the energy you spend. At certain points during the catabolism of carbohydrate, fat, and protein, energy is needed to power a reaction that otherwise would not occur. At each of these points, a molecule of ATP is split into ADP + P to push the reaction.

You can see that catabolism is not a cost-free process. Energy (ATP) must be spent at certain points to keep catabolism going. However, the amount of ATP generated during catabolism is greater than the amount consumed, so that in the end there is a net gain. The catabolism of acetyl CoA is the most efficient energy-yielding process in the body, estimated to capture about 66 percent of the total initial energy.

• *ATP provides energy for anabolism.* As already mentioned, anabolic processes require ATP. To make a protein chain, one ATP is split for each amino acid added to the chain; to make glycogen, one ATP provides the energy to add each glucose; to make fatty acids from acetyl CoA, ATP is needed at the rate of one for each acetate added; and so on. To keep the body's metabolic work going on, energy must continuously be supplied.

• *ATP provides energy for muscle movements.* A muscle cell is packed with an orderly array of long, thin protein molecules lined up side by side. To contract a muscle, molecule A and molecule B must combine chemically, moving closer together as they do so. They must then execute another chemical reaction that slides them even closer together. The reactions that make muscles move are powered by energy carriers similar to ATP. For peristalsis, for the beating of the heart muscle, for the inhalation of air into the lungs, and for many other automatic muscular actions, these reactions do the necessary work.

• *ATP provides energy for the transmission of nerve impulses.* Even during sleep, the brain and nerves are active. At the molecular level,

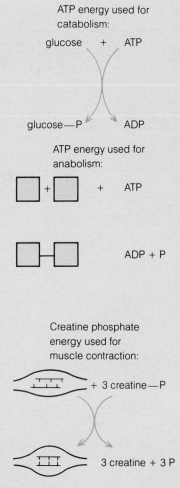

ATP energy used for catabolism:

glucose   +   ATP

glucose—P   ADP

ATP energy used for anabolism:

☐ + ☐   +   ATP

☐—☐   ADP + P

Creatine phosphate energy used for muscle contraction:

+ 3 creatine—P

3 creatine + 3 P

Lipid in muscle. The lipid droplets are stored close to the muscle fiber (bottom), and the mitochondria, which generate energy from fatty acids, crowd around these droplets. This was photographed under an electron microscope at a magnification of 47,000X.

From D. W. Fawcett, *An Atlas of Fine Structure*, (Philadelphia: Saunders, 1966), Fig. 60. Courtesy of the author and publisher.

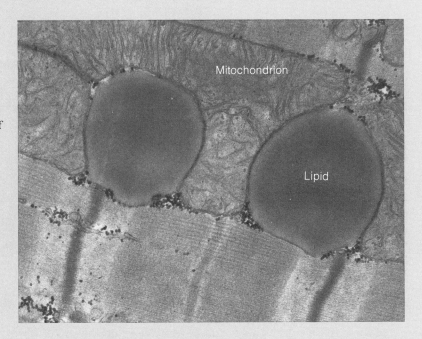

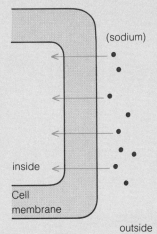

During the transmission of a nerve impulse, sodium rushes into the cell, depolarizing it. (Potassium rushes out: not shown.)

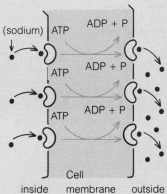

ATP energy is then used to repolarize the cell membrane.

the membranes of the nerve cells, which contain protein pumps, maintain an electrical charge by pumping sodium ions out and potassium ions in. When a nerve impulse travels along these cells, they depolarize: Sodium rushes in and potassium out. To regain the readiness to fire, the membrane pumps go to work to repolarize the cell, sorting out the potassium and sodium ions again. Each protein pump splits one molecule of ATP each time it transfers an ion across the membrane.

These few examples show the uses of ATP-carried energy for basal metabolic activities. If you wish to use additional energy to compose a poem, knit a sweater, or jog a mile, additional ATP must be available for the extra nervous and muscular activities that are involved.

Completing the Picture

This Highlight concludes one of nutrition's major stories: how the four principal types of atoms found in food and the energy that bonds them flow into the body, undergo rearrangements there, and ultimately flow out again. It may be satisfying to you to realize that you can now follow any of these atoms, or the energy connecting them, through the complete cycle around which they flow. Just for fun, let's imagine painting a carbon atom red and watching it travel through its cycle. Let's begin at the point where the carbon atom forms part of a molecule of carbon dioxide in the air.

This particular molecule of carbon dioxide enters a potato leaf. There, sparked by a photon from the sun, it is combined with water to become part of a molecule of glucose. This glucose then travels to the root, where it is attached to other glucose molecules to make starch. The starch is stored in the potato until you eat it. After you have swallowed it, the red carbon atom appears in your intestine, where the starch is hydrolyzed to glucose again; the glucose enters your bloodstream and is carried to a cell. Inside the cell, the glucose is broken down into two three-carbon compounds, and the red carbon atom finds itself in one of them.

Let's suppose that the three-carbon compound loses a carbon to carbon dioxide, leaving the red one in acetyl CoA. The acetyl CoA may be used to synthesize body fat, in which case the red carbon atom will be trapped in a fat cell for a while, or it may be used to synthesize an amino acid and become part of a protein such as hemoglobin and as such travel in a red blood cell throughout the circulatory system.

Now let's suppose that the body's primary need is for energy and that the acetyl CoA is further broken down to two molecules of carbon dioxide and water. Released in one of these carbon dioxide molecules, the red carbon atom finds its way back into the blood. Ultimately it is freed into air spaces in the lungs and breathed back into the atmosphere.

Around again the red carbon atom goes, possibly cycling back through another potato plant and into you again. But it is far more likely that it will go elsewhere next time—into an acorn on an oak tree, perhaps, and later into a chipmunk's cheek. And around again.

It may prove satisfying to you to follow the path of a hydrogen atom or an oxygen atom in the same way. There is also a nitrogen cycle, although the complete outlines are not apparent from the discussions of nitrogen that have been presented here. But let us take one more example of one of nature's shifting scenes—energy flow.

Energy is born in the sun. It enters a potato leaf and is captured into glucose. As part of the bonds in glucose, it enters your body. When the glucose is broken apart, energy is freed. It may be used to combine a molecule of ADP with phosphate to make ATP. Some energy therefore stays in your body when the carbon with which it was associated is breathed out. Later, the energy in the ATP is either spent or stored. Let's assume in this case that it is spent.

The ATP is broken apart, releasing some energy to help move a muscle or to transmit a nerve impulse. Some of the energy ends up as work accomplished and heat radiated away. You cannot say that this energy is lost; it is just no longer available to do work.

Energy changes forms, unlike atoms—which can cycle again and again through the atmosphere, to plants, and back to the atmosphere, always remaining recognizable. Originating in the sun, energy may exist for a while as part of a chemical bond and later as heat energy. This heat energy, although still in the same amount as when it came from the sun, cannot be used again by plants or animals to fuel their

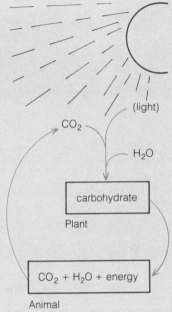

The carbon cycle.

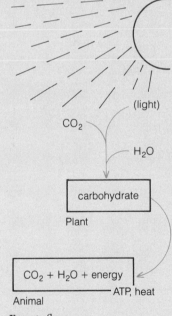

Energy flow.

The downhill flow of energy is not a cycle.

work. Thus life on earth can go on only for as long as the sun continues to burn and flood our plants with light.

This discussion has taken us far from the problems of nutrition, although you may agree that the concept of energy must be understood if the very real nutritional problems of underweight and obesity are to be dealt with. Ironically, although energy weighs almost nothing, you weigh more when you store energy. The reason this is so is clear from the Tinker Toy analogy, in which energy is represented by the sticks. The sticks weigh nothing but in order to keep them in place you must attach them to wheels, which do weigh something. To capture energy and store it in your body, you must trap it in molecules of fat. Thus the more energy you store, the heavier you become. Fat also takes up space, and so the more energy you store, the bulkier you become. The problems of energy excess, which causes overweight and obesity, and energy deficit, which causes underweight and kcalorie malnutrition, result from this arrangement. The practical considerations relating to these problems are taken up in Chapter 8.

Summing Up

The energy in food resides in the chemical bonds that hold nutrient molecules together. In the body, when these bonds are broken, some of this energy is released as heat; but much of the energy is captured through coupled reactions into energy-carrier molecules such as ATP. When ATP is broken down to ADP and phosphate, the energy is again released and used to anabolize body compounds. ATP-like compounds power all of the energy-requiring processes in the body.

The cell's most efficient means of generating ATP are the sequences of reactions known as the TCA cycle and the electron transport chain. In the TCA cycle, acetyl CoA (from carbohydrate, fat, or protein) is attached to oxaloacetate to form citrate, and citrate is processed in a series of reactions that convert it back to oxaloacetate. During these reactions, two carbon dioxide molecules are released, and energy is transferred into other carrier compounds. The major carrier is NAD^+. Each NAD^+ molecule receives two high-energy electrons to become $NADH + H^+$ and then transfers them to a series of other carriers. This is the electron transport chain. At each step the electrons lose energy. At several of these steps the energy is transferred, in a coupled reaction, to ATP. The electrons are finally donated to oxygen, yielding water.

The ATP generated in the electron transport chain carries a large amount of energy in its terminal phosphate group. Thus, it can participate in other coupled reactions to do the body's work. Among its contributions are energy to power the first step in the catabolism of glucose; energy to synthesize glycogen, fatty acids, and proteins; and energy for muscle movements and for repolarizing nerve cells after the transmission of nerve impulses. After the energy originally found in food has been transferred into ATP and used for these purposes, it leaves the body as heat or work accomplished and is no longer usable.

Thus although carbon and the other atoms present in nutrients cycle repeatedly through living things, energy flows downhill, being gradually dissipated as heat. Although no net energy is lost in this process, heat energy is not reconvertible to chemical bonds; hence a new supply of usable energy must flow constantly from the sun, through plants, and into animals and human beings. This explains the need for food to sustain life.

Energy storage involves the capture of energy that chemically binds organic molecules together and therefore entails storage of matter that occupies space and has weight. The problem of storing more energy than is needed therefore becomes a problem of storing more weight.

To Explore Further

A brief and clear explanation in paperback of the ways energy flows through living things is:

● Lehninger, A. L. *Bioenergetics: The Basis of Biological Energy Transformations*, 2nd ed. New York: Benjamin-Cummings, 1971.

A more technical but clear and highly accurate treatment of the biochemical pathways, including the TCA cycle and the electron transport chain, is:

● Lehninger, A. L. *Biochemistry*, 2nd ed. New York: Worth, 1975.

Nutrition and Adaptation

For an organism to remain viable, it is essential that not only its extracellular milieu be maintained constant, but also the capacity of its tissues to do their work must be adequate. In order for this second-order homeostasis to occur, large changes in enzyme activity may be necessary.

R. E. OLSEN

The term *adaptation* has some meaning to everyone. When you say that you have adapted to a situation, you mean that something inside you has changed so that you can handle the situation better. You might be astonished to learn how literally it is true that adapting means something inside you changes.

In nutrition, adaptation has specific meanings, and understanding what they are provides the health professional with the insight necessary to provide help tailored to a patient's needs. When we say, "He isn't adapted to such a rich diet yet, let's build up to it gradually," or "Before we attempt surgery on this patient we had better build her up nutritionally; she isn't equipped to withstand it at this point," we are speaking of concrete physical realities. Also, adaptation explains otherwise incomprehensible everyday happenings. Why is it, for example, that a person can drink large amounts of alcohol on one occasion without getting drunk, while on another he can't? How is it that a woman can absorb 30 percent of the iron she ingests when she is pregnant or iron-deficient, but only 10 percent when she is not? Why does a prescription drug work so much more powerfully in the body of a person who hasn't eaten for two days than in the same person when he is well fed?

Nutrition books often make vague statements about the state of the body. They say that the body's response to stress, or to illness, or to medication, drugs, or nutrients depends on its "prior nutritional history," or its "health" or "physiological state." These statements mean something, and this Highlight is intended to help you understand the meaning.

For any change to come about, the body's machinery — its proteins — have to be changed, and this can be brought about in two ways. First, the rate at which the proteins work can be either speeded up or slowed down. Second, the number of working protein units can be increased or decreased. The first kind of change, the change in rate of action, makes possible quick responses to short-term needs. The second, the change in number of working protein units, brings about adjustments to longer-term, more gradual changes in demand.

The second kind of change is the subject of this Highlight. Whenever a demand is placed on the body such that its ordinary responses (rate changes) are not enough to rise to the occasion, there is a need to alter the body's physical equipment (number of protein molecules needed to do the job). The ability to respond to this need has been referred to as a kind of "second order homeostasis" (see quote at beginning of Highlight).

The equipment inside a cell, then, is different in a major way from that in a factory, and the difference makes the cell much more adaptable to changing circumstances than the factory. A factory is built of heavy, permanent equipment, which can turn out a specific number of products — say, cars — per day for as long as it is operated. Should demand increase, a major renovation would have to be undertaken to enlarge the factory or build a new one; should demand decrease, some of the equipment could be idled; but in either case a certain amount of inefficiency would be inevitable. The factory is inelastic; it is

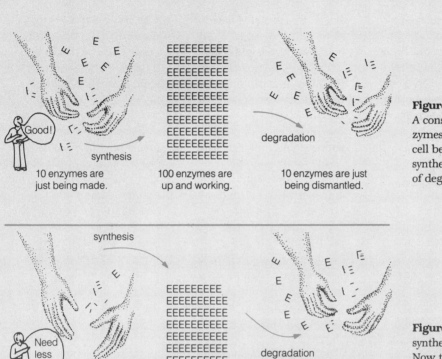

Figure 1a Steady state. A constant number of enzymes is present in the cell because the rate of synthesis equals the rate of degradation.

10 enzymes are just being made.

100 enzymes are up and working.

10 enzymes are just being dismantled.

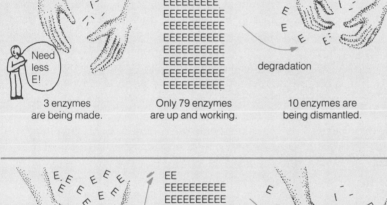

Figure 1b The rate of synthesis has been slowed. Now there is a smaller, and declining, number of enzymes working in the cell.

3 enzymes are being made.

Only 79 enzymes are up and working.

10 enzymes are being dismantled.

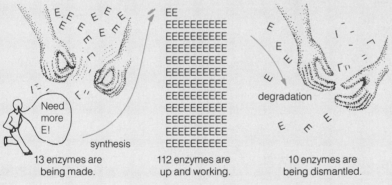

Figure 1c The rate of synthesis has been speeded up. Now there is a greater, and increasing, number of enzymes working in the cell.

13 enzymes are being made.

112 enzymes are up and working.

10 enzymes are being dismantled.

Figure 1 Enzyme adaptation. The number of enzymes at work is normally constant (A), not because the same molecules are always there but because new ones are appearing as fast as the old ones are disappearing. The number can be changed by changing the rate of synthesis (B and C) or by changing the rate of degradation (not shown).

not prepared to shrink or grow as a cell can do. But in a cell, the protein machinery itself is being replaced all the time anyway — every hour — and so to alter its nature or extent is no big deal.

To explain how this replacement takes place: Most of the body's machinery is composed of protein — enzymes, transport proteins, "pumps," membrane receptors, and the like. Each type of machinery is represented by a population of identical molecules, each with a certain life expectancy. At any point in time, a study of this population of protein molecules would reveal that some of its members are newly made and just beginning to work, others are established and hard at work, still others are at the end of their useful lives and about to be dismantled and their parts recycled. The making and the taking apart balance so that the number of protein molecules present and working remains constant (Figure 1). These rates may be very fast (9 out of every 10 protein molecules in the population may be replaced every hour) or very slow (1 out of every 10 may be replaced in a month.)

The rate at which a cell replaces any particular set of proteins determines the *half-life* of the proteins — a term that characterizes the stability of their population

size. Some proteins have a short half-life, some a long one. Under constant conditions, the difference between the two kinds is not obvious, but if a disturbance arises, the differing half-lives have a marked effect. For example, suppose protein synthesis suddenly shuts down (perhaps an essential amino acid is missing). The proteins with short half-lives will rapidly disappear from the cell because they are still being rapidly degraded, while those with long half-lives will linger and continue to work because their degradation is proceeding very slowly.

The explanation just given has presented several concepts that biochemists usually express in technical terms. They speak not only of the *half-life* of proteins, but of the *rate of synthesis* and the *rate of degradation.* Using these terms they devise precise mathematical formulas to describe quantitatively exactly what is going on within a cell or organ system. The description given here in everyday terms, however, should suffice to permit understanding of the kinds of changes that take place in the body as it continuously adapts to its changing environmental circumstances. The examples that follow should deepen that understanding.

The Body Exposed to Alcohol The first time a person takes a drink, he may not be able to handle it very well. He feels it "go to his head," as if there were no way for the body to get rid of it. However, on repeated drinking, a person finds it easier to tolerate alcohol, and in the heavy drinker there is a marked adaptation that has an effect on many other aspects of the person's health. Ordinarily everyone possesses a certain number of alcohol-metabolizing enzymes in the liver, enough to metabolize about one drink's worth of alcohol every hour and a half. These enzymes are constantly being replaced. In response to repeated heavy drinking the liver establishes and maintains a larger population of enzymes to metabolize alcohol, so that after many weeks, months, or years, the heavy drinker is able to handle alcohol almost twice as fast as he could at first. This is an adaptive response, and in the sense that alcohol is toxic, it confers an advantage on the body; but it has some consequences.

The liver's adaptation to alcohol happens to affect its ability to handle certain drugs as well, because some of the alcohol-metabolizing enzymes also work on drugs. With all of these additional enzymes manufactured and inserted into its membranes, the liver can now metabolize *both* alcohol and drugs faster than a normal liver can do. Now, when the physician prescribes a drug, it disappears from the body faster than the doctor might expect. You can see how it is that a person prescribing drugs for someone would have to be aware of the previous drug and alcohol use history of that person in order to prescribe correctly. (See Highlight 9 for more details on the liver's alcohol-metabolizing systems.) And perhaps you can generalize from this to see that many other aspects of the prior "chemical history" of a patient will determine what his body is ready for, how much he can handle, and the rate at which he will handle it. The patient's prior nutrition is relevant to these questions also.

The Child With Advanced Protein Deficiency   In the last stages of kwashiorkor, when the disease has become very severe, the digestive system shuts down and the pancreas stops producing digestive enzymes. In this case adaptation involves making *less* of something. This confers a survival advantage on the child, because energy and building blocks are thereby conserved to serve higher

---

Miniglossary

atrophy (ATT-tro-fee): growing smaller. Atrophy of an organ reflects a decreased rate of synthesis or an increased rate of degradation of enzymes and other proteins; cells parts; and even whole cells.

a = without
trophy = growth

degradation: breaking down. Enzymes may break things down but enzymes and other proteins are also broken down themselves, normally at a constant rate that is characteristic for each protein. By changing the *rate of degradation* of a particular protein, the cell can change the total number of molecules of that protein that will be present at any given time.

half-life: the length of time it takes for half of a population (in this case, of protein molecules) to disappear after synthesis of new members has stopped. Under these circumstances, the half-life depends on the rate of degradation. The term *half-life* is a shorthand way of describing how fast a population of proteins can change in size.

hypertrophy (high-PURR-tro-fee): growing larger. Hypertrophy of an organ reflects an increased rate of synthesis or a decreased rate of degradation of enzymes and other proteins, cell parts, and sometimes even whole cells. See also *atrophy*.

hyper = more, too much

induction (of enzymes): the process by which an enzyme is made to appear in response to a need for it. A signal (perhaps a hormone, perhaps the substance the enzyme itself works on) arrives at the portion of DNA, or gene, that codes for that enzyme; the gene's information is copied into molecules of messenger RNA, and these are sent out to the cell's protein-making bodies (ribosomes) where the enzyme is made.

synthesis: making. Enzymes may synthesize substances, but they are also themselves synthesized. In this Highlight the synthesis of enzymes and other proteins is under discussion. The synthesis of proteins proceeds at a rate that is characteristic for each protein. Alteration of the *rate of synthesis* of a particular protein can alter the number of molecules of that protein that is present in the cell.

---

priority purposes such as maintaining the brain, heart, and lung tissue and their minimum vital functions. The making of less equipment for the GI tract and

pancreas is reflected in the atrophy of those organs. They lose so much protein (and associated supporting lipid and other material) that they become physically smaller.

The intestinal villi shrink, and the areas of the pancreas that produce digestive enzymes disappear.

When a kwashiorkor child has been brought into the hospital very near death and the attempt is being made to save the child, the person responsible for feeding the child has to take care to go slowly, because the child is not equipped — literally does not have the equipment — to digest food. The first choice is simple carbohydrate in small quantities, with only a very little protein, sufficient to engage the available enzymatic machinery. If this little can be digested, then the body will begin to adapt to eating protein again (make more digestive enzymes, using the newly supplied amino acids and energy). Now, more foods containing protein, and finally fat, can be supplied. The body will not produce fat-digesting enzymes and the proteins necessary for carrying fat from place to place in the body until the many other proteins have first been made which are of higher priority for recovery.

Not all children with kwashiorkor can recover. In some, the process of degeneration goes too far. Originally, the body has the resources to adapt, but they can be exhausted.

This example shows that, as far as possible, the body is directly responsive to the

tasks it is given to do. The exact enzymes the pancreas produces in malnutrition at each stage have not been studied in the human being, but it is likely that they are exactly those it has to have to take care of its needs most efficiently. In kwashiorkor, carbohydrate has been present in the diet, so the pancreas has probably kept on producing the enzyme amylase to digest it. Fat has not been present, so production of pancreatic lipase has probably been halted. Providing kcalories in the usable form — as carbohydrate — lifts the constraints from the making of digestive enzymes, and providing just a little fat at first gives the signal for the pancreas to start making the lipase enzyme again. Step by step, nutritional therapy can then build up to a normal diet, but if too much were given too soon, the system would be overwhelmed and the child might die. A diet manual might say only, "Avoid whole milk during the first week, because fat is poorly tolerated at the start," but the person reading with an understanding of enzyme adaptation might see deeply into this simple statement to the underlying reality: The enzymes aren't there at first. (They come back slowly, in response to being presented with the material they work on, a phenomenon the biochemists call enzyme *induction*.)

The Child Fed Too Much Protein   At the end of Chapter 3, a page was devoted to protein overload; we said: "Animals fed high-protein diets experience . . . hypertrophy of their livers and kidneys." The reason may be obvious after the example of adaptation given previously. What should jump to mind is: "That means proteins. The liver and kidneys must be making additional enzymes to manage all the additional amino acids that are flooding the system." In fact, amino acids are metabolized in the liver. A large and active group of enzymes is necessary to perform this metabolism. Their presence is reflected in an enlarged liver. The kidneys have grown because they have built additional nitrogen-excreting machinery.

The Vitamin C Megadoser   When a pregnant woman takes megadoses of Vitamin C, her body adapts by accelerating its destruction and excretion of the vitamin. So does the fetus's body. Both mother and fetus produce large amounts of a vitamin C-destroying enzyme. These adaptations are all very well — until the baby is born. The baby now has greatly overdeveloped vitamin C-destroying machinery, but only a normal intake of the vitamin. The result: scurvy, the vitamin

HIGHLIGHT 7B ADAPTION **251**

C-deficiency disease. The intake is normal but the infant's nutrition history has brought about an abnormal state of apparent need. (See Chapter 10 for more about vitamin C dependence and withdrawal.) What was adaptive in the womb has proved maladaptive after birth. The baby's body will readjust but it will take time — how long depends on the half-life of the proteins involved.

The High Consumer of Cholesterol The person who consumes just *enough* cholesterol to supply his body's needs can afford to maintain fewer cholesterol-making enzymes in his liver. A person who consumes *no* cholesterol whatever has to maintain enzymes to make it. And a person who eats *excess* cholesterol maintains few or no cholesterol-making enzymes; in fact his liver has to produce enzymes that will destroy the cholesterol brought back from depots around the body where it has been rejected for lack of need. Thus three apparently similar people who eat differently may have quite different cellular machinery at work in their bodies. One makes few enzymes either for manufacturing, or for destroying, cholesterol. The second makes enzymes to manufacture his own cholesterol. The third makes enzymes to destroy it. (We are

not talking here about the person who has inherited a defective gene for the cholesterol-destroying proteins so that his intake has to be carefully controlled.)

This is still another way in which adaptation takes place, and should clinch the point of this Highlight. Any protein the body can make is a candidate for regulation. A protein can be made or degraded rapidly, slowly, or not at all. Normally the steady state prevails — a comfortable rate of synthesis accompanied by a matching rate of degradation — but when circumstances change, the responses can be as finely orchestrated as a symphony.

Thus it is that whenever the doctor, nurse, or other health professional approaches a person with therapy, whether it be nutrition, drug, exercise, or whatever, he is not approaching a body that can be assumed to have a certain fixed set of characteristics. Depending on what that person did yesterday or ate last week or is accustomed to eating or drinking or smoking or breathing, his body may be equipped with considerably different enzymatic and other protein machinery than that of the patient in the next bed in the same hospital room. The very number of molecules devoted to serving each of the body's multitude of different purposes differs from one individual to the next. It is hoped

that this Highlight has made you "see" these differences so that you have a deeper insight than you might otherwise have of what is meant by such vague phrases as those quoted at the start: "prior nutrition history," "health," and "physiological state." Seeing the impact of a person's nutrition history on his present health will help equip you to practice wise diet therapy, and also, hopefully, will persuade you that what you eat and drink today will affect your health tomorrow and in the months and years to come.

To Explore Further

This Highlight has dealt informally with a subject that has received highly organized treatment elsewhere. A technical but brief and clear presentation of the subject is:

● Olson, R. E. Introductory remarks: nutrient, hormone, enzyme interactions. *American Journal of Clinical Nutrition* 28 (1975):626-637.

Olson also makes the point, not made here, that while most of the changes the body undergoes help it to maintain normality, there comes a time when its adaptability is exhausted and the further changes that then take place are pathological.

If you'd like an in-depth look into the kind of research involved in developing pictures of how the body works (like the picture presented in this Highlight), take a look at the following review:

● Ott, D. B., and Lachance, P. A. Biochemical controls of liver cholesterol biosynthesis. *American Journal of Clinical Nutrition* 34 (1981):2295-2306.

This review cites 68 individual research reports, each of which represents hundreds of hours of experimentation. It happens to be about cholesterol, but each of the adaptation phenonena described here merits the same amount of attention.

Energy Output

This Self-Study provides two methods for determining your daily energy output. The detailed method involves computing the energy you spend on the three components — basal metabolism, muscular activity, and the assimilation of food — and then adding the three together. The shortcut method involves making estimates of these factors.

Detailed Method   First: Determine from your body surface area the energy you need to support your basal metabolic rate.

a. Use Figure 1 to determine your surface area. Draw a straight line from your height (left column) to your weight (right column). The point at which that line crosses the middle column shows your surface area in square meters. For example, a person 5 feet 3 inches tall, weighing 110 pounds, has a surface area of 1.5 square meters.

b. Use Table 1 to find the factor for your sex and age, and multiply your surface area by this factor. For a nineteen-year-old male, the factor is 40.5 kcal per square meter per hour. This multiplied by 1.5 square meters equals 61 kcal per hour. (Notice that we round off at each step; this method is not so accurate that using many decimal places is meaningful.)

c. Multiply the product by 24 hours per day to find your basal metabolic energy needs per day. Using our example, 61 kcal/hour times 24 hours per day equals 1464 kcal/day. Enter the number you arrived at into Space A on Form 3.

Second: Determine the energy you need for your muscular activities. The following is an accurate method, provided that the day you select is typical. Keep a 24-hour diary of your activities. Record them on Form 1, and specify the length of

Table 1. Basal Metabolic Rate*

Age (yr)	Males (kcal/sq m/hr)	Females (kcal/sq m/hr)	Age (yr)	Males (kcal/sq m/hr)	Females (kcal/sq m/hr)
3	60.1	54.5	26	38.2	35.0
4	57.9	53.9	27	38.0	35.0
5	56.3	53.0			
6	54.0	51.2	28	37.8	35.0
7	52.3	49.7	29	37.7	35.0
			30	37.6	35.0
8	50.8	48.0	31	37.4	35.0
9	49.5	46.2	32	37.2	34.9
10	47.7	44.9			
11	46.5	43.5	33	37.1	34.9
12	45.3	42.0	34	37.0	34.9
			35	36.9	34.8
13	44.5	40.5	36	36.8	34.7
14	43.8	39.2	37	36.7	34.6
15	42.9	38.3			
16	42.0	37.2	38	36.7	34.5
17	41.5	36.4	39	36.6	34.4
			40-44	36.4	34.1
18	40.8	35.8	45-49	36.2	33.8
19	40.5	35.4	50-54	35.8	33.1
20	39.9	35.3			
21	39.5	35.2	55-59	35.1	32.8
22	39.2	35.2	60-64	34.5	32.0
			65-69	33.5	31.6
23	39.0	35.2	70-74	32.7	31.1
24	38.7	35.1	75+	31.8	
25	38.4	35.1			

*From W.M. Boothby, in *Handbook of Biological Data*, ed. W.S. Spector (1956), reprinted courtesy W.B. Saunders Company, Philadelphia.

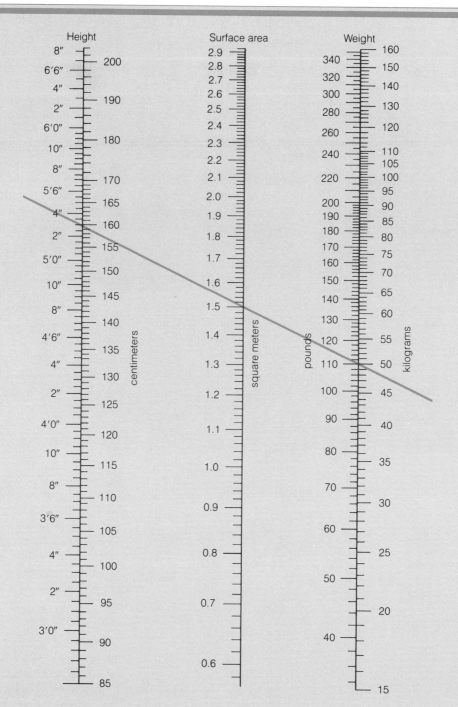

Figure 1 Chart for determination of surface area. A line is drawn between height (5 feet 3 inches) and weight (110 pounds) to yield 1.5 square meters as the surface area.

Adapted from W. M. Boothby, J. Berkson, and H. L. Dunn, Studies of the energy of normal individuals: a standard for basal metabolism, with a nomogram for clinical application, *American Journal of Physiology* 116(1936):468–484.

Form 1. Minutes Spent at Each Energy Level

Clock time	Total minutes	Activity	Energy level*							
			a	b	c	d	e	f	g	h
7:00–7:45	45	Dressing			23	22				
7:45–8:15	30	Eating		26	4					
8:15–9:00	45	Bike to School			4	25	16			
Total										

*See Table 2 for an explanation of these levels.

time *in each activity* that you spent at various energy levels. Table 2 lists the levels and their energy cost. Every minute of the day should be accounted for (1,440 minutes in all).

Treat flights of stairs specially. Record the time spent on stairs as "walking," and put it down as such on the form. But keep a separate record of the number of flights you climbed up and down (count fourteen to fifteen steps as one flight of stairs).

For example, suppose you got up at seven o'clock and spent the first 45 minutes of the day moving about quietly, dressing and getting ready for breakfast. You also went down a flight of stairs to get the newspaper, back up again, and then downstairs for breakfast. You might enter this 45-minute period on one line of Form 2 as shown, recording 8 minutes of it as activity at Level b (sitting or standing still), 23 minutes as Level-c activity (very light), and 14 minutes as Level-d activity (light). You would also note the stair climbing separately ("down twice, up once"). Continue until you have made a complete record for 24 hours.

Be careful not to overestimate the energy levels of your activities. Remember, the kcalories you spend on them depend on the extent and vigor of your muscular movements, not on how "busy" you feel while engaging in them or how tired you get performing them.

Add up the minutes you spent at each energy level to reach totals at the bottom of Form 1, and transfer these totals to Form 2. (Notice that there is a place at the bottom of this form to compute the extra energy spent climbing stairs.) You have now calculated the total energy spent in the day *for muscular activities.* Enter this number into Space B on Form 3.

Third: Calculate your estimated total energy requirement for the metabolic needs incurred by eating food. If you know how many kcalories you ingested that day, use 10 percent of the kcalories (the first alternative for Space C Form 3). Or use the second alternative for Space C, as shown on the form.

Table 2. Energy Levels and Their Energy Cost*

Energy level	Type of activity	Energy (kcal/kg/min)† woman	man
a	Sleep or lying still, relaxed‡	0.000	0.000
b	Sitting or standing still (includes activities like sewing, writing, eating)	0.001-0.007	0.003-0.012
c	Very light activity (like driving a car, walking slowly on level ground)	0.009-0.016	0.014-0.022
d	Light exercise (sweeping, eating, walking normally, carrying books)	0.018-0.035	0.023-0.040
e	Moderate exercise (fast walking, dancing, bicycling, cleaning vigorously, moving furniture)	0.036-0.053	0.042-0.060
f	Heavy exercise (fast dancing, fast uphill walking, hitting tennis ball, swimming, gymnastics)	0.055	0.062

† Measured in kcalories per kilogram per minute above basal energy. Where ranges are given, pick the midpoint within the range, unless you have reason to believe you are unusually relaxed or energetic when performing the activity. For example, for "sitting," a man should normally pick 0.007; if he is sitting very relaxed, 0.003; if very tense, 0.012.

‡ For purposes of this exercise, these are assumed to be at the basal level of activity.

* Adapted from J. V. G. A. Durnin and R. Passmore, *Energy, Work and Leisure* (London: Heinemann Educational Books, 1976).

Last: Add all three figures — (A) metabolic needs per day, (B) energy needs for activities, and (C) energy for SDE — to obtain the total energy you spent in a 24-hour period. This figure represents the best estimate you can easily obtain of the number of kcalories you need to eat each day to maintain your weight. The RDA tables and the Canadian Dietary Standard provide recommendations for energy intake for people in your age-sex category (see Appendix O), but the figure you have arrived at here is your "personalized recommended energy intake." You will want to use this figure for the Self-Study at the end of the next chapter.

Form 2. Energy Cost for Activities (exclusive of basal metabolism and the effect of food)

Energy level	Total minutes spent		Energy cost per minute (kcal/kg/min)				Total energy cost per kg (kcal/kg)
a		×	(women) 0.000		(men) 0.000	=	0.000
b		×	0.001 −0.007	or	0.003 −0.012	=	
c		×	0.009 −0.016	or	0.014 −0.022	=	
d		×	0.018 −0.035	or	0.023 −0.040	=	
e		×	0.036 −0.053	or	0.042 −0.060	=	
f		×	0.055	or	0.062		

Subtotal   1,440

Extra energy spent on stairs:

flights down		+	0.012		=
flights up		+	0.036		=

Total kcal/kg/24 hours

Now multiply by body weight (kg) to arrive at   × _____

Total energy spent on activities for the day: =   [   ]

kcal/day

Shortcut Method As an alternative to the previous exercise, estimate your total energy expenditure by using the following short method:

a. Estimate the energy you spend on basal metabolism by using the figure 1.0 kcal/kg/hr (for men) or 0.9 kcal/kg/hr (for women).
b. Estimate the energy you spend on physical activities by using the following guidelines. For sedentary (mostly sitting) activity (typing), take 20 percent of the energy spent on basal metabolism (**a**). For light activity (teach-ing), take 30 percent. For moderate activity (nursing), take 40 percent. Or for heavy work (roofing), use 50 percent or more.

c. Estimate the energy spent on metabolizing food as *either* 10 percent of your typical kcalorie intake for a day *or* 10 percent of (**a** plus **b**).

Now add these three figures together.

Example: Estimate the energy needs of a woman who weighs 150 pounds.

a. First, change pounds to kilograms:

150 lb × 1 kg/2.2 lb = 60 kg

Then multiply weight in kilograms by the factor for women:

68 kg × 0.9 kcal/kg per hr = 61 kcal/hr

Then multiply the kcalories used in one hour by the hours in a day:

61 kcal/hr × 24 hr/day = 1,464 kcal/day

Energy used for basal metabolism (a) is 1464 kcal/day.

Form 3. Estimation of Total Energy Expenditure

A. Calculate energy spent on basal metabolism using the factor 1 kcal/kg/hour (for men) or 0.9 kcal/kg/hour (for women).

_____ kcal/kg/hour × _____ kg × 24 hours = A. _____ kcal
(round off to whole number)

B. Transfer from Form 2 the total kcalories you sent on muscular activities in 24 hours exclusive of basal metabolism.

B. _____ kcal
(round off to whole number)

C. To figure the specific dynamic energy, add A + B and take 10 percent of the total:
(A. _____ kcal + B. _____ kcal) × .10

C. _____ kcal
(round off to whole number)

Total energy expenditure for 24 hours = A + B + C = _____ kcal

This is your personalized "RDA" for energy.

b. Now, suppose the woman is a typist, engaged in sedentary activity. Multiplying the metabolic energy by 20 percent gives:

1,464 kcal/day × 0.20
= 293 kcal/day

Energy used for muscular activities (b) is 293 kcal/day.

c. If we know that this woman normally eats about 1,900 kcal/day, we can estimate the metabolic need generated by eating this much at 10 percent of that, or 190 kcal. Alternatively, we can take 10 percent of the sum of (a) and (b):

(1,464 kcal/day + 293 kcal/day) × 0.10 = 176 kcal/day

Answer: Her energy expenditure for a day is (a) + (b) + (c), or 1,464 + 293 + 190 (or 176) kcal. The total is 1,947 (or 1,933) kcal. The exact figure is based on several estimates, so it's probably best to express her needs as falling within a range: say, 1,920 to 1,960 kcal/day.

Form 4. Foods Eaten in One Day

Food I ate	Serving size	Exchange group	Number of exchanges
Banana	1 medium	fruit	2

Optional Extras

1. If you worked the detailed calculations suggested above, you can now classify your lifestyle. Compare your activity energy (Space B on Form 4) with your metabolic energy (Space A). Express B as a percentage of A. Percentages correspond to activity levels as follows:

20% = sedentary
30% = lightly active
40% = moderately active
50% = very active

How active are you? Example: My basal metabolic energy is 1,200 kcal/day. My activity energy is 300 kcal/day. 300 is 25% of 1,200, so I would be classed as a lightly active person.

2. Practice estimating kcalorie amounts in meals, using the exchange system as demonstrated in this chapter. List the foods you ate on one day of your record-taking (Introduction Self-Study) on Form 4. Then translate them into exchanges, using Appendix L for reference. For foods not listed in the exchange system, estimate exchange groupings and kcalorie amounts. Then collect your exchanges into the next form (Form 5), and figure your total kcalories for the day.

You will find that this system works well if you ate mostly protective foods (those listed in the exchange system), but it fails to take into account the less nutritious or empty-kcalorie foods, such as candy, cola beverages, alcoholic beverages, and the like. How closely does your kcalorie estimate agree with the calculated amount you have already arrived at? Would a greater familiarity with the exchange system be useful to you in estimating your nutrient and kcalorie intakes? If so, repeat this exercise using the second and third days' records of your Self-Study.

Form 5. kCalories Consumed in One Day (based on exchanges)*

Exchange group	Total exchanges	kCalories
Milk		
Vegetables		
Fruit		
Bread		
Meat		
Fat		
Total kcalories		

*If you used whole milk, add two fat exchanges for each milk exchange that you drank. If you used medium- or high-fat meat, add fat exchanges as indicated in the exchange lists.

CHAPTER 8

CONTENTS

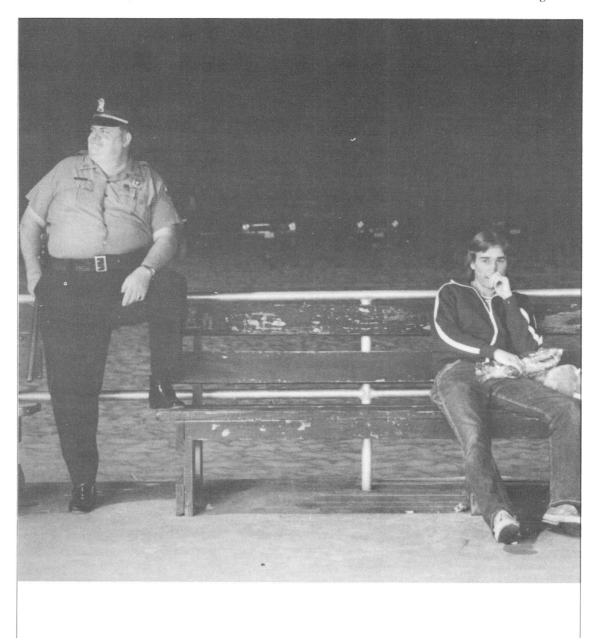

OVERWEIGHT AND UNDERWEIGHT

No matter how much you huff and puff, you can't just shake it off, rock it off, roll it off, knock it off or bake it off. . . . The only way is to eat less and exercise more.

AMERICAN MEDICAL ASSOCIATION

Obesity is a major malnutrition problem. It is simultaneously one of the most important and least understood areas in the science of nutrition. Everyone knows roughly what it is: If you are too fat, you are overweight; if much too fat, you are obese. But why and how obesity occurs and what can be done about it are matters for much speculation, debate, and frustration. For the obese person who has earnestly tried every known means of losing weight only to fail, frustration can turn to despair.

Less well recognized is the problem of underweight, which can be equally mysterious. A "skinny" person finds it as hard to gain a pound as a fat person does to lose one.

This chapter emphasizes the problems of overweight and obesity, partly because they have been more intensively studied and partly because they are a more widespread health problem in the developed countries. This does not imply that the underweight person faces a less difficult problem. The concluding section shows that what we know about the one extreme sometimes applies equally well to the other.

Overweight and underweight both result from unbalanced energy budgets. The overweight person has consumed more food energy (kcalories) than he has expended and has banked the surplus in his fat cells. The underweight person has not consumed enough and so has depleted his fat stores. Energy itself doesn't weigh anything and can't be seen, but when it exists in the form of chemical bonds in nutrients or body fat, the material that it holds together is both heavy and visible.

The amount of fat you might deposit or withdraw from "savings" on any given day depends on your energy balance for that day—the amount you consume (energy-in) versus the amount you expend (energy-out). And as Chapter 7 shows you can reduce your fat deposits by withdrawing more energy from them than you put in. A pound of body fat stores 3,500 kcal. To lose a pound (of body fat) you must experience a deficit: The kcalories you take in must be 3,500 less than the kcalories you expend. To lose that pound in a week, you would need to achieve an average deficit of 500 kcal a day. Repeat: Fat loss always obeys the rule that a person losing weight (fat) must experience a deficit of 3,500 kcal for every pound lost.

This cruel fact is one many of us would like to circumvent. Isn't there an easier way? No, the hard truth is that

> The only way to lose body fat is to cut kcalories.

Magical alternatives that have been offered time and again over the centuries—ways to "shrink the stomach," to eat "negative kcalories," to "eat all you want and lose weight"—prove to be born of wishful thinking. They are effective only when they indirectly affect the kcalorie balance. The success of these plans is not in achievement of their goals but in their popularity. They sell easily to susceptible people who want something for nothing, who become enthusiastic practitioners (but only briefly), and who pass on the word to the next person. This type of reaction reflects a human characteristic that for all our scientific rationality we have failed to outgrow: We love magic. Many writers of fallacious books on diets and sellers of fraudulent diet pills and formulas use this characteristic to their advantage.

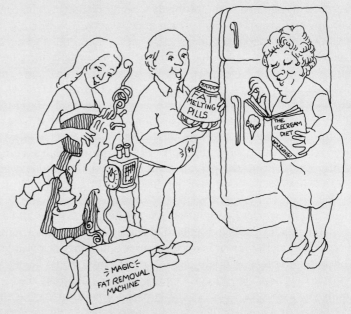

A FLAG SIGN OF A SPURIOUS CLAIM
IS THE USE OF:

Magical thinking
The promise of something for nothing

Ideal Weight and Body Fatness

How fat is too fat? And how thin is too thin? It isn't always possible to tell from the bathroom scales, because body weight says nothing about body composition. The relative amounts of lean and fat tissue vary widely from one person to the next. A dancer or an athlete, whose muscles are well developed and whose bones have become dense from constant stress, may weigh much more than a sedentary person with the same figure. What is needed is a measure of body fatness—not of body weight. Ideally, by a very rough approximation, fat makes up about 18 percent of a man's body weight and about 22 percent of a woman's, with the remainder being contributed by water (55 to 60 percent), muscle and other lean tissue (10 to 20 percent), and bone minerals (6 to 8 percent). But there is no easy way to look inside a person and see the bones and muscles.

Several laboratory techniques for estimating body fatness have been developed. One way is to determine the body's density (weight/volume). Lean tissue is denser than fat tissue, so the more dense a person's body is, the more lean tissue it must contain. Weight is easy to measure with a scale, but volume measurement involves submerging the whole body in water and measuring the amount of water displaced; this requires a large tank and takes up too much space to be practical for use in, say, a doctor's office. Another way is to inject a substance like radioactive potassium or heavy water (deuterium oxide) and allow it to penetrate into the lean tissues (these substances do not dissolve into the fat tissues). A blood sample will show the extent to which the substance has been diluted, providing an estimate of the amount of lean tissue.

A direct measure of the amount of body fat can be obtained by lifting a fold of skin from the back of the arm, from the back, or from other body surfaces and measuring its thickness with a caliper that applies a fixed amount of pressure. A skinfold over an inch thick indicates overfatness; under a half inch reflects underweight. The fat under the skin in these regions is roughly proportional to total body fat. This technique—the skinfold test—is a practical diagnostic tool in the hands of trained people and is in increasingly wide use.

A still simpler test is the mirror test: Undress and stand before a mirror. If you look too fat, you may be too fat. (A notoriously poor judge of this test, however, is the teenage girl who thinks any amount of fat, no matter how small, is a serious blemish. It may be that she needs to change her self-image—not to go on a diet.)

The scales are not necessarily an accurate indicator of body fatness, then, but you most probably use them anyway. After weighing yourself, you turn to the so-called ideal weight tables published by the insurance companies (see inside back cover). You then discover that for a person your height and sex, three weight ranges are suggested: one for a person with a small frame, one for medium, and one for a person with a large frame. Don't forget your shoes: women are assumed to be wearing two-inch heels; men, one-inch heels. (Thus a man who stands 5 feet 10 inches tall in his bare feet would look up the range for a man 5 feet 11 inches in shoes.) Finally, if you weigh yourself nude, you must adjust for

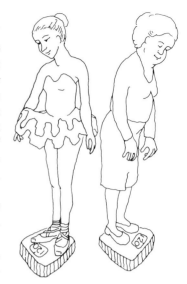

ideal weight: a misnomer, not the desirable but the average weight given in insurance tables for persons of a given sex and height in the United States—not necessarily ideal for a given individual.

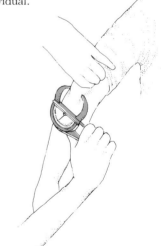

skinfold test: clinical test of body fatness in which the thickness of a fold of skin on the back of the arm (triceps), below the shoulder blade (subscapular), or in other places is measured using an instrument called a caliper. A new and better term for this is **fatfold test.**

frame size: the size of a person's bones and musculature. This is a vague term; frame-size standards were not established by the insurance companies. A recent attempt is reported on page 683, Chapter 18).

A "rule of thumb" method of estimating ideal weight is on the inside back cover.

overweight: body weight more than 10 percent above "ideal" weight.

obesity: excessive body fatness; often loosely defined as a condition of being overweight by 15 or 20 percent or more.

underweight: body weight more than 10 percent below normal or average ("ideal") weight.

clothing (the tables assume 2 to 4 pounds for clothes).

All these steps involve a lot of guesswork. How do you decide on your frame size, for example? As of 1983, no validated standards had yet been provided.[1] A common sense method is available, however: Compare your wristbone with several other people's, and judge for yourself.

After finding the applicable table weight, you have to apply the most important judgment factor of all. Ask yourself whether the weight range you have singled out is really ideal for *you*. At what weight are you most healthy? Does your family tend to be healthy at the heavier, or lighter, end of the weight ranges? A recent reinterpretation of the insurance company statistics suggests that many people are healthiest at weights *above* those thought to be ideal in the past (see Highlight 8).

Ideal weight probably changes with age. Many people typically become less active as they grow older. Their muscles get smaller, and their bones decrease in density. Thus a person who at 25 was lean and muscular might weigh the same at 65 and yet have become considerably fatter. Such a person should either gradually lose weight as time goes on or, preferably, maintain a program of vigorous physical activity to preserve muscle and bone strength. Not much is known about ideal weights at older ages, but clearly, people do tend to gain about 20 to 30 pounds during adulthood. This may not be inconsistent with good health unless it precipitates high blood pressure.

With all of their limitations, the ideal-weight tables are often used to draw arbitrary lines between too much and too little body weight. A person who is more than 10 percent above the weight on the table is considered overweight; if 20 percent or more, he is considered obese. (Some authorities say obesity is 15 percent above the ideal weight, some say 25 percent.) Similarly, a person who is more than 10 percent below the table weight is considered underweight.

The Problem of Obesity

juvenile-onset obesity: obesity arising in childhood; also called developmental obesity.

adult-onset obesity: obesity arising after adolescence; sometimes called reactive obesity if it appears to arise in response to a specific traumatic or stressful life event.

However you define it, obesity does occur to an alarming extent and is increasing in the developed countries. For example, in the United States some 10 to 25 percent of all teenagers and some 25 to 50 percent of all adults are obese.

Some people become fat in childhood and others later on. Few of either type lose the excess weight. There is no specific age that divides juvenile-onset obesity from adult-onset obesity, but as the terms imply, there is a distinction between the two types. A child who is obese will develop sturdy muscles and bones as she grows, to support her excess

---

[1]A. Keys and F. Grande, Body weight, body composition and calorie status, in *Modern Nutrition in Health and Disease*, 5th ed., eds. R. S. Goodhart and M. E. Shils (Philadelphia: Lea and Febiger, 1973), pp. 1-27. A whole new method of estimating frame sizes from wrist measurements is available in Grant's *Nutritional Assessment Guidelines*, cited at the end of Chapter 9, but the validity of this method has not been determined.

weight. Thus as an adult she will have more lean body mass and more body fat than the average person and will likely always be stocky, even after losing her excess fat. People who become obese as children are also less likely to be able to reduce successfully than people who become obese as adults.

Research on fat cells suggests a possible reason why early-onset obesity is especially resistant to treatment. Simply stated, early overfeeding stimulates fat cells to increase abnormally in *number*. The number of fat cells becomes fixed by adulthood. Thereafter, a gain in weight can take place only by increasing the *size* of the fat cells. The number of fat cells regulates hunger in some way, so a person with an abnormally large number of fat cells will be abnormally hungry and will always tend to overeat. On the other hand, a person who gains weight in adulthood has a normal number of fat cells and needs only to reduce the size of the cells.

This theory has been heavily criticized on several grounds.[2] But even the critics agree that there are certain periods in life when body fat increases more rapidly than lean tissue: early infancy (up to about two years), again during preadolescence (and throughout adolescence in girls), and possibly again during the third trimester of pregnancy. These are critical periods, in the sense that what happens at these times may be irreversible and crucial to the person's later physical fate. Prevention of obesity would thus be most important during these times. There is also agreement that fat is hard to lose no matter when it was gained.

Hazards of Obesity   Insurance companies report that fat people die younger from a host of causes including heart attacks, strokes, and complications of diabetes. In fact, gaining weight often appears to precipitate diabetes. Fat people more often suffer high levels of blood fat, hypertension, coronary heart disease, postsurgical complications, gynecological irregularities, and the toxemia of pregnancy. The burden of extra fat strains the skeletal system, causing arthritis—especially in the knees, hips, and lower spine. The muscles that support the belly may give way, resulting in abdominal hernias. When the leg muscles are abnormally fatty, they fail to contract efficiently to help blood return from the leg veins in the heart; blood collects in the leg veins, which swell, harden, and become varicose. Extra fat in and around the chest interferes with breathing, sometimes causing severe problems. Gout is more common and even the accident rate is greater for the severely obese.[3]

"Fat people" means *very* fat people. Some degree of overweight, by today's strict standards, may be healthy. See Highlight 8.

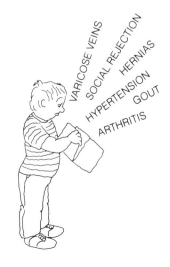

VARICOSE VEINS
SOCIAL REJECTION
HERNIAS
HYPERTENSION
GOUT
ARTHRITIS

---

[2]E. M. Widdowson and M. J. Dauncey, Obesity, in *Nutrition Reviews' Present Knowledge in Nutrition*, 4th ed. (Washington, D.C.: Nutrition Foundation, 1976), pp. 17-23.

[3]Keys and Grande, 1973; K. M. West, Prevention and therapy of diabetes mellitus, in *Nutrition Reviews' Present Knowledge in Nutrition*, 4th ed. (Washington, D.C.: Nutrition Foundation, 1976), pp. 356-364; B. B. Blouin, Diet and obesity (news digest), *Journal of the American Dietetic Association* 70 (1977):535; R. A. Seelig, Obesity: A review, reprint by United Fresh Fruit and Vegetable Association (Washington, D.C., 1976); and C. F. Gastineau, Obesity: Risks, causes, and treatment, *Medical Clinics of North America* 56 (July 1972):286-293.

A linear (straight-line) relationship:

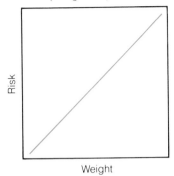

The actual relationship of risk to weight:

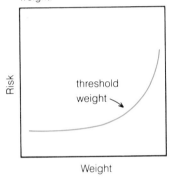

Adapted from C. C. Seltzer, Some re-evaluations of the *Build and Blood Pressure Study, 1959* as related to ponderal index, somatotype and mortality, *New England Journal of Medicine* 274 (1966):254-259.

As if all this were not enough, there are also social and economic disadvantages. A fat person is less often sought after for marriage, pays higher insurance premiums, meets discrimination when applying for a job, can't find attractive clothes so easily, and is limited in his choice of sports. Fat girls have only a third the chance of being accepted into college that lean girls have. The fat child often suffers ridicule from her classmates and the unbearable humiliation of having the captain of the team choose her last.

The many disadvantages justify our calling obesity a severe physical handicap. However, it is unlike other handicaps in two important ways. First, mortality risk is not linearly related to excess weight. Instead, there is a threshold at which risk dramatically increases. Being only a few pounds above this threshold weight may cause blood pressure, blood glucose, and blood lipids to zoom upwards. The concept of a danger zone of weight, which is relatively new, is illustrated in the margin. Second, obesity is reversible, and if it is corrected in time, some of its risks are too.[4] Mortality rates (from insurance data) are no higher for the formerly obese than for the never obese.[5]

Ideally a person would never have to struggle with the problem of obesity, because he would never have become obese to begin with. Preventive efforts are needed, especially in vulnerable groups: infants, preadolescents, adolescents, and women before they are pregnant. (This is in no way meant to imply that a woman who is pregnant should attempt to lose weight. Weight loss during pregnancy is even more hazardous than obesity.) Where prevention has failed, treatment is urgently needed. But how to treat? Before turning to the matters of diet, drugs, exercise, and other means of attacking the problem, it is necessary to try to figure out what causes it.

Causes of Obesity

kCalories are not stored in fat until the body's other energy needs have been met. Excess body fat can accumulate only when kcalories are eaten beyond those needed for the day's metabolic, muscular, and digestive activities. To put it bluntly, obesity results from overeating.

This fact, however, neither explains the cause of obesity nor indicates the cure. Why do people overeat? Is it a hunger problem? An appetite problem? A satiety problem? Is it genetic? Metabolic? Environmental? Is it a matter of habits learned in early childhood? Is it psychological? Would you believe that all of these factors may play a role? To tell the truth, we do not know the cause. The following paragraphs only offer ideas that are presently being considered.

[4]E. Eckholm and F. Record, *Worldwatch Paper 9: The Two Faces of Malnutrition* (Washington, D.C.: Worldwatch Institute, 1976).

[5]Gastineau, 1972.

Hunger, Appetite, and Satiety   The theories of how food intake is regulated could not be summarized in fewer than 50 pages.[6] It may be that the brain monitors blood glucose concentration and signals "eat" when glucose gets too low; the obese individual may have an insensitive monitor. Food intake may be regulated by fat cells, which send hormonal signals to the brain when they have been fed enough—and obese people may have too many fat cells. Then again, they may not.[7] Centers outside the brain may also initiate feeding behavior.[8] It may be that food tastes better to some people than to others, although recent experiments suggest there is no difference between the obese and nonobese in this respect.[9]

Hunger is said to be physiological—an inborn instinct—whereas appetite is psychological—a learned response to food. Possibly obese people have learned to enjoy eating for reasons other than to satisfy the hunger drive. We have all experienced appetite without hunger: "I'm not hungry, but I'd love to have a piece." The too-thin person may often experience the reverse, hunger without appetite: "I know I'm hungry, but I don't feel like eating."

The clue in some cases may lie in the fact that the obese person doesn't know when to stop: She goes on eating when she is full. One theory of food intake regulation states that feeding behavior is turned on all the time and that a neural or hormonal switch is supposed to turn it off whenever the body's physiological need has been met.[10] The stomach is known to be able to signal to the brain when nutrients have arrived. The satiety theory suggests that the obese person's "set point" is too high or is malfunctioning and that the underweight person's is too low. But the exact nature of the satiety signal is unknown.

External Cues   Some obese people are unconscious eaters. Rather than respond only to internal, visceral hunger cues, they respond helplessly to such external factors as the time of day ("It's time to eat") or the availability, sight, and taste of food.[11] This is the basis of the external cue theory.

hunger: the physiological need to eat.

appetite: the desire to eat, which normally accompanies hunger.

satiety (sat-EYE-uh-tee): the feeling of fullness or satisfaction at the end of a meal; it prompts a person to stop eating.

external cue theory: the theory that some people eat in response to such external factors as the presence of food or the time of day rather than to such internal factors as hunger.

[6]An example is S. Lepkovski, Regulation of food intake, *Advances in Food Research* 21 (1975):1-69.

[7]Widdowson and Dauncey, 1976.

[8]E. M. Stricker, N. Rowland, C. F. Saller, and M. I. Friedman, Homeostasis during hypoglycemia: Central control of adrenal secretion and peripheral control of feeding, *Science* 196 (1977):78-81.

[9]C. L. Hamilton, Physiologic control of food intake, *Journal of the American Dietetic Association* 62 (1973):35-40; and D. A. Thompson, H. R. Moskowitz, and R. G. Campbell, Taste and olfaction in human obesity, *Physiology and Behavior* 19 (1977):335-337.

[10]Keys and Grande, 1973; A. J. Stunkard, Eating patterns and obesity, *Psychiatric Quarterly* 33 (1959):284-295; P. H. Linton, M. Conley, C. Kuechenmeister, and H. McClusky, Satiety and obesity, *American Journal of Clinical Nutrition* 25 (1972):368-370; and M. Cabanac, R. Duclaux, and N. H. Spector, Sensory feedback in regulation of body weight: Is there a ponderostat? *Nature* 229 (1971): 125-127.

[11]J. F. Schumaker and M. K. Wagner, External-cue responsivity as a function of age at onset of obesity, *Journal of the American Dietetic Association* 70 (1977):275-279.

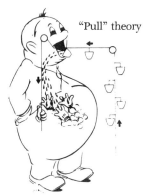

"Pull" theory

The "pull" theory of obesity proposes that a subtle metabolic disorder increases food intake either by affecting hunger-satiety signals transmitted to a "satiety center" or by altering the sensitivity of the satiety center to such signals.

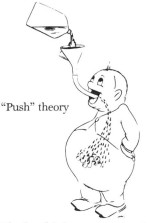

"Push" theory

The "push" theory proposes that the obese person "force-feeds" himself, overeating for non-physiological reasons.

Adapted from T. B. Van Itallie and R. G. Campbell, Multidisciplinary approach to the problem of obesity, *Journal of the American Dietetic Association* 61(1972):385-390.

Of interest in this connection is the report of an experiment in which lean and fat people in a metabolic ward were offered their meals in monotonous liquid form from a feeding machine. The lean people ate enough to maintain their weight, but the fat people drastically reduced their food intake and lost weight. When kcalories were added to the formula, the lean people adjusted their intake to continue maintaining weight as if they had an internal, unconscious kcalorie counter. The obese people were insensitive to the change, continued drinking the same amount of formula as before, and stopped losing weight.[12]

For the person who responds to external cues, today's environment provides abundant cues to promote eating behavior. Restaurants, TV commercials, the display of food in our markets, vending machines in every office building and gas station—all prompt us to eat and drink high kcalorie foods. There are no "vegetable houses" on our main streets, only steakhouses. Kitchen appliances such as the hamburger cooker and the doughnut maker make high kcalorie foods easy to prepare and thus quickly available.

Psychology: Emotional Needs   The psychiatrist Dr. Hilde Bruch, who has devoted as much attention to the human hunger drive as Freud did to the sex drive, states that hunger and appetite are understandably mixed up together because both are intimately connected to deep emotional needs. Two factors that she finds most important in this connection are the fear of starvation and "the universal experience in the early life of every individual that food intake requires the cooperation of another person." Feeding behavior is a response not only to hunger or appetite but also to more complex human sensations, such as "yearning, craving, addiction, or compulsion."[13]

Others agree that food is widely used for non-nutritive purposes, especially in a culture like ours where food is abundant. An emotionally insecure person, who feels unsure of acceptance by other people, might eat as a substitute for seeking love or friendship. Eating is less threatening than calling a friend and risking rejection. Often, especially in adolescent girls, eating is used to relieve boredom. And one researcher has found that eating helps ward off depression.[14]

Obesity as a Response to Stress   Animals under stress have been observed to substitute one instinctive behavior for another. During a confrontation, for example, one animal may suddenly stop posturing

[12]T. B. Van Itallie and R. G. Campbell, Multidisciplinary approach to the problem of obesity, *Journal of the American Dietetic Association* 61 (1972):385-390.

[13]H. Bruch, Role of the emotions in hunger and appetite, *Annals of the New York Academy of Sciences* 63, part 1 (1955):68-75.

[14]R. I. Simon, Obesity as a depressive equivalent, *Journal of the American Medical Association* 183 (1963):208-210.

and begin to groom itself intensively. It is possible that people also displace one behavior with another when they are threatened. Rather than fight or flight, the activity they select may be eating.

The hormones secreted in response to physical stress favor the rapid metabolism of energy nutrients to fragments that can be used to fuel the muscular activity of fight or flight. Under emotional stress the same hormones are secreted. If a person fails to use the fuel in violent physical exertion, the body has no alternative but to turn these fragments to fat.[15] If blood glucose has been used this way, then the lowered glucose level will signal hunger, and the person will eat again soon after. Stress eating may appear in different patterns: Some people eat excessively at night when feeling anxious, others characteristically go on an eating binge during an emotional crisis.[16] The overly thin often react oppositely. Stress causes them to reject food and thus become thinner.

Metabolic Obesity It may be that some people have inherited a greater tendency to accumulate body fat than others. One researcher speculates that some people might tend to use carbohydrate (from blood glucose and liver glycogen) more extensively to meet certain energy needs, whereas others might tend to use blood lipid. The glycogen users would experience lowered blood glucose more readily and so would be hungry more often.[17] A difference like this could be due to a difference in the amount of a particular hormone or enzyme involved in fat production and conceivably might imply that a low-carbohydrate diet is needed. Dozens of theories are presently being tested. Doubtless some will explain at least a few specific cases of obesity.

Insulin Insensitivity Once a person has become obese, the situation tends to perpetuate itself. The enlarged fat cells become resistant to insulin, the hormone that promotes glucose uptake into cells and its conversion to fat. The excess glucose remains in the bloodstream and stimulates the insulin-producing cells of the pancreas to multiply and secrete more insulin. This promotes further fat storage.[18] As if this were not enough, the enlarged fat cells are also less sensitive to other

Insulin: see also Chapter 1 and Highlight 2.

---

[15]This response to stress has been studied in animals. An example of such a study is C. D. Berdanier, R. Wurdeman, and R. B. Tobin, Further studies on the role of the adrenal hormones in the responses of rats to meal-feeding, *Journal of Nutrition* 106 (1976):1791-1800.

[16]Stunkard, 1959.

[17]W. H. Griffith, Food as a regulator of metabolism, *American Journal of Clinical Nutrition* 17 (1965):391-398.

[18]J. Mayer, as quoted by M. Kernan, Inactivity places burden of obesity on America's youth, *St. Petersburg Times*, 12 August 1973.

hormones that promote fat breakdown.[19] Weight loss restores insulin levels to normal, but it first has to be achieved against these odds.

Heredity versus Environment   Hormones and enzymes are under the control of genes, and genes are inherited. In some animal strains, obesity is inherited as predictably as hair or eye color. Is human obesity inherited? One way to test this possibility is to study identical twins raised in different families, one family fat and the other thin. If genes determine fatness, then both twins will become equally fat or thin. But if the environment is responsible, the twins will resemble their respective families. Another approach is to study adopted children, to see whether they resemble their natural or adoptive parents. Studies of both kinds suggest that the tendency to obesity is inherited.[20] But the environment is permissive; that is, it can allow obesity to develop when the potential is there.

Inheritance of the tendency to obesity is probably very complex and governed by many different genes. To complicate the situation further, these genes probably occur with different frequencies in different populations.[21]

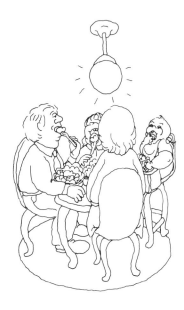

Habits: Learned Responses to Food   If a person can inherit the potential to become obese, the environment can doubtless help it become real. Food-centered families encourage such behaviors as overeating at mealtimes, rapid eating, excessive snacking, and eating to meet needs other than hunger. Children readily imitate overeating parents, and their behavior at the table persists outside the home. Obese children have been observed to take more bites of food per interval of time and to chew them less thoroughly than their nonobese schoolmates.[22]

People who eat small but frequent meals may tend to store less fat than those who eat large meals at irregular intervals.[23] Thus families that allow their children to skip meals may be promoting obesity.

Inactivity   The many possible causes of obesity mentioned so far all relate to the input side of the energy equation. What about output? A

---

[19]*Obesity '73: A Report from the Geigy Symposium on Obesity, Its Problems and Prognosis* (New York: Ardsley, 1973).

[20]J. Mayer, Obesity, in *Modern Nutrition in Health and Disease*, 5th ed., eds. R. S. Goodhart and M. E. Shils (Philadelphia: Lea and Febiger, 1973), pp. 625-644.

[21]A. Montagu, Obesity and the evolution of man, *Journal of the American Medical Association* 195 (1966):105-107.

[22]R. S. Drabman, D. Hammer, and G. J. Jarvie, Eating rates of elementary school children, *Journal of Nutrition Education* 9 (1977):80-82.

[23]P. Fabry, Metabolic consequences of the pattern of food intake, in *Handbook of Physiology*, section 6, ed. C. F. Code (Washington, D.C.: American Physiological Society, 1967), pp. 31-49; and G. A. Leveille and D. R. Romsos, Meal eating and obesity, *Nutrition Today*, November/December 1974, pp. 4-9.

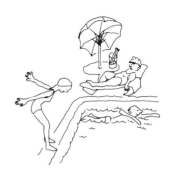

person may be obese because he eats too much, but another possibility is that he spends too little energy. It is probable that the most important single contributor to the obesity problem in our country is under-activity.[24] The control of hunger/appetite actually works quite well in active people and only fails when activity falls below a certain minimum level.[25] Obese people under close observation are often seen to eat less than lean people, but they are sometimes so extraordinarily inactive that they still manage to have a kcalorie surplus. One authority has noted that normal people actually swim 35 minutes during "an hour of swimming," whereas obese people swim only 7 minutes. Most of their time is spent sitting, standing, or lying in the sun.[26]

Individuality   No two people are like either physically or psychologically, and no doubt the causes of obesity are as varied as the people who are obese. Many causes may contribute to the problem in a single person. Given this complexity, it is obvious that there is no panacea. The top priority should be prevention, but where prevention has failed the treatment of obesity must involve a simultaneous attack on many fronts.

Treatments of Obesity: Poor Choices

The only means of reducing body fat is to shift the energy budget so that energy-in is less than energy-out. This is most effectively done by eating less and exercising more. A later section of this chapter addresses these strategies, but because rumors of other means fly about, they will first be dispensed with briefly.

Water Pills   For the obese person, the idea that excess weight is due to water accumulation may be an attractive one. Indeed, temporary water retention, seen in many women around the time of the menstrual period, may make a difference of several pounds on the scale. Oral contraceptives may have the same effect. (They may also promote actual fat gain in some women. A woman who has this problem should consult her physician about switching brands.) In cases of severe swelling of the belly, as much as 20 pounds of excess body water may accumulate.[27]

If water retention is a problem, it can be diagnosed by a physician, who will prescribe a diuretic (water pill) and possibly a mild degree of

---

[24]Keys and Grande, 1973.

[25]J. Yudkin, Prevention of obesity, *Royal Society of Health Journal* (July 1961), pp. 221-224.

[26]Mayer as quoted by Kernan, 1973; B. Bullen, as quoted in R. A. Seelig, 1976.

[27]Keys and Grande, 1973.

salt restriction. But the obese—that is, overfat—subject has a smaller percentage of body water than the person of normal weight. If she takes a self-prescribed diuretic, she has done nothing to solve her fat problem, although she may lose a few pounds on the scale for half a day and suffer from dehydration.

Diet Pills   Some doctors prescribe amphetamines ("speed") to help with weight loss (the best known are dexedrine and benzedrine). These reduce appetite—but only temporarily. Typically the appetite returns to normal after a week or two, the lost weight is regained, and the user then has the problem of trying to get off the drug without gaining more weight. It is generally agreed that these drugs cause a dangerous dependency and are of little or no usefulness in treating obesity.[28] No known drug is both safe and effective, and many are hazardous. The only effective appetite-reducing agent to which tolerance does not develop in time is cigarette smoking, which of course entails hazards of its own too numerous to mention.

Health Spas   One of the biggest money-making schemes that profits from people's desires to lose weight the easy way is the health spa. Equipped with hot baths, massaging machines, health drinks, and the like, these places provide programs for the unsuspecting public to improve their figures while putting forth a minimum of effort. They can be used to advantage. People who really exercise there reap the expected benefits. But health spas can be extremely costly, and most of the gimmicks offer no real health advantage other than the psychological boost the consumer herself supplies. Hot baths do not speed up the basal metabolic rate so that pounds can be lost in hours. Steam and sauna baths do not melt the fat off the body, although they may dehydrate a person so that his weight on the scales changes dramatically. Machines intended to jiggle parts of the body while the person leans passively on them provide pleasant stimulation but no exercise and so no expenditure of kcalories.

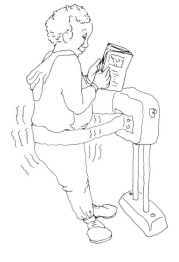

cellulite (SELL-you-leet): supposedly a lumpy form of fat; actually, a fraud.

Some people believe there are two kinds of body fat: regular fat and "cellulite." Cellulite is supposed to be a hard and lumpy fat that yields to being "burned up" only if it is first broken up by methods like the massage or the machine typical of the health spa. The notion that there is such a thing as cellulite received wide publicity with the publication of a book by a certain Madam R of Paris, which sold widely during the 1970s. The *Journal of the American Medical Association* has published the statement that cellulite does not exist.[29]

---

[28]L. Eisenberg, The clinical use of stimulant drugs in children, *Pediatrics* 49 (1972):709-715; G. R. Edison, Amphetamines: A dangerous illusion, *Annals of Internal Medicine* 74 (1971):605-610; and B. Lucas and C. J. Sells, Nutrient intake and stimulant drugs in hyperactive children, *Journal of the American Dietetic Association* 70 (1970):373-377.

[29]D. C. Fletcher, What is cellulite? (letter to the editor), *Journal of the American Medical Association* 235 (1976):2773.

Books like the one by Madam R are often written to make money, and they vary widely in reliability. Madame R probably earns a sizable income from the proceeds of her spa, and her book has enticed many people to spend their money there. She is under no legal obligation to publish only confirmed research findings, and she has not done so: She has published misinformation. Yet she can't be sued unless a customer of hers can prove that her book has caused him bodily harm.

The First Amendment, which guarantees freedom of the press, makes it possible for people like Madame R to express whatever views they like, whether sound or unsound or even dangerous. This freedom is a cornerstone of the U.S. Constitution, and to deny it would be to move hazardously near to totalitarianism. But it puts the burden on consumers to read books skeptically and critically and to use their own judgment in evaluating them. Quacks may hesitate to sell *products* that are outright frauds, because they can readily be punished for misrepresentation, but they do not hesitate to sell *books*.

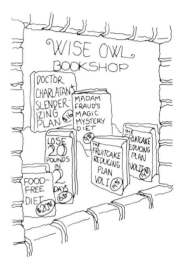

CAUTION WHEN YOU READ!

Seeing a statement in the pages of a book is no guarantee that it is a fact.

The public is not generally aware that books on nutrition are so unreliable that most professional organizations have had to form committees to combat the misinformation they publish. An example is the Committee on Nutritional Misinformation of the Food and Nutrition Board, National Academy of Sciences/National Research Council. If there is a reward for working on these committees, it is not a dollar reward. On the contrary, it costs time and energy for people to serve on them and money to the organizations to publish their statements.

What about textbooks? Perhaps we, the authors, stand too close to the subject to speak without bias about them, but it is our impression that they sell better if other professors find them factual and reliable. We also stand close enough to know that science professors who write textbooks welcome, even seek, criticism from others in the field. One of the sources of our motivation is plain curiosity, which drives us to keep reading and studying in the hope of getting satisfactory answers to our own and our students' questions.

By far the most reliable of all publications on nutrition are the scientific journals. But even among these there are differences. Those that we rely on most heavily are what we call reputable journals. They are the publications of such organizations as the American Medical Association and the American Dietetic Association, which require confirmed credentials and training for membership. Articles are published in them only after a rigorous review by peers of the authors, people who know how to do research and who are familiar with the area under study. The general reader may find journal articles unspeakably dull and boring, but the motivated reader finds them a gold mine of information. Once the purposes and methods are understood, a journal article can be more exciting than a detective story.

Hormones   Because hormones are powerful body chemicals and many affect fat metabolism, it has long been hoped that a hormone might be found that would promote weight loss. Several have been tried. With testing, all have proven ineffective and often hazardous as well. Thyroid hormone, in particular, causes loss of lean body mass and heart problems except when medically prescribed for the correction of a thyroid deficiency—and thyroid deficiency is very seldom the cause of obesity.[30]

human chorionic gonadotropin (core-ee-ON-ic go-nad-o-TROPE-in) **(HCG):** a hormone extracted from the urine of pregnant women; believed (incorrectly) to promote fat breakdown.

Among the hormones advertised as promoting weight loss is HCG (human chorionic gonadotropin), a hormone extracted from the urine of pregnant women. HCG has legitimate uses; for example, it can stimulate ovulation in a woman who has had difficulty becoming pregnant. But it has no effect on weight loss and does not reduce hunger.[31] A rash of "clinics" run by "doctors" that sprang up on the West Coast during 1976 and 1977 advertised tremendous success using HCG in the treatment of obesity. These outfits seem to have had one element in common: They prescribed an extremely rigid low-kcalorie diet, which accounted for their apparent effectiveness. The American Medical Association and the California Medical Association have concluded that the claims made for HCG are groundless and that the side effects are unknown and probably dangerous.[32]

Surgery   Sheer desperation prompts some obese patients to request bypass surgery, an operation in which a portion of the small intestine is

[30]Current concepts of obesity, reviewed by M. R. C. Greenwood and J. Hirsch, *Dairy Council Digest* 46 (1975).

[31]U.S. Department of Health, Education, and Welfare, Food and Drug Administration, *FDA Consumer Memo*, HEW publication no. (FDA) 77-3035 (Washington, D.C.: Government Printing Office, 1977).

[32]HEW, 1977.

removed or disconnected. Then the patient can continue overeating but will absorb considerably fewer kcalories. Side effects from this procedure are many and highly undesirable, including liver failure, massive and frequent diarrhea, urinary stones, intestinal infection, and malnutrition. Reports of mortality range from 2 to 10 percent. Still, in the United States surgery has been reported to be effective more than half the time for treating the massively obese where all other methods have failed.[33] It should probably be attempted only in otherwise healthy and cooperative patients under 30 who weigh more than 300 pounds and who have tried everything else.[34]

Highlight 23 offers more information on bypass surgery for the obese.

The Successful Treatment of Obesity

It seems that the only realistic and sensible way for the obese person to achieve and maintain ideal weight is to cut kcalories, to increase activity, and to maintain this changed lifestyle to the end of his life. This is a tall order. Fewer than a third of those who lose weight manage to keep it off over the long run. To succeed means modifying all of the attitudes and behaviors that have contributed to the problem in the first place, sometimes against physiological pressures that can't be changed. Still, it can be and has been done successfully, as many former "fatties" can attest. A three-pronged approach usually accounts for their success: diet, exercise, and behavior modification.

The way a particular person loses weight is a highly individual matter. Two weight-loss plans may both be successful and yet have little or nothing in common. To heighten the sense of individuality, the following sections are written in terms of advice to "you." This is not intended to put you under pressure to take it personally but to give you the illusion of listening in on a conversation in which an obese person (with, say, 50 pounds to lose) is being competently counseled by someone familiar with the techniques known to be effective. Notes in the margin highlight the principles involved.

Diet   No particular diet is magical, and no particular food must either be included or avoided. You are the one who will have to live with the diet, so you had better be involved in its planning. Don't think of it as a diet you are going "on"—because then you may be tempted to go "off." The diet can be called successful only if the pounds do not return. Think of it as an eating plan that you will adopt for life. It must consist of foods that you like, that are available to you, and that are within your means.

Diet Counseling Principles:

Involve the person.

[33]*American Journal of Clinical Nutrition*, January 1977. This entire issue was devoted to surgery for the obese.
[34]*Geigy Symposium*, 1973.

Planning a Weight Loss Diet

When you are maintaining weight on, say, 2,400 kcalories a day, the following balance is suggested:

15 percent of kcalories from protein
30 percent or less from fat
55 percent or more from carbohydrate

These kcalorie amounts translate into grams as follows:

Protein, 360 kcal or 90 g
Fat, 720 kcal or about 80 g
Carbohydrate, 1,320 kcal or 330 g

Now suppose you want to reduce weight. You could cut your kcalorie amount in half, to 1,200 kcal per day. To avoid getting too hungry, for "satiety value," you must have ample protein and fat. But for health reasons, fat should not supply more than about a third of your kcalories. You must therefore cut the fat grams in half. For maximum satiety, then, leave the protein amount as is. (Protein intake, of course, should never be cut much below the recommended intake.)

So far, you have:
Protein, 90 g or 360 kcal
Fat, 40 g or 360 kcal

This gives a total of 720 kcal and therefore leaves only 480 to be supplied by carbohydrate. This means:

Carbohydrate, 120 g or 480 kcal

Thus you have had to cut your carbohydrate down to about a third of what it was formerly. This balance is typical of successful, nutritious weight-loss plans.[35] The protein may even be raised and the carbohydrate lowered a little more to deliver a nearly perfect 1/3-1/3-1/3 balance of kcalories from the three energy nutrients. In terms of exchanges, such a plan might be designed as on the next page:

Adopt a realistic plan.

Choose a kcalorie level you can live with. If you maintain your weight on 2,000 kcal a day, then you can certainly lose at least a pound a week on a 1,200 kcal diet. A deficit of 500 kcal a day for seven days is a 3,500-kcal deficit—enough to lose a pound of body fat. But let's make a larger deficit, just to be sure. There is no point in hurrying, because you will never go off the diet—and nutritional adequacy can't be achieved on fewer than about 1,200 kcal—1,000 at the very least.

Make the diet adequate.

Put diet adequacy high on your list of priorities. This is a way of putting yourself first. "I like me, and I'm going to take good care of me"

[35]A. J. Vergroesen, Physiological effects of dietary linoleic acid, *Nutrition Reviews* 35 (January 1977):1-5.

Table 1 A Sample Balanced Weight-Loss Diet*

Exchange group	Number of exchanges	Carbohydrate (g)	Protein (g)	Fat (g)
Milk (skim)	2	24	16	0
Vegetables	4	20	8	0
Fruit	3	30	0	0
Bread	2	30	4	0
Meat (lean)	11	0	77	33
Fat	2	0	0	10
Total		104	105	43

*In this diet, carbohydrate supplies 34 percent of the kcalories, protein 34 percent, and fat 32 percent. The protein kcalories are higher than needed for maintenance. When the dieter returns to a maintenance plan by adding (mostly) carbohydrate foods, the ratio will resemble the recommended 15 percent protein, 30 percent fat, 55 percent carbohydrate.

This diet is one of many that offers the needed balance. Another could be higher in bread and fat and lower in meat exchanges.

The design of a weight-reduction diet—with all the protein, half the fat, and only a third the carbohydrate of a regular diet—may be responsible for many people's belief that cutting carbohydrate is necessary for weight loss. In a sound weight-loss diet, however, carbohydrate kcalories are not cut below about a third of the total. To eliminate carbohydrate altogether would be to invite a host of health hazards. Nor should you fast, except under a doctor's supervision.

A diet of 1,200 kcalories or less should be supplemented with a standard daily multivitamin-mineral preparation. Megadoses are unnecessary; RDA amounts are appropriate.

is the attitude to adopt. This means including low-kcalorie foods that are rich in valuable nutrients—tasty vegetables and fruits, whole-grain breads and cereals, and a limited amount of lean protein-rich foods like poultry, fish, eggs, cottage cheese, and skim milk. Within these categories, learn what foods you like and use them often. If you plan resolutely to include a certain number of servings of food from each of these groups each day, you may be so busy making sure you get what you need that you will have little time or appetite left for high-kcalorie or empty-kcalorie foods.

About a third of the kcalories in your diet should come from fat, to make your meals more satisfying. At least a third of the fat should be

Emphasize high nutrient density.

Individualize: Use foods you like.

Stress do's, not don'ts.

polyunsaturated fat—soft margarine, salad dressing, mayonnaise, or the like. Read the label to be sure of the kind of fat. And measure your fat with extra caution: A slip of the butterknife adds even more kcalories than a slip of the sugar spoon. And speaking of empty kcalories, omit sugar, pure fat/oil, and alcohol altogether—if you are willing. Let your carbohydrate come from starchy foods and your fat from protein-rich foods. Table 1 shows how you can plan a diet using the exchange system.

If at all possible, give up alcohol altogether until you have reached your goal, then add a conservative amount to your daily maintenance plan. If you insist on including alcohol in your diet plan, limit it strictly to no more than 150 kcal a day (see Table 2). Add this amount on top of your diet plan and reconcile yourself to a slower rate of weight loss. On no account should the empty kcalories of alcohol be allowed to displace the nutritious kcalories of the foods in the plan.

Eat regularly, and if at all possible, eat before you are very hungry. When you do decide to eat, eat the entire meal you have planned for yourself. Then don't eat again until the next meal. Save "free" or favorite foods or beverages for the end of the day, in case you are hungry once more.

You may have blamed yourself for eating compulsively in the past. That very character trait can work to your advantage: Compulsive people finish what they have started. So diet compulsively. Keep a record of what you have eaten each day for at least a week or two until your habits are beginning to be automatic.

It may seem at first as if you have to spend all your waking hours thinking about and planning your meals. Such a massive effort is

Eat regular meals, no skipping—at least 3 a day.

Take a positive view of yourself.

Table 2.   kCalories in Alcoholic Beverages and Mixers

Beverage	Amount (oz)	kCalories
Beer	12	150
Gin, rum, vodka, whiskey (86 proof)	1 1/2	105
Dessert wine	3 1/2	140
Table wine	3 1/2	85
Tonic, ginger ale, other sweetened carbonated waters	8	80
Cola, root beer	8	100
Fruit-flavored soda, Tom Collins mix	8	115
Club soda, diet drinks	8	1

100 proof means 50 percent alcohol; 86 proof means 43 percent.

One oz is 28 g, 1 1/2 oz is 42 g.

One gram alcohol = 7 kcal.

always required when a new skill is being learned. (You spent hours practicing writing the alphabet when you were in the first grade.) But after about three weeks, it will be much easier. Your new eating pattern will become a habit. Many sound and helpful books and booklets are available to help you get started, some of which are listed in this chapter's To Explore Further.

Visualize a changed future self.

Weigh yourself only once every week or two and always on the same scale, so that you can see clearly the progress you are making. Although 3,500 kcal roughly equals a pound of body fat, there is no simple relationship between kcalorie balance and weight loss over short intervals. Gains or losses of a pound or more in a matter of days reverse themselves quickly; the smoothed-out average is what is real. Don't expect to lose continuously as fast as you did at first. A sizable water loss is common in the first week, but it will not happen again.

Take well-spaced weighings to avoid discouragement.

If you see a gain in weight and you know you have strictly followed your diet, this probably represents a shift in water weight. Many dieters experience a temporary plateau after about three weeks—not because they are slipping but because they have gained water weight temporarily while they are still losing body fat. The fat you are hoping to lose must be combined with oxygen (oxidized) to make carbon dioxide and water if it is to leave the body. The oxygen you breath in combines with the carbons of the fat to make carbon dioxide and with the hydrogens to make water. The carbon dioxide will be breathed out quickly. But the water stays in the body for a longer time. The water takes a while to leave the cell, then enters the spaces between the cells, then works its way into the lymph system, and finally enters the bloodstream. Only after the water arrives in the blood will the kidneys "see" it and send it to the bladder for excretion. While water is making its way into the blood, you have a weight gain, because the water weighs more than the fat that was oxidized.[36] If you faithfully follow your diet plan, one day the plateau will break. You can tell from your frequent urination.

Anticipate a plateau (realistic expectations from the start).

You may find it helpful to control your environment, to avoid situations that prompt you to eat. Begin at the grocery store. Shop when you aren't hungry, and buy only the foods you plan to use on your diet. Purge from your pantry all forbidden items. If you must keep them on hand for other members of your family, surrender them into someone else's possession and ask that they be kept out of your sight as much as possible. Have low-kcalorie foods ready to eat; prepare ahead. To help further with your motivation, mount a mirror on the refrigerator door.

Control external cues.

It is easier to exclude a food than to exercise away its kcalories. To remind yourself of the reality that kcalories eaten must be spent in physical activity, post the following table conspicuously in a place where you might otherwise be tempted to eat:

Discourage magical thinking.

[36]Water weight accumulates during fat oxidation because one fatty acid weighing 284 units leaves behind water weighing 324 units, 14 percent more.

Table 3.   Activity Equivalents of Food kCalorie Values*

Food	kCalories	Activity equivalent to work off the kcalories (minutes)		
		Walk[†]	Jog[‡]	Wait[§]
Apple, large	101	19	5	78
Beer, 1 glass	114	22	6	88
Cookie, chocolate chip	51	10	3	39
Ice cream, 1/6 qt	193	37	10	148
Steak, T-bone	235	45	12	181

*Adapted from M. V. Krause and M. A. Hunscher, *Food, Nutrition and Diet Therapy*, 5th ed. (Philadelphia: Saunders, 1972), p. 431.

[†]Energy cost of walking at 3.5 mph, for a 70-kilogram person is 5.2 kcal per minute.

[‡]Energy cost of running is 19.4 kcal per minute.

[§]Energy cost of reclining is 1.3 kcal per minute.

After losing 20 to 30 pounds, expect to reach a stable plateau.[37] Take this as a good sign. It means that you have lost so much weight that you now require fewer kcalories to maintain your weight. Take a deep breath (you knew this was coming and you are courageous) and institute a change: Increase your activity, cut your kcalories further, or both.

Use positive reinforcement. Never blame, never punish.

If you slip, don't punish yourself. Positive reinforcement is very effective at changing behavior, but punishment seldom works. If you ate an extra 1,000 kcal yesterday, don't try to eat 1,000 fewer kcalories today. Just go back to your diet. On the other hand, you can plan ahead and budget for binges. If you want to celebrate your birthday with cake and ice cream, cut the necessary kcalories from your bread and milk allowance for several days *beforehand*. Again, if you do this compulsively, your weight loss will be as smooth as if you had stayed with the daily plan.

Identify your problem and correct it.
Watch serving sizes.

You may have to get tough with yourself if you stop losing weight or start gaining unexpectedly. You may be slipping on serving sizes. Many a dieter has let herself, in time, measure out her meat exchanges too carelessly—and added an extra 500 kcal to the day's intake. Equally common is the "just this once" substitution of high-fat meat like steak for a fish fillet that was in the plan. You can get away with this only if you scrupulously omit the right amount of fat from other foods the same day. Ask yourself honestly (no one is listening in), "What am I doing wrong?" Very, very seldom does an unpredicted weight plateau of any duration have no explanation in the dieter's own choices.

Learn kcaloric values and fat contents of foods.

[37]Keys and Grande, 1973; and L. Haimes, E. Harrison, H. A. Jordan, P. G. Lindner, and J. Rodin, Applying behavioral techniques in a bariatric practice, part 1, *Obesity and Bariatric Medicine* 6 (January/February 1977):10-16.

Finally, if you stop losing weight or begin to gain, be aware that you may be choosing to stop. Your weight is under your control, and you are entirely free to gain if you wish. You may find you are choosing to take a break, to go into a holding pattern, and to get adjusted before going on. Rather than letting yourself suffer from guilt feelings and feelings of failure, hold your head high and take the attitude, "This is me, and this is the way I am choosing to be right now."

Stress personal responsibility.

Honor the individual.

Exercise   Weight loss is possible without exercise. Obese people often—and very understandably—do not enjoy moving their bodies very much. They feel heavy, clumsy, even ridiculous. The choice of whether to exercise regularly, informally, or not at all is a strictly individual matter. But even if you choose not to alter your habits at first, let your mind be open to the possibility that you will want to take up sports, dancing, or another activity later on. As the pounds come off, moving your body becomes a pleasure, as does letting others see you move. And the health advantages of regular exercise are well documented. It can truly make you look, feel, and be healthier.

Pave the way for later changes.

You must keep in mind that if exercise is to help with weight loss, it must be active exercise—voluntary moving of muscles. Being moved passively, as by a machine at a health spa or by a massage, does not increase kcaloric expenditure. The more muscles you move, the more kcalories you spend.

If you are very inactive, you may find yourself stuck at a plateau after a while unless you undertake some form of regular muscular activity. As with foods, let the activity be one that you enjoy—or that you feel you can most likely learn to enjoy in time. What fits best with your self-image: Rapid walking? Bicycling? Running errands for friends? Many people find that after two or three weeks of effort, exercise becomes as habitual as binge eating was before: You can get addicted to it.

Behavior Modification   Everybody is different, but people who overeat are often seen to behave in certain ways at the table. Hence the need for behavior modification. Most of us are only faintly aware of our eating behavior and can find it interesting, even funny, to observe ourselves. Notice your own table style and compare it to someone else's. How often do you put down your fork (if at all)? How often do you interrupt your eating to converse with a friend? How fast do you chew your food? Do you always clean your plate? Several good books and other resources (check To Explore Further) can help you not only to observe yourself closely but also to set about systematically and effectively retraining yourself to eat like a thin person.

For many people, learning to eat slowly is one of the most important behavior changes to adopt. The satiety signal indicating that you are full is sent after a 20-minute lag. You may eat a great deal more than you need before the signal reaches your brain. Conversely, underweight people need to learn to eat more food within the first 20 minutes of a meal.

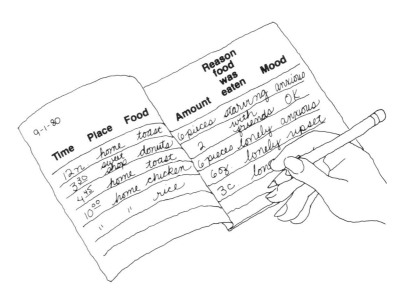

You may find it helpful to join a group such as TOPS (Take Off Pounds Sensibly) or Weight Watchers. A modest expenditure for your own health and well-being is well worth while (but avoid expensive, quick-weight-loss, "magical" ripoffs, of course). Many dieters find it helpful to form their own self-help groups structured around some of the resources already mentioned.[38] Sometimes it also helps to enlist a family member's participation and cooperation.[39] Correspondence groups are also available.[40]

Keep records to increase your personal investment in success.

In case you are a person who eats in response to external cues rather than internally felt hunger, you may need to keep a record for a while of all the circumstances surrounding your eating—the time, the place, the person you are with, the emotions you have at the time, the physical sensations, and other things. An example of such a record is shown above. Looking back, you can see what stimulates you to eat and learn to control these stimuli. If you find that you are indeed eating for the "wrong" reasons—for example, boredom—this discovery will pave the way for adopting behaviors better suited to your needs than compulsive eating. You can begin to make rules for yourself, like "Never eat when you're upset."

If you are especially sensitive to pressure from your family or friends or hosts (can't say no), it will help to have some assertiveness training. Learning not to clean your plate might be one of your first objectives.

[38]H. A. Jordan and L. S. Levitz, Behavior modification in a self-help group, *Journal of the American Dietetic Association* 62 (1973):27-29.

[39]L. S. Levitz, Behavior therapy in treating obesity, *Journal of the American Dietetic Association* 62 (1973):22-26.

[40]An example is described in A. R. Marston, M. R. Marston, and J. Ross, A correspondence course behavioral program for weight reduction, *Obesity and Bariatric Medicine* 6 (July/August 1977):140. Abstract cited in *Journal of the American Dietetic Association* 71 (1977):462.

From all the behavior changes available to you, you can choose the ones to begin with. Don't try to master them all at once. No one who attempts too many changes at one time is successful. Set your own priorities: Pick one trouble area that you think you can handle, start with that, practice your strategy until it is habitual and automatic. Then you can select another trouble area to work on.

Enjoy your new, emerging self. Inside of every fat person a thin person is struggling to be freed. Get in touch with—reach out your hand to—your thin self, and help that self to feel welcome in the light of day.

Use small-step modification.

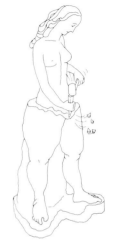

The Problem of Underweight

Much of what has been said about obesity applies to underweight as well, although its hazards are not so great. In fact, the only causes of death seen more often in thin people than in normal-weight people are infections such as tuberculosis. (Suicide is more common among underweight people, but the underweight is not thought to be a cause. The severe depression probably came first and caused anorexia, or lack of appetite.)

The causes of underweight may be as diverse as those of overeating. Hunger, appetite, and satiety irregularities may exist; there may be contributory psychological factors in some cases and metabolic ones in others. Clearly there is a genetic component as well. Early underfeeding may limit the number of fat cells in the same way overfeeding may increase it—although an episode of undernutrition sometimes precipitates later overeating and obesity. Habits learned early in childhood, especially food aversions, may perpetuate the problem. The demand for kcalories to support physical activity and growth often contributes: An extremely active boy during his adolescent growth spurt may need more than 4,000 kcal a day to maintain his weight. Such a boy may be too busy to take the time to eat that much. The underweight person states with justification that it is as hard for him to gain a pound as for an obese person to lose one. So much energy may be spent adapting to a higher food intake that it may take as many as 750 to 800 extra kcalories a day for the underweight person to gain a pound a week.[41]

Strategies recommended for weight gain center mostly on increasing food intake, using foods that provide as many kcalories in as small a volume as possible so as not to get uncomfortably full. Recommended are nutritious, high-kcalorie milkshakes; liberal servings of meat, bread, and starchy vegetables; and desserts. Whereas the weight loser is urged to select the lowest kcalorie items from each food group, the gainer is encouraged to pick the highest-kcalorie items from those same

anorexia (an-o-REX-ee-uh): lack of appetite.

an = not
orexis = appetite

---

[41]Questions doctors ask . . . , *Nutrition and the MD*, June 1978.

groups. Often she may need to resort to systematic between-meal snacking in addition to regular meals. No known pill, shot, hormone, or surgical procedure will increase weight safely, and a reduction in activity is not recommended unless the condition is associated with illness or is so severe as to threaten overall health.

As with weight loss, the person attempting a weight gain must anticipate a plateau, at which time a further increase in food intake will be necessary to continue the gain.[42]

anorexia nervosa (nerv-OH-sah): a severe self-imposed limitation of food intake sometimes seen in adolescents; a dangerous condition requiring skilled professional treatment.

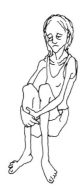

Chapter 16 describes the course of anorexia nervosa.

Anorexia Nervosa   An extreme underweight condition is sometimes seen, usually in young women who claim to be exercising self-denial in order to control their weight. They actually go to such an extreme that they become severely undernourished, finally achieving a body weight of 70 pounds or even less. The distinguishing feature of the anorexic, as opposed to other very thin people, is that she intentionally starves herself. Often there is a whole cluster of accompanying "typical" characteristics of the family and the girl's attitudes.[43]

Anorexia nervosa is a serious condition that demands treatment by an experienced doctor or clinic. Even if temporarily reversed by forced feeding, it can reappear. If the underlying cause is not successfully dealt with, this illness can result in permanent brain damage or death. Strategies for successful treatment are well worked out, and recent advances have been encouraging.[44]

Summing Up

People of the same sex, age, and height may differ in weight due to differing densities of their bones and muscles. The weight compatible with good health depends on the individual. A person whose body fat contributes significantly more than about 10 percent over ideal body weight is considered overweight. Weight tables based on height give an approximation of the weight ranges found to be average for the population as a whole. Body fatness, and therefore body weight, should normally decline with age as metabolism and activity decline.

Obesity is sometimes defined as body weight more than 20 percent above desirable weight. More precisely, obesity is excessive body fatness, which can be accurately diagnosed using the skinfold test. Some 10 to

[42]Keys and Grande, 1973.

[43]H. Bruch, ed., Anorexia nervosa: A review, *Dietetic Currents, Ross Timesaver* **4** (March/April 1977).

[44]Articles describing successful recovery are Bruch, 1977; B. J. Stordy, V. Marks, F. R. C. Path, R. S. Kalucy, and A. H. Crisp, Weight gain, thermic effect of glucose and resting metabolic rate during recovery from anorexia nervosa, *American Journal of Clinical Nutrition* **30** (1977):138-146; and K. C. Fox and N. M. James, Anorexia nervosa: A study of 44 strictly defined cases, *New Zealand Medical Journal* **84** (27 October 1976):309. Abstract cited in *Journal of the American Dietetic Association* **70** (1977):660-661.

25 percent of the young people in the United States and some 25 to 50 percent of its adults are obese by these standards.

Obesity sometimes arises in early life (juvenile onset) and sometimes later (adult onset); the former is harder to correct and both need to be prevented. Possible reasons for the irreversibility of juvenile-onset obesity include overmultiplication of fat cells in response to overfeeding and establishment of the wrong metabolic set point for hunger or satiety.

Obesity entails a host of health hazards, including heart and blood vessel disease, diabetes, complications in pregnancy or after surgery, arthritis, abdominal hernias, varicose veins, respiratory problems, and gout, in addition to social and economic disadvantages. By contrast, underweight (weight more than 10 percent below desirable weight) is associated with an increased risk of infection. Mortality risk in obesity is not linear and is reversible.

Causes of obesity are a matter for much speculation and may include abnormalities in hunger or satiety regulation, in fat-cell number, in responsiveness to external cues that prompt eating behavior, in reactions to emotions and stress, in metabolism, in heredity, or in learned eating habits. An important contributor to obesity in this country is the extreme physical passivity and inactivity that characterize a sedentary lifestyle. However, causes differ widely among different people; treatment must therefore be individualized and multifaceted.

Ineffective and dangerous treatments include the use of diuretics ("water pills"), amphetamines ("diet pills"), hormones, and—except as a last resort for the intractably and morbidly obese—surgery. The most important step in successful treatment is the adoption of a balanced and nourishing low-kcalorie diet, and fat loss is greatly enhanced by regular exercise and behavior modification. Major criteria for success are a permanent change in eating habits and maintenance of the goal weight over the long term.

Diet can also help the underweight person. Behavior modification and other strategies that facilitate weight loss can be adapted to promote weight gain. But the special case of anorexia nervosa requires skilled professional attention. In all weight-control problems—obesity, underweight, and anorexia—real success is achieved only when new, adaptive eating and coping behaviors have permanently replaced the old ones.

To Explore Further

Recommended references on all nutrition topics are listed in Appendix J. In addition, we selected many to cite in this chapter's notes.

A brief review of the concepts of hunger, appetite, drive, and satiety and of the roles of fat cells and the hypothalamus in controlling food intake appears in:

● Lepkovski, S. Regulation of food intake. *Advances in Food Research* 21 (1975):1-69.

A touching personal account by a woman who lost seventy pounds and recorded her thoughts and feelings throughout the experience:

● LeShan, E. *Winning the Losing Battle: Why I Will Never Be Fat Again.* New York: Bantam Books, 1981.

One of the most useful and well written books we've seen to help with behavioral control of obesity is:

● Nash, J. D., and Long, L. O. *Taking Charge of Your Weight and Well-Being.* Palo Alto, Calif.: Bull Publishing Company, 1978.

It presents a complete program with step-by-step instructions and forms for eighteen weeks' worth of record-keeping.

Another excellent — and much smaller — book of the same kind advertises itself "for teenagers only" but is highly recommended for adults whose eating habits are the same as they were in the teen years:

● Ikeda, J. *Change Your Habits, Change Your Shape.* Palo Alto, Calif.: Bull Publishing Company, 1978.

A highly recommended weight-loss guide for young people is:

● Berg, F. *How to Lose Weight the Action Way.* Hettinger, N. D.: Flying Diamond Books, 1980.

A paper describing the ways in which a spouse can be helpful in the weight-control efforts of an obese person is:

● Brownell, K. D., Heckerman, C. L., Westlake, R. J., Hayes, S. C., and Monti, P. M. The effect of couples training and partner cooperativeness in the behavioral treatment of obesity. *Behavioral Research and Therapy* 16 (1978):323-333.

One of many recent popular books to help people learn to be more assertive is:

● Smith, M. J. *When I Say No, I Feel Guilty.* New York: Bantam Books, 1975 (paperback).

The possibility that fiber and its interplay with insulin may have an important role to play in satisfying appetite and so controlling food intake is discussed in:

● Heaton, K. W., ed. *Dietary Fibre: Current Developments of Importance to Health.* Westport, Conn.: Food and Nutrition Press, 1979.

Weight Watchers, Inc., publishes several cookbooks, all based on the exchange system, that present a very sensible, nutritious, balanced diet for weight loss.

A diet book that uses the exchange system—and includes exchanges for fast foods—is:

● Better Homes and Gardens' *Eat and Stay Slim*, 2nd ed. Des Moines, Iowa: Meredith, 1979.

The 1979 price was $3.95

Consumer Guide put out a booklet in 1979 entitled *Diets '79*, which rated the Scarsdale Diet, the "Mayo Clinic" Diet, the Pritikin program, and many others as to whether they work, how safe they are, and how permanent their effects are. The booklet was so successful it will very likely be followed by another like it every now and then. Watch for these.

The entire issue of *Nutrition and the MD*, November 1979 (six pages), was devoted to obesity: its causes, treatment, incidence in children, and so forth.

The *American Journal of Clinical Nutrition* published a supplement issue in February 1980, entirely devoted to surgical and other drastic procedures for morbid obesity.

The *International Journal of Obesity* began publication in 1977. Volume 1 of an even newer journal, *Appetite*, appeared in 1980.

For the serious reader who wants more in-depth information, Mayer's chapter on obesity in Goodhart and Shils' *Modern Nutrition in Health and Disease* is recommended; see Appendix J for the complete reference.

Another major reference containing voluminous recent research and scholarly reflection is:

● Stunkard, A. J., ed. *Obesity.* Philadelphia: Saunders, 1980.

A thought-provoking short film shows a woman reacting to frustration and anxiety by eating a whole chocolate cake. Called *Crumb and Punishment*, the film is useful to stimulate discussion on the need for behavior change. It is available from R. L. Korschun, R. D., 7000 S.W. 62nd Avenue, Penthouse J, Miami, FL 33413.

Metropolitan Life Insurance Company produced a film in the 1970s that has enjoyed a wide showing and has helped many people get a handle on weight control. *Song of Arthur* is available free, and makes enjoyable viewing for about twenty minutes of class time.

The Body's Set Point

This Highlight offers insight into a new area of research and thinking in relation to body weight. It shows current thinking on how the body goes about deciding what it wants to weigh, and how it maintains that weight.

The Set Point for Weight
The reality of the set point is not debated. Many experiences with both humans and animals testify to its existence. For example, when subjects in an experiment are made to overeat so that they gain weight, they spontaneously lose weight back to whatever is normal for them as soon as the experiment is over. And when animals undergo surgical removal of fat tissue, they compensate afterwards by depositing more fat until they are back where they started from.[1] Children recovering from malnutrition grow faster than their age-mates for a spell of "catch-up growth"; then as soon as they are at the right weight, they grow at the normal rate. People who give up smoking often gain a fixed amount of weight — say, 20 pounds — and then stop gaining and maintain their weight at the newly set level. All these examples illustrate the body's tendency to settle at a weight plateau for long periods of

[1]G. A. Bray and L. A. Campfield, Metabolic factors in the control of energy stores, *Metabolism* 24 (1975):99-117.

The energy needs of individuals, or the efficiency with which individuals utilize energy, vary greatly and cannot be predicted on the basis of current knowledge.

D. M. HEGSTED (1976)

time. The plateau may change from time to time with changed circumstances, but the new level then tends to stay as fixed as the old one did.

How the Body Maintains its Weight To maintain weight or to achieve a smooth rate of gain as in catch-up growth or pregnancy, the individual must somehow adjust kcalorie input and output so that they balance just so. Many people think this is managed primarily by regulating appetite (if you spend more energy, you eat more food; if you spend less energy, you eat less food), and to some extent it is managed this way. But surprisingly, the body can also balance its energy budget by changing the output side (if you eat more food you spend more

energy). It does this by increasing not only physical activity but, more importantly, metabolic activity in some mysterious and fascinating ways. Let's look at this less known side of the balancing act first.

How the Body Adjusts its Energy Output Ms. A stays healthy and active on a starvation diet; Mr. B eats immense quantities of food and stays thin. Both weigh 140 pounds and both are equally active. The difference lies in their metabolism: Mr. B "burns" more fuel to do the same amount of work. Or to put it another way, Mr. B spends a lot of his energy on metabolic pathways in which energy nutrients are oxidized without their energy being used or captured and stored as fat, while Ms. A uses every kcalorie she consumes to do work or to put into storage, and wastes none. To put it in still another way: Mr. B's metabolism is wasteful, Ms. A's is conservative. So she gets by on fewer kcalories, and if she ate more — even if she stayed very active — she'd get fat. Much study is being invested, today, in metabolic pathways to see which enzymes are the wasteful ones.[2]

[2]The First Ross Conference on Medical Research included a number of papers touching on this problem. For example: J. S. Garrow, Energy balance in obesity, in *Report of the First Ross Conference*, ed. J. Kinney (Columbus, Ohio: Ross Laboratories, 1980), pp. 134-138.

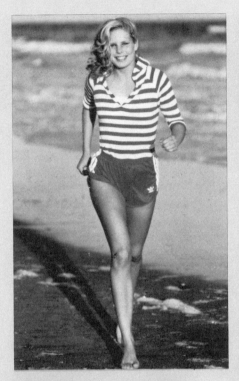

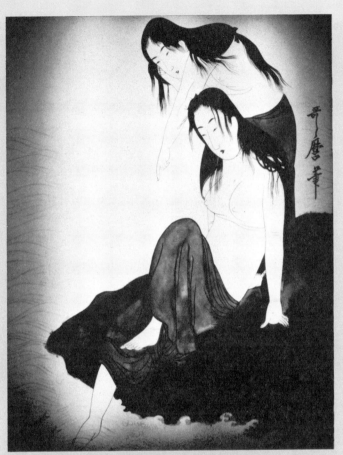

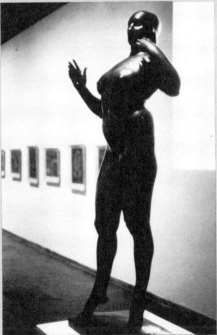

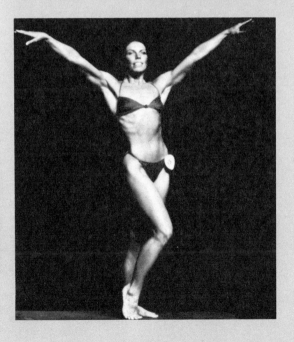

Each of these women is considered beautiful by the standards of her culture. Which do you suppose are healthy? Perhaps all of them?

The same individual may use energy with different efficiency at different times, depending partly on how much the person weighs at the time, and partly on other factors. Sometimes, for example, you may lose more weight than you might predict from your food intake; this may be explained by an increase in energy wastage that occurs during stress — even the "good" stress, exercise.[3] You might have said, when you felt this was going on, "I'm burning up a lot of kcalories in nervous energy," or "My metabolism has been racing lately." What you are sensing is that the kcalorie-bearing nutrients from the food you have eaten are not being efficiently converted to usable energy currency like fat as they normally are. By

[3]E. A. Newsholme, A possible metabolic basis for the control of body weight (Sounding Board), *New England Journal of Medicine* 302 (1980):400-405.

analogy: You could put a package on an elevator and send it up to the eighth floor; or for the same cost in electricity you could send the elevator up part way and back down to the first floor. In the first case, work is accomplished; the package has been delivered to the eighth floor (this is analogous to the storing of fat). In the second case, an equal amount of energy has been spent but no work has been accomplished (no fat has been stored). So one person eats and stores fat; another eats and does not.

There is a chemical explanation for the difference. The first person's body's enzymes have smoothly converted the nutrients eaten to other substances while efficiently extracting and storing all the energy from them. The second person's body's enzymes have converted the nutrients to some substance, then to another, then back to the

first, then back to the second. (Chemists call this action shuttling. Each of the chemical reactions entails a loss of energy as heat; nothing is stored.

This metabolic difference between people also fits the analogy of a water wheel. When water turns the wheel, the wheel turns a gear that operates machinery inside the mill. Work is done. Some of the enzymes in cells operate very much as if they were connected by gears. They are situated in complexes next to each other, and when one acts, it drives its neighbor to act. The reactions these enzymes perform are called *coupled reactions* (see Highlight 7A). But the gears can be disconnected so that the wheel will continue turning without operating any machinery inside the mill. As with the elevator: energy is now being "wasted," not stored. Chemically, this is known as *uncoupling:* The

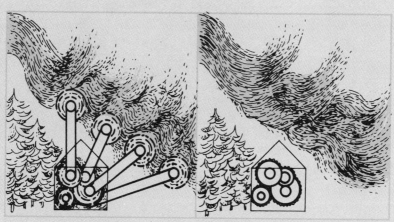

In both cases the same amount of energy is being spent, but only when the gears are engaged is work done. (In the body, fat is stored only when the metabolic gears are engaged. Sometimes kcalories are taken from food without fat storage.)

reaction that spends energy keeps on going without driving the reaction that stores energy. With such a disruption of the normally conservative system, a person can seem to be breaking the rules — that is, can eat kcalories and not store fat.

Within one person, metabolism may shift, being efficient and conservative at one time, inefficient and wasteful at another. The thyroid hormone, which regulates the body's metabolic rate, works by bringing about changes from one kind of metabolism to the other. In the cold, for example, the body produces more heat. People say their metabolism speeds up. Actually, the thyroid hormone signals the metabolic pathways to uncouple at key places to generate heat rather than to store energy.

The thinking reader may perceive an application implied by these facts: Why not use thyroid hormone to make people lose weight? This ingenious solution to the stubborn problem of obesity has been tried, and it works. Thyroid hormone does uncouple the using of kcalories from fat storage, but unfortunately the benefits are outweighed by hazards in the form of lean body tissue damage, including heart damage.[4]

[4]*Physicians' Desk Reference*, 34th ed. (Oradell, N.J.: Medical Economics Company, Litton Industries, 1980), pp. 570, 1302, 1616, and others.

Natural selection, too, has used these facts to meet the needs of hibernating animals, who need to use their body fat at one time to support activities (work) and at another to provide heat. These animals actually make two kinds of fat — white fat, which fuels work, and brown fat, which only releases heat. Humans, too — although they don't hibernate — possess some brown fat as well as white fat, and it is possible that the type of fat a person possesses determines whether that person is an energy conserver (fat type) or energy waster (thin type).[5]

Whatever the case may be, all of these examples show that body cells have ways of choosing whether to store or spend energy. This may provide a clue to the way the body maintains its weight. If you eat more than usual on a given day, you may metabolize it faster (more wastefully) than usual, so that you don't gain weight as you might expect. Conversely, if you eat less than usual, you may conserve more of it than usual, so that you don't lose weight as you might expect. If this is so, it helps to explain why gaining and losing weight are equally hard to do (if you are at your "set point"), and may also ac-

[5]N. J. Rothwell and M. J. Stock, Regulation of energy balance, in *Annual Review of Nutrition*, ed. W. J. Darby, H. P. Broquist, and R. E. Olsen, vol. 1 (Palo Alto: Annual Reviews, Inc., 1981), pp. 235-256.

count for the mysterious plateaus at which both weight gainers and weight losers tend to get stuck.

It has long been suspected that obese people's metabolism in some sense "slows down" whenever they go on a diet. The facts being presented here may explain why this happens. At least some fat people may have a high set point. In counseling them, the diet advisor may have to think as follows:

Fat Person: I'd like to lose two pounds a week. I lose no weight when I eat 2,000 kcalories a day.

Advisor: Well, then, perhaps you should cut back your intake by 1,000 kcalories a day. That's supposed to be enough to lose two pounds a week.

Fat Person: OK, I'll eat 1,000 kcalories a day.

Advisor: (mutters to himself): No, well, as soon as you cut back, your metabolism will slow down by, maybe, 15 percent. Right now, your metabolism probably costs about 1,500 kcalories a day. Your diet will reduce that by up to 300 kcalories. So . . . hm . . . your stay-even level will not be 2,000 while you're dieting, it'll only be 1,700, and that means . . . ahem . . . to lose a pound a week you'll have to eat 700 . . . oh, dear, that's hardly enough to keep a stressed body alive, much less healthy.

Advisor (aloud): Tell you what: How about aiming for one pound a week, rather than two? Theoretically, you should be able to do that on 1,500 kcalories a day, but I think you'd better cut back to 1,200 kcalories a day. (Thinks to himself: "Later I'll suggest exercise, too.")

This is bad news for the dieter. It sounds like hard work, which it is. It is often enough to drive the dieter away in search of easier-appearing remedies and promises of magic. But it's the hard truth that has to be faced in many cases.

This section has shown that the body can alter its energy output by invisible means, by changing the activity of its enzymes, so that kcalories taken in end up sometimes stored in fat and sometimes dissipated into the air as radiated heat. The body also alters its energy intake, by deciding how much food to ask you to eat. How it does this is the subject of the next section.

Altered Intake: Hunger

How do you decide how much to eat? Do you ever say, "Well, let's see: I spent about 600 kcalories this afternoon so I'll eat about 600 kcalories for dinner"? Many people count the kcalories they *eat*, but if anyone consciously counts the kcalories they *spend*, that person has yet to confess to it. Yet you are

---

Miniglossary

brown fat: fat cells whose enzymes oxidize fat without using the energy released to do work (see *uncoupling*); the energy is released as heat. In humans, the predominant type of fat is **white fat**, in which fat breakdown is coupled to the making of usable energy-carrying compounds that can do work.

catch-up growth: the rapid rate of growth seen in a child or young animal fed adequately after a period of deprivation.

coupled reaction: a pair of chemical reactions that occur simultaneously; one drives the other. (Some of the energy released by one reaction is consumed by the other.)

coupling: see *coupled reaction.*

set point: the point at which controls are set (for example, on a thermostat). In the case of body weight, the set point is that point above which the body tends to lose, and below which it tends to gain, weight.

shuttling: going back and forth. In a metabolic pathway in which (for example) A is converted to B, B to C, and C to D, shuttling might occur as follows: A to B to C to B to C to B to C to D.

uncoupling: the separation of a coupled reaction so that all the energy released is lost without doing any work (see also *coupled reaction*).

---

somehow counting kcalories unconsciously; and the result is the magnitude of your hunger. All that emerges to consciousness is a thought like: "Pass the butter," or "No thanks, I'm just not hungry tonight." But what governs hunger?

To answer this question would be to win the Nobel Prize. Many attempts are presently being made. Evidently many factors are involved. Over the short term, hunger is responsive to cues from the stomach and the brain; over the long term, hunger seems to be responsive to the amount of heat the body is generating (thermostatic control), the amount of glucose that is circulating in the blood (glucostatic control), and the amount of fat the body has stored (lipostatic control). All of these types of control are believed to work so that an individual eats just enough, but not too much, to achieve or maintain the body's set-point weight.

Short-term regulation refers to the signals that tell you when to stop eating a particular meal. As soon as you start eating, hunger begins to decrease. Several things are happening at once: The stomach is getting full and its stretch-sensitive nerves are sending messages to the brain; the brain's hypothalamus is detecting raised blood glucose; heat is being generated; glycogen and fat are being manufactured and stored in the cells. Somewhere in the interplay of all these processes, one or more events finally flip the switch that turns off eating behavior and you stop eating.

When you end a meal, you may have eaten just enough to compensate for the kcalories you spent prior to the meal. But if you didn't, then long-term control mechanisms would enter the picture to adjust your intakes on the next few days. Let's say you ate too much; then these controls ensure that your next few meals are more widely spaced; that you eat less often. Or, you may find yourself compensating by eating a smaller meal the next time or two.

How do these long-term controls work? To choose just one of the possibilities, suppose the brain keeps track of the body's total fat content. It could do this by making a certain amount of a hormone — one that is soluble in fat — and sending this hormone out to the body tissues. Some of this hormone would dissolve in the body fat and stay there. By measuring the amount that came back, the brain would have an indirect measure of the body fat. It could then adjust appetite accordingly — and, for that matter, it could send signals to "waste more energy" or "conserve more energy," whichever the need might be. Thus, it could adjust both what you eat (intake) and what you spend (output).

The Balance Between Intake and Output   The preceding example was given in purely theoretical terms because it is too early to know how long-term controls really operate to manage body weight. It is important to understand from all this, however, the point that we do *not* understand how body weight is regulated. But it clearly is, and many factors seem to be working together in this regulation. The system deserves respect. To tinker with it without a full understanding is to take unknown risks.

For example: Suppose the body, for whatever reason, "has" to maintain a certain amount of fat in proportion to its lean. Suppose further that in some people, this set amount of fat is quite high, so that they tend to be obese. Now suppose such a person tries to lose weight. It will be difficult, because all the systems just described will oppose the effort. Hunger will persist, and metabolic conservation measures will make the body tend to hang onto its fat. Still, if the person exerts immense willpower and tries to starve him/herself, some measure of "success" (weight loss) may be registered on the scale. But what will that weight loss reflect? What tissue do starving people lose? Lean, protein tissue, working metabolic tissue, the very part of the body's materials the obese person can least afford to

lose. The lean body mass is the body's kcalorie-*spending* part, and to lose it means to make it even harder to burn up kcalories.

This description of the bind one might get into if one tried to lose weight below one's set point is not entirely fanciful. Genetically obese rats, when forced to lose weight, lose body lean tissue in proportion to the fat they lose. If they are forced to reach the same weight as normal rats, they develop extremely skinny lean bodies underneath their fat, as if they were sacrificing lean tissue in order to maintain fat.[6] This is malnutrition hidden in a cloak of fat, and is probably as unhealthy as, or more so than, the original state of obesity. It may be best in such cases to choose a middle ground — that weight, whatever it is, at which the *lean body* is most healthy.

Implications for Ideal Weight   While researchers have been attempting to discover what makes the body stick at a certain weight, insurance companies have been asking what weight is best for health. In 1900 it was thought that to be thin was dangerous, because of the risk of tuberculosis; but by 1920 it was evident that to be fat was also unhealthy because of the increased risk of

[6]Regulation of food intake in fatty and lean growing Zucker rats, *Nutrition Reviews* 35 (1977):181-183.

Table 1. Average Weights of U.S. Citizens — 1980*

Height (in)	Weight (lb) Age 18-24	Age 25-34	Age 35-44	Age 45-54	Age 55-64	Age 65-74	Height (in)	(Weight (lb)) Age 18-24	Age 25-34	Age 35-44	Age 45-54	Age 55-64	Age 65-74
Men							**Women**						
62	130	141	143	147	143	143	57	114	118	125	129	132	130
63	135	145	148	152	147	147	58	117	121	129	133	136	134
64	140	150	153	156	153	151	59	120	125	133	136	140	137
65	145	156	158	160	158	156	60	123	128	137	140	143	140
66	150	160	163	164	163	160	61	126	132	141	143	147	144
67	154	165	169	169	168	164	62	129	136	144	147	150	147
68	159	170	174	173	173	169	63	132	139	148	150	153	151
69	164	174	179	177	178	173	64	135	142	152	154	157	154
70	168	179	184	182	183	177	65	138	146	156	158	160	158
71	173	184	190	187	189	182	66	141	150	159	161	164	161
72	178	189	194	191	193	186	67	144	153	163	165	167	165
73	183	194	200	196	197	190	68	147	157	167	168	171	169
74	188	199	205	200	203	194							

*From the HANES Survey, 1980. For comparison, look on the inside back cover at the "ideal weights" published by the insurance companies. Also notice that weights are given for older age groups. The insurance company tables assumed that the weight that was ideal at 25 would be ideal throughout life; this table permits weight gain to take place until middle age.

heart attacks, strokes, and other causes of death associated with obesity. "Ideal weights" were set at the levels at which insured people were most likely to live the longest. The "ideal weight tables" on the inside back cover are the result of this effort.

As of 1983, however, the table weights were being revised upwards as the result of a discovery. "Insured people" are not the same as "all people." People who apply for insurance are more likely than others to have high blood pressure, and obesity raises the blood pressure further, shortening their average lifespans. But for people who don't have high blood pressure, being fat, within reason, does not shorten life. A broad range of

weight is compatible with good health and long life.[7]

The new ideal weights are shown on the inside back cover. They are higher than the old ones. In fact, they are close to the average weights for the whole U.S. population, shown in Table 1. For many people, this means that the body's set-point weight — the weight at which it tends to stay — is actually its ideal weight, too, in terms of health and life expectancy.

[7]A. Keys, Overweight, obesity, coronary heart disease and mortality, *Nutrition Reviews* 38 (1980):297-307. This lecture was also published in *Nutrition Today*, July/August 1980, pp. 16-22.

It is too early to know how many people this idea may apply to, but certainly it does not apply to people who are unhealthy because of their present weight. People who have high blood pressure, especially, can benefit by losing weight and should make the effort to do so. Someone who feels stuck at a very high weight should not feel that weight loss is impossible. A way, not discussed here, to change your set point is to increase lean body mass by exercise. Dieting will also pay off, if you persist for a long time using the sound principles outlined in the chapter. Don't give up.

If you ever have to go to the hospital, and if you are fortunate enough to go to a hospital in which nutrition assessment and care receive the attention they deserve, you may be asked these questions on admission:

- What is your height? (Better: The questioner will measure your height.)
- What is your weight? (Better: The questioner will weigh you.)
- What is your *usual weight?*

The concept of usual body weight is so useful in clinical nutrition that it is given the abbreviation UBW and is used as one of the parameters in nutrition assessment (see Chapter 18).

This Highlight has presented a new idea: that a moderate degree of fatness may be "ideal" in many cases — if health rather than fashion-model beauty defines "ideal." This concept may be difficult for many young people, especially young women, to accept. They are likely to react "Well, sure, I know that's OK for my health, but it's not so beautiful to be so fat. For fashion's sake, I have to be thin." And it's true: "Thin" is still "in," as of 1982, in the fashion world. But fashions are changing. The time may come when it is stylish to be healthy, and the conflict between the natural, set point weight and the ideal weight will melt away.

To Explore Further

The new concepts presented here about regulation of body weight were reviewed with great insight and clarity by:

- Rothwell, N. J., and Stock, M.J. Regulation of energy balance, in *Annual Review of Nutrition,* ed. W. J. Darby, H. P. Broquist, and R. E. Olson, vol. 1. Palo Alto: Annual Reviews, Inc., 1981, pp. 235-256.

An early, but still comprehensive and valid, review of how hunger works is:

- Lepkovsky, S. Regulation of food intake. *Advances in Food Research* 21 (1975):1-69.

Some later thoughts on how hunger may be regulated have been contributed by:

- Van Itallie, T. B., Smith, N. S., and Quartermain, D. Short-term and long-term components in the regulation of food intake: evidence for a modulatory role of carbohydrate status. *American Journal of Clinical Nutrition* 30 (1977):742-757.

The researcher who first explained to the nutrition community how the new ideal weights were arrived at published his remarks in:

- Keys, A. Overweight, obesity, coronary heart disease and mortality. *Nutrition Reviews* 38 (1980):297-307. This lecture was also published in *Nutrition Today,* July/August 1980, pp. 16-22.

A discussion of Keys' impact on the ideal weight concept and the bases for the new tables appeared in:

- Controversy 8: Ideal Weight, in Hamilton, E. M. N., and Whitney, E. N. *Nutrition: Concepts and Controversies,* 2nd ed. St. Paul: West, 1981, pp. 246-251.

Among the many references showing the anomalies and discrepancies in people's energy balances and body weights are two excellent reviews:

- Hegsted, D. M. Energy needs and energy utilization.
- Barnes, R. H. Energy.

These reviews appear as Chapters 1 and 2 (pp. 1-9 and 10-16) in *Nutrition Reviews' Present Knowledge in Nutrition,* 4th ed. Washington, D.C.: Nutrition Foundation, 1976.

Diet Planning

The exchange system can be used to plan diets for weight loss, weight gain, or maintenance. For practice in the use of this convenient system, try planning two diets, one for weight maintenance or gain, the other for weight loss. Use your own "personalized RDA for energy," derived in the Chapter 7 Self-Study, as a baseline for planning.

This is not, incidentally, a "make-work" exercise. Although the use of the exchange system takes practice, it is well worth the time spent. Anyone who needs to plan or follow a diet, for any reason, will find that it soon becomes *easier* through use of the exchange system than it would be any other way.

Diet for Weight Maintenance or Gain

1. Set your daily kcalorie level. If you choose to maintain weight, it should be equal to your "personalized RDA." If you wish to gain weight, it should be at least 500 kcal above your "RDA."
2. Decide on the ratio of protein:fat:carbohydrate kcalories to be delivered by the diet. A suggested ratio is:

about 10 to 15 percent of the kcalories from protein, not more than 30 percent from fat, and the rest from carbohydrate. Given the daily kcalorie level you chose, how many kcalories will you allot to each nutrient?
3. Translate these kcalorie amounts into grams. (Remember, 1 g protein or carbohydrate = 4 kcal; 1 g fat = 9 kcal.) Enter these gram amounts at the top of Form 1.
4. Now decide how many exchanges of milk, vegetables, and fruit you'd like to have each day; enter these numbers in the form; and compute the number of grams of carbohydrate, protein, and fat they will deliver (don't compute kcalories

Form 1.   Diet Planning by Exchange Groups

Exchange group	Number of exchanges*	Amounts to be delivered†			
		Carbohydrate (g)	Protein (g)	Fat (g)	Energy‡ (kcal)
Milk					
Vegetable					
Fruit					
Bread					
Meat					
Fat					
	Total actually delivered				

*From steps 4, 5, 6.
†From step 3.
‡From step 7.

yet). See p. 39 or Appendix L for the exchange system values. (Caution: Use pencil. You'll want to change these numbers several times before you finalize your plan.)

Only one more group of foods — the bread exchanges — contribute any carbohydrate to the diet. Select the number of bread exchanges that will bring your total carbohydrate intake close to the amount you want. Adjust the numbers of these four exchanges until they seem reasonable to you.

(Suggestions: Diets for adults should include two to three milk exchanges daily, two or more vegetable exchanges, and at least two and preferably more fruit exchanges. The number of bread exchanges is variable, but the bread list includes many nutritious foods containing complex carbohydrates. It is not unusual for women's diets to include four to six bread exchanges and for men's to include twice as many or even more. High-kcalorie diets can have many more of all of these carbohydrate-containing exchanges.)

If you have a special fondness for sugar or sugar-containing foods, add a line to Form 1 under Bread, and allow yourself some "sugar exchanges" (see p. 40). At the end of this step, you should have a carbohydrate gram total within about 10

percent of the number you planned in step 3.

5. Subtotal the protein grams delivered by these four groups of foods. Only one more group of foods — the meat exchanges — will contribute any protein to the diet. Select the number of meat exchanges you need to bring your total protein intake close to what you planned in step 3.

Note: The recommended intake of carbohydrate is high compared to what many people are used to. Planners often find that once they have completed step 4 of this procedure they have already used up their protein allowance and must therefore drastically limit their meat consumption. If it works out this way for you, you have two choices. You can accept the dictates of this pattern and resolve to limit your meat intake accordingly. Or you can increase the number of protein grams you will allow yourself (step 3) and reduce carbohydrate and/or fat to keep the kcalorie level within bounds.

At the end of this step, you should have a protein gram total that agrees (within 10 percent) with your plan of step 3.

6. Subtotal the fat grams delivered by these five groups of foods. Now use the fat exchanges to bring your total fat intake up to the level planned in step 3.

7. Fill in the kcalorie amounts contributed by the exchanges you have selected, and check to see that the total agrees (within 10 percent) with the kcalorie level you set in step 1. The completed form now indicates the total exchanges of each type that you will consume on each day of your diet.

8. Distribute the exchanges you have selected into a meal pattern like that of Form 2. You may want to plan four to six meals a day or to have three meals and one snack; if so, or if you have other preferences, make your own form.

9. Finally, to see how your diet plan might work out on an actual day, make a sample menu. Look over the exchange groups and choose foods you would like to eat in each category that fit the pattern you worked out in step 8. For example:

My meal pattern for breakfast specifies:
    1 fruit
    2 bread
    1 milk
    1 sugar
    1 fat
So I might choose:
    1/2 c orange juice
    3/4 oz dry cereal and
      1 slice bread, toasted
    1/2 c milk on the cereal
and
    1/2 c milk in a glass
    1 tsp sugar on the cereal
    1 pat margarine on the
      toast

Diet for Weight Loss

1. Set your daily kcalorie level. If you wish to lose a pound a week, set it 500 kcal per day below your "personalized RDA." You could set it higher or lower than this, but on no account should you set it below 1,000 kcal per day.

2. Decide on the ratio of protein:fat:carbohydrate kcalories to be delivered by the diet. A suggested ratio is that offered in Table 1 of Chapter 8: about 33 percent of the kcalories from each energy nutrient.

3. Translate these kcalorie amounts into grams, as in the previous diet plan.

4. Now decide on the number of carbohydrate-containing exchanges you'll have, as in step 4 of the preceding exercise. Try to include two milk, two vegetable, and at least two fruit exchanges, and make up the rest of your carbohydrate intake with bread exchanges. Allow no sugar unless you really can't do without it. At the end of this step you should have a carbohydrate gram total within about 10 percent of the number you planned in step 3.

5. Now subtotal the protein grams you have so far, and bring your total protein intake up to the level of your plan by adding meat ex-

changes. At the end of this step, you should have a protein gram total that agrees (within 10 percent) with your plan of step 3.

6. Now subtotal the fat grams you have so far, and add fat exchanges to bring your total fat intake up to the level planned in step 3.

7. Fill in the kcalorie amounts contributed by the exchanges you have selected, and check to see that the total agrees (within 10 percent) with the kcalorie level you set in step 1.

8. Distribute the exchanges into a meal pattern, using Form 2 or your own form based on your own preference.

Form 2.   Meal Patterns

Exchange group	Total exchanges consumed daily*	Exchanges consumed at each meal				
		Breakfast	**Lunch**	**Snack**	**Dinner**	**Snack**
Milk						
Vegetable						
Fruit						
Bread						
Meat						
Fat						

*From Form 1, column 2.

9. Make a day's sample menus, as in step 9 of the preceding exercise.

Adding Exercise to the Diet Plan

Just to make sure you lose weight, plan to spend an hour a day three times a week engaging in some activity. Study the table presented here and find your favorite activity. Using your actual weight as the basis for calculation, figure how many kcalories you'd spend on an hour of that activity. How many, then, would you spend in three hours a week? How many days would it take you to lose a pound from participating in this activity? Plan to spend an hour three days a week, and estimate the number of pounds' difference this will make in a year.

Table 1. Approximate Energy Expenditure by a 150-Pound Person in Various Activities*

Activity	Energy (kcal/hr)
Lying down or sleeping	80
Driving an automobile	120
Standing	140
Domestic work	180
Walking, $2\ 1/2$ mph	210
Bicycling, $5\ 1/2$ mph	210
Gardening	220
Golf; lawn mowing, power mower	250
Bowling	270
Walking, $3\ 3/4$ mph	300
Swimming, $1/4$ mph	300
Square dancing, volleyball, roller skating	350
Wood chopping or sawing	400
Tennis	420
Skiing, 10 mph	600
Squash and handball	600
Bicycling, 13 mph	660
Running, 10 mph	900

*From the USDA/USDHHS Dietary Guidelines. Based on material prepared by Robert E. Johnson, M.D., Ph.D., and colleagues, University of Illinois.

PART TWO

VITAMINS, MINERALS, AND WATER

INTRODUCTION

CONTENTS

SUPPORTING ACTORS

The introduction to Part One identified the nutrients: carbohydrate, lipid, protein, vitamins, minerals, and water. The eight chapters in Part One were devoted entirely to the first three of these—the principal actors—whose presence in the body accounts for what you are (you are literally made of these three materials and compounds derived from them) and for what you do (because they supply the energy for all your activities).

As you saw, each of those three nutrients is a giant by molecular standards. A single molecule of carbohydrate may be composed of 300 glucose units, each containing 24 atoms, for a total of some 7,000 atoms. Lipids and proteins are similar in size. Even when they are broken down during digestion, they are absorbed as sizable units—and these are often reassembled in the cells back into macromolecules. Only if they are oxidized for fuel do they diminish in size to tiny molecules of carbon dioxide and water (three atoms each). If this occurs, they release tremendous quantities of energy for your use.

Furthermore, you eat (by molecular standards) tremendous quantities of these three nutrients: a hundred or so grams a day of each. If you could purify the carbohydrate, lipid, and protein in your daily diet, they would fill two or three cups.

The second three nutrients—vitamins, minerals, and water—differ profoundly from the first three in almost every way: in their size and shape, in the roles they play in the body, in the amounts you consume. Perhaps the only characteristics they share with the first three are that they are vital to life and that they are available in food.

Chapters 9 to 14 are devoted to these nutrients: three to the vitamins, two to the minerals, and one to water. A few generalizations presented here will help you put these supporting actors in perspective.

Carbohydrate, fat, and protein: large organic molecules.

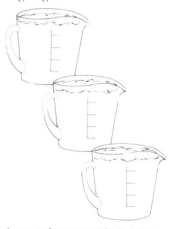

Amount of energy nutrients eaten daily
Carbohydrate, fat, and protein: 50-200 g a day of each.

Vitamins: small organic molecules.

Vitamins: yield no energy.

vitamin: an organic compound vital to life, needed in minute amounts. (The first vitamins discovered were amines.)

vita = life

amine = containing nitrogen

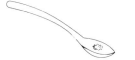

Amount of vitamins eaten daily

Organic: see p. 5.

Vitamins

The vitamins are organic compounds generally much smaller than the energy nutrients. A molecule of vitamin C, for example, is comparable in size to a single glucose unit. Vitamins are never strung together to make body compounds (although each may be attached to a protein), and if they are broken down they yield no usable energy. You consume minute amounts of vitamins daily—a few micrograms (millionths of a gram) or milligrams (thousandths of a gram) or, at the very most, a few grams. Yet they are vital; in fact, they were named for this characteristic. As you will see in Chapters 9 to 11, they serve as helpers, making possible the processes by which the first three nutrients are digested, absorbed, and metabolized in the body. There are some 15 different vitamins, each with its own special roles to play.

Vitamins as Organic Substances   The fact that vitamins are organic has several consequences. For one, vitamins are destructible. They can be broken down, oxidized, altered in shape. They must therefore be handled with care. Your body makes special provisions to absorb them, providing several of them with custom-made protein carriers like those provided for the lipids. A vitamin may be useful in one form here and another there, so special enzymes are also provided that can slightly alter the form of a vitamin to make it active in a given role.

> Many vitamins exist in several related forms.

The destructibility of vitamins also has implications for their handling outside the body. Food handlers and cooks are well-advised to be aware of the vulnerability of the vitamins in foods and to treat them with respect.

> Vitamins are destructible.

Fat-Soluble and Water-Soluble Vitamins   As you may recall, some organic compounds are hydrophilic (water-loving), because positive and negative charges abound on their surfaces and so attract them to the positive (H^+) and negative (OH^-) ions of water. Others are hydrophobic (water-avoiding) and are attracted into the neighborhood of the uncharged, fat-loving compounds. Carbohydrates and proteins are in the first and lipids in the second category. The vitamins are divided between these classes: some are water-soluble (the B vitamins and vitamin C) and others are fat-soluble (vitamins A, D, E, and K).

> Water-soluble vitamins: B complex and C.
> Fat-soluble vitamins: A, D, E, K.

This fact has several implications for vitamin absorption, transport, storage, and excretion.

Absorption of Vitamins The digestive system absorbs these two types of substances differently. Water-soluble substances cross the intestinal and vascular walls directly into the blood, but fat-soluble substances are handled laboriously. Except for the short-chain fatty acids, fat-soluble substances must be emulsified and carried across the membranes of the intestinal cells associated with fat and often with bile. They cannot cross the blood vessel walls to enter the bloodstream directly but must be transported by way of the lymph, from which they later enter the bloodstream.

Lymphatic system: see pp. 181-182.

> Water-soluble vitamins: absorbed into blood.
> Fat-soluble vitamins: absorbed into lymph with fat.

Transport of Vitamins The body's principal transportation system—the bloodstream—is a system of waterways. Water-soluble vitamins travel freely dissolved in blood; fat-soluble vitamins must be made soluble in water by being attached to protein carriers.

> Water-soluble vitamins: free in blood.
> Fat-soluble vitamins: carried by proteins.

Storage and Excretion of Vitamins Once the fat-soluble vitamins have been absorbed and transported to cells of the body, they tend to become sequestered there, associated with fat. The water-soluble vitamins, on the other hand, are not held so firmly in place. If they are not in use, they circulate freely among all organs of the body, including the kidneys.

The body's principal excretion medium is also water. The kidneys are sensitive to high concentrations of substances in the blood that flows through them. They selectively remove those substances in excess and pass them into the urine. The kidneys detect and remove excess water-soluble vitamins, but they less readily detect excess fat-soluble vitamins, because these do not accumulate in the blood; they tend to be hidden away in fat-storage places in the body.

> Water-soluble vitamins: excesses excreted.
> Fat-soluble vitamins: excesses stored.

This difference has two implications. First, excess vitamin A eaten today may be stored to meet next month's needs, and blood levels will remain normal. But if too much vitamin C is in the blood, the kidneys respond by excreting the excess, and tomorrow's needs will be met by depleting the vitamin C pool in the blood. Thus vitamin A can be eaten in large amounts once in a while and still meet your body's needs over the interval. But vitamin C must be eaten in smaller amounts more frequently.

> Water-soluble vitamins: needed in frequent small doses.
> Fat-soluble vitamins: can be taken in larger doses less often.

The B vitamin riboflavin is a yellow compound so bright that it is easy to see in a water solution. Since excesses of the B vitamins are excreted, bright yellow urine may signify the presence of this vitamin. If you are in the habit of taking a multivitamin supplement "to avoid deficiencies" and your diet is otherwise adequate, you may notice this effect.

Some vitamin supplements are inexpensive, but others entail costs far above the value they confer on you in preventing possible deficiencies. As you read on, you may discover that it is easy to make your diet adequate by eating nutritious foods alone and that you do not need a vitamin supplement. If you do consume an adequate diet, the following statement may apply to you:

> Overdosing with B vitamins may not hurt you, but it will do nothing for you except to increase the dollar value of your urine.

The difference in the body's handling of excess fat-soluble and water-soluble vitamins has a second implication: Because the water-soluble vitamins are excreted almost as rapidly as they are taken in, toxicity from overdoses occurs transiently if at all. The fat-soluble vitamins, however, can accumulate and reach toxic levels in body stores. This is known to occur with vitamins A and D in particular.

If you help yourself to a second piece of pecan pie at dinner, you are aware that you are eating more food. The sheer bulk of the energy nutrients and water in the pie makes you feel full. You know, too, that you are eating more kcalories. But excess vitamin intakes can be undetectable. The amount of vitamin A you need, in pure form, is but a droplet a day. Ten times as much is still only a few drops. This means that it is far easier to take an overdose of vitamins, especially in pure form (pills or drops), than of energy nutrients.

> Water-soluble vitamins: toxicity unlikely.
> Fat-soluble vitamins: toxicity likely.

Vitamins and the Four Food Group Plan   Throughout Part One, we made frequent reference to the exchange system of grouping foods, because that system is based on the carbohydrate-fat-protein composition of foods. Now that the vitamins are under consideration, the Four Food Group Plan becomes more useful. The grouping of foods in this plan is based largely on their protein, vitamin, and mineral contents. The first group, milk and milk products, includes the foods that make outstanding contributions of the vitamin riboflavin and the mineral calcium, as well as protein. The second group, meats and meat substitutes, is notable for its contributions of several B vitamins and the mineral iron, besides protein. Because of their high concentrations of riboflavin and calcium and their low concentrations of iron, the cheeses (which in the exchange system were treated as meat substitutes) are classified with milk and milk products in this plan. The third group, the vegetable and fruit group, is notable for its vitamin A and C contents, and the fourth, the grain products, adds important B vitamins and iron to the total. A review of the description of the Four Food Group Plan in Chapter 1 is recommended before you proceed with the chapters to come.

Minerals

As Chapters 12 and 13 will explain, the minerals are inorganic compounds, smaller than vitamins and found in still more simple forms in foods. Table salt, for example, is the principal source of the minerals sodium and chlorine; it enters the body as a two-atom pair (NaCl). Some minerals may be put together into building blocks for structures such as bones and teeth — but only with the help of the lively enzymes, which arrange them in orderly arrays. When minerals are withdrawn from bone and excreted, they yield no energy. They may also float about in the fluids of the body, by their presence giving the fluids certain characteristics, but they are not metabolized — arranged and rearranged — in the complicated ways or to the same extent as the energy nutrients are. You consume only small amounts of minerals daily, comparable to the amounts of vitamins in your diet. There are some 20 or 30 different minerals important in nutrition.

Minerals: small inorganic molecules.

Na and Cl: symbols for sodium and chlorine (see Appendix B).

Minerals: yield no energy.

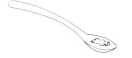

Amount of minerals eaten daily

Minerals as Inorganic Substances   The minerals are elements — like carbon, hydrogen, oxygen, and nitrogen of which the energy nutrients are composed — and so are simpler than the vitamins, which are compounds. Because they contain no carbon, minerals are inorganic; they need never have been part of a living thing. This means that the variety of forms they may take is more limited than for the vitamins; that is, minerals cannot have different chemical structures. Calcium, for example, enters the body as an ion with two positive charges. It may be combined with any of a number of negative ions

Element and compound: see Appendix B.

Ion: see Appendix B.

salt: a compound composed of two ions other than H^+ and OH^-, such as $CaCl_2$ or $NaCl$ ($Ca^{++}Cl_2{}^-$ or Na^+Cl^-), held together by an ionic bond (electrostatic attraction). See Chapter 14 and Appendix B.

ionic state: the number of positive or negative charges that an ion may carry. The two states of iron are explained in Appendix B.

(phosphate, sulfate, and the like) to form salts in foods. The calcium may be more absorbable in these combinations, but in the body these dissociate, and the calcium ion itself is what is used. Some minerals, however, do play key roles as part of large organic complexes. For example, the iron in hemoglobin is responsible for that protein's oxygen-carrying function, and many minerals are responsible for the specificity of enzymes. Still, even in these associations, the minerals remain distinct.

Minerals exist as inorganic ions.

The Indestructibility of Minerals An atom of iron may exist in two different ionic states, and it may be combined with a variety of other ions in salts, but it never loses its identity. It is always iron. Cooking it, exposing it to air or acid, or mixing it with other substances has no effect on it. In fact, if you burn a food until only the ash is left and eat the ash, you will be eating all the minerals that were in the food before it was burned. Once they have entered your body they are there until excreted; they cannot be changed into anything else.

Minerals retain their chemical identity.

Because they are indestructible, minerals in food need no special handling to preserve them. You need only make sure that you don't soak them out of the food or throw them away in cooking water. As long as they are kept in the food, they may be handled in any way whatever without any effect on the amount of the mineral present.

Minerals and Water By virtue of being ionic, minerals tend to associate with water and thus tend to form either acidic or basic solutions.

Mineral ions are water-soluble.

Acid-base balance: see p. 127 and Chapter 14.

Water balance: see p. 125 and Chapter 14.

Because minerals are water-soluble, they influence the acid-base balance of the body. In associating with other ions in the body fluids, they affect the distribution of water into the various body compartments.

Absorption, Transport, and Excretion of Minerals Like the water-soluble vitamins, some minerals are readily absorbed into the blood, transported freely, and readily excreted by the kidneys. There are exceptions, however. Each mineral differs in the amounts the body can absorb and in the extent to which it must be handled specially and transported by protein or other organic carriers.

> Minerals vary in the amounts absorbed and in the routes and ease of excretion.

Like fat-soluble vitamins, some minerals must have carriers to be absorbed and to travel in the blood. Others travel freely as ions.

> Some minerals require carriers.

Some are stored like the fat-soluble vitamins and like them are therefore toxic if taken in excess. Because their presence is not obvious in foods, overdosing with toxic minerals is a real possibility.

> Some minerals are toxic in excess.

Toxic in excess: iron, copper, chlorine, magnesium, manganese, iodine, fluorine, and others.

Other minerals do not accumulate in the body but are readily excreted; toxicity with these is not a risk.

In publishing its 1980 recommendations, the U.S. Committee on RDA gave ranges of safe intakes for many of the trace minerals and made a point of saying that the upper limits should not habitually be exceeded.

Minerals in the Diet The amount of minerals needed in the daily diet varies from a few micrograms for minerals like cobalt to a million times as much, a gram or more, for minerals like calcium, phosphorus, and sodium. The amount of each mineral found in the body varies equally widely. Thus many authorities divide them into two categories: the major minerals (Chapter 12) and the trace minerals (Chapter 13). A diet made up of a wide variety of foods is certain to provide enough minerals in both categories.

Water

Water is abundant, indispensable, and often ignored—because like air, it is everywhere and we take it for granted. Water is inorganic, a single molecule being composed of three atoms (H_2O).[1] The amounts you must consume relative to the other nutrients are enormous: 2 to 3 l a day. That's 2,000 to 3,000 grams, about ten times the amount of energy nutrients you need. Of course, you need not drink water as such in these quantities; it comes abundantly in foods and beverages. The specific ways that the body uses water are described in Chapter 14.

Water: small inorganic molecule.

Water: yields no energy.

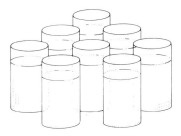

Amount of water needed daily

[1]A more accurate way to describe how water is organized would be to say that, although we know that the ratio of hydrogen atoms to oxygen atoms is 2:1, we do not know that water exists as discrete molecules.

CHAPTER 9

CONTENTS

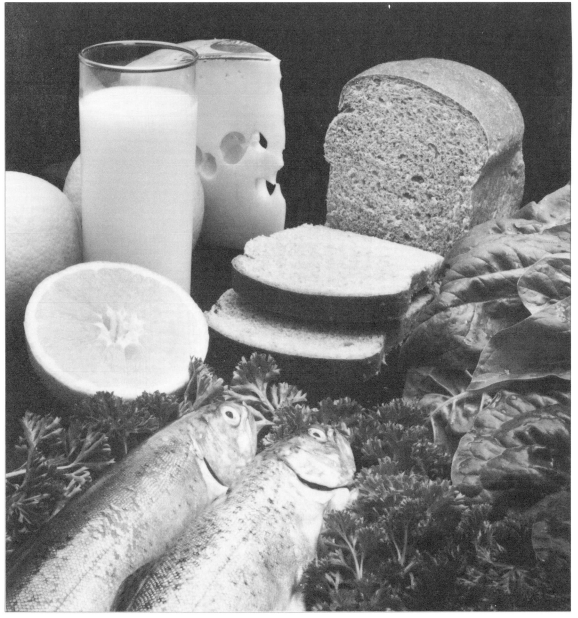

Foods rich in B vitamins.

THE B VITAMINS

Tests were initiated by the results of my studies on a chicken disease similar to beriberi. I was able to establish that that disease is caused by feeding certain grains, especially rice. Only polished rice (raw or boiled) proved to be harmful; unpolished rice was tolerated quite well by the chickens. . . . From these experiments I drew the conclusion that the cuticles probably contain a substance or substances which neutralize the harmful influence of the starchy nutriment. . . .

C. EIJKMAN, 1897

A television commercial broadcast widely some years ago shows a middle-aged businessman shuffling weakly out of his bedroom with his bathrobe slung loosely around his sagging paunch. He sinks into his chair at the breakfast table and wearily lifts the morning paper to screen his face from the daylight and from his bright-eyed, energetic wife. As she places his coffee cup before him, she observes sympathetically, "Sweetie, you look so tired. Did you forget to take your vitamin pill today?" (Fadeout, with the voice of the announcer saying, "Are you tired in the morning? Do you hate to face the day? What you need is Brand A Vitamins.") Repeat: The same man, transformed, trim and bouncy, waltzes into the breakfast nook, pirouettes gaily around the table, kisses his sweet wife affectionately, takes two hasty sips of coffee, and strides humming out the door. She turns cheerfully to the camera and smiles, "Brand A Vitamins have done wonders for my Harry."

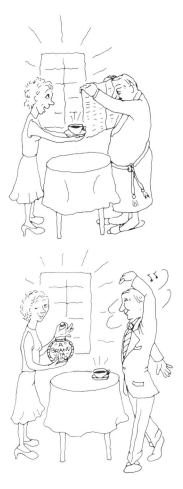

True? No. Poor Harry. If he tries to live on only coffee and vitamins, he will remain a wreck. Like all of the organic nutrients found in foods, the B vitamins are composed of carbon, hydrogen, oxygen, and other atoms linked together by chemical bonds. Of course, these bonds contain energy, but that energy cannot be used to fuel activities or to do the body's work. The energy Harry needs comes from carbohydrate, fat, and protein; the vitamins will only help him burn the fuel if he has the fuel to burn.

It is true, however, that without B vitamins you would certainly feel tired. You would lack energy. Why is this? Some of the B vitamins serve as helpers to the enzymes that release energy from the three energy nutrients—carbohydrate, fat, and protein. The B vitamins stand alongside the metabolic pathways and help to keep the disassembly lines moving. In an industrial plant they would be called expediters. Some of them help manufacture the red blood cells, which carry oxygen to the body's tissues; the oxygen must be present for oxidation and energy release to occur.

313

So long as B vitamins are present, their presence is not felt. Only when they are missing does their absence manifest itself as a lack of energy. A child who learned this defined vitamins on a test as "what if you don't eat you get sick." The definition is one of the most insightful we've seen.

Coenzymes

coenzyme (co-EN-zime): small molecule that works with an enzyme to promote the enzyme's activity. Many coenzymes have B vitamins as part of their structure.

co = with

prosthetic (pros-THET-ic) **group:** a coenzyme that is physically part of (attached to) its enzyme.

prosth = in addition to

active site: that part of the enzyme surface on which the reaction takes place.

To review the structures and functions of enzymes, see Chapter 3.

The B vitamins are entitled to individual attention, but the whole array of them is presented here first to show you the "forest" in which they are the trees. They come together in foods, they work together in the body, and there is much to be learned from viewing them as a group.

Each of the B vitamins is part of an enzyme helper known as a coenzyme. A coenzyme is a small nonprotein molecule that associates closely with an enzyme. Some coenzymes form part of the enzyme structure, in which case they are known as prosthetic groups; others are associated more loosely with the enzyme. Some participate in the reaction being performed and are chemically altered in the process, but they are always regenerated sooner or later. Others are unaltered but form part of the active site of the enzyme. Thus although there are differences in details, one thing is true of all: Without the coenzymes, the enzymes cannot function.

The consequences of a failure of metabolic enzymes can be catastrophic, as you will realize if you restudy the central pathway of metabolism by which glucose is broken down. The nicknames for some of the coenzymes that keep the processes going (NAD^+, TPP, FAD, and CoA) are listed beside the reactions they facilitate.

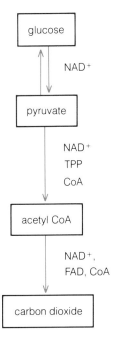

B-Vitamin Terminology

Many of the vitamins have both names and numbers, a mixture of terminologies that confuses newcomers to the study of nutrition. As of 1979, a single set of names for the vitamins had been agreed on and was published,[1] and those names are used in this book. Still, to read the many worthwhile writings published prior to 1979, you have to be aware of the alternative names:

Correct name	Other names commonly used (see also Appendix C)
thiamin	vitamin B_1
riboflavin	vitamin B_2
niacin	nicotinic acid, nicotinamide, niacinamide
vitamin B_6	pyridoxine, pyridoxal, pyridoxamine
folacin	folate, folic acid
vitamin B_{12}	cobalamin
pantothenic acid	(none)
biotin	(none)

(These examples of coenzyme functions are intended to illustrate the way these little molecules work to facilitate enzymatic reactions. It is not necessary to memorize the details in order to understand this principle. The idea is that each has a specific, vital job to perform to keep life processes going.)

Look at the first step. Some of the enzymes involved in the breakdown of glucose to pyruvate require the coenzyme NAD^+. Part of this molecule is a structure the body cannot make, hence it must be obtained from the diet; it is an *essential nutrient*. This essential part is the B vitamin called niacin.

niacin (NIGH-uh-sin): a B vitamin. Niacin can be eaten preformed or can be made in the body from one of the amino acids (see pp. 328-330).

In other words, to take glucose apart the cells must have certain enzymes. For the enzymes to work, they must have the coenzyme NAD^+. To make NAD^+, the cells must be supplied with niacin (or a closely related compound they can alter to make niacin). The rest of the coenzyme they can make without outside help.

The next step in glucose catabolism is the breakdown of pyruvate to acetyl CoA. The enzymes involved in this step require NAD^+ plus another coenzyme, TPP. The cells can manufacture the TPP they need from thiamin, but thiamin is a compound they cannot synthesize, so it must be supplied in the diet. Thiamin is the vitamin part.

thiamin (THIGH-uh-min): a B vitamin.

Another coenzyme needed for this step is coenzyme A, or CoA for short. As you have probably guessed, the cells can make CoA except for an essential part of it that must be obtained in the diet. This essential part — the vitamin part — is pantothenic acid.

pantothenic (PAN-to-THEN-ic) **acid:** a B vitamin.

[1] The vitamin names used here are those published in Nomenclature policy: Generic descriptors and trivial names for vitamins and related compounds, *Journal of Nutrition* 112 (1982):7-14.

riboflavin (RIBE-o-flay-vin): a B vitamin.

The above 4 B vitamins are parts of coenzymes in the glucose-to-energy pathway. Some of these coenzymes have other functions too.

For want of a nail, a horseshoe was lost.

For want of a horseshoe, a horse was lost.

For want of a horse, a soldier was lost.

For want of a soldier, a battle was lost.

For want of a battle, the war was lost,

And all for the want of a horseshoe nail!

—Mother Goose

The next step in glucose catabolism is breakdown of acetyl CoA to carbon dioxide. The enzymes involved in this process require two of the three coenzymes mentioned above — NAD^+ and coenzyme A — and, in addition, another — FAD. Again, FAD is synthesized in the body, but part of its structure, the vitamin riboflavin, must be obtained in the diet.

Now suppose the body's cells lack one of these B vitamins — niacin, for example. Without niacin, the cells cannot make NAD^+. Without NAD^+, the enzymes involved in every step of the glucose-to-energy pathway will fail to function. Since it is from these steps that energy is made available for all of the body's activities, everything will begin to grind to a halt. This is no exaggeration. The symptoms of niacin deficiency are the devastating "four Ds": dermatitis, which reflects a failure of the skin to maintain itself; dementia (insanity), a failure of the nervous system; diarrhea, a failure of digestion and absorption; and death. These are only the most obvious, observable symptoms. Every organ in the body, being dependent on the energy pathways, is profoundly affected by niacin deficiency. As you can see, niacin is a little like the horseshoe nail for want of which a war was lost.

The complete breakdown of amino acids and fat, as well as that of glucose, depends on the coenzymes just described. You may remember that a major product of the breakdown of amino acids and fat is acetyl

Coenzyme action. Each coenzyme is specialized for certain kinds of chemical reactions. NAD^+ (containing niacin), for example, can accept hydrogen atoms removed from other compounds and can lose them to compounds that ultimately pass them to oxygen (see Highlight 7A). There are many steps during the catabolism of glucose in which hydrogens are removed and NAD^+ participates in this way. A model of the way NAD^+ works with an enzyme to remove hydrogens is shown here.

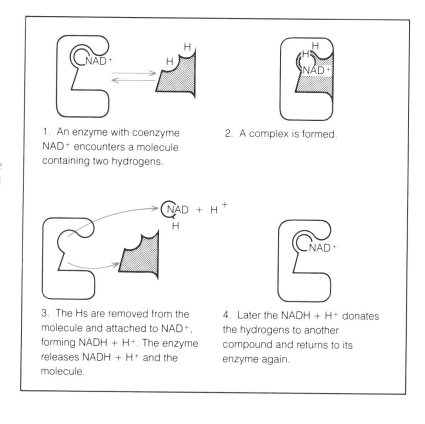

1. An enzyme with coenzyme NAD^+ encounters a molecule containing two hydrogens.

2. A complex is formed.

3. The Hs are removed from the molecule and attached to NAD^+, forming $NADH + H^+$. The enzyme releases $NADH + H^+$ and the molecule.

4. Later the $NADH + H^+$ donates the hydrogens to another compound and returns to its enzyme again.

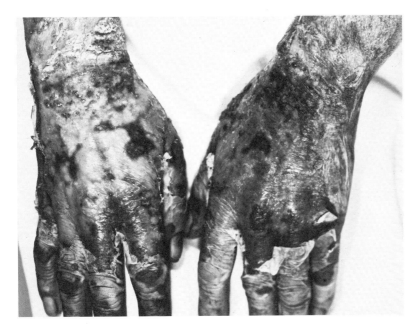

The dermatitis of pellagra. The skin darkens and flakes away as if it were sunburned. In kwashiorkor there is also a "flaky paint" dermatitis but the two are easily distinguishable. The dermatitis of pellagra is bilateral and symmetrical, and occurs only on those parts of the body exposed to the sun.

Courtesy of Dr. Samuel Dreizen, D.D.S., M.D.

CoA and that this product is processed in exactly the same way as the acetyl CoA from glucose. Thus the release of energy from all foods depends on the same vitamins.

Not only the breakdown (catabolism) but also the building (anabolism) of compounds in the body requires coenzymes. For example, one step in the manufacture of a nonessential amino acid is the step in which the nitrogen-containing amino group is attached to a carbon skeleton—a process called transamination. Enzymes performing this function require a coenzyme made from the essential nutrient vitamin B_6.

Two other B vitamins—folacin and vitamin B_{12}—are involved in building the units that form part of DNA and RNA. Whenever a cell divides, it must make a whole new copy of its DNA; thus these two coenzymes are necessary for making all new cells. They also serve other functions. (Folacin, for example, is a coenzyme in the reaction shown on p. 102, in which one amino acid is converted to another by removing a CH_2OH group.)

Finally, biotin, another B vitamin, serves as helper in many reactions in which acid groups are shifted from one structure to another. This activity is needed in making fatty acids.

In summary, these eight B vitamins play many specific roles in helping the enzymes to perform thousands of different molecular conversions in your body. They are active in carbohydrate, fat, and protein metabolism and in the making of DNA and thus new cells. They are found in every cell and must be present continuously for the cells to function as they should. It must now be abundantly clear why

transamination: the transfer of an amino group from one compound to another, as when nonessential amino acids are manufactured in the body.

vitamin B_6: a family of compounds that act as part of the coenzymes in amino acid metabolism. The step that begins the breakdown of stored glycogen to glucose also depends on these coenzymes.

folacin (FOLL-uh-sin) and **vitamin B_{12}:** two B vitamins that act as part of the coenzymes in the manufacture of new DNA and new cells.

biotin (BY-o-tin): a B vitamin; a coenzyme involved in fat synthesis.

poor Harry needs the B vitamins to make him feel well, even though by themselves they do nothing for him. No matter what he eats, he needs B vitamins to help him process it.

B Vitamins and Prescription Drugs

Like the coenzymes, drugs are small but potent molecules, and they often work in the body by altering the actions of its proteins. However, although the body is equipped by eons of evolutionary time to accommodate the vitamins and to use them appropriately, it has had no such long experience with drugs. Most of the prescription drugs are new compounds, synthesized in the laboratory, which by chance have effects on body functions that may be useful when disease threatens. But many drugs have side effects: While they work in one area to counteract the disease process or to correct an abnormality, they may also work in other areas to interfere with normal body processes. Sometimes they interfere with the action of the B vitamins.

For example, a potent drug that blocks the action of the tuberculosis bacterium, nicknamed INH,[2] has saved countless lives because of its efficacy against tuberculosis. But INH is also a vitamin B_6 antagonist: It binds and inactivates the vitamin, inducing a deficiency. Whenever INH is used to treat tuberculosis, supplements of vitamin B_6 are given as a precautionary measure.

Another example is aspirin, the most frequently prescribed pain reliever. It is very effective against pain, but it also interferes with the absorption of folacin from the GI tract and so can cause a deficiency. (It has similar effects on vitamin C and iron.) This doesn't imply that aspirin should never be used but rather that people using drugs and physicians prescribing them should be aware that they may have nutritional consequences and take the appropriate measures to find out and correct them.

It is important for someone new to the study of nutrition to be reminded at this point that this part of the book is about healthy people only. The nutrient needs of people who are ill or who are using large amounts of drugs — including nonprescription drugs like alcohol — are not discussed here. Nor are the special needs of people with inborn genetic defects that may greatly increase their individual needs for certain nutrients. The recommended intakes and the statements about foods that provide the recommended amounts apply to most people, normally, but there are exceptions that are outside our province. Parts Four and Five are addressed to the problems of nutrition in disease, and Highlight 9 is devoted to the special effects of alcohol.

[2] Isonicotinic acid hydrazide, or isoniazid.

B-Vitamin Deficiency

Removing a number of "horseshoe nails" can have such disastrous and far-reaching effects that it is difficult to imagine or predict the results. Oddly enough, although we know a great deal about their individual molecular functions, we are unable to say precisely why a deficiency of one B vitamin produces the disease beriberi whereas the deficiency of another produces pellagra. We do know, however, that with the deficiency of any B vitamin, many body systems become deranged, and similar symptoms may appear.

A B-vitamin deficiency seldom shows up in isolation. After all, people do not eat nutrients singly; they eat foods, which contain mixtures of nutrients. If a major class of foods is missing from the diet, the nutrients contributed by that class of foods will all be lacking to varying extents. In only two cases have dietary deficiencies associated with

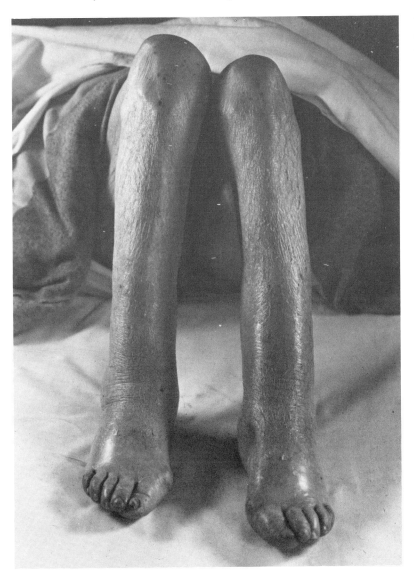

The edema of beriberi. Thiamin deficiency also sometimes produces a "dry" beriberi, without edema, for reasons not well understood. Another marked symptom is inability to walk, manifested by collapse of the lower limbs when the person tries to stand.

Courtesy of Dr. Samuel Dreizen, D.D.S., M.D.

beriberi: the thiamin-deficiency disease; pointed the way to discovery of the first vitamin, thiamin.

For a history of discoveries of the vitamins, see Appendix A.

pellagra (pell-AY-gra): the niacin-deficiency disease.

pellis = skin
agra = seizure

single B vitamins been observed on a large scale in human populations, and deficiency diseases have been named for them. One of these diseases, beriberi, was first observed in the Far East when the custom of polishing rice became widespread. Rice contributed 80 percent of the kcalories consumed by the people of those areas, and rice hulls were their principal source of thiamin. When the hulls were removed, beriberi spread like wildfire. It was believed to be an epidemic, and medical researchers wasted much time and energy seeking a microbial cause before they realized that the problem was not what was present but what was absent.

The other disease, pellagra, became widespread in the U.S. South in the early part of this century, when people subsisted on a low-protein diet whose staple grain was corn. This diet was unusual in that it supplied neither enough niacin nor enough of its amino acid precursor to make up the deficiency.

Even in these cases, the deficiencies were not pure. When foods were provided containing the one vitamin known to be needed, the other needed vitamins that may have been in short supply came as part of the package.

Significantly, these deficiency diseases were eliminated by supplying foods—not pills. Although both diseases were attributed to single B vitamins, both were likely to have been B-complex deficiencies in which one vitamin stood out above the rest. Giving one B vitamin to patients with a B-complex deficiency may make overt latent deficiencies of other B vitamins.

Pushers of vitamin pills make much of the fact that vitamins are vital and indispensable to life. But life went on long before there were vitamin pills, and human beings thrived on exactly the same kinds of foods as are available now. If your diet lacks a vitamin, the natural solution is to adjust it so that food supplies that vitamin.

Pushers of so-called natural vitamins would have you believe that their pills are the best of all because they are purified from real foods rather than synthesized in a laboratory. But if you think back on the course of human evolution, you may conclude that it really is not natural to take any kind of pills at all. In reality, the finest, most complete vitamin "supplements" available are meat, legumes, milk and milk products, vegetables, fruits, and grain products.

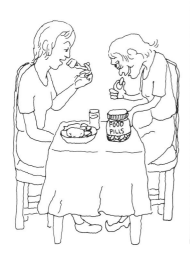

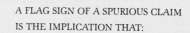

A FLAG SIGN OF A SPURIOUS CLAIM
IS THE IMPLICATION THAT:

Vitamin needs should be met by taking pills.

Once vitamin research was well under way and other B vitamins had been discovered, the clarification of their function was often greatly helped by laboratory experiments in which animals or human volunteers were fed diets devoid of one vitamin. The effects of the deficiency of that vitamin could then be studied to determine what functions it normally performed. Other deficiency diseases were discovered in this way and have since been observed to occur outside the laboratory.

Table 1 sums up a few of the better-established facts about vitamin B deficiency. A look at the table will make another generalization possible. Different body systems depend to different extents on these vitamins. Processes in nerves and in their responding tissues, the muscles, depend heavily on glucose metabolism and hence on thiamin; thus paralysis sets in when this nutrient is lacking. The replacement of old red blood cells with new ones occurs at a rapid pace, and the making of new cells depends on folacin and vitamin B_{12}, so one of the first symptoms of a deficiency of either of these nutrients is a type of anemia. But again, each nutrient is important in all systems, and these lists of symptoms are far from complete.

The skin and the tongue appear to be especially sensitive to vitamin B deficiencies, although the listing of these items in Table 1 may give them undue emphasis. Remember that in a medical examination these are two body parts that the doctor can easily observe. The skin is a visible body tissue, and if it is degenerating, there may well be other tissues beneath it that are also manifesting ill effects. Similarly, the

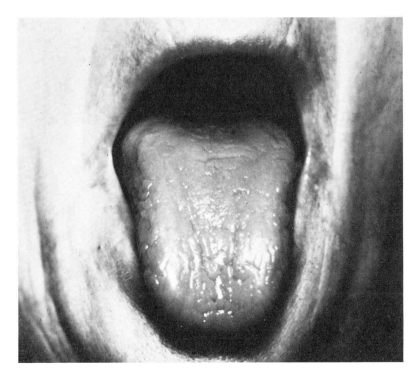

Tongue symptom of B-vitamin deficiency. The tongue is smooth due to atrophy of the tissues (glossitis). This person has a folacin deficiency.

Courtesy of Dr. Samuel Dreizen, D.D.S., M.D.

Table 1. Vitamin B-Deficiency Symptoms

Vitamin	Disease	Deficiency syndrome		Technical terms for symptoms
		Area affected	**Main effects**	
Thiamin	beriberi	nervous system	mental confusion peripheral paralysis	
		muscles	weakness wasting painful calf muscles	
		cardiovascular system	edema enlarged heart death from cardiac failure	
Riboflavin	ariboflavinosis	facial skin	dermatitis around nose and lips cracking of corners of mouth	**cheilosis** (kee-LOH-sis)
		eyes	hypersensitivity to light reddening of cornea	**photophobia**
Niacin	pellagra	skin	bilateral symmetrical derma- titis, especially on body parts exposed to sun	
		tongue	smoothness (atrophy of surface structures)	**glossitis** (gloss-EYE-tis)
		GI tract	diarrhea	
		nervous system	irritability mental confusion, progressing to psychosis or delirium	
Vitamin B$_6$	(no name)	skin	dermatitis cracking of corners of mouth irritation of sweat glands	**cheilosis**
		tongue	smoothness (atrophy of surface structures)	**glossitis**
		nervous system	abnormal brain wave pattern convulsions	
Folacin	(no name)	tongue	smoothness (atrophy of surface structures)	**glossitis**
		GI tract	diarrhea	
		blood	anemia (characterized by large cells)	**macrocytic anemia**
Vitamin B$_{12}$	pernicious anemia	blood	anemia (characterized by large cells)	**macrocytic anemia**
		nervous system	degeneration of peripheral nerves	
Pantothenic acid	(Deficiency observed only in animals)			
Biotin	(Deficiency observed in humans only under experimental conditions)			

mouth and tongue are the visible parts of the digestive system; if they are abnormal, there may well be an abnormality throughout the GI tract. What is really happening in a vitamin deficiency happens inside the cells of the body; what the doctor sees and reports are its outward manifestations.

It is more and more apparent that you cannot observe a symptom and automatically jump to a conclusion regarding its cause. This warning was given earlier (in Chapter 2) about dermatitis: A symptom is not a disease. As you have seen, deficiencies of linoleic acid, riboflavin, niacin, and vitamin B_6 can all cause dermatitis. A deficiency of vitamin A can too. Because skin is on the outside, where you and your doctor can easily look at it, it is a useful indicator of things-going-wrong-in-cells. But by itself a skin symptom tells you nothing about its possible cause.

The same is true of anemia. We often think of anemia as being caused by an iron deficiency, and often it is. But anemia can also be caused by a folacin or vitamin B_{12} deficiency, by digestive tract failure to absorb any of these nutrients, or by such nonnutritional causes as infections, parasites, or loss of blood. So caution: A little knowledge is a dangerous thing.

A FLAG SIGN OF A SPURIOUS CLAIM
IS THE IMPLICATION THAT:

A specific nutrient will cure a given symptom.

A person who feels chronically tired may be tempted to diagnose herself as having anemia. Knowing only enough to associate iron deficiency with this condition, she may decide to take an iron supplement. But the iron supplement will relieve her tiredness only if the symptom is caused by iron-deficiency anemia. If she has a folacin deficiency (and folacin deficiency may be the most widespread vitamin deficiency in the world), taking iron will only prolong the period in which she receives no relief. If she is better informed, she may decide to take a vitamin supplement with iron, covering the possibility of a vitamin deficiency. But now she is forgetting that there may be a nonnutritional cause of her symptom. If the cause of her tiredness is actually hidden blood loss due to cancer, the postponement of a diagnosis may be equivalent to suicide.

fortification: the addition of nutrients to a food, often in amounts much larger than might be found naturally in that food.

enrichment: now considered synonymous with fortification but previously referred to the addition of specific nutrients to refined breads and cereals in the United States.

whole-grain products: grain products made from the whole grain, including the bran, the germ, and the endosperm.

bran: the nutrient-rich coat of a wheat grain.

germ: the nutrient-rich part of the wheat grain, which provides nutrients for the plant's growth.

endosperm: the starchy, relatively nutrient-free bulk of the wheat grain.

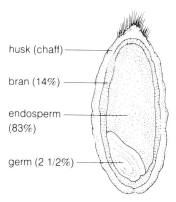

husk (chaff)

bran (14%)

endosperm (83%)

germ (2 1/2%)

A kernel of wheat.

refined grain products: products made of grain that has been milled, losing most of the bran and the germ in the process and containing only the endosperm.

Major, epidemic-like deficiency diseases such as pellagra and beriberi are no longer seen in the United States and Canada, but lesser deficiencies of nutrients, including the B vitamins, sometimes are observed. They occur in people whose food choices are poor because of poverty, ignorance, illness, or poor health habits like alcohol abuse. They are especially likely if the staple grain food is refined, as were most bread and cereal products chosen by U.S. consumers during the 1930s. One way to protect these people is to add nutrients to their staple food, a process known as fortification or enrichment. The enrichment of refined breads and cereals, required by law in the United States since the early 1940s, has increased many people's B-vitamin intakes. Thus before noting which foods are the richest sources of the individual B vitamins, you need to know what enrichment means.

Refined, Enriched, and Whole-Grain Bread

The part of the wheat plant that is made into flour and then into bread and other baked goods is the kernel. About 50 kernels cluster in the head of the plant, on top of the stem, where they stick tightly until fully ripe. In the milling process these kernels are first separated from the stem and then further broken apart.

The wheat kernel (whole grain) has three main parts: the germ, the bran, and the endosperm. The germ is the part that reproduces when planted, and so it contains concentrated food to support the new life. It is especially rich in iron, vitamin E, and the B vitamins thiamin, riboflavin, and niacin. The bran, a protective coating around the kernel similar to the shell of a nut, is also rich in nutrients. In addition, the bran is a source of valuable fiber. The endosperm is the soft inside portion of the kernel containing starch and proteins (including gluten, which is used for making white flour). The husk, commonly called chaff, is unusable for most purposes.

People interested in nutrition are concerned about the loss of nutrients from the wheat kernel during the milling process. In earlier times the kernel was milled by grinding it between two stones to expose the endosperm and then blowing or sifting out the inedible chaff. Much of the bran and germ were included in the final product.

As improvements were made in the machinery for milling, a whiter, smoother-textured flour resulted. Consumers liked this flour better than the former crunchy, dark brown, "old-fashioned" flour. But to produce white flour, millers use only the endosperm. (To produce whole-wheat flour, millers grind the entire kernel.) Thus during the further processing of refined, white flour for the market, additional nutrients are lost. The bran layers and other parts of the kernel that remain after white flour is milled are used as livestock and poultry feed. These parts of the grain actually contain more protein, minerals, and vitamins than the endosperm does.

As white flour became more popular for making breads, bread eaters suffered a tragic loss of needed nutrients. A survey conducted in the United States in 1936 revealed that people were suffering from the loss of the nutrients iron, thiamin, riboflavin, and niacin, which they had formerly received from their unrefined bread. The Enrichment Act of 1942 required that these lost nutrients be returned to the flour. Thus enriched bread restores iron and the vitamins thiamin and niacin to the level of whole wheat; riboflavin is added to a level about twice that in whole grain.

To a great extent, the enrichment of white flour eliminated the deficiency problems that had been observed in people who depended on bread for most of their kcalories but who were unwilling to use the whole-grain product. Today you can almost take it for granted that all refined bread, grains like rice, wheat products like macaroni and spaghetti, and cereals like farina have been enriched. The law provides that all grain products that cross state lines must be enriched. A look at Table 2 shows to what levels whole-grain bread, unenriched white bread, and enriched white bread contains these four nutrients.

enrichment: with respect to breads and cereals in particular, this term refers to the process by which four specific nutrients lost during refinement are added back to refined grain products at levels specified by law: thiamin, niacin, and iron at levels about equal to those in the original whole grain; riboflavin at a level about twice that in the original whole grain.

A wheat plant.

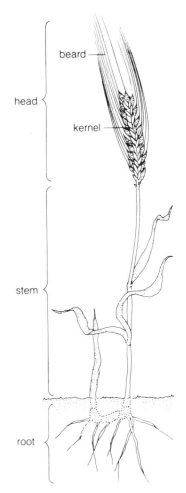

Table 2.   Nutrient Levels of 1-lb Loaves of Bread

Item number*	Type of bread	Iron (mg)	Thiamin (mg)	Riboflavin (mg)	Niacin (mg)
368	Whole-wheat	13.6	1.36	0.45	12.7
346	Italian, unenriched	3.2	0.41	0.27	3.6
345	Italian, enriched	10.0	1.32	0.91	11.8

*As listed in Appendix H.

But the food composition tables don't tell the whole story. When the grain is refined, many nutrients not listed in the tables are also lost. As more and more foods are refined and processed, other nutrients may begin to be lost from our diet. Evidence is piling up that fiber needs are increasing as fiber is lost from many refined foods, not just from bread and cereal. Some experts have attributed the new cases of chromium-deficiency diabetes to the increased use of processed foods. Therefore, although the enrichment of wheat and other cereal products restores four of the lost nutrients, there is increasing evidence that we should return to the use of the whole grain in order to restore trace minerals and fiber to our diet. *Nutrition and the MD* reports: "Whole grain items are preferred over enriched products because they contain more magnesium, zinc, folacin, and vitamin B_6 than enriched bread and cereals."[3]

[3]Improving on the basic four, *Nutrition and the MD*, October 1977.

The B Vitamins in Food

The preceding sections have shown both the great importance of the B vitamins in promoting normal, healthy functioning of all body systems and the severe consequences of deficiency. Now you may want to know how to be sure you are getting enough of these vital nutrients. This chapter concludes with some practical pointers regarding food intake.

First, a Caution   One way to discover whether your intake of a vitamin is sufficient is to calculate the amount you are consuming each day in the foods you eat and to compare your intake with the recommended intake (RDA or Canadian Dietary Standard. See the Self-Study that follows Highlight 9). This is an informative exercise, and some 15 nutrients can be studied this way. However, there are more accurate means of determining whether a deficiency exists, and there are other distinct limitations on the dietary record method. First, you have to assume that the recommended intake applies to you. People's needs for nutrients vary over a wide range; you may not be typical. Of course, you may need much less, but you may also need more. Second, you have to assume that your body's handling and absorption of the vitamin is normal. If your digestive system is disturbed, if you are ill (especially with diarrhea), or if you are emotionally upset, your absorption of certain nutrients may be impaired. Third, when you look up the foods you eat in a table of food composition, you have to assume that the food you ate contained the amount of the nutrient listed in the table. But foods vary too. Not all 200-g tomatoes contain exactly 1.3 mg of niacin. The nutrient contents of foods are averages. Furthermore, the professionals who make up the tables make still a fourth assumption—that the foods are stored and prepared in a way that minimizes losses of vitamins. So there are at least four possible sources of error in assuming that your nutrient intakes compared with your nutrient needs this way are meaningful.

The table of food composition most often used is given in Appendix H.

Still, the dietary record is the simplest way to check on a person's nutrient status and is the way most often used by the average person. **Some more precise means of assessing nutrition status (physical examination, body measurements, and biochemical tests) are described in Chapter 18.**

With the above cautions in mind, let us examine the foods for their B-vitamin content. Only six of the B vitamins are discussed in detail here—those for which the contents of foods have been relatively well analyzed and for which the Canadian and U.S. governments have set dietary standards. Once a diet has been planned to meet the needs for these vitamins, it meets the general description of "a balanced and varied diet" and is therefore likely to ensure adequacy for other nutrients not considered here.

Thiamin   The recommended daily thiamin intake for adults is about 1.5 mg for men and about 1.0 mg for women (plus an extra half milligram during pregnancy). Infants require about half a milligram and children about three-fourths.

Because thiamin is used for energy production, more is needed when energy expenditure is high. (In fact, the thiamin requirement can be stated in terms of milligrams per 1,000 kcal.) Provided that you are consuming enough kcalories to meet your energy needs—and obtaining those kcalories from thiamin-containing foods—your thiamin intake will adjust automatically to your need. However, people who derive a large proportion of their kcalories from empty-kcalorie items like sugar or alcohol may suffer thiamin deficiency. A person who is fasting or who has adopted a very low-kcalorie diet needs the same amount of thiamin as he did when he was eating more; needs remain unchanged during fasting because they are proportional to energy expenditure, not to energy intake.[4]

Table 3 shows the thiamin contents of 50 common foods. If you study the table while thinking about your own food habits, you will probably conclude that many of the foods you like and eat daily contribute some thiamin, but none by itself can meet your total need for a day. A useful guideline is to eliminate empty-kcalorie foods from your diet and to include ten or more different servings of nutritious foods each day, assuming that on the average each serving will contribute about 10 percent of your need. Foods chosen from the bread and cereal group should be either whole-grain or enriched. Thiamin is not stored in the body to any great extent, so daily intake is best.

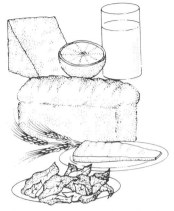

Thiamin: Most nutritious foods contribute about 10 percent of daily need per serving.

Riboflavin   The recommended daily riboflavin intake for adults is about 1.4 to 1.8 mg for men and about 1.1 to 1.3 mg for women (plus about 0.3 mg during pregnancy), depending on how much energy they expend daily. (Like thiamin, riboflavin needs can be stated in terms of milligrams per 1,000 kcal.) Young children's needs begin at about 1 mg a day and rise rapidly during their growing years. Teenagers, because they are very active, need more riboflavin than adults.

Unlike thiamin, riboflavin is not evenly distributed among the food groups. Table 4 shows the riboflavin contents of 50 common foods; the concentration of 1s and 5s in the left-hand column shows that the major contributors are milk and meat. The need for riboflavin provides a major reason for including milk in some form in every day's meals; no other food that is commonly eaten can make such a substantial contribution toward meeting the day's needs. People who don't use milk products can substitute generous servings of dark-green leafy vegetables, because a cup of greens—collards, for example—provides about the same amount of riboflavin as a cup of milk. Among the meats, liver and heart are the richest sources, but all lean meats, as well as eggs, provide some riboflavin. Most people derive about half their riboflavin from milk and milk products, about a fourth from meats,

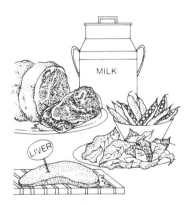

Riboflavin: Milk contributes about 50 percent, meat about 25 percent, enriched breads and cereals additional amounts. The person who does not drink milk should substitute greens.

[4]M. Brin and J. C. Bauernfeind, Vitamin needs of the elderly, *Postgraduate Medicine* 63 (3) (1978):155-163.

Table 3. Thiamin Contents of 50 Common Foods*

Ex-change group[†]	Food	Serving size[‡]	Thia-min (mg)	Ex-change group[†]	Food	Serving size[‡]	Thia-min (mg)
5L	Lean pork roast	3 oz	.91	1	Whole milk	1 c	.07
5L	Ham	3 oz	.40	1	Yogurt (from whole milk)	1 c	.07
5L	Oysters	3/4 c	.25	4	Corn muffin	1	.07
5M	Liver, beef	3 oz	.23	4	Bran flakes	1/2 c	.07
4	Green peas	1/2 c	.22	4	Puffed rice	1 c	.07
5M	Beef heart	3 oz	.21	4	Muffin	1	.07
4	Lima beans	1/2 c	.16[§]	5M	Hamburger	3 oz	.07
2	Collard greens	1/2 c	.14	2	Cooked tomatoes	1/2 c	.06
3	Orange	1	.13	2	Tomato juice	1/2 c	.06
4	Dried beans	1/2 c	.13	2	Brussels sprouts	1/2 c	.06
5L	Lamb, leg	3 oz	.13	3	Pineapple	1/2 c	.06
2	Dandelion greens	1/2 c	.12	4	White bread	1 slice	.06
4	Rice, enriched	1/2 c	.12	4	Whole-wheat bread	1 slice	.06
2	Asparagus	1/2 c	.12	4	Hamburger bun	1/2	.06
3	Orange juice	1/2 c	.11	4	Potato chips	15	.06
5L	Veal roast	3 oz	.11	4	French fried potatoes	8	.06
1	2% fat fortified milk	1 c	.10	5L	Chipped beef	3 oz	.06
4	Spaghetti, enriched	1/2 c	.10	2	Mustard greens	1/2 c	.06
4	Macaroni, enriched	1/2 c	.10	2	Broccoli	1/2 c	.06
4	Cooked cereal	1/2 c	.10	5M	Egg	1	.05
4	Corn on cob	1 small	.09	3	Pink grapefruit	1/2	.05
1	Skim milk	1 c	.09	2	Summer squash	1/2 c	.05
4	Potato	1 small	.08	2	Green beans	1/2 c	.05
4	Mashed potato	1/2 c	.08	5L	Chicken, meat only	3 oz	.05
1	Powdered skim milk	1/3 c	.08	5L	Lean beef roast	3 oz	.05

*These are not necessarily the best food sources but are selected to show a range of thiamin contents. Note the presence of all food groups except fat in the left-hand column.

†The numbers refer to the exchange lists: 1 is milk; 2, vegetables; 3, fruit; 4, bread; 5L, lean meat; 5M, medium-fat meat.

‡Serving sizes are the sizes listed in the exchange lists, except for meat.

§One serving of any of the first six foods contains at least 10 percent of the RDA (for an adult male) of 1.5 mg.

and most of the rest from leafy green vegetables and whole-grain or enriched bread and cereal products.

Riboflavin is light-sensitive; it can be destroyed by the ultraviolet rays of the sun or of fluorescent lamps. For this reason milk is seldom sold and should not be stored in transparent glass containers. Cardboard or plastic containers protect the riboflavin in the milk from ultraviolet rays.

Niacin Recommended niacin intakes are stated in "equivalents," a term that requires explanation. Niacin is unique among the B vitamins because it can be obtained from another nutrient source—protein. The amino acid tryptophan can be converted to niacin in the body: 60 mg of

niacin equivalents: the amount of niacin present in food, including the niacin that can theoretically be made from the tryptophan present in the food.

Table 4.   Riboflavin Contents of 50 Common Foods*

Exchange group[†]	Food	Serving size[‡]	Riboflavin (mg)	Exchange group[†]	Food	Serving size[‡]	Riboflavin (mg)
5M	Beef liver	3 oz	3.60	2	Brussels sprouts	1/2 c	.11
5M	Beef heart	3 oz	1.04	2	Spinach	1/2 c	.11
1	2% fat fortified milk§	1 c	.52	5L	Canned tuna	3 oz	.10
1	Skim milk	1 c	.44	2	Mustard greens	1/2 c	.10
1	Canned evaporated milk	1/2 c	.43	4	Lima beans	1/2 c	.09
1	Whole milk	1 c	.41	4	Green peas	1/2 c	.09
1	Dry skim milk	1/3 c	.40	4	Pumpkin	3/4 c	.09
1	Yogurt (whole milk)	1 c	.39	4	Muffin	1	.09
5L	Oysters	3/4 c	.30	4	Corn muffin	1	.08
5L	Chipped beef	3 oz	.30	3	Strawberries	3/4 c	.08
5L	Veal roast	3 oz	.26	2	Summer squash	1/2 c	.08
5L	Leg of lamb	3 oz	.23	4	Corn on cob	1 small	.08
5L	Lean roast beef	3 oz	.19	4	Dried beans	1/2 c	.07
2	Collard greens	1/2 c	.19	3	Pear	1	.07
5M	Hamburger	3 oz	.18°	4	Spaghetti, enriched	1/2 c	.06
5L	Sardines	3 oz	.17	4	Macaroni, enriched	1/2 c	.06
5L	Ham	3 oz	.16	3	Raspberries	1/2 c	.06
5L	Chicken, meat only	3 oz	.16	4	Pancake	1	.06
5L	Canned salmon	3 oz	.16	2	Green beans	1/2 c	.06
2	Dandelion greens	1/2 c	.15	4	White bread	1 slice	.05
5M	Egg	1	.15	2	Cauliflower	1/2 c	.05
5M	Cheese, creamed cottage	1/4 c	.15	4	Mashed potatoes	1/2 c	.05
4	Winter squash	1/2 c	.14	3	Orange	1	.05
2	Asparagus	1/2 c	.13	3	Peach	1	.05
2	Broccoli	1/2 c	.12	4	Hamburger bun	1/2	.04

*These are not necessarily the best food sources but are selected to show a range of riboflavin contents. Note in the left-hand column that the 1s and 5s cluster at the top and that the 2s near the top all represent 1/2-c servings of dark-green leafy vegetables.

†The numbers refer to the exchange lists: 1 is milk; 2, vegetables; 3, fruit; 4, bread; 5L, lean meat; 5M, medium-fat meat.

‡Serving sizes are the sizes listed in the exchange lists, except for meat.

§2% milk appears above skim milk because it is fortified with dry powdered milk, not because of the fat in it (riboflavin is water-soluble). Canadian 2% milk has only vitamin D added.

°One serving of any of the foods to this point contains at least 10 percent of the RDA (for an adult male) of 1.7 mg.

tryptophan yields 1 mg of niacin. Thus a food containing 1 mg niacin and 60 mg tryptophan contains the equivalent of 2 mg niacin, or 2 mg equivalents.

Recommended daily intakes for men are about 15 to 20 mg equivalents and for women about 12 to 15 (plus 2 to 5 mg equivalents during pregnancy and lactation). Infants', children's, and teenagers' needs are proportional not to their size but to their energy output.

Tables of food composition list only the preformed niacin in foods, although people actually derive the vitamin from both niacin itself and dietary tryptophan. However, tryptophan is also used to build needed

A compound that can be converted to a nutrient in the body is known as a **precursor** of that nutrient. Thus tryptophan is a precursor of niacin.

To obtain a rough approximation of your niacin intake:

1. Calculate total protein consumed (g).
2. Subtract your protein requirement to obtain "leftover" protein usable to make niacin (g).
3. Divide by 100 to obtain the amount of tryptophan in this protein (g).
4. Multiply by 1,000 to express this amount of tryptophan in milligrams (mg).
5. Divide by 60 to get niacin equivalents (mg).
6. Finally, add the amount of niacin obtained preformed in the diet (mg).

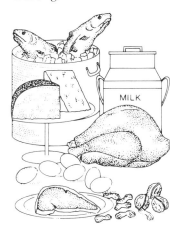

Niacin is adequate if protein is adequate.

schizophrenia (skitz-oh-FREN-ee-uh): a kind of mental illness.

schizo = split
phren = mind

orthomolecular psychiatry: a branch of psychiatry that attempts to treat mental illness by correcting nutrient imbalances and deficiencies.

ortho = right

body proteins, so not all of it is available for making niacin. Thus calculating the amount of niacin available from the diet is a complicated matter. A means of obtaining a rough approximation is shown in the margin, but the simplest assumption is that if the diet is adequate in complete protein, it will supply enough niacin equivalents to meet the daily need.

Milk, eggs, meat, poultry, and fish contribute about half the niacin equivalents consumed by most people, and about a fourth come from enriched breads and cereals. Vegetarians are well advised to emphasize nuts and legumes in their diets, as these are good sources of niacin and protein. A look at the nutrient contents of foods (in Appendix H) will reveal other good sources.

Most people in Canada and the United States presently consume a lot of animal protein, so niacin deficiency is a problem only where protein deficiency occurs. The widespread pellagra that was seen during the early part of this century in the U.S. South was due to the fact that the predominantly cornmeal/salt pork/molasses diet of the people of that area was lacking in both niacin and protein; what little protein they consumed was unusually low in tryptophan. Symptoms of niacin deficiency are no longer observed very often, except in people like alcoholics and undernourished hospital patients, whose protein intakes are unacceptably low.

At the time that pellagra was widespread in the South, half the cases in insane asylums were caused by niacin deficiency.[5] Unfortunately, not all insanity is caused by a lack of niacin; if it were, it would be wonderfully easy to cure. Insanity induced by niacin deficiency has symptoms very like those of schizophrenia, but it clears up miraculously when niacin or tryptophan is given. The hope that large doses of niacin would also cure schizophrenia has led to some important research and a whole new area of study—orthomolecular psychiatry—but the results so far have been disappointing. There is no evidence that large doses of niacin have any effect whatever on mental disease other than the dementia of pellagra.[6]

Large doses of niacin have been observed, however, to lower blood cholesterol levels in some cases, and for a while interest ran high in exploring the possible value of niacin therapy in the prevention of atherosclerosis. Both niacin and niacinamide (an alternative form of the vitamin) have been extensively tested for their cholesterol-lowering effects, but both have been found disappointing. Niacin causes irritation of the intestines and possibly liver damage, and niacinamide

[5]H. N. Munro, Impact of nutritional research on human health and survival, *Federation Proceedings* 30 (July/August 1971), reprinted in *The Nutrition Crisis: A Reader*, ed. T. P. Labuza (St. Paul: West, 1975), pp. 5-13.

[6]Task Force on Vitamin Therapy in Psychiatry, American Psychiatric Association, Megavitamin and orthomolecular therapy in psychiatry, pp. 44-47. Excerpts reprinted in *Nutrition Reviews/Supplement: Nutrition Misinformation and Food Faddism*, July 1974, pp. 67-70.

is ineffective altogether.[7] Research into the possible benefits of niacin therapy for atherosclerosis has largely given way to other, more promising approaches.

One problem with large therapeutic doses of niacin (ten times the normal intake) is that they produce flushed skin and a painful, stinging sensation that may be alarming, although megadoses seem to cause no permanent harm if taken only a few times. Some people who believe in the therapeutic power of niacin even like this "niacin flush." Those who don't like the reaction can take niacinamide.

Vitamin B$_6$ Because the vitamin B$_6$ coenzymes play many roles in amino acid metabolism, dietary needs are roughly proportional to protein intakes. Adults need about 2 mg of vitamin B$_6$ a day; this is enough to handle 100 g of protein. Pregnant and lactating women need about half a milligram more. Infants probably receive enough B$_6$ either from breast milk or cow's milk formula. There is some possibility that older people have a greater need for vitamin B$_6$ than young adults.

Pregnant women often show low blood concentrations of B$_6$ even though their diets are ample in the vitamin. It is thought that this is due to the high demand for B$_6$ by the fetus, whose blood normally has about five times more B$_6$ than the mother's. Vitamin B$_6$ is often prescribed for relief of the nausea and vomiting of pregnancy as well as for depression felt by women taking oral contraceptives.[8]

Convenient reference tables showing vitamin B$_6$ contents of foods are not available. However, by this time you must have realized that the B vitamins are found for the most part in the same groups of foods. Thus the only workable strategy for meeting B-vitamin needs is to eat a variety of nutritious foods. In the case of vitamin B$_6$, the richest food sources seem to be muscle meats, liver, vegetables, and whole-grain cereals.

Folacin Folacin occurs in foods in both bound and free forms; the free form is better absorbed. Canada's recommendation for daily intake, stated in terms of "free folate (folacin)," is 200 μg a day for adults, with 50 μg added for pregnancy. The U.S. recommendation for adults is stated in terms of all forms of folacin and is 400 μg a day. The need for folacin rises dramatically during pregnancy, more than the need for any other nutrient, even protein; the RDA doubles the folacin intake to 800 μg a day during pregnancy. This increased need reflects the role folacin plays in cell multiplication. The blood volume in a pregnant woman nearly doubles, for example, and the folacin

megavitamin therapy: the administration of huge doses of vitamins in the attempt to cure disease.

mega = huge

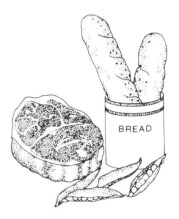

Vitamin B$_6$ is found in meats, vegetables, and whole-grain cereals.

Note: Recommended folacin intakes are stated in micrograms (μg). A microgram is a thousandth of a milligram or a millionth of a gram. The RDA for folacin, 400 μg, can also be stated as 0.4 mg.

[7]M. K. Horwitt, The Vitamins, Section G: Niacin, in *Modern Nutrition in Health and Disease*, 5th ed., eds. R. S. Goodhart and M. E. Shils (Philadelphia: Lea and Febiger, 1973), pp. 198-202.

[8]B. S. Worthington, J. Vermeersch, and S. R. Williams, *Nutrition in Pregnancy and Lactation* (St. Louis: Mosby, 1977), p. 185.

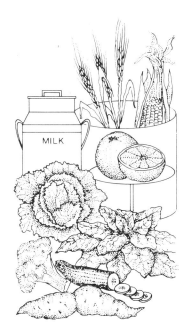

Folacin is the "foliage" vitamin.

coenzymes are used to manufacture the new blood cells. The typical diet in the United States probably delivers about 600 μg daily.

Tables of the folacin contents of foods are now being developed and probably soon will be incorporated into the standard table of food composition. The best food sources of this vitamin are organ meats (such as liver), green, leafy vegetables (the name of the vitamin is related to the word *foliage*), beets, and members of the cabbage family (such as cauliflower, broccoli, and brussels sprouts). Among the fruits, oranges, orange juice, and cantaloupe are the best sources; among the starchy vegetables, corn, lima beans, parsnips, green peas, pumpkin, and sweet potato are good sources. Whole-wheat bread, wheat germ, and milk also supply folacin.

The presence of folacin in dark-green leafy vegetables is one reason for the Four Food Group Plan recommendation that these vegetables be included in the diet at least every other day. Some forms of folacin are readily destroyed by cooking, hence the advisability of including raw vegetables like salad greens and fruits like citrus fruits in daily menus.

Folacin deficiency may result from an inadequate intake, impaired absorption, or unusual metabolic need for the vitamin. A significant number of cases of anemia develop from these causes, especially among pregnant women. Among the poor and in other parts of the world, folacin deficiency due to inadequate intake is probably the most common vitamin deficiency.

The risks of overdosing with folacin are greater than those for the other B vitamins discussed so far. They arise from the close relationship between folacin and vitamin B_{12} (see next section).

Note: Recommended vitamin B_{12} intakes are stated in micrograms.

Vitamin B_{12} is adequate if animal foods are included in the diet. Among vegetable products only a few (those that include microorganisms) contain B_{12}, most notably yeast and fermented soy products.

Lacto-ovo-vegetarians: see p. 140.

intrinsic: inside the system. The intrinsic factor necessary to prevent pernicious anemia is now known to be a mucopolysaccharide, made in the stomach, that aids in the absorption of vitamin B_{12}.

Vitamin B_{12}   According to both the U.S. and Canadian recommendations, adults need about 3 μg of vitamin B_{12} a day (plus 1 μg during pregnancy). This is the tiniest amount imaginable—three-millionths of a gram, and a gram would not even fill a quarter-teaspoon. The ink in the period at the end of this sentence probably weighs about 3 μg. But what seems like such a tiny amount to the human eye contains billions of molecules of vitamin B_{12}, enough to provide coenzymes for all the enzymes that need its help.

Vitamin B_{12} is unique among the nutrients in being found almost exclusively in animal flesh and animal products. Anyone who eats meat is guaranteed an adequate intake, and lacto-ovo-vegetarians (who use milk, cheese, and eggs) are also protected from deficiency. But strict vegetarians must use vitamin B_{12}-fortified soy milk or other such products or take B_{12} supplements.

A second special characteristic of vitamin B_{12} is that it requires an "intrinsic factor"—a compound made inside the body—for absorption from the intestinal tract into the bloodstream. The design for this factor is carried in the genes. The intrinsic factor is now known to be synthesized in the stomach, where it attaches to the vitamin; the complex then passes to the small intestine and is gradually absorbed.

Certain people have in their genetic makeup a defective gene for the intrinsic factor and so cannot make it; this defect usually becomes manifest in midlife. Without the intrinsic factor, they can't absorb the vitamin even though they are taking enough in their diets, and so they develop deficiency symptoms. In such a case, or when the stomach has been injured and cannot produce enough of the intrinsic factor, vitamin B_{12} must be supplied to the body by injection, thus bypassing the block in the intestinal tract.

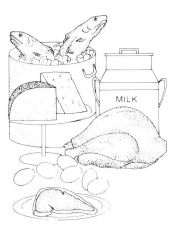

One of the most obvious B_{12}-deficiency symptoms is the kind of anemia characterized by large, immature red blood cells identical to those seen in folacin deficiency. Either vitamin B_{12} or folacin will clear up this condition. However, vitamin B_{12} also functions in maintaining the sheath that surrounds and protects nerve fibers and in promoting their normal growth, as well as in producing mature red blood cells. Thus a deficiency of vitamin B_{12} also causes a creeping paralysis of the nerves and muscles, which begins at the extremities and works inward and up the spine. This paralysis cannot be remedied by administering folacin, so early detection and correction of the B_{12} deficiency is necessary if permanent nerve damage and paralysis are to be avoided. Hence the name "pernicious" anemia: The vitamin B_{12} deficiency has a hidden, sneaky, and frightening symptom. Because of the danger of a high level of folacin masking a lack of B_{12}, the amount of folacin in over-the-counter vitamin preparations is limited by law to 400 μg, an amount too low to have this effect.[9]

The way folacin masks pernicious anemia underlines a point already made several times: It takes a skilled diagnostician to make a correct diagnosis and the risk you take when you diagnose yourself on the basis of a single observed symptom is clearly a serious one.

A second point should also be underlined here. Since B_{12} deficiency in the body may be caused by either a lack of B_{12} in the diet or a genetically caused inability to absorb the vitamin, a change in diet alone may not correct it. You might wish to think about this **in relation to the cautions offered on p. 63 and 323.**

Strict vegetarians are at special risk for unchecked B_{12} deficiency for two reasons: first, because they receive none in their diets; and second, because they consume large amounts of folacin from the vegetables they eat. The amount of vitamin B_{12} that can be stored in the body is 1,000 times the amount used each day, so it may take years for a deficiency to develop in a new vegetarian. When it does, it may be masked by the high folacin intake. Sometimes the damage is first seen in the breast-fed infant of a vegan mother.[10]

Vegan: see p. 140.

[9]Committee on Safety, Toxicity, and Misuse of Vitamins and Trace Minerals, National Nutrition Consortium, *Vitamin-Mineral Safety, Toxicity, and Misuse* (Chicago: The American Dietetic Association, 1978).

[10]Vitamin B_{12} deficiency in the breast-fed infant of a strict vegetarian, *Nutrition Reviews* 37 (May 1979):142-144.

The history of the discovery of vitamin B_{12} makes an intriguing story and epitomizes the fascination of vitamin research. In the early years, all that was known about pernicious anemia was that it could be controlled but not cured by eating large amounts of calf liver. (Researchers concluded that liver contained a factor—the "extrinsic factor"—needed to prevent the disease, and later they identified the factor as vitamin B_{12}.) The concentration of B_{12} in liver was so great that some was absorbed even without the help of the intrinsic factor. At one time people suffering from pernicious anemia had no choice but to eat several pounds of liver a day, but now they can be cured by the injection of a few micrograms of the purified vitamin every three weeks.

extrinsic: outside the system. The extrinsic factor first detected in raw liver and found necessary to prevent pernicious anemia is now known to be vitamin B_{12}.

Other B Vitamins The six best-known B vitamins have already been discussed. Two other B vitamins—pantothenic acid and biotin—are needed for the synthesis of coenzymes that are active in a multitude of body systems. These are just as important for normal body function as the vitamins discussed so far, but little is known about the human requirements for them. Both pantothenic acid and biotin are widespread in foods, and there seems to be no danger that people who consume a variety of foods will suffer deficiencies. Claims that they are needed in pill form to prevent or cure disease conditions are at best unfounded and at worst intentionally misleading.

Pantothenic acid and biotin: deficiencies not seen in humans.

Another pair of compounds sometimes called B vitamins are inositol and choline. These are probably not essential nutrients for humans, although deficiencies can be induced in laboratory animals in order to study their functions. Like the B vitamins described above, they serve as coenzymes in metabolism. Even if they were essential for humans, supplements would be unnecessary, because they are abundant in foods.

Possible B vitamins:

inositol (eye-NOSS-i-tall)
choline (KO-leen)

Health food purveyors make much of inositol and choline, insisting that we must supplement our diets with them. This incorrect notion arises from an unjustified application of findings from animal studies to human beings.

CAUTION WHEN YOU READ!

To weigh the reliability of nutrition information, ask yourself, Has the finding been proved applicable to human beings?

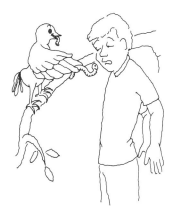

Highlight 11 enlarges on this theme, which has been a major problem with recent publicity about vitamin E.

B Vitamins That Are Not A newcomer among vitamin frauds is "vitamin B_{15}," pangamic acid. First isolated in 1951 from rice bran, brewer's yeast, and horse liver, pangamic acid was thought to be a B vitamin because of its presence in common foods. Many physiological functions were attributed to it. It is not known, however, whether humans or animals can synthesize pangamic acid, and no specific disease state can be attributed to a deficiency of it. No person who eats a balanced and varied diet need fear a deficiency, and no person who does not eat a balanced and varied diet will benefit significantly by adding purified pangamic acid to her vitamin pill collection.

Preparations sold as vitamin B_{15} may contain any mixture of chemicals; their contents are not controlled by the government of either the United States or Canada because in both nations vitamin B_{15} is considered an illegal drug.[11] *Nutrition and the MD* has nominated B_{15} for the title "quack nutrient of the year."[12]

Two other compounds deserve mention here, if only to say that they are not vitamins: the bioflavonoids and laetrile. The bioflavonoids are natural body constituents to which vitaminlike characteristics have been attributed. Sold in some stores in purified form as "vitamin P," they have made much money for store owners. However, despite much work, no bioflavonoid deficiency has been induced in animals or discovered in humans, and there is therefore no need to make special efforts to include them in the diet. They were disqualified as vitamins by the American Institute of Nutrition and the American Society of Biological Chemists in 1950.[13] As for laetrile (also called amygdalin and dubbed "vitamin B_{17}" by its enthusiasts), it has been proclaimed a cancer cure by the general public. However, it has never been shown by any kind of reliable testing to cure cancer.[14] Thus the FDA labels laetrile a hoax.

Not vitamins:
vitamin B_{15} (pangamic acid)
The story of vitamin B_{15} is told in Highlight 17.

vitamin P (bioflavonoids)

vitamin B_{17} (laetrile, amygdalin)

Much of the success of products like vitamin P and vitamin B_{17} is due to their emotional appeal. We have called the trick of inducing people to believe in miracle cures magical thinking. In the case of laetrile, another kind of emotional appeal is also used: scare tactics. People fear cancer, perhaps more than they fear any other disease. Laetrile proponents have capitalized on this fear by scaring the public into believing that the medical establishment frowns on

[11]K. McNutt, Vitamin B_{15}—pangamic acid—what is it?, unpublished statement from the National Nutrition Consortium, June 1978.

[12]Pangamic acid . . . "vitamin B_{15}," *Nutrition and the MD*, December 1978.

[13]R. S. Goodhart, The vitamins, Section M: Miscellany, in *Modern Nutrition in Health and Disease*, 5th ed., eds. R. S. Goodhart and M. E. Shils (Philadelphia: Lea and Febiger, 1973), pp. 259-267.

[14]Controversy 15: The FDA, in E. M. N. Hamilton and E. N. Whitney, *Nutrition: Concepts and Controversies* (St. Paul: West, 1979), pp. 362-364.

laetrile for dishonest reasons. "The doctors don't care if you die," they say, "so long as you pay huge sums for their services." Wanting to trust someone, wanting to hope that a cure is possible, the victim of cancer and her friends and relatives fall easy prey to this deception. The deception is all the more cruel because the victim yields to it out of love of life, and her relatives go along because they care about her and are willing to try anything to help her get well.

A FLAG SIGN OF A SPURIOUS CLAIM IS:

Scare tactics.

Putting It All Together   If you wanted to plan a diet that was adequate for the six B vitamins discussed above, you would be well advised to consume daily 2c or more of milk or dairy products (for riboflavin and niacin equivalents); two or more servings of meat, fish, poultry, or eggs, including liver and pork occasionally (for thiamin, riboflavin, niacin, and vitamin B_6); whole-grain breads and cereals (for thiamin, riboflavin, niacin, and vitamin B_6); and green, leafy vegetables (for folacin). The animal products would supply vitamin B_{12}, and all would supply thiamin. What foods would then be missing? Other vegetables, fruits, and fats—but as you will see in the following chapters, these latter foods are rich in vitamins A, C, D, E, and K. The conclusion is unavoidable: A balanced and varied diet is the best guarantee of adequacy for the essential nutrients. Such a diet would include selections from all the food groups.

Minimizing Losses in Food Handling

The B vitamins are all water-soluble. Whenever a vegetable is soaked or cooked in water and the water is thrown away, significant losses of these vitamins occur. In addition, each of the B vitamins is sensitive to heat to some extent, and riboflavin can be destroyed by light.

Bad advice

Moralizing is tiresome. For fun, we will play the devil's advocate instead and tell you how to maximize *losses* of the B vitamins. First, cook meats at high temperatures for long periods of time and throw away the juices that leak out of them. Leave milk in a transparent container on the countertop in the sunlight for several hours to destroy the riboflavin before storing it in the refrigerator. When baking, bake at high temperatures for long periods of time, using unenriched refined flour for your recipes. Buy unenriched bread and cereal products. When buying vegetables, select those that are several days old and that have been sitting at room temperature in the market since they came in. On bringing them home, put them in the sink, cover them with water, and let them soak for half a day before washing them. When cooking them, slice them thinly, cover them completely with water, bring the water slowly to a boil, and cook them for a long time. Discard the cooking water. If leftover vegetables are to be reheated, pour off the old water and add fresh water. Up to 50 or 60 percent of the B-vitamin content of foods can be lost in this way.

Lest you fear that we will offer no practical, positive suggestions about storing and cooking foods containing water-soluble vitamins, you may be reassured to learn that we provide these at the end of Chapter 10. Of all the water-soluble vitamins, vitamin C is the most vulnerable—to losses in cooking water, to heat, and to several other agents as well. Recommendations for the preservation of this most sensitive of the vitamins apply to the B vitamins too.

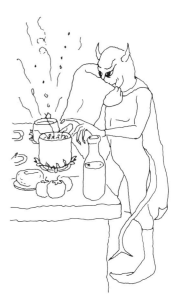

Summing Up

The B vitamins serve as coenzymes assisting many enzymes in the body. Thiamin, riboflavin, niacin, and pantothenic acid are especially important in the glucose-to-energy pathway; they are active in the coenzymes TPP, FAD, NAD^+, and CoA respectively. Vitamin B_6 facilitates amino acid transformations and thus protein metabolism; folacin and vitamin B_{12} are involved in pathways leading to the synthesis of new cells, and biotin is involved in lipid synthesis. These are only examples of the coenzymes' roles; there are many others.

B-vitamin deficiencies seldom occur in isolation; all have multiple symptoms affecting each body organ and tissue in proportion to the roles they play there. A lack of thiamin causes beriberi; a lack of niacin (unless compensated for by its amino acid precursor tryptophan) causes pellagra; a lack of vitamin B_{12} causes pernicious anemia. Human deficiencies of the other B vitamins, although not given names, have been observed for riboflavin, vitamin B_6, and folacin. The anemia of folacin deficiency resembles that of B_{12} deficiency because it produces large immature red blood cells; a key difference between the two, however, is that B_{12} deficiency also causes nerve damage and paralysis.

Vitamin deficiencies cannot be confirmed by inspection of an individual's food intake alone, although food intake provides some clues. The comparison of calculated nutrient intakes with recommendations rests on several assumptions: (1) that the individual is average (that the recommendations are applicable), (2) that body absorption is normal, (3) that the foods consumed are typical (that nutrient values found in tables of food composition are accurate), and (4) that the food has been prepared with reasonable care. Biochemical assessments of nutrition status are more accurate means of pinpointing nutrition problems. These cautions are meant to provide you with a context for considering food sources and nutrient intakes.

Thiamin is widely distributed in foods, but no food contributes a very great amount of it; a balanced and varied diet of nutritious food will best assure an adequate amount of this nutrient. Riboflavin is primarily concentrated in milk and secondarily in meats, which makes eating members of these two food groups advisable. Niacin is found wherever protein is found and can also be made from the amino acid tryptophan; it is therefore supplied in proportion to the amounts of protein in all common foods, except corn (which is low in tryptophan). These three vitamins (and iron) are added to all enriched breads and cereals. Vitamin B_6 is most abundant in meats, vitamin B_{12} is found only in animal products, and folacin is supplied best by green, leafy vegetables. Any diet plan that includes moderate amounts of all these foods assures probable adequacy for these nutrients.

To Explore Further

The complete terminology for the vitamins, together with their popular names and the correct chemical structures, were agreed on by the relevant scientific societies and published in:

● Nomenclature policy: Generic descriptors and trivial names for vitamins and related compounds. *Journal of Nutrition* 112 (1982):7-14.

Douglas Ramsey, who was captured by the Vietcong in 1966 during the Vietnamese War, personally experienced severe beriberi and scurvy and lived to tell the story in a moving account:

● Seven years in captivity as Douglas K. Ramsey tells it. *Nutrition Today*, May/June 1973, pp. 14-21.

A useful reference for the advanced student of nutrition is the review on choline, the lead article in *Nutrition Reviews* 36 (1978):201-207.

The principal hazards of overdosing with vitamins and minerals have been reviewed and published by the National Nutrition Consortium in a 1978 booklet available from the American Dietetic Association (see Appendix J):

● *Vitamin-Mineral Safety, Toxicity, and Misuse.*

Those who are interested in the history of nutrition discoveries may want to read the original report on the treatment of pernicious anemia using liver, republished from the 1926 *Journal of the American Medical Association:*

● Minot, G. R., and Murphy, W. P. Treatment of pernicious anemia by a special diet (Nutrition Classics). *Nutrition Reviews* 36 (February 1978):50-52.

The most authoritative (and still readable) book on the interactions of drugs with nutrients, including the vitamins, is:

● Roe, D. A. *Drug-Induced Nutritional Deficiencies.* Westport, N.Y.: Avi Publishing, 1976.

Another useful book for detecting the influence of drugs on nutrition status, which should be on every clinical nutritionist's desk, is:

● Grant, A. *Nutritional Assessment Guidelines*, 2d ed., 1979.

It is available from Anne Grant, Box 25057, Northgate Station, Seattle, WA 98125 ($7.50 plus $1.00 for postage and handling).

If liver cells could talk, they would describe the alcohol of intoxicating beverages as demanding, egocentric, and disruptive of the liver's normally efficient way of running its business. For example, liver cells prefer fatty acids as their fuel, but when alcohol is present, they are forced to use alcohol and let the fatty acids accumulate in huge stockpiles.

Brain cells would make the same criticisms. They expect to use glucose for fuel, and they need niacin and thiamin to free its energy. When alcohol enters the body it grabs all the available supply of

Glucose, the typical physiological sugar, is urgently important to the brain. The brain draws it from the blood. . . to use at once. . . . Narcotics diminish the oxidation of sugar by the brain. When the quantity of sugar supplied to the brain by the blood is less the oxidative turn-over is less owing to the lack of oxidative food. Without vitamin B the brain cannot make proper use of glucose as a food. Thought and behavior alter. If the conditions be prolonged, unconsciousness ensues, and if prolonged further the brain-cells are permanently damaged.

SIR CHARLES SHERRINGTON

getting rid of it. What liver cells have that other cells do not have is the ability to make alcohol-processing machinery — namely, the enzyme alcohol dehydrogenase and the MEOS described below. Alcohol dehydrogenase can convert alcohol to acetaldehyde, which can in turn be converted to acetyl CoA, the compound that all energy nutrients become on their way to being used as fuel. But we are getting ahead of our story. Let's start at the beginning, when alcohol first enters the body in a beverage, and follow it until it leaves or is made into useful acetyl CoA.

Alcohol Enters the Body

To the chemist, *alcohol* refers to a class of compounds containing reactive hydroxyl (OH) groups. The glycerol to which fatty acids are attached in triglycerides is an example of a chemist's alcohol. But to the average person, *alcohol* refers to the intoxicating ingredient in beer, wine, and hard liquor (distilled spirits). The chemist's name for this particular alcohol is *ethanol*. Glycerol has three carbons with three hydroxyl groups attached; ethanol has only two carbons and one hydroxyl group. For the remainder of this Highlight we will be discussing "alcohol," but you will know that we are really talking about a particular alcohol — ethanol.

$$
\begin{array}{c}
H \\
| \\
H - C - OH \\
| \\
H - C - OH \\
| \\
H - C - OH \\
| \\
H
\end{array}
$$

Glycerol is an alcohol.

$$
\begin{array}{c}
H \\
| \\
H - C - H \\
| \\
H - C - H \\
| \\
OH
\end{array}
$$

Ethanol is the alcohol in beer, wine, and distilled spirits.

these two B vitamins, so that the glucose remains idle and unused. The work of the brain cells thus slows down for lack of glucose energy.

The most dramatic evidence of alcohol's disruptive behavior appears in the liver. This is the only organ whose cells can burn alcohol for fuel to any great extent. All other cells are affected by the presence of alcohol but can do practically nothing about

339

From the moment alcohol enters the body in a beverage, it is treated as if it has special privileges. Foods sit around in the stomach for a while, but not alcohol. The tiny alcohol molecules need no digestion; they can diffuse as soon as they arrive, right through the walls of the stomach. You can feel euphoric right away when you drink, especially if your stomach is empty. When your stomach is full of food, the molecules of alcohol have less chance of touching the walls and diffusing through, so you don't feel the effects of alcohol so quickly. (If you don't want to become intoxicated at parties, then, eat the snacks provided by the host. High-fat snacks are best suited for slowing alcohol absorption because of their stomach-slowing effect.)

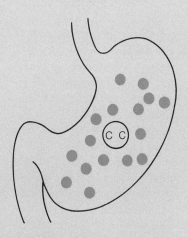

The alcohol (C-C) in a stomach filled with food has a low probability of touching the walls and diffusing through.

When the stomach contents are emptied into the duodenum, it doesn't matter that plenty of food is mixed with the alcohol. The alcohol is absorbed rapidly, "as if it were a V.I.P."[1] (Here again, high-fat snacks help moderate the effects of alcohol. Fat delays the emptying of the stomach, and so keeps the alcohol from entering the bloodstream so rapidly.)

Alcohol Arrives in the Liver   The capillaries that surround the digestive tract merge into the veins that carry the alcohol-laden blood to the liver. Here the veins branch and rebranch into capillaries that touch every liver cell. As already mentioned, liver cells are the only cells in the body that possess many molecules of alcohol dehydrogenase, the enzyme that can convert alcohol to a compound the body can use.

Alcohol dehydrogenase converts alcohol to acetaldehyde. Simultaneously it converts a molecule of NAD^+ to $NADH + H^+$. (You may recall that the N in NAD^+ is a form of niacin, one of the B vitamins.) Acetaldehyde uses another NAD^+ and TPP (the T stands for thiamin) to be converted to acetyl CoA, the compound that enters the TCA cycle to generate energy. Each molecule of alcohol

[1] F. Iber, In alcoholism, the liver sets the pace, *Nutrition Today*, January/February 1971, pp. 2-9.

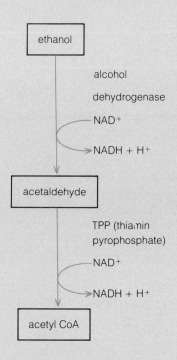

that enters the capillaries of the liver, then, will tie up two molecules of niacin and one of thiamin while being processed. A well-nourished person probably has enough niacin and thiamin to take care of a moderate amount of alcohol, but there is still a limit to the amount of alcohol anyone can process in a given time. This limit is set by the number of molecules of the enzyme alcohol dehydrogenase that reside in the liver. If more molecules of alcohol arrive at the liver cells than the enzymes can handle, the extra molecules of alcohol re-enter the general circulation and move on past the liver. From the liver they are carried to all parts of the body, circulating again

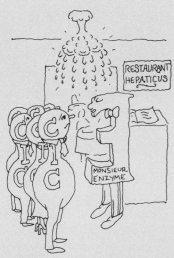

"I have places for only four of you."

and again through the liver until enzymes are available to convert them to acetaldehyde.

The amount of alcohol dehydrogenase is the rate-limiting factor in the body's handling of alcohol. The amount of enzyme that is produced varies with individuals and is controlled by heredity. Some racial groups, particularly Orientals and native Americans, do not have the genetic information for producing alcohol dehydrogenase. This difference has been offered as an explanation for why some persons, particularly Orientals, do not become heavy drinkers; they are made too uncomfortable by drinking to become addicted. In those who can make the enzyme, production is increased (up to the inherited limits) the more frequently it is stimulated. Thus a frequent drinker has

an abundant supply of alcohol dehydrogenase, which makes possible quick recovery from the effect of a drink. This may be how addiction occurs: A person consumes ever more alcohol to achieve the same euphoria. (An experienced drinker who has abstained for a while, however, loses the ability to metabolize alcohol rapidly. On starting to drink again, this person may be taken unawares at the stunning effect of even one drink.)

The amount of alcohol dehydrogenase is also affected by whether you eat or not. Fasting for as little as a day causes degradation of the enzyme (protein) within the cells, and can reduce the rate of alcohol metabolism by half. Drinking on an empty stomach thus not only lets the drinker feel the effects more promptly but also brings about higher blood alcohol levels for longer periods of time and increases the effect of alcohol in anesthetizing the brain.

As more and more alcohol is converted first to acetaldehyde and then to acetyl CoA, the available supply of niacin and thiamin is depleted. This has a profound effect on every cell in the entire body. There may be abundant glucose going past the cells to fuel their work, but cells need niacin and thiamin to make use of the glucose. Brain cells are especially vulnerable to a deficit of niacin and thiamin, because they rely solely on glucose for their energy.

Figure 1 is a drawing of the pathway from glucose to energy, showing the many places along the way that require niacin (NAD^+) and thiamin (TPP). The drawing of pathways like this one seems to be a favorite pastime of chemists and a most unfavorite kind of activity for beginning nutrition students. If you are such a student, take a moment with us to look carefully at this map, which shows how to get from here to there chemically.

Maps can be simple or complex, according to need. Sometimes when you ask for directions, the directing person will say simply, "There's construction up that street, so turn left at the second stoplight." He knows, and you do too, that there is no need to know the names of the streets you are passing but certainly you need to be told of possible obstacles. In Figure 1, we have named only the "streets" that are crucial to your understanding, but we have drawn in places where there may be "construction" that will cause traffic to back up or necessitate an alternate route.

This map is intended to show you that for glucose to get from "here to there," niacin and/or

Figure 1   A simplified version of the glucose-to-energy pathway, showing the entry of ethanol into the pathway. The coenzymes that are the active forms of thiamin and niacin are the only ones included. (For a more detailed diagram, see the figure on p. 236).

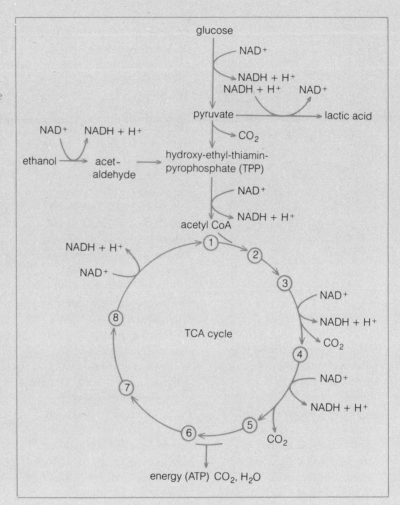

Acetyl CoAs are blocked from getting into the TCA cycle by the high level of NADH. Instead of being used for energy, they become building blocks for fatty acids.

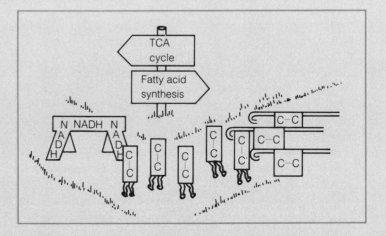

thiamin must be present. If they are not (and when alcohol is present they may not be), the road will be blocked and traffic will back up — or an alternate route will be taken. There are physical consequences to such changes in the normal flow of traffic from glucose to available energy. Think about some of these as you follow the diagram.

If all the body's niacin and thiamin are tied up, no energy will be produced even if there is plenty of glucose. (A shortage of glucose affects the brain, creating confusion and a change in behavior.) In each step where NAD+ is converted to NADH + H+, hydrogen ions accumulate. (As a result, the acid-base balance shifts toward acid; this is dangerous.) If there is not enough niacin to carry the compounds through the TCA cycle, acetyl CoA will build up. The excess acetyl CoA then takes the route to the synthesis of fatty acids. (Fat clogs the liver so it cannot function.[2]) As thiamin is depleted, more and more pyruvate builds up; it is converted to lactic acid, because

there is a surplus of NADH + H+, which this reaction can put away into temporary storage. The conversion of pyruvate to lactic acid relieves the accumulation of NADH + H+, but creates new problems: A lactic acid buildup has serious consequences of its own (it adds to the body's acid burden and interferes with the excretion of uric acid, causing goutlike symptoms).

When the liver lays aside important functions to attend to alcohol, there are other consequences. Protein synthesis nearly halts, because the liver cells use available resources to make alcohol dehydrogenase. As a re-

Pyruvate is converted to lactic acid if the pathway to acetyl CoA is blocked.

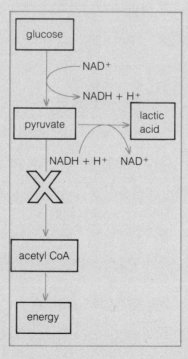

sult there is less protein for wrapping up the triglycerides to be carried through the blood. The consequent accumulation of fat in the liver can be seen after a single night of heavy drinking. Some important antibodies and other proteins essential to the health of the body are not synthesized either.

The synthesis of fatty acids is stepped up, because the acetyl CoA from the energy nutrients can not get into the TCA cycle while alcohol is being processed (here again alcohol has V.I.P. treatment). Thus the amount of fat stuck in the liver increases further. Fatty liver, the first stage of liver deterioration seen in heavy drinkers, interferes with the distribution of nutrients and oxygen to the liver cells. If the condition lasts long enough, the liver cells will die and the area will be invaded by fibrous scar tissue — the second stage of liver deterioration called fibrosis. Fibrosis is reversible with good nutrition and abstinence from alcohol, but the next (last) stage — cirrhosis — is not.

The liver's V.I.P. treatment of alcohol is reflected in its handling of drugs, as well as nutrients. In addition to the enzyme alcohol dehydrogenase, the liver possesses an enzyme system that metabolizes *both* alcohol and drugs — any compounds that have certain chemical features in common. Called the MEOS (microsomal

[2]C. S. Lieber, Liver adaptation and injury in alcoholism, *New England Journal of Medicine* 288 (1973):356-361.

ethanol oxidizing system), this system handles only about one fifth of the total alcohol a person consumes, but the MEOS also enlarges if repeatedly exposed to alcohol, so that it can handle more alcohol in shorter periods of time. When this system enlarges, it changes the body's responses to drugs as well as to alcohol. This can make it confusing and tricky to work out the correct doses of medications.

The doctor may prescribe sedatives every four hours, for example, assuming the patient does not drink, and expecting the MEOS to dispose of the drug at a certain predicted rate. Well and good; but if the patient does drink and uses the drug at the same time, the drug will be much more potent. The MEOS is busy disposing of alcohol, the drug can't be handled till later; and the dose may build up to where it greatly oversedates, even kills, the patient.

The opposite kind of thing can happen if the prescription is written for a drinker whose liver is adapted to metabolizing large quantities of alcohol. When this patient takes the drug (and does *not* drink simultaneously), the drug's effects wear off unexpectedly fast, leaving the patient undersedated. Imagine the doctor's alarm if the patient wakes up on the table during an operation! (Such an occurrence is rare with a skilled

---

Miniglossary

alcohol dehydrogenase: an enzyme found in the liver that converts ethanol to **acetaldehyde** (ass-et-AL-duh-hide).

antidiuretic hormone (ADH): a hormone produced by the pituitary gland in response to dehydration (or a high sodium concentration in the blood); stimulates the kidneys to reabsorb more water and so excrete less. This ADH should not be confused with the enzyme alcohol dehydrogenase, which is sometimes also abbreviated ADH.

cirrhosis (seer-OH-sis): advanced liver disease, in which liver cells have died, hardened, and turned orange; usually associated with alcoholism.

   cirrhos = an orange

euphoria (you-FORE-ee-uh): a feeling of great well-being, often sought by humans through the use of drugs such as alcohol.

   eu = good
   phoria = bearing

fatty liver: an early stage of liver deterioration seen in several diseases including kwashiorkor and alcoholic liver disease. Fatty liver is characterized by accumulation of fat in the liver cells; the fat would normally be carried away in lipoproteins.

fibrosis: an intermediate stage of liver deterioration seen in several diseases including viral hepatitis and alcoholic liver disease. In fibrosis the liver cells lose their function and assume the characteristics of connective tissue cells (fibers).

gout: accumulation of uric acid crystals in the joints.

MEOS (microsomal ethanol oxidizing system): a system of enzymes in the liver that oxidize not only alcohol but also several classes of drugs. (The **microsomes** are tiny particles of membranes with associated enzymes that can be collected from broken-up cells.)

   micro = tiny
   soma = body

narcotic (nar-KOT-ic): any drug that dulls the senses, induces sleep, and becomes addictive with prolonged use.

necrosis (neck-RO-sis): death of tissue.

V.I.P. (Very Important Person): a person with special privileges.

---

anesthesiologist in charge, but then a skilled anesthesiologist always asks the patient about his drinking pattern before putting him to sleep.)

Ethanol Arrives in the Brain   Alcohol is a narcotic. It was used for centuries as an anesthetic because of its ability to deaden pain. But it wasn't a very good anesthetic, because one could never be sure how much a person would need and how much would be a lethal dose. As new, more predictable anesthetics were discovered, they quickly replaced alcohol.

However, alcohol continues to be used today as a kind of anesthetic in social conditions, to help people relax or to relieve anxiety. People think that alcohol is a stimulant, because it seems to make people lively and uninhibited at first. Actually, though, the way it does this is by sedating inhibitory nerves; it acts as a depressant.

When alcohol flows to the brain it reaches the frontal lobe first, the reasoning part. As the alcohol molecules diffuse into the cells of this lobe, they interfere with reasoning and judgment. If additional molecules continue to enter the bloodstream from the digestive tract before the liver has had time to oxidize the first ones, then the speech and vision centers of the brain become narcotized, and the area that governs reasoning becomes more incapacitated. Later the cells of the brain responsible for large-muscle control are affected; at this point, people "under the influence" stagger or weave when they try to walk. Finally, the conscious brain is completely subdued and the person "passes out." Now, luckily, he can drink no more; if he could, he could die, if the anesthetic effect reached the deepest brain centers that control breathing and heartbeat.

In one way, you might consider it lucky that the brain centers are organized as they are, and respond to alcohol

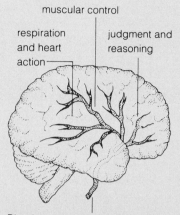

muscular control

respiration and heart action

judgment and reasoning

Blood carrying alcohol enters here.

in the order just described: One passes out before one can drink a lethal dose. It is possible, though, to drink fast enough that the effects of alcohol continue to accelerate after one has gone to sleep. The occasional death that takes place during a drinking contest is attributed to this effect. The drinker drank enough to kill before being put to sleep.

Liver cells are not the only cells that die with excessive exposure to alcohol; brain cells are particularly sensitive. When liver cells have died, others may later multi-

ply to replace them, but there is no regeneration of nerve cells. Hence the permanent brain damage observed in some heavy drinkers.

With these changes in mind, it is time to take a look at alcohol consumption from the social view and at the malnutrition that results from excessive drinking.

Drinking and Drunkenness   If you want to drink socially, you should drink with food and should sip, not gulp, your drinks. If you drink this way, the alcohol molecules will dribble into the liver cells, and the enzymes will be able to handle the load. Spacing of drinks is important too: It takes about 1-1/2 hours to metabolize one drink, depending on your body size, on previous drinking experience, on how recently you have eaten, and on how you are feeling at the time.

If a friend has drunk too much and you want to help him sober up, there is no

Alcohol Doses and Brain Responses

Number of drinks	Blood alcohol	Effect on brain
2 drinks	.05%	judgment impaired
4 drinks	.10%	control impaired
6 drinks	.15%	muscle coordination and reflexes impaired
8 drinks	.20%	vision impaired
12 drinks	.30%	drunk, out of control
14 drinks or more	.50-.60%	amnesia, finally death

reason to wear yourself out walking him around the block. The muscles have to work harder, but since they can't metabolize alcohol, they can't help clear the blood. Time is the only thing that will do the job; each person has a particular level of the enzyme alcohol dehydrogenase, and it clears the blood at a steady rate. This is not true for most nutrients. If you bring in more of a nutrient, generally the body steps up its metabolism rate. But not with alcohol.

Nor will it help your friend to give him a cup of coffee. Caffeine is a stimulant, but it won't speed up the metabolism of alcohol. The police say ruefully, "If you give a drunk a cup of coffee you won't make him sober, but you may make him a wide-awake drunk."

So far we have mentioned only one way that the blood is cleared of alcohol — metabolism by the liver. However, about 10 percent of the alcohol is excreted through the breath and in the urine. This fact is the basis for the breathalyzer test for drunkenness administered by the police. The amount of alcohol in the breath is in proportion to that still in the bloodstream. In most states legal drunkenness is set at 0.15 percent, although many states are lowering the criteria to 0.10 percent — especially as statistics accumulate that show a relationship between alcohol use and industrial and traffic accidents.

The lack of glucose for the brain's function and the length of time needed to clear the blood of alcohol are responsible for some diverse consequences of drinking. Responsible aircraft pilots know that they must allow 24 hours for their bodies to clear alcohol completely and refuse to fly any sooner. Major airlines enforce this rule. Women who may become pregnant are warned to abstain from the use of alcohol because the lack of glucose may interrupt the development of the fetus's central nervous system. This could occur even before the woman is aware that she is pregnant.

You may have heard the story of the country woman who kept saying "Amen!" as the preacher ranted about one sin after another; but when he got to her favorite sin, she whispered to her husband that the preacher had "quit preachin' and gone to meddlin'." We've tried to stick to scientific facts, so the only "meddlin'" that we will do is to urge you to look again at the accompanying drawing of the brain and note that judgment is affected first when someone drinks. When you hear someone say he is a better driver or a better salesman when he has had one drink, you can be sure he is ignorant of alcohol's action in the brain. What has really happened is that his judgment has been altered by one drink so that he *thinks* he is a better driver or salesman. If he really did perform better, it was because the alcohol depressed his inhibitions or muted his self-criticisms or tensions. He needs to look for a more healthful way to achieve these effects.

Drinking and Malnutrition   It has been estimated that more than 9 million people in the United States abuse alcohol to the point that their personal relationships, their jobs, or their health is impaired. One of the health hazards is malnutrition. Alcohol depresses appetite by the euphoria it produces as well as by its attack on the mucosa of the stomach, so that heavy drinkers usually eat poorly if at all. With a large portion of their kcalories coming from the empty kcalories of alcohol, it is difficult for them to obtain the essential nutrients. Thus some of their malnutrition is due to lack of food. If they eat well during the times they are not drinking, they may survive for many years without clinical evidence of deficiencies. Another cause of malnutrition, as already mentioned, is the B-vitamin depletion that plagues the long-time drinker.

Protein deficiency also develops, partly from the poor diet but also from the depression of protein synthesis in the cells. Normally the cells would at least use the amino acids that a person happens to eat, but the drinker's liver deaminates the amino acids and channels their carbon backbones into fat or into the TCA cycle to be used for energy. Alcohol's interference with glucose metabolism tends to increase the body's use of amino acids for energy, and eating well does not protect the drinker from protein depletion. One has to stop drinking alcohol for complete protection.

Two additional deficiencies that research has uncovered even in well-nourished alcoholics are iron deficiency[3] and folacin deficiency.[4] Abstaining from alcohol cures both deficiencies very quickly; at the most it takes only two or three days while a person eats an ordinary hospital diet. But with continued use of alcohol, even with extra supplementation, the deficiencies persist.[5] So although it may help to take vitamin supplements, this measure too is not enough to prevent the malnutrition seen in the heavy drinker.

Alcohol depresses antidiuretic hormone (ADH). All people who drink have observed the increase in urination that accompanies drinking, but they may not realize that they can easily get into a vicious cycle as a result. Loss of body water leads to thirst. Thirst leads to more drinking — but drinking of what? The only fluid that will bring relief of this thirst is water. The smart drinker, then, either drinks beer (which contains plenty of water), or drinks wine or hard liquor with mixers or chasers. If a person tries to use concentrated alcoholic beverages to quench thirst, it only becomes worse.

The water loss caused by depression of antidiuretic hormone involves loss of more than just water and some alcohol. With water loss there is a loss of such important minerals as magnesium, potassium, and zinc (see Chapter 14). These minerals are vital to the maintenance of fluid balance and to many chemical reactions in the cells, including muscle contraction. Repletion therapy has to be instituted early in the recovering alcoholic to bring magnesium and potassium levels back to normal as quickly as possible.

In summary, ethanol interferes with many chemical and hormonal reactions in the body. In particular, this disruptive molecule depresses protein synthesis, increases fatty acid synthesis, increases

mineral loss through increased urinary excretion, and interferes with the metabolism of glucose to energy by grabbing the available niacin and thiamin for its own metabolism. Its kcalories are useful only to the liver cells, and it effectively blocks the utilization of glucose by the rest of the body. Protein, the B vitamins, and minerals are the principal nutrient deficiencies found in heavy drinkers.

To Explore Further

In both of the following articles, the metabolism of alcohol in the body is clearly described and explained. Iber's article is especially well suited for the general reader:

● Lieber, C. S., The metabolism of alcohol. *Scientific American* 234 (1976):25-33.

● Iber, F., In alcoholism, the liver sets the pace. *Nutrition Today*, January/February 1971, pp. 2-9.

A clear, advanced, and up-to-date description of alcohol's metabolic and nutritional effects is presented in:

● Shaw, S., and Lieber, C. S. Nutrition and alcoholism, in *Modern Nutrition in Health and Disease*, 6th ed., ed. R. S. Goodhart, and M. E. Shils, Philadelphia: Lea and Febiger, 1980, pp. 1220-1243.

A teaching aid, *Alcoholic Malnutrition* by F. Iber, is a set of 16 slides illustrating the way the liver sets the pace in the nutritional troubles that beset the alcoholic. This aid can be ordered from the Nutrition Today Society (address in Appendix J).

[3]E. R. Eichner, The hematologic disorders of alcoholism, *American Journal of Medicine* 54 (1973):621-630.

[4]E. B. Southmayd, The role of the dietitian in team therapy for chronic alcoholism, *Journal of the American Dietetic Association* 64 (1974):184-186.

[5]Eichner, 1973.

B Vitamins

Exercises 1 to 3 make use of the information you recorded on Forms 1 to 3 in the Self-Study at the end of the Introduction to Part One.

1. Look up and record your recommended intake of thiamin (from the RDA tables on the inside front cover or from the Canadian Dietary Standard in Appendix O). Also record your actual intake, from the average derived on Form 2 (p. 14). What percentage of your recommended intake did you consume? Was this enough? What foods contribute the greatest amount of thiamin to your diet? If you consumed more than the recommendation, was this too much? Why or why not? In what ways would you change your diet to improve thiamin intake?

2. Repeat Exercise 1 using riboflavin as the subject.

3. Estimate your niacin intake using the method outlined on p. 330. Did you consume enough niacin preformed in foods to meet your recommended intake? If not, did you consume enough extra protein to bring your intake up to the recommendation? What do you suppose are the limitations on this means of estimating niacin intake?

Optional Extras

4. Find alternative sources of B vitamins for the person who doesn't drink milk. Many nonwhites avoid milk products because of lactose intolerance or personal preference. How can these people meet their riboflavin needs without drinking milk? Plan a day's menus around the foods popular in the U.S. South (pork, fish, chicken, corn bread, hominy grits, and sweet potatoes) to provide adequacy for thiamin and riboflavin. Be sure not to exceed the appropriate kcalorie level. Is it necessary to eat enriched corn bread and grits in order to get enough of these nutrients? Show your calculations.

5. Explode some of the myths surrounding the vitamins. Go to a health food store and interview the owner or salesperson about the virtues of the products being sold there. Jot down these claims and the evidence cited to substantiate them. Which claims would you be inclined to believe on the basis of the evidence? Which are examples of the spurious claims that we have identified with flag signs?

6. Discover how many kcalories alcohol contributes to your diet. You can use Appendix H to compute this. For example, 12 ounces of beer contain 150 kcalories, 1 gram of protein, no fat, and 14 grams of carbohydrate. Therefore, this beer derives 4 of its kcalories from protein (4 kcalories from 1 gram protein) and 52 of its kcalories from carbohydrate (14 grams times 4 kcalories per gram). The remaining 94 kcalories must come from alcohol. Now you can add a line for alcohol energy to the table above and work out what percentage of your kcalories comes from alcohol. What percentage of your total kcalories does this number represent? Example: I consume 1,800 kcal total. 94 kcal are from alcohol. (94 ÷ 1,800) × 100 = 5.2 percent.

One drink means one of the following:

- 12 oz beer
- 5 oz regular wine
- 3 oz sherry or port wine
- 1 1/2 oz whiskey
- 1 highball or cocktail

Guidelines for appropriate and safe alcohol consumptions: For the adult whose energy expenditure permits an intake of 1,800 kcal/day or more, two drinks a day are a generous allowance of about 10 percent of the total kcalories. For a person consuming fewer kcalories the energy intake from alcohol must be proportionately less. And for the pregnant woman, no alcohol consumption is advisable.

CHAPTER 10

CONTENTS

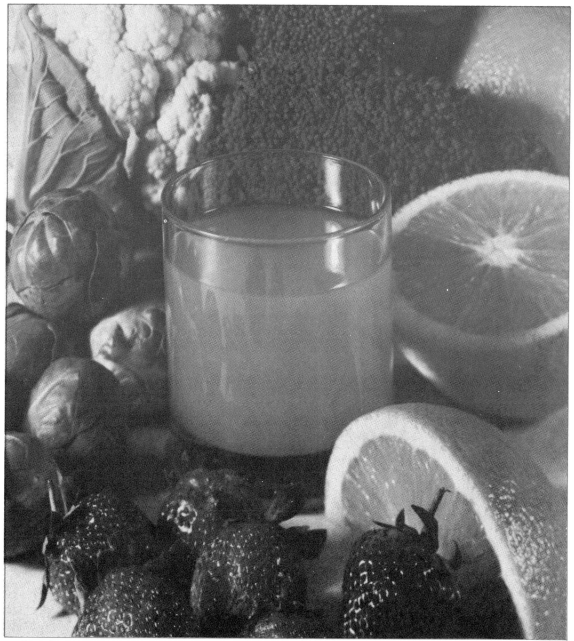

Foods rich in C vitamins.

VITAMIN C: Ascorbic Acid

It is often felt that only the discovery of a microtheory affords real scientific understanding of any type of phenomenon, because only it gives us insight into the inner mechanism of the phenomenon, so to speak.

C. G. HEMPEL and P. OPPENHEIM

Two hundred years ago, any man who joined the crew of a seagoing ship knew he had only half a chance of returning alive—not because he might be slain by pirates or die in a storm but because he might contract the dread disease scurvy. As many as two-thirds of a ship's men might die of scurvy on a long voyage. Only ships that sailed on short voyages, especially around the Mediterranean Sea, were safe from this disease. It was not known at the time that the special hazard of long ocean voyages was that the ship's cook used up his provisions of fresh fruits and vegetables early and relied for the duration of the voyage on cereals and live animals brought along as provisions.

The first nutrition experiment conducted on human beings was devised in 1747 to find a cure for scurvy. Dr. James Lind, a British physician, divided 12 sailors with scurvy into six pairs. Each pair received a different supplemental ration: vinegar, sulfuric acid, sea water, orange, lemon, or none. The ones receiving the citrus fruits were cured within a short time. Sadly, it was 50 years before the British Navy made use of Lind's experiment by requiring all vessels to carry sufficient limes for every sailor to have lime juice daily. British sailors are still derisively called "limeys" as a result of this tradition.

The anti-scurvy "something" in limes and other foods was dubbed the antiscorbutic factor. Nearly 200 years later, the factor was isolated from lemon juice and found to be a six-carbon compound similar to glucose. It was named ascorbic acid.[1] Shortly thereafter it was synthesized, and today hundreds of millions of vitamin C pills are produced in pharmaceutical laboratories each year and sold for a few dollars a bottle.

Human needs for vitamin C are the subject of much disagreement among experts. The publication of Linus Pauling's controversial book *Vitamin C and the Common Cold* thrust this vitamin into the limelight in 1970 and persuaded thousands of readers that they should be taking

scurvy: the vitamin C-deficiency disease.

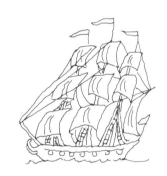

antiscorbutic factor: the original name for vitamin C.

anti = against
scorbutic = causing scurvy

ascorbic acid: one of the two active forms of vitamin C (see Figure 1). Many people consistently refer to all vitamin C by this name.

a = without
scorbic = having scurvy

---

[1]The agreed-on term for this vitamin, which has often been referred to as ascorbic acid, is vitamin C: American Institute of Nutrition, Committee on Nomenclature, Nomenclature policy: Generic descriptors and trivial names for vitamins and related compounds, *Journal of Nutrition* 109 (1979):8-15.

Doses of 10 to 20 or more times the recommended intake of a nutrient are termed **megadoses**. In the case of vitamin C, any amount over 1 g (1,000 mg) is considered a megadose.

doses much higher than the 30 or so milligrams a day cited as adequate in published recommended intakes. Highly respected nutritionists and other scientists have taken positions at both extremes on this issue. The controversy over the common cold has largely died down in the popular press (see Highlight 10), but the question of how much is enough is still being hotly debated.

There is also a controversy over the risks of taking large doses of vitamin C. Some argue for megadoses on the grounds that the risks are negligible but the risks of deficiency are great. Others argue against megadoses because the risk of deficiency is negligible but the risks of toxicity are great. Both positions are based on reasoning from small amounts of evidence and large numbers of words.

We face a difficult task in trying to sort out what is known about vitamin C, what is possible, and what claims are clearly unfounded. This chapter deals with the vitamin's known roles and debunks the obvious myths, leaving matters that are in the realm of uncertainty to Highlight 10.

Metabolic Roles of Vitamin C

Vitamin C is a mysterious vitamin. Like all the vitamins, it is a small organic compound needed by human beings in minute amounts daily. Being organic, it is convertible to several different forms, two of which are active (see Figure 1). Like the B vitamins, it is water-soluble, and so it is excreted rapidly when excesses are taken and is not stored for long in the body. But unlike the B vitamins (which for the most part have clearly defined metabolic roles as coenzymes), vitamin C acts in ways that are imperfectly understood. It plays many different important roles in the body, and the secret may be that its mode of action is different in each case. In some settings it may act as a coenzyme or cofactor, assisting a specific enzyme in the performance of its job. In others, it may act in a more general way—for example, as an antioxidant. Often the conclusion reached by investigators researching vitamin C is that it has to "be present" for certain reactions to occur but that the mechanism of its action will require further research.

Figure 1 Active forms of vitamin C. The reduced form can lose two hydrogens with their electrons, becoming oxidized. The electrons may then reduce some other compound.

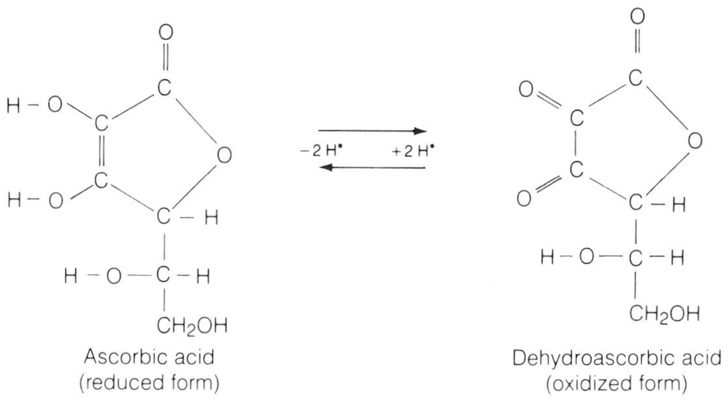

Ascorbic acid
(reduced form)

Dehydroascorbic acid
(oxidized form)

Collagen Formation The best-understood metabolic role of vitamin C is its function in helping to form the protein collagen. Brief mention was made of this protein in Chapter 4; it is the single most important protein of connective tissue. It serves as the matrix on which bone is formed and is the material of scars. When you have been wounded, collagen forms, and glues the separated tissue faces together, making a scar. The cement that holds cells together is largely made of collagen (and calcium); this function is especially important in the artery walls, which must expand and contract with each beat of the heart, and in the walls of the capillaries, which are thin and fragile and must withstand a pulse of blood every second or so without giving way.

Collagen, like all proteins, is formed by stringing together a chain of amino acids. An unusual amino acid found in abundance in collagen is hydroxyproline. After the amino acid proline has been added to the chain, an enzyme adds an OH group to it, making hydroxyproline. This step, which completes the manufacture of collagen, requires oxygen and a special form of iron—the ferrous ion. This iron has a tendency to convert to another form (ferric ion), which the enzyme can't use. Vitamin C stands by to catch ferric ions and reconvert them to the

collagen: a water-insoluble protein; the characteristic protein of connective tissue.

kolla = glue
gennan = to produce

Collagen is unique among body proteins, because it contains large amounts of the amino acid proline and has OH groups attached to this amino acid.

Ion: see Appendix B. Iron is an atom that can exist in two ionic states, ferric (Fe^{+++}, lacking 3 electrons) or ferrous (Fe^{++}, lacking 2).

1. Amino acids are strung together in a chain that includes many prolines.

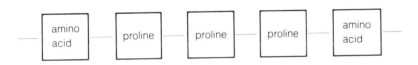

Figure 2 How vitamin C helps form collagen.

2. An enzyme, with the help of iron (Fe^{++}), adds OH groups to the prolines. Vitamin C stabilizes the iron in the ferrous form.

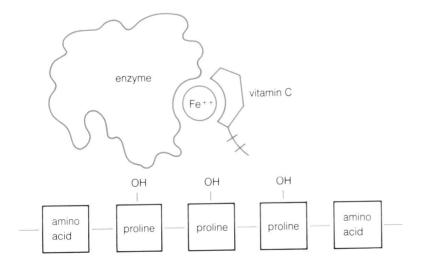

3. The completed collagen molecule contains many hydroxyproline units.

ferrous form so that the enzyme can keep on working.[2] Figure 2 shows how this process is believed to occur.

Antioxidant Action Chemists call the two forms of iron just described oxidized and reduced iron. The oxidized (ferric) form has lost electrons (see Appendix B); the reduced (ferrous) form has regained them. Any substance that can donate electrons to another is a reducing agent; when it donates its electrons it reduces another compound and simultaneously becomes oxidized itself. Vitamin C is such a compound.

The technicalities of oxidation-reduction reactions are not within our province, and the object of mentioning them is only to make one point clear: Many substances found in foods and important in the body can be altered or even destroyed by oxidation. (An example in Chapter 2 was oils that turn rancid when exposed to air.) Vitamin C—because it can be oxidized itself—can protect other substances from this destruction. Vitamin C is like a bodyguard for oxidizable substances: It stands ready to sacrifice its own life to save the life of another. Unemotionally, the chemists call such a bodyguard an antioxidant.

Because of its antioxidant property, vitamin C is sometimes added to food products, not only to improve their nutritional value but also to protect important constituents from oxidation. In the intestines, it protects ferrous iron in this way. In the cells and body fluids, it probably helps to protect other molecules, including the fat-soluble compounds vitamin A, vitamin E, and the polyunsaturated fatty acids, by maintaining their watery neighborhood in the appropriately reduced state.[3] Vitamin E and the polyunsaturated fatty acids are very important constituents of cell membranes, and these membranes house much of the cells' machinery. This machinery must be meticulously maintained so that the cells can live and work and so that they will discriminate successfully among the things that should enter them (cross their membranes) and those that should be excluded. Vitamin C—perhaps by way of its ability to alternate between the oxidized and the reduced state—helps maintain these vital functions.

The Absorption of Iron Vitamin C eaten at the same time as iron helps to promote the absorption of this mineral. It is not yet known how the vitamin performs this service, but one intriguing possibility is entitled to a paragraph of explanation.

You can't pick up a screw with a screwdriver—unless the screwdriver is magnetic. Even then, the screw may fall off at the slightest jolt. You can pick up a screw with a pair of pliers, but then you have to hold it tightly or it will fall out of their grip. But if you have a magnetic pair

For a picture of the way oxygen destroys the double bonds in an unsaturated fatty acid, see p. 64.

antioxidant: a compound that protects others from oxidation by being oxidized itself.

Chemists describe this action of vitamin C as maintaining the "oxidation-reduction equilibrium" or "redox state" and as participating in "electron transport."

---

[2]The role of ascorbic acid in the hydroxylation of peptide-bound proline, *Nutrition Reviews* 37 (January 1979):26-28.

[3]R. E. Hodges and E. M. Baker, The vitamins, Section K: Ascorbic acid, in *Modern Nutrition in Health and Disease*, 5th ed., eds. R. S. Goodhart and M. E. Shils (Philadelphia: Lea and Febiger, 1973), pp. 245-255.

of pliers, you can hold the screw so securely that the only problem may be that you can't let it go. A chelating agent is the molecular equivalent of a magnetized pair of pliers, and vitamin C is an outstanding example of such a molecule. These molecules are especially good at holding onto ions that have two positive charges, like ferrous iron (Fe^{++}). Vitamin C can grab and hold such an ion because it has two arms with negative charges on them (see the diagram in the margin). Thus vitamin C can not only reduce iron but can also stabilize it in the reduced form. The complex, iron-chelated-by-vitamin-C, may be much more easily absorbed by the intestinal cells than iron alone.[4]

Whatever the mechanism, it is now well known that eating foods containing vitamin C at the same meal with foods containing iron can double the absorption of iron. This strategy is highly recommended for women and for children, whose kcalorie intakes are not large enough to guarantee that they will get enough iron from the foods they typically eat.

chelating (KEE-late-ing) **agent:** a molecule that can assume a form suitable for trapping ions with two positive charges.

The typical U.S. diet supplies only 5-6 mg iron in every 1,000 kcal. Children need 10 mg per day, and women need 18 mg (see Chapter 13).

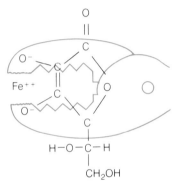

Chelation. The negatively charged "arms" of the chelating agent stabilize the two positive charges of the ferrous ion and hold the ion in place.

The Chinese have for centuries employed the strategy of serving vitamin C-rich fruits or vegetables and iron-rich meats in the very same dishes: loquat chicken, beef with broccoli, sweet-and-sour pork (including pineapple), chop suey (meat with cabbage), and dozens of others. Westerners are more likely to serve foods singly, although it is traditional to accompany certain meats with certain fruits: turkey with cranberries or pork with applesauce. These combinations are especially desirable if you choose to reduce your meat consumption in line with recent recommendations. To get the maximum iron value from small servings of iron-rich foods, serve a vitamin C-rich food at every meal.[5]

Some people try to protect the body from overwork by serving it different foods separately so that it can concentrate on handling those foods one at a time. Some evidence against this notion is presented in Chapter 5. The cooperation between vitamin C and iron, which seldom appear together in any one food, provides another argument against this simplistic notion.

A FLAG SIGN OF A SPURIOUS CLAIM
IS THE NOTION THAT:

Foods should be ingested singly to ease the body's work.

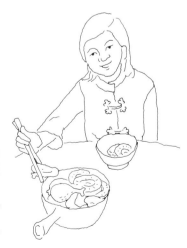

---

[4]We are indebted to Professor Stanley Winter of Golden West College, Huntington Beach, California, for pointing out this possible role of vitamin C to us.

[5]M. Balsley, Soon to come: 1978 Recommended Dietary Allowances, *Journal of the American Dietetic Association* 71 (1977): 149-151.

> On the contrary: Multicolored, mixed dishes are probably those to which the body, as well as the eye and the palate, responds most gratefully.

Amino Acid Metabolism   Vitamin C is involved in the metabolism of several amino acids. In at least some instances it probably functions as it does during collagen formation, by keeping iron or copper in a reduced state to aid an enzyme in adding OH groups to other compounds. Some of these amino acids may end up being converted to hormones of great importance in body functioning, among them norepinephrine and thyroxin.

The adrenal gland contains a higher concentration of vitamin C than any other organ in the body, and during stress it releases large quantities of the vitamin together with the stress hormones epinephrine and norepinephrine. What the vitamin has to do with the stress reaction is unclear, but it is known that stress increases vitamin C needs.

Epinephrine and norepinephrine were formerly called adrenaline and noradrenaline.

Vitamin C is also needed for the synthesis of the thyroid hormone, thyroxin, which regulates the rate of metabolism. The metabolic rate speeds up under extreme stress and also when you need to produce more heat—for example, when you have a fever or when you are in a very cold climate. Thus infections and exposure to cold increase your needs for vitamin C. Perhaps its involvement in the fever response to infection explains the vitamin's possible effects on cold prevention and symptoms, although there are other possibilities (see Highlight 10).

In scurvy, protein metabolism may be altered, incurring a negative nitrogen balance.[6] No one knows why this occurs, but the involvement of vitamin C with amino acids provides a notable example of the way nutrients of different classes cooperate with one another to maintain health.

Vitamin C and Other Nutrients   Some evidence suggests that vitamin C in some way aids the body in using folacin and vitamin B_{12}. It also interacts with calcium. Bones and teeth were long believed to be inert, like stones, but they are actually very active. Calcium is continuously being withdrawn and redeposited in these structures, another process for which vitamin C is essential. In scurvy, the teeth become loose in the jawbone and fillings may become loose in the teeth, reflecting loss of tooth material faster than it can be replaced.

[6]Hodges and Baker, 1973.

Vitamin C Deficiency

In both the United States and Canada, vitamin C deficiency is still seen despite the past century's explosion of nutritional knowledge. In the United States, the Ten-State Survey (see Chapter 18) showed evidence of unacceptable serum levels of vitamin C in about 15 percent of all age groups studied, with symptoms of outright scurvy showing up in 4 percent. Especially in infants, teenagers, and people over 60 years of age, intakes of vitamin C were much lower than the RDA (less than 50 percent). In Canada, many Eskimos and Indians and some members of the general population have deficiency symptoms. Evidently all we need is to be alerted to the symptoms that can result and to make efforts to obtain enough of this vitamin.

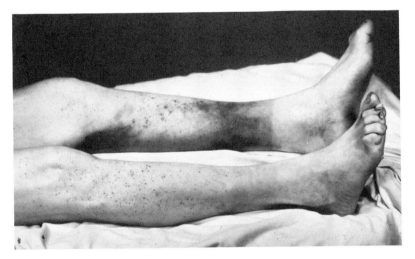

Early skin symptom of scurvy. There is a tiny hemorrhage around each hair follicle. These pinpoint hemorrhages are called **petechiae** (pet-EEK-ee-eye).

Photo courtesy of Dr. Samuel Dreizen, D.D.S., M.D.

With an adequate intake, the body maintains a fixed pool of vitamin C and rapidly excretes any excess in the urine. With an inadequate intake, the pool becomes depleted at the rate of about 3 percent a day. Obvious deficiency symptoms don't begin to appear until the pool has been reduced to about a fifth of its optimal size, and this may take two months or more to occur. Thus the first sign of an incipient vitamin C deficiency is a lowered serum or plasma vitamin C concentration.[7] A low intake as revealed by the diet history is the cue that prompts the diagnostician to request a clinical test to measure the body's vitamin C levels.

As the pool size continues to fall, latent scurvy appears. Two of the earliest signs have to do with the role of the vitamin in maintaining

Clinical tests: see discussion on p. 689.

latent: the period in disease when the conditions are present but before the symptoms have begun to appear.

latens = lying hidden

overt: out in the open, full-blown.

ouvrire = to open

[7]Vitamin C shifts unpredictably between the plasma and the white blood cells known as leukocytes; thus a plasma or serum determination may not accurately reflect the body's pool. The appropriate clinical test may be a measurement of leukocyte vitamin C. A combination of both tests may be more reliable than either one alone.

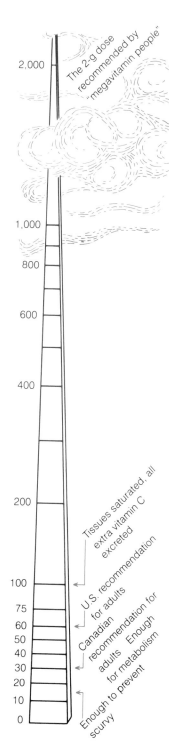

The 2-g dose recommended by "megavitamin people"

2,000

1,000

800

600

400

200

Tissues saturated, all extra vitamin C excreted

100 — U.S. recommendation for adults
75 — Canadian recommendation for adults
60 — Enough for metabolism
50
40
30
20
10 — Enough to prevent scurvy
0

Recommendations for vitamin C intake (mg).

capillary integrity: The gums bleed easily, and spontaneous breakage of capillaries under the skin produces pinpoint hemorrhages. If the vitamin levels continue to fall, the full set of symptoms of overt scurvy appears. Failure to promote normal collagen synthesis causes further hemorrhaging. Muscles, including the heart muscle, may degenerate. The skin becomes rough, brown, scaly, and dry. Wounds fail to heal because scar tissue will not form. Bone rebuilding is not maintained; the ends of the long bones become softened, malformed, and painful, and fractures appear. The teeth soften, and may become loose in the jawbone. Anemia is frequently seen, and infections are common. There are also characteristic psychological signs, including hysteria and depression. Sudden death is likely, perhaps because of massive bleeding into the joints and body cavities.

Once diagnosed, scurvy is readily reversed by giving vitamin C. It can be cured within about five days. Moderate doses in the neighborhood of 100 mg per day are all that are needed.[8]

Recommended Intakes of Vitamin C

How much vitamin C is enough? Allowances recommended by different nations vary from as low as 30 mg per day in Britain and Canada to 60 mg per day in the United States and 75 mg in Germany. The requirement—the amount needed to prevent the appearance of the overt deficiency symptoms of scurvy—is well known to be only 10 mg, but larger intakes raise the pool size. At about 60 mg per day the pool size becomes stable and does not respond to further increases. At an intake of 100 mg per day, 95 percent of the population probably reach the maximum pool size.[9]

It may seem strange that of the United States and Canada, two similar industrialized nations, one should recommend twice the vitamin C intake of the other. In view of the wide range of possible intakes, however, the Canadian and U.S. recommendations are not so far apart. Both are generously above the minimum requirement, and both are well below the level at which toxicity symptoms might appear. The range of possible intakes, illustrated in the margin from the perspective of people who espouse megadoses, shows that the Canadian and U.S. allowances are in the same ballpark. In contrast, the recommendation by Pauling and others that people should take 2 to 4 g a day (or even 10 g!) is clearly 'way up in the clouds.

It is important to remember that recommended allowances for vitamin C, like those for all the nutrients, are amounts intended to maintain health in healthy people, not to restore health in sick people.

[8]Hodges and Baker, 1973.

[9]A. Kallner, D. Hartmann, and D. Hornig, Steady-state turnover and body pool of ascorbic acid in man, *American Journal of Clinical Nutrition* 32 (1979):530-539.

Unusual circumstances may increase nutrient needs. In the case of vitamin C, a variety of stresses deplete the body pool and may make intakes higher than 50 or so mg desirable. Among the stresses known to increase vitamin C needs are infections; burns; extremely high or low temperatures; cigarette smoking; toxic levels of heavy metals such as lead, mercury, and cadmium; and the chronic use of certain medications, including aspirin, barbiturates, and oral contraceptives.[10] After a major operation (such as removal of a breast) or extensive burns, when a tremendous amount of scar tissue must form during healing, the amount needed may be as high as 1,000 mg (1 g) a day or even more.

Remember the distinction between the *requirement* and the recommended *allowance* or *standard* (see pp. 108-110).

Vitamin C Toxicity

The easy availability of vitamin C in pill form and the publication of Pauling's book recommending intakes of over 2 g a day have led thousands of people to take vitamin C megadoses. Not surprisingly, instances have surfaced of vitamin C causing harm.

Some of the suspected toxic effects of megadoses have not been confirmed for doses up to 3 g or more per day. Among these are formation of stones in the kidneys, upset of the body's acid-base balance, and destruction of vitamin B_{12} resulting in a deficiency. Research and reasoning have demonstrated that these effects are theoretically possible, but no cases of their actual occurrence in human beings have yet been seen.

When vitamin C is inactivated and degraded, a product along the way is oxalate. People sometimes have oxalate crystals in their kidneys that are not due to vitamin C overdoses.[11]

Other toxic effects, however, have been seen often enough to warrant concern. Nausea, abdominal cramps, and diarrhea are often reported. Several instances of interference with medical regimens are known. The large amounts of vitamin C excreted in the urine obscure the results of tests used to detect diabetes, giving a false positive result in some instances and a false negative result in others. Patients taking medications to prevent their blood from clotting may unwittingly abolish the effect of these medicines if they also take massive doses of vitamin C.

The anti-clotting agents with which vitamin C interferes are such anticoagulants as warfarin and dicoumarol.

People of certain genetic backgrounds are more likely to be harmed by vitamin C megadoses than others. Some black Americans, Sephardic Jews, Orientals, and certain other ethnic groups have an inherited enzyme deficiency that makes them susceptible to any strong reducing agent. Megadoses of vitamin C can make their red blood cells burst, causing hemolytic anemia. At least one person has died from this

[10]F. Clark, Drugs and vitamin deficiency, *Journal of Human Nutrition* 30 (1976):333-337; and Committee on Safety, Toxicity, and Misuse of Vitamins and Trace Minerals, National Nutrition Consortium, *Vitamin-Mineral Safety, Toxicity, and Misuse* (Chicago: The American Dietetic Association, 1978).

[11]*Vitamin-Mineral Safety*, 1978.

gout (gowt): a metabolic disease in which crystals of uric acid precipitate in the joints.

sequence of events. Those with the sickle-cell trait may also be more vulnerable to megadoses of vitamin C. In sickle-cell anemia, the hemoglobin protein is abnormal; it responds to a reducing agent by assuming a shape that distorts the red blood cells, making them clump, and clog capillaries. A case of this kind has also been reported. Those who have a tendency toward gout and those who have a genetic abnormality that alters the way they break down vitamin C to its excretion products are theoretically more prone to forming stones if they take megadoses of C, although no instances of either of these two events have yet been reported.

The proponents of vitamin C megadoses argue that these conditions are very rare and that the "normal" person need not worry about them. Opponents angrily retort that they are *not* rare and that nobody is "normal." The enzyme abnormality mentioned in the paragraph above is found in about 13 percent of black Americans and in a higher percentage of Sephardic Jews and Orientals.[12] If you have few acquaintances among these ethnic groups, then this condition may seem rare to you, but if you know more than ten such people, or if you are a member of any of these ethnic groups yourself, the risks of taking massive doses of vitamin C may apply directly to you or to one of your friends.

No two people have the same genetic heritage. Nobody has a complete set of "normal" genes and enzymes. No two people's nutrient needs are exactly alike. There are doubtless some people whose need is for vitamin C much higher than the average, and there are also some for whom the risks of taking large doses are much more severe than they are for others. Perhaps the greatest risk in speculating about megadosing with vitamin C or any other nutrient is the risk of generalizing. What is safe for your friend may not be safe for you.

CAUTION WHEN YOU READ!

A statement that applies to nearly all people does not apply to all people.

[12]The risks of vitamin C overdosing for special genetic types are spelled out by V. Herbert, Facts and fictions about megavitamin therapy, *Journal of the Florida Medical Association* 66 (April 1979):475-481.

The body of a person who has taken large doses of vitamin C for a long time adjusts by destroying and excreting more of the vitamin than usual. If the person then suddenly reduces her intake to normal, the accelerated disposal system can't put on its brakes fast enough to avoid causing a deficiency: It destroys too much. Some case histories have shown that adults who discontinue megadosing develop scurvy on intakes that would protect a normal adult. They have developed a temporary vitamin C dependency. An innocent victim of this kind of error is the newborn baby of a megadoser. In his mother's womb he has adjusted to high levels of vitamin C; once born into an environment providing much smaller amounts, he develops scurvy.[13]

The experience of a person who stops megadosing and then experiences a vitamin C deficiency on a normal intake may lead him to the wrong conclusion. "I took 3 g a day," he may say, "and then when I stopped my gums started to bleed and I knew I was vitamin C-deficient. Don't you see, that proves that I need very high doses? The recommended 30 to 60 mg are not nearly enough for me."

In reality, this person has deceived himself. To see whether the recommended, moderate intake of vitamin C is sufficient, he will have to taper off, reducing his large intakes gradually and allowing his body to adjust back to the normal condition. The emergence of withdrawal symptoms from drug doses of vitamin C does not prove a need any more than the emergence of withdrawal symptoms in a person using heroin or alcohol proves that he needs heroin or alcohol. The addict's body appears to need the drug only because it has adapted in order to cope with the drug, not because the drug is an essential nutrient. In these cases, as in hundreds of others, the consequences of drug abuse cannot be used to justify continued drug use. And in these cases, as in hundreds of others, medical help may be needed to assist in withdrawal.

After reviewing the published research on large doses of vitamin C, the National Nutrition Consortium reported in 1978 that there are probably very few instances in which taking more than 100 to 300 mg a day is beneficial. Adults may not be exposing themselves to very severe risks if they choose to dose themselves with 1 to 2 g a day, but above 2 g "genuine caution should be exercised," and amounts above 8 g per day may be "distinctly harmful. It is irresponsible and inexcusable to

vitamin C dependency: a temporary condition manifested by the withdrawal symptoms experienced by the person who stops overdosing; the body has adjusted to a high intake and so "needs" a high intake until it can readjust.

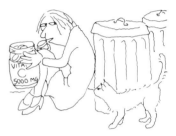

A pharmacological dose is higher than the intake needed to prevent deficiency symptoms and may have unexpected effects, as it may be working by a different mechanism than that by which the preventive or physiological dose works. See the discussion on pp. 453-454.

withdrawal reaction: a reaction to withdrawal (usually of a drug) that reveals that the user has become dependent, as for example when an infant born of a mother who took massive doses of vitamin C develops scurvy on an intake that would be adequate for the average infant, or when an infant born of an alcoholic mother suffers from the symptoms of withdrawal from alcohol (fetal alcohol syndrome).

---

[13]Two cases of this kind have been reported: *Vitamin-Mineral Safety,* 1978.

proclaim that ascorbic acid is safe in any amounts that may be ingested."[14]

In conclusion, the range of safe vitamin C intakes seems to be broad, as is typical for the other water-soluble vitamins. Between the absolute minimum of 10 mg a day and the reasonable maximum of 1,000 mg, nearly everyone should be able to find a suitable intake. People who venture outside these limits do so at their own risk.

Vitamin C in Fruits and Vegetables

The inclusion of intelligently selected fruits and vegetables in the daily diet guarantees a generous intake of vitamin C. Even those who wish to ingest amounts well above the recommended 30 to 60 mg can easily meet their goals. If you drink a cup of orange juice at breakfast, choose a salad for lunch, and include a stalk of broccoli and a potato on your dinner plate, you will exceed 300 mg even before counting the contributions made by incidental other sources. Clearly, then, you would have no need for vitamin C pills unless you wanted to join the ranks of the megadosers.

Table 1 shows the vitamin C contents of 50 common foods and reveals that the citrus fruits are rightly famous for their C-rich nature. But certain vegetables and some other fruits are in the same league: broccoli, brussels sprouts, cantaloupe, and strawberries. A single serving of any of these provides more than 30 mg of the vitamin.

staple: a food kept on hand at all times and used daily or almost daily in meal preparation.

The humble potato is an important source of vitamin C in Western countries, not because a potato by itself meets the daily needs but because potatoes are such a popular staple and are eaten so frequently that overall they make substantial contributions. They provide about 20 percent of all the vitamin C in the U.S. diet. Some young men report french fries as their only regular source of vitamin C, and yet because they eat so many, they receive the recommended amounts.

Foods that contain vitamin C are sometimes classified as "excellent," "good," or "fair" sources. The "excellent" category includes several dark-green vegetables and sweet peppers, as well as some of the foods already mentioned. The "good" category includes cauliflower and several more varieties of greens. The "fair" group includes asparagus, green peas, lima beans, turnip, tomatoes, lettuce, and many other plant foods. You might want to skim the fruit and vegetable sections of Appendix H to see which of your favorite foods are the best vitamin C contributors. Some of the items may prove a pleasant surprise.

Vitamin C contents of individual foods vary widely, as a look at various types of oranges (Appendix H) will show. One factor influencing the amount of vitamin C found in a fruit or vegetable is the

[14]*Vitamin-Mineral Safety*, 1978.

Table 1.   Vitamin C Contents of 50 Common Foods*

Exchange group[†]	Food	Serving size[‡]	Vitamin C (mg)	Exchange group[†]	Food	Serving size[‡]	Vitamin C (mg)
2	Brussels sprouts	1/2 c	68	4	Winter squash	1/2 c	14
3	Strawberries	3/4 c	66	3	Pineapple	1/2 c	12
3	Orange	1	66	2	Spinach	1/2 c	12
3	Orange juice	1/2 c	60	2	Summer squash	1/2 c	11
2	Broccoli	1/2 c	52	4	French-fried potatoes	8	10
3	Grapefruit juice	1/2 c	48	2	Radishes	4	10
3	White grapefruit	1/2	44	4	Mashed potatoes	1/2 c	10
3	Pink grapefruit	1/2	44	3	Blueberries	1/2 c	10
2	Collard greens	1/2 c	44	4	Pumpkin	3/4 c	9
2	Mustard greens	1/2 c	34	2	Green beans	1/2 c	8
2	Cauliflower	1/2 c	33	4	Sweet potato	1/4 c	8
3	Cantaloupe	1/4	32§	4	Corn on cob	1 small	7
3	Tangerine	1	27	3	Pear	1	7
2	Cabbage	1/2 c	24	3	Peach	1	7
5M	Beef liver	3 oz	23	2	Onions	1/2 c	7
2	Cooked tomatoes	1/2 c	21	3	Pineapple juice	1/3 c	7
2	Tomato juice	1/2 c	20	3	Banana	1/2 med	6
2	Asparagus	1/2 c	19	4	Potato chips	15	5
4	Green peas	1/2 c	17	2	Beets	1/2 c	5
2	Turnips	1/2 c	17	2	Carrots	1/2 c	5
2	Dandelion greens	1/2 c	16	4	Corn	1/3 c	4
3	Raspberries	1/2 c	16	1	2% fat fortified milk	1 c	2
4	Potato	1 small	15	1	Skim milk	1 c	2
3	Blackberries	1/2 c	15	1	Whole milk	1 c	2
4	Lima beans	1/2 c	15	1	Yogurt	1 c	2

*These are not necessarily the best food sources but are selected to show a range of vitamin C contents. Note in the left-hand column the clustering of 2s and 3s at the top and 1s and 4s at the bottom. No grains appear among the 4s, and there is a marked lack of 5s (meats) and a total absence of 6s (fats).

†The numbers refer to the exchange lists: 1 is milk; 2, vegetables; 3, fruit; 4, bread; 5L, lean meat; 5M, medium-fat meat.

‡Serving sizes are the sizes listed in the exchange lists, except for meat.

§One serving of any of the foods to this point contains the Canadian standard of 30 mg vitamin C, equal to half the RDA for adults (60 mg).

amount of sun it is exposed to. The reason for this may be clear to you if you recall that the vitamin, being a hexose, is a member of the carbohydrate family and that carbohydrates are produced by photosynthesis. No vitamin C is found in seeds, only in growing plants. Thus grains (breads and cereals) contain negligible amounts of the vitamin. Milk is also a notoriously poor source, and this is why orange juice is added early to an infant's diet.

Hexose: see p. 24.

No animal foods other than the organ meats contain vitamin C. For this reason, if for no other, fruits and vegetables must be included in any diet to make it nutritionally adequate.

Protecting Vitamin C

Vitamin C is an organic compound synthesized and broken down by enzymes found in the fruits and vegetables that contain it. Like all enzymes, these have a temperature optimum: They work best at temperatures at which the plants grow, normally about 70° F (25°C), which is also the room temperature in most homes. When a fruit has been picked, synthesizing activity (which has depended on a continued influx of energy from sunlight) largely stops; degradative activity, which releases energy, continues. Chilling the fruit slows down these processes. To maximize and protect vitamin C content, fruits and vegetables should be sun-ripened, chilled immediately after picking, and kept cold until they are used.

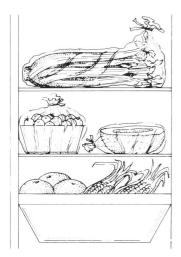

Because it is an acid and antioxidant, vitamin C is most stable in an acid solution, away from air. Citrus fruits, tomatoes, and many fruit beverages containing the vitamin are acid enough to favor its stability. As long as the skin is uncut or the can is unopened, the vitamin is protected from air. If you store a cut vegetable or fruit or an opened container of juice, you should cover it tightly with a wrapper that excludes air and store it in the refrigerator.

Being water-soluble, vitamin C readily dissolves into water that vegetables are washed or boiled in. If the water is discarded, the vitamin is poured down the drain with it. Cooking methods that minimize this kind of loss are steaming vegetables over water rather than in it or boiling them in a volume of water small enough to be reabsorbed into the vegetables by the time they are cooked. Of course, if the water soaks back into the food, as in making preserves or fruit pies, a larger volume of water can be used.

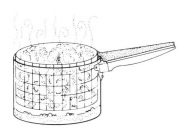

High temperatures and long cooking times should be avoided, to minimize the exposure of vitamin C to oxygen. Iron destroys vitamin C by catalyzing its oxidation, but perhaps the benefits of cooking with iron utensils outweigh this disadvantage (see Chapter 12). Another agent that destroys C is copper.

All of these factors represent legitimate concerns to which industrial food processors rightly pay attention. Awareness of them has brought about changes in many commercial products: fortification of instant mashed potatoes with vitamin C to replace that lost during processing, quick freezing of vegetables to minimize losses, and display of fresh produce in crushed-ice cases in grocery stores. Saving a small percentage of the vitamin C activity in foods can mean saving several hundred pounds of the vitamin a day; when some of it goes to people whose intakes are otherwise marginal, this can make a crucial difference.

Meanwhile, in your own kitchen, a law of diminishing returns operates. Vitamin C losses under reasonable conditions are not catastrophic. (For example, reconstituted orange juice typically retains 80 percent of its original vitamin C activity after eight days of storage.) You have other things to do besides hovering over your precious ascorbic acid, shielding it from all harm. If you turn the devil loose in your kitchen, as suggested in Chapter 9, you can indeed suffer undesirably high losses of this nutrient, but you can tolerate some losses if you make sure to start with plenty of foods containing ample amounts of vitamin C. To be on the side of the angels, perhaps all you need is a little common sense.

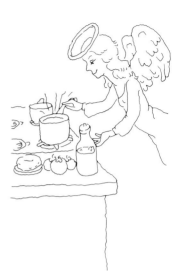

Summing Up

Vitamin C acts as an antioxidant in the body, helping to maintain iron in its reduced (ferrous ion) form and thus cooperating with enzymes that require this form of iron as a cofactor. The vitamin also helps regulate the overall oxidation-reduction state of the body cells and fluids, probably protecting vitamins A and E and the polyunsaturated fatty acids in this manner. In cooperation with iron it promotes the formation of the protein collagen, which is needed for scar tissue, intercellular cement, connective tissues (especially those of capillaries and other blood vessels), and the matrix of bones and teeth. It is involved in the metabolism of several amino acids, including the amino acid precursors of the hormones norepinephrine and thyroxin. It may also be involved in the absorption and utilization of folic acid and vitamin B_{12}, and it aids in the absorption of the mineral calcium.

Deficiency of vitamin C causes scurvy, characterized by bleeding from capillaries in the gums and under the skin, degeneration of muscles, failure of wounds to heal, malformations of bones and teeth, anemia, and ultimately death. Scurvy is prevented by the daily intake of only 10 mg of vitamin C and can be cured by a few days of 100-mg doses.

Recommended daily intakes of vitamin C range from 30 mg (Canada) to 60 mg (United States) or slightly higher (Germany). Stresses such as cigarette smoking or chronic aspirin use increase needs somewhat. Therapeutic doses used to aid recovery from scurvy, major operations, burns, or fractures range from 100 mg to not more than 1,000 mg (1 g). Toxic effects of megadoses (3 to 10 g) have been reported. The sudden discontinuance of megadoses may unveil an induced dependency, and scurvy may occur when intake is reduced to normal.

The best food sources of vitamin C are the citrus fruits, strawberries and cantaloupe, broccoli and other members of the cabbage family, and greens. Important "fair" sources include tomatoes, green peas, and (because they are eaten frequently by many people) potatoes. Preparation of foods to protect their vitamin C contents is best done away from air and alkaline solutions and without the use of large volumes of water. The inclusion of intelligently selected fruits and vegetables in the daily diet makes it easy to ingest well over 100 mg of vitamin C and unnecessary for healthy people to take any kind of vitamin C supplements.

To Explore Further

The American Dietetic Association has made available a cassette on vitamin C, Cassette-a-Month 7-78. The Association's address is in Appendix J.

A thoughtful and informative 1978 update on vitamin C appears in a publication by the National Nutrition Consortium:

● *Vitamin-Mineral Safety, Toxicity, and Misuse.*

This also is available from the American Dietetic Association.

The entire September 1975 issue of the *Annals of the New York Academy of Sciences* (vol. 258) was devoted to vitamin C; it contains 51 important articles reviewing recent research. Even the general reader might take this volume off the shelf and skim through it just to see how involved and extensive the work on this little vitamin really is.

On cooking to conserve nutrients, see:

● Seelig, R. A.   Conserving nutrients in fresh fruits and vegetables. United Fresh Fruit and Vegetable Association (address in Appendix J).

Vitamin C: Rumors versus Research

When Dr. Linus Pauling published his book *Vitamin C and the Common Cold* in 1970, he started a storm of controversy that raged for a decade.[1] Newspaper headlines screamed VITAMIN C CURES COLDS; others yelled back VITAMIN C NO EFFECT. One "famous scientist" said this, another that. Meanwhile, behind the scenes, teams of researchers in laboratories and hospitals across the world went to work designing and execut-

[1]L. C. Pauling, *Vitamin C and the Common Cold* (San Francisco: W. H. Freeman, 1970).

I have seen a paper with some writing on it strung round the neck heal such illness of the whole body and in a single night. I have seen a fever banished by pronouncing a few ceremonial words. But such remedies do not cure for long. We have to be on the watch. Illness can be fictitious, so also can cure. Human nature is perverse.

PLATO

ing experiments to determine whether in fact vitamin C has any therapeutic or preventive effect against the viruses that cause the myriad disorders collectively called the cold.

Since then some hundreds of articles have been published in the research journals, numbering several thousands of pages. Hundreds of people have been tested in a variety of experimental designs and still the answer is not completely clear. Meanwhile, Pauling has gone on to make additional claims for vitamin C; he urges that any patient diagnosed with cancer should immediately start taking 10 grams a day.[2] More research studies have followed, and the cancer question is generating as much controversy as the common cold.

The purpose of this Highlight is twofold. First, it is intended to make you aware of the difficulties inherent in attempting to discover whether a nutrient (or any therapeutic approach) remediates symptoms or cures a disease. The second purpose — because vitamin C may actually be involved in some way with cures of colds and cancer —

[2]Pauling, L. Vitamin C therapy of advanced cancer (a letter to the editor), *New England Journal of Medicine* 302 (1980):694; N. Horwitz, Now Japanese report 6-fold survival jump in terminal cancer with ascorbate megadoses, *Medical Tribune*, 22 (July 1981).

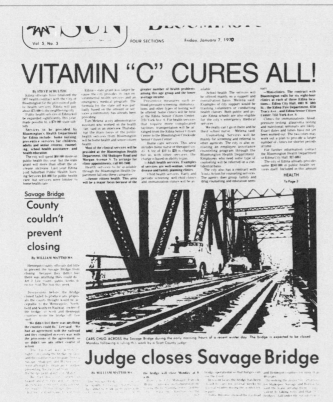

VITAMIN "C" CURES ALL!

Judge closes Savage Bridge

is to show you the kinds of research questions that will have to be answered before we can know what it does.

In most studies on the efficacy of vitamin C, two groups of people were selected. Only one group was given vitamin C; both were followed to determine whether the vitamin C group did better in terms of colds or cancer than the control group. A number of pitfalls are inherent in an experiment of this kind; they must be avoided if the results are to be believed.

Controls First, the two groups must be similar in all respects except for vitamin C dosages. Most important, both must be equally well to rule out the possibility that an observed difference might have occurred anyway. (If group A gets twice as many colds as group B anyway, then the fact that group B happened to receive the vitamin proves nothing.) Also, in experiments involving a nutrient it is imperative that the diets of both groups be similar, especially with respect to the nutrient. (If those in group B were receiving less vitamin C from their diet, this fact might cancel the effects of the supplement.) Similarity of the experimental and control groups is one of the characteristics of a well-controlled experiment and is accomplished by *randomization*, a process of choosing

the members from the same starting population by throws of the dice or some such method involving chance.

Sample Size To ensure that chance variation between the two groups does not influence the results, the groups must be large. (If one member of a group of five people catches a bad cold by chance, he will pull the whole group's average toward bad colds; but if one member of a group of 500 catches a bad cold, it will not unduly affect the group average.) In reviewing the results of experiments of this kind, a question to ask is always, Was the number of people tested large enough to rule out chance variation? Statistical methods are useful for determining the significance of differences between groups of various sizes.

Placebos If a person takes vitamin C for a cold and believes it will cure him, his chances of recovery are greatly improved. The administration of any pill that the taker believes is medicine hastens recovery in about half of all cases.[3] This phenomenon, the effect of faith on healing, is known as

---

[3]This finding is widely agreed on; it is discussed, among other places, in the debate on vitamin C in *Nutrition Today* (March/April 1978). See To Explore Further at the end of this Highlight.

the placebo effect. In experiments designed to find out whether vitamin C actually affects prevention of or recovery from colds or cancer, this mind-body effect must rigorously be ruled out.

To control for this effect, the experimenters must give pills to all participants, some containing vitamin C and others, of similar appearance and taste, containing an inactive ingredient (placebos). All subjects must believe they are receiving the vitamin so that the effects of faith will work equally in both groups. If it is not possible to convince all subjects that they are receiving vitamin C, then the extent of unbelief must be the same in both groups. An experiment conducted under these conditions is called blind.

Double Blind The experimenters, too, must not know which subjects are receiving the placebo and which are receiving the vitamin C. Being fallible human beings and having an emotional investment in a successful outcome, they tend to hear what they want to hear and so to interpret and record results with a bias in the expected direction. This is not dishonest but is an unconscious shifting of the experimenters' perception of reality to agree with their expectations. To avoid it, the pills given to the subjects must be coded by a third party, who does not reveal to the experimenters which subjects received which medication until all results have been recorded quantitatively.

Replication Repeating an experiment and getting the same results is called replication. The skeptical scientist, on hearing of a new, exciting finding will ask, "Has it been replicated yet?" It it hasn't, he will withhold judgment regarding its validity.

In discussing all of these subtleties of experimental design, our intent is not to make a research scientist

CAUTION WHEN YOU READ!

Before concluding that an experiment has shown that a nutrient cures a disease or alleviates a sympton, ask yourself:

Was there a control group similar in all important ways to the experimental group?

Was the sample size large enough to rule out chance variation?

Was a placebo effectively administered (blind)?

Was the experiment double blind?

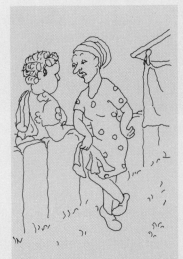

out of you but to show you what a far cry real scientific validity is from the experience of your neighbor Mary (sample size, one; no control group), who says she takes vitamin C when she feels a cold coming on and "it works every time." (She knows what she is taking, and she has faith in its efficacy.) These are a few of the important variables involved in researching a "cure." With them in mind, let us review the literature to see how successfully Dr. Pauling's vitamin C theory has stood the test of experimentation.

Reviewing the Evidence
Thomas C. Chalmers, a physician, reviewed the data from 14 clinical trials of vitamin C in the treatment and prevention of the common

cold.[4] Of the 14 clinical trials reviewed, 5 were poorly controlled, in Chalmers's judgment; and 8 were reasonably well controlled in that the subjects given vitamin C and those given placebos were randomly chosen. In addition, these 8 studies were double blind. When the data from these 8 studies were pooled, there was a difference of 1/10 of a cold per year and an average difference in duration of 1/10 of a day per cold in those subjects taking vitamin C over those taking the placebo. In two studies, the effects of vitamin C seemed to be more striking in girls than in boys.

In one study, a questionnaire given at the conclusion revealed that a number of the subjects had correctly guessed the contents of their capsules. A reanalysis of the results showed that those who received the placebo *who thought they were receiving vitamin C* had fewer colds than the group receiving vitamin C *who thought they were receiving the placebos!*

Other reviewers who have assembled and looked at all the evidence, as Chalmers

[4]T. C. Chalmers, Effects of ascorbic acid on the common cold, *American Journal of Medicine* 58 (1975):532-536. An independent 1975 review that covered the same experiments and reached the same conclusions was M. H. M. Dykes and P. Meier, Ascorbic acid and the common cold: Evaluation of its efficacy and toxicity, *Journal of the American Medical Association* 231 (1975):1073-1079.

did, have reached the same conclusions. At the end of the 1970s, reports of additional experiments were still coming out, and most were consistent with previous findings. The balanced picture emerging from the reviews seems to indicate that the effects of the vitamin, if any, are small.

The writer of popular science articles rarely reports on such reviews of literature because they are cold, objective, and give many viewpoints, rarely stressing one. They are not, therefore, sensational enough to sell in the marketplace. Who wants to read a scholarly, conservative, textbooklike report in a newspaper? What usually appears in the newspaper or in the TV news is the report of one experiment that obtained a significant result. "Professor So-and-So of the Such-and-Such Lab at the Etcetera University," the commentator may say, "has found that vitamin C does make a difference after all, at least for little girls. In a double-blind, co-twin study, in which one of each pair of twins received vitamin C and the other a placebo, the youngest girls receiving vitamin C had significantly shorter and less severe illnesses than their twins. . . ."

If you chose to look up the source of the report,

you would probably find that the study had been conducted as described and that the little girls had indeed had fewer colds than the little boys.[5] But the researchers themselves did not jump to the conclusion that vitamin C makes a difference. They pointed out very carefully that they had seen such a difference in their experiment, and in an admirable effort to put their finding in perspective, they went on to say: "One should be aware that, as the number of tests increases, the possibility of obtaining a 'significant' result by chance alone is also increased." In other words, the experiment would have to be repeated and the same result seen several times more before it could be accepted as real. The general public may be made uneasy by scientists who admit that their results are inconclusive, but the scientific community prefers total honesty to dogmatic statements.

The scientist who reports a "significant" finding from a single experiment is not being dishonest. Her purpose is simply to tell how she did it and what she saw, add-

ing a piece to the total picture. To get the total picture, you must look at many experiments.

Another kind of scientific reporting is useful for this purpose: reviews of literature, such as Chalmers's review referred to in this Highlight. These articles are just what their name implies — candid, objective reviews of all or nearly all of the experimental work on a theory that has been reported in the professional journals. The purpose of a review is to present a balanced picture of the research in an area. Probably the section of a review of literature that students most appreciate is the list of references. Without having to research the indexes on a topic, they can find a large number of references (perhaps as many as 50 or 60) listed in one place and in addition may read a critique of each (see Figure 1).

CAUTION WHEN YOU READ!

To weigh the reliability of nutrition information, ask yourself:

Is this one viewpoint? Or is it a balanced picture?

[5]J. Z. Miller, W. E. Nance, J. A. Norton, R. L. Wolen, R. S. Griffith, and R. J. Rose, Therapeutic effect of vitamin C: A co-twin control study, *Journal of the American Medical Association* 237 (1977):248-251.

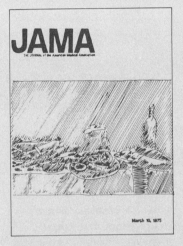

Journals

Reports of single experiments are presented in journals like the *Journal of the American Medical Association*.

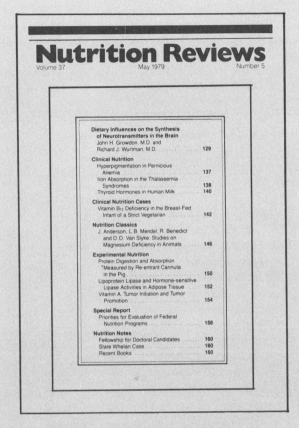

Reviews

To find a critique of all the important work on a subject, you can turn to a journal of reviews like the one shown here. One major review appears in *Nutrition Reviews* every month. It is followed by a bibliography that provides references to all of the original work reviewed.

Index

You can look up a large number of experiments on a single topic in an index of abstracts. The part of a page shown here, from *Biological Abstracts*, lists all recently published titles containing the word *vitamin C* and gives each one a reference number. The number refers to a short summary of the reported work, which also tells exactly where it was published. The indexes will lead you to reports of experiments in many different journals. New volumes of *Biological Abstracts* come out semimonthly. *Nutrition Abstracts and Reviews*, a monthly publication, would also contain titles including the word *vitamin C*.

Subject Context	▼ Keyword	Ref. No.
HABILITY/ INFLUENCE OF	VITAMIN B-6 UPON REPRODUCTION AND	50647
VITAMIN B-1 VITAMIN B-2	B-6 VITAMIN A VITAMIN C VITA	18486
AGNESIUM COPPER ZINC	B-6 VITAMIN B-12 AND FOLIC-A	69163
ASTIC-DRUG VITAMIN B-1	B-6 VITAMIN B-12 DIAGNOSIS L	23040
E CHANGES VITAMIN B-1	B-6 VITAMIN B-12 METABOLIC-D	49852
M VITAMIN A VITAMIN B-1	B-6 VITAMIN B-12 VITAMIN C P	7317
ITAMIN K FOLACIN NIACIN	B-6 VITAMIN B-12 VITAMIN C P	24026
VITAMIN B-1 VITAMIN B-2	B-6 VITAMIN B-12 VITAMIN C/	24030
VITAMIN B-1 VITAMIN B-2	B-6 VITAMIN C VITAMIN P EPIN	43638
E METABOLIC-DRUG ANTI	B-6 4 AMINO BUTYRATE 2 OXO	62889
ROL BILE ACID VITAMIN C	B-6/ EFFECT OF THE ALIMENTAR	42968
LORIDE IN RAT JEJUNUM	B-6/ IN-VIVO ABSORPTION AND	7806
BROMINE THEOPHYLLINE	BIOGENIC AMINE PSYCHOTROPIC	75520
UCTIVITY IN COWS GRASS	BUTTER FAT/ EFFECT OF A MICR	51809
SYNERGISTIC EFFECT OF	C AND ASPIRIN ON GASTRIC LES	12698
ENTATION OF DIETS WITH	C AND ASPIRIN TO IMPROVE THE	57020
T FOOD/ NITRATE NITRITE	C AND IN-VITRO MET HEMO GLO	25613
TH ON PECTIN ESTERASE	C AND PROTEIN CONTENTS OF T	63379
ATURAL COMPOUNDS OF	C AND THE POSSIBILITY OF ITS	71403
NTENTS OF DRY MATTER	C AND VITAMIN B-1 THERMOLABI	8724
M/ INHIBITING EFFECT OF	C AND VITAMIN B-12 ON THE MI	62091
PONSE TO A MIXTURE OF	C AND VITAMIN E AND CHOLINE	69403
LOVECH BULGARIA WITH	C AND VITAMIN P BY THE METH	57246
IN B-2 VITAMIN D-3 AND	C BY DENSITOMETRY OF THIN LA	24199
RATE CALCIUM THIAMINE	C CALORIC VALUE/ NUTRIENT C	53439
FLAVINE PYRIDOXINE AND	C CHILD VITAMIN K VITAMIN D	43033
RMONE DRUG VITAMIN A	C COENZYME Q-10 ZYMOSAN P	4081
TION ON VITAMIN A AND	C CONTENT OF WHEY SOY DRIN	30295
NEY HYDROXY PROLINE/	C DEFICIENCY IN GUINEA-PIGS	62414
YPER CHOLESTEROLEMIA	C DEFICIENCY, FUNCTION OF VI	68530
SED CONDITIONS HUMAN	C DEFICIENT GUINEA-PIGS INFL	32645
ISEASE CZECHOSLOVAKIA	C DRY MATTER SPECIFIC GRAVIT	22052

Figure 1 Sources of reliable nutrition information.

The reviews and experiments on vitamin C and the cold have provided one answer that still has to be cautiously phrased: The statistical effect of vitamin C on colds in the kinds of populations studied has been small. Meanwhile, what has the research on cancer shown so far?

Vitamin C and Cancer   In 1976, Pauling and his associate Cameron reported that they had administered vitamin C to 100 cancer patients in the Vale of Leven, Scotland, and had prolonged their survival rate. As compared with 1,000 similar patients who had been in the same hospital in earlier years and who had had only 50 days left to live, these patients lived 210 days.[6] In response, a group of researchers at the Mayo Clinic in Rochester, Minnesota, conducted a study to test the validity of this finding. The Mayo Clinic researchers criticized the earlier study on several grounds. It was not legitimate to use former patients as controls; most importantly, they said the control subjects should have been chosen randomly from the *same* population as those

given vitamin C to make sure they were similar. They therefore conducted a randomized, controlled, double-blind trial, giving vitamin C to 60 patients and a placebo that tasted and looked similar, to 63 patients. Both groups of patients worsened at the same rate and died at the same times. The authors concluded, "We cannot recommend the use of high-dose vitamin C in patients with advanced cancer who have previously received irradiation or chemotherapy."[7]

Pauling angrily jumped on the authors for their conclusion, pointing out that they had not fairly tested his hypothesis. His patients had relatively strong immune systems because they had not had the debilitating cancer treatments (radiation, chemotherapy) that the Mayo patients had had. The question whether large doses of vitamin C prolong survival time in cancer patients whose immune systems are not already severely damaged remains to be tested in a randomized, controlled, double-blind trial.[8]

[6]E. Cameron and L. Pauling, Supplemental ascorbate in the supportive treatment of cancer: Prolongation of survival times in terminal human cancer, *Proceedings of the National Academy of Science USA* 73 (1976):3685-3689.

[7]E. T. Creagan, C. G. Moertel, J. R. O'Fallon, A. J. Schutt, M. J. O'Connell, J. Rubin, and S. Frytak, Failure of high-dose vitamin C (ascorbic acid) therapy to benefit patients with advanced cancer, *New England Journal of Medicine* 301 (1979):687-690.

[8]Pauling, 1980.

Miniglossary

control: in any experiment in which a variable (see p. 453) is being tested, one group of subjects must be studied for the effect of that variable while a second group is followed — the **control group**, which is similar in all respects to the first except for that variable.

double-blind experiment: an experiment in which neither the subjects nor the investigators know which subjects are members of the experimental group and which are serving as control subjects, until after the experiment is over.

indexes: books in which the articles published in journals are listed by author, title, or topic (see Figure 1).

placebo (pla-SEE-bo): an inert, harmless medication given to provide comfort and hope.

placebo effect: the healing effect that faith in medicine, even inert medicine, often has.

randomization: the selection of control and experimental groups from a population using throws of the dice or some such method that ensures the members will be chosen by chance; helps ensure that the groups will be similar.

replication: repeating an experiment and getting the same results, a crucial test of the validity of an experimental finding.

Since the Mayo study a few other reports have trickled in, relating to the vitamin's effect on cancer. According to the *Medical Tribune* (a newspaper, not a journal), a Japanese researcher administered various doses of vitamin C to 99 terminal cancer patients who were "untreatable by any conventional forms of cancer therapy." Those receiving 5 to 30 g a day lived an average of 6.1 times longer than those receiving 4 g a day or less.[9] No mention was made of whether the study was double blind, so its validity is impossible to assess. It is mentioned here in hopes that the reader will be reminded to view it, and all other such studies, with skepticism unless the full details are given and stand up to close inspection. The question remains open whether vitamin C helps with cancer at all, but one result is entirely clear from the Mayo study. It did not help with advanced cancer patients who had received radiation or chemotherapy.

As this is written, a further attempt to define the effect of vitamin C, if any, on cancer is being made using a randomized, controlled, double-blind design. Because cancer takes too long (20 years) to develop, the researchers are studying a cancer precursor instead:

[9]Horwitz, 1981.

polyps in the colon. Within a few years, enough data should be in to indicate whether the vitamin C approach to cancer is a hopeful one.[10]

The big questions — Does vitamin C prevent/cure colds? Does it relieve cancer victims? — remain to be answered. Obviously there is more to come before the whole story will be known. Researchers are hard at work in many labs and clinics pursuing greater understanding of what the vitamin does and doesn't do. This Highlight can not give a final answer on a subject of such ongoing research. But this Highlight has fulfilled its two promises: to make you aware of the difficulties inherent in this kind of research, and to show you the kinds of research questions that will have to be answered before we know what vitamin C does. While you await reports of the next controlled, double-blind studies on carefully defined and randomized groups of patients, you may wonder what doses of vitamin C to take, yourself, in the light of what is already known. The decision is entirely up to you, but in case you should choose to aim for an intake of several hundred milligrams a day (say, 10

[10]W. R. Bruce, G. M. Eyssen, A. Ciampi, P. W. Dion, and N. Boyd, Strategies for dietary intervention studies in colon cancer, *Cancer* 47 (1981):1121-1125.

times the RDA), this reminder is in order: You can easily obtain this amount of vitamin C by including many C-rich vegetables and fruits in your daily diet. There is no need to take any kind of pills.

To Explore Further

Pauling's latest book is:

● Pauling, L. *Vitamin C, the Common Cold and the Flu.* W. H. Freeman, 1976.

L. Pauling's ingenious and thought-provoking arguments in favor of taking large doses of vitamin C are presented in:

● Pauling, L. Are recommended daily allowances for vitamin C adequate? *Proceedings of the National Academy of Sciences* 71 (1974):4442-4446.

Most of the March/April 1978 issue of *Nutrition Today* was devoted to a lively debate between Dr. Pauling and several prominent nutrition authorities. The debate brings out the major issues surrounding Pauling's new ideas about vitamin C and the differences in attitude among people attempting to assess the validity of his theories.

The most famous and fascinating story about vitamin C is the story of how Norman Cousins, the *Saturday Review* editor, recovered from a supposedly incurable disease. Cousins researched some of the medical literature, decided that vitamin C would cure him, removed himself from the hospital, and got well with the help of vitamin C megadoses and laughter. His account of the experience is intriguing and thought-provoking, telling how the patient's attitude, relief from stress, and faith affect healing. Highly recommended:

● Cousins, N. Anatomy of an illness (as perceived by the patient). *Nutrition Today,* May/June 1977, pp. 22-28; reprinted from the *New England Journal of Medicine.*

The sequel, which explores further the attitude of doctors and patients and the importance of the patient's involvement in his own cure, is also stimulating reading:

● Cousins, N. What I learned from 3,000 doctors. *Saturday Review,* February 18, 1978, pp. 12-16.

The American Dietetic Association makes available a cassette:

● Herbert, V. Megavitamin therapy. *CAM,* May 1977 (address in Appendix J).

Vitamin C

1. Look up and record your recommended intake of vitamin C (from the RDA tables on the inside front cover or from the Canadian Dietary Standard in Appendix O). Also record your actual intake, from the average derived on Form 2 in the Self-Study at the end of the Introduction to Part One (p. 14). What percentage of your recommended intake did you consume? Was this enough? What foods contribute the greatest amount of vitamin C to your diet. If you consumed more than the recommendation, was this too much? Why or why not? In what ways would you change your diet

to improve it in this respect?

Optional Extras

2. Find a substitute for fruit sources of vitamin C. Suppose a person dislikes fruits but likes vegetables. How much of a serving of greens would she have to consume daily to meet her recommended intake for vitamin

C? How many servings of potatoes would meet the recommended intake?

Cabbage is a favorite vegetable of the Chinese. How much cabbage must a person eat to consume the recommended intake of vitamin C?

Mexicans eat citrus fruits infrequently but use chili peppers and tomatoes daily. Can they meet their vitamin C needs this way?

3. Return to the health food store and ask about the virtues of vitamin C supplements. Jot down the claims and the evidence cited to substantiate them. Which claims are you inclined to believe? Which seem spurious?

CHAPTER 11

CONTENTS

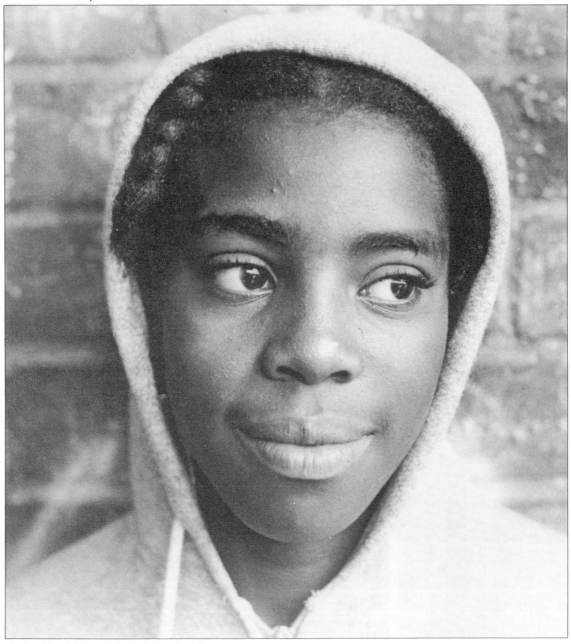

The health of the eyes depends on vitamin A.

THE FAT-SOLUBLE VITAMINS: A, D, E, and K

I remember well the time when the thought of the eye made me cold all over.

CHARLES DARWIN

Has it ever occurred to you how remarkable it is that you can see things? As an infant you were enchanted with the power this gave you. You closed your eyes and the world disappeared. You opened them and made everything come back again. Later you forgot the wonder of this phenomenon, but the fact remains: Your ability to see brings everything into being for you, more so than any of your other senses. Light reaching your eyes puts you in touch with things outside your body, from your friend sitting on the couch near you to stars in other galaxies.

Has it ever occurred to you how extraordinary it is that a child grows? From a mere nothing, a speck so tiny that it is invisible to the naked eye, each person develops into a full-size human being with arms and legs, teeth and fingernails, a beating heart and tingling nerves. Years go into the making of an adult human being, with each day bringing changes so gradual they seem undetectable. Only if you are absent during a part of this process do you notice it on your return and remark to a child, "My, how you've grown!"

And when did you last think about your breathing? In, out, in, out, day and night, year after year, you take in the oxygen you need and release it, disposing of the used-up carbons whose energy moves you and keeps you alive. The nutrients discussed in this chapter—vitamins A, D, E, and K—are vital for these and other processes that you may often take for granted.

The Roles of Vitamin A

Vitamin A has the distinction of being the first fat-soluble vitamin to be recognized. It may also be one of the most versatile, because of its role in several important body processes.

Vision   At the place where light hits the retina of the eye, profoundly informative communication occurs between the environment and the person. The eye receives the signal—light—and transforms it into informational signals that travel to the interior of the brain. There a

retina (RET-in-uh): the layer of light-sensitive cells lining the back of the inside of the eye; consists of rods and cones.

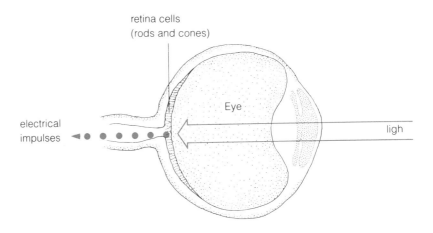

retina cells
(rods and cones)

Eye

electrical
impulses

ligh

pigment: a molecule capable of absorbing certain wavelengths of light, so that it reflects only those that we perceive as a certain color.

rhodopsin (ro-DOP-sin): the light-sensitive pigment of the rods in the retina.

iodopsin (eye-o-DOP-sin): the light-sensitive pigment of the cones in the retina. Both rhodopsin and iodopsin contain retinal; the proteins are different.

retinal (RET-in-al): an active form of vitamin A.

cones: the cells of the retina that respond to light by day.

rods: the cells of the retina that respond to light by night.

mental picture forms of what the light conveys. For this to happen, the eye performs a remarkable transformation of light energy into nerve impulses. The transformers are the molecules of pigment (rhodopsin, iodopsin, and others) in the cells of the retina.

Experts have written whole volumes about the eye, but it is not our intent to convey more than the briefest summary of the way its intricate machinery works. From the standpoint of nutrition, what is important is to know that this extraordinary capability, like so many others already discussed, depends first on the perfect structures and functions of protein and other molecules, which are synthesized following instructions coded in the genes, and depends second on obtaining in the diet pieces of those molecules that the body cannot synthesize—the essential nutrients. The description that follows identifies the cells in the retina, which respond to light by day and by night; the pigments within those cells, which absorb the light; and the way they convert light into nerve impulses, which are interpreted in the brain as a picture. The punchline is that a portion of each pigment molecule is the compound retinal, a compound the body can synthesize only if vitamin A or its relatives are supplied by the diet.

A mechanical genius could not have designed such a system better. Light itself cannot be conducted through the solid material of the brain, so it is changed into signals transmitted by nerves. But light comes in different colors (wavelengths), which reveal a lot about the environment. To keep the colors sorted out, the eye uses different light-sensitive cells (cones) to receive them. Blue light is absorbed by one set of cells, green by another, and yellow-red by a third. By day, combinations of these give the full range of color vision. By night, the light entering the eye is of low intensity, and the set of cells (rods) that can receive this light are of one kind only, so that by night a person can normally discern only the presence of light but not its color.

What absorbs the light is the pigment molecules inside the cells. Each pigment molecule is composed of a protein called opsin bonded to a molecule of retinal. When a particle of light (a photon) enters the eye, it is absorbed into the retinal molecule, which responds by changing shape (it actually changes color too, becoming bleached). In its altered form retinal cannot remain bonded to opsin and so is released. This disturbs the shape of the opsin molecule.

This shape change is used to send a message saying, in effect, "Light has entered here." By a mechanism not completely understood, the cell membrane is disturbed by the pigment's change in shape and permits charged ions to enter and leave the cell. The cell hyperpolarizes (that is, the electrical charge across its membrane changes), and an electrical impulse is generated that travels along the cell's length. At the other end of the cell, the impulse is transmitted to a nerve cell, which conveys it deeper into the brain. Thus the message is sent.

Meanwhile, back in the retina and once again in the dark, the changed molecule of retinal is converted back to its original form and rejoined to opsin to regenerate the pigment rhodopsin. Many molecules of retinal are involved in this process. There are about 6 to 7 million cone cells and 100 million rod cells in the retina, and each cell contains about 30 million molecules of visual pigment. Repeated small losses incurred by visual activity necessitate the constant replenishment of retinal or its precursors from the blood, which brings a new supply of these compounds from the body stores. Ultimately, vitamin A and its relatives in food are the source of all the retinal in the pigments of the eye.

Bright light seen at night destroys much more retinal than light seen by day, for three reasons. First, the pupil is wide-open at night, to allow as much light as possible to enter the eye. Second, there is an adaptation in the retina itself: A shadowing pigment protects the rods by day (they are not needed in bright light) but withdraws at night, leaving them exposed. Third, there are many more rods than cones. Hence if a bright light suddenly shines at night through the wide-open pupil onto the unprotected rods, much of the pigment in them is bleached and momentarily inactivated. More retinal than usual is freed, and more is lost. A moment passes before the pigments regenerate and sight returns. You no doubt have experienced this phenomenon when you were "blinded" by a flashlight shining directly into your eyes. People who must do a lot of night driving, facing headlights from oncoming cars, thus need an increased amount of vitamin A.

The eye is not designed for night driving or, in general, for accommodating itself to bright light at night. The mechanisms of vision evolved over millions of years, before humankind had harnessed electricity and lit up the night with headlights, beacons, and streetlights. In nature, animals in the wilderness have no need to adapt to sudden flashes of bright light at night, because they occur so seldom.

Vitamin A is undeniably an important nutrient, if for no other reason

opsin (OP-sin): the protein portion of the visual pigment molecule (rhodopsin) in the rods.

photon (FOE-ton): a particle of light energy. Depending on its wavelength, a photon conveys different colors of light.

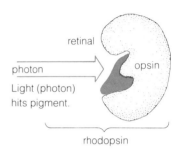

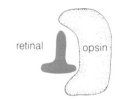

Retinal changes shape and is released from opsin. Opsin changes shape.

than that it plays a vital role in vision. But only one-thousandth of the vitamin A in the body is in the retina. It does other things as well.

mucosa (myoo-COH-suh): the membranes, composed of cells, that line the surfaces of body tissues.

urethra (you-REE-thruh): the tube through which urine from the bladder passes out of the body.

The cells on the body surfaces are known as **epithelial** (ep-i-THEE-lee-ul) **cells**.

mucus (adjective **mucous**): a substance secreted by the epithelial cells of the mucosa; mucopolysaccharide (see also p. 154).

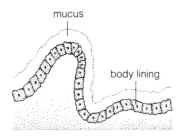

keratin (KAIR-uh-tin): a water-insoluble protein; the normal protein of hair and nails. Keratin may be produced under abnormal conditions by cells that normally produce mucus.

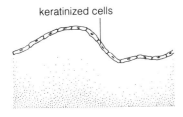

Body lining in vitamin A deficiency.

Maintenance of Linings Fortunately for you, your mucosa are all intact. You may not properly appreciate what these membranes do for you, but consider how important it is that each of these surfaces should be smooth: the linings of the mouth, stomach, and intestines; the linings of the lungs and the passages leading to them; the linings of the urinary bladder and urethra; the linings of the uterus and vagina; the linings of the eyelids and sinus passageways. The cells of all these surfaces—epithelial cells—secrete a smooth and slippery substance (mucus) that coats and protects them from invasive microorganisms and other harmful particles. The mucous lining of the stomach also shields its cells from digestion by the gastric juices. In the upper part of the lungs, these cells also possess little whiplike hairs (cilia), which continuously sweep the coating of mucus up and out, so that any foreign particles that chance to get in are carried up and away by the flow. (When you clear your throat and swallow, you are excreting this waste by way of your digestive tract.) In the vagina, similar cells sweep the mucus down and out. During an infection in any of these locations, these surface cells secrete more mucus and become more active, so that a noticeable discharge occurs; when you cough it up, blow your nose, or wash it away, you help to rid your body of the infective agent.

Vitamin A plays a role in maintaining the integrity of all these membranes. When vitamin A is not present, the cells cannot produce the carbohydrate normally found in mucus and produce a protein called keratin instead. As you might predict, greater losses of vitamin A occur during infection than under normal conditions.

The mucous membranes line an area within the body larger than a quarter of a football field, so this function of vitamin A accounts for most of the body's vitamin A need. And as if this weren't enough, vitamin A is also essential for healthy skin, another one or two square meters of body surface. Thus all surfaces, both inside and out, are maintained with the help of vitamin A.

Besides its roles in vision and in the maintenance of internal and external linings, vitamin A has an important part to play during growth.

Bone Growth "Growth is when everything gets bigger all together" is the definition given by a five-year-old. Certainly that is how it looks from the outside. A baby's hands, feet, arms, legs, and internal organs are all baby-size; an adult's are all relatively larger. Actually, however, the organs and body parts all grow at different rates and experience growth spurts at different times. The brain, for instance, reaches 80 percent of its adult size by the time a child is two, but the testes are still baby-size when a male first enters his teens. Furthermore, body parts do not just "get bigger"; bones are a case in point.

To enlarge the interior of a brick fireplace, the first thing you have to do is remove some of the old bricks. Similarly, to make a bone larger requires remodeling, as the picture in the margin shows. To convert a small bone into a large bone, the bone-remodeling cells must "undo" some parts of the small bone as they go.

It is in the undoing that vitamin A is involved. Some of the cells involved in bone formation are packed with sacs of degradative enzymes that can take apart the structures of bone. With the help of vitamin A in a carefully controlled process, these cells release their enzymes, which gradually eat away at selected sites in the bone, removing the parts that are not needed as the bone grows longer. (A similar process occurs when a tadpole loses its tail and becomes a frog. As you know, the tail doesn't simply fall off; rather it is resorbed, "growing" shorter and shorter until it disappears. As a fetus you also had a tail and lost it, a process that depended on vitamin A.)

Vitamin A's role in promoting good night vision, the health of mucous membranes and skin, and the growth of bone are well known although still not completely understood. Others, less well understood, include roles it plays in reproduction, in maintaining the stability of cell membranes, in helping the adrenal gland to synthesize a hormone (corticosterone), in helping to ensure a normal output of thyroid hormone (thyroxin) from the thyroid gland, in helping to maintain nerve cell sheaths, in assisting in immune reactions, in helping to manufacture red blood cells, and many others. Vitamin A research still in progress is yielding many new answers to the questions of how this nutrient functions in the body

Vitamin A Deficiency

Up to a year's supply of vitamin A may be stored in the body, 90 percent of it in the liver. If you stop eating good food sources of the vitamin, deficiency symptoms will not begin to appear until after your stores are depleted. Then, however, the consequences are profound and severe. Table 1 itemizes some of them. Some have to do with the role of vitamin A in vision, some with its functions in epithelial tissue, some with its part in growth; others are as yet unexplained.

Impaired Night Vision If sufficient retinal is not available (from the blood bathing the cells of the retina) to rapidly regenerate visual pigments bleached by light, then a flash of bright light at night will be followed by a prolonged spell of night blindness. This is one of the first detectable signs of vitamin A deficiency. Because night blindness is easy to test, it is a symptom that aids in diagnosis of the condition. (Of course it is only a symptom and may indicate some condition other than vitamin A deficiency.)

These sacs of degradative enzymes are **lysosomes** (LYE-so-zomes).

lyso = to break
soma = body

The cells are osteoclasts (see p. 387).

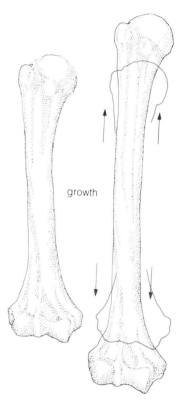

growth

As bone lengthens, vitamin A helps remove old bone.

night blindness: slow recovery of vision after flashes of bright light at night; an early symptom of vitamin A deficiency.

Night blindness.

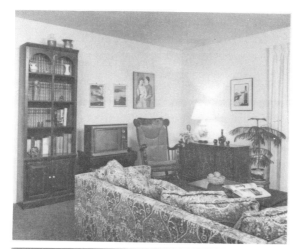

In bright light you can see all the details in this room.

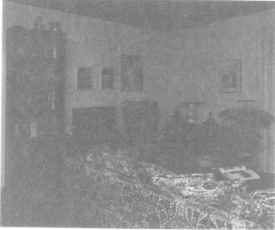

When the lights are turned out, you are momentarily blinded.

normal
night
vision

defective
night
vision

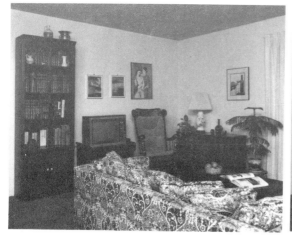

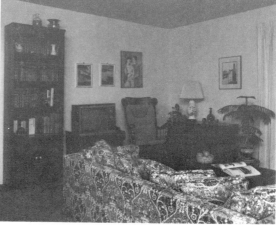

Then you recover your vision and can again see the details in the semidarkness.

A vitamin A deficiency makes this recovery of night vision impossible.

Table 1.   Vitamin A Deficiency

Area affected	Main effect	Technical name for symptoms
Eye		
retina	night blindness	
membranes	failure to secrete mucopolysaccharide causes changes in epithelial tissue and keratinization	
general*	drying (mildest form) irreversible drying and degeneration of the cornea causing blindness (most severe)	**xerosis** **keratomalacia**
Skin	hair follicles plug with keratin forming white lumps	**hyperkeratosis**
GI tract	changes in lining; diarrhea	
Respiratory tract	changes in lining; infections	
Urogenital tract	changes in lining favor calcium deposition resulting in kidney stones, bladder disorders	
Bones	bone growth ceases; shapes of bones change	
Teeth	enamel-forming cells malfunction, teeth develop cracks and tend to decay; dentin-forming cells atrophy	
Nervous system	brain and spinal cord grow too fast for stunted skull and spine; injury to brain and nerves causes paralysis	
Blood	anemia, often masked by dehydration	

*The eye's symptoms of vitamin A deficiency are collectively known as xerophthalmia.

enamel: the hard mineral coating of the outside of the tooth, composed of calcium compounds embedded in a fine network of keratin fibers.

dentin: the softer material underlying the enamel of the tooth, composed of calcium compounds embedded in a network of collagen fibers.

For a picture of tooth structure, see p. 457.

Roughened Surfaces   Instead of staying smooth and well-rounded and producing normal mucus, the epithelial cells flatten and harden with vitamin A deficiency, losing their protective mucous coating and filling with keratin instead. In the eye this process leads to drying and hardening of the cornea, which may progress to blindness. In the

The epithelial cells fill with keratin in a process known as **keratinization.** The progression of this condition to the extreme is **hyperkeratosis.**

hyper = too much

In the eye, the symptoms of vitamin A deficiency are collectively known as **xerophthalmia** (zer-off-THAL-mee-uh).

xero = dry
ophthalm = eye

An early sign is **xerosis** (drying of the cornea); the latest and most severe is **keratomalacia** (KAIR-a-toe-ma-LAY-shuh), total blindness.

malacia = softening, weakening

cornea (KOR-nee-uh): the transparent membrane covering the outside of the front of the eye.

The accumulation of this hard material, keratin, around each hair follicle is **follicular hyperkeratosis.**

follicle (FOLL-i-cul): a group of cells in the skin from which a hair grows.

mouth, drying and hardening of the salivary glands makes them susceptible to infection; failure of mucous secretion in the mouth may lead to loss of appetite. Mucous secretion in the stomach and intestines is reduced, hindering normal digestion and absorption of nutrients, causing diarrhea, and so indirectly worsening the deficiency. Infections of the respiratory tract, the urinary tract, and the vagina are also made more likely by vitamin A deficiency. On the outer body surface, the cells also harden and flatten, making the skin dry, rough, scaly, and hard. Around each hair follicle an accumulation of hard material makes a lump.

Abnormal Growth   Because growth and development of the brain and eyes are most rapid in the unborn and in the very young baby, the effects of vitamin A deficiency are most severe in and around the time of birth. For example, in a child of one or two, abnormal growth of the skull may cause crowding of the brain (which is growing rapidly at that age). Tooth growth may also be abnormal. Crooked teeth in a child may reflect a vitamin A deficiency suffered by its mother while its jawbones were forming during her pregnancy. Damage to the eyes is also most pronounced in the young, with blindness the result in thousands of cases of vitamin A deficiency throughout the world. Vitamin A deficiency is second only to protein-kcalorie malnutrition as a nutrition problem afflicting the young of the world.

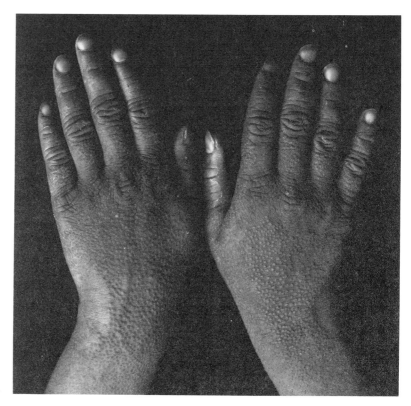

Follicular hyperkeratosis.

Photo courtesy of Parke-Davis & Company.

Naivete on the part of the well-intentioned can cause more harm than good, as is often observed when attempts are made to remedy the problem of malnutrition in the underdeveloped countries. An awareness of the way nutrients function in the body and of their interdependence must precede efforts to correct malnutrition problems, as the case of vitamin A illustrates.

Vitamin A depends on proteins for its functions and transport in the body. In protein-kcalorie malnutrition, when vitamin A stores are also low, there is a balance of a kind. But when protein is given without supplemental vitamin A, protein carriers that may be synthesized deplete the liver of the last available stores of vitamin A, thus precipitating a deficiency.[1] Administration of protein has been observed to cause an epidemic of blindness, as when skim milk was offered by UNICEF to children in Brazil (in 1961). Vitamin A capsules were supplied with the milk, but the parents often ate the capsules or sold them, giving only the milk to the children.[2]

The mineral zinc is also needed for the body to use vitamin A properly. An apparent vitamin A deficiency may reflect an underlying zinc deficiency that must first be corrected.

> Knowledge of nutrition must accompany the giving of nutritional help.

In the United States as well, the problem of vitamin A deficiency is all too common. The Ten-State Survey revealed that a third of the children under six who were examined had less than the recommended vitamin A intakes.[3] Spanish-Americans and blacks exhibited the most pronounced evidence of deficiency. Some subgroups of the Canadian population are also deficient, notably Canadian and Eskimo women, especially during their pregnancies.

A major source of vitamin A is the vegetable group, and a probable reason for widespread deficits of vitamin A in children is their refusal to eat these foods. A section of Chapter 16 emphasizes the importance of encouraging children to like vegetables and suggests practical ways to ease their acceptance.

[1] O. A. Roels and N. S. T. Lui, The vitamins, Section A: Vitamin A and carotene, in *Modern Nutrition in Health and Disease*, 5th ed., eds. R. S. Goodhart and M. E. Shils (Philadelphia: Lea and Febiger, 1973), pp. 142-157.

[2] O. A. Roels, Vitamin A physiology, *Journal of the American Medical Association* 214 (1970):1097-1102.

[3] U.S. Department of Health, Education, and Welfare, *Ten-State Nutrition Survey, 1968-1970*, publication no. (HSM) 72-8130 (Atlanta: Center for Disease Control, 1972).

Recommended Intakes of Vitamin A

Vitamin A terminology is in a period of transition. Vitamin A occurs in a number of different forms, and these convert to the active forms in the body with different efficiencies. Now that the chemistry and conversion rates of most of these compounds are known, it makes sense to state the recommended amounts of vitamin A and the amounts found in foods in terms of the total activity available from the various forms after they have been converted to the active form. The active form used for reference is retinol, and the recommended amounts of vitamin A are stated in terms of retinol equivalents (RE). As of 1980, both U.S. and Canadian authorities were using this terminology and were recommending 1,000 RE per day for adult men and 800 RE for women.

The amounts of vitamin A found in *foods*, however, are reported using an older system of measurement, international units (IU), which are based on some assumptions that are now known to be not completely correct. In the future, tables of food composition will report the vitamin A activity of foods in RE, but until they do, you will have to do some computing. If you wish to use a table like Appendix H or Table 3 in this chapter to compute your vitamin A intake, you will have to remember both terms, RE and IU, and the fact that 1 RE is roughly equivalent to 5 IU. Some additional guidelines for interpreting vitamin A measures given in IU are offered after the next section.

Vitamin A Toxicity

Vitamin A toxicity is not likely if you depend on foods for your nutrients, but if you take pills or supplements containing the vitamin, toxicity is a real possibility. Overdoses have serious effects on many of the same body systems that vitamin A helps when ingested in proper amounts (see Table 2). Children are most likely to be affected, because they need less, they are smaller and more sensitive to overdoses, and it is easy to make the mistake of giving them too much in pill form or in other concentrates. The availability of breakfast cereals, instant meals, fortified milk, and chewable candy-like vitamins each containing 100 percent of the recommended daily intake of vitamin A makes it possible for a well-meaning parent to provide several times the daily allowance of the vitamin to a child in a few hours. Serious toxicity is seen in small infants when they are given more than ten times the recommended amount every day for weeks at a time. A child herself may also overdose: Liking vitamin pills and thinking of them as candy, she may eat several.

There is a wide range of vitamin A intakes in which neither deficiency nor toxicity symptoms appear. Recommended intakes in both the United States and Canada are set at about double the minimum

retinol: one of the active forms of vitamin A, similar to retinal. Retinol is an alcohol; retinal is an aldehyde (see pp. 339 and 64).

RE (retinol equivalent): a measure of vitamin A activity; the amount of retinol that a vitamin A compound will yield after conversion.

IU (international unit): a measure of vitamin A activity, determined by such biological methods as feeding a given compound to vitamin A-deprived animals and measuring the number of units of growth produced. IUs were used to measure vitamin A before chemical analysis of the vitamin A compounds and their precursors was possible.

1 RE ~ 5 IU. More accurately, 1 RE = 3.33 IU from animal foods or 10.0 IU from plant foods.

Table 2.   Vitamin A Toxicity

Disease	Area affected	Main effects
Hypervitaminosis	bones	increased activity of osteoclasts causes decalcification, joint pain, fragility, stunted growth, thickening of long bones; pressure increases inside skull, mimicking brain tumor.
	blood	red blood cells lose hemoglobin and potassium; menstruation ceases; clotting time slows; bleeding is easily induced
	nervous system	loss of appetite, irritability, fatigue, restlessness, headache, nausea, vomiting, muscle weakness, interference with thyroxin
	GI tract	nausea, vomiting, abdominal pain, diarrhea, weight loss
	skin	dryness, itching, peeling, rashes, dry scaling lips, loss of hair, brittle nails
	liver	jaundice, enlargement
	spleen	enlargement
Hypercarotenemia	skin	yellow color

osteoclasts: the cells that destroy bone during its growth. Those that build bone are **osteoblasts.**

osteo = bone
clast = break
blast = build

jaundice: yellowing of the skin; a symptom of liver disease, in which bile and related pigments spill into the bloodstream.

necessary to prevent deficiency. Doubtless, many people need not consume amounts this high. The exact upper limit of safety can't be determined exactly, because people's tolerances to overdoses vary. Probably the amount of added vitamin A that anyone can tolerate depends on the length of time he takes it and on how much of the vitamin has already accumulated in his body stores before he begins to overdose.

In one case, only one month of daily doses of 10 times the recommended intake has been reported as having toxic effects,[4] but in others it may take 40 times the recommended intake for several months to elicit symptoms of toxicity.[5] The National Nutrition Consortium advises that adults should avoid daily intakes of more than 5 to 10 times the recommended amounts to ensure safety.[6] In general, it makes sense to get your vitamin A from natural, mostly plant, sources.

[4]S. J. Yaffe and L. J. Filer, Jr., American Academy of Pediatrics, Joint Committee Statement on Drugs and on Nutrition, The use and abuse of vitamin A, *Pediatrics* 48 (1971):655-656.

[5]D. R. Davis, Using vitamin A safely, *Osteopathic Medicine* 3 (October 1978):31-43.

[6]Committee on Safety, Toxicity, and Misuse of Vitamins and Trace Minerals, National Nutrition Consortium, *Vitamin-Mineral Safety, Toxicity, and Misuse* (Chicago: The American Dietetic Association, 1978).

Acne: see also zinc, pp. 455-456.

Adolescents should be warned that massive doses of vitamin A taken internally will have no beneficial effect on acne but may cause the miseries itemized in Table 2. The belief that vitamin A cures acne arises from the knowledge that it is needed for the health of the skin. As with all nutrients, however, the vitamin promotes health when enough is supplied; more than enough has no further beneficial effects.

However, a relative of vitamin A, vitamin A acid does sometimes help relieve the symptoms of acne when applied directly to the skin surface. The acid helps loosen the plugs that may accumulate in pores, allowing the skin to cleanse itself naturally. Such a treatment should of course be undertaken only on a doctor's recommendation.[7]

preformed vitamin A: vitamin A in its active form. See vitamin A (below).

precursor: a compound that can be converted into active vitamin A (see also p. 63).

beta-carotene: a vitamin A precursor found in plants (see provitamin A carotenoids, below).

vitamin A: the family of compounds found in animal foods, similar to and including retinol and retinal, which have high vitamin A activity.

provitamin A carotenoids: the family of compounds found in plant foods, similar to and including beta-carotene, which have less vitamin A activity and convert relatively inefficiently to vitamin A.

It is possible to suffer toxicity symptoms only when excess amounts of the preformed vitamin from animal foods or supplements are taken. The precursor, beta-carotene, which is available from plant foods, is not converted to vitamin A rapidly enough in the body to cause toxicity but is instead stored in fat depots as carotene. Being yellow in color, it may accumulate under the skin to such an extent that the overdoser actually turns yellow.

Vitamin A in Foods

Most of the vitamin A compounds found in animal foods have activities similar to that of retinol, and these are known as the vitamin A family. There is another family of compounds found in plant foods that have considerably less activity but can convert to active vitamin A with a low efficiency. For example, 6 μg of the plant pigment beta-carotene can convert to 1 μg of retinol in the body. The family of plant pigments similar to beta-carotene is known as the provitamin A carotenoids.[8]

[7]For further information on nutrition and acne, read Controversy 18: Acne, in E. M. N. Hamilton and E. N. Whitney, *Nutrition: Concepts and Controversies* (St. Paul: West, 1979), pp. 445-446.

[8]This terminology was agreed on by several nutrition, biochemistry, and medical societies and published in 1979: American Institute of Nutrition, Committee on Nomenclature, Nomenclature policy: Generic descriptors and trivial names for vitamins and related compounds, *Journal of Nutrition* 109 (1979):8-15.

In earlier years it was thought that the carotenoids had greater activity than we now know they have. (It was thought that about two units of carotene converted to one unit of vitamin A; now the ratio appears to be closer to six to one.[9]) The vitamin A "activity" listed in the food tables we still use today used the older, incorrect assumption. Thus the vitamin A contents of the *plant* foods shown in Appendix H and Table 3 of this chapter look bigger than they really are. If you seek to meet the recommended intake for vitamin A using plant foods, you might well aim high. Since the carotenoids are not toxic, there is probably no harm in daily intakes of about 15,000 IU for adults.

Table 3 shows the vitamin A contents of 50 common foods. If we could show you a color photograph of these foods, you would notice immediately that the top 15 items are all brightly colored—green, yellow, orange, and red. Any food with significant vitamin A activity must have some color, since the vitamin and its plant precursor carotene are colored compounds themselves (vitamin A is a very pale yellow; carotene is a rich, deep yellow, almost orange). The dark-green leafy vegetables contain abundant amounts of the green pigment chlorophyll, which masks the carotene in them. A skilled hostess or restaurateur knows that an attractive meal includes foods of different colors that complement one another but may not be aware that such a meal probably ensures a good supply of vitamin A as well.

On the other hand, food with a yellow or orange color does not invariably have vitamin A or carotene. Many of the compounds that give foods their colors, such as the yellow and red xanthophylls, are unrelated to vitamin A and have no nutritional value.

On the third hand (this chapter has three hands), if a food is white or colorless, it contains little or no vitamin A. Notice that many of the foods at the bottom of Table 3 are in this category.

About half of the vitamin A activity in foods consumed in the United States comes from fruits and vegetables, and half of this comes from the dark leafy greens (not iceberg lettuce or green beans) and the yellow or orange vegetables, such as yellow squash, carrots, and sweet potatoes. The other half comes from milk, cheese, butter and other dairy products, eggs, and meats. Since vitamin A is fat-soluble, it is lost when milk is skimmed. Skim milk is often fortified with 5,000 IU (the intake recommended for men) of vitamin A per quart to compensate.[10] The butter substitute, margarine, is usually fortified with 15,000 IU per pound.[11]

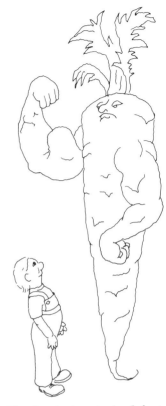

The vitamin A contents of plant foods may look greater than they really are.

chlorophyll: the green pigment of plants, which absorbs photons and transfers their energy to other molecules, initiating photosynthesis.

photosynthesis: the synthesis of carbohydrates by plants from carbon dioxide and water, using the sun's energy.

[9]Other reasons for considering the vitamin A activity of plant foods presently listed in tables to be an overstatement: The carotenoids other than beta-carotene are less than half as active; many are less well absorbed (perhaps only a third as well), and individual variability makes some of them still less well utilized by some individuals.

[10]In Canada, 1,500 IU per liter.

[11]Milks and margarines are also usually fortified with vitamin D.

Table 3.   Vitamin A Contents of 50 Common Foods*

Exchange group[†]	Food	Serving size[‡]	Vitamin A (IU)	Exchange group[†]	Food	Serving size[‡]	Vitamin A (IU)
5M	Beef liver	3 oz	45,420	1	Yogurt (made with whole milk)	1 c	340
4	Pumpkin	3/4 c	10,943§	2	Green beans	1/2 c	340
2	Dandelion greens	1/2 c	10,530	4	Corn on cob	1 small	310
2	Carrots	1/2 c	7,610	3	Orange juice	1/2 c	275
2	Spinach	1/2 c	7,200	3	Orange	1	260
2	Collard greens	1/2 c	5,130°	6	Cream, light	2 tbsp	260
4	Winter squash	1/2 c	4,305	4	Lima beans	1/2 c	240
4	Sweet potatoes	1/4 c	4,250	6	Cream, heavy	1 tbsp	230
2	Mustard greens	1/2 c	4,060	4	Corn	1/3 c	230
3	Cantaloupe	1/4	3,270	1	2% fat fortified milk	1 c	200
2	Broccoli	1/2 c	2,363	5L	Sardines	3 oz	190
3	Dried apricots	4 halves	1,635	6	Soft margarine	1 tsp	156
3	Peach	1	1,320	3	Blackberries	1/2 c	145
2	Cooked tomatoes	1/2 c	1,085	3	Banana	1/2 med	115
2	Tomato juice	1/2 c	970	5M	Creamed cottage cheese	1/4 c	105
2	Asparagus	1/2 c	605	4	Corn muffin	1	100
5M	Egg	1	590	3	Raspberries	1/2 c	80
5L	Oysters	15, 3/4 c	555	5L	Chicken, meat only	3 oz	80
3	Pink grapefruit	1/2	540	4	Yellow grits	1/2 c	75
4	Green peas	1/2 c	430	4	Pancake	1	70
2	Summer squash	1/2 c	410	5L	Canned tuna	3 oz	70
2	Brussels sprouts	1/2 c	405	3	Blueberries	1/2 c	70
1	Canned evaporated milk	1/2 c	405	3	Strawberries	3/4 c	68
3	Tangerine	1	360	5L	Canned salmon	3 oz	60
1	Whole milk	1 c	350	3	Pineapple	1/2 c	50

*These are not necessarily the best food sources but are selected to show a range of vitamin A contents. Note how many 2s and 3s are at the top of the left-hand column and how many 5s are at the bottom.

†The numbers refer to the exchange lists: 1 is milk; 2, vegetables; 3, fruit; 4, bread; 5L, lean meat; 5M, medium-fat meat; 6, fats and oils.

‡Serving sizes are the sizes listed in the exchange lists, except for meat.

§Vitamin A activity reported in plants may be spuriously high. The actual amount of active vitamin A derived from plants depends on the body's conversion of the precursor, carotene, to the active vitamin.

°One serving of any of the first six foods contains the RDA (for an adult male) of 5,000 IU.

The safest and easiest way to meet your vitamin A needs, then, is to consume generous servings of a variety of dark-green, deep-orange, and other richly colored vegetables and fruits. A 1-c serving of carrots, sweet potatoes, or dark greens such as spinach would provide such liberal amounts of carotenoids that, even allowing for inefficient absorption and conversion, intake would be sufficient. Alternatively, a diet including more or larger servings of medium sources would ensure an ample intake. No doubt you can find food sources of the vitamin that appeal to you and can easily calculate the minimum amounts you should eat in order to meet your needs.

The fruit and vegetable family is one of the Four Food Groups. Its importance for meeting vitamin A needs is reflected in the recommendation that adults have at least four servings a day, including "at least one dark-green or deep-orange" item every other day.

Fast foods are notable for their *lack* of vitamin A.[12] Anyone who dines frequently on hamburgers, french fries, shakes, and the like is well advised to emphasize vegetables heavily at other meals.

One animal food notable for its vitamin A content is liver. A moment's reflection should reveal the reason for this: Vitamin A not needed for immediate use is stored in the liver.[13] Some nutritionists recommend that people include a serving of liver in their diets every week or two, partly for this reason. Because the vitamin A in liver is preformed, active vitamin A, an intake of 5,000 IU in this form is probably equivalent to an intake of at least 15,000 IU in plant carotenoids.

People sometimes wonder if vitamin A toxicity can result from using liver too frequently. This problem has never been observed except in the Arctic, where explorers who have eaten large quantities of polar bear liver have become ill with symptoms probably indicating vitamin A toxicity. Liver is an extremely nutritious food, and its periodic use is highly recommended.

Recall that one of the B vitamins—folacin—is found most abundantly in dark-green vegetables.

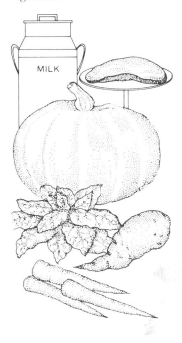

The Bone Vitamin: D

Vitamin A helps to remodel bones; vitamin D helps to grow them. Vitamin A is versatile and important in many body systems; vitamin D seems to play its part only in connection with the minerals of the bone system. That part is considerable, however, and vitamin D is indispensable to keep the system working during periods of bone growth or remodeling. Vitamin D is a member of a large and cooperative bone-making and maintenance team made up of nutrients and other compounds, including vitamins C and A; the hormones parathormone and calcitonin; the protein collagen, which precedes bone; and the minerals calcium, phosphorus, magnesium, fluoride, and others, of which the bone is finally composed.

Blood calcium is very active metabolically. It has been estimated that about a fourth of the calcium in the blood is exchanged with bone calcium every minute. The special function of vitamin D is to help make calcium and phosphorus available in the blood that bathes the bones so that they can be deposited there as the bones grow (harden or mineralize).

Parathormone and calcitonin: see p. 413.

Collagen: see p. 353.

mineralization (calcification): the process in which calcium, phosphorus, and other minerals crystallize on the collagen matrix of a growing bone, hardening the bone.

[12]C. P. Greecher and B. Shannon, Impact of fast food meals on nutrient intake of two groups, *Journal of the American Dietetic Association* 70 (1977):368-372.

[13]Liver is not the only organ that stores Vitamin A. The kidneys, adrenals, and other organs also perform this function, but liver is the only one that is usually eaten.

Vitamin D raises blood concentrations of these minerals in three ways: by stimulating their absorption from the gastrointestinal tract; by helping to withdraw calcium from bones into the blood; and by stimulating calcium retention by the kidneys. The star of this particular show is calcium itself; vitamin D is a supporting actor. A description of how calcium moves from food into the blood and into and out of bone is reserved for Chapter 12, where a closer view of the whole system is provided. The object here is to make you aware of the importance of vitamin D, the risks of deficiency and toxicity, and the ways in which it can be obtained from foods.

A note should be made here of one way this nutrient is unique: The body can synthesize its own vitamin D in the skin with the help of sunlight. In this sense vitamin D is not an essential nutrient. Given enough sun, you need consume no vitamin D at all in the foods you eat. Rather, it is like a hormone—a compound manufactured by one organ of the body that has effects on another.

The precursor of vitamin D made in the liver is 7-dehydro-cholesterol, which is made from cholesterol. This is one of the body's many "good" uses for cholesterol.

The liver manufactures a vitamin D precursor, which is released into the blood and circulates to the skin. When ultraviolet rays from the sun hit this compound, it is converted to previtamin D_3, which works its way back into the interior of the body. Slowly, then, over the next 36 hours, the previtamin is converted with the help of the body's heat to vitamin D_3. Two more steps occur before the vitamin becomes fully active: The liver adds an OH group and then the kidney adds another at specific locations to produce the active vitamin.[14]

The technical name for the final product, active vitamin D, is 1,25-dihydroxycholecalciferol (die-hi-DROX-ee-COAL-ee-cal-SIFF-er-all) — dihydroxy vitamin D for short.

There are thus two ways to meet your vitamin D needs: self-synthesis and consumption of foods containing the preformed vitamin—chiefly animal foods.[15]

Vitamin D Deficiency and Toxicity

Both inadequate and excessive vitamin D intakes take their toll in the United States, despite the fact that the vitamin has been known for decades to be essential for growth and toxic in excess. The Ten-State Survey revealed that nearly 4 percent of the children under six who were examined showed evidence of vitamin D deficiency, with several cases of overt rickets. The National Nutrition Survey in Canada revealed low intakes of vitamin D in women and children but no overt cases of rickets—although they may exist in persons not tested. Worldwide, rickets still afflicts large numbers of children.

rickets: the vitamin D-deficiency disease in children.

A rare type of rickets, not caused by vitamin D deficiency is known as **vitamin D-refractory rickets.**

[14]The whole story is told by one of the principal investigators in this area, whose meticulous work has revealed many more details than are presented here. See DeLuca (1979) in this chapter's To Explore Further.

[15]A plant version of vitamin D (ergosterol) may also yield an active compound, vitamin D_2 (calciferol), on irradiation, but less is known about the body's further use of this compound. Thus animal sources of vitamin D are considered the only reliable ones.

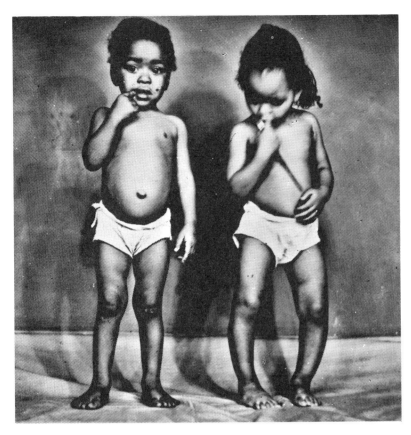

Rickets.

Photo courtesy of Parke-Davis & Company.

The symptoms of an inadequate intake of vitamin D are those of calcium deficiency, as shown in Table 4. The bones fail to calcify normally and may be so weak that they become bent when they have to support the body's weight. A child with rickets who is old enough to walk characteristically develops bowed legs, often the most obvious sign of the disease.

Adult rickets, or osteomalacia, occurs most often in women who have little exposure to sun and who go through repeated pregnancies and periods of lactation. The bones of the legs may soften to such an extent that a woman who was tall and straight before her first pregnancy becomes bent, bowlegged, and stooped after her second or third.

Vitamin D deficiency depresses calcium absorption and results in low blood calcium levels and abnormal mineralization of bone. An excess of the vitamin does the opposite, as shown in Table 5: It increases calcium absorption, causing abnormally high concentrations of the mineral in the blood, and promotes return of bone calcium into the blood as well. The excess calcium in the blood tends to precipitate in the soft tissues, forming stones. This is especially likely to happen in the

osteomalacia (os-tee-o-mal-AY-shuh): the vitamin D-deficiency disease in adults.

osteo = bone
mal = bad (soft)

Osteomalacia may also occur in calcium deficiency; see Chapter 12.

Bowing of the ribs causes the symptom known as **pigeon breast.** The beads that form on the ribs resemble rosary beads; thus this symptom is known as **rachitic** (ra-KIT-ik) **rosary** (the rosary of rickets).

fontanel: the open space in the top of a baby's skull before the skull bones have grown together.

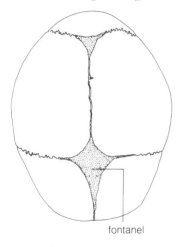

fontanel

thorax: the part of the body between the neck and the abdomen.

alkaline phosphatase: an enzyme in blood.

Table 4. Vitamin D Deficiency

Disease	Area affected	Main effects
Rickets	bones	faulty calcification resulting in misshapen bones (bowing of legs) and retarded growth
		enlargment of ends of long bones (knock-knees)
		deformities of ribs (bowed, with beads or knobs)
		delayed closing of fontanel results in rapid enlargement of head
	blood	decreased calcium and/or phosphorus
	teeth	slow eruption; teeth not well-formed; tendency to decay
	muscles	lax muscles resulting in protrusion of abdomen
	excretory system	increased calcium in stools, decreased calcium in urine
	glandular system	abnormally high secretion of parathyroid hormone
Osteomalacia	bones	softening effect: deformities of limbs, spine, thorax, and pelvis; demineralization; pain in pelvis, lower back, and legs; bone fractures
	blood	decreased calcium and/or phosphorus, increased alkaline phosphatase
	muscles	involuntary twitching, muscle spasms

kidneys, which concentrate calcium in the effort to excrete it. Calcification or hardening of the blood vessels may also occur. This process is especially dangerous in the major arteries of the heart and lungs, where it can cause death.

The range of safe intakes of vitamin D is narrower than that of vitamin A. Half the recommended intake is too little, but over a few

Table 5.   Vitamin D Toxicity

Disease	Area affected	Main effects
Hypervitaminosis D	bones	increased calcium withdrawal
	blood	increased calcium and phosphorus concentration
	nervous system	loss of appetite, headache, excessive thirst, irritability
	excretory system	increased excretion of calcium in urine; kidney stones; irreversible renal damage
	tissues	calcification of soft tissues (blood vessels, kidneys, lungs), death

times the recommended intake may be too much. Intakes of 4,000 IU per day cause high blood calcium levels in infants, but some are sensitive to lower doses than this. Intakes of 10,000 IU per day for four months or 200,000 IU per day for two weeks cause toxicity in children and, if further prolonged, in adults. The amounts of vitamin D found in foods available in the United States and Canada are well within these limits, but pills containing the vitamin in concentrated form should definitely be kept out of the reach of children.

Vitamin D activity was previously expressed in international units (IU) but as of 1980 is expressed in micrograms of cholecalciferol. To convert, use the factor:

100 IU = 2.5 μg
400 IU = 10 μg.

Vitamin D from Sun and Foods

In rapidly growing children, an intake of close to 400 IU of vitamin D a day is recommended; mature adults need half as much. Only a few animal foods supply significant amounts of the vitamin, notably, eggs, liver, and some fish, and even these vary greatly, depending on the animal's exposure to sun and on its consumption of the vitamin in its foods. The fortification of milk with 400 IU per quart (360 IU per liter in Canada) is the best guarantee that children will meet their vitamin D needs and underscores the importance of milk in children's diets.

The RDA for vitamin D for adults over 22 is 5 μg cholecalciferol (200 IU).

Canadian Dietary Standard: 2.5 μg cholecalciferol.

Significant amounts of vitamin D can be made with the help of sunlight. No exact measures have been made, but it is generally agreed that most adults, especially in the sunnier climates, need not make special efforts to obtain vitamin D in food. However, people of all ages need vitamin D; if you are not outdoors much or if you live in a northern or predominantly cloudy or smoggy area, you are advised to make sure your milk is fortified with vitamin D, to drink at least 2 c a day, and to make frequent use of eggs and periodic use of liver in menu planning.

Exposure to sun should be reasonable. Excessive exposure to sun may cause skin cancer.

Vitamin E

Antioxidant: see p. 354.

oxidant: a compound (such as oxygen itself) that oxidizes other compounds.

As we stated at the start, this book is intended to give you a sense of what to believe and what not to believe, presenting well-known and documented research in the chapters and reserving recent, speculative, and controversial material for the Highlights. Much of what is presently being said about vitamin E is too uncertain to have won the security of a textual presentation and so is addressed in Highlight 11. However, there is one role vitamin E plays—as an antioxidant—that is quite well understood.

Like vitamin C, vitamin E is readily oxidized. If there is plenty of vitamin E in a mixture of compounds exposed to an oxidant, chances are this vitamin will take the brunt of the oxidative attack, protecting the others. Because it is soluble in fat, vitamin E is found in fat-rich fluids and tissues of the body in association with the lipids of cell membranes and with the other fat-soluble vitamins. Because of this and its relative abundance in the diet, it is especially effective in preventing the oxidation of vitamin A and the polyunsaturated fatty acids. It also helps vitamin A to be absorbed.

erythrocyte hemolysis (eh-REETH-ro-cite he-MOLL-uh-sis): the vitamin E-deficiency disease in human beings.

erythrocyte: red blood cell.
  erythro = red
  cyte = cell

hemolysis: bursting of red blood cells.
  hemo = blood
  lysis = breaking

Of 12 possible diseases associated with vitamin E deficiency in animals, only one has been demonstrated in human beings. When the blood concentration of vitamin E falls below a certain critical level, the red blood cells tend to break open and spill their contents, probably due to oxidation of the polyunsaturated fatty acids (PUFAs) in their membranes. (Cell membranes are rich in PUFAs, and those of the red blood cells in particular are exposed to high concentrations of oxygen because of their repeated circulation through the lungs.) In animals, this action tends to occur more readily if the diet is high in PUFAs, suggesting that it is indeed vitamin E's role in protecting PUFAs from oxidation that prevents the deficiency disease. A person's need for vitamin E may therefore depend on the amount of PUFAs consumed. Fortunately, vitamin E and the polyunsaturates tend to occur together in the same foods.

Vitamin E is readily destroyed by heat processing and oxidation, so fresh or lightly processed foods are preferable as sources of this vitamin. The processed and convenience foods often used by the elderly and nursing homes may contribute to a vitamin E deficiency if their use continues over several years.[16]

Vitamin E is the only one of the fat-soluble vitamins for which toxicity symptoms are unknown in humans; even prolonged intakes of many times the recommended intake have few observable effects. Sensitive individuals may complain of nausea and intestinal discomfort, but the general impression seems to be that for most people intakes from pills of up to 300 IU per day are harmless—and useless.[17]

[16]H. H. Koehler, H. C. Lee, and M. Jacobson, Tocopherols in canned entrees and vended sandwiches, *Journal of the American Dietetic Association* 70 (1977):616-620.

[17]For more information on vitamin E myths and realities, read Controversy 20: Vitamin E, in E. M. N. Hamilton and E. N. Whitney, *Nutrition: Concepts and Controversies* (St. Paul: West, 1979), pp. 481-482.

About 60 percent of the vitamin E in the diet comes directly or indirectly from vegetable oils in the form of margarine, salad dressings, and shortenings; another 10 percent comes from fruits and vegetables; smaller percentages come from grains and other products. Soybean oil and wheat germ oil have especially high concentrations of E; cottonseed, corn, and safflower oils rank second, with a tablespoon of any of these supplying more than 15 mg of the vitamin. Other oils contain less (for example, peanut oil supplies about half as much per tablespoon). Animal fats such as butter and milk fat have negligible amounts of vitamin E.

The RDA for vitamin E for adults: 10 mg for men, 8 mg for women. Canadian Dietary Standard: 8-9 mg for men, 6 mg for women.

Vitamin E units: 1 mg = 1 IU.

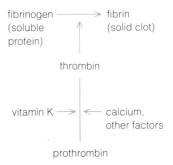

The clotting process

The Blood-Clotting Vitamin: K

Like vitamin D, vitamin K seems to be limited in its versatility. But like D, its presence can make the difference between life and death. At least 13 different proteins and the mineral calcium are involved in making a blood clot, and vitamin K is essential for the synthesis of at least 4 of these proteins, among them the protein thrombin.

When any of these factors is lacking, blood cannot clot and hemorrhagic disease results; if an artery or vein is cut or broken under these circumstances, bleeding goes unchecked. (As usual, this is not to say that the cause of hemorrhaging is always vitamin K deficiency. Another cause is hemophilia, which is not curable by vitamin K.) Deficiency of vitamin K may occur under abnormal circumstances when absorption of fat is impaired (that is, when bile production is faulty or in diarrhea). The vitamin is sometimes administered preoperatively to reduce bleeding in surgery but is only of value at this time if a vitamin K deficiency exists. Toxicity can result when too much vitamin K is given, especially to an infant or to a pregnant woman.

Again, like vitamin D, vitamin K is made within your body—but not by you. In your intestinal tract there are billions of bacteria, which normally live in perfect harmony with you, doing their thing while you do yours. One of their "things" is synthesizing vitamin K that you can absorb. You are not dependent on bacterial synthesis for your K, however, since many foods also contain ample amounts of the vitamin, notably, green leafy vegetables, members of the cabbage family, and milk.

Brand new babies are commonly susceptible to a K deficiency, for two reasons. First, a baby is born with a sterile digestive tract; he has his first contact with intestinal bacteria as he passes down his mother's birth canal, and it takes the bacteria a day or so to establish themselves in the baby's intestines. Second, a baby may not be fed at the very outset (and breast milk is a poorer source of vitamin K than cow's milk). A dose of vitamin K (usually in a synthetic form similar but not identical to the natural vitamin) may therefore be given at birth to prevent

K stands for the Danish word *Koagulation* (coagulation or clotting).

Thrombin: see p. 130.

hemorrhagic (hem-o-RAJ-ik) **disease:** the vitamin K-deficiency disease.

hemophilia: a hereditary disease having no relation to vitamin K but caused by a genetic defect that renders the blood unable to clot because of lack of ability to synthesize certain clotting factors.

The bacterial inhabitants of the digestive tract are known as the **intestinal flora.**

flora = plant inhabitants

Provisional RDA for vitamin K (1980): 70-140 μg.

sterile: free of microorganisms, such as bacteria.

The synthetic substitute usually given for vitamin K is **menadione** (men-uh-DYE-own).

hemorrhagic disease of the newborn; it must be administered carefully to avoid toxic overdosing. People taking sulfa drugs, which destroy intestinal bacteria, may also become deficient in vitamin K.

Putting It All Together

This chapter concludes the treatment of the vitamins. Another look at diet adequacy and balance is in order at this point. For the B vitamins, meat, milk, breads, cereals, and vegetables are good sources; for vitamin C, the fruits are important. With this consideration of the fat-soluble vitamins, the sixth group of foods in the exchange system, namely the fat group, assumes significance. The diagram that follows shows how the selection of foods from all six exchange groups ensures that each nutrient discussed so far will be consumed in the recommended amounts. The individual lines of the web may be of interest, but the main point of the figure is that it is a web: Different foods supply different assortments of nutrients, so that a wide and varied selection is the best guarantee of adequacy for all.

Note: Some vitamins known to be essential in human diets have not been studied sufficiently to permit setting recommended intakes. Food sources of these nutrients are less well known. However, the variety of

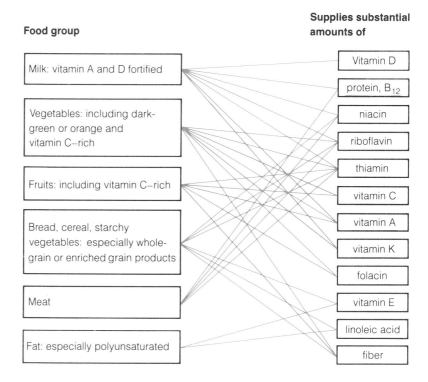

Food group

Milk: vitamin A and D fortified

Vegetables: including dark-green or orange and vitamin C–rich

Fruits: including vitamin C–rich

Bread, cereal, starchy vegetables: especially whole-grain or enriched grain products

Meat

Fat: especially polyunsaturated

Supplies substantial amounts of

Vitamin D

protein, B$_{12}$

niacin

riboflavin

thiamin

vitamin C

vitamin A

vitamin K

folacin

vitamin E

linoleic acid

fiber

selections suggested above is so great that chances are good they will supply most nutrients in amounts sufficient to meet the needs of virtually all members of a healthy population. This diagram will be repeated at the end of Chapter 13, where it will be shown that some modifications are necessary to ensure adequacy for certain minerals.

Summing Up

Vitamin A as part of the visual pigment rhodopsin is essential for vision, especially in dim light. Vitamin A is involved in maintaining the integrity of mucous membranes throughout the internal linings of the body and thus in promoting resistance to infection. It helps maintain the health of the skin and is essential for the remodeling of bones during their growth or mending; it also plays a part in cell membrane functions, in hormone synthesis, in reproduction, and other functions.

Deficiency of vitamin A causes night blindness due to the failure to regenerate rhodopsin; a failure of mucous secretion, which can lead by way of keratinization of the cornea to blindness; disorders of the respiratory, urogenital, reproductive, and nervous systems; and abnormalities of bones and teeth. Toxicity symptoms are caused by large excesses (10 times the recommended intake or more) taken over a prolonged period and result only from the preformed vitamin (from supplements or animal products such as liver)—not from the precursor carotene and its relatives, the yellow pigments found in plants.

The recommended intake for vitamin A (800 RE for women, 1,000 RE for men) is easily met by periodically consuming the vitamin's richest food sources, such as liver or dark-green leafy vegetables, or by consuming other concentrated sources daily, such as carrots, cantaloupe, yellow squash, or broccoli. All food sources of vitamin A or the carotenoids have some color.

Vitamin D promotes intestinal absorption of calcium, mobilization of calcium from bone stores, and retention by the kidneys and is therefore essential for the calcification of bones and teeth. Given reasonable exposure to sun, humans can synthesize this vitamin in the skin from a precursor manufactured by the liver. Deficiency of vitamin D causes the calcium deficiency diseases (rickets in children and osteomalacia in adults); excesses cause abnormally high blood calcium levels, due to excessive GI absorption and withdrawal from bone, and result in deposition of calcium crystals in soft tissues, such as the kidney and major blood vessels. The recommended intake of 400 IU (2.5 μg cholecalciferol) per day is best met by drinking fortified milk; food sources of vitamin D are unreliable. However, exposure to sunlight probably ensures vitamin D adequacy for the average adult.

The best-substantiated role of vitamin E in humans is as an antioxidant that protects vitamin A and the polyunsaturated fatty acids

(PUFAs) from destruction by oxygen. Although many vitamin E-deficiency symptoms have been observed in animals, only one has been confirmed in humans: hemolysis of red blood cells due to oxidative destruction of the PUFAs in their membranes. The recommended intake of about 6 to 10 mg per day for adults is more than adequate to prevent this. The human requirement for vitamin E is known to vary with PUFA intake; since the vitamin occurs with PUFAs in foods, it is normally supplied in the needed amounts. Deficiences are seldom observed but there is some concern that the overuse of processed foods may make deficiences more likely. Toxicity symptoms are rare.

Vitamin K, the coagulation vitamin, promotes normal blood clotting; deficiency causes hemorrhagic disease. The vitamin is synthesized by intestinal bacteria and is available from foods such as green vegetables and milk. Deficiency is normally seen only in newborns, whose intestinal flora have not become established, in people taking sulfa drugs, or in people whose fat absorption is impaired.

Adequate intakes of all the nutrients discussed so far are ensured by selecting a variety of foods from all six of the food exchange groups, as shown in the diagram on p. 398; inclusion of polyunsaturated oils promotes ample intakes of both linoleic acid and vitamin E.

To Explore Further

The vast problem of vitamin A deficiency throughout the world is summarized in an 88-page booklet available from the World Health Organization (address in Appendix J):

- WHO/USAID Joint Meeting. *Vitamin A Deficiency and Xerophthalmia.* Technical Report Series 590. Albany, N.Y.: Q Corporation, 1976.

Vitamin A deficiency may be implicated in some kinds of cancer. The story is still far from complete, but you might like to look up these three articles:

- Basu, T. K. Vitamin A and cancer of epithelial origin. *Journal of Human Nutrition* 33 (February 1979):24-31.

- Sporn, M. B., Dunlop, N.M., Newton, D.L., and Smith, J. M. Prevention of chemical carcinogenesis by vitamin A and its synthetic analogs (retinoids). *Federation Proceedings* 35 (1976):1332-1338.

- Vitamin A, tumor initiation and tumor promotion. *Nutrition Reviews* 37 (1979):153-156.

Recent research on vitamin D is summarized by one of the major investigators in the area in a featured article in *Nutrition Reviews:*

- DeLuca, H. F. The vitamin D system in the regulation of calcium and phosphorus metabolism. *Nutrition Reviews* 37 (1979):161-193.

This would make stiff reading for the general reader, but is recommended to anyone who wants to gain an appreciation of all the complexities. Of special interest is the new hope this research brings to renal patients, whose bone disease was untreatable until the kidney's role in vitamin D metabolism was understood.

A two-page summary of vitamin E myths and realities, assembled by a committee of experts, is available free from General Mills (address in Appendix J):

● Expert Panel on Food Safety and Nutrition, Committee on Public Information, Institute of Food Technologists. Vitamin E. *Contemporary Nutrition* 2 (November 1977).

Other interesting and useful information on the vitamins can be found in the general references listed in Appendix J.

HIGHLIGHT 11

Vitamin E: A Cure-All?

Is it likely that the RDA Committee is grossly in error about the amounts of vitamin E needed for optimum health? One "common sense" way of approaching such questions (which might be called a "biological" approach) is to consider that mankind evolved on the food it could readily obtain, and that one should not expect to find large natural barriers blocking access to foods needed for health. Let us see what one would have to eat to get 1,500 IU of vitamin E each day. . . . [It] would require some eight or nine pounds of oil, something over a gallon a day.

RONALD M. DEUTSCH

You are watching a movie about the early days in the Old West. A wagon is parked in the woods. A man is mixing a batch of something in a washtub and then ladling it into medicine bottles. The man is now dressed in a high silk hat and swallow-tailed coat and is hawking the "medicine" from a makeshift stage on the rear of the wagon. The camera shows the faces in the crowd, mesmerized by the man's tale of the wonderful cures this medicine has effected. "Step right up, folks, and buy this time-tested medicine, only a dollar for the giant bottle, and it will cure lumbago, the ague, and rheumatism." The faces in the crowd register concern over some private ailment they wish could be cured by this magical medicine. As you watch the film, you wonder how the people could have been duped by such a show.

Today's magical medicine barkers don't wear high silk hats or mix their potions in washtubs. Those props have gone out of style along with the ailments the old barkers sought to cure. Only the faces in the crowd remain the same. They listen avidly now as the authors of a book on vitamin E hawk their wares on a television talk show. The authors sound knowledgeable, sure of the truth of what they are saying.

There must be some reasonable explanation for the fact that so many people honestly believe the many claims made for the curative powers of vitamin E, especially since research shows that human beings are rarely deficient in this vitamin. Let's examine what is known about this vitamin, which has caught the public's fancy as a cure for everything from impotence in males to the healing of burns.

Animal Research Male rats deprived of vitamin E cease to manufacture sperm. Their testes become atrophied, brownish, and flabby. The rabbit, dog, and monkey show similar damage, but the mouse seems remarkably resistant, taking a great deal longer to exhibit these signs.[1]

[1] M. K. Horwitt: Vitamin E, in *Modern Nutrition in Health and Disease*, 6th ed., ed. R. S. Goodhart and M. E. Shills (Philadelphia: Lea and Febiger, 1980), pp. 181-191.

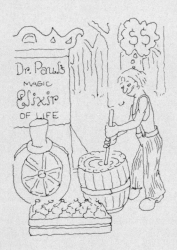

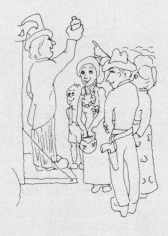

In pregnant female rats on a diet lacking vitamin E, the fetus dies after the first week. If vitamin E is restored to the diet during the first week of pregnancy, the fetus can be saved, indicating that a vitamin E deficiency damages the blood supply between the uterus and the placenta.[2]

In animals on a vitamin E-deficient diet, the muscles become weak and a kind of muscular paralysis sets in; this too can be reversed by restoring the vitamin to the diet. The extent of the paralysis seems to be related to the amount of polyunsaturated fat in the tissues. The heart muscles of rabbits, sheep, and cattle (plant-eating animals) seem to be especially vulnerable. Fatal heart attacks are not uncommon, and they take place before overt signs of the deficiency have developed.[3]

These results of studies of vitamin E-deficient animals indicate a possible role for the vitamin in prolonging virility in males, carrying a fetus to full term in females, and keeping muscles healthy, particularly heart muscles. The next logical quest is to see if the vitamin is necessary for maintenance of these functions in human beings.

The search to find such a role for vitamin E in humans has continued for over 30 years, but thus far it has

[2]Horwitt, 1980.
[3]Horwitt, 1980.

produced only negative results. However, the "faces in the crowd" continue to look to vitamin E as the potion that will prolong virility, abolish miscarriages, and cure muscular weakness like that in muscular dystrophy.

Why is it that laboratory findings on vitamin E deficiencies in animals cannot be applied to humans? To answer this question, we must examine nutrition research on animals.

Animal Research Methods   Two steps are necessary in both animal and human research to show that lack of a nutrient is causing a certain symptom. First, a diet lacking that nutrient and only that nutrient must be fed. The administration of this diet must result consistently in the appearance of the deficiency symptom. Then, when the nutrient is returned to the diet, the deficiency symptom must disappear. Furthermore, in nutrient research using animals, several preparatory steps must be taken.

● An animal must be found that does not synthesize the nutrient. For example, vitamin C-deficiency research cannot be carried out on rats, because rats synthesize vitamin C. Guinea pigs have to be used instead.

● A laboratory feed must be prepared that contains all the essential nutrients except the

one under study. This is not the simple task of finding a food for the animal; it entails mixing the nutrients in the correct proportion. The result is usually a mixture of synthetic nutrients, since natural foods would very likely contain traces of the nutrient being excluded. Moreover, chemical analysis must show that the mixture is indeed free from the nutrient and that it is not lacking in another essential nutrient. (Alternatively an antinutrient can be used to bind, inactivate, or compete with the nutrient in question, but then the researcher must distinguish between the effects of the nutrient's lack and those of the antinutrient's presence.)

● The animals must have a common heredity and be maintained on similar diets for the same length of time prior to the start of the experiment.

● Other variables may need to be controlled. For example, it has been shown in other work that a nutrient's absorption is under seasonal hormone control,[4] so that fact will need to be considered in the design of the experiment.

When the deficiency symptom has been produced in

[4]H. Weindling and J. B. Henry, Laboratory test results altered by "the pill," *Journal of the American Medical Association* 229 (1974):1762-1768.

the laboratory animal and alleviated with the addition of the missing nutrient, researchers can say they have found that the lack of that particular nutrient, in that species, caused a particular symptom. When other laboratories have replicated these results, they are accepted — for that species. Until laboratory research has shown this relationship to be true for another species of animal, researchers can only theorize that the relationship may be true in both.

Applications to Humans

It is much trickier to apply knowledge gained from research with laboratory animals to humans than to transfer knowledge gained from one species to another in the laboratory. The experimental animal is caged, thus assuring that feed, fluid, temperature, and most of the factors in his environment will be controlled. It is also possible to allow the experiment to continue until death intervenes, after which an autopsy can show the effects of the nutrient deficiency on the internal organs.

In research with humans, the intake of food and fluid cannot be controlled except in very short-term experiments. In addition, there is no way of knowing that each subject is in a similar state prior to the beginning of the experiment. This fact necessi-

> **Miniglossary**
>
> **ague** (AY-gyoo): a chill, a fit of shivering; an old-fashioned term.
>
> **lumbago** (lum-BAY-go): rheumatic pain in the joints, an old-fashioned term.
>
> **muscular dystrophy** (DIS-tro-fee): a hereditary disease in which the muscles gradually weaken; its most debilitating effects arise from weakening of the respiratory muscles.
>
> *dys* = bad, difficult
> *trophy* = growing
>
> **nutritional muscular dystrophy:** a vitamin E-deficiency disease of animals, characterized by gradual paralysis of the muscles. Not the same as the hereditary muscular dystrophy seen in humans.
>
> **rheumatism:** pain in the joints, an old-fashioned term.

tates the use of large numbers of human subjects so that the results can be averaged. Finding a large enough population hinders the launching of such an experiment and adds to the cost. Experimentation on human beings must also depend on subjects who are free to break the restrictions of the diet or to drop out of the experiment at any time, even if they are being paid to be subjects.

In the case of vitamin E research on human beings, there have been some unique obstacles in addition to these.[5]

● Vitamin E is widely distributed in foods. It is, therefore, difficult to compose a diet totally devoid of it.

● Vitamin E is one of the fat-soluble vitamins and as such is stored in abundance in the tissues of the body, particularly in adipose tissue. Therefore, a deficiency state has to be maintained for a long time before the body becomes depleted.

Another type of study that can be carried out with humans is that in which results from many case studies involving a possible vitamin E deficiency are pooled to see if there is a common thread of truth. For the most part, these efforts have been unproductive. Vitamin E has been shown to be ineffective in the treatment of such diseases as muscular dystrophy, reproductive failure, and heart disease. It seems that these conditions in humans are not the result of vitamin E deficiency.[6]

[5]Committee on Nutritional Misinformation, Food and Nutrition Board, NAS/NRC, Who needs vitamin E? *Journal of the American Dietetic Association* 64 (1974):365-366.
[6]Editorial: Vitamin E in clinical medicine, *Lancet* 1 (1974):18.

When a symptom has been shown to be caused by a deficiency of a nutrient in several species of laboratory animals, this fact can be used as a pointer toward the existence of the same relationship in humans. However, until a deficiency symptom can be produced in human subjects by a diet lacking the nutrient and then cured by the restoration of that nutrient, it cannot be claimed that the symptom is caused by the lack of that nutrient.

The amount of misinformation that has arisen out of the public's failure to understand these distinctions and the profit-making incentive of those who promote misunderstandings of this kind has cost the public millions of dollars every year.

A FLAG SIGN OF A SPURIOUS CLAIM IS THE USE OF:

Animal research findings misapplied to humans.

The Appeal of Myths

There would seem to be another factor operating in the public's ready acceptance of claims that cannot be substantiated in human beings. The areas where animal research suggests a possible role for vitamin E in the human body are the same that currently are of the greatest concern to people. Emotional appeals for belief in the efficacy of vitamin E fall on willing ears when it is claimed that supplements of it will cure, for example, muscular dystrophy. *Hereditary muscular dystrophy* is a disease afflicting children, who usually die at an early age when their respiratory muscles cease to function properly. *Nutritional muscular dystrophy*, however, is the muscular weakness produced in many animals by a deficiency of vitamin E.[7] This deficiency leads to atrophy of the muscles; it can be cured by reintroducing vitamin E into the diet. At no time has there been any evidence in reliable literature that links this condition to hereditary muscular dystrophy.

It is easy to understand how the public might be confused by the use of these similar terms for separate conditions, but a nutritionist should be aware of the dif-

[7] A. Davis, *Let's Eat Right to Keep Fit* (New York: Harcourt Brace Jovanovich, 1970), chap. 20.

ference. Some years ago a popular writer on nutrition published in her book an account of a child with muscular dystrophy being cured through early administration of vitamin E. Throughout the several pages devoted to vitamin E, it was apparent that she was not aware of the difference between muscular dystrophy and nutritional muscular dystrophy. The cruelty of such a promise to parents of children with the disease is unconscionable.

In this discussion of vitamin E we have focused on the inadequacy of animal research for finding out about human nutrition. If we were to present a more balanced picture of the research on vitamin E, we would include several other kinds of studies. Research into the well-known antioxidant effect of the vitamin is finding application in a variety of disease conditions in humans such as sickle-cell anemia and liver poisoning. Studies on the effects of megadoses have been revealing that they are more harmful than the public realizes. The list of suggested readings at the end of this Highlight points to these and other areas of active recent research.

While the details of our knowledge continue to change, however, the principles remain the same. This Highlight has shown how carefully research into the roles of a nutrient has to be conducted, how useful animals are in the quest for knowledge, and how conservatively the information from animal studies has to be interpreted. While the work goes on, the public continues to want final answers now, or at least to make decisions based on what is now known.

With all of the uncertainty regarding people's vitamin E status, and with the public's belief in the dire effects of deficiencies, many people are resorting to the use of supplements "as an insurance measure." Luckily, none of the work that has been done indicates that vitamin E toxicity develops in humans at the levels usually taken in supplements. It may be that a person's belief that vitamin E is helping to alleviate a condition — for instance, sexual impotence — may provide a psychological boost that in itself is worth the price of the vitamin. There is one dangerous aspect that should be noted, however: If taking a vitamin lulls a user into avoiding the correct diagnosis and treatment of a serious condition, the vitamin supplement may cost more than anyone can afford to pay. In the meantime, the modern-day hawkers of vitamin E supplements get richer, but as far as we know, no one gets any healthier.

To Explore Further

For a concise summary of what's new in vitamin E research, we recommend:

● Controversy 15: Vitamin E, in Hamilton, E. M. N., and Whitney, E. N. *Nutrition: Concepts and Controversies*, 2nd ed. St. Paul: West, 1979, pp. 518-520.

As that summary shows, moderate doses (200 IU/day) of vitamin E protect human red blood cells from oxidizing air pollutants. It also shows that up to 1981, research had still not demonstrated any beneficial effect of vitamin E on atherosclerosis, high blood lipid levels, or a variety of symptoms of aging.

Vitamin E therapy can be effectively used in a variety of medical situations, and these have been reviewed by:

● Horwitt, M. K. Therapeutic uses of vitamin E in medicine. *Nutrition Reviews* 38 (1980):105-113.

Some day it may be possible to interpret the significance for humans of some work with rats showing a beneficial effect of vitamin E on cataracts. So far, however, it has been evident that the vitamin plays no obvious role with human cataracts:

● Another use for vitamin E? (Medical News). *Journal of the American Medical Association* 243 (1980):1025.

Among the demonstrated ill effects of vitamin E megadoses are white blood cell damage, interference with the clotting action of vitamin K, slowing of wound healing, and damage to various body organs. The white blood cell effects are shown in:

● Prasad, J. S. Effect of vitamin E supplementation on leukocyte function. *American Journal of Clinical Nutrition* 33 (1980):606-608.

Some of the others are reviewed in:

● Herbert, V. Vitamin E report (a letter to the editor). *Nutrition Reviews* 35 (1977):158.

SELF-STUDY

The Fat-Soluble Vitamins

Exercises 1 to 3 make use of the information you recorded on Forms 1 to 3 in the Self-Study at the end of the Introduction to Part One.

1. Look up and record your recommended intake of vitamin A (from the RDA tables on the inside front cover or from the Canadian Dietary Standard in Appendix O). Note that this recommendation is stated in RE units.

2. Estimate your actual intake of vitamin A by restudying Form 1 (p. 000) in light of what you now know from reading Chapter 11. List all the foods you ate during your three-day self-study period that contributed more than 100 IU of vitamin A. Sort the amounts of vitamin A they contributed into two columns: one for animal foods, the other for plant foods. Add up these two columns separately. Now, using the rule of thumb that 10 IU of vitamin A from plant foods or 3.33 IU from animal foods is approximately equivalent to 1 RE, divide the amount in your plant-food column by 10. Divide the amount in your animal-food column by 3.33.

Then add the two columns together to express your three-day vitamin A intake in RE. Finally, divide this number by 3 (days) to derive your average estimated intake of vitamin A per day in RE.

3. What percentage of your recommended intake of vitamin A did you consume? Was this enough? What foods contribute the greatest amount of vitamin A to your diet? What percentage of your intake comes from plant foods? If you consumed more than the recommendation, was this too much? Why or why not? In what ways would you change your diet to improve it in these respects?

Optional Extras

Tables of food composition do not show vitamins D, E, and K, but you can guess at the adequacy of your intake.

4. For vitamin D, answer the following questions: Did you drink fortified milk (read the label)? Eat eggs? Fortified breakfast cereals? Liver? Are you in the sun frequently? (Remember, though, that excessive exposure to sun can cause skin cancer in susceptible individuals.)

5. For vitamin E, consider the foods you ate in 24 hours. Vitamin E often accompanies linoleic acid in foods. Did you consume enough linoleic acid? (The recommendation is 3 percent of total kcalories from linoleic acid, as specified in the Chapter 2 Self-Study.)

6. For vitamin K, does your diet include 2 c of milk or the equivalent in milk products every day? Does it include leafy vegetables frequently (every other day)? Do you take antibiotics regularly (which inhibit the production of vitamin K by your intestinal bacteria)?

7. Return to the health food store and ask some more questions, this time about the fat-soluble vitamins. Does the salesperson try to alert you to the risks of overdosing with these vitamins?

CHAPTER 12

CONTENTS

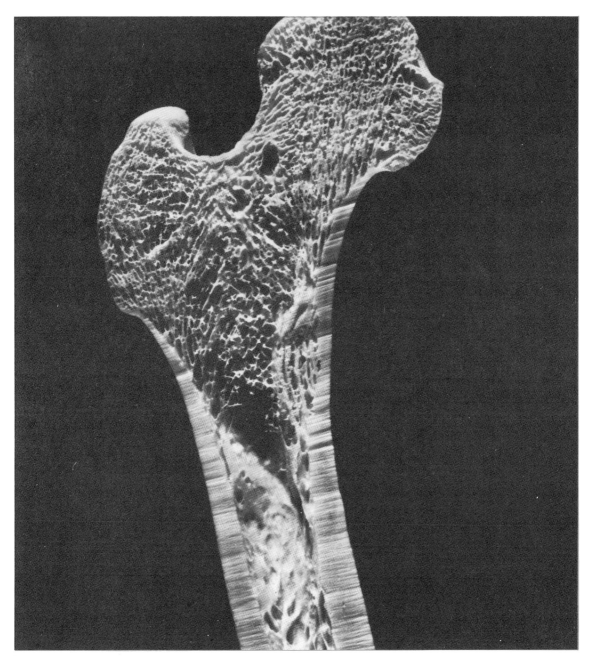

Cross section of bone, showing trabeculae.

THE MAJOR MINERALS

Chapters 1 to 11 have been devoted to the first four of the six classes of nutrients: carbohydrates, fat, protein, and vitamins. Now we move on to the minerals. A few generalizations about minerals that distinguish them from vitamins were presented in the introduction to Part Two. (You may want to review those points before you continue.)

Because the amounts of the minerals found in the body and needed in the diet vary so widely, many authorities have divided them into two categories: the major minerals (sometimes called macrominerals) and the trace minerals (sometimes called microminerals).

Major minerals:	Trace minerals:
calcium	iron
phosphorus	iodine
potassium	zinc
sulfur	selenium
sodium	manganese
chlorine	copper
magnesium	molybdenum
	cobalt
	chromium
	fluorine
	silicon
	vanadium
	nickel
	tin
	arsenic (?)
	cadmium (?)

The major minerals are sometimes called the **macrominerals.** They are needed in amounts on the order of 0.1 g or more each day. They comprise 0.1% of the body weight or more.

The trace minerals are sometimes called the **microminerals.** They are needed in amounts on the order of 0.01 g or less each day and comprise 0.01% of the body weight or less.

Figure 1 shows how much the human body needs of some of these minerals.

Figure 1   The amounts of minerals in a 60-kilogram human body. A line separates the major minerals from the trace minerals. The major minerals are those present in amounts larger than 5 g (a teaspoon). A pound is about 454 g; thus only calcium and phosphorus appear in amounts larger than a pound. There are more than a dozen trace minerals, although only four are shown here; not shown are fluoride, silicon, vanadium, chromium, cobalt, nickel, zinc, selenium, molybdenum, and tin.

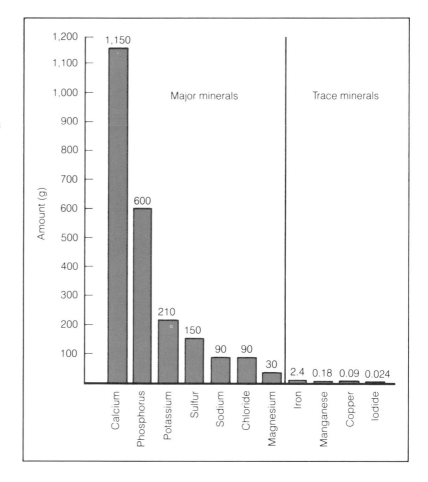

The influence of the minerals on the acid-base balance of the body fluids is proportional to the amounts found in the body. Thus the major minerals have a much greater effect than the trace minerals on this balance. The special roles of minerals in regulating the pH of body fluids depend on their interaction with water, the last nutrient to be discussed in this book. Chapter 14 is reserved for a discussion of these roles, and Table 1 in that chapter shows the major minerals divided into the acid- and base-forming classes.

In addition to the mineral elements listed above, most of which have long been familiar to nutritionists, others that are needed in the daily diet in very tiny amounts have recently come to light. The list of needed mineral elements is still growing longer as research continues. Perhaps 30 or more minerals will eventually prove to be essential in the human diet. This means that the amount of information available on the minerals, like that on the vitamins, is overwhelmingly great and cannot be treated exhaustively in an introductory textbook. What is probably most important is for you to be aware of the minerals that are presently known to be lacking in the diets of significant numbers of people. Those most needing emphasis by this criterion are calcium, iron, iodine, zinc, and fluorine. Calcium will be emphasized most heavily in this chapter; the others, being trace minerals, will be discussed in Chapter 13.

Calcium

A popular book on nutrition that has enjoyed wide sales over the past 30 years makes extravagant claims for calcium.[1] The writer implies that even a very slight decrease in dietary intake causes these symptoms: air swallowing and indigestion; insomnia and other forms of the inability to relax; irritability of the muscles, including cramps and spasms; menstrual cramps; hypersensitivity to pain; a tendency to hemorrhage; cataracts; tooth decay; and complications in childbirth. Since there is hardly anyone in the world who is free of all of these symptoms, the naive reader might be led to believe that calcium is a virtual cure-all and that people must make special efforts to procure adequate amounts of this extremely important, even miraculous, nutrient.

The claims made for this wonderful nutrient are based on a misunderstanding of the facts about the roles it plays in the body. A deficiency of calcium caused by failure of the *body* to maintain a proper concentration can cause some of these symptoms, but a *dietary* deficiency cannot. In fact, a dietary calcium deficiency has little or no effect on its blood concentration or on the functions mentioned above.

The Roles of Calcium Calcium's most obvious role is as a component of bones and teeth: 99 percent of the calcium in the body is found in these structures. The remaining 1 percent circulates in the watery fluids of the body, where it performs a number of important functions. Some calcium is found in close association with cell membranes; it appears to be essential for their integrity. The calcium found between and among cells is essential for keeping them in association with one another. In some way it helps to support or maintain the intercellular cement—collagen. In association with cell membranes, calcium helps to regulate the transport of other ions into and out of cells. In association with the membranes of muscle cells, calcium is essential for muscle relaxation and so helps maintain the heartbeat. Calcium must be present between nerve and nerve, and between nerve and muscle, for the transmission of nerve impulses.

Collagen: see pp. 130, 353.

The mineral must also be present if blood clotting is to occur, because it is one of the 14 factors directly involved in this process. (The other 13 are proteins; vitamins, such as vitamin K, are also needed for the synthesis of some of these proteins.) Calcium is also needed as a cofactor for several enzymes, acting like a coenzyme.

cofactor: a mineral element that, like a coenzyme, works with an enzyme to facilitate a chemical reaction.

Coenzyme: see p. 314.

[1] A. Davis, *Let's Eat Right to Keep Fit* (New York: Harcourt Brace Jovanovich, 1970), chap. 21. This and other unreliable books are on a list of nutrition books that are not recommended, available on request from the American Medical Association (address in Appendix J).

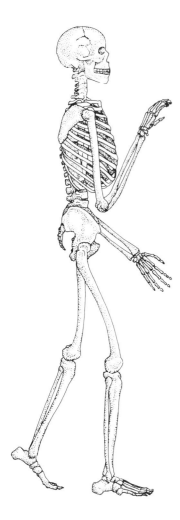

An awareness of all these functions might lead you to believe that a deficiency of calcium in food would cause nerve and muscle irritability and possibly nervous tension, hemorrhaging, and the other symptoms mentioned earlier. Yet in fact none of these things happens with a dietary deficiency of calcium. The reason for this is that the amount of calcium found in the blood remains remarkably constant over a wide range of dietary intakes; a deficiency affects the calcium stores in bones.

Why the Blood Calcium Level Does Not Change   It is an axiom of nature that if a function is vital to life it will be maintained against tremendous odds. Breathing is such a function; there is no way you can stop breathing voluntarily, as you may remember learning when you were a very small child. A child having a tantrum will make furious efforts to hold his breath until he is blue in the face. But even as he starts to lose consciousness, his automatic, instinctive reflexes take over and he begins to breathe again. In the same way, if the beating of the heart is stopped by a heart attack, which affects the node of cells in the heart muscle known as the pacemaker, a second node of cells nearby takes over and keeps the heartbeat going—albeit at a slower pace. Or if the secretion of pancreatic enzymes fails, a second set of enzymes similar to the pancreatic ones, produced by the small intestine, continue to work so that some digestion will still proceed.

These examples could be multiplied many hundreds of times to show that wherever there is a vital function, backup systems provide for it to be carried out in emergencies. You can tell how important a body function is for survival by observing how many different systems serve the backup function. By this criterion it is obvious that maintenance of the blood's calcium concentration is extremely important for overall health and even life, for calcium is the most closely regulated ion in the body.

The bones hold the body upright, but from the blood's point of view, this is not their primary role. The bones serve as a "bank" for calcium and other minerals. The minerals can be readily withdrawn from bone when blood levels begin to fall, and they can be redeposited into bone if blood levels rise too high. The 99 percent of the body's calcium stored in bone constitutes a tremendous "savings account."

The concentration of ionic calcium in the blood is maintained within very narrow limits, around 10 mg/100 ml of blood. If it falls or rises ever so slightly, it is immediately corrected. Four separate systems serve to maintain the blood calcium level. Some calcium in the blood itself is reversibly bound to such blood proteins as the albumins and globulins. The first line of defense against falling blood calcium is the release of this bound calcium from the proteins. The other three systems are regulated with the help of vitamin D and hormones.

One of these systems is the absorption system. A calcium-binding protein is made by the intestinal cells with the help of vitamin D, and

albumins (al-BYOO-mins) and **globulins** (GLOB-yoo-lins): two major classes of blood proteins.

more of this protein is made if more calcium is needed. Thus you will absorb more when you need more. This system is most obviously reflected in the increased absorption by a pregnant woman. She may drink the same amount of milk that she did before she was pregnant but absorbs 50 percent of the calcium from it; formerly she absorbed only 30 percent. Thus her body's calcium supply almost doubles, even if her food intake does not change at all. Similarly, growing children absorb 50 or 60 percent of ingested calcium; when their growth slows or stops (and their bones no longer demand a net increase in calcium content each day), their absorption falls to the adult level of about 30 percent.

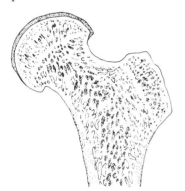

trabeculae (tra-BECK-you-lie), singular **trabecula:** lacy filaments inside bone that serve as a storage site for calcium and phosphorus. They are readily broken down and built up again in response to the body's changing needs for these minerals.

The second system is a storage system. Calcium is reversibly stored in the trabeculae of the bones. When blood calcium concentration rises, more is put away inside these lacy filaments. When calcium is needed in the blood, the trabeculae break down again. The photograph at the opening of this chapter shows the exquisite architecture of bone.

The third system involves the kidneys. The kidneys are sensitive to blood calcium concentrations and excrete more when blood calcium rises above the acceptable level and less when it falls.

These three systems are regulated by two hormones, one secreted by the parathyroid glands and the other secreted by both the thyroid and the parathyroid glands. The first, parathormone, is released whenever blood calcium falls below 7 mg/100 ml. Parathormone affects all three systems, stimulating increased absorption in the intestines, release of calcium from bone trabeculae, and increased retention by the kidneys. The other hormone, calcitonin, is secreted by both the thyroid and parathyroid glands when blood calcium rises above tolerance. Calcitonin inhibits the release of calcium from bone. For these reasons, blood calcium concentrations are very little affected by varying dietary intakes.

To say that food calcium never affects blood calcium is not to say that blood calcium never changes. In fact, sometimes blood calcium does rise above normal, causing a condition known as calcium rigor. When this happens, the muscle fibers contract and cannot relax. Similarly, calcium levels may fall below normal in the blood, causing calcium

parathyroid (para-THIGH-royd) **glands:** 4 small glands situated on the surface of the thyroid gland, 2 on each side; they produce the hormones parathormone and calcitonin.

thyroid glands: 2 glands in the neck, one on each side; they produce the hormones thyroxin (see p. 223) and thyrocalcitonin (see below).

parathormone (para-THOR-mone): hormone secreted by the parathyroid glands in response to low blood calcium concentrations; causes increased intestinal absorption, release from bones, and increased renal resorption of calcium.

calcitonin (cal-si-TONE-in): one form, **thyrocalcitonin**, is secreted by the thyroid glands in response to high blood calcium concentration, inhibiting release of calcium from bone; the other is secreted by the parathyroid.

calcium rigor: hardness or stiffness of the muscles.

calcium tetany: intermittent spasms of the extremities due to nervous and muscular excitability.

tetany—also a situation characterized by uncontrolled contraction of muscle tissue, due to a change in the stimulation of nerve cells. These conditions do not reflect a dietary lack or excess of calcium but are due to a lack of vitamin D or to glandular malfunctions resulting in abnormal amounts of the hormones that regulate blood calcium concentration.

On the other hand, a chronic dietary deficiency of calcium or a chronic deficiency due to poor absorption can, over the course of years, diminish the savings account in the bones. It is the bones, not the blood, that are depleted by calcium deficiency.

rickets: the calcium- (or vitamin D-) deficiency disease in children.

Calcium Deficiency   The disease rickets has been mentioned in connection with vitamin D deficiency. Often in rickets the amount of calcium in the diet is adequate, but it passes through the intestinal tract without being absorbed into the body, leaving the bones undersupplied. Vitamin D deficiency, by depressing the production of the calcium-binding protein, is the most common cause of rickets. (The symptoms have been described in Table 4 of Chapter 11.) In children, the failure to deposit sufficient calcium in bone causes growth retardation, bowed legs, and other skeletal abnormalities. In adults, the disease may set in after a normal childhood, during which calcium intake and absorption were adequate, and after the skeleton has become fully calcified. Prolonged inadequate calcium uptake during adulthood, often due to vitamin D deficiency, may cause the gradual and insidious removal of calcium from the bones, resulting in altered composition or reduced density of the bones in old age, which makes them fragile.

Altered composition of the bones is reflected in **osteomalacia**, the condition in which the bones become soft (see p. 393).

Reduced density of the bones results in **osteoporosis** (oss-tee-oh-pore-OH-sis), literally porous bones.

The fragility of the bones is most severe in the pelvic bone, which may become so brittle that it breaks when the person is walking. You may have heard of an old person who fell and broke her hip. What often actually happens is that her hip breaks while she is walking, and then she falls. The pelvic bone may shatter into countless fragments, so that it can never be repaired but has to be replaced with an artificial hip.

Many older people are severely afflicted with osteoporosis. The causes seem to be multiple, but a calcium deficiency during the growing years is a factor always present. This fact underscores the importance of prevention: Drink plenty of milk while you are young to have strong bones in later life.

A net calcium loss occurs in many adults, especially in women after menopause or hysterectomy, suggesting that hormonal changes are responsible. Many minerals and vitamins are required to form and stabilize the structure of bones, including magnesium, fluoride, vitamin A, and others. Any of these may be essential for preventing osteoporosis. One obvious line of defense, however, is to maintain a lifelong adequate intake of calcium.

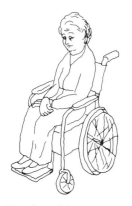

The RDA for calcium: 800 mg.

Canadian Dietary Standard: 800 mg for men, 700 mg for women.

Food Sources of Calcium   The recommended intake of calcium, arrived at by way of balance studies, is 700 to 800 mg (0.7 to 0.8 g) per day for adults in both the United States and Canada. Adults can stay in balance on intakes lower than this if they adapt over a long period of time to lower intakes, and the World Health Organization recommends only 400 to 500 mg per day for adults. However, high phosphorus intakes increase calcium excretion, and in the United States and Canada, where the diets are rich in phosphorus-laden protein, 700 to 800 mg seems to be a protective recommendation.

Calcium is found almost exclusively in a single class of foods—milk and milk products—as shown in Table 1. For this reason, if for no other, members of this group must be included in the diet daily. Because a cup of milk contains almost 300 mg calcium, an intake of 2 c milk provides an amount nearly adequate for most people. The other dairy food that contains comparable amounts of calcium is cheese. One

Table 1. Calcium Contents of 50 Common Foods*

Exchange group[†]	Food	Serving size[‡]	Calcium (mg)	Exchange group[†]	Food	Serving size[‡]	Calcium (mg)
5L	Sardines with bones	3 oz	372	6	Cream, light	2 tbsp	30
1	2% fat fortified milk	1 c	352	4	Winter squash	1/2 c	29
1	Canned evaporated milk	1/2 c	318	2	Turnips	1/2 c	27
1	Skim milk	1 c	296	5M	Egg	1	27
1	Dry skim milk	1/3 c	293	2	Summer squash	1/2 c	26
1	Whole milk	1 c	288	3	Dried fig	1	26
1	Yogurt	1 c	272	2	Onions	1/2 c	25
5L	Oysters	3/4 c	170	4	Whole wheat bread	1 slice	25
5L	Canned salmon with bones	3 oz	167	2	Brussels sprouts	1/2 c	25
2	Collard greens	1/2 c	145	4	Mashed potato	1/2 c	24
2	Dandelion greens	1/2 c	126	2	Carrots	1/2 c	24
2	Spinach	1/2 c	106	3	Blackberries	1/2 c	23
2	Mustard greens	1/2 c	97	4	White bread	1 slice	21
4	Corn muffin	1	96[§]	3	Pink grapefruit	1/2	20
5M	Creamed cottage cheese	1/4 c	58	3	White grapefruit	1/2	19
4	Pancake	1	58	4	Rye bread	1 slice	19
3	Orange	1	54	4	Green peas	1/2 c	19
2	Broccoli	1/2 c	49	5M	Peanut butter	2 tbsp	18
4	Dried beans	1/2 c	45	3	Strawberries	3/4 c	17
4	Pumpkin	3/4 c	43	5L	Chipped beef	3 oz	17
4	Muffin	1	42	2	Asparagus	1/2 c	15
4	Lima beans	1/2 c	40	4	Hamburger bun	1/2	15
3	Tangerine	1	34	3	Raspberries	1/2 c	14
2	Cabbage	1/2 c	32	3	Cantaloupe	1/4	14
2	Green beans	1/2 c	32	4	Sweet potatoes	1/4 c	14

*These are not necessarily the best food sources but are selected to show a range of calcium contents. Study of the left-hand column will help you to generalize about which foods contain the most calcium.

[†]The numbers refer to the exchange lists: 1 is milk; 2, vegetables; 3, fruit; 4, bread; 5L, lean meat; 5M, medium-fat meat; 6, fats and oils.

[‡]Serving sizes are the sizes listed in the exchange lists, except for meat.

[§]To this point, all foods supply at least 10 percent of the recommended intake (for a man) of 800 mg.

slice of cheese (1 oz) contains about two-thirds as much calcium as a cup of milk. For people who don't drink milk, greens are an important food; a 1-c serving provides as much calcium (and riboflavin) as a cup of milk.

The absurdity of attempting to meet calcium needs in any way other than by consuming two servings a day of these foods can be demonstrated by listing the amounts of other foods you would have to consume instead: 6 heads of iceberg lettuce, 10 c of cooked green beans, 12 oranges or eggs, or 20 c of strawberries!

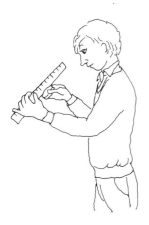

The amount of calcium recommended for the daily diet is so great that it cannot be packaged in a single pill that could be swallowed. To be absorbed, calcium is combined into an organic salt such as calcium gluconate or calcium lactate—a process that makes the pill extremely bulky. To get 600 mg of calcium in this salt you would have to take six pills the diameter of a quarter and the thickness of four quarters. You therefore never find significant amounts of calcium in vitamin-mineral supplements of the type that are to be taken once a day. Many vitamin-mineral supplements do contain some calcium, however.

There are two ways to read a label: One is to read what it contains, and the other is to read how much. A list of the ingredients in a pill that contains calcium might mislead unaware consumers into believing that their calcium needs would be met by the pill. However, often the label lists the calcium content of each pill as 10 mg. Only when you compare this amount with the recommended intake (800 mg) do you realize that you would have to take 80 of these pills to meet your calcium needs. This discussion should remind you of a point made once before (p. 141): Use a yardstick.

It is important to remember, too, that pills do not supply the relative amounts of nutrients that are in the best balance for your overall health. A typical calcium supplement, for example, is labeled with the instructions to take six a day. Yet six pills a day supply less than 50 percent of the recommended intake of calcium and 500 percent of the vitamin D. (Vitamin D is added to the pill to enhance the absorption of calcium.)

On the other hand, 2 c of vitamin A & D-fortified skim milk would supply the following percentages of the nutrients an adult man needs: calcium, 60 percent; vitamin D, 50 percent; protein, 40 percent; vitamin A, 50 percent; thiamin, 12 percent; riboflavin, 50 percent; plus 24 g carbohydrate in the form of lactose. You will recall from Chapter 6 that calcium absorption is enhanced by some of these other nutrients. Once again, a point made previously (p. 6) is relevant: There are fringe benefits to eating a nutrient in a natural food as opposed to a purified nutrient preparation.

For most people, the obvious way to meet calcium needs is to include milk and milk products in the diet daily. This is especially important for pregnant or lactating women and for children in the growing years (their calcium balance must be positive to permit good skeletal growth). Adults concerned with feeding children who dislike milk may find it helpful to learn how to conceal milk in foods. Ice cream, ice milk, and yogurt are acceptable substitutes for regular milk, and puddings, custards, and baked goods can be prepared in such a way that they also contain appreciable amounts of milk. Powdered skim milk, which is an excellent and inexpensive source of protein, calcium, and other nutrients, can be added to many foods (such as cookies and meatloaf) in preparation. For children with a milk allergy, a calcium-rich substitute such as fortified soy milk must be found. Butter and cream contain negligible calcium, because calcium is not soluble in fat.

The word *daily* should be stressed with respect to food sources of calcium. Because of its limited ability to absorb calcium, the body cannot handle massive doses periodically but instead needs frequent opportunities to take in small amounts.

Calcium must be soluble if it is to be absorbed. The hydrochloric acid in the stomach increases solubility, as do vitamin C and some of the amino acids. But a high-fat diet may inhibit the absorption of calcium by forming insoluble soapy scums with calcium, which are then excreted in the feces. This may be the case in any of the diseases that affect the absorption of fat, leaving a high fat content in the intestine to combine with calcium.

The lactose in milk forms a soluble compound with calcium. This enhances the value of milk as one of the best food sources of calcium. (Remember, too, that milk is chosen as the vehicle for fortification with vitamin D.) Calcium levels are lower in breast milk than in cow's milk, but babies absorb it better from breast milk, probably because of the higher lactose content of breast milk.

An important relationship exists between calcium and phosphorus. Each is better absorbed if they are ingested together. Authorities differ on the ratio that might best favor health, but it seems probable that most would agree on a 1:1 ratio; perhaps any ratio from 3:1 to 1:3 is all right.

Some foods contain certain compounds, called binders, that combine chemically with calcium (and other minerals such as iron and zinc) to prevent their absorption, carrying them out of the body with other wastes. For example, phytic acid and oxalic acid render the calcium, iron, and zinc in certain foods "unavailable." Phytic acid is found in oatmeal and other whole-grain cereals, and oxalic acid in peanuts, rhubarb, and spinach, among other foods.[2] The calcium-binding properties of these binders in no way affect the overall value of the foods. Whole grains and greens are nutritious for so many reasons that no one should hesitate to include them in menu planning.

The Four Food Group Plan recommends daily milk servings:

Children under 9	2-3 c
Children 9-12	3+ c
Teenagers	4+ c
Adults	2 c
Pregnant women	3+ c
Lactating women	4+ c
Older women	3 c

milk allergy: the most common food allergy; caused by the protein in raw milk. Milk allergy is sometimes overcome by cooking the milk to denature the protein, sometimes "cured" by abstinence from and gradual reintroduction to milk. See also the discussion of lactose intolerance, p. 30.

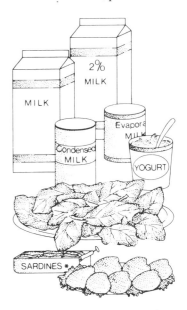

binders: chemical compounds occurring in foods that can combine with nutrients (especially minerals) to form complexes that the body cannot absorb. **Phytic** (FIGHT-ic) and **oxalic** (ox-AL-ic) **acids** are examples of such binders.

[2]Oxalate content of common foods, *Nutrition and the MD*, September 1979.

A generalization that has been gaining strength throughout this book is supported by the information given here about calcium: A balanced diet that supplies a variety of foods is the best guarantee of adequacy for all essential nutrients. All food groups should be included, and none should be overused. Calcium is found lacking wherever milk is underemphasized in the diet—whether through ignorance, simple dislike, lactose intolerance, or allergy. By contrast, iron is found lacking whenever milk is overemphasized, as Chapter 13 shows.

Phosphorus

Phosphorus is the mineral in second largest quantity in the body. About 85 percent of it is found combined with calcium in the crystals of the bones. Its concentration in blood plasma is less than half that of calcium: 3.5 mg/100 ml plasma. But as part of one of the body's major acids (phosphoric acid), it is a part of the structure of all body cells.

The average person hears very little about phosphorus, even though it plays a critical part in all cell functions. This lack of publicity in popular nutrition writing is probably due to the fact that deficiencies are unknown. Phosphorus is widespread in foods in association with calcium and protein; if these nutrients are adequate in the diet, then phosphorus is too.

Phosphorus is intimately associated with the calcium in bones and teeth as calcium phosphate, one of the compounds in the crystals that give strength and rigidity to these structures.[3] It is also a part of DNA and RNA, the genetic code material present in every cell. Thus phosphorus is necessary for all growth, because DNA and RNA provide the instructions for new cells to be formed.

Phosphorus plays many key roles in the cells' transfers of energy. Many enzymes and the B vitamins become active only when a phosphate group is attached. The B vitamins, you will recall, play major roles in energy metabolism. Again, phosphorus is critical in energy exchange. ATP itself, the energy carrier of the cells, contains three phosphate groups and uses these groups to do its work.

Some lipids contain phosphorus as part of their structure. These phospholipids help to transport other lipids in the blood; they also form a part of the structure of cell membranes, where they affect transport of nutrients into and out of the cells.

Phosphorus in the plasma is one of the most important buffers. A diagram in Chapter 14 shows how a buffer works in a solution such as blood to maintain the required acid-base balance.

Animal protein is the best source of phosphorus, because phosphorus is so abundant in the energetic cells of animals. People in the developed countries eat large quantities of animal protein and so

[3]The suffix *ate* in *calcium phosphate* indicates that oxygen is bound to the phosphorus.

excrete more phosphorus than people who consume a protein-poor diet. The extra phosphorus they excrete carries some calcium with it. This is why the recommended intakes for calcium in the United States and Canada are higher than they are for other countries. The recommended intakes for phosphorus are the same as those for calcium: 700 to 800 mg per day for adults.

The RDA for phosphorus: 800 mg.

Canadian Dietary Standard: 800 mg for men, 700 mg for women.

Sodium

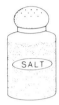

Sodium is the positive ion in the compound sodium chloride, ordinary table salt. Salt has been known throughout recorded history. The Bible's saying, "You are the salt of the earth," means that a person is valuable. If, on the other hand, "you are not worth your salt," you are worthless. Even the word *salary* comes from the word *salt.* Carnivores generally do not travel to find salt, because they get it from eating other animals, but a grazing animal will travel many miles to a salt lick, driven by its body's need for sodium.

There is seldom a sodium shortage in the diet. Foods usually include more salt than is needed, and it enters the body fluids freely. The kidneys filter the surplus out of the blood into the urine. They can also sensitively conserve salt and return it to the blood in the event of a deficiency, which might occur during heavy sweating or starvation. Intakes vary widely, especially because of cultural differences in diets. Orientals, who use a great deal of soy sauce and monosodium glutamate (MSG or Accent) for flavoring, consume the equivalent of about 30 to 40 g of salt per day; most people in the United States average about 6 to 18 g. Vegetarians probably consume much less than this.

The total amount of fluid in the body depends primarily on the sodium and potassium ions present. Cells can move these ions across their membranes, and they work constantly to keep sodium on the outside and potassium on the inside. Nerve transmission and muscle contraction depend on the cells' permitting a temporary exchange of sodium and potassium ions across their membranes. About 30 to 45 percent of the body's sodium is thought to be stored on the surface of the bone crystals, where it is easy to recover if the blood level drops.

The activity of the kidney in regulating the body content of sodium is remarkable. Sodium is absorbed easily from the intestinal tract, then travels in the blood, where it ultimately passes through the kidney. The kidney filters all the sodium out, then with great precision returns to the bloodstream the exact amount needed. Normally, the amount excreted equals the amount ingested that day.

If the blood level of sodium rises, as it will after a person eats heavily salted foods, the thirst receptors in the brain will be stimulated. The fluid intake will increase to make the sodium-to-water ratio constant. Then the extra fluid will be excreted by the kidneys along with the extra sodium.

Dieters sometimes think that eating too much salt or drinking too much water will make them gain weight, but this is not the case. Excess water is excreted immediately. Excess salt is excreted as soon as enough water is drunk to carry the salt out of the body. From this perspective, then, the way to keep body salt (and "water weight") under control is to drink more, not less, water.

If the blood level of sodium drops, as it does during vomiting, diarrhea, or heavy sweating, both water and sodium must be replenished. If only water is replaced, the blood concentration of sodium drops and water migrates into the cells. This results in symptoms of water intoxication: muscle weakness, apathy, nausea, and loss of appetite. Times when such a condition might exist are during athletic contests or heavy physical work in the heat, after extensive burns, or following accidents or surgery that involve loss of blood. Overly strict use of low-sodium diets in the treatment of kidney or heart disease may also deplete the body of needed sodium. The symptoms quickly vanish with the return of both sodium and water.

Estimated safe and adequate daily dietary intake of sodium (Committee on RDA): 1.1-3.3 g (1,100-3,300 mg).

No recommendation needs to be made for daily sodium intake, because of the sensitive controls operating in the body. Furthermore, cooks add salt generously in food preparation, and diners add more from the salt shaker on the table. The highest concentrations in foods are in cured ham, bacon, pickles, potato chips, and cold cuts, where the salt acts as a preservative. Pregnant women should normally not restrict their salt intake (see Chapter 15).

High blood pressure is often called **hypertension.** People sometimes confuse hypertension with stress, but hypertension is an internal and stress an external condition. Stress may cause hypertension in sensitive people, however.

5 g of salt would be about 2 g of sodium.

1 g salt = 1/5 tsp

The use of highly salted foods may contribute to high blood pressure. This may be true only for those who have a genetic tendency to develop high blood pressure. Black Americans are especially at risk in this respect. With a high sodium level in the blood, the volume of the blood increases. As this greater volume courses through the arteries, it expands them and puts their walls under tension. The heart then must work harder to pump the extra fluid throughout the system. It is presently recommended that we reduce our sodium intake by cutting our salt intake to not more than 5 g added salt a day (that is, salt added by manufacturers and consumers above and beyond that already in the food as grown). In practice, this would mean avoiding highly salted foods and removing the salt shaker from the table. (Appendix I shows the sodium contents of foods.)

Public water can contribute significant sodium to people's intakes. In some areas, where the water supply contains more than 100 mg of sodium per liter, some people's blood pressure is affected. Where highways are salted in winter to melt the snow, the runoff may contribute to this problem by adding more salt to the underground water. A sodium standard for public water of perhaps 20 mg per liter might need to be adopted in these areas.[4]

Chlorine

The element chlorine occurs naturally as a poisonous gas, but when it combines with sodium in salt, it is not poisonous but is part of a life-giving compound. It occurs in salt as the negative chloride ion.

The chloride ion is the major negative ion of the fluids outside the cells, where it is found mostly in association with sodium. Chloride can move freely across membranes and so is also found inside the cells in combination with potassium.

In the stomach, the chloride ion is part of hydrochloric acid. This is what maintains the strong acidity of the stomach. The cells that line the stomach continuously expend energy to push chloride into the stomach fluid. One of the most serious consequences of vomiting is the loss of chloride ions from the stomach, which upsets the acid-base balance of the body.

A chlorine compound is added to public water to sterilize it before it flows through pipes into people's homes. Turning to the deadly poisonous gas chlorine, it kills dangerous microorganisms that might otherwise spread disease, and then evaporates, leaving the water safe for human consumption. The addition of chlorine to public water is one of the most important public health measures ever introduced in the developed countries and has eliminated such water-borne diseases as typhoid fever, which once ravaged vast areas, killing thousands of people.

Estimated safe and adequate daily dietary intake of chloride (Committee on RDA): 1.7-5.1 g (1,700-5,100 mg).

Potassium

Potassium is critical to maintaining the heartbeat. The sudden deaths that occur in severe diarrhea, and in children with kwashiorkor may often be due to heart failure caused by potassium loss. As the principal positively charged ion inside body cells, it plays a major role in maintaining water balance and cell integrity. In water loss from the body in which sodium is lost, the ultimate damage comes when potassium is pulled out of the cells and excreted. Dehydration is especially scary, because potassium deficiency affects the brain cells early, making the victim unable to decide that she needs water.

[4]E. J. Calabrese and R. W. Tuthill, A review of literature to support a sodium drinking water standard, *Journal of Environmental Health* 40 (September/October 1977):80-83.

During nerve transmission and muscle contraction, potassium and sodium briefly exchange places. Nerve and muscle cells, then, are especially rich in potassium, but all cells must contain some. Potassium is also known to play a catalytic role in carbohydrate and protein metabolism, but the exact nature of this role is not known.

A deficiency of potassium from getting too little in the diet is unlikely. Abnormal conditions like diabetic acidosis or loss of large volumes of water can cause potassium deficiency, however. One of the earliest symptoms is muscle weakness.

Estimated safe and adequate daily dietary intake of potassium (Committee on RDA): 1,875-5,625 mg (1.9-5.6 g).

The warning implied by this information is that water loss from the body can be a grave danger. Adults are warned not to take diuretics (water pills) except under the direction of a physician; if another physician is consulted for a different health problem, he should be alerted to the fact that a diuretic is in use.

Gradual potassium depletion can occur when a person sweats profusely day after day and fails to replenish his potassium stores. A study of this effect shows that up to about 3 g of potassium can be lost in a day. The average diet in this country supplies about 1.5 to 2.5 g. If a person sweats heavily and often, the authors of this study recommend that he eat about five to eight servings of potassium-rich food each day.[5]

Potassium-rich foods include bananas, orange juice and many other fruit juices, and potatoes, tomatoes, and many other vegetables. For details, see Appendix I.

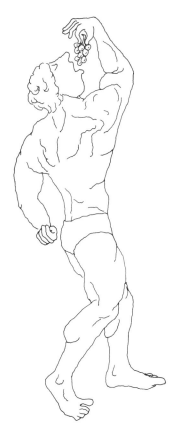

It has been pointed out several times previously that there are advantages to eating food instead of taking supplements. Salt tablets contain sodium and chloride, but foods contain a multitude of minerals. The body evolved in dependence on foods, not supplements. Men who think fruit is only for dainty ladies might take note that because of the potassium it contains, fruit may do more for their muscles than meat.

A borderline food is the liquid "sweat replacer," such as Gatorade, designed especially for athletes like football players. In choosing one of these, the buyer should look for potassium on the label.

The principal sources of potassium among foods commonly eaten are orange juice, bananas, dried fruits, and potatoes. Potassium supplements are not advisable except when prescribed, because too much potassium is as dangerous as too little. Even salt substitutes containing potassium should be avoided, especially by heart patients, except as recommended by a physician.

[5]H. W. Lane and J. J. Cerda, Potassium requirements and exercise, *Journal of the American Dietetic Association* 73 (1978):64-65.

Sulfur

Sulfur is present in all proteins and plays its most important role in determining the contour of protein molecules. Sulfur helps the strands of protein to assume a particular shape and hold it—and so to do their specific jobs, such as enzyme work. Some of the amino acids contain sulfur in their side chains, and once built into a protein strand, these amino acids can link to each other by way of sulfur-sulfur bridges. The bridges stabilize the protein structure. Skin, hair, and nails contain some of the body's more rigid proteins, and these have a high sulfur content.

You can see some **disulfide bridges** in the picture of insulin on p. 98.

There is no recommended intake for sulfur, and no deficiencies are known. Only if a person lacks protein to the point of severe deficiency will he lack the sulfur-containing amino acids.

Magnesium

Magnesium barely qualifies as a major mineral. Only about 1 3/4 oz are present in the body of a 130-pound person. Most of this is in the bones. Bone magnesium seems to be a storage reservoir to ensure that some will be on hand for vital reactions regardless of recent dietary intake.

Magnesium also acts in all the cells of the soft tissues, where it forms part of the protein-making machinery and where it is necessary for the release of energy. Its major role seems to be as a catalyst in the reaction that adds the last high-energy phosphate bond to ATP. Magnesium also helps relax muscles after contraction and promotes resistance to tooth decay by holding calcium in tooth enamel.

A dietary deficiency of magnesium does not seem likely, but deficiency may occur as a result of vomiting, diarrhea, alcoholism, or protein malnutrition; in postsurgical patients who have been fed incomplete fluids into a vein for too long; or in people using diuretics.

It is interesting to note that in areas with a high magnesium content in the water supply, there is a lower incidence of sudden death from heart failure.[6] A severe deficiency causes tetany, an extreme and prolonged contraction of the muscles very much like the reaction of the muscles when calcium levels fall. Magnesium deficit is also thought to cause the hallucinations experienced by alcoholics during withdrawal from alcohol.

Recommended intakes of magnesium are 300 to 350 mg a day for adult males, 250 to 300 mg for females. The amounts in foods have not been thoroughly studied as yet, but good food sources include nuts, legumes, cereal grains, dark-green vegetables, seafoods, chocolate, and cocoa. The kidney acts to conserve magnesium; that not absorbed is excreted in the feces.

The RDA for magnesium: 350 mg for men, 300 mg for women.

Canadian Dietary Standard: 300 mg for men, 250 mg for women.

[6]M. S. Seelig and H. A. Heggtreit, Magnesium interrelationships in ischemic heart disease: A review, *American Journal of Clinical Nutrition* 27 (1974):59-79.

Summing Up

Of the major minerals—calcium, phosphorus, potassium, sulfur, sodium, chlorine, and magnesium—calcium was selected for emphasis in this chapter because the risks of deficiency are the greatest. About 99 percent of the body's calcium is a structural component of the bones and teeth; these structures, in addition to their obvious roles, serve as a reserve to help maintain blood calcium at a constant concentration. The 1 percent of body calcium found in body fluids helps maintain cell membrane integrity, intercellular cohesion, transport of substances into and out of cells, and transmission of nerve impulses. It is also an essential factor for blood clotting and acts as a cofactor in some enzyme systems.

Ionic calcium concentration in the blood is held constant by equilibrium between free and bound calcium and by the hormones parathormone and calcitonin (with the help of vitamin D). Abnormal calcium concentrations in blood reflect abnormal amounts of these hormones or of vitamin D in the system; a lack of dietary calcium has its impact on bone, not blood.

Calcium deficiency in the body may be caused directly by inadequate calcium intakes over a prolonged period of time or indirectly by vitamin D deficiency, which suppresses calcium absorption. The diseases that result are rickets, osteomalacia, and osteoporosis, which are described in Chapter 11.

The recommended calcium intake is easily met by consuming 2 c or more of milk or equivalent dairy products such as cheese; fortified soy milk is an alternative in the case of milk allergy or lactose intolerance. The only other rich food source of calcium is dark-green leafy vegetables, 1 c cooked greens being equivalent to 1 c milk in calcium content. Daily consumption of calcium-containing foods is preferable to infrequent large amounts.

Phosphorus, another major mineral, is abundant in foods, and therefore deficiencies are highly unlikely. It participates with calcium in forming the crystals of bone and therefore composes a large proportion of the minerals found in the body.

Sodium is also abundant in the diet, as part of salt, and is efficiently handled by the body. Deficiencies are rare except in dehydration. Genetically sensitive people may develop high blood pressure in response to too-high sodium intakes; control of dietary salt is recommended for these people. Chlorine, also part of salt, contributes to the formation of the stomach's hydrochloric acid. Both sodium and potassium are important in body fluids (see Chapter 14).

Potassium, which can also form salts, is primarily involved in the working of nerve and muscle cells. A deficiency caused by protein deprivation or dehydration can stop the heart; excess potassium is also dangerous.

Sulfur, like phosphorus, is a major mineral constituent of body tissues. It is abundant in the diet, and deficiencies are unknown.

Magnesium plays a role in the synthesis of body proteins and so is in a key position with respect to all body functions. It is seldom found lacking in human beings, except in conditions that aggravate dietary protein deficiency, such as kwashiorkor and alcoholism. A deficiency of magnesium causes severe neuromuscular and cardiovascular disorders.

To Explore Further

The general references listed in Appendix J contain additional information on all the minerals covered in this chapter, and they also lead to further reading.

A booklet on sodium in foods is available:

● Marsh, A. C., Klippstein, R. N., and Kaplan, S. D. "The Sodium Content of Your Food," published by the USDA (booklet no. 233 in the Home and Garden Bulletin Series), available for $2 from the U.S. Government Printing Office (address in Appendix J). Mention stock number 001-000-04179-7 when ordering.

A concise and informative review of the recent information explosion about the role of zinc in nutrition is:

● Swanson, C.A., and King, J.D. Human zinc nutrition. *Journal of Nutrition Education* 11 (October-December 1979):181-183.

[If a] shopper is thought-ful,... [he] scratches his head. How much thiamin, he asks himself, is .09 mg?

RONALD M. DEUTSCH

If you want to buy good nutrition, you have to know what's in the foods you choose. Whether your nutritional goal is to decrease your fat intake, to trade sugars for starch and fiber, to obtain the RDA for protein, to meet your vitamin and mineral needs, to avoid salt, or whatever, it helps to be able to read food labels. The smart consumer not only reads the label but reads between the lines. This Highlight offers all you need to know to become such a consumer.

Claims and Information on Labels First of all, all labels must state:

● the common name of the product

● the name and address of the manufacturer, packer, or distributor

● the net contents in terms of weight, measure, or count

● the ingredients listed in descending order of predominance by weight

This information has to be prominently displayed, and must be expressed in ordinary words. That's all there is to the required label — but if you know how to read the front of a package you're already a step ahead of the naive buyer. This is particularly true in regard to the ingredient list. Whatever is listed first is what the package contains the largest amount of. Consider the following ingredient lists:

● an orange powder that contains "Sugar, citric acid, orange flavor . . ." versus a juice can that contains "Wa-

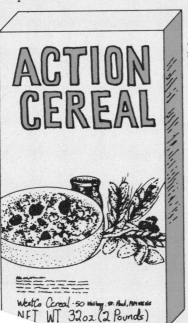

WestCo Cereal · 50 Holbay · St. Paul, MN 55165
NET WT 32 oz. (2 Pounds)

...ackage must always ...ame, the name ...ompany, the weight ... ingredients.

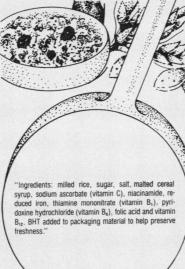

"Ingredients: milled rice, sugar, salt, malted cereal syrup, sodium ascorbate (vitamin C), niacinamide, reduced iron, thiamine mononitrate (vitamin B₁), pyridoxine hydrochloride (vitamin B₆), folic acid and vitamin B₁₂. BHT added to packaging material to help preserve freshness."

NUTRITION INFORMATION

Serving size	¼ cup (1 oz)	
Servings per container	32	with ½ cup vitamin D fortified whole milk
Calories	130	210
Protein	3g	7g
Carbohydrate	18g	24g
Fat	5g	9g

PERCENTAGE OF U.S. RECOMMENDED DAILY ALLOWANCES (%U.S.RDA)

Protein	4	10
Vitamin A	*	2
Vitamin C	*	*
Thiamine	4	8
Riboflavin	10	20
Niacin	2	2
Calcium	2	15
Iron	4	4
Vitamin D	*	10

*Contains less than 2% of the U.S. RDA for this nutrient

The nutrition information panel tells you the nutrients in a serving. Now all you have to know is how to read "percent of U.S. RDA."

ter, tomato concentrate, concentrated juices of carrots, celery . . ."

● or a cereal that contains "Puffed milled corn, sugar, corn syrup, molasses, salt . . ." versus one that contains "100% rolled oats"

● or a canned fruit that contains nothing but "Apples, water"

If you read the label, you know what you're getting, and what the main ingredient is.

Labels often tell you more than the minimum, however. If a nutrient is added to a food (for example, vitamin D to a breakfast drink), or if an advertising claim is made (like saying that orange juice is a good source of vitamin C), then the package must provide an information panel that complies *fully* with the nutrition labeling requirements. Without a complete information panel, nutrition claims could deceive the consumer about the true nutritional value of a food.

Several types of claims on labels are forbidden:

1. that a food is effective as a treatment for a disease
2. that a balanced diet of ordinary foods cannot supply adequate amounts of nutrients (excepting the iron requirements of infants, children, and pregnant or lactating women)
3. that the soil on which food is grown may be responsible for deficiencies in quality
4. that storage, transportation, processing, or cooking of a food may be responsible for deficiencies in its quality
5. that a food has particular dietary qualities when such qualities have not been shown to be significant in human nutrition
6. that a natural vitamin is superior to a synthetic vitamin[1]

The nutrition labeling section of the law then states that, if

[1]M. Stephenson, Making food labels more informative, *FDA Consumer* 9 (8) (1975):13-17.

any nutrition information or claim is made on the label of a food package, it must conform to the following format under the heading "Nutrition Information":

● serving or portion size
● servings or portions per container
● kcalorie content per serving
● protein grams per serving
● carbohydrate grams per serving
● fat grams per serving
● protein, vitamins, and minerals as percentages of the U.S. RDAs. (No claim may be made that a food is a significant source of a nutrient unless it provides at least 10 percent of the U.S. RDA of that nutrient in a serving.)

To fully understand the meaning of this part of the label, you must be able to interpret statements about vitamins and minerals made in terms of the U.S. RDA, which is not quite the same as the RDA.

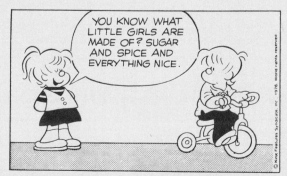
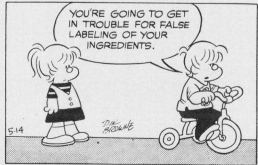

© King Features Syndicate, Inc. and Dick Browne.

The U.S. RDA The U.S. RDA table is shown on the inside *back* cover. It was designed from the RDA tables of 1968, in order to set standards for labeling. The RDA tables (see inside *front* cover) give different recommendations for each age group. But the designers of the U.S. RDA decided to use one recommended amount for each nutrient: whichever was the highest of the regular RDAs (not counting the RDAs for pregnant and lactating women, which are too high to use as a general standard). Thus in picking a U.S. RDA for iron, the decision makers chose the woman's RDA of 18 mg, which is higher than that for any other person. In setting a U.S. RDA for magnesium they chose 400 mg — the RDA of males age 15 to 18 — because it is the highest RDA for any age group. The only exceptions to this rule were for calcium and phosphorus — set a little lower than the very highest because needs vary so widely — and for four nutrients that did not appear in the RDA tables of 1968: biotin, pantothenic acid, copper, and zinc. These were already known to be essential for human beings, and so tentative U.S. RDAs were set for them so manufacturers could list them if they wished. Regular RDAs have since been set for these four nutrients; they are not different enough from the 1968 estimates to cause concern and so the U.S. RDAs have not been changed.

The U.S. RDA table includes two values for protein. If the protein is of high quality, less is needed, and the U.S. RDA is 45 g. If it is of lower quality, then the U.S. RDA is 65 g. This rule enables the consumer to "buy protein" in appropriate amounts, without having to understand the concept of protein quality.

In the years since 1968, when the U.S. RDAs were published, the RDA tables have been revised three times and the values for most of the nutrients have changed somewhat. However, the U.S. RDAs have not been revised for several reasons. For one thing, the 1968 RDAs are generally higher than the later versions, but they are safe to consume. The most likely mistake the public will make is to think of them as maximum amounts ("I must get *up to* 100% of the U.S. RDA") — so it's better to let them be a little high than a little low.

Also, it would cost the industry and therefore the consumer a lot of money to relabel all the food packages now ready for distribution. A third reason is the confusion that would result for foods labeled as either "enriched" or "fortified." Nutrients inserted at levels higher than 50 percent of the U.S. RDA in a food have to be labeled as "supplements." If the U.S. RDA were lowered to agree with the 1980 RDAs, some "enriched" and "fortified" foods would end up as "supplements" and then would have to comply with further regulations and definitions.

With this understanding of the U.S. RDAs, you can extract a lot of information from a nutrition label. If you just want to know generally what amounts of nutrients are in the package, the percent-of-U.S. RDA will tell you that without your having to do any calculating. If you read, for example, that a serving of breakfast cereal provides "Vitamin A — 25%," then you can be sure it provides at least a quarter of *your* vitamin A allowance for a day (unless you are pregnant or lactating). If you want to know exactly how many units of vitamin A are in a serving, you can look at the U.S. RDA table (inside back cover), find out that the U.S. RDA is 1,000 RE, and figure 25 percent (a quarter) of that is 250 RE.[2] For the nutrients included in the RDA tables, then, all the information is there that most consumers might want.

Labeling laws also require that any food claiming to be "low in calories" must state

[2]Vitamin A RDA for women is 800 RE; for men, 1,000 RE. For this one nutrient, you then may have to calculate further, using the factor 1RE-5IU, for comparison with food composition tables. For all the other nutrients it's simple.

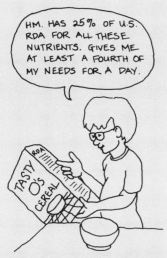

HM. HAS 25% OF U.S. RDA FOR ALL THESE NUTRIENTS. GIVES ME AT LEAST A FOURTH OF MY NEEDS FOR A DAY.

If it delivers 25% of the U.S. RDA for a nutrient, then it delivers at least 25% of *your* RDA for that nutrient. (For your RDA, see inside front cover. For U.S. RDA, see inside back cover.)

the absolute number of kcalories per serving. Any food calling itself a "reduced calorie" food must be at least a third lower in kcalories than the food it most closely resembles and must carry a nutrition label. Furthermore, wherever additives are listed on labels, their functions must be stated.

The information just presented helps you with ordinary foods labeled "fish" or "beans," and with foods that present information panels like breakfast cereals. But what about foods that simply say "TV dinner" or "macaroni and cheese"?

Nutrients in Convenience Foods The FDA has devised "nutritional quality guidelines" for the nutrient contents of many kinds of convenience foods: frozen dinners, breakfast cereals, meal replacements, non-carbonated vitamin C-fortified fruit- or vegetable-type beverages, and main dishes such as macaroni and cheese or pizza. If a product complies with the nutritional quality guidelines, it may carry on its label the statement that it "provides nutrients in amounts appropriate for this class of food as determined by the U.S. government." For example, frozen dinners must contain one or more sources of protein from meat, poultry, fish, cheese, or eggs, and these must make up at least 70 percent of the total protein; they must include one or more vegetables or vegetable mixtures other than potatoes, rice, or cereal-based products; and they must have a certain minimum nutrient level for each 100 kcalories, as shown in Table 1.

What if the label says nothing more than a name, such as *mayonnaise?* For some items the law provides Standards of Identity and excuses manufacturers from the requirement of listing ingredients. Standards of Identity exist for such foods as bread and mayonnaise — common foods that at one time were often prepared at home, so that the basic recipe was understood by almost everyone. Certain ingredients must be present in a specific percentage before the food may use the standard name. Any product like mayonnaise, for example, may use that name on the label only if it contains 65 percent by weight of vegetable oil, either vinegar or lemon juice, and egg yolk. The FDA does not have the authority to require

Table 1.   Required Nutrient Content of Highly Processed Foods Such as Frozen Dinners*

Nutrient	For Each 100 Calories Required Components	For the Combined Required Components Regardless of Calories
Protein, grams	4.60	16.0
Vitamin A, IU	150.00	520.0
Thiamin, mg	0.05	0.2
Riboflavin, mg	0.06	0.2
Niacin, mg	0.99	3.4
Pantothenic acid, mg	0.32	1.1
Vitamin B_6, mg	0.15	0.5
Vitamin B_{12}, µg	0.33	1.1
Iron, mg	0.62	2.2

*Stephenson, M.: Making food labels more informative. *FDA Consumer* 9(8):13-17, 1975.

that ingredients be listed for these foods, but it urges manufacturers to give the consumer more detailed information, and many manufacturers do so voluntarily.

Imitation Foods Still another class of foods that concerns consumers are inferior foods developed in imitation of, and as substitutes for, familiar foods. A section of the law requires that, if a food is an imitation of a traditional food, this fact must be stated on its label. With the new food technology, however, many imitation food products on the market may very well be superior to traditional foods; it is misleading to the consumer to imply that they are inferior. For this reason, the regulation now requires that the word *imitation* must be used on the label only if the product is "a substitute for and resembles another food but is nutritionally inferior to the food imitated. . . . Nutritional inferiority is defined as a reduction in the content of an

essential vitamin or mineral or of protein that amounts to 10 percent or more of the U.S. RDA."

Thus if you read *imitation* on a label, you may conclude that it is a poor imitation nutritionally. This may be of no consequence when the item is an incidental item in your diet, like vanilla, because you do not depend on vanilla for any nutrients. But if it's a fruit drink that you drink daily, and if you usually include no other items from the fruit and vegetable group in your diet, then the label may alert you to a needed change.

Up to this point you have learned you can tell from a food label:

● what the ingredients are

● whether anything has been added

● the number of kcalories

and often:

● the amount of protein, fat, and carbohydrate, and of the vitamins and minerals listed in the RDA tables

You also have a feel for the nutrient contributions that are made by processed and convenience foods, and by imitation foods. But the discerning reader may still ask, "Is this enough information? What else do I need to know?" The questions are worthwhile because nutrition-minded people are still concerned about several aspects of food labeling.

Misleading Labels As they presently appear, food labels provide useful information. But labels can be improved further. The law still allows loopholes through which can slip certain kinds of true but misleading claims. You might be interested in trying your skill at selecting from the following the two claims that are misleading even though true (all three claims are true):

1. A label says one serving of food provides 35 times as much iron as an 8-oz glass of whole milk.
2. A label says a fortified product contains "more vitamin C than fresh orange juice."
3. A label says that a brand of instant nonfat dry milk has "all the calcium, protein, B vitamins of whole milk."[3]

Check the bottom of the page for the answers.[4] Two other ways a consumer might be led off the track are shown in the following examples:

4. A label claims that an artificially constituted food or

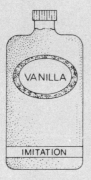

[3]L. Schwartzberg, C. George, and M. C. Phillips, Issues in food advertising: The nutrition educator's viewpoint, *Journal of Nutrition Education* 9 (1977):60-63.

[4]1. True but misleading, because milk is recognized as a poor source of iron. 2. True but misleading, because orange juice contains so many *other* nutrients by virtue of being a natural food. 3. True and responsible.

dietary supplement contains all of the vitamins and minerals known to be essential in human nutrition, in amounts equal to the U.S. RDA wherever this has been established. This implies a completeness that may be overestimated. A critic points out that "it is often not appreciated that we really do not know everything that should be included in artificially constituted foods."[5]

5. A breakfast bar or snack food label gives nutrition information showing that the protein, fat, carbohydrate, and certain vitamin and mineral contents are the same as those found in a milk, egg, and toast breakfast with orange juice. This fails to mention that the carbohydrate is sugar (versus the complex carbohydrate in toast), that the fat is saturated fat (versus the oil the egg might have been fried in), or that there is considerable salt in the food. Proposals under consideration for new labeling laws would require listing added sugar and salt in a prominent place on the label.

Consumers are putting pressure on legislatures to provide labeling laws that will make such misleading claims illegal.

"Fortified" versus "Nutritious" Foods   Another area of concern has to do with fortified foods. Suppose a label lists only a few nutrients, and claims to supply a large amount of each of them. The label makes the food appear to be nutritious, but if the few nutrients listed are the only ones in the food, then the food is really not all that nutritious. (Remember, nearly 40 nutrients are essential for humans.) Also, if the food is very high in kcalories, it may be a poor choice even though it has substantial amounts of certain nutrients in it. Labels should help consumers to distinguish between truly nutritious foods and nutrient-empty foods that may have been fortified with one or two nutrients just for appearance' sake. The concept of nutrient density — nutrients per kcalories — may be expressed in terms used on labels in the future to make such distinctions[6] (see Self-Study at the end of this Highlight).

Sugar and Salt   Another problem still to be resolved in nutrition labeling has to do with the amounts of sugar and salt in foods. Consumers

want, and are entitled to, this information but food producers are concerned that the labels not put them at an unfair disadvantage, so the exact requirements for labeling still have to be worked out. What should be called "sugar," for example: all mono- and disaccharides including those found naturally in the food; or all added sugars including honey, corn syrup, etc; or only added sucrose? How should sugar contents be listed? If in grams per serving, then the amount of sugar in a cola beverage will be seen to be more than that in a serving of sugar-coated cereal; but if sugar is stated as a percentage, then the amount in the cereal will appear very high because it isn't diluted by water.

As for salt, should it be listed as salt, or as sodium? Should just the added salt or sodium be listed, or should that occurring naturally in the food be included? If the sodium occurring naturally in the food is included, how much expense should the manufacturer sustain in trying to make sure the amounts are accurate? The amount of sodium varies from one shipment of produce to the next. While no official decision has been made, all of the major companies have voluntarily started sodium labeling in line with current practices (in mg/serving).

[5]A. M. Schmidt, Food and drug law: A 200-year perspective, *Nutrition Today* 10 (4) (1975):29-32.

[6]H. A. Guthrie, Concept of a nutritious food, *Journal of the American Dietetic Association* 71 (1977):14-19; A. J. Wittwer, A. W. Sorenson, B. W. Wyse, and R. G. Hansen, Nutrient density — evaluation of nutritional attributes of foods, *Journal of Nutrition Education* 9 (1), January-March 1977, pp. 26-30.

Regulations proposed by FDA, if approved, may ease the consumer's task in sizing up the sodium amounts in foods. The regulations define under what conditions manufacturers may use the terms "sodium free," "low sodium," "reduced sodium," and "moderately low sodium" on product labels. Basically the regulations define maximum levels of sodium content per serving that can be contained in a product when certain claims are made on a label.

The proposed regulations also provide for product comparative statements as long as the sodium reduction is at least 10 percent. A label could say, for example, "This product contains 25 percent less sodium than our regular product." They also permit use of the terms "unsalted," "without salt added," and "no salt added" when no salt has been added during the processing of the food and when the product substitutes for another food that normally is processed with salt. When these terms are used on the label, sodium content also must be listed.

While nutrition labeling would have to include a sodium listing under rules proposed today, manufacturers could continue to make salt and sodium statements on labels without triggering full nutrition labeling requirements.

FDA also recommends that potassium content be listed in nutrition labeling. This is because people with kidney and other diseases who must control their sodium intake also must control their potassium intake and because potassium often is used in place of sodium by people who must reduce their sodium intake to help treat high blood pressure and related health problems.[7]

Whatever decisions are finally made, the labels that include such information will benefit consumers who wish to limit their intakes of these substances. It isn't enough to stop using the sugar bowl and the salt shaker, because only about one-third of your total intake of these additives is sprinkled on foods by you. The other two-thirds is added during processing. When you eat processed foods, your intake of these items is involuntary. That's why they were called *additives* above. The next Highlight raises and tries to answer some of the important questions people ask about additives.

To Explore Further

The best source for the general reader of the latest information on labeling laws, regulations governing additives, and all other areas under the province of the FDA is the *FDA Consumer* magazine which comes out monthly. Your library probably subscribes, or you can get a subscription of your own (see Appendix J).

For the exact wording of the laws relating to the food supply, and of proposals now under consideration, dig into the *Federal Register*, which arrives weekly at your library. Back issues may be found in the U.S. Government documents section.

For a comprehensive scoring of many foods on the basis of their nutrient density, *Nutrition and the MD* recommends:

● Hanse, R. G. *Index of Nutritional Quality Food Profiles*. This 184-page book is available for $10.80 from the Utah State University Bookstore, Utah State University, UMC 01, Logan, UT 84322.

For help in reading labels, many booklets are available. One we like is:

● Inside information about the outside of the package, a pamphlet available free from Pillsbury Company, 1177 Pillsbury Bldg., 608 Second Avenue South, Minneapolis MN 55402.

A helpful cassette is *A Practical Nutrient Density-Nutritional Quality Index for Food*, by B. Wyse, R. G. Hansen, and A. W. Sorenson, available from the American Dietetic Association (address in Appendix J). The Association also makes available a cassette, *Food Labeling*, prepared by M. Robinson.

---

[7]The last four paragraphs are quoted verbatim from *HHS News*, 15 June 1982, a newsletter from the Department of Health and Human Services.

1. Look up and record your recommended intake of calcium (from the RDA tables on the inside front cover or from the Canadian Dietary Standard in Appendix O). Also record your actual intake, from the average derived on Form 2 (p. 14). What percentage of your recommended intake did you consume? Was this enough? What foods contribute the greatest amount of calcium to your diet? If you consumed more than the recommendation, was this too much? Why or why not? In what ways would you change your diet to improve it in this respect?

Optional Extras

2. Compute your sodium intake, using Appendix I. A dietary goal quoted in Chapter 12 is to restrict added salt intake to 5 g a day or less. This means 2 g (2,000 mg) added sodium, because sodium contributes 40 percent of the weight of the sodium chloride molecule. (By "added salt," we mean salt added by the manufacturer in processing or by you in cooking or at the table. It is assumed that foods you eat already contain about 3 g naturally occurring salt. So in calculating, count only the sodium you find in processed foods and in the salt shaker.)

Is your salt intake ample? Excessive? Should you consider making any changes, and if so, what kind?

Some authorities feel that the dietary goal for sodium should not apply to normal people but only to those who already have hypertension or some form of heart disease. A compromise is to recommend sodium restriction just for those normal people who have a hereditary tendency toward hypertension. Is this condition characteristic of your family?

3. Find alternative calcium sources for someone who doesn't drink milk. Plan a day's menus around this person's favorite foods.

4. Consider nature's arrangement of nutrients in foods: Phosphorus is critical in the transfer of energy, the structure of genetic material, the transport of substances across cell membranes, the structure of the skeleton, and the maintenance of the acid-base balance. It is so widespread in foods that we need not worry about suffering a deficiency. Why is this? Can you see any evolutionary reason why this vital nutrient should happen to be so abundant in the animal and plant tissues that we use as food?

Nutrient Density

Highlight 12 describes food labels and the need for consumers to know how nutritious the foods are that they buy. The concept of nutrient density helps people estimate the nutritional value of foods. Using this concept, you can decide which of your favorite foods are the most nutritious.

Pick a food, any food you are curious about, and follow this procedure using Form 1 to record the information:

1. Record your recommended kcalorie intake and your recommended intakes for protein, vitamins, and minerals from the inside front cover or from Appendix O. (The Self-Study at the end of Highlight 7 directed you to calculate how much energy you need for a typical day. You could use this personalized calculation in place of your recommended kcalorie intake if you feel it is more accurate.)

2. Look up in Appendix H the number of kcalories and the amounts of protein, vitamins, and minerals provided by a serving of the food you are interested in, and list these numbers under your recommended intakes.

3. Determine what percentage of your recommended intake for kcalories a serving of the food provides. This will be your comparison number.

4. Determine what percentage of your recommended intake a serving of the food provides for each nutrient.

5. Divide each percentage derived for the nutrients by

Form 1. Nutrient Density of a Food

Food chosen for analysis: _____

	Energy (kcal)	Pro-tein (g)	Cal-cium (mg)	Iron (mg)	Vita-min A (IU)	Thia-min (mg)	Ribo-flavin* (mg)	Vita-min C (mg)
① Your recommended intake								
② Amount provided by one serving of the food								
Percentage of recommended intake provided by 1 serving	③ Com-parison number	④						④
⑤ Nutrition score								
⑥ Is the food nutritious? _____

*A complete calculation would include niacin, but we have omitted it because of the difficulty in estimating niacin derived from tryptophan (see Chapter 9).

the comparison number to give each nutrient a score.

6. By one suggested standard, the food is nutritious if it receives a score greater than 1 for each of four nutrients or greater than 2 for each of two. By this standard, how nutritious is the food you selected? Repeat this procedure several times to study a variety of the foods in your diet that you are curious about.

7. Finally, review your food records (p. 12) and list from them the foods that made the major contributions to your kcalorie intakes on the days you studied. Jot down by each food your reason for choosing it:

- personal preference or familiarity (I like it; I often eat it)
- social pressure (it was offered; I couldn't refuse)
- availability (I was hungry and it was the only food offered)
- economy (it was the only food I could afford)
- convenience (I was too rushed to prepare anything else)
- nutritional value (I thought it was good for me)
- other (explain)

From what you know now, you can make a good guess about the nutritive value of each of these foods. In

some cases you will find that a food chosen primarily because it tastes good to you is also nutritious — a happy surprise. In others, you may find that a food you thought was nutritious is not especially noteworthy in this sense. Such insights can help guide you toward food selections that meet your needs for pleasure as well as for good nutrition.

Optional Extras

8. Practice translating the nutrition panel of a label, which is expressed in percentages of the U.S. RDA, into the actual amounts of nutrients delivered by a serving of a food. Use the example in the margin, or copy from the label of a food you use in your home. First, look up the U.S. RDA for each nutrient listed, and take the indicated percentage of it. This is the

number of units of that nutrient you will get from a serving of the food. Then answer this question: How much of *your* RDA would a serving of the food deliver?

Example: 25 percent of the U.S. RDA for Vitamin A is 25 percent of 5,000 IU or 1,250 IU. My RDA for vitamin A is 4,000 IU, so I would receive 1,250/4,000, or about 31 percent of my RDA from a serving of the food.

9. Practice your skill in evaluating foods from what's on their labels. The following two lists of ingredients are from foods advertised as meal substitutes. *Both* provide 25 percent of the U.S. RDA for every nutrient. But one is fat and sugar; the other more nearly resembles a food, and its fat is more polyunsaturated. Which is which? What other differences do you see between the two? Which is the more desirable meal substitute?

Percentage of U.S. Recommended Dietary Allowances (U.S. RDA)

	One serving (10 fluid oz)
Protein	25%
Vitamin A	25%
Vitamin D	25%
Vitamin E	25%
Vitamin C	25%
Folic Acid	25%

The first one is a pair of bars of pastry, like brownies, which contains 25 percent of all the U.S. RDAs, 275 kcalories, and this ingredient list:

Hydrogenated vegetable oils (coconut and palm kernel oil), sugar, milk protein, enriched flour [flour, niacin, iron, thiamine mononitrate (vitamin B_1), riboflavin (vitamin B_2)], almonds preserved with BHA, natural and artificial flavor, vital wheat gluten, salt, enzyme modified milk, artificial color, vegetable lecithin, baking soda, magnesium oxide, ascorbic acid (vitamin C), vitamin E acetate, vitamin A palmitate, niacinamide, iron, calcium pantothenate, vitamin D_2, vitamin B_6 hydrochloride, riboflavin (vitamin B_2), thiamin mononitrate (vitamin B_1), folic acid, potassium iodide, vitamin B_{12}.

The second one is a canned sweet drink similar to chocolate milk, which contains 25 percent of all the U.S. RDAs, 225 kcalories, and this ingredient list:

Skim milk, sugar, sodium caseinate, corn oil, malted milk, cocoa, artificial flavors, magnesium sulfate, purified cellulose, salt, disodium phosphate, calcium phosphate, potassium citrate, sodium ascorbate, carboxymethyl cellulose, calcium carrageenan, ferric orthophosphate, vitamin E acetate, zinc sulfate, niacinamide, artificial color, calcium pantothenate, copper sulfate, vitamin A palmitate, pyridoxine hydrochloride, thiamine hydrochloride, riboflavin, folic acid, biotin, potassium iodide, vitamin B_{12}, vitamin D_2. (Hint: sodium caseinate is the same as milk protein.)

CHAPTER 13

CONTENTS

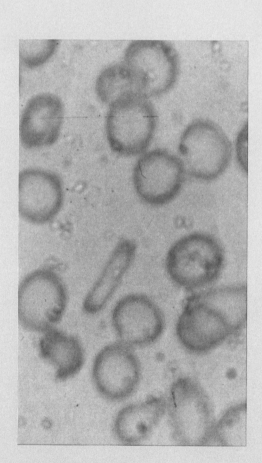

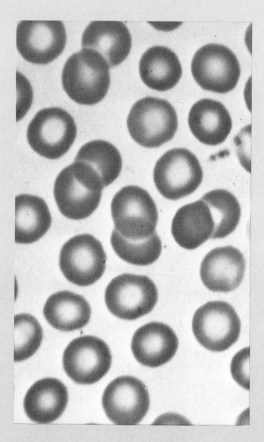

Blood cells in iron-deficiency anemia.

Normal blood cells.

THE TRACE MINERALS

"Although erythrocytes occupy less than fifty percent of the volume of the blood fluid, they can absorb seventy-five times more oxygen than can possibly be dissolved in the plasma itself."

"[Hemoglobin] must be a tricky substance," said Mr. Tompkins thoughtfully.

GEORGE GAMOW and MARTYNAS YCAS, *Mr. Tompkins Inside Himself*

If you could remove all of the trace minerals from your body, you would have only a bit of dust, hardly enough to fill a teaspoon. You would also die instantly. Although present in tiny quantities, each of the trace minerals performs some vital role for which no substitute will do. A deficiency of any of them may be fatal, and an excess of many is equally deadly. Remarkably, the way you eat and the way your body handles these minerals enables you to maintain a supply that is just sufficient for health and within the limits of toxicity.

Laboratory techniques developed in the past two decades have enabled scientists to detect the minute quantities of trace minerals in living cells for the first time. Study of the "new" trace elements, using animals, is one of the most active areas of research in nutrition today. An obstacle to determining the precise role of a trace element lies in the nearly impossible task of providing an experimental diet devoid of that element. Even the dust in the air or the residue left on laboratory equipment by the rinsing water may contaminate the feed enough to prevent a deficiency. Thus research in this area is limited to the study of small laboratory animals, which can be fed highly refined, purified diets in an atmosphere free of all contamination.

The best-known trace elements—iron, iodine, and zinc—have been so thoroughly studied that we can describe many of their roles with certainty. Government authorities have established recommended daily intakes for these three. For six others, the Committee on RDA published tentative ranges for safe and adequate daily intakes for the first time in 1980. Five others are known to be essential nutrients, but the amounts needed are so tiny that they have not yet been measured. Many others are presently under study to determine whether they too perform indispensable roles in the body.

Whole books have been published just on the trace minerals.[1] In selecting the information to present in this chapter we have chosen to give most attention to those that are likely to have the greatest impact on your health. Iron, for example, is often deficient in the diets of

[1] For example, E. J. Underwood, *Trace Elements in Human and Animal Nutrition*, 4th ed. (New York: Academic Press, 1977).

people the world over, and an iron deficiency profoundly hurts the quality of life. Iodine is easy to obtain in adequate amounts, but simple ignorance can precipitate a deficiency, with tragic and irreversible consequences. Until recently, zinc and chromium deficiencies were unheard of, but now that we know of their existence and their effects, we see the need to help people protect themselves from these conditions too. No doubt the years to come will bring new knowledge of equal importance about some of the other trace elements, but an acquaintance with these few can enable you to take action—to select a diet composed of protective foods that will ensure adequacy for all the essential nutrients.

protective foods: foods known to be naturally rich in some nutrients and therefore presumed to be rich in others as well. The Four Food Group Plan identifies these as milk, milk products, meat, poultry, fish, eggs, legumes, nuts, vegetables, fruits, and grains.

Iron

Of all the trace minerals, iron deserves the most attention. It is a problem nutrient for millions of people. If you want to plan and consume a diet adequate in iron, you must be well informed.

Iron in the Body Iron is found in every cell, not only of the human body but of all living things, both plant and animal. It occurs in many vital proteins, including those involved in cell respiration and DNA synthesis. It is part of many major enzymes.

Most of the iron in the human body is a component of the proteins hemoglobin and myoglobin. Both these proteins carry oxygen and release it. As the cells' environments change, ionized iron can change from a +2 charge to +3 and back again, thereby releasing or holding on to oxygen, which has a −2 charge.

hemoglobin: the oxygen-carrying protein of the red blood cells.

hemo = blood
globin = globular protein

myoglobin: the oxygen-carrying protein of the muscle cells.

myo = muscle

The **ferrous** ion has a +2 charge; **ferric** iron has a +3 charge.

Hemoglobin is the oxygen carrier in the red blood cells, and its iron can have either charge. Myoglobin is in the muscle cells, and its iron can have only a +2 charge. Myoglobin therefore has a greater holding capacity for oxygen and so serves as a reservoir for oxygen; its presence in the muscle cells seems to draw oxygen into them. The muscle cells use this oxygen as the receiver for used-up carbon and hydrogen atoms flowing down the glucose-to-energy pathway. These atoms combine to make carbon dioxide and water, the final waste products of metabolism. Thus oxygen keeps the energy-yielding pathway open so that the muscles can remain active. As the muscles use up and excrete their oxygen (combined with carbons and hydrogens), the red blood cells shuttle between muscles and lungs to maintain fresh supplies.

The average red blood cell lives about four months. When it has aged and is no longer useful, it is removed from the blood by liver cells, which take it apart and prepare many of the degradation products for excretion. Its iron, however, is attached to a protein carrier. The iron is returned to the bone marrow, where new red blood cells are constantly being produced. Thus although red blood cells are born, live, and die within a four-month cycle, the iron in the body is recycled through each new generation. Only tiny amounts of iron are lost, principally in urine, sweat, and shed skin.

About 75 percent of the iron in the body is in the red blood cells, so iron losses are greatest whenever blood is lost. For this reason, "women need more iron," as a well-known television commercial proclaims: Menstruation incurs losses that make a woman's iron needs up to twice as great as a man's.

To replace the lost iron, the body provides special proteins to absorb it from food and carry it to the liver, bone marrow, and other blood-manufacturing sites. Iron absorbed into the intestinal cells from food is captured by a blood protein, transferrin, that carries it to tissues throughout the body. Each tissue takes up the amount of iron that it needs: The bone marrow and liver take large quantities, other tissues take less. In a pregnant woman, the placenta is avid for iron, devouring large quantities for delivery to the fetus even if this means depriving the mother's tissues of iron. Should there be a surplus, special storage proteins in the bone marrow and other organs store it.

transferrin (trans-FURR-in): the body's iron-carrying protein.

The storage proteins are **ferritin** (FAIR-i-tin) and **hemosiderin** (heem-oh-SID-er-in).

Iron routes in the body.

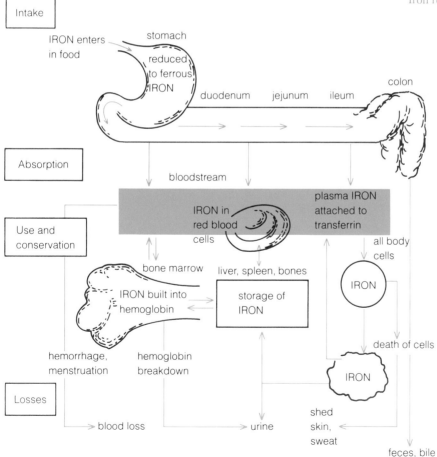

Iron clearly is the body's gold, a precious mineral to be hoarded and closely guarded. The number of special provisions for its handling show that it is as vital as calcium. At the receiving end, in the intestines, another provision shows this even more clearly. Normally only about 10 percent of dietary iron is absorbed. But if the body's supply is diminished or if the need increases for any reason, absorption increases. More transferrin (the carrier that picks up iron from the intestines) is produced so that more than the usual amount of iron can be absorbed. Only if this measure fails and the stores are used up do the red cells become depleted. Then anemia sets in.

Iron absorption responds to the body's need. (This figure does not show how the intestinal cells also help to regulate iron absorption.)

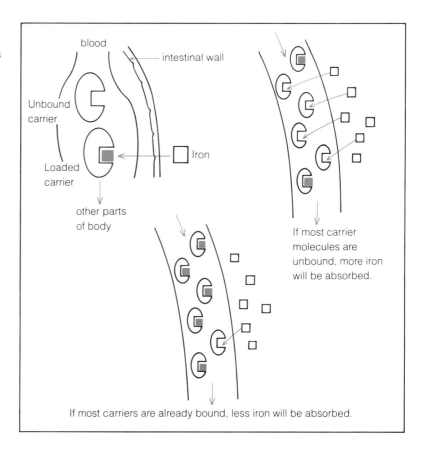

blood

intestinal wall

Unbound carrier

Loaded carrier

Iron

other parts of body

If most carrier molecules are unbound, more iron will be absorbed.

If most carriers are already bound, less iron will be absorbed.

The most common tests for iron deficiency are measures of the number and size of the red blood cells and of their hemoglobin concentration. But before these levels fall, at the very beginning of an iron deficiency, the transferrin concentration *rises*. There is a sensitive test that will detect a developing iron deficiency before it is full-blown; it tests the amount of transferrin in the blood and the amount of iron that it is carrying.

Technically, this technique is known as measuring the total iron-binding capacity (TIBC) and the transferrin saturation.

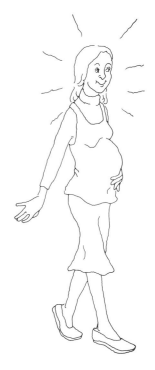

For women only: You are often told that you need more iron, yet you may often have had your blood cell count or hemoglobin level pronounced normal. Does this mean that you don't need more iron? Not necessarily. The difference between you and the men you know is a difference in your body stores of iron, which doesn't show up in these tests. Most men eat more food than women do, because they are bigger, and so their iron intakes are higher. Besides, women menstruate, and so their iron losses are greater. These two factors—lower intakes and higher losses—put you much closer to the borderline of deficiency. Even though you may never have been diagnosed as iron-deficient, you are likely to be deficiency-prone. Should you lose blood for any reason (even by giving a blood donation) or become pregnant (so that your blood volume would need to increase), you would need to pay special attention to your diet in an effort to maintain your iron stores. The information about iron in foods, which appears later in this chapter, is especially important for you.

Iron-Deficiency Anemia   If iron stores are exhausted, the body cannot make enough hemoglobin to fill its new red blood cells. Without enough hemoglobin, the cells are small. Since hemoglobin is the bright red pigment of the blood, the skin of a fair person who is anemic may become noticeably pale. A sample of iron-deficient blood examined under the microscope shows smaller cells that are a lighter red than normal (see the photograph at the start of this chapter). The undersized cells can't carry enough oxygen from the lungs to the tissues, so energy release in the cells is hindered. Every cell of the body feels this effect; the result is fatigue, weakness, headaches, and apathy.

Long before the mass of the red blood cells is affected, however, a developing iron deficiency may affect other body tissues, including the brain. As researchers have become better acquainted with iron, they have learned that it plays roles in the body, including brain functions, not earlier appreciated. For example, iron works with an enzyme that helps to make neurotransmitters, the substances that carry messages from one nerve cell to another. Children deprived of iron show some psychological disturbances, such as hyperactivity, decreased attentiveness, and even reduced IQ. These symptoms are among the first to appear when the body's iron level begins to fall and among the first to disappear when iron intake is increased again.[2]

In a dark-skinned person, this symptom can be observed by looking in the corner of the eye. The eye lining, normally pink, will be very pale, even white.

Iron-deficiency anemia is a **microcytic** (my-cro-SIT-ic) **hypochromic** (high-po-KROME-ic) **anemia.**

micro = small
cytic = cells
hypo = too little
chrom = color

[2]R. L. Leibel, Behavioral and biochemical correlates of iron deficiency: A review, *Journal of the American Dietetic Association* 71 (1977):399-404; and E. Pollitt and R. L. Leibel, Iron deficiency and behavior, *Journal of Pediatrics* 88 (1976):372-381.

Maximum treadmill work time in women with different hemoglobin levels. The numbers within the bars show how many women were tested at each level. The chart shows that the lower a woman's hemoglobin level, the less muscular work she can perform.

Adapted from G. W. Gardner, V. R. Edgerton, B. Senewiratne, R. J. Barnard, and Y. Ohira, Physical work capacity and metabolic stress in subjects with iron deficiency anemia, *American Journal of Clinical Nutrition* 30 (1977):910-917. Courtesy of the authors and publisher.

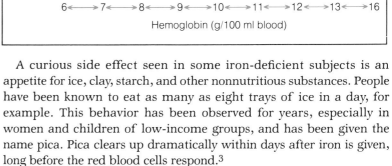

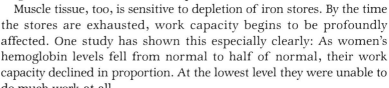

A curious side effect seen in some iron-deficient subjects is an appetite for ice, clay, starch, and other nonnutritious substances. People have been known to eat as many as eight trays of ice in a day, for example. This behavior has been observed for years, especially in women and children of low-income groups, and has been given the name pica. Pica clears up dramatically within days after iron is given, long before the red blood cells respond.[3]

Muscle tissue, too, is sensitive to depletion of iron stores. By the time the stores are exhausted, work capacity begins to be profoundly affected. One study has shown this especially clearly: As women's hemoglobin levels fell from normal to half of normal, their work capacity declined in proportion. At the lowest level they were unable to do much work at all.

pica (PIE-ka): a craving for unnatural substances.

picus = woodpecker or magpie

Many of the symptoms described here are easily mistaken for "mental" symptoms. A restless child who fails to pay attention in class might be thought contrary. An apathetic homemaker who has let her housework pile up unattended-to might be thought lazy. But the possibility is real that both these persons' problems are nutritional.

No responsible nutritionist would ever claim that all mental problems are caused by nutritional deficiencies. But nutrition is always a possible cause or contributor to problems like these. When you are seeking the solution to a behavioral problem it makes sense to check the adequacy of the diet and to have a routine physical examination before going the more expensive and involved route of consulting a mental health professional.

---

[3]Leibel, 1977.

It is conventional to measure the body's iron status by measuring the amount of hemoglobin (in grams per 100 milliliters of blood). The normal level is considered 14 to 15 g/100 ml for adult men, 13 to 14 g/100 ml for women. Yet many people who have values lower than this have no obvious symptoms. American blacks have average values about half a gram lower than these; it is not known whether this is a racial characteristic or is due to insufficient iron intakes. Some women have no symptoms of anemia—at least as measured by the performance of mental tasks—at levels as low as 10 g or even 8 g.[4] Doubtless people vary: One man may feel miserable with a hemoglobin of 12 g, another may feel no effects at a drastically low level of, say, 6 g: "Who, me? Anemic?"[5] Still, such symptoms as fatigue, weakness, and the like are often seen at levels not much below the standards.

When hemoglobin begins to fall, it is a sign that a long period of depletion of body stores has already occurred. In view of this fact and in light of the behavioral effects of iron deficiency in children, it seems reasonable to aim at "normal" hemoglobin levels for the general population: 14 to 15 for men, 13 to 14 for women. Values much below these represent a real hazard to health and to the quality of life.

Norms for children:

Ages 2-5	11 g/100 ml
Ages 6-12	11.5 g/100 ml

Note that hemoglobin is measured in grams per 100 ml, but we often just use the number alone in speaking of it: "Hemoglobin, 14."

A low hemoglobin level may represent a dietary iron deficiency, and if it does, the doctor may prescribe iron supplements. But the cause of an iron deficiency may be something else. For example, a vitamin B_6 deficiency can indirectly cause anemia, because B_6 is required to make the iron-containing portion of the hemoglobin molecule. A vitamin E deficiency can cause anemia by making the red blood cell membranes so fragile that the cells lose their hemoglobin. A vitamin B_{12} or folacin deficiency can cause it, because these vitamins are used in making new red blood cells to replace the old ones as they die. A vitamin C deficiency can cause it by reducing the absorption of iron.[6] Recently it has been learned that vitamin A, too, is involved in the making of red blood cells and that some people's low hemoglobin levels can be corrected only by administering vitamin A.[7]

Feeling fatigued, weak, and apathetic is a sign that something is wrong but does not indicate that you should take iron supplements. It indicates that (you guessed it!) you should consult your doctor. The doctor herself must use all her knowledge to diagnose correctly

[4]P. C. Elwood and D. Hughes, Clinical trial of iron therapy on psychomotor function in anaemic women, *British Medical Journal* 3 (1970):254-255.

[5]W. H. Crosby, Current concepts in nutrition: Who needs iron? *New England Journal of Medicine* 297 (1977):543-545.

[6]R. H. Matthews and M. Y. Workman, Nutrient content of selected baby foods, *Journal of the American Dietetic Association* 72 (1978):27-30.

[7]R. E. Hodges, H. E. Sauberlich, J. E. Canham, D. L. Wallace, R. B. Rucker, L. A. Mejia, and M. Mohanram, Hematopoietic studies in vitamin A deficiency, *American Journal of Clinical Nutrition* 31 (1978):876-885.

secondary nutrient deficiency:
one caused indirectly—not by
inadequate intake but by the
deficiency of another nutrient,
interference with absorption,
disease, or other causes.

the primary cause of a secondary anemia; you don't have a chance at making this kind of diagnosis. In fact, taking iron supplements may be the worst possible thing you could do, because they may mask a serious medical condition, such as hidden bleeding from cancer or an ulcer. Once again, this caution deserves repeating:

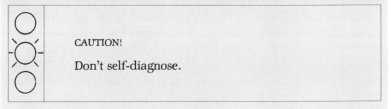

CAUTION!

Don't self-diagnose.

However, the role of all these nutrients in making and maintaining red blood cells dictates a preventive measure: Eat right! A study of over 200 older adults in Boston provides evidence to support this recommendation. These people all had moderately low hemoglobin levels (below 13 g/100 ml) to begin with. Two-thirds were given iron-fortified foods; the other third received foods without added iron. At the end of the study, *all* had higher hemoglobin levels. Food made a difference, iron supplements did not.[8] The appropriate risk-free "supplements," then, are nutritious foods.

By these criteria, iron-deficiency anemia is a major health problem in both the United States and Canada and even more so in the rest of the world. It is especially common in older infants, children, women of childbearing age, and people in low-income and minority groups. The incidence of iron deficiency in these groups ranges from 10 to over 50 percent.[9] It tends to cluster with other indicators of low socioeconomic status, such as family instability, little money spent on food, little attention given to children.[10] But no segment of society is free of iron-deficiency anemia, and these groups are not the only ones affected. For example, 1 out of every 20 Canadian men is at moderate risk (hemoglobin 12 to 14), and 1 out of every 100 is at high risk (hemoglobin below 12).[11]

[8]S. N. Gershoff, O. A. Brusis, H. V. Nino, and A. M. Huber, Studies of the elderly in Boston: I. The effects of iron fortification on moderately anemic people, *American Journal of Clinical Nutrition* 30 (1977):226-234.

[9]M. Winick, Nutritional disorders of American women, *Nutrition Today*, September/October-November/December 1975, pp. 26-28.

[10]D. M. Czajka-Narins, T. B. Haddy, and D. J. Kallen, Nutrition and social correlates in iron deficiency anemia, *American Journal of Clinical Nutrition* 31 (1978):955-960.

[11]Z. I. Sabry, J. A. Campbell, M. E. Campbell, and A. L. Forbes, Nutrition Canada, *Nutrition Today*, January/February 1974, pp. 5-13.

Iron Overload   Iron toxicity is rare but not unknown. The body protects itself against absorbing too much iron by setting up a "block" in the intestinal cells. A protein traps extra absorbed iron and holds it until it can be shed from the body when the mucosal cells are shed. The average life of an intestinal cell is only three days, so this method efficiently removes excess iron from the system. Still, the mucosal block can be overwhelmed, and iron overload is the result.

Two kinds of iron overload are known. One is caused by a hereditary defect, the other by ingesting too much iron. Tissue damage, especially to the liver, occurs in both, but it is most severe in those who also drink large quantities of alcohol.[12] Alcohol increases the absorption of ferric iron, and wines contain substantial amounts of iron, so the overconsumption of wine is particularly risky.

Iron overload is more common in men than in women. An argument against the fortification of foods with iron to protect women is that it might put more men at risk of overload. Indeed, there is some evidence from Sweden, where foods are generously fortified with iron, that this measure has increased the incidence of iron overload in men. It is too bad that a measure meant to promote the health of one sex might put the other sex at risk.

The ingestion of massive amounts of iron can cause sudden death. The second most common cause of accidental poisoning in small children is ingestion of iron supplements or vitamins with iron (the first is aspirin).[13] As few as 6 to 12 tablets have caused death in a child.[14] A child suspected of iron poisoning should be rushed to the hospital to have his stomach pumped; 30 minutes may make a crucial difference.

Iron in Foods   The usual Western mixed diet provides only about 5 to 6 mg of iron in every 1,000 kcal. The recommended daily intake for an adult man is 10 mg and most men require more than 2,000 kcal, so a man can easily meet his iron needs without special effort. The recommendation for a woman, however, is 14 to 18 mg per day. Because women typically consume fewer than 2,000 kcal per day, they understandably have trouble achieving this intake. A woman who wants to meet her iron needs from foods must increase the iron-to-kcalorie ratio of her diet so that she will receive about double the

mucosal block to iron absorption: the provision of a binding protein (ferritin) in the mucosal cells which captures and holds unneeded iron until it is shed with the cells.

iron overload: toxicity from iron overdose.

hemochromatosis (heem-oh-crome-a-TOCE-iss): iron overload characterized by deposits of iron-containing pigment in many tissues, with tissue damage; an inborn error (see p. 116).

hemosiderosis (heem-oh-sid-er-OH-sis): iron overload characterized by excessive iron deposits in hemosiderin, the normal iron-storage protein.

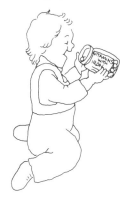

[12]The detection of early hemochromatosis, *Nutrition Reviews* 36 (March 1978):76-79; and C. V. Moore, Major minerals, Section C: Iron, in *Modern Nutrition in Health and Disease*, 5th ed., eds. R. S. Goodhart and M. E. Shils (Philadelphia: Lea and Febiger, 1973), pp. 297-323.

[13]W. H. Crosby, Prescribing iron? Think safety, *Archives of Internal Medicine* 138 (1978):766; abstract in *Journal of the American Dietetic Association* 73 (1978):344.

[14]Committee on Safety, Toxicity, and Misuse of Vitamins and Trace Minerals, National Nutrition Consortium, *Vitamin-Mineral Safety, Toxicity, and Misuse* (Chicago: The American Dietetic Association, 1978).

Recommended intakes of iron:

Men   10 mg/day
Women   14 mg/day (Canada)
        18 mg/day (U.S.)

How recommended daily intake for iron is calculated (for example, for an adolescent girl):

Losses from urine and shed skin: 1/2-1 mg

Losses through menstruation (about 15 mg total averaged over 30 days):   1/2 mg

Net for growth: 1/2 mg

Average daily need (total):
                             1 1/2-2 mg

Only 10 percent of ingested iron is absorbed, so this girl must ingest 15-20 mg per day.

Meeting iron needs from food (example):

Food choice	Iron (mg)	Energy (kcal)
1 egg	1.1	80
3 oz beef	2.9	245
3 slices bread	1.5	165
1/2 c tomatoes	0.6	25
1/2 c broccoli	0.6	40
1 small apple	0.4	70
1/2 small banana	0.4	50
1 sweet potato	1.0	155
2 c milk	0.4	320
Total	8.9	1,150

This example shows that selection of a variety of nutritious foods according to the Four Food Group Plan rule—without any added butter, margarine, or sugar—uses up 1,150 of a woman's 2,000 kcal and supplies fewer than 10 mg of iron.

average amount of iron—at least 10 mg per 1,000 kcal. This means she must emphasize the most iron-rich foods in every food group.

In considering which foods are the best sources of iron it is important to know that iron is absorbed differently from various foods. **The average amount of iron absorbed is 10 percent, but up to 40 percent of the iron in meat-fish-poultry and soybeans may be** absorbed. Less than 10 percent of the iron in eggs, whole grains, nuts, and dried beans is absorbed. At the bottom of the list is spinach: Only 2 percent of its iron is absorbed. The listing of common foods in Table 1 does not take iron's varying absorbability into account, but even so, meat-fish-poultry are at the top. Obviously, then, a woman who includes some meat in everyday meal planning will get a head start toward meeting her iron needs, especially if she makes periodic use of liver and other organ meats.

Foods in the milk group do not appear in Table 1 at all. Milk and cheese are notoriously poor iron sources, as poor in iron as they are rich in calcium. Although these foods are an indispensable part of the diet, they should not be overemphasized. In considering the grain foods,

Meat-fish-poultry contain about half their iron bound into molecules of **heme** (HEEM), the nonprotein part of the hemoglobin and myoglobin proteins. Heme iron is much more absorbable than nonheme iron. Meat-fish-poultry also contain a factor other than heme that promotes the absorption of iron, even of the iron from other foods eaten at the same time as the meat.

Overconsumption of milk is a common cause of iron deficiency in children; the resulting anemia is known as **milk anemia**.

Table 1. Iron Contents of 50 Common Foods*

Ex-change group[†]	Food	Serving size[‡]	Iron (mg)	Ex-change group[†]	Food	Serving size[‡]	Iron (mg)
5L	Oysters	3/4 c	10	3	Dried apricots	4 halves	.8
5M	Beef liver	3 oz	8	4	Winter squash	1/2 c	.8
4	Bran flakes, enriched	1/2 c	6.2	4	Whole-wheat bread	1 slice	.8
5M	Beef heart	3 oz	5	3	Blackberries	1/2 c	.7
5L	Chipped beef	3 oz	4	4	Pumpkin	3/4 c	.7
5L	Lean beef roast	3 oz	2.9	5L	Canned salmon	3 oz	.7
5L	Veal roast	3 oz	3	4	Cooked cereal	1/2 c	.7
5M	Hamburger	3 oz	2.7	3	Blueberries	1/2 c	.7
3	Prune juice	1/4 c	2.6	4	Spaghetti, enriched	1/2 c	.7
5L	Sardines	3 oz	2.5	4	Macaroni, enriched	1/2 c	.7
4	Dried beans	1/2 c	2.5	2	Broccoli	1/2 c	.7
2	Spinach	1/2 c	2.4	4	Potato chips	15	.6
4	Lima beans	1/2 c	2.2	3	Raspberries	1/2 c	.6
5L	Ham	3 oz	2.2	5M	Peanut butter	2 tbsp	.6
5L	Canned tuna	3 oz	1.6	4	White bread	1 slice	.6
2	Dandelion greens	1/2 c	1.6	3	Dried fig	1	.6
4	Green peas	1/2 c	1.5	4	Muffin	1	.6
5L	Leg of lamb	3 oz	1.4	4	Corn muffin	1	.6
5L	Chicken, meat only	3 oz	1.4	3	Applesauce	1/2 c	.6
2	Mustard greens	1/2 c	1.3	2	Cooked tomatoes	1/2 c	.6
3	Strawberries	3/4 c	1.1	4	French-fried potatoes	8	.6
5M	Egg	1	1.1	4	Popcorn, no fat	3 c	.6
2	Tomato juice	1/2 c	1.1[§]	3	Pear	1	.5
4	Rice, enriched	1/2 c	.9	4	Potato	1 small	.5
2	Brussels sprouts	1/2 c	.9	4	Corn on cob	1 small	.5

*These are not necessarily the best food sources but are selected to show a range of iron contents. Note the preponderance of 5s at the top of the left-hand column and the total absence of 1s in this table. Remember, too: Iron is better absorbed from meat-fish-poultry and soybeans than from other foods.

[†]The numbers refer to the exchange lists: 1 is milk; 2, vegetables; 3, fruit; 4, bread; 5L, lean meat; 5M, medium-fat meat. Note that milk exchanges (1) are missing.

[‡]Serving sizes are those in the exchange lists, except for meat.

[§]To this point, all foods supply at least 10 percent of the recommended intake (for a man) of 10 mg.

remember that iron is one of the enrichment nutrients. Whole-grain or enriched breads and cereals—not refined, unenriched pastry products—are the best choices. Finally, among the vegetables, the legume family and the dark greens are the most iron-rich; among the fruits, dried fruits are the best. A set of guidelines, then, for planning an iron-rich diet:

enrichment: the addition of iron, thiamin, riboflavin, and niacin to refined grain products to restore approximately their original contents (see p. 324).

- *Milk and cheese.* Don't overdo these foods (but don't omit them either; you need them for calcium). Drink skim milk to free up kcalories to be invested in iron-rich foods.

- *Meat.* Use liver and other organ meats frequently, perhaps every week or two. Meats, fish, and poultry are excellent iron sources.

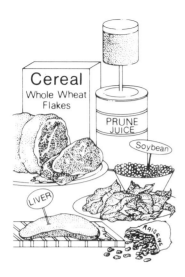

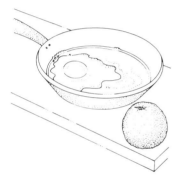

fortification: the addition of nutrients to a food—but not necessarily the nutrients that were originally found there.

● *Meat substitutes.* Don't forget legumes: A cup of peas or beans can supply up to 5 mg iron.

● *Breads and cereals.* Use only whole-grain, enriched, and fortified products.

● *Vegetables.* The dark-green leafy vegetables are rich in iron.

● *Fruits.* Dried fruits like raisins, apricots, peaches, and prunes are high in iron.

Knowledgeable cooking and menu planning can enhance the amount of iron delivered by your diet. The iron content of 100 g of spaghetti sauce simmered in a glass dish is 3 mg, but it's 87 mg when the sauce is cooked in an unenameled iron skillet. Even in the short time it takes to scramble eggs, their iron content can be tripled by cooking them in an iron pan. Foods containing 25 mg or more of vitamin C can more than double the amount of iron absorbed from iron sources eaten at the same meal.[15] Therefore, two additional suggestions are:

● Cook with iron skillets whenever possible.

● Serve vitamin C-containing foods at every meal.

Even after taking all of these precautions, a woman may not accumulate enough storage iron to prepare her for the increased demands of pregnancy and childbirth. In 1974 the Committee on RDA acknowledged for the first time that pregnant women might need supplemental iron. The Canadian Dietary Standard also includes this statement. However, the iron from supplements is far less well absorbed than that from food, and the doses have to be as high as 50 mg per day. Absorption of iron from supplements can be improved by taking them with meat or with vitamin C-rich foods or juices.

The use of fortified foods is another option. Some breakfast cereals boast that they contain 100 percent of the recommended daily intake of iron. The use of these may indeed boost the day's iron intakes, even though absorption of the iron used in them is poor. A number of proposals have been made for further fortification. Canada is considering adding iron to milk;[16] other ideas are to add it to coffee, to junk foods, even to salt. At present, 25 percent of all the iron consumed in the United States derives from fortified foods. A proposal to increase further the iron level in enriched bread has been defeated.[17] Ultimately, it is up to the consumer herself to see that she gets enough iron.

[15]M. Balsley, Soon to come: 1978 Recommended Dietary Allowances, *Journal of the American Dietetic Association* 71(1977):149-151; and J. D. Cook and E. R. Monsen, Vitamin C, the common cold, and iron absorption, *American Journal of Clinical Nutrition* 30 (1977):235-241.

[16]D. Rosenfield, Nutritional optimization of new foods (commentary), *Journal of the American Dietetic Association* 72 (1978):475-477.

[17]For a full description of the disagreements surrounding this decision, see Controversy 13: Iron Superenrichment, in E. M. N. Hamilton and E. N. Whitney, *Nutrition: Concepts and Controversies* (St. Paul: West, 1979), pp. 292-294.

Iodine

Iodine occurs in the body in an infinitesimally small quantity, but its principal role in human nutrition is well known and the amount needed is well established. Iodine is a part of thyroxin, a hormone secreted by the thyroid gland. Thyroxin is responsible for the basal metabolic rate. The hormone enters every cell of the body to control the rate at which the cell uses oxygen. This is the same as saying that thyroxin controls the rate at which energy is released.

Thyroxin: see also p. 223.

Iodine must be available for thyroxin to be synthesized. The amount in the diet is variable and generally reflects the amount present in the soil in which plants are grown or on which animals graze. Iodine is plentiful in the ocean, so seafood is a completely dependable source. In the United States, in areas where the soil is iodine-poor (most notably the Plains states), the use of iodized salt has largely wiped out the iodine deficiency that once was widespread.

> People sometimes wonder whether sea salt, made by drying ocean water, is preferable to purified sodium chloride for use in the salt shaker. Sea salt does contain trace minerals, but it loses its iodine during the drying process. Thus in a region where goiter is a risk, iodized sodium chloride is the salt to choose.

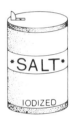

When the iodine level of the blood is low, the cells of the thyroid gland enlarge in an attempt to trap as many particles of iodine as possible. If the gland enlarges until it is visible, it is called a simple goiter. Goiter is estimated to affect 200 million people the world over. In all but 4 percent of these cases the cause is iodine deficiency. Furthermore, 8 million people have goiter because they overconsume plants of the cabbage family and others that contain an antithyroid substance whose effect is not counteracted by dietary iodine.[18] The goitrogens present in plants serve as a reminder that food additives may not be such great offenders as some natural components of foods (see Highlight 13).

goiter (GOY-ter): an iodine-deficiency disease. Goiter caused by iodine deficiency is **simple goiter**.

goitrogen: a thyroid antagonist found in food; causes **toxic goiter**.

In addition to causing sluggishness and weight gain, an iodine deficiency may have serious effects on the development of an infant in the uterus. Severe thyroid undersecretion during pregnancy causes the extreme and irreversible mental and physical retardation known as cretinism. A cretin has an IQ as low as 20 and a face and body with

cretinism (CREE-tin-ism): an iodine-deficiency disease characterized by mental and physical retardation.

[18]F. M. Strong, Toxicants occurring naturally in foods, in *Nutrition Reviews' Present Knowledge in Nutrition*, 4th ed. (Washington, D.C.: Nutrition Foundation, 1976), pp. 516-527.

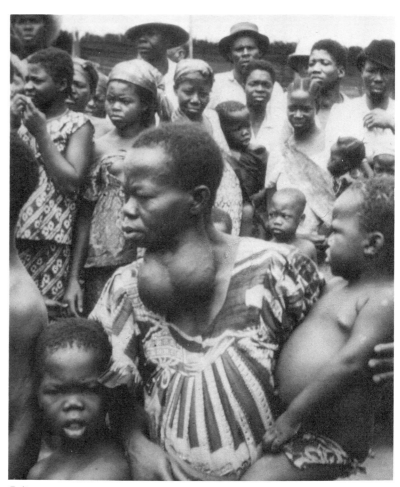

Goiter.

Courtesy of FAO.

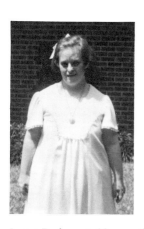

Laura Drake, age 38, a cretin.

abnormalities like those shown in the margin. Much of the mental retardation associated with cretinism can be averted by early diagnosis and treatment.

The iodization of salt in the Plains states eliminated the widespread misery caused by goiter and cretinism in the local people during the 1930s. Once these scourges had disappeared, a new generation of children grew up who never saw the problem and so had no appreciation of its importance. Rejecting iodized salt out of ignorance, they allowed iodine deficiences to creep back into their lives. Hopefully, now, education is keeping them informed of the need to continue using iodized salt.

The recommended intake of iodine for adults is 100 to 150 μg a day, a miniscule amount. Like chlorine, iodine is a deadly poison in large amounts, but traces of it are indispensable to life. The need for iodine is easily met by consuming seafood, vegetables grown in iodine-rich soil, and (in iodine-poor areas) iodized salt. In the United States, you have to read the label to find out whether salt is iodized; in Canada all table salt is iodized.

The RDA for iodine: 150 μg.

Canadian Dietary Standard: 140-150 μg for men, 100-110 μg for women.

Many of the minerals share with the fat-soluble vitamins the characteristics of being toxic in excess. Iodine, in particular, is notorious in this respect. The skull and crossbones on the iodine bottle warns the user that this substance is a deadly poison and that it must be kept out of the reach of children.

Much of the prejudice against iodized salt and fluoridated water arises from the conclusion that these minerals must be avoided altogether because they are dangerous when used in excess. This misconception raises an important point about all the nutrients and many other substances: They may work one way at a high concentration and another at a low concentration. There is not a simple linear relationship between the dose level and its effects.

Let's take three examples—a hormone, a vitamin, and a drug. The hormone insulin, at physiological doses, lowers blood glucose concentrations by facilitating the transport of glucose into cells. At a much higher dose (100 or 1,000 times more than is normally found in the body), insulin seems to *raise* blood glucose concentrations. When the insulin dose exceeds a threshold level, the body responds by secreting an antagonistic hormone (glucagon) in such large amounts that a backlash occurs; the normal effects are reversed.

The distinction being made here is that between normal doses and massive doses of the same compound; that is, the distinction between a pharmacological dose and a physiological dose. At the high level used in some experiments the vitamin acts as a drug, overwhelming body systems that at normal concentrations are impervious to it. It is as if a different compound altogether were acting in the body.

Drugs are similar. The antibiotic streptomycin works by interfering with protein synthesis in growing cells. Since protein synthesis must occur for growth to occur and since bacterial cells grow rapidly, the drug rapidly kills these cells without affecting the more slowly growing cells of the human digestive tract. At a higher dose level, the drug would also kill the cells of the human body.

Thus if you read or hear one report of a certain substance having a certain effect on people, you cannot necessarily conclude that the substance is "good" or "bad." You must ask what dose was used and whether the same effect would have been observed if the substance had been used at a higher or lower concentration. Two corollaries to this observation might be the following:

linear relationship: a relationship between two variables in which one increases in direct proportion to the other.

nonlinear relationships:

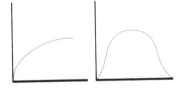

A **variable** is a factor that can vary, such as age, height, dose. One variable may depend on another; for example, the height of the average child depends on age. One variable may be independent of another; for example, the intelligence of a child is independent of height.

physiological dose: a dose equivalent to the amount of a nutrient (or hormone) normally found in the body.

pharmacological dose: a much higher dose, at which unexpected, druglike effects are often observed.

> ☀ CAUTION WHEN YOU READ!
>
> What is a poison at a high concentration may be an essential nutrient at a low concentration. (What is "bad" high may be "good" low.)
>
> What is a needed nutrient at a low concentration may be toxic at a high concentration. (More is not necessarily better.)

Additives proven to cause cancer at any dose are prohibited. See discussion of the Delaney Clause in Highlight 13.

Laboratory scientists responsible for investigating the effects of additives in foods have discovered these facts over the years. They have realized that it is necessary to demonstrate that an additive causes harm *at the dose level we can realistically expect to find in our foods* before concluding that it is dangerous. If the general public understood this, many of the scares that appear from time to time in the media would lose their impact. For many reasons, massive doses of many substances have undesirable effects, but in the real world of real people, effects like these are not so often felt.

In the interest of selling a product or an idea, promoters sometimes appeal to emotions; a most powerful emotion is fear. "This additive causes cancer, and they are using it in bread." When you feel physically threatened you may not stop to reason and seek out the evidence; you may just do what you are told—in this case avoid the grocery store product and buy the promoter's product instead because it makes you feel safe. Yet the additives in foods are extensively tested before they are approved for general use, and the laws that regulate their use are well enforced. Each additive is there for a reason.

The situation is complex and requires an understanding of many subtleties. To be fair, no simple statement can be made about the effects of all the additives. Each must be investigated individually. Still, it should be clear from this Digression that you need not feel fear each time someone claims that our foods are being contaminated with poisons.

A FLAG SIGN OF A SPURIOUS CLAIM IS:

Scare tactics

To balance this discussion, remember that sometimes you are right to be scared. An occasional outbreak of food poisoning does occur, for example, showing that the inspection system failed to catch a hazard in time. Occasionally a food product is removed from the market when a previously unsuspected side effect of one of its constituents becomes evident. The rarity of these occurrences, however, testifies to the overall effectiveness of the consumer protection agencies. Highlight 13 is devoted to some further aspects of consumer protection and additives.

Zinc

Zinc occurs in a small quantity in the body (about 2 g) but is a helper for some 20 enzymes and forms part of the structure of bone. High concentrations of zinc appear in the eye, liver, muscles, and male reproductive organs. It is involved in DNA and protein synthesis, the action of insulin, the immune reactions, and the utilization of vitamin A. With all of these vital roles, it is not surprising that zinc is necessary for the healing of wounds; a deficiency of zinc can seriously retard this process. Zinc is also required for a normal sense of taste. The impressive accumulation of new information about zinc in recent years has led to the conclusion that this mineral is as important as protein in the normal processes of growth and maintenance of body tissues.

A deficiency of zinc was first observed in humans in the 1960s in the Middle East, where a diet high in cereal and low in animal protein was common. Cereal grains, although rich in zinc, contain fibers and phytic acid, which hinder the absorption of zinc. The zinc deficiency was marked by growth retardation, especially of sexual organs, and loss of taste; these symptoms responded to the administration of zinc. Since then, zinc deficiencies have also been identified in schoolchildren in at least one U.S. city (Denver), and are suspected to exist among preschoolers, older people, hospital patients, and other populations whose protein intakes may be limited.

Animal foods are good sources of zinc, with the richest being oysters, herring, milk, and egg yolks. Among plant foods, whole grains are richest in zinc, but it is not so well absorbed from them as from meat. The recommended intake of 9 to 15 mg a day for adults is probably easily met by the diet of the average middle-class person, but deficiency is likely if animal protein is underemphasized. As a rule of thumb, two small servings of animal protein a day will provide sufficient zinc.

Teenagers and young college students who are concerned about acne may learn that zinc has been effective in its treatment in cases where vitamin A has not been.[19] However, self-dosing with zinc can cause

The Egyptian boy in this picture is seventeen years old but is only four feet tall, like a seven-year-old in the United States. His genitalia are like those of a six-year-old. The retardation is ascribed to zinc deficiency.

Reproduced with permission of *Nutrition Today* magazine, P.O. Box 1829, Annapolis, Maryland, 21404, March 1968.

Phytic acid: see p. 417.

The RDA for zinc: 15 mg.

Canadian Dietary Standard: 10 mg for men, 9 mg for women.

[19] G. Michaëlsson, L. Juhlin, and A. Vahlquist, Effects of oral zinc and vitamin A on acne, *Archives of Dermatology* 113 (1977):31-36.

toxicity with severe consequences: muscle incoordination, dizziness, drowsiness, lethargy, renal failure, anemia, and others.[20] As with all the nutrients, and especially the trace minerals, overdoses of zinc are dangerous. The appropriate strategy would be to consult a physician about using zinc for acne.

The "Newer" Trace Elements

Iron, iodine, and zinc are the best known of the trace elements, but six others have recently become better recognized through inclusion in the RDA tables. They deserve a bit of individual attention.

Copper The body contains about 75 to 100 mg of copper, which performs several vital roles. As a catalyst in the formation of hemoglobin, it helps to make red blood cells. It is involved in the manufacture of collagen and helps to maintain the sheath around nerve fibers. Most of what is known about copper is from animal research, which has provided clues about its possible roles in humans. Copper's critical roles seem to have to do with helping iron shift back and forth between its +2 and +3 states. This means that copper is needed in many of the reactions related to respiration and the release of energy.

Estimated safe and adequate daily dietary intake of copper (adults): 2-3 mg.

A copper deficiency is rare but not unknown. It has been seen in children with kwashiorkor and with iron-deficiency anemia and can severely disturb growth and metabolism.

The best food sources of copper include grains, shellfish, organ meats, legumes, dried fruits, fresh fruits, and vegetables—a long list showing that copper is available from almost all foods. About a third of the copper taken in food is absorbed, and the rest is eliminated in the feces.

Manganese The human body contains a tiny 20 mg of manganese, mostly in the bones and glands. Still, this represents billions on billions of molecules. Animal studies suggest that manganese cooperates with many enzymes, helping to facilitate dozens of different metabolic processes. Manganese deficiency in animals deranges many systems, including the bones, reproduction, the nervous system, and fat metabolism.

Estimated safe and adequate daily dietary intake of manganese (adults): 2.5-5.0 mg.

Deficiencies of manganese have not been seen in humans, but toxicity may be severe. Miners who inhale large quantities of manganese dust on the job over prolonged periods show many of the symptoms of a brain disease, with frightening abnormalities of appearance and behavior: "Facial expression is mask-like, the voice

[20]Questions doctors ask . . . , *Nutrition and the MD,* October 1978.

monotonous; and intention-tremor, muscle rigidity and spastic gait appear."[21]

The example of manganese underlines again the fact that toxicity of the trace elements occurs at a level not far above the estimated requirement. Thus it is as important not to overdose as it is to have an adequate intake. The Committee on RDA underscores this point by adding the special warning to its trace-mineral table, not to exceed the upper end of the range of recommended intakes. The National Nutrition Consortium, too, worries that now more trace minerals are known, they will be added to vitamin-mineral pills, making toxic overdoses more likely. The FDA is not permitted to enforce limits on the amounts of trace minerals added to supplements, so this is an area in which the consumer himself has to be careful and aware.[22]

CAUTION:

Beware of supplements containing trace minerals.

It is safer to consume a diet that provides foods from a variety of sources than to try to put together, without causing toxicity, a combination of pills that will meet all your needs.

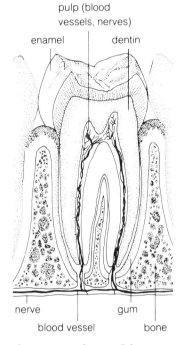

pulp (blood vessels, nerves)

enamel

dentin

nerve

gum

blood vessel

bone

The outer two layers of the teeth, enamel and dentin, are composed largely of calcium compounds, including hydroxyapatite and fluorapatite.

Fluoride   Only a trace of fluoride occurs in the human body, but studies have demonstrated that where diets are high in fluoride, the crystalline deposits in bones and teeth are larger and more perfectly formed. When bones and teeth become calcified, first a crystal called hydroxyapatite is formed from calcium and phosphorus. Then fluoride replaces the hydroxy (OH) portions of the crystal, rendering it insoluble in water and resistant to decay.

Drinking water is the usual source of fluoride, although fish and tea may supply substantial amounts. Where fluoride is lacking in the water supply, the incidence of dental decay is very high. Dental problems can

hydroxyapatite (high-droxy-APP-uh-tite): the major calcium-containing crystal of bones and teeth.

fluorapatite (fleur-APP-uh-tite): the stabilized form of bone and tooth crystal, in which fluoride has replaced the hydroxy groups of hydroxyapatite.

[21]T. K. Li and B. L. Vallee, Trace elements, Section B: The biochemical and nutritional role of trace elements, in *Modern Nutrition in Health and Disease*, 5th ed., eds. R. S. Goodhart and M. E. Shils (Philadelphia: Lea and Febiger, 1973), pp. 372-399.

[22]Annual report from the National Nutrition Consortium (update), *Journal of the American Dietetic Association* 70 (1977):538-540.

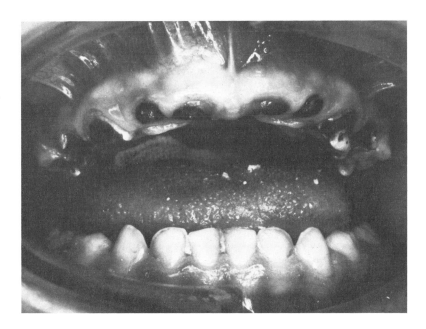

Unprotected teeth decay extensively. This child's teeth were frequently bathed with apple juice.

Courtesy of H. Kaplan and V. P. Rabbach.

cause a multitude of other health problems, affecting the whole body. Fluoridation of community water where needed, to raise its fluoride concentration to one part per million (1 ppm), is thus an important public health measure. Fluoridation of community water is presently practiced in more than 5,000 communities across the United States, and about 100 million people are drinking it (see Figure 1).

fluorosis (fleur-OH-sis): mottling of the tooth enamel; due to ingestion of too much fluoride during tooth development.

osis = too much

In some communities the natural fluoride concentration in water is high, 2 to 8 ppm, and children's teeth develop with mottled enamel. This condition, called fluorosis, is not harmful (in fact, these children's

Figure 1   Fluoridation in the United States.

From D. P. DePaola and M. C. Alfano, Diet and oral health, *Nutrition Today,* May/June 1977, pp. 6-11, 29-32. Courtesy of the authors and of *Nutrition Today* magazine, 703 Giddings Avenue, Suite 6, Annapolis MD 21401, © May/June 1977.

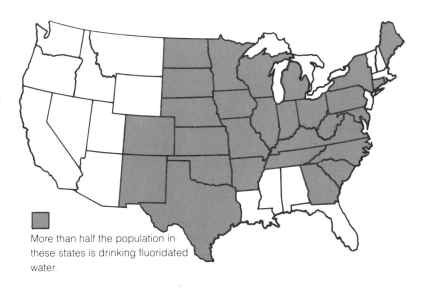

More than half the population in these states is drinking fluoridated water.

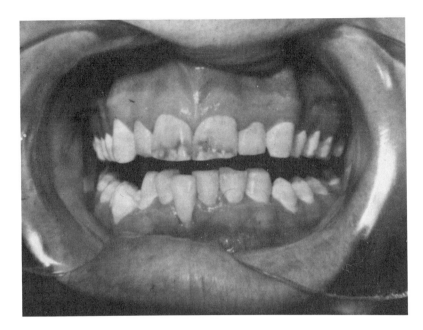

Fluorosis.

Courtesy of H. Kaplan and V. P. Rabbach.

teeth are extraordinarily decay-resistant), but violates the prejudice that teeth "should" be white. Fluorosis does not occur in communities where fluoride is added to the water supply.

Not only does fluoride protect children's teeth from decay, but it makes the bones of older people resistant to the degeneration of osteoporosis. Fluoride is also required for growth in animals and is an essential nutrient for humans; in fact, the continuous presence of fluoride in body fluids is desirable. Luckily, all normal diets include fluoride. It is toxic in excess, but toxicity symptoms appear only after chronic intakes of 20 to 80 mg a day over many years. The amount consumed from fluoridated water is typically about 1 mg a day. Despite its value and the limited possibility of receiving excessive fluoride in the water supply, violent disagreement often surrounds the introduction of fluoride to a community.

People in unfluoridated communities need to find alternative means of protecting their children's teeth. The best temporary solution seems to be to use fluoride toothpastes and/or to have children obtain a topical fluoride application yearly. Fluoride tablets are also available. For infants there are vitamin drops with fluoride in them, but their effectiveness is limited.

Chromium The element chromium has been shown to remedy impaired carbohydrate metabolism in several groups of older people in the United States.[23] Experiments on animals have shown that

Osteoporosis: see p. 414.

Estimated safe and adequate daily dietary intake of fluoride (adults): 1.5-4.0 mg.

topical: a surface application.

[23]K. M. Hambidge, Chromium nutrition in man, *American Journal of Clinical Nutrition* 27 (1974):505-514.

chromium works closely with the hormone insulin, facilitating the uptake of glucose into cells and then the breakdown of that glucose with the release of energy. When chromium is lacking, the effectiveness of insulin is severely impaired, and a diabetes-like condition results.

Like iron, chromium can have two different charges: The $+3$ ion seems to be the most effective in living systems. It also occurs in association with several different complexes in foods. The one that is best absorbed and most active is a small organic compound named the glucose tolerance factor (GTF). This compound has been purified from brewer's yeast and pork kidney and is believed to be present in many other foods. It may be that when more is known the GTF, rather than chromium, will be dubbed an essential nutrient and classed among the vitamins.

Depleted tissue concentrations of chromium in human beings have been linked to adult-onset diabetes and growth failure in children with protein-kcalorie malnutrition.

GTF (glucose tolerance factor): a small organic compound containing chromium.

Estimated safe and adequate daily dietary intake of chromium (adults): 0.05-0.2 mg.

selenium (se-LEEN-ee-um)

Estimated safe and adequate daily dietary intake of selenium (adults): 0.05-0.2 mg.

Selenium   Selenium, too, is a trace element that functions as part of large molecules, especially certain enzymes. It also acts alone as an antioxidant and can substitute for vitamin E in some of that vitamin's antioxidant activities. Deficiencies are unknown, and food sources are abundant.

molybdenum (mo-LIB-duh-num)

Estimated safe and adequate daily dietary intake of molybdenum (adults): 0.15-0.5 mg.

Molybdenum   Finally, molybdenum has also been recognized as an important mineral in human and animal physiology. It functions as a working part of several enzymes, some of which are giant proteins. One, for example, contains two atoms of molybdenum and eight of iron. Deficiencies of molybdenum are unknown in animals and humans, because the amounts needed are miniscule—as little as 0.1 part per million parts of body tissue. Excess molybdenum causes toxicity in animals, but this effect has not been seen in humans.

These six "newer" trace minerals have not been known for long. Others are even more recent newcomers. Nickel is now recognized as important for the health of many body tissues, and deficiencies cause harm to the liver and other organs. Silicon is known to be involved in bone calcification, at least in animals. Tin is necessary for growth in animals and probably in humans. Vanadium, too, is necessary for growth and bone development and also for normal reproduction; human intakes of vanadium may be close to the minimum needed for health. Cobalt is recognized as the mineral in the large vitamin B_{12} molecule; the alternative name for B_{12}, cobalamin, reflects the presence of cobalt. In the future we may discover that many other trace minerals also play key roles: silver, mercury, lead, barium, cadmium. Even arsenic—famous as the poisonous instrument of death in many

The intricate vitamin B_{12} molecule contains one atom of cobalt.

murder mysteries—may turn out to be an essential nutrient in tiny quantities.[24]

As research on the trace minerals continues, many interactions between them are also coming to light. An excess of one may cause a deficiency of another. A slight manganese overload, for example, may aggravate an iron deficiency. And a deficiency of one may open the way for another to cause a toxic reaction. Iron deficiency, for example, makes the body much more susceptible than normal to lead poisoning. The continuous outpouring of new information about the trace minerals is a sign that we have much more to learn.

[24]The "newer" trace elements, *Nutrition and the MD*, November 1975.

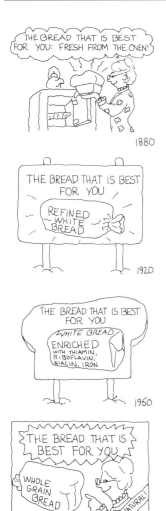

Putting It All Together

One reason the trace minerals are receiving increased attention today is that the food supply has increasingly been refined. As more people turn to refined, processed, and prepared foods and away from the crude products of the farm, they enjoy a saving in convenience and time but suffer a loss of the richness and variety of nutrients that occur in less-pure foods. As a result, deficiencies crop up where the existence of a needed nutrient might never before have been suspected. A case in point is chromium, which is lost when sugar and whole grains are refined. Humans need unbelievably small amounts of chromium, but when it is lacking, severe disorders in body physiology occur. Another case is zinc, which is lost when cereal grains are refined. Deficiencies of zinc are no longer unknown in the United States, and their effects can be devastating. The increasing use by the wealthy nations of highly refined, processed foods concerns nutritionists; they fear that the advice to consume "a balanced diet" no longer is enough to protect people against serious nutritional deficiencies and imbalances.

A "balanced diet," as recommended by the Four Food Group Plan (see Appendix M), consists of (for an adult):

- Milk or milk products, 2 cups
- Meat or meat substitutes, 2 servings
- Fruits and vegetables (1 C-rich, 1 A-rich), 4 servings
- Breads and cereals (whole-grain or enriched), 4 servings

But the optimum diet may need to be more carefully defined than this. Meat substitutes, for example, may lack the iron sorely needed by groups at risk for iron deficiency. Legumes, being rich in iron, and especially soybeans, whose iron is well absorbed, may be acceptable meat substitutes—but other meat substitutes made from other vegetable proteins may be iron-poor. Breads and cereals that have been refined and then enriched may be good sources only of the nutrients on the label; overusing enriched breads may mean risking deficiencies of chromium, zinc, and other minerals. In the case of two other nutrients—iodine and fluorine—food sources are so unreliable in some geographical locations that the definition of an adequate diet must be expanded to include iodized salt and fluoridated water or fluoride supplements.

A diagram at the end of Chapter 11 demonstrated that foods from all six exchange groups are necessary for an adequate diet. With the qualifications made here, that diagram has to be modified. If you are curious about the adequacy of your diet, you might ask yourself if you have all your nutrient bases covered by using the following diagram as a checklist:

☑

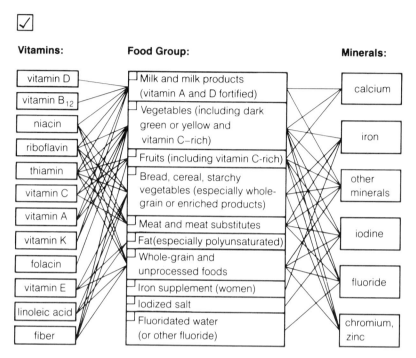

Vitamins:

vitamin D

vitamin B$_{12}$

niacin

riboflavin

thiamin

vitamin C

vitamin A

vitamin K

folacin

vitamin E

linoleic acid

fiber

Food Group:

Milk and milk products (vitamin A and D fortified)

Vegetables (including dark green or yellow and vitamin C–rich)

Fruits (including vitamin C-rich)

Bread, cereal, starchy vegetables (especially whole-grain or enriched products)

Meat and meat substitutes

Fat (especially polyunsaturated)

Whole-grain and unprocessed foods

Iron supplement (women)

Iodized salt

Fluoridated water (or other fluoride)

Minerals:

calcium

iron

other minerals

iodine

fluoride

chromium, zinc

Summing Up

Iron is found principally in the red blood cells, where it comprises part of the oxygen-carrier protein hemoglobin. When red blood cells die and are dismantled in the liver, the iron is retrieved and transported by iron-carrier proteins back to bone marrow, where new red blood cells are synthesized. There is no route of excretion for iron; losses are small except when blood is lost, as in menstruation or hemorrhage. Thus women's needs for iron are greater than men's (14 to 18 mg a day for women, 10 mg for men).

Iron-deficiency anemia, one of the world's most widespread malnutrition problems, is most common in women and children; it causes weakness, fatigue, headaches, and pallor. Food sources of iron for women must be chosen carefully if even two-thirds of the recommended intake is to be met within a kcalorie allowance that is not excessive. The enrichment of breads and cereals somewhat improves women's iron intakes, but iron enrichment or fortification of other foods may produce iron overload in men. Addition of an iron supplement to the diet may be advisable for some women.

Foods relatively rich in iron include (in roughly descending order) liver and other organ meats, soybeans, dried beans and legumes, red meats, and dark-green vegetables. Other significant contributors are enriched breads and cereals, eggs, and dried fruits such as raisins and prunes. Iron is better absorbed from meats and soybeans than from other foods, and its absorption is enhanced by eating vitamin C at the same meal. Milk and milk products are notable for their lack of iron.

Zinc is necessary for normal development, including sexual development, and for wound healing and the sense of taste. Deficiencies of zinc have been observed in some children in the United States as well as in children in the Middle East. Diets in the Middle East are high in whole-grain cereals, which contain absorption-inhibiting fiber and phytic acid.

Iodine forms part of the thyroid hormone; deficiency causes goiter (enlargement of the thyroid gland), slowed metabolism, and stunted growth and mental retardation in children. Addition of iodine to salt in **minute quantities protects against deficiency, provided iodized salt is used. Education must accompany this measure to make it effective.**

Copper is important for red blood cell formation, collagen synthesis, and central nervous system function. Manganese aids many body enzymes, but its safe range is narrow, with toxicity causing a severe brain-disease syndrome in humans.

The fluoride ion combines with calcium and phosphorus to stabilize the crystalline structure of bones and teeth against resorption or decay. In communities where the water contains fluoride, dental caries and osteoporosis are less prevalent than in communities where the water supply is low in fluoride.

Chromium, as part of the glucose tolerance factor, works with insulin in promoting glucose uptake into cells and normal carbohydrate metabolism. Chromium deficiency is now believed to have a significant incidence among older people and to be responsible for some cases of maturity-onset diabetes; it may cause growth failure in children as well.

Other trace minerals include selenium, important as an antioxidant and in fat metabolism, and molybdenum, a part of several enzyme systems. Many other trace minerals are under investigation.

In light of the increased use of refined, highly processed foods by the wealthy nations, a balanced diet (as outlined by the Four Food Group Plan) may not provide adequacy for all the trace minerals. Some women may need iron supplements, and it may be desirable as well to use whole-grain rather than refined (even enriched) products for their chromium and zinc, to use iodized salt in iodine-poor areas, and to use fluoride supplements in unfluoridated communities.

To Explore Further

A technical reference which tells how to estimate the amount of iron you actually get from your foods, taking the vitamin C and meat effects into consideration, is:

● Monsen, R. R., Hallberg, L., Layrisse, M., Hegsted, D. M., Cook, J. D., Mentz, W., and Finch, C.A. Estimation of available dietary iron. *American Journal of Clinical Nutrition* 31 (1978):134-141.

The superenrichment debate was covered in a lively issue of *Nutrition Today*, July/August 1977. A more general debate over the question whether to fortify foods or to educate consumers about diet appears in:

● T. P. LaBuza, ed., *The Nutrition Crisis: A Reader.* St. Paul: West, 1975, pp. 129-145.

For an insight into the subtle effects of early iron deficiency, read:

● Leibel, R. L. Behavioral and biochemical correlates of iron deficiency: A review. *Journal of the American Dietetic Association* 71 (1977):399-404.

On diet and oral health, an excellent review is:

● DePaola, D. P., and Alfano, M. C. Diet and oral health. *Nutrition Today*, May/June 1977, pp. 6-11, 29-32.

A well researched review of the health benefits of fluoridation is:

● Richmond, V. L. Health effects associated with water fluoridation. *Journal of Nutrition Education* 11 (April-June 1979):62-64.

This and the letters to the editor, together with the author's response that appeared in the October-December issue of the *Journal* (pp. 162-168) are highly recommended reading.

A teaching aid with slides, *Iron*, by C. A. Finch, can be ordered from the Nutrition Today Society (address in Appendix J).

A cassette tape, *Trace Elements in Nutrition* by D. Fletcher (CAM 2-75), can be ordered from the American Dietetic Association (address in Appendix J). Also available is *Iron Nutrition—An Update* by H. S. White (CAM 9-77).

Additional information on all the trace elements is presented in the general references recommended in Appendix J.

Food Additives

If you are curious to know what substances are in the foods you eat and what they do, you can't help wondering about additives. Reading labels is all very well (Highlight 12), but it takes you only so far. The most a label tells you about additives is what they do to the foods they are in — but what do they do to *you?* This question may especially concern you if you have heard some of the stories that implicate additives in the causation of cancer, birth defects, and other frightening conditions.

For example: Cyclamate, a widely used artificial sweetener, was banned from use in 1969 because of some tests suggesting that it could cause cancer. Since then five other substances have been banned for similar reasons: red dye #2, violet #1, carbon black, diethylpyrocarbonate, and salts of cobalt (used in beer).

All substances are poison. The right dose differentiates a poison and a remedy.

PARACELSUS

Two others, saccharin and nitrite, have also been banned, but the bans have been suspended — a situation some consumers find confusing and troubling. And some 20 other substances have been challenged as unsafe, including salt, sugar, xylitol, caffeine, MSG (monosodium glutamate), and all synthetic colors and flavors.[1] People wonder what they might be consuming now that will be banned in the future, and what harm it may be doing.

A public paranoia has thus developed that has destroyed many consumers' confidence in the safety of the food supply. This is doubly ironic. The public's mistrust has stemmed from the presence in foods of substances that were put there to make the foods safer, more attractive, or in other ways beneficial to consumers. And the banning of some of these substances has resulted from the requirement that they be tested, that the tests be closely monitored, and that the whole process be open to public view.

[1] M. Foster, How safe are our foods?, *Nutrition Reviews/Supplement*, January 1982, pp. 28-34.

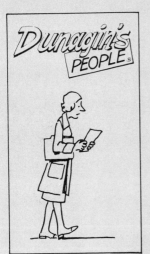
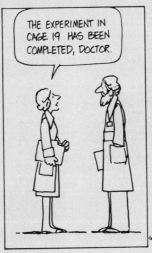
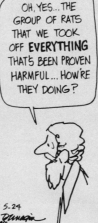
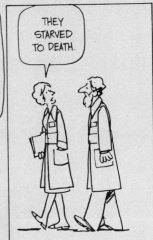

DUNAGIN'S PEOPLE by Ralph Dunagin ©1981 Field Enterprises, Inc.   Courtesy of Field Newspaper Syndicate.

Before getting into some of the down-to-earth facts about additives, it is important to make a distinction and to offer a perspective. Harmful substances do occur in foods. Sometimes they are even put there intentionally, by people who haven't realized the potential harm they may cause. But a greater danger by far comes from harmful substances that get into foods accidentally by way of contamination with disease-causing microorganisms or with unwanted substances from packaging or processing materials or environmental pollution. In other words, the term *additive* is too loose. We should distinguish between *intentional additives*, put there on purpose after a rational thinking process, and *incidental* or *indirect additives*, which find their way into foods by accident.

This Highlight is about intentional additives, and comes to a not very alarming conclusion. The next Highlight is about contamination of foods and shows where some serious hazards may exist. To get a balanced picture of the possible hazards in the food supply, you should really read them both.

Terminology   To begin at the beginning, then, intentional food additives are substances put into foods to give them some desirable characteristic: color, flavor, texture,

stability, or resistance to spoilage. Some additives are nutrients added to foods to increase their nutritional value, such as vitamin C added to fruit drinks or potassium iodide added to salt. The most common ones, roughly in order of the quantities used, are listed in the accompanying miniglossary. In addition, there are numerous additives used in still smaller quantities for miscellaneous other purposes.

Regulations Governing Additives   The agency charged with the responsibility of deciding what additives shall be in foods is the Food and Drug Administration (FDA). FDA's authority over additives hinges primarily on their safety. The procedure a manufacturer has to go through to get permission to put a new additive in food puts the burden on him to prove the additive is safe, and may take several years. First he has to test it chemically to satisfy the FDA that:

● it is effective (it does what it is supposed to do)

● it can be detected and measured in the final food product

Then he has to feed it in large doses to animals and prove that:

● it is safe (it causes no cancer, birth defects, or other injury)

The manufacturer can't do just any animal tests. The doses are specified; two kinds of animals (usually rodents and dogs) must be used; and the time periods must be long. Finally, the manufacturer must submit all his test results to FDA.[2]

FDA responds to the manufacturer's petition by announcing a public hearing. Consumers are invited to participate at these hearings, where experts present testimony for and against the acceptance of the additive for the proposed uses. Thus the consumer's rights and responsibilities are written into the provisions for deeming additives safe.

If FDA approves the additive's use, that doesn't mean the manufacturer can add it in any amount to any food. On the contrary: FDA writes a regulation establishing limits for the use of the additive. The regulation states in what amounts, and in what foods, the additive may be used. No additives are permanently approved; all are periodically reviewed.

Many substances were exempted from complying with this procedure at the time the law came into being, because there were no known hazards in their use. These substances, some 700 in all,

[2] P. Lehman, More than you ever thought you would know about food additives, *FDA Consumer*, April 1979 (reprint).

Miniglossary

additive: a chemical substance added to food, either intentionally, in processing, or incidentally (as an accident such as contamination from the environment or packaging material). See *intentional food additive; incidental food additive.*

botulism (BOTT-you-lism): a form of food poisoning caused by **botulinum toxin**, a toxin produced by bacteria that grow in meat.

carcinogen (car-SIN-oh-jen): a cancer-causing agent.

carcinos = cancer
gennan = to produce

Delaney Clause: a clause in the Food Additive Amendment to the Food, Drug, and Cosmetic Act that states that no substance shall be added to foods that is known to cause cancer in animals or humans at any dose level, no matter how small.

GRAS (Generally Recognized as Safe) list: a list of food additives, established by the Food and Drug Administration (FDA), that had long been in use and were believed safe. The list is subject to revision as new facts become known.

hazard: state of danger; used to refer to any circumstance in which toxicity is possible under normal conditions of use. See also *toxicity.*

incidental additive: see *indirect additive.*

indirect additive: an additive unintentionally added to a food by an accident of contamination such as packaging materials or chemicals used during processing.

intentional food additive: an additive intentionally added to food, such as nutrients or colors.

margin of safety: as used when speaking of food additives, a zone between the concentration normally used and that at which a hazard exists. For common table salt, for example, the margin of safety is 1/5 (five times the concentration normally used would be hazardous).

nitrite: a salt added to food to prevent botulism.

nitrosamine (nigh-TROHS-uh-meen): a derivative of nitrite that can be formed in the stomach when nitrite combines with an amine; a carcinogen.

paranoia (para-NOY-uh): excessive or irrational suspiciousness and distrustfulness; unjustified fear.

para = beyond
nous = mind

toxicity: the ability of a substance to be toxic (cause harmful effects). All substances are toxic if high enough concentrations are used. See also *hazard.*

Miniglossary of Additives

Emulsifiers, stabilizers, thickeners: to give texture, smoothness, or other desired consistencies.

Nutrients: to improve nutritive value.

Flavoring agents: to add or enhance flavor.

Leavening (neutralizing) agents: to control acidity or alkalinity.

Preservatives, antioxidants, sequestrants, antimyotic agents: to prevent spoilage, rancidity of fats, and microbial growth.

Coloring agents: to increase acceptability and attractiveness.

Bleaches: to whiten foods such as flour and cheese and to speed up the maturing of cheese.

Humectants, anticaking agents: to retain moisture in some foods and to keep others (such as salts and powders) free-flowing.

were put on what is known as the GRAS list (Generally Recognized as Safe). However, any time substantial scientific evidence or public outcry has questionned the safety of any of the substances on the GRAS list, a special reevaluation has been made. Meanwhile, the entire GRAS list has been systematically and intensively reevaluated, and all substances about which any legitimate question was raised have been removed or reclassified. A set of 2,100 flavoring agents is similarly being reviewed, as well as some 200 coloring agents.[3]

One of the criteria an additive must meet to be placed on the GRAS list is that it must not have been found to be a carcinogen (a cancer-causing agent) in any test on animals or humans. The Delaney Clause (a part of the law on additives) is uncompromising in addressing carcinogens in food and drugs and has been under fire in recent years for being too strict. This brings us to the questions of what laws are appropriate in regulating food additives, and what changes should be made.

The Delaney Clause is criticized because it does not allow for the different effects on the body of varying dose levels of an additive. For example, when the artificial sweetener cyclamate was banned in 1969, it was estimated that a human would

[3]Lehman, 1979.

have to drink, each day, at least 138 12-ounce bottles of soft drinks containing cyclamates to ingest an amount of cyclamate comparable to the quantity given animals in the tests that caused the ban.[4] The FDA was criticized for banning the use of cyclamates, but under the law it had no alternative. The Delaney Clause does not give FDA the right to make a judgment on dose levels of carcinogens or on the applicability of animal research to humans or even on the reproducibility of an experiment.

At present, a similar controversy centers on saccharin. Some animal tests have suggested that saccharin may be a weak carcinogen; thus it has had to be automatically banned. But while consumers were grateful in 1969 when cyclamate was banned, they were upset and resentful in 1977 at the proposed banning of saccharin, the only familiar artificial sweetener remaining on the market. To satisfy both the law and the consumers, Congress passed the ban and then suspended it; as of 1983 saccharin was still being sold, but with a warning label: "Use of this product may be hazardous to your health. This product contains saccharin which has been determined to cause cancer in laboratory animals."

[4]R. D. Middlekauf, Legalities concerning food additives, *Food Technology* 28 (May 1974):42-49.

Nitrites, which are added to smoked meats such as hot dogs and cold cuts, have suffered a similar fate. A test on rats, published in 1978, suggested they caused cancer, and again an automatic ban had to be invoked. But the case of nitrites had a new twist: They are not added to meats "just" for flavor or eye appeal. They prevent bacterial spoilage, and in particular, the growth of the deadly bacterial species that produces botulinum toxin, the most potent biological poison known. An amount as tiny as a single crystal of salt can kill a person within an hour, and in survivors, troublesome after-effects linger for months. If nitrites were banned, the risk to users of these products would be intolerable; no other preservative was known that could do nitrite's job; and the only alternative seemed to be to take all smoked meats off the market.

The ban on nitrite was therefore suspended, pending further investigation. Not long after, the experiment connecting nitrites to cancer was heavily criticized, and its validity is doubtful. The risk to users of products containing nitrites is probably slight in comparison to other risks (see box, "Nitrates, Nitrites, Nitrosamines"), but consumers have been shaken by the alarms raised, and are more inclined to be mistrustful of all additives as a result.

Another additive, which had much of the public

Nitrates, Nitrites, Nitrosamines

Q: What are the risks associated with these additives?

A: Wait a minute. You've asked the question wrong. These compounds aren't additives. Nitrates and nitrites are all salts that contain the nitrate or nitrite ions. Nitrosamines are compounds in which the nitrite ion has combined with an amine. All of these compounds occur naturally in the environment; nitrates are used as fertilizer and are present in the water supply, and nitrites are present in high concentrations in many vegetables. But it's true that nitrates and nitrites are *used* as additives.

Q: OK, so what are the risks associated with their use?

A: Well, again, whether they are added to food or present there naturally, or present in drinking water, the risks are the same. There is a chance that nitrates may cause cancer (we don't know for sure yet), and nitrosamines are known to do so. The main problem is that nitrates and nitrites can both be converted to nitrosamines during cooking, or in the human stomach.

Q: Nitrosamines *do* cause cancer, you say. Are nitrosamines ever added to foods?

A: No, never.

Q: How serious is the risk of cancer from nitrates and nitrites added to food?

A: That's a hard question to answer. It is not known for sure whether nitrosamines do form in the stomach when you eat nitrates and nitrites in foods. And it's not known whether they cause cancer in humans. They do, in animals.

Q: Can I avoid using nitrites if I want to?

A: Not very easily. FDA has estimated that they are present in 7 percent of our food supply. You could avoid using all products to which they are added — bacon, hot dogs, ham, processed poultry, fish, and meat — but even if you became a strict vegetarian, you'd get them in the vegetables you eat.

Q: How do the amounts in vegetables compare with those in meats?

---

alarmed during the late 1970s, was Yellow No. 5 (tartrazine), a color additive that in occasional rare instances causes an allergic reaction in people who are also allergic to aspirin. Tartrazine was for a while blamed for causing many (some people said most) cases of hyperactivity in children, and a special diet (the "Feingold" diet), composed entirely of additive-free foods, was recommended for these children. By 1980 it was clear that the majority of cases of hyperactivity are not caused by tartrazine or other additives, but legislation is now in force requiring that tartrazine must be mentioned on all labels of foods that contain it so that consumers can avoid it if they wish.

The Public's Fears about Additives   Another reason for the public's sometimes unreasonable fear of additives is a generalized fear of anything "chemical" or "synthetic." Many deadly

A: Well, bacon is permitted to have 120 parts per million (ppm) of nitrite as sold in the store. Other meats can have 200 ppm, but most have less than 50 ppm. Smoked fish can have 500 ppm nitrate and 200 ppm nitrite. Some vegetables contain up to 3,000 ppm nitrates, and even drinking water sometimes has several hundred ppm.

Q: So I have to avoid all processed meats and — oh, dear, which vegetables must I exclude from my diet?

A: Wait a minute, I didn't suggest you do any such thing. Remember, every move you make in life involves some risk, and every food can be toxic if taken in excess. I suggest you adopt a strategy of minimizing the risks.

Q: How can I minimize the risks?

A: Well, first of all, remember: Variety ensures dilution. I mean, whenever you switch from food to food, you are diluting whatever's in one food with what's in the other. So eat *some* processed meats, but don't eat them all the time. And don't give up any vegetables; they're all good; you need them in your diet for many positive reasons.

Q: OK, the meat I'll choose to have occasionally is bacon; that's my favorite. How can I minimize the risks associated with bacon?

A: Good question. There are at least three things you can do. First, always consume a vitamin C source at the same meals, like orange juice or lettuce and tomatoes. Vitamin C is thought to prevent the formation of nitrosamines in the stomach. Second, don't fry the bacon too crispy. When it starts to burn, that's when the nitrosamines may be being formed. And third, don't re-use the bacon fat, because that's where they tend to be concentrated.

Q: Well, thanks for all the answers. I feel a little better informed. I wish I could say I feel reassured, too, but I don't. In fact I feel nervous about everything I eat these days.

A: I know how you feel. It takes a while to get comfortable with the idea of living with a certain amount of risk. I hope it won't be long before you feel OK about it.

poisons are "natural" substances found in foods or produced by living organisms (consider mushrooms). Ironically, contrary to the public's suspicions, it is the processing of food and the introduction of additives that removes toxic substances, prevents the growth of dangerous microorganisms, and makes the food safe for our use. Foods are made of chemicals anyway, as the humorous display of Figure 1 demonstrates. It has been argued that the food industry has not only the right but also the responsibility to educate the public about the safety of food additives. From this point of view, a food packager who advertises "no additives is not doing the public a favor. By implying that there is something wrong with additives, he is exploiting the public's emotionalism rather than helping educate.[5]

[5] M. J. Sheridan and E. M. Whelan, "Consumerism" and the American food industry, *ACSH News and Views* 1 (April 1980):1, 14-15.

People who sell foods, like people who sell anything, may be inclined to take advantage of their customers in unfair ways, as we have often said before. A realistic (not necessarily cynical) view of this tendency helps protect you, the consumer, from being "taken." Take a close look, sometime, at the foods that claim to contain "NO ADDITIVES, NO PRESERVATIVES." Are they beneficial, nutritious foods? How do they resist spoilage — or do they? Do they contain large amounts of salt? (Salt is really an additive too, but not commonly thought of as one. In fact it is a very effective preservative — but is it preferable to other preservatives in terms of its effects on human health?) What is the motivation behind the claim on the label? Is the intention to reveal to you the unadorned truth about the contents of the package? Or is it trying to imply a health-promoting property that is really not unique to the food in the package — with or without additives?

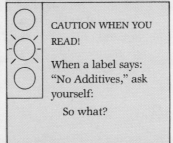

CAUTION WHEN YOU READ!

When a label says: "No Additives," ask yourself:
    So what?

While thinking about motivation, you might ask yourself another question, too. Would a manufacturer put an additive in his food that he knew would harm human health? Even if he was an uncaring, unscrupulous, selfish individual, would he dare? In light of all the rules and safeguards surrounding additives, wouldn't he surely get caught and have to go to punitively great expense in removing the additive, losing sales, and so forth? Thinking purely selfishly, wouldn't it be in his best interest to do his best to make sure no harmful substances get into the food he sells?

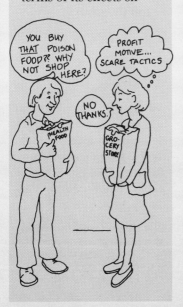

Another reason why the public has become scared about what's in foods is — ironically — because chemists are so much better at their jobs than they used to be, and the analytical techniques they use are so much more powerful than they were in the past. Where once they would say there were no detectable levels of a substance in food "down to one part per million," now they have ways of detecting the same substance at one part per billion. This makes it seem as if new substances are appearing in our foods while in fact they may have been there all the time but are only now being seen. And the concentrations are so extremely low as to be insignificant. It is ironic, too, that the removal of substances from the GRAS list, which has improved the safety of those permitted, so alarmed the public that the effect seems to have been to make them mistrustful of the entire process. But the main reason for exaggerated alarm about additives is the public's failure to understand the difference between toxicity and hazard.

Toxicity versus Hazard
Toxicity — the capacity of a chemical substance to harm living organisms — is a general property of matter; hazard is the capacity of a chemical to produce injury under conditions of use. All substances are potentially

Toast & Coffee Cake
Gluten
Amino acids
Amylose
Starches
Dextrins
Sucrose
Pentosans
Hexosans
Triglycerides
Monoglycerides and
  diglycerides
Sodium chloride
Phosphorus
Calcium
Iron
Thiamin (vitamin B_1)
Riboflavin (vitamin B_2)
Niacin
Pantothenic acid
Vitamin D
Methyl ethyl ketone
Acetic acid
Propionic acid
Butyric acid
Valeric acid
Caproic acid
Acetone
Diacetyl
Maltol
Ethyl acetate
Ethyl lactate

Scrambled Eggs
Ovalbumin
Conalbumin
Ovomucoid
Mucin
Globulins
Amino acids
Lipovitellin
Livetin
Cholesterol

Lecithin
Choline
Lipids (fats)
Fatty acids
Lutein
Zeaxanthine
Vitamin A
Biotin
Pantothenic acid
Riboflavin (vitamin B_2)
Thiamin (vitamin B_1)
Niacin
Pyridoxine (vitamin B_6)
Folic acid (folacin)
Cyanocobalamin
  (vitamin B_{12})
Sodium chloride
Iron
Calcium
Phosphorus

Chilled Cantaloupe
Starches
Cellulose
Pectin
Fructose
Sucrose
Glucose
Malic acid
Citric acid
Succinic acid
Anisyl propionate
Amyl acetate
Ascorbic acid (vitamin C)
B-carotene (vitamin A)
Riboflavin (vitamin B_2)
Thiamin (vitamin B_1)
Niacin
Phosphorus
Potassium

Coffee
Caffeine

Methanol
Ethanol
Butanol
Methylbutanol
Acetaldehyde
Methyl formate
Dimethyl sulfide
Propionaldehyde
Pyridine
Acetic acid
Furfural
Furfuryl alcohol
Acetone
Methyl acetate
Furan
Methylfuran
Diacetyl
Isoprene
Guaiacol
Hydrogen sulfide

Tea
Caffeine
Tannin
Butanol
Isoamyl alcohol
Hexanol
Phenyl ethyl alcohol
Benzyl alcohol
Geraniol
Quercetin
3-galloyl epicatechin
3-galloyl epigallocatechin

Sugar-Cured Ham
Myosin
Actomyosin
Myoglobin
Collagen
Elastin
Amino acids
Creatine
Lipids (fats)

Linoleic acid
Oleic acid
Lecithin
Cholesterol
Sucrose
Glucose
Pyroligneous acid
Phosphorus
Thiamin (vitamin B_1)
Riboflavin (vitamin B_2)
Niacin
Cyanocobalamin
  (vitamin B_{12})
Pyridoxine (vitamin B_6)
Sodium chloride
Iron
Magnesium
Potassium

Cinnamon Apple Chips
Pectin
Hemicellulose
Starches
Sucrose
Glucose
Fructose
Malic acid
Lactic acid
Citric acid
Succinic acid
Ascorbic acid (vitamin C)
B-carotene (vitamin A)
Cinnamyl alcohol
Cinnamic aldehyde
Potassium
Phosphorus
Acetaldehyde
Amyl formate
Amyl acetate
Amyl caproate
Geraniol

Good Morning

Your "Breakfast Chemicals"

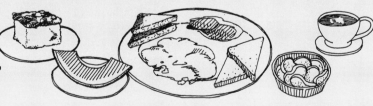

Figure 1. *These chemicals are found naturally in foods. There are no additives present! The chemical listings are not necessarily complete.*

Kindly supplied by the Manufacturing Chemists' Association.

toxic, but are hazardous only if consumed in sufficiently large quantities."[6]

People often fail to understand the distinction between toxicity and hazard, and so become overly afraid of dangers that are real, but small enough to ignore. For example: if you eat a bucketful of sand, it can kill you. (Anything — even water — is toxic if you take enough of it.) But this doesn't mean you should be afraid to eat a sandwich at the beach because it might have one grain of sand in it. In contrast, though, you had *better* be afraid to eat spoiled meat that might contain botulinum toxin. The question to ask is, "Is it dangerous like sand or water — where there's no chance I'll get enough to hurt me? Or is it dangerous like botulinum toxin — where the amount I actually consume can hurt me?" Food additives, if they are dangerous at all, are dangerous like water or sand. They are allowed in foods only with a wide margin of safety.

This distinction is readily accepted in other areas — such as air travel: "We fly in airplanes because they are "safe," but 'safe' is defined by the low number of deaths per million passenger miles, not the total absence of risk."[7] When chemicals are involved, however, there seems to be an added scare factor.

To see food additives in the correct perspective, then, it is necessary to understand the concept of margin of safety. Most additives that involve risk are allowed in foods only at levels 100 times below those at which the risk is still known to be zero; their margin of safety is 1/100. Experiments to determine the extent of risk involve feeding test animals the substance at different concentrations throughout their lifetimes. The additive is then permitted in foods at 1/100 the level that can be fed under these conditions without causing any harmful effect whatever. In many foods, naturally occurring substances appear at levels such that the margin of safety is closer to 1/10. Even nutrients, as you have seen, involve risks at high dosage levels. The margin of safety for vitamins A and D is 1/25 to 1/40; it may be less than 1/10 in infants.[8] For some trace elements, it is about 1/5. Common table salt is consumed daily by people in amounts only three to five times less than those that cause serious toxicity.[9]

The margin of safety concept also applies to nutrients when they are used as additives. Iodine has been added to salt to prevent iodine deficiency, but it has had to be added with care because it is a deadly poison in excess. Similarly, iron has been added to refined bread and other grains (enrichment), and has doubtless helped prevent many cases of iron-deficiency in women and children who are prone to that disease. But the addition of too much iron could put men (who usually have enough) at risk for iron overload. The margin of safety for iron, too, is not so generous, and the upper limit has to be remembered. The moral of these stories is that things have to be looked at in their contexts.

All of the additives just named are in foods for a reason, of course. They offer benefits, beside which the risks are deemed small enough to ignore, or worth taking. When the benefit to be gained from an additive is less, as in the case of color additives that "only" enhance the appearance of foods but do not improve their health value or safety, then the risks may be deemed not worth taking. Only 31 of a possible 200 color additives are now

[6]F. M. Strong, Toxicants occurring naturally in foods, in *Nutrition Reviews' Present Knowledge in Nutrition*, 4th ed. (Washington, D.C.: Nutrition Foundation, 1976), pp. 516-527.

[7]A. M. Schmidt, Food and drug law: A 200-year perspective, *Nutrition Today*, 10 (4) (1975):29-32.

[8]J. M. Coon, Natural food toxicants: A perspective, in *Nutrition Reviews' Present Knowledge*, 1976, pp. 528-546.

[9]Strong, 1976.

approved for use by FDA.

It is also the manufacturers' responsibility not to use more of an additive than they have to, to get the needed effect. The case of nitrites, where higher dose levels could conceivably be associated with a risk, is an obvious example. Additives should also *not* be used:

- to disguise faulty or inferior products
- to deceive the consumer
- where they significantly destroy nutrients
- where their effects can be achieved by economical, sound manufacturing processes[10]

Additives in Perspective
All that has been said so far has been reassuring. The use of additives in the food supply seems to be justified, in many cases, by the benefits we gain from them; the risks associated with their use are small. All intentional additives are, and will doubtless continue to be, closely regulated and monitored. Furthermore, in many cases, combinations of additives are no more harmful than additives used singly, and may even be beneficial. Giving further reassurance, the FAO/WHO Expert Committee on Food Additives has concluded that "an increase in the number of food additives on a permitted list does

not imply an over-all increase in the [total amount of] additives used; the different additives are largely used as alternatives . . . there is *less* likelihood of long exposure, or of high or cumulative dose levels being attained if a wide range of substances is available for use" (emphasis ours).[11]

Finally, it should be noted that the safety of food additives is not first, or even third, on FDA's list of priority concerns; it is sixth. In order of concern, hazards within the FDA's areas of responsibility are:

- food-borne infection, which is increasing because of large-scale operations and multiple transfers involving handling
- nutrition, which requires close attention as more and more artificially constituted foods appear on the market
- environmental contaminants, which are increasing yearly in number and concentration and whose consequences are difficult to foresee and forestall
- naturally occurring toxicants in foods, which occur randomly in arbitrary levels and constitute a hazard whenever people turn to consuming single foods either by choice (fad diets) or by necessity (famine)
- pesticide residues
- intentional food additives, listed last "because so much is known about them, and all

are now, and surely will continue to be, well regulated."[12]

The top item on this list is food poisoning, a real and frequent hazard to people who consume food that has been contaminated by toxic microorganisms during processing, packaging, transport, storage, or preparation in the home.

Deaths from food-borne infection can occur whenever batches of contaminated foods escape detection and are distributed. Close monitoring of processing, preparation, and distribution of food is extraordinarily effective, but individual consumers must be vigilant and knowledgeable in order to protect themselves against occasional hazards. Batch numbering makes it possible to recall all food items from a contaminated batch through public announcements on TV and radio. In the kitchen, the consumer must obey the rules of proper preparation and storage of foods to avoid the dangers of food poisoning (see To Explore Further).

Second on the above list is nutrition, the subject to which this entire book is addressed; third is contamination, the subject of Highlight 14. Fourth is naturally occurring toxicants in foods, a much more serious and real hazard than most consumers realize. This deserves a paragraph of attention.

Many commonly used

[10]The use of chemicals in food production, processing, storage and distribution, *Nutrition Reviews* 31 (1973):191-198.

[11]Coon, 1976.

[12]Schmidt, 1975.

plants and plant products contain naturally occurring toxicants. Mushrooms were mentioned earlier as a familiar example; but did you know of these others? A number of common foods have been observed to cause genuine toxic effects in people who consume them:

● Cabbage, mustard, and other plants contain goitrogens, which can enlarge the thyroid gland.

● Potatoes contain solanine, a powerful inhibitor of nerve impulses; the margin of safety, assuming ordinary consumption of potatoes, is 1/10.

● Spinach and rhubarb contain oxalates, tolerable as usually consumed; but one normal serving of rhubarb contains 1/5 the toxic dose for humans.[13]

● Honey can be a host to the botulinum organism just described, and can accumulate enough toxin to kill an infant.[14]

There are 700 other examples of plants that — as used — have caused serious illnesses or deaths in the Western hemisphere.[15] At the same time, there has been no case of a death or illness caused by an additive as used at legally permitted levels in food.[16] A well known environmental scientist has said, "One can predict that if the standards used to test manmade chemicals were applied to 'natural' foods, fully half of the human food supply would have to be banned."[17]

The fifth item on the list of FDA's hazards is pesticide residues, another issue touched on in the next Highlight, and sometimes a serious problem. In view of all this, the subject of this Highlight, FDA's problem number 6, would seem to have been given enough space here.

In summary, then, the ideas presented here have been:

● All foods are composed of chemicals, even if they have no additives in them.

● Additives that might be toxic do not constitute a hazard at the concentrations used.

● Additives are allowed in foods only because they con-fer a benefit in comparison to which the risk, if any, is insignificant.

● The presence of several additives in foods is not more hazardous than the presence of any one of them.

● If rank-ordered among the problems related to the food supply, the risk from additives falls last below a number of more significant factors.

People who are concerned about the levels of various additives and pollutants in the food supply would be well advised to eat as wide a variety of foods as possible so as to dilute the amount of any one substance. "The wider the variety of food intake, the greater the number of different chemical substances consumed, and the less is the chance that any one chemical will reach a hazardous level in the diet."[18]

Finally, it is important to remind you that this discussion has not dealt with the pollutants and contaminants in foods. Highlight 14 continues with that discussion.

To Explore Further

A leaflet is available free from the American Medical Association to help you learn to prepare foods safely in your kitchen:

● Foodborne illness: The consumer's role in its prevention. Chicago: American Medical Association, 1976. The AMA's address is in Appendix J.

[13]Middlekauf, 1974.

[14]I. B. Vyhmeister, What about honey? *Life and Health*, August 1980, pp. 5-7; R. W. Miller, Honey: Making sure it's pure, *FDA Consumer* 13 (September 1979):12-13.

[15]A. Brynjolfsson, Food irradiation and nutrition, *Professional Nutritionist*, Fall 1979, pp. 7-10.

[16]M. W. Pariza, Food safety from the eye of a hurricane, *Professional Nutritionist*, Fall 1979, pp. 11-14.

[17]R. Dubos, The intellectual basis of nutrition science and practice, an article presented at the NIH conference on the Biomedical and Behavioral Basis of Clinical Nutrition, June 19, 1978, in Bethesda, Maryland, and reprinted in *Nutrition Today*, July/August 1979, pp. 31-34.

[18]Coon, 1976.

Richard Wilson has written a delightful, light-hearted, and also technically sophisticated 6-page demonstration of risk analysis. He compares the risks of eating a peanut-butter sandwich, walking next to a brick wall, smoking a cigarette, and others:

● Wilson, R. Analyzing the daily risks of life. *Technology Review* 81, February 1979; reprint available from Alumni Association, Massachusetts Institute of Technology, Cambridge, MA 02139.

A handy summary of FDA's laws and regulations is available in the 72-page paperback booklet:

● *Requirements of Laws and Regulations Enforced by the U.S. Food and Drug Administration*, U.S. Department of Health, Education, and Welfare publication no. (FDA) 79-1042 (Washington, D.C.: Government Printing Office, 1979).

The complete National Academy of Sciences' 276-page report on food safety became available in 1979 (write to the NAS at the address in Appendix J):

● National Academy of Sciences. *Report on Food Safety.*
The report includes case histories of saccharin, mercury, nitrites, and aflatoxin.

The review of GRAS list additives was summarized:

● Yesterday's additives — generally safe. *FDA Consumer*, March 1981, pp. 14-15.
Of the 415 GRAS substances, 305 were found to be without hazard; 68 without hazard as used; 19 without hazard as used but needing further investigation; 18 unevaluatable. Only 5

required the setting of safer usage conditions. The complete report of the select committee on GRAS substances is available for $6 from the National Technical Information Service, Springfield, VA 22161. The report includes the reassessment of all food and color additives. Ask for PB 80203789.

FDA's own report on the current uses and status of additives is a brief and crystal clear discussion:

● Lehman, P. More than you ever thought you would know about food additives. *FDA Consumer*, April 1979 (reprint).
Of the 200 possible food colors, Lehman says, 31 are presently approved for use.

A general review of all color additives and how the FDA regulates them:

● Damon, G. E., and Jannsen, W. F. Additives for eye appeal. *FDA Consumer*, July/August 1973, pp. 15-18.

The issues surrounding the use of additives in foods are raised in an interesting symposium reported in *Nutrition Reviews*, January 1980. W. J. Darby addresses the question how "benefit" from additives can be quantified; V. O. Wodicka talks about risk and responsibility; and FDA's S. A. Miller discusses "the new metaphysics" — the problem of defining "zero risk".

● Risk versus benefit: The future of food safety. Underwood-Prescott Award Symposium Papers presented at Massachusetts Institute of Technology, Cambridge, Massachusetts, September 25, 1979. *Nutrition Reviews* 38

(1980):33-64.

On food-coloring agents, a recent, highly technical review is:

● Parkinson, T. M., and Brown, J. P. Metabolic fate of food colorants. *Annual Review of Nutrition* 1 (1981):175-205.

The interesting conclusion to this article is that synthetic coloring agents have been studied more thoroughly than their natural counterparts and therefore their safety is known, while the safety of natural coloring agents (such as the pigments of plants) cannot be assumed on the basis of present knowledge.

The American Council on Science and Health has prepared a short report outlining its position that the Delaney Clause should be modernized. The report is available as an 11-page pamphlet, "The U.S. Food Safety Laws: Time for a Change?" from ACSH (address in Appendix J).

Three big books of food additives are available:

● *CRC Handbook: Regulatory Status of Direct Food Additives.* Boca Raton, Fl.: CRC Press, 1981.

● *Food Chemicals Codex*, 3rd ed. Washington, D.C.: National Academy Press.

● Taylor, R. J. *Food Additives.* Somerset, N.J.: Wiley, 1980.

The Nutrition Today Society makes available a teaching aid, Additives, by R. L. Hall (address in Appendix J).

FDA also makes available a free 15-minute slide show that traces the history of color, flavor, and other additives, shows their uses, and explains FDA's regulation of them: "What About Food Additives?"

1. Look up and record your recommended intake of iron (from the RDA tables on the inside front cover or from the Canadian Dietary Standard in Appendix O). Also record your actual intake, from the average derived on Form 2 in the Self-Study at the end of the Introduction to Part One (p. 14). What percentage of your recommended intake did you consume? Was this enough?

Which of the foods you eat supply the most iron? Rank your top five iron contributors: How many were meats? Legumes? Greens? Did any of them fall outside these classes? If so, what were they? How much of a contribution does enriched or whole-grain bread or cereal make to your iron intake? Are there refined bread/cereal products in your diet, such as pastries, that you could replace with enriched or whole-grain products to increase your iron intake?

Optional Extras

2. Investigate iron sources. If you have a need to learn more about individual foods and their contributions of iron to the diet, look up some of the following in Appendix H: different kinds of liver; different green, leafy vegetables; various breads and cereals (do enriched breads have more or less iron than whole-grain breads, or are they about the same?); nuts and legumes; dried fruits; molasses and other sugar sources. Pay particular attention to the foods you eat. Then plan several days' menus you would enjoy that provide your recommended intake.

3. Consider your iodine need. Are you in an area of the country where the soil is iodine-poor? If so, do you use iodized salt? There's a digression in Chapter 18 about people getting more than enough iodine. Are you in this category?

4. Remind yourself of fluoride. Is the water in your county fluoridated? If not, how do you and your family ensure that your intakes of fluoride are optimal?

5. Check your diet for its balance of refined versus whole foods. Review your three-day food record (Introduction Self-Study) and separate the foods you ate into two categories: predominantly natural, unprocessed foods like those on the exchange lists (Appendix L) and highly processed foods, such as TV dinners, pastries, and potato chips. By each food, record its kcalorie value. How many total kcalories did you consume in three days? Of these, what percentage came from highly processed foods? In light of the discussion of trace elements in Chapter 13, what implications do you suppose this estimate has for the nutritional adequacy of your diet?

Scoring Your Diet against the Four Food Group Plan

The best guidelines for a nutritious diet are those a well-informed individual chooses for personal use. There is no one right way. However, if a single guide is sought, a serviceable and long-lived one is the Four Food Group Plan. Representatives of all four food groups appear in the diets of almost all the world's people. Wherever all four groups are represented by their most nutritious members, there is likely to be adequate nutrition.

To help people discover how well planned their own diets are, nutrition educators sometimes employ a scorecard like that shown here (Form 1). Such a scorecard can be most helpful, especially in instances where a person's diet planning is based on the Four Food Group system. If you recorded your diet for the first Self-Study as directed, you can now try this quick scoring system. Some people find that they can rely entirely on a nutrition scorecard like this. Others find it too simple to be satisfactory.

The scorecard can be misleading in two ways. A high score can be belied by poor nutrient intakes if the particular selections from the food groups are poor. This may mean you should

reexamine the food groups to find better sources of the nutrients you lack. Conversely, your diet can supply adequate amounts of all of the nutrients without scoring well on the scorecard. If this is the case, you may want to note and remember what special foods are meeting your nutrient needs.

The scorecard illustrates a point that is important in diet planning. Notice that it allows points for foods from each of the four food groups to a maximum of twenty-five. The only way you can score a perfect one hundred is to choose from all four groups. The message is to diversify your investment. Don't overdo any one food or food group; don't leave one out either, without compensating carefully. This way you will reap the benefits, not only of the nutrients you know are in the foods you choose, but also of those that are unlisted — vitamin D, zinc, vitamin

B_6, iodine, folacin, and some thirty others. A diet that provides an abundance of all the familiar nutrients is virtually guaranteed to supply the others equally generously.

Optional Extra

This chapter's Highlight was on additives. Today's highly complex food industry could not have developed without the introduction of additives to ensure stability. Without them, it would be impossible to produce food in one part of the world and have it survive processing, packaging, transportation over great distances, and many months of storage before it is consumed. If these additives were suddenly eliminated, chaos and widespread starvation would result before another system could be evolved.

To dramatize this point for yourself, walk through the supermarket and read the package labels to see what additives are present in the foods there. Remember that the processed meats also contain additives to prevent spoilage. Now imagine that all the additives had suddenly ceased to exist and you were revisiting the same supermarket a year later. What differences would you see?

Form 1. Food Selection Scorecard

Food group and recommended intake	Your score	Your intake from group (specify food and amount)
Fruits & vegetables—4 or more servings (1/2 c cooked edible portion or 3-4 oz, 100 g, raw); at least one raw daily		
One serving vitamin A-rich dark green or deep orange fruit or vegetable (any food with more than your RDA) = 10 points (no more than 10 points allowed)		
One serving vitamin C-rich fruit or vegetable (any food with more than your RDA) = 10 points (no more than 10 points allowed)		
Other fruits and vegetables, including potatoes = 2.5 each		
Subtotal (no more than 25 points allowed)		
Breads & cereals—4 or more servings of whole-grain or "enriched" (1 oz dry-weight cereal or 1-oz slice bread or equivalent grain product)		
One serving cereal or 2 bread equivalents = 10 points (no more than 10 points allowed)		
Other bread equivalents = 5 points each		
Subtotal (no more than 25 points allowed)		
Milk & milk products—2 or more servings (8 oz fluid milk; calcium equivalents are 1 1/3 oz hard cheese, 1 1/3 c cottage cheese, 1 pint ice milk or ice cream)		
One serving = 12.5 points		
Subtotal (no more than 25 points allowed)		
Meat & meat substitutes—2 or more servings (2-3 oz cooked lean meat, fish, poultry; protein equivalents are 2 eggs, 2 oz hard cheese, 1/2 c hard cheese, 1/2 c cottage cheese, 1 c cooked legumes, 4 tbsp peanut butter, 1 oz nuts or sunflower seeds); count cheese either in milk group or in meat group, not both		
One serving = 12.5 points		
Subtotal (no more than 25 points allowed)		
GRAND TOTAL (no more than 100 points)		

The above are FOUNDATION FOODS. ADDITIONAL FOODS are those that do not fit into the above groupings but add flavor, interest, variety, and (often) kcalories. List those eaten:

_____   _____   _____

_____   _____   _____

_____   _____   _____

CHAPTER 14

CONTENTS

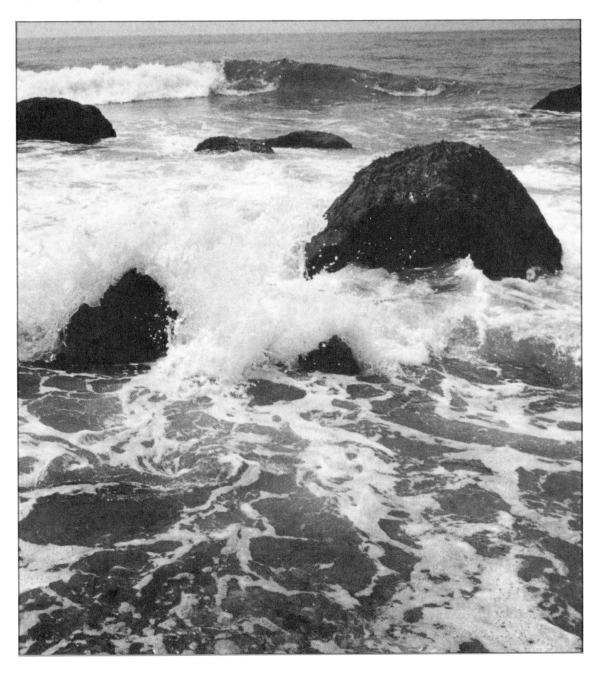

WATER AND SALTS

It was assuredly not chance that led Thales to found philosophy and science with the assertion that water is the origin of all things.

LAWRENCE J. HENDERSON

Water and salts provide the medium in which nearly all of the body's reactions take place, participate in many of them, and supply the means for transporting vital materials to cells and waste products away from them. Every cell in the body is bathed in water of the exact composition that is best for it. The fluid found in the eye contains the dissolved materials necessary for the health of the rod and cone cells; the fluid inside the spinal column is perfectly constituted for nerve cell function; the fluid at each point along the GI tract is ideal for the activities of the cells in that part of the tract — and so on.

Each of these fluids is constantly undergoing loss and replacement of its constituent parts as cells withdraw nutrients and oxygen from them and excrete carbon dioxide and other waste materials into them. Yet the composition of the body fluids in each compartment remains remarkably constant at all times. We have provided details about two examples of this constancy: the regulation of blood glucose concentration (Chapter 1) and that of blood calcium (Chapter 12). On closer examination, it becomes apparent that every important constituent of body fluids is similarly regulated. The interstitial fluid, for example, always has a high concentration of sodium and chloride ions and lower concentrations of about eight other major ions. The intracellular fluid always has high potassium and phosphate concentrations and lower concentrations of other ions. These special fluids regulate the functioning of cells; the cells in turn regulate the composition and amount of the fluids. The entire system of cells and fluids remains in a delicate but firmly maintained state of dynamic equilibrium.

The maintenance of this balance is so important that it is credited with our ability and that of other animals to live on land. Our single-celled ancestors depended totally on the sea water they lived in to provide nutrients and oxygen and to carry away their waste. We have managed over the course of our 2-billion-year evolutionary history to internalize the ocean — to continue bathing our cells in a warm nutritive fluid that keeps them alive. It is interesting to note that the amounts of salts in our body fluids, and their temperature, are believed to be the same as in the ocean — not as it is now, but as it was at the

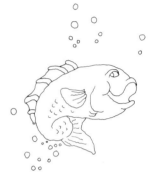

We, too, live in water.

Ionic compounds: see Appendix B.

dynamic equilibrium: a state of balance in which rapid exchange is taking place. For example, body fluids, bones, and fat maintain a constant composition but exchange materials continuously with their surroundings. As opposed to a condition of **static equilibrium**, dynamic equilibrium is a condition of **homeostasis** (see p. 47).

Salt does not refer only to sodium chloride but also to ionic compounds, as defined in Appendix B.

time when our ancestors emerged onto land. The ocean has since become more salty, but we still carry the ancient ocean within us.

The Uniqueness of Water

Water in the body is not simply a river coursing through the arteries, capillaries, and veins, carrying the heavy traffic of nutrients and waste products. Some of the water is a part of the chemical structure of compounds that form the cells, tissues, and organs of the body. For example, protein holds water molecules within its structure. This water is locked in and is not readily available for any other use.

> The water held in protein molecules often discourages the very obese person who has starved himself and lost lean body mass. When he first eats a small amount of food, restoring even a pound of his protein tissue brings with it the retention of 4 lb water. Small wonder that the obese person thinks that any tiny amount of food causes him to gain enormous amounts of weight. As a result, he concludes that dieting is futile for him.

Water also participates actively in many chemical reactions, instead of being merely the medium in which they take place. A good example of this is the splitting of two glucose units (a disaccharide). Water participates by being split, with a hydrogen going to one glucose and an oxygen and hydrogen going to the other. By this action, the bond that held the two glucose units together is broken.

As the medium for the body's chemical traffic, water is very nearly a universal solvent. Luckily for our body integrity, this is not quite the case, but water does dissolve amino acids, glucose, minerals, and many other substances needed by the cells. Fatty substances are specially wrapped in water-soluble protein so that they too can travel freely in the blood and lymph. Water thus makes an ideal transportation medium.

Another important characteristic of water is its incompressibility: Its molecules resist being crowded together. Thanks to this characteristic, water acts as a lubricant around joints. For the same reason, it can protect a sensitive tissue, such as the spinal cord, from shock. The fluid that fills the eye serves in a similar way to keep optimal pressure on the retina and lens. The unborn infant is cushioned against blows by the bag of water it develops in. Water also lubricates the digestive tract and all tissues moistened with mucus.

Still another of water's special features is its heat-holding capacity. This characteristic of water is well known to coastal dwellers, who know that land surrounded by water is protected from rapid and wide variations in temperature from day to night. Water itself changes temperature slowly; at night, when the land cools, the water holds its heat and gives it up gradually to the air, moderating the coolness of the night. In contrast, the desert has a wide variation in temperature from day to night because of the lack of water on the land and in the air. In our bodies, water helps to maintain our temperature at a constant 98.6° F (37° C) by resisting fluctuations in temperature.

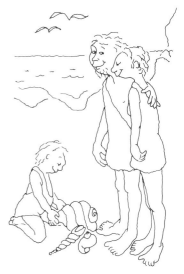

Related to this characteristic is the fact that a great deal of heat is required to change water from a liquid to a gas. This serves the body when cooling is needed. In a very hot environment, we sweat: Water is brought to the body surface through the sweat glands. When the sweat evaporates, it carries off all the absorbed heat and so cools the body.

Another fascinating characteristic of water that makes life possible on earth is the fact that it contracts as it gets colder but that, unlike other substances, it expands as it freezes. (It is most dense at 4° C.) Ice is thus lighter than cold water and so floats instead of sinking. This protects the water beneath from the coldness of the air. Thus pond water below a protective sheet of ice can remain unfrozen, and living things in a pond can survive through hard winters, even when the temperature of the air falls many degrees below freezing.

The expansion of water during freezing explains why packages of frozen food tell you "Do not refreeze." As it freezes, the water disrupts the structure of the food and so changes its texture. People sometimes wonder if there is any danger in eating a twice-frozen food. Provided that they haven't let it spoil while it was thawed, the only problem is that the food may be less appealing. Its nutrient content is not affected by refreezing.

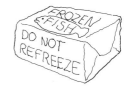

The Constancy of Body Water

Water constitutes 55 to 60 percent of your body weight, and it is fortunate that the total amount of water remains constant. That it does so is a consequence of two delicate balancing systems that regulate both its intake and its excretion.

Water Intake: Thirst   When you need water, you drink. Everybody knows that, but it takes a thinking physiologist to ask why. The evidence from experiments with thirst points to the possibility that several mechanisms operate in its regulation. One is in the mouth itself: When the blood is too salty (having lost water but not salts), water is withdrawn from the salivary glands into the blood. The mouth becomes dry as a result, and you drink to wet your mouth. Another thirst mechanism is in a brain center, where cells sample and monitor

Water follows salt, moving in the direction of higher osmotic pressure (see p. 488).

The brain center described here is the **hypothalamus** (hy-po-THAL-a-mus).

the salt concentration in the blood. When they find it too high, they initiate impulses that travel to brain centers that in turn stimulate drinking behavior. The stomach may also play a role. Thirsty animals drink until nerves in their stomachs, known as stretch receptors, are stimulated enough to turn off the drinking. More must be learned about these mechanisms, but it is clear from what we know already that thirst is finely adjusted to provide a water intake that exactly meets the need.

Water Excretion   This mechanism is better understood. The cells of the hypothalamus, which monitor salt concentration in the blood, stimulate the pituitary gland to release a hormone, ADH, whenever the body's salt concentration is too high. ADH stimulates the kidneys to hold back (actually reabsorb) water, so that it recirculates in the body rather than being excreted. Thus the more water you need, the less you excrete. There are also cells in the kidney itself that are responsive to the salt concentration in the blood passing through them. When they sense a too-high salt concentration, they too release a substance. By a

---

Two mechanisms control the way the kidney retains water: the ADH mechanism and the aldosterone mechanism.

The ADH mechanism directly causes water retention by the kidneys.

ADH (antidiuretic hormone): a hormone released by the pituitary gland in response to high osmotic pressure of the blood. Target organ: the kidney, which responds by reabsorbing water.

Hormone: see p. 82.

For more details, see Highlight 2.

The aldosterone mechanism indirectly causes water retention by the kidney:

1. The kidney releases renin in response to high osmotic pressure of the blood.
2. The renin converts angiotensinogen in the blood to angiotensin I and II.
3. The angiotensins stimulate the adrenal gland to release aldosterone.
4. Aldosterone stimulates the kidney to reabsorb sodium.
5. Water follows sodium and is reabsorbed.

aldosterone (al-DOSS-ter-OWN): a hormone released by the adrenal gland in response to the presence of angiotensin. Target organ: the kidney, which responds by reabsorbing sodium.

roundabout route, this substance causes the adrenal gland to release a hormone—aldosterone—that in turn causes the kidneys to retain more water. Again, the effect is that when more water is needed, less is excreted.

These renal excretion mechanisms cannot work by themselves to maintain water balance unless you drink enough. This is because the body must excrete a minimum amount of water each day—the amount necessary to carry out of the body the waste products generated by the day's metabolic activities. Above this minimum (about 900 ml a day), the amounts of water you excrete can be adjusted to balance your intake. The urine merely becomes more dilute. Hence drinking plenty of water is never a bad idea.

Metabolic wastes: ketones and urea (see pp. 212, 206).

But consider sweating (see p. 422).

Water Imbalance   Water deficiency, or dehydration, occurs whenever there is a massive loss of body water (as in kidney malfunction, blood loss, vomiting, or diarrhea) or when water becomes unavailable. Since the consequences are related to losses of the salts that accompany the water, this phenomenon is discussed below. Excess water in the body is reflected in the symptoms of edema, hypertension, or both; these too are related to the body's salt retention.

Massive loss of body water through the kidneys is **diuresis** (dye-yoo-REE-sis).

Losses from lungs and skin are called **insensible water losses.**

The Constancy of Total Body Water   In addition to the obvious dietary source, water itself, all foods contain water (as a look back at the figures on p. 5 will remind you). In addition, water is generated from the energy nutrients in foods (recall that the Cs and Hs in these nutrients combine with oxygen during metabolism to yield CO_2 and H_2O). Daily water intake from these three sources totals about 2 1/2 liters.

In addition to the water excreted via the kidneys, some water is lost from the lungs as vapor, some in feces, and some from the skin. The losses of all of these also total about 2 1/2 liters a day.

2 1/2 l is about 2 1/2 qt.

How Salts Behave

The regulation of body water distribution and transportation is intimately associated with the regulation of salt distribution. A closer look at the way the body handles this problem will pave the way for an understanding of the causes and consequences of imbalances.

Interestingly enough, the very minerals that are most important in regulation of the water balance—sodium, chlorine, phosphorus, and potassium—are those that are most abundant in the diet and thus are very rarely deficient in humans. This is no coincidence. The regulation of water balance is so vital that our bodies have evolved to use these abundant elements for this purpose. Any other course would have brought the process of evolution to a dead halt.

Water intake:

Liquids	950—1,500 ml
Food	700—1,000 ml
Metabolic water	200— 300 ml
	1,850—2,800 ml

Water output:

Kidneys	900—1,400 ml
Lungs	350 ml
Feces	150 ml
Skin	450— 900 ml
	1,850—2,800 ml

Na = sodium

Cl = chlorine

salt: a compound composed of charged particles (ions). However, a compound in which the cations are H^+ is an acid; a compound in which the anions are OH^- is a base.

cation (CAT-eye-un): a positively charged ion.

anion (AN-eye-un): a negatively charged ion.

For a closer look at ions, see Appendix B.

chloride: the ionic form of chlorine.

dissociation: physical separation of the ions in an ionic compound. A salt that partly dissociates in water is an **electrolyte**.

electrolyte solution: a solution that can conduct electricity.

milliequivalent: a number of ions equal to the number of H^+ ions in a milligram of hydrogen. This is a useful measure, because when we are considering ions we are usually interested in the number of positive or negative charges present in a solution rather than in their weight.

This force is known as the **osmotic pressure** of a solution. Water flows in the direction of the higher osmotic pressure. Whatever is dissolved in the water, that creates this pressure, is the **solute** (SOLL-yute).

To understand how cells regulate the amount of water they contain, it is necessary to take a closer look at the minerals as ions, the form in which cells use minerals for water regulation. Cell membranes are freely permeable to water, which flows back and forth across them all the time. Yet they neither lose all their water, shrinking down and collapsing, nor do they overfill with water, swelling up and bursting like balloons. Along the evolutionary path they have contrived a method of keeping their water constant; they do this beautifully by employing the salts to assist them. They make use of the principle that water follows salt.

Chemists use the term *salt* to include many inorganic substances, not just the ordinary table salt most of us are familiar with. To denote table salt, the chemist refers to it as sodium chloride, NaCl. Sodium chloride is a good example to use in a discussion of salts. In the white crystalline substance the sodium and chlorine atoms are bound together by strong electrostatic forces in a rigid crystalline structure. Outwardly, the crystals exhibit no electrical charge. However, when dissolved in water, the rigid structure relaxes. Some of the sodium moves about freely as positively charged ions, and some of the chloride also dissociates and moves about as negatively charged ions. The salt thus reveals itself as a compound composed of charged particles. The positive ions are cations; the negative, anions.

A salt that partly dissociates in water, as sodium chloride does, is known as an electrolyte. Since the fluids of the body are composed of water and partly dissociated salts, they are electrolyte solutions.

Electrolyte solutions are always electrostatically balanced. There is no such thing as a test tube filled with sodium ions. Sodium ions are always positvely charged, and so they cannot exist apart from negatively charged ions. Therefore, in any fluid with dissolved electrolytes there will always be the same number of positive and negative ions. For instance, in the extracellular fluid, the numbers of cations and anions both equal 155 milliequivalents per liter (mEq/l). Of the cations, sodium ions make up 142 mEq/l, and potassium, calcium, and magnesium ions make up the remainder. Of the anions, chloride ions number 104 mEq/l, bicarbonate ions number 27 mEq/l, and the remainder is provided by phosphate ions, sulfate ions, organic acids, and protein. If an anion enters a cell, a cation must accompany it or another anion must leave so that electroneutrality will be maintained.

We stated above that water follows salt. More precisely, there is a force that moves water into a place where a solute, such as sodium chloride, is concentrated. This force can operate only if the divider separating the two fluid solutions is permeable to water but not permeable (or less freely permeable) to the solute. The following figure shows this force in operation. In the top part, equal amounts of solute on both sides of the divider cause the amounts of water to be equal also. In the bottom part, the presence of more solute on side B has drawn water across the divider so that the *concentration* of solute on both sides becomes equal.

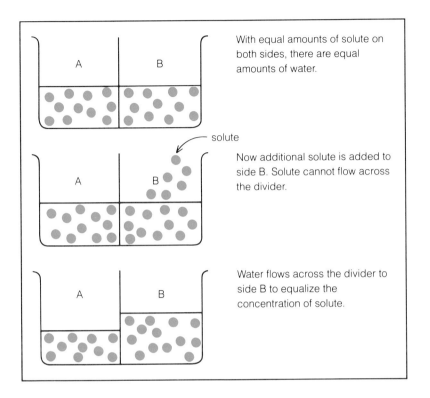

With equal amounts of solute on both sides, there are equal amounts of water.

solute

Now additional solute is added to side B. Solute cannot flow across the divider.

Water flows across the divider to side B to equalize the concentration of solute.

You have seen this force at work if you have ever salted a lettuce salad an hour before eating it. When you came back to the salad, the lettuce was wilted and there was water in the salad bowl. The high concentration of salt (and therefore low concentration of water) on the outside of the lettuce cells caused water to leave the inside of the cells. They collapsed (the lettuce wilted), and the water puddled in the salad dish. Sugar would have caused the same reaction as the salt. There is one way you could have prevented this (here's a cooking lesson for the novice): You could have coated the lettuce lightly with oil, then salted it or put salad dressing containing salt on it; the oil would have acted as a barrier against the salt, keeping the lettuce crisp.

The Body's Use of Salts

With the previous diagram in mind, you can see how the living cell manages to move water in and out as it needs to. It is obvious how vital salts are to the body's well-being.

Water Balance The divider between the water inside and outside of a cell is the cell membrane. The cell cannot pump water directly across its membrane, but it does have proteins in its membrane that can

Other terms used to describe electrolyte solutions:

isotonic: having the same osmotic pressure as a reference solution. For example, a saline solution may be made isotonic to human blood.

hypertonic: having a higher osmotic pressure than a reference solution.

hypotonic: having a lower osmotic pressure than a reference solution.

The salty water on the outside of the lettuce cells is hypertonic to the water inside the cells, so it attracts water out of the cells.

The cell membrane is **semipermeable:** more permeable to some substances (such as water) than to others. This is the condition necessary for osmotic pressure to operate.

For more about the cell-membrane pumps, see pp. 129, 178.

attach to sodium ions and move them from one side of the membrane to the other. When these sodium pumps are active, they pump out sodium faster than it can diffuse into the cell. Water follows the sodium. When potassium pumps are active, they pump in potassium, and water follows this ion. By maintaining a certain concentration of sodium outside and potassium inside, the cell can exactly regulate the amount of water it contains.

Acid-Base Balance In addition to regulating the amount of water found in each body compartment, the body uses its ions to regulate the acidity (pH) of its fluids. The major minerals are most important in this regard, since they are present in the highest concentrations. The chloride ion, for example, shifts back and forth across the membranes of the red blood cells, helping the blood fluid to maintain the proper degree of acidity as the blood travels to and from the lungs. As the blood leaves the lungs bearing red blood cells loaded with oxygen, the chloride ion travels in the plasma. When the cells deliver their oxygen, the plasma picks up carbon dioxide from the tissues and carries it as bicarbonate ions. Thus the plasma's bicarbonate concentration rises. The chloride ions then shift into the red blood cells to keep the total acidity constant. After the blood has passed through the lungs and the bicarbonate level has been lowered, the chloride ions shift back into the blood fluid to maintain the acid-base balance.

The electrolyte mixtures in the body fluids, as well as the proteins, also protect the body against changes in acidity by acting as buffers—substances that can accommodate excess plus or minus charges. The action of a buffer is shown in Figure 1.

Acid- and Base-Formers Some of the major minerals are acid-formers; others are base-formers. Table 1 divides these minerals into the acid- and base-forming classes. Foods, too, can be classified as acid- or base-formers, depending on which of these minerals predominate in them. Grains contain the acid-forming minerals; fruits and vegetables contain base-formers.

The chloride ion, Cl^-, is a negatively charged, acid-forming ion.

The bicarbonate ion, HCO_3^-, is also a negatively charged, acid ion.

buffer: a substance or mixture capable in solution of neutralizing both acids and bases and thereby capable of maintaining the original concentration of hydrogen ions (pH) in the solution.

The base-forming nature of fruits may come as a surprise to people who think of fruits as being acid. You may have heard someone say, for example, "I can't eat oranges; they're too acid for me." In truth, although fruits may taste sour or acid in the mouth, their ash is composed of base-forming minerals. After the *organic* acids have been digested, metabolized, and excreted, only the base-forming minerals are left. Therefore fruits and vegetables are ultimately alkaline to the body as a whole.

A buffer is a large molecule, usually protein, that can accommodate excess plus or minus charges (ions).

Figure 1   Action of a buffer.

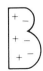

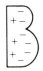

A buffer can be neutral (an equal number of plus and minus charges).

A buffer can be acidic (an excess of plus charges).

A buffer can be alkaline, or basic (an excess of minus charges).

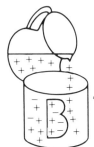

In a solution, a buffer helps the solution keep its acid-base balance by soaking up excess plus or minus charges or by giving them up to the solution.

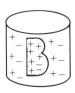

If the solution receives excess plus charges, tending to make it acidic,

If the solution loses plus charges, tending to make it alkaline (basic),

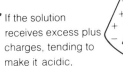

the buffer will pick these up. The solution keeps its acid-base balance.

the buffer will give up its plus charges. The solution keeps its acid-base balance.

Table 1   The Major Minerals*

Acid-formers	Base-formers
Chlorine	Calcium
Sulfur	Magnesium
Phosphorus	Sodium
	Potassium

*The task of remembering each of these seven elements as either an acid-former or a base-former is somewhat simplified if you are aware that each of these elements forms a common compound whose name reveals its role. For example, a compound of calcium is calcium hydroxide. Hydroxides are bases—and thus calcium is a base-former. With phosphorus, a common compound is phosphoric acid; thus phosphorus is an acid-former. The compound of sulfur, sulfuric acid, tells you that sulfur is an acid-former. The rule is consistent: For chlorine, remember hydrochloric acid; for magnesium, sodium, and potassium, the hydroxides.

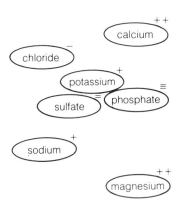

Major mineral ions.

Table 2   Acid- and Base-Forming Foods

Acid-forming foods	Base-forming foods
Meat, fish, poultry	Milk
Eggs	
Cheese	Vegetables
Grains (breads and cereals)	Fruits (except cranberries, prunes, and plums)
Fruits (cranberries, prunes, and plums only)	

Meat, eggs, poultry, and fish contain the acid-forming minerals. Milk and milk products contain both acid- and base-formers. The breakdown of the protein in milk does produce some acid temporarily, but the large amounts of calcium cause milk to be classified as a base-former in the body. Table 2 shows the acid- and base-forming foods.

The Constancy of Total Body Salts

Surprisingly, although one person may eat more base-forming foods and another more acid-forming foods, the body's total content of electrolytes remains constant. The job of regulating the body's salt population is largely delegated to the kidneys, under the supervision of several monitoring systems, notably the adrenal and pituitary glands. The net effect of all the homeostatic balancing systems is to ensure that output balances intake. A person who eats a lot of table salt, for example, excretes more sodium and chloride in his urine than one who eats only a little. Thus the *body's* total electrolytes remain constant, and it is the composition of the *urine* that is affected by what you eat.

If the kidneys are asked to excrete very high concentrations of minerals, or if some part of their intricate machinery is damaged by poison or a mistake in heredity, they may develop stones—deposits of

adrenal glands: the two small glands nestled into the tops of the kidneys. Among the hormones secreted by these glands are the stress hormones (see p. 85) and aldosterone (pp. 86, 486).

ad = on top
renal = of the kidney

pituitary gland: the master gland in the brain; secretes many hormones, including ADH (see pp. 82, 486).

Kidney stones are deposits of minerals that have crystallized within the kidney. Technically, they are termed **renal calculi** (REE-nul CAL-kyoo-lie).

renal = of the kidney
calculus = a small stone

minerals that they were unable to dissolve in water and excrete. A person who has alkaline stones (for example, calcium stones) in her kidneys may be told to eat an "acid ash diet" so that her urine will be acidic, to prevent the further precipitation of such stones. She would be told, then, to cut down on her fruit and vegetable intake and to eat more grains and protein-rich foods (except milk). A person with acid stones (for example, uric acid) would be put on an alkaline ash diet.

Kidney disorders impair the body's ability to regulate its fluid and electrolyte balances. To keep a renal patient alive, the physician may have to resort to the use of a kidney machine, a large apparatus connected directly to the patient's blood supply that filters it and adjusts the concentrations of its dissolved materials. Between sessions with the machine, the burden falls on the dietitian to regulate the renal patient's intakes of electrolytes. The dietitian may have to calculate a diet that precisely specifies the sodium, potassium, calcium, water, and many other constituents. (A dietitian in this very sophisticated medical specialty requires several years of schooling.)

It is not known whether any regulating system other than the kidneys governs the body's salt contents. We have thirst, to govern our intake of water, but do we have a salt hunger to govern our intake of sodium? Salt hunger is well known in plant-eating animals like cattle, which will travel long distances to a salt lick when they have been depleted of sodium. The tongue, in both animals and humans, is equipped with taste receptors that respond only to salt, hence the ability to distinguish a salty taste. Animals know instinctively when to seek this stimulus, but humans may seek it when they have no need. Future research may determine whether a true salt hunger operates in humans.

Water and Salt Imbalances

You are well protected from imbalances of water and electrolytes. Through intake and excretion, your whole body can achieve the optimal levels of fluid and electrolytes over a wide range of different conditions. By these mechanisms your body's cells are supplied with the total amounts of sodium, potassium, and other ions that they need in order to maintain their own local balances. However, you may be thrown into situations that your kidneys, thirst instinct, and cell membranes cannot compensate for. This is the case when large amounts of fluid and electrolytes are lost in an emergency. The most familiar conditions in which this happens are discussed below. As you read, remember that sodium and chloride are the principal cation and anion outside the cell and that potassium and phosphate are the principal cation and anion inside the cell.

Losses of Water and Salt   When you vomit, you lose large amounts of water and hydrochloric acid from your stomach. This leaves you

acid ash diet: a diet of acid-forming foods (foods that, if burned to ash, would be found to contain acid-forming minerals). Such a diet contributes to acidity of the urine, because the kidney collects the excess acid-forming minerals into the urine for excretion.

alkaline ash diet: a diet of base-forming foods.

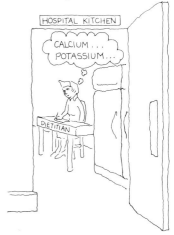

There are 4 kinds of taste receptors on the tongue: those sensitive to salt, sweet, sour, and bitter flavors.

Technically, these kinds of imbalances are known as **fluid-and-electrolyte imbalances**.

Alkalosis, acidosis: see p. 127.

dehydrated and, because of the loss of acid, may initially throw you into alkalosis. If you have a prolonged attack of diarrhea, you lose a more alkaline fluid from the lower portion of the GI tract, consisting largely of sodium ions. This too can leave you dehydrated but will throw you into acidosis. Both vomiting and diarrhea reflect losses of fluid from one body compartment—the gastrointestinal tract.

When either vomiting or diarrhea occurs, an astonishing amount of fluid is involved. One cannot help but wonder where it all comes from. Normally we are not conscious of the large amount of fluid involved in the digestive process, because our bodies are so wonderfully made that we don't have to drink the fluid necessary for digestion. You may recall from Chapter 5 that water is added to the GI tract contents at each step along the way—via saliva, via gastric, intestinal, and pancreatic juices, and via bile—but then is normally reabsorbed in the colon and recycled. The amount of digestive secretions put forth in the average adult has been estimated at over 9 liters/day, or more than three times as much as the water taken in with food and drink and produced during metabolism. It is obvious that replacement of this fluid is of prime importance in the medical and nutritional management of diarrhea and vomiting. Over half of the deaths in children under four are due to diarrhea.

Normally the ratio of mineral particles to water particles (the concentration) is the same on both sides of cell membranes:

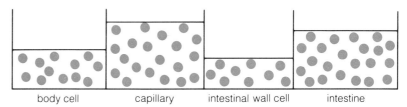

body cell   capillary   intestinal wall cell   intestine

If diarrhea occurs, water flows from the intestinal wall to replace the water lost from the intestine:

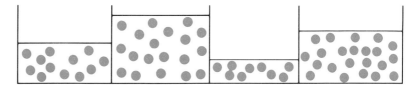

Eventually water flows out of every cell. This is dehydration:

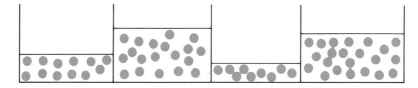

A domino effect operates when the body attempts to maintain water balance: Each fluid compartment is affected in turn by a change in the concentration of the fluids of adjacent compartments. For instance, in prolonged diarrhea, when a large amount of sodium has been lost from the GI tract, sodium and water move into the tract from the nearby interstitial and intravascular spaces. These spaces are continuous throughout the body, and their loss of sodium causes cells all over the body to compensate by shifting potassium out into the interstitial space. Meanwhile, since the whole fluid volume of the blood has decreased, the kidneys are experiencing dehydration and are attempting to retrieve needed water. Their principal means of doing this is to retain sodium, because water travels with sodium. The kidneys thus return sodium from the urine filtrate back to the blood. As the sodium enters, potassium must be exchanged; thus, potassium is lost in the urine. The end result, then, is excretion of potassium that came from cells far removed from the site of the original disturbance. The loss of potassium ions severely affects intracellular functions and, if great enough, can lead to cardiac arrest, since potassium ions are needed for the contractions of the heart muscle.

The examples of vomiting and diarrhea illustrate the body's responses to major fluid losses. If you understand the principles, you can predict what will happen in other fluid-loss situations. For example, when you sweat excessively, you are losing fluid largely from the interstitial space. The dehydration that results affects not only this space but also the vascular and intracellular spaces and other imbalances follow. If you replace the lost water without replacing the salt, you may suffer a severe depletion of your body sodium and chloride. Since these are the major electrolytes lost in sweat, the Food and Nutrition Board offers a rule of thumb: If you have drunk more than about 3 liters of water in a day to replace water lost in heavy sweating, you should take two or more grams of sodium chloride with each additional liter.

One additional example will illustrate another class of fluid loss: loss from the intracellular space, as when a person is severely burned. In this instance, the electrolytes potassium and phosphate and others are lost. Since the salts lost in this case are the chemist's salts, and not the single compound sodium chloride, their replacement must be managed by a physician. The physician's first and most important concern in treating a burn patient is to assess the fluid and electrolyte balance and to plan a careful replacement that will not upset the balance further.

Excess Salt   As you have probably anticipated, there is a risk of overcompensating. Excessive salt intake can be as serious as insufficient intake. (As you know, people lost at sea will die sooner if they drink the salt water.) To excrete excess sodium, the kidneys must excrete a certain amount of water along with it. Thus too much salt can as readily cause dehydration as too little water. When the kidneys are diseased, a moderate salt intake is especially critical. Unexcreted salt accumulates

A liter is roughly the same size as a quart. A U.S. quart is a little smaller and a Canadian (imperial) quart a little bigger than a liter.

1 g of sodium chloride = 1/5 tsp salt

Salt tablets are often 1 g each.

Edema: see also p. 126.

High blood pressure is the same as hypertension.

Still another fluid-loss situation has been described: the taking of diuretics (p. 273). This discussion shows why self-prescribed diuretics are dangerous.

in extracellular fluids and so may cause either edema or high blood pressure or both.

The details of electrolyte balance are among the most important ones that medical students must learn. Mastery of the details is appropriately left to them and to their medical associates. For the general reader and the student of nutrition, it is necessary only to appreciate the importance of this balance and the principles by which it is maintained and to be aware of the situations that threaten it. When any of these gets out of control, a red-hot medical emergency may exist. The most appropriate action is to call the doctor. The water and salts, which we take for granted and usually ignore, are more vital to life than any of the other nutrients considered in this book.

The Water Supply

When you draw water from the tap into a glass and drink it, it is not only water that you are drinking. Chlorine may have been added to it, to kill microorganisms that might otherwise convey disease. Fluoride may have been added to it, if your community has adopted fluoridation (see p. 458). In addition, it contains naturally occurring minerals, toxic heavy metals, live microorganisms, and a miscellany of organic compounds. Most people in the more developed countries take their water supply for granted and assume that it is pure water, and is safe. At the same time, they may be very much concerned over the presence of incidental additives in food. Actually water, too, may contain "incidental additives" of considerable significance to nutrition.

The quality of water varies, depending on its source. It may carry large quantities of dissolved minerals or very few. It may be hard or soft (see below), pure or contaminated. To learn about the water in your particular area, you may want to consult your local health department. The information given here may help you decide what questions to ask. The variables affecting water fall into four groups: minerals, heavy metals, microorganisms, and organic compounds.

Minerals in Water All of the 20 major and trace minerals discussed in the last two chapters are present in various ground waters in different concentrations. Often they make significant contributions as nutrients to the health of the people who drink the water. A case in point is fluoride, which in some areas occurs naturally at the same concentration as in the ocean where our ancestors evolved. Thus it precisely meets the human nutritional need for fluoride.[1] Few communities have yet analyzed their water supplies completely enough to state which mineral needs they may be helping to meet, but most at least have information about the major minerals.

The distinction between hard and soft water, which has some

[1]W. D. Keller, Drinking water: A geochemical factor in human health, *Geological Society of America Bulletin* 89 (March 1978):334-336.

important health implications, is based on three of these minerals. Hard water usually comes from shallow ground, and it contains high concentrations of the cations calcium and magnesium. Soft water usually comes from deep in the earth, and its principal cation is sodium. Well water is hard or soft, depending on the area. Most people distinguish between these two types of water in terms of their practical experience: Soft water dissolves soap better and leaves less of a ring on the tub; hard water leaves a residue of rocklike crystals in the teakettle after a while, and it turns clothes gray in the wash. Hence consumers often consider soft water to be the more desirable and may even purchase water-softening equipment, which removes magnesium and calcium and replaces them with sodium. However, as far as we know today, hard water seems to have a more favorable impact on health.

Soft water can contribute a lot of sodium to people's diets, and thus it appears to contribute to a higher incidence of high blood pressure and heart disease in areas where it is used. The National Academy of Sciences has suggested a standard for public water allowing no more than 100 mg sodium per liter. This limit would ensure that the water supply would add not more than 10 percent to the average person's total sodium intake. The American Heart Association has recommended a more conservative standard of 20 mg per liter, to protect heart and kidney patients whose sodium intakes must be restricted. At present, about half of the U.S. population drinks water containing more than 20 mg per liter. Where snowy roads are salted, the salt running off into the water supply may raise its sodium content considerably higher than this.[2]

Soft water also dissolves certain metals, such as cadmium and lead, from pipes. Cadmium is not an essential nutrient. In fact, it can harm the body, affecting at least some enzymes by displacing zinc from its normal sites of action. Cadmium has been found in high concentrations in the kidneys and urine of patients with high blood pressure and is suspected of having some causal connection with the condition. A normal intake of zinc may protect against cadmium-induced high blood pressure. Lead is another toxic metal, and the body seems to absorb it more readily from soft than from hard water—possibly because the calcium in hard water protects against its absorption.[3]

The examples just given show that the choice to install a water softener in your home may be unwise, especially if your family may be heart-disease prone. (One family we know solves the problem by connecting the water softener only to the hot-water line, then using only hot water for washing and bathing, and only cold water for cooking and drinking.) These examples also show that the minerals in water interact in unpredictable ways. Someday we may be able to fortify our water with the ideal amounts of trace minerals for human

hard water: water containing high concentrations of calcium and magnesium.

soft water: water containing a high sodium concentration.

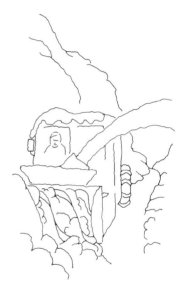

The serious problems of poisoning with lead and other heavy metals are described in Highlight 14.

[2]E. J. Calabrese and R. W. Tuthill, Sources of elevated sodium levels in drinking water . . . and recommendations for reduction, *Journal of Environmental Health* 41 (1978):151-155.

[3]Soft water and heart disease, *Nutrition and the MD*, November 1975.

consumption.[4] But before that time arrives, we have much to learn about what is in the water already and what is ideal for humans.

Toxic Metals in the Water Supply In the wilderness, water cycles rapidly through living systems, undergoing a natural purifying process in every cycle. Animal waste excreted onto the earth is filtered out by the soil before the water arrives underground. Pollutants entering rivers quickly disappear back into the earth as the river flows along, leaving the water pure. But neither the earth nor its rivers can purify completely the heavily polluted water expelled as city sewage or industrial waste. Water leaving a factory may contain concentrations of toxic metals so high that some are still present when it is recycled to become drinking water. And if the water is cycled through the same factory again, it will contain still higher concentrations the next time around.

Human technology bears the burden of purifying water contaminated by human technology. The Public Health Service sets drinking water standards, upper limits for the amounts of toxic metals permitted in water, and public law distributes the responsibility for adhering to these standards among the industries and the water-processing plants.

The metals of greatest concern are mercury, cadmium, and lead. These metals may be absorbed into the body, where they change cell membrane structure, alter enzyme or coenzyme functions, or even change the structure of the genetic material, DNA, causing cancer or birth defects. If they happen to affect the DNA in the germ cells (eggs or sperm), the changes (mutations) will become hereditary. When combined into complexes with organic compounds, these metals may be especially rapidly absorbed and may become even more effective against body tissues.[5]

Mercury is one of the rarer elements in the earth's crust but has been mined extensively for industrial use, and so it is present in our environment in unnaturally high concentrations. Much of it ends up in the water supply as mercury compounds. By far the most toxic of these is methyl mercury, which is efficiently (90 percent) absorbed in the GI tract and accumulates in red blood cells, the brain, and the nerves. In a pregnant woman, methyl mercury becomes concentrated in the growing fetus. Thus it can cause mental and physical defects in the newborn even though the mother has shown no symptoms.

Nerve damage occurs with mercury intakes as low as 300 μg per day, so the Food and Drug Administration has set a limit of one-tenth that amount on the permissible mercury levels in foods and drugs. The acceptable mercury content of water is 0.5 μg per liter.[6] (Monitoring mercury concentrations in water is a task of the public health agencies, such as the Environmental Protection Agency.) Two serious outbreaks

[4]Keller, 1978.

[5]M. M. Varma, S. G. Serdahely, and H. M. Katz, Physiological effects of trace elements and chemicals in water, *Journal of Environmental Health* 39 (1976):90-100.

[6]U.S. Public Health Service standard, in Varma, Serdahely, and Katz, 1976.

of mercury poisoning have occurred in Japan, where people have eaten fish that grew near industrial plants that discharged mercury wastes into the water. Rising levels of environmental mercury have been observed in other industrial countries, including the United States.

Cadmium has already been mentioned in connection with heart disease but has its most toxic effects in the kidney, causing chronic renal disease; in the lungs, causing emphysema; and in the bones, causing osteoporosis and osteomalacia. It has been in commercial use since 1910 and has caused severe outbreaks of disease in Japan. Cadmium in contaminated water can be absorbed into vegetables and grains and so can find its way into human consumers of these foods.[7]

Lead, another highly toxic metal, enters the water supply mostly by being captured in rain falling from atmospheres polluted with automobile exhaust. It is a metabolic poison that prevents hemoglobin formation and the action of several enzymes. Symptoms of mild lead poisoning include lowered hemoglobin, intestinal cramps, fatigue, and kidney abnormalities. These may be reversible if exposure stops. More severe exposure causes irreversible nerve damage, paralysis, mental retardation in children, abortions, and death.[8]

These are only three examples of metal pollutants, but they are enough to illustrate how the purity of the water supply can be threatened by industrial use. Both government and consumer environmental protection groups have to be vigilant in detecting, reporting, and preventing dangerous levels of contamination, because our water is a vital resource.

Microorganisms Many harmless, even beneficial, bacteria dwell in the human digestive tract and are excreted into sewage. If these were the only inhabitants of sewage, there would be no concern about their presence in drinking water. But disease organisms are also excreted into sewage, and others are introduced into it by flies and other carriers. Before a sewage treatment plant releases its effluent into the water supply, it must reduce the bacterial count enough so that further dilution will make recycled water safe for human use.

An efficient secondary sewage plant may remove 99 percent of the bacteria in the water, which sounds pretty good for a start. But there are typically 10 million bacteria in a milliliter (1/5 tsp) of sewage. After 99 percent removal there will still be 100,000 left. Chlorination then kills another 99 percent, leaving 1,000 bacteria per milliliter. Most of these are harmless, and the few that are harmful can be diluted below the danger point if the water leaving the plant enters a large river.[9] Alternatively, the treatment plant may give the water tertiary treatment, sprinkling it over a large land area so that it will be filtered before re-entering the general water supply.

High standards for sewage treatment in the developed countries

The first step in sewage treatment allows the solids to settle out. This is **primary treatment**.

secondary treatment: removes the suspended matter, including bacteria and some viruses.

tertiary treatment: removes dissolved compounds, both organic and inorganic.

[7]Varma, Serdahely, and Katz, 1976.

[8]Varma, Serdahely, and Katz, 1976.

[9]K. Kawata, Water and other environmental interventions: The minimum investment concept, *American Journal of Clinical Nutrition* 31 (1978):2114-2123.

potable (POTE-uh-bul): suitable for drinking.

potare = to drink

An example of an organic pollutant from insecticide is DDT. A very toxic pollutant is PCB, polychlorobenzene (from the plastics industry). Another potent by-product of industrial processes is chloroform.

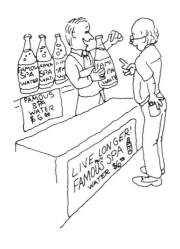

ensure that most people have potable water, but for the rest of the world, microbial contamination remains the primary cause of human diseases and epidemics. Two of the most basic needs of the world's people are safe drinking water and an acceptable standard of waste disposal.[10]

Organics   The fourth class of substances that may occur in water are the organic compounds from sewage, insecticides, petroleum-based and other industries, and other sources. Research on these is less than 20 years old, and few of them have been identified, but many are known to be toxic. Some cause birth defects, some are carcinogenic, some cause permanent alterations of the inherited genetic material.[11] Many contain chlorine, and some may be formed during the chlorination of water. No information is available on the risks now presented by water containing these compounds; standards are only now being established, and new filtering systems may be called for if public water exceeds these standards.[12] The study of organics in the water supply is an increasingly important research area.

Bottled Water   In some regions, consumers have become sufficiently alarmed about their local water supplies to turn to buying bottled water for their own personal consumption. The choice is an individual matter, and we take no position regarding its appropriateness. However, in buying water, as in buying any other product, the consumer needs to be alert to fraudulent claims. Mineral waters sold from "famous spas" offer no known health advantages and may be undesirably high in sodium.[13] On the other hand, bottled water sold in the United States must be tested by the producers once a year for safety and must meet standards set by the Food and Drug Administration for its contents of many chemical substances.[14]

The matter of water quantity still must be discussed. Is there enough to meet our needs? Water is an abundant, natural resource, and until recently its availability has been unquestioned. But the use of water in the industrial countries may put a strain on the supply. Used by agriculture for irrigating and by industry for transporting, dissolving, washing, rinsing, cooling, flushing away waste, and many other purposes, water in huge quantities is diverted from its original, ordinary uses. In the future the water supply may limit human progress. It has been estimated, for example, that if the U.S. population increases by another 20 percent or so, the water supply will be unable to continue meeting all the demands placed on it. We will therefore have to compromise our living standards in order to meet the

[10]Kawata, 1978.

[11]Varma, Serdahely, and Katz, 1976.

[12]N. Wade, Drinking water: Health hazards still not resolved (news and comment), *Science* 196 (1977):1421-1422.

[13]Keller, 1978.

[14]D. C. Fletcher, Safety standards for bottled drinking water (answer to a reader's question), *Journal of the American Medical Association* 238 (1977):2072.

top-priority need for safe, pure water for individual human use.[15]

This book is about individual nutrition and has dealt little with the economic and ecological problems of worldwide supply and demand. This discussion of water brings those problems into the foreground. To continue surviving and to maintain a desirable quality of life in an increasingly crowded and complicated world may mean making some hard choices in the near future.

Summing Up

Water in the body forms part of such chemical compounds as protein, participates in many chemical reactions, and serves as a solvent, transportation medium, and lubricant. Its heat-holding character helps regulate body temperature. Water makes up 55 to 60 percent of the body's weight.

Fluids and electrolytes provide the environment that supports the life of all the body's cells. Their concentration and composition are regulated to remain as constant as possible. Total body water is kept constant by regulating intake and excretion. Intake occurs when the osmotic pressure (solute concentration) of the blood is high, causing withdrawal of water from the salivary glands. The resultant dryness of the mouth stimulates thirst. High osmotic pressure of the blood also stimulates the kidneys to retain water through two hormonal mechanisms, one regulated by the antidiuretic hormone, the other by aldosterone. Excretion occurs whenever body water exceeds needs.

The principal electrolytes in body fluids are sodium, chloride, phosphorus, and potassium; each of these is maintained at a constant concentration by means of renal excretion. Sodium and chloride are the major extracellular electrolytes, and potassium and phosphorus are the major intracellular electrolytes. The electrolytes are involved in moving body water from place to place (by being moved themselves across cell membranes), thus maintaining the water balance. They also determine the pH of body fluids, maintaining the acid-base balance. The total concentrations of electrolytes in all the body compartments are maintained in a vital equilibrium, the electrolyte balance.

In maintaining pH, some major minerals act as base-formers, others as acid-formers. The presence of minerals in foods determines whether the food is an acid-forming or a base-forming food. Thanks to the specialized filtering work of the kidneys, changes in the relative proportions of these foods in the diet alter the acidity of urine but not of the body fluids. In renal disease, dietary concentrations of the major minerals must be strictly controlled.

Fluid and electrolyte imbalances occur when large amounts of fluid

[15]R. W. Phillips, Future programs for increasing food production with reference to the pre-school child, in *Pre-School Child Malnutrition: Primary Deterrent to Human Progress,* an international conference on prevention of malnutrition in the pre-school child, Washington, D.C., December 1964, publication 1282 (Washington, D.C.: National Academy of Sciences, National Research Council, 1966).

are lost, as in vomiting, diarrhea, or sweating. Loss of extracellular fluid occurs in these conditions; intracellular fluid then shifts out of cells to compensate, causing abnormal distribution of electrolytes across cell membranes and consequent cellular malfunction. In the case of sweating, the principal electrolytes that are lost are sodium and chloride. Replacement is achieved by increasing water and salt intake. The imbalances caused by vomiting and diarrhea, burns, and hemorrhages are medical emergencies; replacement should be managed by a physician.

Public water may contain significant quantities of minerals, depending on the source and locale. Hard water is rich in calcium and magnesium; soft water is rich in sodium. The relationship of soft water to heart disease has led to the suggestion that an upper limit be established for the amount of sodium permissible in drinking water.

Discharging industrial waste into the environment may add toxic heavy metals like mercury, cadmium, and lead to the water supply, creating a health hazard. A second threat to water is microbial contamination, which can be controlled by sewage treatment that includes chlorination. Nevertheless, contamination of water remains the primary cause of disease in the underdeveloped countries. A third concern is that highly toxic organic compounds may enter the water supply from agricultural and industrial use; little is known about these. As more and more water is diverted to industrial purposes, there is a need for stringent regulation of its use. There may be a need in the future to limit technological uses of water in order to continue providing a sufficient and safe supply to sustain human life.

To Explore Further

Both of the following are classics in the literature of the history of life on earth, revealing, facets of the intimate relationship between environmental water and the life of cells. Oparin's book is available in paperback:

- Oparin, A. I. *Origin of Life.* New York: Dover, 1938.

- Wald, G. The origin of life. *Scientific American* 190 (August 1956):44-53 (also Offprint No. 47).

A teaching aid, *Nutrient Metabolism: Water, the Essential Nutrient* by J. Robinson, can be ordered from the Nutrition Today Society (address in Appendix J).

The following references are also recommended:

- Calabrese, E. J., and Tuthill, R. W. Sources of elevated sodium levels in drinking water . . . and recommendations for reduction. *Journal of Environmental Health* 41 (1978):151-155.

- Keller, W. D. Drinking water: A geochemical factor in human health. *Geological Society of America Bulletin* 89 (March 1978):334-336.

- Varma, M. M., Serdahely, S. G., and Katz, H. M. Physiological effects of trace elements and chemicals in water. *Journal of Environmental Health* 39 (1976):90-100.

Contaminants in Food

In regard to acute illness, man's food supply probably is safer today than at any time in recorded history . . . [At the same time,] unexpected hazards might arise from unfortunate combinations of circumstances in which only man is at fault or in which nature plays a role over which man has no control. . . . [The stage is set] for improved controls and pertinent research that promise greater assurance of the long-range safety of our food supply.

J. M. COON and J. C. AYRES

The last Highlight (13) dealt with intentional food additives and concluded that as a hazard to consumers, they were greatly overrated. This Highlight deals with indirect additives — things that get into food by mistake — and concludes that they are a matter for real concern. Intentional additives are sixth and last on FDA's priority list of areas of concern; contaminants are third on that same list (see page 475), even when food poisoning and pesticide residues are set aside and considered separately.

What are contaminants, and why are they considered so dangerous? A few examples will help to answer this question.

In 1953 a number of people in Minamata, Japan, became ill with a disease no one had seen before. By 1960, 121 cases had been reported, including 23 in infants. Mortality was high; 46 died, and in the survivors the symptoms were ugly: "progressive blindness, deafness, incoordination, and intellectual deterioration."[1] The cause was ultimately revealed to be methylmercury contamination of fish these people were eating from the bay they lived on. The infants who contracted the disease had not eaten any fish but their mothers had, and even though the mothers exhibited no symptoms during their pregnancies, the poison had been affecting their unborn babies. Manufacturing plants in the region were discharging mercury into the waters of the bay, the mercury was turning to methylmercury on leaving the factories, and the fish in the bay were accumulating this poison in their bodies. Some of the families who were affected were eating fish from the bay every day.[2]

In 1910, Dr. Alice Hamilton of the United States began documenting her observations of the toxicity to humans of another environmentally derived heavy metal, lead. Factory workers intoxicated with lead poisoning experienced a wide variety of symptoms, she said, including anemia, constipation, loss of appetite, abnormal kidney function, jaundice due to liver damage, "wrist drop" (loss of muscular control of the hand), irritability, drowsiness, stupor, and coma. Mothers exposed to lead more often had abortions and stillbirths, and their children were more often sick.[3] Lead also finds its way into food, as will be shown below.

In 1973, in Michigan, 1,000 pounds of polybrominated biphenyl (PBB), a toxic chemical, were accidentally mixed into some livestock feed that was distributed throughout the state. The chemical found its way into millions of animals and then into humans. The seriousness of the accident began to come to light when dairy farmers reported their cows going dry, aborting their calves, and developing abnormal growths on their hooves. Although more than 30,000 cattle, sheep, and swine and more than a million chickens were destroyed, effects on people were not prevented. By 1982 it was estimated that 97 percent of Michigan's residents had become contaminated

[1] W. A. Krehl, Mercury, the slippery metal, *Nutrition Today*, November/December 1972, pp. 4-15.

[2] Krehl, 1972.

[3] M. A. Wessel and A. Dominski, Our children's daily lead, *American Scientist* 65 (1977):294-298.

with PBB. Among the effects in exposed farm residents were nervous system aberrations, and alterations in the liver and immune systems.[4]

Mercury and lead are both heavy metals and PBB is an organic halogen. These two classes of chemicals are among the most toxic and widespread in our environment. A list of the chemical contaminants of greatest concern in foods is presented in Table 1.

On first studying this subject, a reader is likely to want the question answered, "How serious is all this — how dangerous is it for *me?*" Yet no one who has pursued the subject realistically expects to have that question answered in any simple way. It may be a negligible problem in your particular area, today, but tomorrow it may become a severe one if there is a major spill or other accident. A generalization is a possible answer to that question,

[4]*Tallahassee Democrat*, 16 April 1982.

however: The *hazard* is probably small, because we are generally well protected, but in the event of an accident the *risk* can suddenly become very great. (See Highlight 13 for the meaning of *hazard* as opposed to *toxicity.*)

The number of contaminants we could discuss here, and the amount of information available about them, is far beyond our scope. Instead of dealing superficially with all of them, our choice is to illustrate some principles by presenting only two contaminants in depth: lead and DDT. You can then apply the principles to your study of the others at another time.

Lead   Lead is a metal ion with two positive charges, similar in some ways to nutrient minerals like iron, calcium, and zinc. In fact it competes with them for some of the slots they normally occupy, but then is unable to fulfill their roles. Thus it interferes with many of the body's systems. The

most vulnerable tissues are the nervous system, kidney, and bone marrow. Lead is readily transferred across the placenta and its most severe effects are on the developing nervous system. Absorption of lead is 5 to 8 times greater in children than it is in adults, and it tends to stay in their bodies.[5]

This brings us to the first of several points to be made about contamination. A factor in the potential seriousness of a contaminant of food is the extent to which the contaminant lingers in the body. If it were merely a few particles of sand or blue glass beads (Chapter 5), the contaminant wouldn't even stay in the body long enough to worry about, and would interact with it not at all. If it entered the system and then were rapidly metabolized to some harmless compound, then its ingestion might not give cause for concern. Vita-

[5]Metabolism of vitamin D in lead poisoning, *Nutrition Reviews* 39 (1981):372-373.

Table 1.   Chemical contaminants of concern in foods, U.S., 1970-1980*

Heavy metals	Halogenated compounds	Others
lead	chlorine	asbestos
mercury	iodine	dioxins
cadmium	vinyl chloride	acrilonitrile
selenium	ethylene dichloride	lysinoalanine
arsenic	trichloroethylene	diethylstilbestrol
	polychlorinated biphenyls (PCBs)	heat-induced mutagens
	polybrominated biphenyls (PBBs)	antibiotics (in animal feed)

*From E. M. Foster, How safe are our foods? *Nutrition Reviews/Supplement*, January 1982, pp. 28-34.

min C seems to fall into the category of rapidly metabolized drugs, and this accounts for its relative lack of toxicity in most people. If the contaminant were rapidly and preferentially excreted, then, too, it might be possible for the body to survive a brief exposure time. But if it enters the body, interacts with the body's systems, is not metabolized or excreted, and fools the cells' protein machinery into accepting it as part of their structure, then it will persist. Additional doses will be piled on top of the first ones and it will accumulate. All these things are true of lead and

that's why it's so deadly.

Organic halogens like PBB are, as the term organic says, molecules like vitamin C that could in theory be metabolized and disposed of — but their deadliness is related to the same factors. They are resistant to metabolism either in or outside the body (by microorganisms) and furthermore they accumulate from one species to the next, with a consequent build-up in the food chain (Figure 1).

The anemia caused by lead poisoning is the result of many effects lead has on blood. Besides competing with iron for absorption, lead

interferes with several enzymes that synthesize heme, the iron-containing portion of hemoglobin. Lead also deranges the structure of the red blood cell membrane, making it leaky and fragile. Lead interacts with white blood cells, too, interfering with their phagocytic activity (Highlight 22), and also binds to antibodies, thereby reducing the body's resistance to disease.[6]

[6]Wessel and Dominski, 1977; Nutritional influences on lead absorption in man, *Nutrition Reviews* 39 (1981):363-365; D. Pincus and C. V. Saccar, Lead poisoning, *American Family Physician* 19 (1979):120-124.

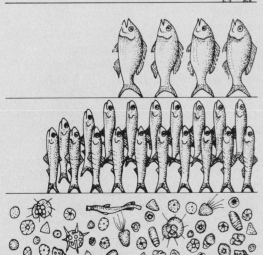
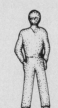

Level 4
a 150-pound person

Level 3
a hundred pounds of fish

Level 2
a few tons of plant-eating fish

Level 1
several tons of
producer organisms

Figure 1   How a food chain works. A person whose principal animal protein source is fish may consume about 100 pounds of fish in a year. These fish will, in turn, have consumed a few tons of plant-eating fish in the course of their lifetimes. The plant eaters, in their lifetimes, will have consumed several tons of photosynthetic producer organisms.

The concern about persistent contaminants is implicit in this pyramid. Assuming 100 percent retention of the contaminant at each level (an oversimplification), a person, being at the top of the food chain, could ingest in a year the amount of contaminant that had accumulated in several tons of producer organisms.

Miniglossary

BHT (butylated hydroxytoluene) (BYOO-til-ate-ed high-DROX-ee-TAHL-you-een): this and its relative **BHA (butylated hydroxyanisole)** (high-DROX-ee-ANN-is-ole) are antioxidants commonly used in bread and other baked products.

heavy metal: any of a number of mineral ions such as mercury and lead, so-called because they are of relatively high atomic weight. Many heavy metals are poisonous.

indirect additive: a substance that can get into food not through its intentional introduction but as a result of its coming in contact with the food during growing, processing, packaging, storing, or some other stage before the food is consumed.

organic halogen: an organic compound containing one or more atoms of a halogen — fluorine, chlorine, iodine, or bromine.

Lead has many other known molecular effects, but these few are enough to illustrate several characteristics of heavy metals. For one thing, all heavy metals act in some of the same ways. If you reread the description of the symptoms of mercury poisoning in Minamata, you can imagine how they, too, arise from interference by mercury with proteins that are trying to do their jobs.

Cadmium, another major environmental contaminant, has similar effects, and the interference of arsenic with respiratory proteins is well known.

You can also see from these examples how interconnected nutrition is with the effects of contaminants. There is more to that story, however, because specific nutrients interact with heavy metals in specific ways. Again, taking lead as an example: Total food intake, fat intake, and calcium, iron, and zinc intakes are known to alter animals' (and probably humans') susceptibility to lead toxicity. Examples:

● A diet low in calcium permits greater amounts of lead to accumulate in the body, probably by permitting more lead to be absorbed.

● Iron deficiency, even mild iron deficiency, permits greater lead intoxication. Iron deficiency in a nursing female makes her milk lead content higher.

● Zinc status affects both tissue accumulation of lead and sensitivity to its effects.[7]

● The absorption of lead is greatest when the stomach is empty.[8]

[7]K. R. Mahaffey, Nutritional factors in lead poisoning, *Nutrition Reviews* 39 (1981):353-362.

[8]M. B. Rabinowitz, J. D. Kopple, and G. W. Wetherill, Effect of food intake and fasting on gastrointestinal lead absorption in humans, *American Journal of Clinical Nutrition* 33 (1980):1784-1788.

The interaction of nutrients with contaminants like lead raises an important point. When an agency is charged with setting the "maximum permissible level" of an environmental contaminant, it sets about testing animals to see what levels bring about detectable ill effects. Usually these animals are being fed the standard laboratory chow — a very nutritious diet — and the only thing varied is their exposure to the contaminant. Healthy, well-nourished animals are likely to have considerably greater resistance to toxicity than they would if they were sick or malnourished. This fact must be remembered when the limits are set.

In 1981, 535,000 U.S. children ages 6 months to 5 years were screened and 22,000 were found with symptoms caused by lead toxicity, reflecting a prevalent national health problem. In the same screening, an almost equal number of children — 23,000 — were identified who needed treatment for iron deficiency, a long-familiar, widespread public health problem. Thus lead toxicity ranks with iron deficiency in prevalence and severity and is more than just a theoretical hazard. One out of every 50 children in rural areas, and more than one out of every 10 inner city children is afflicted with it.[9]

DDT   DDT has aroused concerns typical of those held by consumers about organic insecticides and pesticides in general. DDT is the oldest of the modern insecticides, and has been much studied. It is soluble in fat, and so finds its way into the fat or oil depots of animals or plants. Corn is often sprayed with DDT, so corn oil may contain it; animals fed the corn will then accumulate DDT in their body fat, including the fat of milk and dairy products. Human consumers of corn oil margarine, milk, or dairy products then receive it in

[9]Update: childhood lead poisoning, *Journal of the American Dietetic Association* 80 (1982):592, 594.

their turn — and nursing mothers may then pass it on in their breast milk to their babies. No actual harm to human infants has been documented, but the concentrations of DDT in human milk have often been found to be two or more times higher than the maximum permitted in cows' milk, and it is not known what long-term effects might occur. DDT is known to impair the structure of the material from which birds' eggshells are made, and is partly to blame for the decline of several bird species, including the great bald eagle, the U.S. national emblem.

Opponents of the use of DDT have been very emotional at times: "Every time [the infant] sucks the swollen breasts he gets more DDT than is allowed in cow's milk at the supermarket. Be objec-

tive? Forget it. Objective is for fence posts. How can you be objective in the face of a global insanity that is DDT?"[9] However, others have countered by offering information that makes the DDT contamination of human milk seem less serious than it might at first appear to be.

The point made by those who say "Don't panic" is very important to an understanding of the whole issue of contamination of food with anything potentially harmful to health: that the *amount* of contamination makes all the difference. If it is low enough, then it can be tolerated without ill effects. In the case of DDT, it has been argued that the amount is, indeed, low enough. According to Thomas Jukes, of the Medical Physics Division of the Donner Laboratory at the University of California, Berkeley, the comparison between breast milk and cow's milk DDT levels makes breast milk look bad because the cow's milk level is absurdly low: "Zero tolerance' has been the policy with respect to additives in milk. . . . More than ten years ago, it was evident that the entire stocks of canned milk in the United

[10]Ed Chaney, Information Director of National Wildlife Federation, as quoted by T. H. Jukes, Fact and fancy in nutrition and food science, *Journal of the American Dietetic Association* 59 (1971), reprinted in T. P. Labuza, *The Nutrition Crisis: A Reader* (St. Paul: West, 1975), pp. 456-473.

Table 2.   **DDT at Various Dose Levels: Effects***

Dose	Effects
A dose of 1/2 mg/kg/day	observed to be tolerated by volunteers for 21 months and by workers for 6-1/2 years
1/2 that dose	tolerated by workers 19 years
1/25 that dose	the highest amount found in human breast milk†
1/62 that dose	the amount Indians were receiving in 1964 from their houses, which were sprayed, and from food
1/200 that dose	the amount the general population of the U.S. was receiving, 1953-1954
1/1,250 that dose	the amount the U.S. population was receiving 20 years later

*Adapted from T. H. Jukes, Fact and fancy in nutrition science, from *Journal of the American Dietetic Association* 59 (1971), reprinted in T. P. Labuza, *The Nutrition Crisis: A Reader* (St. Paul: West, 1975), pp. 456-473.

†Assuming the newborn baby would drink 1 1/3 pints of milk per day.

States gave positive tests for DDT. It was, therefore, necessary to face facts, and two choices were available: to ban cows' milk from interstate commerce or to set a tolerance limit."[11] A tolerance limit was therefore set, but it was absurdly low — 140 times lower than the level permitted in most agricultural products.

Table 2 shows that the highest amount a baby would receive from breast milk containing this much DDT would be less than 1/25 as much as people have been seen to tolerate for years without ill effects. Even if infants were ten times more susceptible than adults (and this is highly unlikely), no ill effects could be expected. In all likelihood, infants are more resistant, not more sensitive, than adults to DDT.[12]

Before reaching any conclusions about the acceptability of any amount of DDT in any food, one would have to sift through much more information and make many judgments. *No conclusion has been reached here*, but a point has been made. If it is impossible to have "zero" contamination of food products with toxic substances, this is not necessarily a disaster. Testing can show where the line can be drawn below which doses are acceptable.

DDT can serve as an example of another point, also. Unlike the heavy metals and the persistent halogens, DDT is metabolized in the body, although slowly. It therefore accumulates less rapidly in tissues and builds up less rapidly in the food chain. However, its being metabolized offers a new concern. The question has to be asked: What does this contaminant get metabolized *to*? What are the effects of its metabolites in the body? (You may recall from Highlight 13 the case of nitrites, which may be metabolized to nitrosamines, which may in turn cause cancer.) In mice, DDT is metabolized to DDE, which is a carcinogen.[13] However, this metabolic pathway does not exist in other animals, and DDT has never caused cancer in human beings, even in those who have received DDT for many years at high levels.[14] Obviously, the question is important in each case of a metabolizable contaminant.

It should be noted that sometimes a substance can turn out to be beneficial, not harmful, because of the pathway it follows in the body. For example, the antioxidant BHT, often used in

breads, aroused consumers' fears some years ago on the grounds that it might cause cancer. But among the many tests that were performed on BHT and other additives there were several showing that animals fed large amounts of these substances lived longer than controls. Antioxidants apparently induce the liver to produce enzymes that destroy toxins.[15]

DDT is like lead and probably all other contaminants, in that its toxicity depends on the nutritional state of the animal exposed to it. It depresses liver stores of vitamin A in rats — when they are raised on a particular diet that is deficient in the amino acid methionine (soybeans).[16] It accumulates in body fat, and this leads to some effects that might surprise the observer unaware of the principles of nutrition and metabolism. As long as the animal is well fed, the DDT is tucked away (sequestered) in the body's fat. But if the animal is deprived of food, its body fat starts breaking down, the DDT is mobilized, and it produces blood concentrations potentially toxic to the central nervous system.[17]

[11]Jukes, 1971.
[12]Jukes, 1971.
[13]D. V. Parke, Toxic chemicals in food, *Journal of the Forensic Science Society* 16 (1977):189-196.
[14]T. H. Jukes, How safe is our food supply? *Archives of Internal Medicine* 138 (1978):772-774.
[15]Jukes, 1971.
[16]R. A. Shakman, Nutritional influences on the toxicity of environmental pollutants: A review, *Archives of Environmental Health* 28 (1974):105-113.
[17]Shakman, 1974.

No generalizations can be made as to what specific effects a particular contaminant will have on a particular nutrient in a given species. Similarly, no general statement can be made as to which kind of nutrient imbalance in the diet might most severely handicap an animal or a human in its efforts to resist a pesticide's effect. However, there is a generalization that can be made. Not 100 percent of the time, but more often than not, an adequate diet and optimal health protect against the toxicity of food contaminants and other environmental pollutants.

By this token, it should be repeated, when animal tests are analyzed to determine what levels of a contaminant are acceptable, the analysis should be made with an awareness of the type of diet the test animals were receiving. It cannot be assumed that a dose level that can easily be resisted by healthy, well-nourished animals or people will also be acceptable for their weaker counterparts.

CAUTION WHEN YOU READ!

Toxicity depends on dietary adequacy.

This principle applies generally to actions taken by policymakers and it is taken into account in the margin-of-safety allowances made in setting permissible levels of contamination. But the principle also applies to each individual person. If you want to be well protected against possible exposure to toxic environmental contaminants in the future, you should look to your own health today. If you want your children to be protected, you should make sure that they receive an adequate and varied diet.

Perspective on Contaminants in Foods   It was said, at the start, that the hazard from contamination of food is probably small, and that the risk to individuals is from accidental gross contamination. However, this statement needs qualification. For one thing, lead toxicity is known to be a serious problem in U.S. children today. As for other contaminants, no one knows to what extent the total burden of contaminants accumulating in the environment may be reaching levels that constitute a hazard to human beings. No one knows whether some individuals may be susceptible today to contamination levels already present in some

areas. Another unknown factor is the question of interaction among contaminants. A substance which poses no threat by itself may, in combination with others, present significant danger; an example is the chlorine in drinking water mentioned in Chapter 14. Another unknown is the time factor. Many of the substances of concern have been around for only a short time. What are the effects of prolonged exposure to them? Contaminants are sometimes hard to identify; sometimes it is not even known that they are present; and so they are hard to regulate. There is no systematic procedure for monitoring or controlling their presence in food except in individual cases.[18] It will take vigilance and wisdom to detect and appropriately control these substances. Among the qualifications the people who do this will have to have is an in-depth understanding of nutrition.

To Explore Further

The food supply was the subject of a symposium published in a *Supplement* to *Nutrition Reviews* in January, 1982. Its safety was reviewed in:

● Foster, E. M. How safe are our foods? *Nutrition Reviews/Supplement*, January 1982, pp. 28-34.

[18]S. M. Oace, Diet and cancer, *Journal of Nutrition Education* 10 (1978):106-108.

A recent re-evaluation of the margin of safety for mercury in seafood has reached some reassuring conclusions, which are well worth reading:

● Margolin, S. Mercury in marine seafood: The scientific medical margin of safety as a guide to the potential risk to public health. *World Review of Nutrition and Dietetics* 34 (1980):182-265.

Lead was the subject of several articles in the October 1981 issue of *Nutrition Reviews*. The first article was:

● Mahaffey, K. R. Nutritional factors in lead poisoning. *Nutrition Reviews* 39 (1981):353-362.

The clinical nutrition case for the month described a typical episode of lead poisoning in a child:

● Metabolism of vitamin D in lead poisoning. *Nutrition Reviews* 39 (1981):372-373.

A thought-provoking discussion of other issues related to lead poisoning, not mentioned here, is:

● Wessel, M. A., and Dominski, A. Our children's daily lead. *American Scientist* 65 (1977):294-298.

Diagnosis and treatment of lead poisoning are outlined in:

● Pincus, D., and Saccar, C. V. Lead poisoning. *American Family Physician* 19 (1979):120-124.

Another problem related to lead and not dealt with here is the problem of detecting lead contamination in foods and using an appropriate standard. According to this important article, the standards that have been used to detect lead in foods have themselves been contaminated with lead, so that the amounts people's bodies contain may be much higher that has been thought in the past:

● Settle, D. M., and Patterson, C. C. Lead in albacore: Guide to lead pollution in Americans. *Science* 207 (1980):1167-1176.

Lead poisoning is especially likely in low-income children because they often live in old houses near heavy traffic and are at risk for malnutrition. The WIC program, aimed at remedying nutrition problems in children under 5, is an ideal program for reaching children at risk:

● Preventing lead poisoning: WIC clinics help reach children at risk. *Food & Nutrition* (a USDA publication) 10 (June 1980):4-7.

It is recommended that you not over-use newspaper for grilling food because of the lead content of newsprint:

● Lao, Y. J., and Blackwell, F. O. Potential hazard from newspaper as fuel for grilling food. *Journal of Environmental Health*, January/February 1980, pp. 197-198.

Articles of interest on food contaminants in *FDA Consumer* recently have been:

● Level of PCB's lowered. *FDA Consumer*, September 1979, p. 3.

● Watching the food of animals that produce food, *FDA Consumer*, October 1979, pp. 15-17.

● Corwin, E. On getting the lead out of food, *FDA Consumer*, March 1982, pp. 19-21.

● Better pesticide detection proposed, *FDA Consumer*, December 1979-January 1980, pp. 26-27.

The first article expresses concern over PCB levels in fish in the waters of Colorado, Illinois, Indiana, Massachussetts, Michigan, New Jersey, New York, Ohio, Pennsylvania, and Wisconsin. The second addresses the problem of drug (for example, antibiotic) residues in the flesh of animals given feed containing drugs. The third describes FDA's priorities for reducing lead in the food supply, beginning with canned foods (solder is 98% lead). The fourth proposes better ways of detecting pesticides in foods.

WHO (World Health Organization) has published several dozen booklets on evaluation and testing of additives, contaminants, pesticides, and the like. For example:

● *Pesticide Residues in Food*, Technical Report Series 592, 1976, available from WHO (address in Appendix J).

Diet Rating

With a balanced perspective on foods and a sense of what's important in diet planning and what's not, you can evaluate the many different diets people consume. Here's a summary of the questions you might ask (perhaps you can think of others). Start with 100 points and subtract if any of these criteria are not met:

a. Does the diet provide a reasonable number of kcalories (enough to maintain weight; not too many; and if a reduction diet, not fewer than 1,200 kcalories for an average-size person)? If no, give it a minus 10.

b. Does it provide enough, but not too much, protein (at least the recommended intake or RDA but not more than twice that much)? If no, minus 10.

c. Does it provide enough fat for satiety but not so much fat as to go against current recommendations (say, between 20 and 35 percent of the kcalories from fat)? If no, minus 10.

d. Does it provide enough carbohydrate to spare protein and prevent ketosis (100 grams of carbohydrate for the average-size person)? Is it mostly complex carbohydrate (not more than 10 percent of the kcalories as concentrated

sugar)? If no to either or both, minus 10.

e. Does it offer a balanced assortment of vitamins and minerals — that is, foods from all food groups? If a food group is omitted (for example, meats), is a suitable substitute provided? Count six food groups in all: milk/milk products; meat/fish/poultry/eggs; legumes; fruits; vegetables; grains. For *each* food group omitted and not adequately substituted for, subtract 10 points.

f. Does it offer variety, in the sense that different foods can be selected each day? If you'd class it as "monotonous," give it a minus 10.

g. Does it consist of ordinary foods that are available locally (for example, in the main grocery stores) at the prices people normally pay? Or does the dieter have to buy special, expensive, or unusual foods to adhere to the diet? If you'd class it as "bizarre" or "requiring unusual foods," minus 10.

To apply these criteria to a diet, first make up a day's menus following the diet rules. Then figure out the number of kcalories, the grams of protein, fat, and carbohydrate delivered, and the number of servings of food from each food group. You can do this by looking up each food in the Table of Food Composition, Appendix H. An easier way, however, is to translate the food servings into exchanges, group the exchanges, and add up their contributions of nutrients and kcalories as in Forms 1 and 2. Then figure the percentages of kcalories using Form 3.

Using this system, try evaluating three or more of the following diets:

1. Your own diet.

2. The diet of a local ethnic group other than your own.

3. The vegetarian diet recommended in Highlight 4.

4. Dr. Atkins' Superenergy Diet (unlimited amounts of fatty foods — bacon, mayonnaise, fatty meats, rich cream sauces — and NO fruits, vegetables, potatoes, starches, sugars, breads).

5. The Scarsdale diet (all the lean meat, poultry, and cheese you want; fish, eggs; NO breads, pastries).

6. The ZIP diet (eating no food at all).

7. The Zen macrobiotic diet (the final stage involves eating only brown rice and tea).

8. The Pritikin diet (whole grains, vegetables, legumes, and fruit; NO foods containing fat and cholesterol such as beef and eggs; no milk/milk products).

9. The ice cream diet (all the ice cream you want; nothing else).

10. Any other diet of your choice (what's the latest popular paperback on diet in your local bookstore?).

Form 1. Form for Translating the Day's Menus into Exchanges

Menu item	Serving size	Number of exchanges this serving size represents	Types of exchanges

Form 2. Form for Computing Protein-Fat-Carbohydrate Contributions of the Day's Exchanges

Type of exchange	Number of exchanges	Total protein contributed (g)	Total fat contributed (g)	Total carbohydrate contributed (g)	Total energy contributed (kcal)

Total energy: _____ kcal

Form 3.   Form for Computing Intakes of Protein, Fat, Carbohydrate as Percent of kCalories*

Protein:_____ g × 4 kcal/g = _____ protein kcal.

Carbohydrate:_____ g × 4 kcal/g = _____ carbohydrate kcal.

Fat:_____ g × 9 kcal/g = _____ fat kcal.

Protein kcal as percentage of total kcal:_____ percent.
Carbohydrate kcal as percentage of total:_____ percent.
Fat kcal as percentage of total:_____ percent.

*If you need help with figuring percentages, turn to Appendix D.

PART THREE

NUTRITION THROUGHOUT LIFE

INTRODUCTION

CONTENTS

THE PROCESSES OF GROWTH

"I wish you wouldn't squeeze so," said the Dormouse, who was sitting next to her. "I can hardly breathe."

"I can't help it," said Alice very meekly: "I'm growing."

LEWIS CARROLL, *Alice's Adventures in Wonderland*

The preceding chapters have been addressed to the adult. Wherever nutrition information has been relevant to your needs and concerns, examples and illustrations involving adults have been given, with only occasional references to infants, children, and older people. However, although the principles of nutrition apply throughout the life span, some changes in emphasis are appropriate for these other age groups.

Young people, from infancy through the teen years, are growing — a characteristic not shared by adults. In addition to nutritional needs for maintenance, then, young people have special needs related to the growth process. Furthermore, they are growing psychologically. In considering the nutritional needs and the feeding of infants, children, and teenagers, it is important to keep both kinds of growth in mind.

Growth is not a matter of everything's simply getting bigger all at once. From conception to adulthood, various organs differentiate, grow, and mature at different rates and times, each with its own characteristic pattern. It is helpful to distinguish three growth levels: that of the whole body, that of the organs and tissues, and that of the cells of each organ or tissue. At each level, different considerations become important.

Whole Body Growth Between conception and birth, a human being's weight increases from a fraction of a gram to 3,500 grams. The greatest rate of growth is in the fetal period between eight weeks and term, when weight increases over 500 times. After birth, a baby doubles its weight from 7 to 14 pounds in four months, then slows down somewhat and adds another 7 pounds in the next eight months, reaching about 21 pounds at one year. Thereafter, the growth rate slows to 5 pounds a year or less until adolescence, when it increases dramatically again.

Changes in height follow a similar pattern. From a fifth of a millimeter at three weeks of gestation, the embryo reaches 3 centimeters — just over an inch — at eight weeks, then about 20 inches

The 3 intensive growth periods:

Prenatal period.
First year.
Adolescence.

at birth. Thereafter, the increase in height is greatest during the first year (10 in), half that much the second year (5 in), and then slower still (2 to 3 in) until the adolescent growth spurt. At that time, a sudden increase of some 6 to 8 inches is achieved in a two- to two-and-a-half-year period.

What is important to notice about all this is that growth does not proceed at a steady pace, that the maximal rate of growth is in the prenatal period, and that the two postnatal periods during which growth is fastest are the first year and the teen years.

Growth of Organs and Tissues   The growth of each organ and tissue type has its own characteristic pattern and timing. In the fetus, for example, the heart and brain are well developed at 16 weeks, even though the lungs are still nonfunctional 10 weeks later. During the first year after birth, the brain doubles in weight, but it increases only about 20 percent thereafter. In contrast, the muscles will be more than 30 times heavier at maturity than at birth.

Each organ and tissue, then, has its own unique periods of intensive growth. Each organ needs the growth nutrients most during its own intensive growth period. Thus, a nutrient deficiency during one stage of development might affect the heart and at another might affect the developing limbs.

Cell Growth and Critical Periods   The cells of a single developing organ also follow a schedule unique to them. Each organ has its own specific time for cell division. This time may not be obvious, because it often precedes the period of growth in size. An interesting case is that of the brain. During development of the fetal brain, there is an early period when the cells are increasing dramatically in *number*. Each time a cell divides, it produces two that are half its size. These two do not grow but divide again, producing four cells that are still smaller. During this time of rapid cell division, the size of the brain hardly changes at all. Later, the cells begin to grow and also continue dividing, so that their *size and number* increase simultaneously. It is during these first two periods that the total number of cells to be found in the brain is determined for life. Later still, cell division ceases; thereafter, the total number of cells is fixed, but cells continue to increase in *size*. During this last period, the brain's growth in size is obvious. The development of almost every organ in the body follows a similar pattern, but the timing is different for each.

The third period, during which increase in size is taking place, is the time when the most intensive growth appears to be going on. But actually, the most important events are already over. This fact has important implications for nutrition. The period of cell division is a critical period, critical in the sense that the cell division taking place during that time can occur at only that time and at no other. Whatever nutrients and other environmental conditions are needed in this period

The brain and central nervous system are first to reach maturity.

Stages in organ growth:

1. hyperplasia (high-per-PLAY-zee-uh): an increase in cell number.

2. simultaneous hyperplasia and **hypertrophy** (high-PER-tro-fee): hyperplasia accompanied by an increase in cell size.

3. hypertrophy (except for the liver).

The brain also goes through a fourth period, multiplication of cell contacts, which depends on both nutrition and social stimulation (learning).

must be supplied on time if the organ is to reach its full potential. If cell division and the final cell number achieved are limited during a critical period, recovery is impossible. Thus, early malnutrition can have irreversible effects, although they may not become fully apparent until the person reaches maturity.

The effect of malnutrition during critical periods is seen in the shorter height of people who were undernourished in their early years; in the delayed sexual development of those undernourished during early adolescence; in the poor dental health of children whose mothers were malnourished during pregnancy;[1] and in the smaller brain size and brain cell number of children who have suffered from episodes of marasmus or kwashiorkor. The irreversibility of these effects is obvious when abundant, nourishing food fed after the critical time fails to remedy the growth deficit. Among the many Korean orphans adopted by U.S. families after the Korean War, for example, several years of catch-up growth have still not made up for the effects of early malnutrition.[2]

An area of active recent research points strongly to the probability that malnutrition in the prenatal and early postnatal periods also affects learning ability and behavior. Much of the severe mental retardation seen in developed countries such as the United States is of unknown cause, but many cases are thought to be due to protein deficiency during pregnancy.[3] Clearly, then, it is most critical to provide the best nutrition at early stages of life.

critical period: a finite period during development in which certain events may occur that will have irreversible, determining effects on later developmental stages. A critical period is usually a period of cell division in a body organ.

Growth of the Person   The concept of critical periods can also be applied, loosely, to personality growth. From the moment of birth (and perhaps even earlier), the human child is learning what to expect from life and how to cope with life's problems. These learning experiences follow one another in a characteristic sequence, and each must reach some degree of completion before the next can proceed. An infant's earliest impressions mold attitudes that in maturity may still affect behavior. Persons who nurture children must understand what is going on psychologically as well as physically. They must supply the nutrients that children need, and equally important, they must encourage learning and behavior that will help children to develop fully as human beings.

There are many ways of understanding and interpreting psychological growth and development. The one we have elected to follow is that

[1] D. P. DePaola and M. C. Alfano, Diet and oral health, *Nutrition Today,* May/June 1977, pp. 6-11, 29-32.

[2] N. M. Lien, K. K. Meyer, and M. Winick, Early malnutrition and 'late' adoption: a study of the effects on the development of Korean orphans adopted into American families, *American Journal of Clinical Nutrition* 30 (1977):1734-1739.

[3] S. P. Bessman, The justification theory: the essential nature of the non-essential amino acids, *Nutrition Reviews* 37 (1979):209-220.

of Erik Erikson, whose insightful description of the stages of human growth provides a framework for viewing the whole person.[4] Erikson sees human life as a sequence of eight periods. In each, the individual has a new learning task. To the extent that individuals master each successfully, they develop a strong foundation from which to proceed to the next. To the extent that they fail, they are handicapped in mastering the task at the next level. The stages in life and their respective learning tasks, as identified by Erikson, are:

- *Infant.* Trust versus distrust.
- *Toddler.* Autonomy versus shame and doubt.
- *Preschooler.* Initiative versus guilt.
- *School-age child.* Industry versus inferiority.
- *Adolescent.* Identity versus role confusion.
- *Young adult.*Intimacy versus isolation.
- *Adult.* Generativity versus stagnation.
- *Older adult.* Ego integrity versus despair.

Whether you agree with Erikson's view or see human development in some other light, we hope you agree with the principle that understanding the whole person is important, even in the providing of food. The health professional who knows where his or her client is, developmentally, is best able to communicate effectively with the client and efficiently deliver health care.

The chapters that follow are devoted to the special stages in life. Each stage is presented in terms of the physical growth and development it involves, the related nutrient needs, and feeding patterns that will supply the needed nutrients. For each stage, the attempt is made to put nutrient needs in perspective in relation to the needs of the whole person.

Within the chapters of Part Three, the digressions assume a new function. Until now, we have used them to alert you to fads and fallacies in nutrition information presented to the public. From here on, the digressions are used to illustrate real life situations in which you can apply the nutrition knowledge being discussed.

---

[4]We are indebted to S. R. Williams, who showed how Erikson's scheme could be integrated with nutrition principles in her book *Nutrition and Diet Therapy* (St. Louis: Mosby, 1973).

CHAPTER 15

CONTENTS

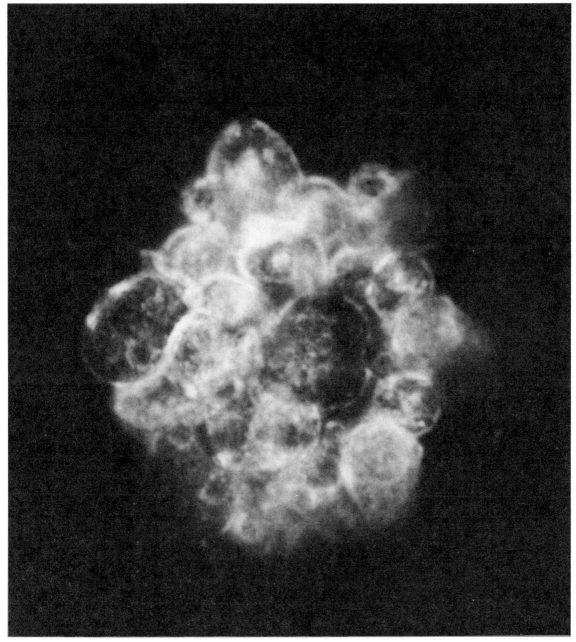

Human embryo three days old.

Courtesy of Landrum B. Shettles.

MOTHER AND INFANT

The Chinese ... credit a child with the age of one year on the day of its birth ... to recognize all the growth and development that has already occurred since the time of conception.

LINDA FERRILL ANNIS

We normally think of nutrition as affecting us here and now: You feel good this afternoon because you ate a good breakfast this morning, and your friend feels sleepy because she had a sweet dessert after lunch. But the effects of nutrition also extend over years. The woman who is expecting a baby and the health professional advising such a woman will be strongly motivated to attend to her nutrition needs if they *see* how critical the nutrients are to the normal course of events in prenatal development.

Pregnancy: The Impact of Nutrition on the Future

The only way nutrients can reach the developing infant in the uterus is through the mother's bloodstream. To convey these nutrients, the mother grows a whole new organ, the placenta, a sort of cushion in which the mother's and baby's blood vessels intertwine and exchange materials — nutrients and oxygen going into the baby's system, wastes leaving it to be excreted by the mother. If the mother's nutrition and stores in early pregnancy are inadequate when she is trying to grow a placenta, then the placenta will be small. No matter how well the mother eats later, her unborn baby will not be able to draw optimum nourishment through an undersized placenta. The infant born from an inadequate prenatal environment will be small and may be unable to attain the full size and health that would otherwise have been possible. A female born of such a pregnancy, even if well nourished throughout her later life, is ill equipped as an adult to grow an ample placenta and so may also bear an undersized or poorly developed infant who also will fail to achieve full adult potential. Thus the poor nutrition of a woman during her early pregnancy can have permanent effects on her *grandchild* even after that child has become an *adult*.[1]

Such effects are impossible to demonstrate directly in people, nor would researchers want to experiment on pregnant mothers to see

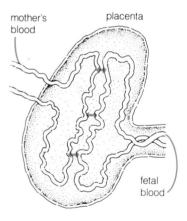

mother's blood   placenta

fetal blood

placenta (pla-SEN-tuh): the organ inside the uterus in which the mother's and fetus's circulatory systems intertwine and in which exchange of materials between maternal and fetal blood takes place. The fetus receives nutrients and oxygen across the placenta; the mother's blood picks up carbon dioxide and other waste materials to be excreted via her lungs and kidneys.

[1] D. B. Coursin, Maternal nutrition and the offspring's development, *Nutrition Today*, March/April 1973, pp. 12-18.

what caused stunting of the body or the brain in their children. But because the questions are important, many of them have been pursued through research using animals. We have every reason to believe that most findings from the animal experiments are applicable to human beings. Some have been inadvertently confirmed in human beings through accidents of history. Hospital records were maintained during the sieges of Holland and Leningrad in World War II, when women were starving before or during their pregnancies. These records showed that poor nutrition *prior* to pregnancy caused more birth defects and stillbirths than poor nutrition during pregnancy.

implantation: the stage of development in which the fertilized egg embeds itself in the wall of the uterus and begins to develop, during the first two weeks after conception.

embryo (EM-bree-oh): the developing infant during its second to eighth week after conception. Before the second week, it is called an **ovum** (OH-vum) or **zygote** (ZYE-goat).

fetus (FEET-us): the developing infant from the eighth week after conception until its birth.

uterus (YOO-ter-us): the womb, the muscular organ within which the infant develops before birth.

amniotic sac (am-nee-OTT-ic): the "bag of waters" in the uterus, in which the fetus floats.

Growth   Conditions in the uterus at the time of conception determine whether the fertilized egg will successfully implant itself in the uterine wall and begin development as it should. During the two weeks following fertilization, in the implantation stage, the egg cell divides into many cells, and these cells sort themselves into three layers. Very little growth in size takes place at this time; it is a critical period that precedes growth. Adverse influences at this time lead to failure to implant or to other disturbances so severe as to cause loss of the fertilized egg, possibly even before the woman knows she is pregnant. Many drugs affect the earliest intrauterine events and later cross the placenta freely. Most health professionals agree that, if possible, a potential mother should take no drugs at all, not even aspirin. Nutrition should be, and should have been, continuously optimal.

The next five weeks, the period of embryonic development, register astonishing physical changes. From the outermost layer of cells, the nervous system and skin begin to develop; from the middle layer, the muscles and internal organ systems; and from the innermost layer, the glands and linings of the digestive, respiratory, and excretory systems. At eight weeks, the three-centimeter-long embryo has a complete central nervous system, a beating heart, a fully formed digestive system, and the beginnings of facial features. Already, an embryonic tail has formed and almost completely disappeared again, and the fingers and toes are well defined.

The last seven months of pregnancy, the fetal period, bring about a tremendous increase in the size of the fetus. Intensive periods of cell division occur in organ after organ.

Meanwhile, the mother's body has been undergoing changes. As already mentioned, she has grown the placenta, which carries nutrients and oxygen to the fetus and carbon dioxide and other wastes to her lungs and kidneys for excretion. The amniotic sac has filled with fluid to cushion the infant. The mother's uterus and its supporting muscles have increased greatly in size, her breasts have changed and grown in preparation for lactation, and her blood volume has almost doubled to accommodate the added load of materials to be carried. The overall gain in weight of mother and child during pregnancy amounts to about 25 to 30 pounds (see Table 1).

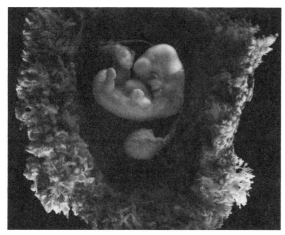

Six-week-old fetus attached to the placenta. At this time the fetus is less than half an inch long.

Courtesy of Dr. Roberts Rugh.

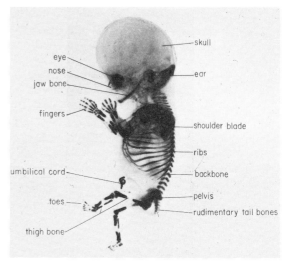

Eight-week-old fetus, showing development of the skeleton. The other tissues were treated so as to be transparent.

Courtesy of Dr. Roberts Rugh.

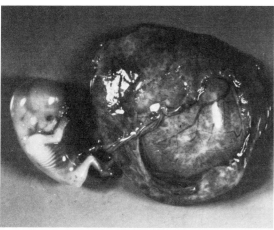

Ten-week-old fetus attached to the placenta. The blood vessels in the umbilical cord are clearly visible.

Courtesy of Dr. Roberts Rugh.

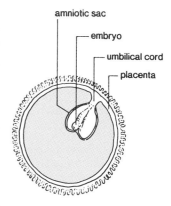

Fetus: 2-9 months.

Human embryo in the amniotic sac. Note the attachment to the placenta by a body stalk which will become the umbilical cord.

A mother's physiology changes during pregnancy, enough so that a naive observer might think that she is ill. She develops an apparent anemia, she may have edema, and her glucose tolerance changes, as if she were diabetic. These and other changes are normal for her altered state, however.

The "physiological anemia of pregnancy" results from the great increase in the mother's blood volume. The red blood cells do not increase as much as the blood fluid, so the number of cells per milliliter is low compared with the nonpregnant state. Values for protein, iron, folacin, and other nutrients are correspondingly lowered, while other values rise (cholesterol and fat-soluble vitamins are examples). The clinician who assesses a pregnant woman's nutrition status therefore uses a set of standards specific for pregnancy (see To Explore Further).

The edema of pregnancy is also "physiological" (that is, expected and normal) — provided that it is not accompanied by indicators of kidney disease such as high blood pressure or protein in the urine. This normal edema results from the raised secretion of the hormone estrogen toward the end of pregnancy, which helps to ready the uterus for delivery.

The altered glucose tolerance of pregnancy is also normal, but could easily be confused, by an untrained observer, with diabetes. These examples are intended to caution the reader who is not familiar with the special standards applicable to pregnancy to jump to no conclusions regarding out-of-line lab test values. The treatment of truly abnormal conditions is the subject of a later section ("Troubleshooting").

Nutrient Needs   Nutrient needs during periods of intensive growth are greater than at any other time and are greater for certain nutrients than for others, as shown in Figure 1. A study of the figure reveals some of the key needs.

Figure 1 Comparison of the nutrient needs of nonpregnant and pregnant women (over 23 years old). The nonpregnant woman's needs are set at 100 percent, the pregnant woman's needs shown as increases over 100 percent. The pregnant woman's iron needs cannot be met by ordinary diets, and she might need to take an iron supplement. (Calculated from the RDA tables, inside front cover.)

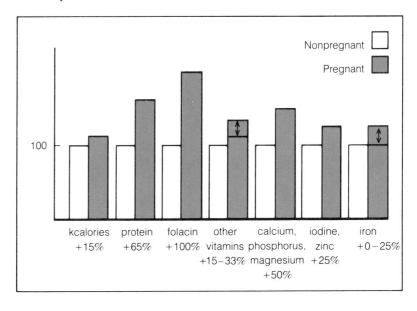

One of the smallest increases apparent is in kcalories; an increase of only 15 percent is recommended for pregnant women, but many individual women may need much more. In each case, enough kcalories are needed to spare protein for its all-important tissue-building work. A recommended average is 40 kcal/kg; and energy intake should never fall below 36 kcal/kg.[2] The increased need for protein is more dramatic — about 75 g/day or more — and generous amounts of carbohydrate are needed to spare the protein. There is no harm in a pregnant woman's taking up to 100 g of protein or even more; in fact, if she has been poorly nourished prior to pregnancy, this may be an ideal intake.

Recommended energy intake: 40 kcal/kg (18 kcal/lb).

Minimum energy intake: 36 kcal/kg (17 kcal/lb).

For a 120-lb woman, this represents at least 2,000 kcal and preferably 2,200 kcal/day.

[2] H. Oldham and B. B. Sheft, Effect of caloric intake on nitrogen utilization during pregnancy, *Journal of the American Dietetic Association* 27 (1951):847-854.

Table 1. Weight Gain during Pregnancy

Development	Weight gain (lbs)
Infant at birth	7 1/2
Placenta	1
Increase in mother's blood volume to supply placenta	4
Increase in size of mother's uterus and muscles to support placenta	2 1/2
Increase in size of mother's breasts	3
Fluid to surround infant in amniotic sac	2
Mother's fat stores	5 to 10
Total	25 to 30

The extraordinary need for folacin in the pregnant woman is due to the doubling of her blood volume. Folacin-deficiency anemia is more often seen in pregnant women than even iron-deficiency anemia, and it is often advisable for the physician to prescribe folacin as a supplement.[3] As you might expect, the vitamin needed in the next highest amount is the other B vitamin associated with the manufacture of red blood cells — B_{12}.

Among the minerals, those involved in building the skeleton — calcium, phosphorus, and magnesium — are in great demand during pregnancy, and increases of about 50 percent are recommended. Intestinal absorption of calcium doubles early in pregnancy, and the mineral is stored in the mother's bones. Later, as the fetal bones begin to calcify, there is a dramatic shift of calcium across the placenta, and the mother's bone stores are drawn upon. Most mothers' intakes have to be increased well above their prepregnancy intakes. If the mother's intake is less than 1.2 g/day, she will pay by losing more calcium from her bones than she has stored for this purpose.[4]

Less is known about the need for zinc during pregnancy, but in animals, zinc deficiency can set in suddenly and cause fetal malformations.[5] The penalty for iodine deficiency — cretinism — is well known.

Recommended protein intake: 75-100 g/day.

Recommended carbohydrate intake: about 50% of energy intake. In a 2,000 kcal/day intake, this represents 1,000 kcal of carbohydrate, or about 250 g. Four cups of milk a day will contribute about 50 g carbohydrate. An apple provides 10 g carbohydrate, and a slice of bread provides 15 g, so this recommendation implies generous intakes of fruit and bread exchanges.

Best food sources of folacin:
green, leafy vegetables.
legumes.
liver.
orange juice and cantaloupe.
other vegetables.
whole wheat products.

Four cups of milk a day will supply 1.2 g calcium. For other food sources, see Chapter 13; for milk substitutes, Highlight 15. The milk should be vitamin D fortified; if it is not, a vitamin D supplement may be needed.

[3]L. B. Bailey, C. S. Mahan, and D. Dimperio, Folacin and iron status in low-income pregnant adolescents and mature women, *American Journal of Clinical Nutrition* 33 (1980):1997-2001; V. Herbert, The vitamin craze, *Archives of Internal Medicine* 140 (1980):173-176.

[4]R. Kumar, W. R. Cohen, and F. H. Epstein, Vitamin D and calcium hormones in pregnancy, *New England Journal of Medicine* 302 (1980):1143-1145.

[5]L. S. Hurley, I. E. Dreosti, H. Swenerton, and J. Gowan, The movement of zinc in maternal and fetal rat tissues in teratogenic zinc deficiency, *Teratology* 1 (1968):216.

Ordinarily, a hemoglobin level below 13 g/100 ml is considered low for a woman (see Chapter 13). In pregnancy, values of 12 g are not unusual, and 11 g is where the line defining "too low" is often drawn.

Best food sources of iron:
  liver, oysters.
  red meat, fish, other meat.
  dried fruits.
  legumes (dried beans, peas, limas).
  dark green vegetables.

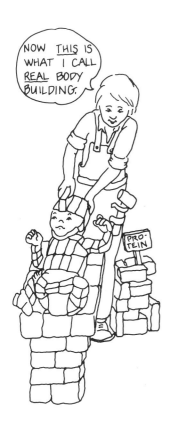

NOW THIS IS WHAT I CALL REAL BODY BUILDING.

PROTEIN

Iron is conserved by the body during pregnancy. Menstruation, which is normally the major route of excretion of iron, ceases; and absorption of iron increases up to threefold. (The blood protein responsible for iron absorption, transferrin, increases.) An additional adjustment is accomplished by the hormones of pregnancy, which act to raise the concentration of iron in the blood, by either increasing absorption still further, or mobilizing iron from its storage places in the bone marrow and internal organs, or both. Thus, a woman *theoretically* needs no more iron during pregnancy than she has needed all along, and the RDA for iron in pregnancy is not higher than for the nonpregnant woman. However, so few women enter pregnancy with adequate stores that the theoretical case hardly ever applies. Most women, even in the United States and Canada, have minimal iron stores; and the demands of pregnancy deplete them to the deficiency point. Even if a woman makes it to the end of pregnancy without falling into frank anemia, she may bleed excessively at delivery — hence the advisability of a prescribed iron supplement to boost her stores. At birth, a baby is supposed to have enough stored iron to last three to six months; this iron must also come from the mother's iron stores. It is considered advisable for almost all pregnant women to take an iron supplement throughout pregnancy and for two to three months after delivery.[6]

Eating Pattern and Weight Gain   If the woman's dietary pattern is already adequate at the start of pregnancy, it can be adjusted to meet changing nutrient needs. The nutrients needing the greatest increase are protein, calcium, phosphorus, magnesium, and folacin; so the foods selected for emphasis should normally be those in the milk, meat, and vegetable categories.

Because kcalorie needs increase less than nutrient needs, the pregnant woman must select foods of high nutrient density. For most women, appropriate choices include foods like skim milk, cottage cheese, lean meats, eggs, liver, dark green vegetables, and whole grain breads and cereals. For vitamin C, she should either increase the size of her one serving of a C-rich food, such as citrus fruit or broccoli, or add a second, fair C source, such as tomatoes. A suggested food pattern is shown in Table 2.

The pregnant woman must gain weight. Ideally, she will have begun her pregnancy at the appropriate weight for her height and will gain about 25 pounds, most of it in the second half of pregnancy. The ideal pattern is thought to be about 2 to 4 pounds during the first three months and a pound per week thereafter. The teenager needs to gain more. A woman who is underweight to begin with should gain more — perhaps 30 pounds — and a woman who is obese at the start of

[6]Committee on Dietary Allowances, *Recommended Dietary Allowances*, 9th ed. (Washington, D.C.: National Academy of Sciences, 1980), p. 138.

pregnancy could perhaps gain less but still should gain between 16 and 24 pounds.[7]

Twenty-five pounds for a normal-weight woman sounds like a lot, but if you look again at the components of the pregnant woman's weight gain (Table 1), you will see that she needs all these pounds — from nutritious kcalories — to provide for the growth of her placenta, uterus, blood, and breasts, as well as for a strong 7 1/2-pound baby. There is little place in her diet, however, for the empty kcalories of sugar, fat, and alcohol, which provide no nutrients to support the growth of these tissues and only contribute to excessive fat accumulation. Much of the weight she gains is lost at delivery; the remainder is generally lost within a few weeks or months, as her blood volume returns to normal and she loses the fluids she has accumulated.

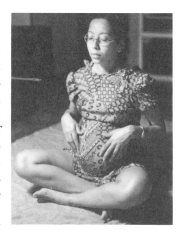

If a woman has gained more than the expected amount of weight early in pregnancy, she should not try to diet in the last weeks. Women have been known to gain up to 60 pounds in pregnancy without ill effects. A *sudden* large weight gain, however, is a danger signal that may indicate the onset of toxemia.

The underweight woman should try to gain weight before she becomes pregnant, to maximize her chance of having a healthy baby. But all women should be attending to their nutrition before they become pregnant. If nutrient supplementation is needed, the family-planning period is a good time to get it started.

[7]Maternal weight gain and the outcome of pregnancy, *Nutrition Reviews* 37 (1979):318-321; California Department of Health, as cited in Nutrition and the pregnant obese woman, *Nutrition and the MD*, January 1978.

Table 2. Daily Food Guide for the Pregnant or Lactating Woman

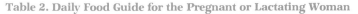

Food	Number of servings		
	Nonpregnant woman	Pregnant woman	Lactating woman
Protein foods			
animal (2-oz serving)	2	2	2
vegetable (at least one serving of legumes)	2	2	2
Milk and milk products	2	4	5
Enriched or whole-grain breads and cereals	4	4	4
Vitamin C-rich fruits and vegetables	1	1	1
Dark-green vegetables	1	1	1
Other fruits and vegetables	1	1	1

California Department of Health, as cited in Nutrition and the pregnant obese woman, *Nutrition and the MD*, January 1978.

If the mother does not gain the full amount of weight recommended, she may give birth to an underweight baby. To the uninitiated, this may seem like no catastrophe, and in some instances it is not. A small mother may give birth to a small, normal, alert, and healthy baby. Nothing is wrong with that. However, a low-birthweight baby is usually also a malnourished baby, one who is more likely to get sick. Such a baby also is likely to be unable to do its job of obtaining nourishment by sucking and to win its mother's attention by energetic, vigorous cries and other healthy behavior. It therefore becomes an apathetic, neglected baby; and this compounds the original malnutrition problem. Such a baby's sickliness is often called "failure to thrive." Thus, for many reasons, babies of normal weight are usually more healthy.

Nutritionists seeking to find a measure by which they can evaluate the outcome of pregnancy have found that birthweight is the most potent single indicator of the infant's future health status. A low-birthweight baby, defined as one that weighs less than 5 1/2 lb (2,500 g), has a statistically greater chance of contracting diseases and of dying early in life. Its birth is more likely to be complicated by problems during delivery than that of a normal baby (defined as weighing a minimum of 6 1/2 lb or 3,000 g). Often, a low-birthweight baby remains underweight throughout life, but surprisingly, one of the problems some of these infants may later encounter is excessive weight gain and obesity.[8] This may be because malnutrition interferes with normal development of that part of the brain that controls food intake.

About 1 in every 15 infants born in the United States is a low-birthweight baby, and about a quarter of them die within the first month of life (see Table 3).[9] Worldwide, it is estimated that one-sixth of all live babies are of low birthweight, more than nine out of ten being born in the underdeveloped countries. Most of them are not premature but are full-term babies; and they are small because of malnutrition. The impact of this malnutrition is further seen in the fact that more than half of all the deaths of children under five years old are caused by low birthweight and nutritional deficiencies.[10]

Low birthweight is often associated with mental retardation, probably by way of deprivation of nutrients and oxygen to the developing brain. It is estimated that about half of all cases of mental retardation could be eliminated by improved programming in

low birthweight (LBW): a birthweight of 5 1/2 lb (2,500g) or less, used as a predictor of poor health in the newborn and as a probably indicator of poor nutritional status of the mother during and/or before pregnancy. Normal birthweight is 6 1/2 lb (3,500 g) or more. Low-birthweight infants are of two different types. Some are **premature;** they are born early and are the right size for their gestational age. Others have suffered growth failure in the uterus; they may or may not be born early but they are **small for gestational age (small for date).**

---

[8]R. L. Huenemann, Environmental factors associated with preschool obesity, 1: Obesity in six-month-old children, *Journal of the American Dietetic Association* 64 (1974):480-487.

[9]National Institute of Child Health and Human Development, Little Babies: Born too soon — born too small, DHEW publication no. (NIH) 77-1079 (Washington, D.C.: Government Printing Office, 1977).

[10]A. Petros-Barvazian and M. Béhar, Low birth weight: What should be done to deal with this global problem? *WHO Chronicle* 32 (June 1978):231-232; *New Trends and Approaches in the Delivery of Maternal and Child Care in Health Services* (sixth report of the WHO Expert Committee on Maternal and Child Health), as cited in *Journal of the American Dietetic Association* 71 (1977):357.

Table 3. Infant Death and Disability in the U.S.

Category	Number
Total births (1974)	3,159,958
Total low-birthweight infants	233,750
Low-birthweight infants who died in first month of life (1960)	56,865
Low-birthweight infants at risk for lifetime disability	about 60,000

*The United States ranks thirteenth among developed nations in infant mortality rate. The death rate of premature infants would be considerably higher if it were not for the superb care available in neonatal intensive care units at major medical centers.

maternal and infant care.[11]

An important consideration for the health of subsequent children is the spacing of offspring to allow the mother's body to regain its nutrient stores. A delay of two to three years between births allows the mother's body to replenish any lost nutrient stores. This is of great benefit to the health of the next child. In the developing countries, where food shortages are common, it is noteworthy that a nonpregnant woman can live three to six months longer than a pregnant woman on the same amount of food.

The profound impact of nutrition during pregnancy on human life is recognized by policy makers all over the world. This recognition has given rise to programs serving pregnant women when education and nutrient supplements were needed. In the United States, the WIC Program (Women's, Infants' and Children's Supplemental Food Program), first funded in 1970, was investing several hundred million dollars a year to help low-income pregnant women during the 1970s and early 1980s. Among the most active nongovernmental agencies is the March of Dimes, which promotes nutrition education for pregnant women as well as other measures to prevent birth defects. Worldwide, most countries have similar programs.

Practices to Avoid   The potential impact of harmful influences during pregnancy cannot be overestimated. Smoking restricts the blood supply to the growing fetus and so limits the delivery of nutrients and removal of wastes. It stunts growth, thus increasing the risk of retarded development and complications at birth.[12] Drugs taken during pregnancy can cause grotesque malformations.

Dieting, even for short periods, is hazardous. Low-carbohydrate diets or fasts that cause ketosis deprive the growing brain of needed glucose and can cause congenital deformity. Most serious may be the invisible effects. For example, carbohydrate metabolism may be rendered

[11]A. C. Higgins, Nutritional status and the outcome of pregnancy, *Journal of the Canadian Dietetic Association* 37 (1976):17-35.

[12]Fetal malnutrition: A risk factor for the pregnant woman who smokes, *Journal of the American Dietetic Association* 75 (1979):121.

permanently defective,[13] or the infant's brain may be permanently damaged.[14]

The consequences of protein deprivation can be severe. This has been observed most frequently in the underdeveloped countries, but it has also been seen among food faddists who adopted an untested vegetarian diet. Their children's height and head circumference were markedly and irreversibly diminished.[15] Iron deficiency during pregnancy in animals has been seen to give rise to offspring whose brain cells could never store the needed iron thereafter.[16]

Most importantly, excessive alcohol consumption can deprive developing nervous tissue of needed glucose and B vitamins and so cause irreversible brain damage and mental and physical retardation in the fetus (fetal alcohol syndrome). The damage can occur with as few as two drinks a day, and its most severe impact is likely to be in the first month, before the woman even is sure she is pregnant. About 1 in every 750 children born in the United States is a victim of this preventable damage.[17]

fetal alcohol syndrome: the cluster of symptoms seen in an infant or child whose mother consumed excess alcohol during her pregnancy; includes mental and physical retardation with facial and other body deformities.

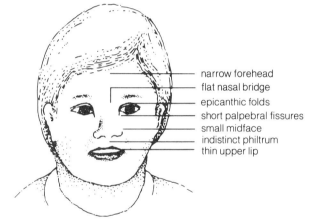

narrow forehead
flat nasal bridge
epicanthic folds
short palpebral fissures
small midface
indistinct philtrum
thin upper lip

These facial traits reflect fetal alcohol syndrome, caused by drinking early in pregnancy. Brain damage and irreversible mental and physical retardation accompany these surface features.

[13] R. M. Pitkin, ed., Nutrition in pregnancy, *Dietetic Currents, Ross Timesaver* 4 (January/February 1977).

[14] C. S. Mahan, Revolution in obstetrics: pregnancy nutrition, *Journal of the Florida Medical Association*, April 1979, pp. 367-372. Children whose mothers, whether diabetic or not, had ketones in their urine during pregnancy are statistically likely to have lower intelligence; J. A. Churchill and H. W. Berendes, Intelligence of children whose mothers had acetonuria during pregnancy (report from the Collaborative Study of Cerebral Palsy, Mental Retardation, and other Neurological and Sensory Disorders of Infancy and Childhood, supported by the National Institute of Neurological Diseases and Stroke of the National Institutes of Health, Bethesda, Maryland), in *Perinatal Factors affecting Human Development*, Scientific Publication No. 185, Pan American Health Organization (Washington, D.C.: World Health Organization, 1969), pp. 30-35.

[15] D. Erhard, The new vegetarians, part 1: Vegetarianism and its consequences, *Nutrition Today*, November/December 1974, pp. 4-12.

[16] R. L. Leibel, Behavioral and biochemical correlations of iron deficiency: A review, *Journal of the American Dietetic Association* 71 (1977):399-404.

[17] K. K. Sulik, M. C. Johnston, and M. A. Webb, Fetal alcohol syndrome: Embryogenesis in a mouse model, *Science* 214 (1981):936-938.

Excessive caffeine consumption (more than 8 cups of coffee a day) has also been thought to cause complications in delivery, but a recent review of the evidence suggests this may have been a false alarm. One or two cups of coffee or tea a day or the equivalent are well within safe limits.[18] Some question exists about the overuse of saccharin, too, and even sugar;[19] a general guideline can be offered: Don't feel obligated to avoid these substances altogether, but use them and all others in moderation.

A table of caffeine amounts in beverages and medications is provided in Chapter 16.

Troubleshooting To avoid the most common problems encountered during pregnancy, some additional measures are helpful. Diabetes is a condition that can make pregnancy more difficult than usual, and sometimes the onset of diabetes occurs when a woman is pregnant. To make sure women with this complication get help, it is recommended that all pregnant women be screened for diabetes at about the sixth month.[20] Thereafter, at every checkup, a woman's urine should be tested for ketones. Ketonuria may indicate the starvation ketosis of ill-advised dieting, a warning sign that permanent brain damage may ensue.[21]

It has been mentioned that a certain degree of edema is to be expected in late pregnancy, but in a poorly nourished woman, it is often part of a larger cluster of symptoms known as toxemia, a condition involving high blood pressure and kidney problems that requires medical attention. Toxemia causes thousands of infant deaths every year, and babies born of toxemic mothers are likely to have retarded growth, lung problems, and other, even more severe birth defects.

Research has shown that toxemia is most common in low-income mothers and pregnant teenagers; it is preventable by good nutrition prior to and in the early stages of pregnancy, because it is most often due to a lack of protein, kcalories, calcium, and/or salt. Adequate calcium is understood to have a direct effect in preventing high blood pressure.[22] To avert toxemia, a pregnant woman should obtain ample protein-rich foods, both meat and milk, in her diet, and her salt intake should be higher than the usual. This doesn't mean that she should add

toxemia (tox-EEM-ee-uh): a cluster of symptoms seen in pregnancy, including edema and often hypertension and kidney complications (*tox* = "poison"; *emia* = "in the blood"). A variety of terms are associated with toxemia. Most common is **eclampsia**; its symptoms include convulsions and coma, associated with high blood pressure, edema, and protein in the urine. Eclampsia may be preceeded by **preeclampsia**, from mild to severe. High blood pressure may also exist throughout pregnancy without toxemia's developing.

[18]S. Linn, S. C. Schoenbaum, R. R. Monson, B. Rosner, P. G. Stubblefield, and K. J. Ryan, No association between coffee consumption and adverse outcomes of pregnancy, *New England Journal of Medicine* 306 (1982):141-145; Third International Caffeine Workshop, *Nutrition Reviews* 39 (1981):183-191.

[19]Coursin, 1973.

[20]C. Borberg, M. D. G. Gillmer, E. J. Brunner, P. J. Gunn, N. W. Oakley, and R. W. Beard, Obesity in pregnancy: The effect of dietary advice, *Diabetes Care* 3 (May/June 1980):476-481; Guidelines for management of the pregnant diabetic woman are given in D. M. Jouganatos and S. G. Gabbe, Diabetes in pregnancy: Metabolic changes and current management, *Journal of the American Dietetic Association* 73 (1978):168-171.

[21]Churchill and Berendes, 1969.

[22]J. M. Belizan and J. Villar, The relationship between calcium intake and edema-, proteinuria-, and hypertension-gestosis: An hypothesis, *American Journal of Clinical Nutrition* 33 (1980):2202-2210.

any salt; the increased need is normally met by the increased food intake. But she shouldn't have to restrict the salt in her diet, either, unless she has a medical condition that makes it necessary to do so. Even after toxemia has set in, it is likely that salt intake should not be reduced, and diuretics (to cause sodium excretion) may be harmful.[23] Good nutrition and rest are the cornerstones of treatment.

Imagine a course of events that goes like this: A pregnant woman notices some puffiness and swelling of her ankles. She consults an advisor who doesn't recognize this as the normal edema of pregnancy and who thinks it is a sign of toxemia setting in. The advisor recommends salt restriction, which is necessary for the edema of severe renal disease or congestive heart failure; but the change in diet imposed on this woman is inappropriate and gradually causes real malnutrition. After two months of taking this precaution, the woman has *true* toxemia.

The message in this story is, of course, not to take advice from anyone who lacks either medical or nutrition knowledge. Consult a doctor about medical conditions; consult a qualified nutrition professional (R.D.) on nutrition. If in doubt, consult both. And, as has been said many times before,

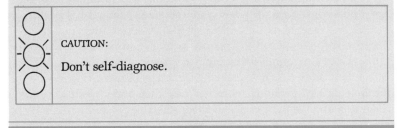

CAUTION:

Don't self-diagnose.

Two anemias are common in pregnancy: iron-deficiency anemia and folacin-deficiency anemia. Both can be missed, for reasons related to the physiology of pregnancy. Iron-deficiency anemia must be diagnosed against the background of the physiological anemia already mentioned. Folacin-deficiency anemia causes nausea (among many symptoms), but the nausea can easily be overlooked because a pregnant woman expects to have morning sickness. It is important to detect and correct, or, better, prevent both anemias; both iron and folacin supplements are often prescribed.

The nausea of morning sickness seems unavoidable, because it arises from the hormonal changes taking place early in pregnancy, but it can be alleviated. A strategy some expectant mothers have found effective

[23]Simple test helps to identify women at risk for toxemia of pregnancy (Medical News), *Journal of the American Medical Association* 237 (1977):1541-1542.

in quelling nausea is to start the day with a few sips of water and a few nibbles of a soda cracker or other bland carbohydrate food, to get something in their stomachs before getting out of bed.

Another problem sometimes seen in pregnancy is vitamin B_6 deficiency, which may in some cases cause depression. Depression can, of course, have other causes, however, so its presence is no indication that a nutritional problem is necessarily present.

Later, as the hormones of pregnancy alter her muscle tone and the thriving infant crowds her intestinal organs, an expectant mother may complain of constipation. A high-fiber diet and a plentiful water intake will help to alleviate this condition. Laxatives should be used only if the doctor orders them, and the type of laxative should be determined by the doctor.

Calcification of the baby teeth begins in the fifth month after conception; for this and for the bones, fluoride is needed. The woman in a county without fluoridated water may need a prescription for a supplement that includes fluoride.

What a lot for a woman to remember! And this is only the briefest summary of the nutrient needs in pregnancy. With all of this to worry about, can a woman relax and enjoy expecting her baby?

Severe, persistent nausea and vomiting **(hyperemesis)** is not normal and may require hospitalization and intravenous feeding to prevent complications.

Nutrition Counseling   In offering nutrition counsel to a pregnant woman, you must be aware of the many physical changes she is undergoing and of her nutrient needs, but it is equally important to be aware of her state of mind and readiness to hear what you have to say. At the outset, it is more important to listen than to talk, to find out answers to questions such as these:

● How does she feel about her pregnancy? (Will she be eager to cooperate or resistant to advice?)

● How much does she already know about nutrition? (Does she already have children? At what level should you begin to instruct her?)

● What sorts of beliefs does she have about pregnancy and childbirth? (Does she hold to myths that you should dispel? Is it important for you *not* to attack her beliefs in order to establish rapport with her?)

● What are her particular questions and concerns?

● What values does she hold dear? (Would she be motivated by the positive ideal of having "a perfect baby"? Or would she more responsive to the negative threat of having to pay expensive medical bills for a child with a birth defect?)

In short, the more you can learn about the particular woman's attitudes, values, and beliefs, the better you can tailor your counseling to effectively deliver nutrition advice and motivate her to abide by it.

A pregnant woman may crave and eat clay, ice, cornstarch, and other nonnutritious substances. This is **pica** (recall Chapter 13) and reflects a need for iron or zinc. The behavior is not adaptive, however, in the sense that the substances she craves do not deliver the nutrients she needs.

Most severe risk factors for malnutrition in pregnancy:
  age 15 or under.
  unwanted pregnancy.
  many pregnancies close together.
  history of poor outcomes.
  poverty.
  food faddism.
  heavy smoking.
  drug addiction.
  alcohol abuse.
  chronic disease
    requiring special diet.
  more than 15% underweight.
  more than 15% overweight.
These factors at the start of pregnancy indicate that poor nutrition is very likely.

Chapter 18 gives pointers on collecting information from clients.

One of your tasks is to dispel myths. The pregnant woman should know that it is *not* true that:

● The fetus is a parasite on the mother and will receive all the nutrients it needs even if she eats poorly. This is true for some nutrients (notably calcium and iron), but in the case of many others (such as protein) a deficiency will harm *both* mother and fetus. She can't eat poorly and expect her baby to do well.

● Mothers know instinctively what to eat during pregnancy; whatever they crave is what they need. The only specific messages the body is known to be able to send to the brain regarding its nutrient needs are for water, possibly salt, and food. Women's tastes for foods do change during pregnancy, and some of the foods they tend to prefer are good for them (milk, for example).[24] Still, in general, the cravings of a pregnant woman seem to be psychological, not physiological.

In counseling, furthermore, it is helpful to dispel fears: It is all right to be nauseated at first, it is natural to have a little puffiness, the constipation of late pregnancy is expected and is a sign that things are going as they should, and so on.

It is important to obtain a clear idea of what the woman typically eats, daily, and what foods she likes in order to advise her on how to adjust her diet for pregnancy in a way she will accept. In advising her about diet, you will be most persuasive if you express her nutrient needs in terms of foods she can visualize herself preparing in her own kitchen. Once she is persuaded that she really should use more vegetables daily, she has to plan their use into her day, shop for them, and cook them. To convince her not only that she *should* have liver once a week but that she will buy it and prepare it, you would ideally prepare it with her in her home. Next best: have her tell you what she plans to buy and how she will cook it, or share a recipe with her, on paper, for her to carry home.

Keep a special lookout for the pregnant vegetarian woman. Vegetarianism, practiced unwisely, poses special risks in pregnancy. The "new" vegetarian who is not knowledgeable about her foodways should be given counsel along the lines suggested in Highlight 4.

Most at risk, however, is the woman with the factors listed in the margin. Such a woman needs intensive nutrition counseling and followup. If, on top of all her other problems, she has a liking for nonnutritious foods (for example, if she is a teenager who identifies herself as a "junk food junkie"), don't tell her not to eat those foods. Help her work out what *to* eat, and then suggest she use her favorite junk foods afterwards to add kcalories.

It is very important to make sure she understands why she needs to gain so much weight to have a healthy pregnancy and realizes that she

---

[24]E. B. Hook, Dietary cravings and aversions during pregnancy, *American Journal of Clinical Nutrition* 31 (1978):1355-1362.

will lose it easily afterwards. (Women who become *fat* during pregnancy from eating the wrong foods may not lose weight easily, but those who achieve a high-*quality* weight gain invested in muscle, blood, fluid, and the like, will have no problem.)

Also, you must deal with negative practices the mother may engage in — smoking, drinking alcohol, and the like. Throughout, it helps to remember that people respond best to positive reinforcement and that you should give as much praise as you can.

The nurse, nutritionist, or other health professional counseling the pregnant woman has to do several kinds of thinking at once during a nutrition counseling session. It is important to safeguard the unborn infant's health, but at the same time it is important to be aware of and to honor the woman's feelings. Two extreme examples will illustrate the kinds of things you have to keep in mind.

At one extreme, there is the woman who (let's say) drinks heavily and has no intention of quitting. Drinking is more important to her than the theoretical possibility of harming an infant she has never seen, doesn't yet love, and hardly can imagine. You certainly owe it to her to give her the information that alcohol causes birth defects, and you should make it as clear as you can that the connection is well established. She should know that the only way to be absolutely sure of excluding the possibility of this kind of retardation is to abstain from drinking altogether throughout the pregnancy. But the choice whether to abstain or not is hers, not yours. As much as you may want her to take your advice, your responsibility ends when you have given her the information. If you push her to make the decision you want, and especially if you act disapproving or judgmental, you may very well "polarize the opposition"— that is, make her stick more firmly to her (wrong) choice. Even if your pushing doesn't have this effect, however, it will probably alienate the woman, who will thereafter be less inclined to talk with you or confide in you. This shuts you off from any opportunities you might have to guide her in her *other* nutrition choices.

In the situation just described, it helps greatly to get a distinction firmly fixed in your own mind: the distinction between what a person *is* and what he or she *does*. You can convey disapproval about what the person *does* (drinking during pregnancy) without alienating the person if you are also clearly conveying respect and esteem for what the person *is* (a person, your equal). If you make the mistake of conveying a feeling that the person *is* something negative (a drunk), you lose the chance to have any beneficial impact at all. It becomes easy to manage situations like this only after you have worked on your own attitudes enough so that you sincerely believe what you are attempting to convey and your esteem for the person, whatever her choice, comes from the heart.

Make the client visualize what's going on in her pregnancy so she will see the importance of eating nutritious foods:

Nurse: Do you know why you need so many meats and eggs and other protein-rich foods?

Patient: Is that what my baby is made of?

Nurse: Yes, that's right. And not only your baby but also all the parts of you that have to grow to take care of the baby — the muscles of your womb, the fluid the baby floats in, the extra blood you make, the placenta, your milk-producing glands . . . you see?

Patient: Yes, I see. Yes, I really see what you're saying.

At the other extreme is the very anxious, insecure woman who has always been very careful of her health but who had a cocktail with some friends once during her early pregnancy before she knew she was pregnant. Now she fears she will bear a baby with a birth defect. How do you counsel her? In such a situation, the chances are very small that harm will have been done. Furthermore, and equally importantly, the episode is in the past and nothing can be done to change it. The choices she can make now affect the present and the future, not the past.

A pregnancy can be a long, suspenseful experience, especially for parents who fear a flawed outcome. The counselor should play down the things that can't be changed and emphasize the positive: what can be done, now and in the weeks to come, to ensure the best possible outcome.

Fetal alcohol syndrome has been recognized only since 1975 as a major cause of birth defects. It is totally preventable by abstention from drinking, but a difference of opinion exists on the question whether a person who drinks one or two drinks a day during pregnancy is risking damaging her baby (see To Explore Further). The jury is still out, but while it is debating, we recommend complete avoidance of alcohol. All women should be informed that there is a risk, that the risk is greater for heavier drinkers, and that the bottom line is not yet known. For a complete guarantee that there will be no damage, a woman can choose not to drink at all. If it is too late to make that choice (if the woman did drink in early pregnancy), the reassurance can be offered that alcohol often does *not* harm the developing infant. Many drinkers, even heavy drinkers, bear normal babies; besides, she didn't know and can't change what's past. What can she do now, beginning today, to support the healthiest possible pregnancy?

Finally, you need to determine whether the mother is planning to breastfeed her baby. If she is, and if it's her first time, she will need instructions to prepare for a successful experience.

Pregnancy for many women is a time of adjustment to major changes. The woman who is expecting to bear a baby is a growing person in more ways than one. Not only physically, but also emotionally, her needs are changing. If it is her first baby, she senses that her lifestyle will have to change as she takes on the new responsibility of caring for a child. Ideally, she will be encouraged to develop this sense of responsibility by caring for herself during pregnancy. According to Erikson, the psychological events of adolescence culminate in the formation of an identity. Experts from many schools of thought agree that one's self-image begins to form early and ideally is strongly positive: "I'm OK!" The expectant mother needs encouragement in thinking of herself as a thoroughly worthwhile and important person with a new and challenging task that she can and will perform well. She is also, as a young adult, still working out her relationship with her mate, and he and she both know that the coming of a first baby will affect that relationship profoundly. There is a need for sensitive communication and understanding on both parts in this time of transition.

It was mentioned earlier that women's cravings during pregnancy do not seem to reflect real physiological needs. Yet women going through this major experience should not be laughed at, and the validity of their feelings should be recognized. If a woman wakes her husband at 2 o'clock in the morning and begs him to go to the nearest all-night grocery to buy her some pickles and chocolate sauce, it is probably not because she lacks a combination of nutrients uniquely supplied by these foods. She is expressing a need, however, as real and as important as her need for nutrients — for support, understanding, and love.

Preparing for Breastfeeding   Toward the end of her pregnancy, a woman who plans to breastfeed her baby should begin to prepare. No elaborate or expensive procedures are necessary; but breastfeeding in humans involves many behaviors and attitudes that require learning, and it usually goes more smoothly for the mother who prepares than for the one who expects it to happen automatically. More is involved than can be discussed in detail here; it is recommended that she read at least one of the books mentioned in Appendix C. Talking with women who have breastfed their babies successfully is also helpful, as is having a family and medical team support system.

As far as possible, the mother should discuss her plans in advance with the members of that support system, whoever they may be — her husband, her mother, her other children, the doctor, the midwife, a nurse. Ideally, there will be classes that she and her husband can attend together before the baby is born. Before the birth time, if possible, she should acquire two or more nursing bras — the kind that give good support and that have drop-flaps so that either breast can be freed for nursing. Also, if her nipples are tender, she should prepare them — again, not by any complicated means but by exposing them to chafing so that they will become tougher. One book says that human nipples tend to be "overprotected" by the clothing we wear and can be toughened by the following means:

● Stop using soap on the breasts for the last three months of pregnancy so that the skin's own protective secretions can make the nipple area strong and resistant to irritation.

● Let the nipples rub against the outer clothing (wear the nursing bra open or cut holes in an older bra for each nipple) so that they will be chafed.

A woman with flat or inverted nipples may want to manipulate her breasts by hand to help correct this condition, or obtain a nipple shield that will help the nipple evert.

Breastfeeding: Nutrition and Counsel

If a mother chooses to breastfeed, her nutrient supplies will continue to support the infant's development as well as her own even after birth. Adequate nutrition of the mother makes a highly significant contribution to successful lactation; without it, lactation is likely to falter or fail. She should continue to eat high-quality foods to the end of her pregnancy, not attempt to restrict her weight gain unduly, and plan to enjoy ample food and fluid at frequent intervals after she has given birth and until lactation is established. At birth, more learning is necessary (see "How to Breastfeed" and "Troubleshooting"), but a few more words about nutrition of the mother are in order first.

Nutrient Needs A nursing mother produces 30 oz milk/day, on the average, with wide variations. At 20 kcal/oz, this milk output amounts to 600 kcal/day. In addition, the energy needed to produce this milk equals some 400 kcal more; so the energy allowance for a lactating woman could be a generous 1,000 kcal/day above her ordinary need. The RDA table suggests that 500 kcal come from added food; and the other 500 kcal from the stores of fat her body accumulated during pregnancy for that purpose.

A comparison between a woman's recommended intakes during pregnancy (second half) and during lactation is shown in Figure 2. The figure reveals that the nursing mother's needs for several nutrients are down, whereas others increase only slightly. Calcium, phosphorus, magnesium, and protein needs continue to be high. These nutrients were going into the baby in the womb; now they are flowing into the baby through the mother's milk. Little iron is secreted in milk; so no

Figure 2 Comparison of the nutrient needs of pregnant and lactating women. The nonpregnant woman's needs are set at 100 percent (calculated from the RDA tables, inside front cover).

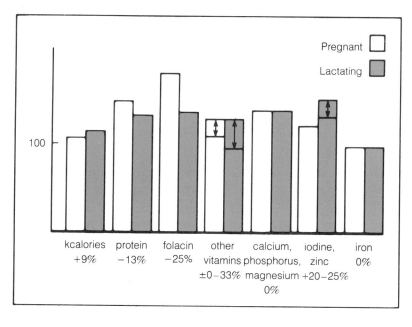

increase in iron intake is needed, provided, of course, that the mother's iron nutrition has been good all along. The folacin requirement falls as the mother's blood volume declines.

Eating Pattern   Logically, because the mother is making milk, she needs to consume something that resembles it in composition. The obvious choice is cow's milk. The nursing mother who can't drink milk needs to find nutritionally similar substitutes such as cheese or soy milk and greens (see Highlight 15). As before, nutritious foods should make up the remainder of the needed kcalorie increase. Because breast milk is a fluid, the mother's fluid intake should be liberal; a busy new mother often forgets this.

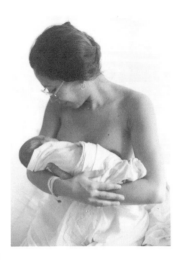

The question is often raised whether a mother's milk may lack a nutrient if she is not getting enough in her diet. The answer differs from one nutrient to the next, but in general the effect of nutritional deprivation of the mother is to reduce the quantity, not the quality, of her milk. For the energy nutrients and most vitamins and minerals, the milk has a constant composition. If one nutrient is in short supply, correspondingly less milk will be produced, but it still will have the proper composition.[25] The mother's diet may make her blood cholesterol higher or lower to some extent but seems not to affect her breast milk cholesterol.[26] For some of the water-soluble vitamins and trace minerals, the composition may be more variable, but most evidence seems to indicate that for these ingredients, too, the breast milk concentrations are constant.[27] Even the taking of a vitamin-mineral supplement seems not to raise nutrient concentrations in the breast milk of an otherwise well-nourished mother.[28] It is best to avoid

[25] L. S. Sims, Dietary status of lactating women I: Nutrient intake from food and from supplements, *Journal of the American Dietetic Association* 73 (1978):139-146.

[26] M. J. Mellies, K. Burton, R. Larsen, D. Fixler, and C. J. Glueck, Cholesterol, phytosterols, and polyunsaturated/saturated fatty acid ratios during the first 12 months of lactation, *American Journal of Clinical Nutrition* 32 (1979):2383-2389.

[27] For example, it seems that the folacin in breast milk is constant, according to T. Tamura, Y. Yoshimura, and T. Arakawa, Human milk folate and folate status in lactating mothers and their infants, *American Journal of Clinical Nutrition* 33 (1980):193-197. So is thiamin, at least with above-adequate intakes; riboflavin may change a little; and copper, iron, and zinc do not seem to vary except that the concentrations change over the course of lactation; P. A. Nail, M. R. Thomas, and R. Eakin, The effect of thiamin and riboflavin supplementation on the level of those vitamins in human breast milk and urine, *American Journal of Clinical Nutrition* 33 (1980):198-204; E. Vuori, S. M. Mäkinen, R. Kara, and P. Kuitunen, The effects of the dietary intakes of copper, iron, manganese, and zinc on the trace element content of human milk, *American Journal of Clinical Nutrition* 33 (1980):227-231. Even fluoride in breast milk appears not to depend on the woman's water supply; O. B. Dirks, J. M. P. A. Jongeling-Eijndhoven, T. D. Flissebaalje, and I. Gedalia, Total free and ionic fluoride in human and cow's milk as determined by gas-liquid chromatography and the fluoride electrode, *Caries Research* 8 (1974):181-186.

[28] M. R. Thomas, S. M. Sneed, C. Wer, P. A. Nail, M. Wilson, and E. E. Sprinkle, III, The effects of vitamin C, vitamin B_6, vitamin B_{12}, folic acid, riboflavin, and thiamin on the breast milk and maternal status of well-nourished women at 6 months postpartum, *American Journal of Clinical Nutrition* 33 (1980):2151-2156.

"megadoses" of vitamins or other nutrients, of course. And to repeat: Water is the major ingredient of milk, and a nursing mother's fluid intake should be ample.

The period of lactation is the natural time for a woman to lose the extra body fat she accumulated during pregnancy. If her choice of foods is judicious, a kcalorie deficit and a gradual loss of weight (1 lb/week) can easily be supported without any effect on her milk output. Fat can only be mobilized slowly, however, and too large a kcalorie deficit will inhibit lactation.[29] On the other hand, if a mother does not breastfeed, she may never lose the fat she gained during pregnancy.[30]

Counseling about Breastfeeding   The choice whether to breastfeed or not is the mother's, and it is usually laden with emotional overtones. The nurse, nutritionist, or whoever counsels the mother has two tasks — to provide accurate information and to provide support. As counselor, your ancillary task is *not* to let your particular prejudices induce you to pressure her to make the choice you would prefer — as one nurse instructor puts it, "Don't lay your trip on her." What is right for you may not be right for her; if you pressure her you may succeed in making her feel guilty but you are not likely to make her more successful in nurturing her infant. The sections "Advantages of Breastfeeding" and "Advantages of Feeding Formula" offer the information that you might share with the mother-to-be who asks for your input into her decision.

Advantages of Breastfeeding   During the first two or three days of lactation, the breasts produce colostrum, a premilk substance whose antibody content is even higher than that of the milk that comes later. Both colostrum and breast milk are sterile as they leave the breast, and the baby cannot contract a bacterial infection from them even if his mother has one. Both contain active white blood cells in the same concentration as in the mother's blood to devour enemy agents such as bacteria and viruses.[31] Thus, colostrum and breast milk protect infants just as modern medicine (vaccinations) and technology (sanitary water supplies) attempt to protect them.

Breast milk is also tailor-made to meet the nutritional needs of the human infant. It offers its carbohydrate as lactose; its fat as a mixture with a generous proportion of the essential fatty acid, linoleic acid; and its protein largely as lactalbumin, a protein the human infant can easily digest. Its vitamin contents are ample. Even vitamin C, for which milk is not normally a good source, is supplied generously by breast milk.

colostrum (co-LAHS-trum): a milklike secretion from the breast, rich in protective factors, that precedes milk during the first day or so after delivery.

lactalbumin (lact-AL-byoo-min): the chief protein in human breast milk, as opposed to **casein** (CAY-seen), the chief protein of cow's milk.

[29]M. J. Whichelow, Success and failure of breast-feeding in relation to energy intake, *Proceedings of the Nutrition Society* 35 (September 1976):62A-63A.

[30]J. C. King and S. Charlet, Current concepts in nutrition — pregnant women and premature infants, *Journal of Nutrition Education*, October-December 1978, pp. 158-159.

[31]J. Mayer, A new look at old formulas, *Family Health/Today's Health*, October 1976, pp. 38, 40, 78.

As for minerals, the calcium-to-phosphorus ratio (2-to-1) is ideal for the absorption of calcium, and both of these minerals and magnesium are present in amounts appropriate for the rate of growth expected in a human infant. Breast milk is also low in sodium. In addition, it contains factors that favor absorption of the iron it contains. On the average, 49 percent of the iron is absorbed from breast milk, as compared with only 4 percent from fortified formula.[32] Zinc, too, is better absorbed from breast milk, which contains a zinc-binding protein necessary for absorption of zinc by the newborn.[33]

Powerful agents against bacterial infection also occur in breast milk. Among them is lactoferrin, an iron-grabbing compound, which keeps bacteria from getting the iron they need to grow on, helps absorb iron into the infant's bloodstream, and also works directly to kill some bacteria.[34]

lactoferrin (lak-toe-FERR-in): a factor in breast milk that binds iron and keeps it from supporting the growth of the infant's intestinal bacteria.

Breast milk also contains antibodies, although not as many as colostrum. These antibodies protect specifically against the intestinal diseases most likely to threaten the infant's life. Entering the infant's body with the milk, these antibodies inactivate bacteria within the digestive tract, where they would otherwise cause harm. Some of the antibodies also "leak" into the bloodstream, because the infant's immature digestive tract cannot completely exclude whole proteins. These antibodies provide additional protection against such diseases as polio.[35] Breast milk also contains a factor (the bifidus factor) that favors the growth of the "friendly" bacteria *Lactobacillus bifidus* in the infant's digestive tract, so that other, harmful bacteria cannot grow there. Another factor present in breast milk stimulates the development of the infant's GI tract.[36]

bifidus factor (BIFF-id-us, by-FEED-us): a factor in breast milk that favors the growth, in the infant's intestinal tract, of the "friendly" bacteria *Lactobacillus* (lack-toh-ba-SILL-us) *bifidus*, so that other, less desirable intestinal inhabitants will not flourish.

As this is written, other factors are still being identified and characterized, including:

- several enzymes.[37]
- a factor that enhances the infant's absorption of folacin.[38]

[32] J. A. McMillan, S. A. Landaw, and F. A. Oski, Iron sufficiency in breast-fed infants and the availability of iron from human milk, *Pediatrics* 58 (1976):686-691.

[33] Acrodermatitis enteropathica, zinc, and human milk, *Nutrition Reviews* 36 (1978):241-242.

[34] R. R. Arnold, M. F. Cole, and J. R. McGhee, A bactericidal effect for human lactoferrin, *Science* 197 (1977):263-265; Probable role of lactoferrin in the transport of iron across the intestinal brush border, *Nutrition Reviews* 38 (1980):256-257.

[35] S. J. Fomon and S. J. Filer, Milks and formulas, in *Infant Nutrition*, 2nd ed., ed. S. J. Fomon (Philadelphia: Saunders, 1974), pp. 359-407.

[36] M. Winick, Infant nutrition: Formula or breast feeding? *Professional Nutritionist*, Spring 1980, pp. 1-3.

[37] These enzymes include RNAse, lipoprotein lipase, and lysozyme, among others. K. M. Shahani, A. J. Kwan, and B. A. Friend, Role and significance of enzymes in human milk, *American Journal of Clinical Nutrition* 33 (1980):1861-1868.

[38] N. Colman, N. Hettiarachchy, and V. Herbert, Detection of a milk factor that facilitates folate uptake by intestinal cells, *Science* 211 (1981):1427-1429.

- several hormones, including LHRH,[39] thyroid hormone,[40] and prostaglandins.[41]

- lipids (in addition to antibodies and white blood cells) that protect the infant against infection.[42]

- a morphine-like compound, perhaps transmitted from food the mother has eaten, for which there are corresponding receptors in the infant's brain.[43]

Much remains to be learned about the composition and characteristics of human milk, but clearly it is a very special substance.

In addition, there are indications that breastfeeding:

- is less likely to produce an obese child.

- promotes better tooth and jaw alignment.

- protects against allergy development during the most vulnerable period.

- favors optimum bonding between mother and child.

It may have other advantages, too; some studies suggest that mothers who breastfeed are less likely to develop breast cancer and to form unwanted clots in the bloodstream after delivery. A woman who wants to breastfeed can derive justification and satisfaction from all of these advantages.

A clot in the bloodstream is a **thrombus** or **embolism**; these terms are sometimes combined as **thromboembolism**.

Advantages of Formula Feeding   The substitution of formula feeding for breastfeeding involves copying nature as closely as possible. A comparison of the nutrient composition of human and cow's milk shows that they differ. Cow's milk is significantly higher in protein, calcium, and phosphorus, for example, to support the calf's faster growth rate. But a formula can be prepared from cow's milk so that it does not differ significantly from human milk in these respects; the formula makers first dilute the milk and then add carbohydrate and nutrients to make it nutritionally comparable to human milk. The antibodies in cow's milk do not protect the human baby from disease (they protect the calf from cattle diseases), but the high level of preventive medical care (vaccinations) and public health measures

The added carbohydrate should be lactose, as this is the sugar of milk, but sometimes sucrose is added instead. See Highlight 15.

[39]E. R. Gonzales, Does breast milk unleash gonadotropins? (Medical News), *Journal of the American Medical Association* 244 (1980):634-635.

[40]Thyroid hormones in human milk, *Nutrition Reviews* 37 (1979):140-141.

[41]Prostaglandins in human milk, *Nutrition Reviews* 39 (1981):302-303.

[42]J. J. Kabara, Lipids as host-resistance factors of human milk, *Nutrition Reviews* 38 (1980):65-73.

[43]E. Hazum, J. J. Sabatka, K. J. Chang, D. A. Brent, J. W. A. Findlay, and P. Cuatrecasas, Morphine in cow and human milk: Could dietary morphine constitute a ligand for specific morphine (mu) receptors? *Science* 213 (1981):1010-1012.

achieved in the developed countries, especially in the United States and Canada, make these considerations less important than they were in the past. Safety and sanitation can be achieved with either mode of feeding by the educated mother whose water supply is reliable.

Like the breastfeeding mother, the one who feeds formula should be supported in her choice. Bearing and nurturing a baby involves much more than merely pouring nutrients in, in whatever form. The mother who offers formula to her baby has valid reasons for making her choice, and her feelings should be honored. She and the baby can benefit in many ways from the supportive approval of those around them.

One of the major advantages of formula feeding is that gained by the mother whose attempts at breast feeding have been beset with frustration. If she truly doesn't want to breastfeed or, worse, if she earnestly does want to and can't, continuing to try is an agonizing course, as hard on the baby as on the mother. When the mother finally accepts the necessity of formula feeding and weans the baby to the bottle, a period of anguish for both may be followed by the onset of peace and the first real opportunity to develop the all-important mother-child love. Other advantages:

● The mother can be sure the baby is getting enough milk; there is no limit to the supply.

● She can offer the same closeness, warmth, and stimulation as the breastfeeding mother does.

● Other family members can get close to the baby and develop a warm relationship in feeding sessions.

● The mother will be free, sooner, to give her time to her other children or to contribute to the family's welfare by returning to work.

The attendant who is asked to advise on breastfeeding versus bottlefeeding should remember the advantages of both. In fact, when addressing any audience, you should remember that some members of that audience will be women who bottle-fed their babies. To praise breastfeeding out of proportion or without qualification can only make them feel guilty or angry.

Many mothers choose to breastfeed at first but wean within the first 1 to 6 months. This is a nice compromise. Even a few weeks of breastfeeding will significantly reduce the likelihood of the baby's developing an allergy to cow's milk, and this advantage alone is important if such an allergy is likely. Furthermore, the baby gets the immunological protection and all the special advantages of breastfeeding during the most critical first few weeks or months. Then the mother can choose in good conscience to shift to the bottle. But it is imperative that she wean the baby onto formula, not onto plain milk of any kind — whole, low-fat, or skim. Only formula contains enough iron (to name but one of many, many factors) to support normal development in the baby's first year.

When Breastfeeding is Preferred It has been stated that a woman should be free to choose the mode of feeding she prefers. This implies that the two modes of feeding are equally beneficial to the infant. However, this is true only for the full-term infant born to a well-educated, financially secure family in a clean, civilized environment. If the infant is premature; if the family is poor, or if other factors act to the baby's disadvantage, then breastfeeding becomes the preferred choice.

Some authorities feel that a premature baby should be fed breastmilk even if the mother can't nurse. That is, if the baby is being kept sealed away in an incubator in the intensive care unit, the mother should milk herself with her hands or a breast pump and carry the milk to the intensive care unit to be fed to the baby. It may make a life-saving difference.[44] Breastfeeding manuals show how to use manual massage or breast pumps to obtain milk.

Some communities maintain breast milk "banks"— storage and delivery facilities for breast milk. Mothers who have milk to spare donate it to the bank; others can purchase it when it is needed. Success and safety in milk banking requires awareness of the need for aseptic technique by the donor and prompt freezing of the milk. Breast milk normally contains bacteria and viruses from the mother's skin and nipple ducts — acceptable for her own baby but not for someone else's. Freezing is necessary to prevent spoilage while preserving the milk's antibodies and other protective factors, which would be destroyed by pasteurization. The current recommendation is that a premature or ill baby's own mother collect, freeze, and transport her milk daily to the hospital and that banked milk only be used temporarily, if there is no better alternative. Breast milk can be stored safely in the freezer for up to 6 months, provided that it stays solidly frozen (below $0°$ F).[45]

A premature baby receiving breast milk may be given a supplement of special formula for prematures, depending on the philosophy of the clinic responsible for its care. Babies not receiving breast milk can be successfully nourished on this formula alone and even on total parenteral nutrition (nutrients delivered directly into a central vein).

In the underdeveloped countries, breastfeeding is indispensable in protecting all infants' lives against the ravages of disease caused by unsanitary conditions, poverty, and ignorance. When artificial feeding is substituted, as when an infant is brought into a clinic for treatment of diarrhea, it will support the infant's life only when accompanied by competent medical care in a sanitary hospital setting. When the infant goes home, the mother will often have nothing but contaminated well water with which to prepare formula and no equipment for sterilizing bottles and nipples. For such a mother to switch to the bottle is to pronounce a death sentence on her baby.[46]

[44]M. W. Choi, Breast milk for infants who can't breast feed, *American Journal of Nursing* 78 (1978):852-855.

[45]Questions readers ask, *Nutrition and the MD*, December 1981.

[46]R. E. Brown, Breast feeding in modern times, *American Journal of Clinical Nutrition* 26 (1973):556-562.

How to Breastfeed   The most important pointers for the breastfeeding mother are presented in list form here, to save space. To help carry them out, the team present at the baby's birth will ideally provide the necessary support. Thereafter, whoever attends the mother should make sure she learns these things. A home visit after a week or ten days is advisable for followup.

1. At the moment of birth, the healthy, full-term infant starts to breathe on its own and within moments makes sucking motions showing readiness to feed. Within the first 30 minutes the sucking reflex is especially strong; nursing the baby right away will get breastfeeding off to a good start. The first 45 minutes are also a critical period for bonding, the formation of a physical and emotional tie between mother and infant that will persist throughout infancy.

If the mother can't nurse right away (if she is sedated), the newborn should wait. He doesn't need the nutrients; he needs the appropriate first impression. Do not give him a bottle, for he can develop an attachment to it and then will resist the breast later.

2. The fluid that flows from the breast at first is colostrum, a thin, yellowy fluid that doesn't look like milk. It is high in antibodies and other protective factors, contains exactly the nutrients the newborn infant needs, and gradually changes to become mature breast milk within the first week.

3. Beginning at the first feeding, the mother should learn how to *relax* and position herself so that she and the baby will both be comfortable and so that the baby can drink without having his breathing obstructed (see Figure 3). She needs to learn how to squeeze the areola between two fingers so that she can slip enough of it into the baby's mouth to achieve good pumping action (Figure 4). She also needs to learn how to make the baby let go: Don't pull! Break the suction by slipping a finger between his gums or holding his nose for a second.

4. The infant's sucking is the stimulus for the release of a hormone that promotes the making of more milk. Therefore, if the infant is hungry he should be allowed to suck longer; this will ensure a greater milk supply at the next nursing. The same hormone promotes the contraction of the uterus, so that it stops bleeding and returns to normal size as quickly as possible after birth — another reason to put the baby to the breast immediately after birth, if possible.

5. The rooting reflex makes the infant turn his mouth towards whichever side of his face is touched. If you want the infant to nurse, you should not touch his other cheek, or he will turn his head away from the nipple toward your hand. Touch his cheek with the nipple so that he will turn and take the nipple.

6. The let-down, or milk-ejection, reflex makes the milk flow when the mother perceives the need. At first, the stimulus for let-down is the baby's actual suckling. Later, when the reflex is well established, the

bonding: the forming of a bond between mother and infant. A critical event in bonding, thought to be mediated by chemical messengers in breast milk, occurs in the first 45 minutes after birth, so this is an especially important time for mother and infant to be close, if possible. However, the tie between mother and infant is strengthened by many other events and behaviors during the early months and years.

We're calling the baby *he* most of the time, because we have to call the mother *she*. But we like girl babies too.

The hormone that promotes milk production is **prolactin**; the one that initiates let-down is **oxytocin**.

rooting reflex: the reflex that makes a newborn turn towards whichever cheek is touched and search for the nipple.

Figure 3   If both mother and baby are positioned so that they are completely
relaxed and comfortable, the milk will flow easily.

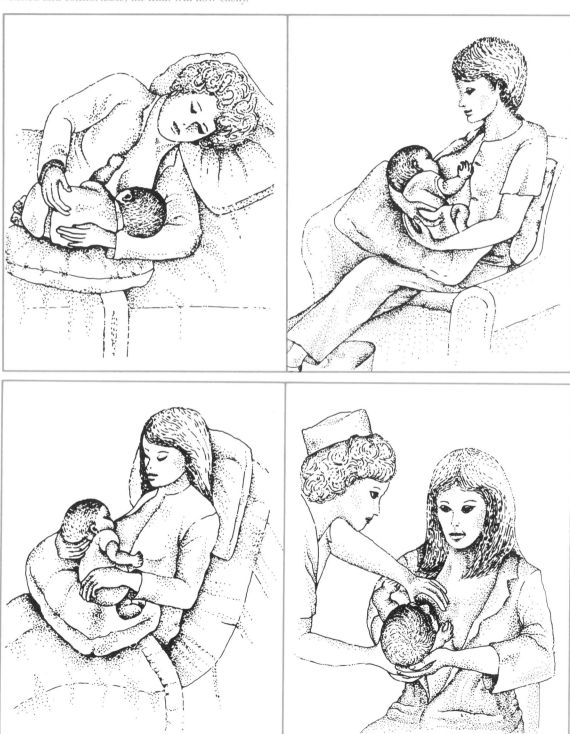

sound of the baby's crying may be enough to trigger it. You can tell it is working when, while the mother is nursing the baby on one breast, milk drips from the other. Let-down has to occur for the baby to obtain milk easily; if it is slow, the baby may struggle and tire before getting enough. The mother must learn to relax and go with the let-down reflex; it may take several weeks for this habit to become established. A glass of water before nursing can help; some people recommend a moderate drink of beer or wine for the late afternoon feeding, when the mother may be tense.

let-down reflex: the reflex that forces milk to the front of the breast when the infant begins to nurse.

7. The draught reflex, which occurs later during a nursing session, draws milk from the hindmost milk-producing glands of the breast after the foremilk has been released. The mother can feel this as a tingly sensation within the breast. The baby should be allowed and encouraged to nurse after the draught has begun, so that he will get enough milk. If feeding is interrupted after the draught reflex has occurred, it may not occur again for some time and the baby may not get enough milk. Hindmilk is richer in fat than foremilk and so provides satiety after the baby has sucked enough to satisfy his sucking need.

draught reflex (DRAFT reflex): the reflex that moves the hind-milk toward the nipple after the infant has drawn off the fore-milk.

8. The sucking and swallowing reflexes work together so that the baby's tongue and jaw pump milk from the breast and the swallow follows. The nipple has to rest well back on the baby's tongue, and his lips and gums have to be pressing on the areola if he is to stimulate milk release successfully and then swallow it (see Figure 5).

satiety (sat-EYE-uh-tee): a feeling of fullness or satisfaction from eating or drinking.

Figure 4   Gently squeeze the areola between two fingers to insert the nipple far enough into the baby's mouth.

areola (a-REE-uh-luh): the colored halo around the nipple. Beneath the areola lie the ducts that bring milk from the mammary glands. Pumping action on the areola promotes flow of milk from the glands through the ducts.

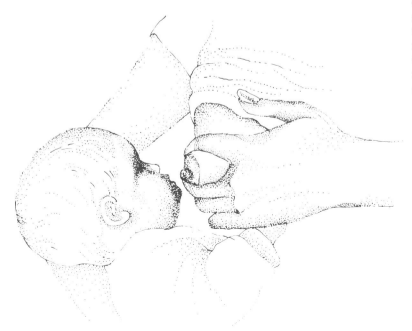

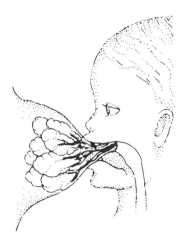

This baby's gums are milking the mammary glands by pressing on the milk ducts; the milk is squirting into the baby's throat.

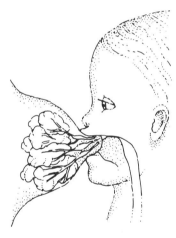

This baby hasn't got an adequate grasp on the nipple and will not get enough milk.

Figure 5 Correct and incorrect grasp of nipple.

9. Although the baby can suck half the milk from the breast within 2 minutes and 80 to 90 percent of it within 4 minutes, he should continue sucking for 10 minutes or more on one breast. The sucking itself, as well as the removal of milk from the breast, is believed to stimulate lactation. After he has put in his 10 minutes or so — his share of the work — the baby can be given the other breast to finish satisfying his hunger. Nursing sessions should normally start on alternate breasts, so that each breast is emptied regularly. When the baby seems to be full, hold him upright to let him expel any swallowed air (burping), and then give him another chance to nurse.

10. For the first ten days, even if everything is going smoothly at home, the nursing mother should ideally have enough help and support so that she can rest in bed for several hours a day. Real rest and a plentiful fluid intake are indispensable to successful lactation.

11. Demand feedings, no fewer than 6 a day, are most likely to promote optimal milk production and infant growth. The infant should be encouraged to nurse; or the milk should be manually pumped out at intervals to keep the supply going. A mother who nurses her baby even 12 times a day during the first two weeks will ensure that supply keeps up with demand and will gain enough practice to maintain successful lactation easily later on. The midnight feeding should not be skipped, even if the baby is inclined to sleep through it. If the mother feels that she is spending immense amounts of time breastfeeding, she should remind herself that the bottlefeeding mother is spending as much or more time washing bottles, sterilizing formula, and feeding her baby. Breastfeeding will not continue to be so time consuming for more than a very few weeks. Remember the advantages; remember that this time will pass; and enjoy it while it lasts.

12. Mothers often want to know if they can skip an occasional feeding, substituting a bottle of formula for the missed feeding. To be sure not to suppress lactation, the mother can express the amount of milk the baby would drink, even if she only throws it away; that way, the breast gets the message to keep on producing that much milk. The mother who is confident that lactation is well established, however, may not bother to do this, and will experience no noticeable diminution of the supply.

A mother who wants to skip one or two feedings daily, for example, if she goes to work outside the home, can substitute formula for those feedings and continue to breastfeed morning and evening. She will probably find that her milk is not adequate to restore those feedings easily (for example, on weekends), but that she and her baby can continue to enjoy the morning and evening feedings for as long as desired.

Troubleshooting Solutions can be found for almost all of the problems that can arise in connection with breastfeeding. Breastfeeding manuals give many further details beyond those listed below (see Appendix C).

1. Sore nipples should be treated kindly, but nursing can continue even if the nipples are bleeding. Air and sunlight between feedings will help to heal them. Getting the let-down reflex going smoothly helps a lot, because then the baby doesn't have to suck hard on the nipple. Nurse on the less-sore breast first; when the milk lets down, switch to the sore one and position the baby to minimize the pain; then, when most of the fast-flowing, early milk from that breast is gone, switch back and let the baby satisfy the sucking need on the other breast.

2. Engorgement can make the breasts so full and hard that the baby can't get his mouth around the nipple. Pump out some of the milk, use a nipple shield, and/or massage or warm the breasts to help let-down get started. They will get smaller and softer, while still producing ample milk, after the first several days of lactation.

3. An inverted nipple can be managed similarly. A nipple shield can be used to press around the nipple and make it poke out so the baby can get hold of it.

4. An undrained sinus can make a hard, uncomfortable lump in the breast. Massage the lump while the baby is nursing, to move the milk toward the nipple where it will join the main supply.

5. Supplemental water can be offered if the baby seems to be thirsty after a long feed, but it is ill advised to offer sugar-water or other supplemental feedings. Infants fed sweetened water in the first few months tend to have a greater preference for sweets later in infancy.[47] Also, sweetened water carries kcalories, which should come to the infant only from the breast. The full extent of the baby's demand should be communicated to the mother's body by way of sucking, so that the milk supply will increase to meet it.

6. Infection of a breast (mastitis) is best managed by *continuing to breastfeed.* By drawing off the milk, the infant helps to relieve pressure in the infected area; he does not become infected because the infection is outside of and in between the milk-producing glands.

7. If the mother wants to be away during a feeding before lactation is securely established, she should express enough milk into a bottle to feed the baby while she is gone. This will communicate the appropriate amount of demand to the breasts so that they will produce the needed milk for the next feeding.

engorgement: overfilling of the breasts with milk so that they become swollen and hard.

You can tell if a nipple is inverted by pressing the areola between two fingers. An inverted nipple folds inward toward the breast. Pushing the areola toward the chest wall (manually or with a shield) everts the nipple.

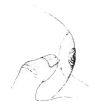

Inverted nipple.

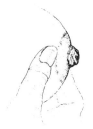

Normal nipple.

Infection of a breast is **mastitis**.

[47]G. K. Beauchamp, Ontogenesis of taste preferences (paper presented at the 5th Congress of the International Organization for the Study of Human Development, Campione, Italy, May 1980), cited in G. K. Beauchamp, M. Bertino, and M. Moran, Sodium regulation: Sensory aspects, *Journal of the American Dietetic Association* 80 (1982):40-45.

8. The baby who seems to be up all night crying for milk and asleep much of the day *may* be getting less milk by day and may therefore be hungry at night. In any case, to rectify the situation, the *mother* should relax and nap during the day, too. (To do this, she must have support, or must be willing to let all but the indispensable chores wait until another day or week.) This way, she'll have more milk during the day and can gradually get the baby turned around. By six weeks, these problems will probably be ironed out.

9. If the mother wants to begin taking an oral contraceptive, she should probably wait until after she has weaned the baby and should use another mode of contraception in the meantime. Oral contraceptives slightly inhibit lactation; further, the hormones are known to reach the baby via the breast milk and can temporarily feminize male infants.

10. Most importantly, if the baby is irritable and wakeful, the mother may fear that her milk supply is inadequate. The baby's small bowel movements may suggest to her that he is not getting enough milk, but she can be reassured that there is little indigestible material in breast milk and therefore little waste. Worrying itself can inhibit lactation. She should be reassured that bottle-fed babies cry, too, and that her own ability to calm down, relax, and let her fears go will help more than any amount of anxiety. However, if she really wants to wean the baby, she can be supported in that choice and congratulated on having nursed for as long as she did. Even feeding for only a few days, so that the baby gets the benefit of the protective factors in colostrum, makes a contribution to the baby's health and development in which the mother can take pride.

Contraindications to Breastfeeding

If a woman has a communicable disease that could threaten the infant's health so that they have to be separated, then of course she cannot breastfeed. Similarly, if she must take medication that is secreted in breast milk and that is known to affect the infant, she must not breastfeed. Drug addicts, including alcohol abusers, are capable of taking such high doses that their infants can become addicts by way of breast milk; in these cases, too, breastfeeding is contraindicated.

Most prescription drugs, however, do not reach nursing infants in sufficiently large quantities to affect them adversely. Moderate use of alcohol and moderate smoking are compatible with breastfeeding. Coffee drinking is fine, in moderation, as is the eating of foods such as garlic and spices. A particular food may affect the baby's liking for the mother's milk, but this is an individual matter. If a woman has an ordinary cold, she can go on nursing without worry. The infant will catch it from her anyway, if he is susceptible, and he may be less susceptible thanks to immunologic protection than a bottle-fed baby would be.

A woman sometimes hesitates to breastfeed because she has heard that environmental contaminants such as DDT may enter her milk and harm her baby. DDT has been reported in the milk of mothers at higher concentrations than are allowed in cow's milk.[48] The significance of these findings is hard to evaluate, and the decision whether to breastfeed on this basis might best be made after consultation with a physician or dietitian familiar with the local circumstances.

Another environmental contaminant that has caused concern is the PCBs, which are found in rivers and waterways polluted by industry. An episode of accidental PCB consumption by pregnant women in Japan arose when they consumed contaminated cooking oil; later they gave birth to abnormally small babies whose skin was unusually dark for a while. PCBs are stored in body fat and remain in the body; they are excreted only in the fat of breast milk.

For more about DDT and PCBs, turn to Highlight 14.

According to the Committee on Environmental Hazards of the American Academy of Pediatrics, women in the United States need not fear contamination of their breast milk with PCBs unless they have eaten large amounts of fish caught in PCB-contaminated rivers such as the Saint Lawrence Seaway or have been directly exposed because of their occupations. Should a woman have any question about PCBs in her breast milk, she should ask the advice of the local state health department.[49]

How to Feed Formula   These are the pointers you need if you are to advise the mother who chooses to feed her baby formula.

1. The choice of formula is usually not critical. Any brand that meets the AAP standards is fine for most babies. For the allergic or ill baby, or for one with an inborn error, however, special formulas are necessary.

AAP (American Association of Pediatrics) standards are shown in Highlight 15, where all the details regarding formula selection are given.

2. The mother who chooses not to breastfeed may experience some discomfort as her own milk dries up. An injection of estrogen or a large dose of vitamin B_6 may be used to hasten the process. (Vitamin B_6 is needed in food, of course, but megadoses can be used to suppress lactation.[50])

3. Formula today in the United States and Canada is often bought premixed and sterile in cans from the store and is easy to feed in presterilized throwaway bottles. But the mother who mixes or bottles her own must learn the rules of safe formula preparation and

[48]Fomon and Filer, 1974.

[49]Committee on Environmental Hazards of the American Academy of Pediatrics, PCBs in breast milk, *Pediatrics* 62 (1978):407.

[50]"Large doses" means over 200 mg pyridoxine, 100 times the RDA. M. D. Foukas, An antilactogenic effect of pyridoxine, *Journal of Obstetrics and Gynecology, British Commonwealth* 80 (1973):718-720; R. G. Marcus, Suppression of lactation with high doses of pyridoxine, *South Africa Medical Journal* 49 (1975):2155-2156.

Formula preparation:
  Liquid concentrate (inexpensive, relatively easy)
    — mix with equal part water.
  Powder formula (cheapest, lightest for travel)
    — read label directions.
  Ready-to-feed (easiest, most expensive) — pour directly into clean bottles.
  Evaporated milk — ask nutritionist or nurse; use *both* vitamins and iron in addition.
  Whole milk — do not use.

administration. Until the baby is strong and clearly resistant to infection (at 2 to 3 months), formula should be prepared with great care, with safe, pure water and fresh, refrigerated, or canned ingredients. It has to be sterilized and kept sterile until it is presented to the baby. (These rules can be relaxed if the total environment is clean and the water supply is pure. Then all that is necessary is to wash bottles and nipples well with soapy water and rinse them throughly before preparing a fresh batch of formula.) If half a bottle is left after a feeding, it should be resterilized immediately if it is to be used again; this shouldn't be a regular practice, however, because nutrient losses are incurred by high temperature treatment. Unsterile formula should never be let stand at room temperature.

The mother should be trained in formula preparation by an experienced person and should be observed and guided at least once as she goes through the steps herself. The less well educated, economically well off, and experienced she is, and the less strong and healthy her baby is, the more important are these safeguards. In poor areas, especially where a sanitary water supply is not dependable, these rules and training are crucial.

4. Formula can be offered warm or cold. The baby may prefer warm formula if accustomed to it, but no harm is done by feeding it cold unless it is refused.

5. Close contact during feeding is important. Infant and mother should both be comfortable and relaxed, and the infant should be positioned so that he can drink easily. His head should be higher than his body so that he will be drinking "downhill." The nipple hole should be large enough to allow one swallow of milk to flow each time the baby sucks; if it is too small, it should be enlarged; and if it is too large, it should be replaced. Check the nipple to make sure the formula is flowing. The bottle should be tilted so that the nipple is full of formula, not air, while the baby is sucking.

6. When the baby stops drinking, he should be sat or held upright and patted on the back to help him bring up any bubbles of air he may have swallowed. Then after he has burped, offer him more formula. But don't try to force him to finish the bottle; like making children clean their plates, this promotes obesity.

7. The feeding schedule can vary but best promotes development if adjusted to the baby's expressed hunger needs at first, within reason. Some babies need to feed much more frequently than others. Remember that a dehydrated baby (feverish, hot) may be thirsty for water, which can be offered in place of formula if the baby cries soon after a feeding.

8. Sterilized formula can be replaced by regular, clean, fresh formula and then by milk as the baby grows older. Chapter 16 gives general suggestions as to timing, but the pediatrician should be consulted in each individual case.

9. Babies love their bottles; the sucking provides needed stimulation as well as nutrients. They should never be allowed to sleep with them, however, because of the potential damage to developing teeth. The bedtime bottle may be the most cherished, but it should be firmly removed. At weaning time (some time around nine months or so, when the baby can sit up and begin to manage a cup), one of the daily bottles can be taken away at a time and replaced by milk in a drinking cup. The last bottle may be the bedtime one, and this could be given up at about a year at the discretion of the parents and pediatrician.

10. Most importantly (to repeat): Hold the baby as closely and lovingly as a breastfeeding mother does. Much more occurs during a feeding than the mere transfer of nutrients into the baby's body. The human warmth and stimulation delivered with the formula do as much as the formula itself to promote normal, healthy development.

Supplements for the Baby

It is unnecessary to give vitamin-mineral supplements to a newborn baby. If he is breastfed, breast milk and his own internal stores will meet his needs until he is well into the second half of his first year, and then the introduction of intelligently chosen juices and foods will keep up with his changing requirements. The only exceptions to this statement have to do with vitamin D and fluoride.

Breast milk does not provide enough vitamin D, and the infant who has little exposure to sunlight is at risk of developing rickets. People often wonder how much sunlight it takes to prevent deficiency. So many variables are involved that no single answer to this question is possible. Among the relevant factors are:

- Latitude (how far from the sun).
- Season (winter versus summer).
- Area of skin exposed (winter versus summer clothes).
- Color of skin (light versus dark).
- City versus country (smog filters out the vitamin D-producing ultraviolet rays of the sun).

A light-skinned baby with just a diaper on in strong summer sun and clear air might make enough vitamin D in a few minutes to meet his daily need. A dark-skinned baby wrapped up for cold weather in a smoggy city might not make enough even if he was outside for several hours.[51]

[51]At particular risk are inner-city black Muslim infants who are breastfed. Not all milks are kind, *Nutrition and the MD*, May 1980; W. F. Loomis, Skin-pigment regulation of vitamin-D biosynthesis in man, *Science* 157 (1967):501-506; R. M. Neer, The evolutionary significance of vitamin D, skin pigment, and ultraviolet light, *American Journal of Physical Anthropology* 43 (1975):409-416.

Also, the fluoride contents of breast milk may be somewhat unreliable.[52] The baby's pediatrician is likely to be well informed on this matter and to prescribe appropriate supplementation.

If the baby is formula-fed, the makeup of the formula determines what further supplementation may be necessary. Vitamins A and D are needed if the formula is not fortified with A and D. Vitamin C is needed if it is not in the formula. Fluoride is needed if the milk does not contain it. Again, the pediatrician is the expert to consult on local needs. Table 1 in the next chapter shows what supplements are needed as the transitions are made from breastfeeding to formula, and formula to milk.

Summing Up

Growth is a major factor influencing the nutritional needs of developing infants and children. The growth rate is fastest during prenatal life, the first year, and the adolescent years. Growth patterns for different organs vary. Most are characterized by critical periods, during which cells divide and nutrition has greater importance than usual. Psychological growth accompanies and facilitates physical growth.

During pregnancy, changes in both mothers' and infants' bodies necessitate increased intakes of the growth nutrients. A pregnant woman should gain about 25 to 30 pounds from foods of high nutrient density. Malnutrition during pregnancy affects the developing fetus: Low-birthweight babies often fail to thrive. Alcohol, smoking, drugs, dieting, and unbalanced nutrient intakes of all kinds should be avoided for the duration of pregnancy. Protein and ample kcalories are especially important. Fluid intake should be ample and salt normally should not be restricted.

The breastfeeding mother needs additional kcalories from foods of high nutrient density and a generous fluid intake. The rapidly growing newborn infant requires milk, preferably breast milk, which provides the needed nutrients in quantities suitable to support the infant's growth. Advantages of breast milk over formula, especially in underdeveloped countries, are that it protects the infant against disease and that it is sanitary, economical, and premixed to the correct proportions. To avoid allergy, all susceptible infants should be breastfed at first, even in developed countries.

Formula feeding matches breastfeeding as closely as possible. The mother should be supported and assisted with whichever mode of feeding she selects. The health professional can greatly benefit the health of both mother and infant by learning what information the mother needs and offering that information in useable terms.

[52]J. C. Gallagher and B. L. Riggs, Nutrition and bone disease, *New England Journal of Medicine* 298 (1978):193-195.

To Explore Further

Many of the references suggested in Appendix J include good sections or chapters on nutrition of pregnant and lactating women. In addition, the following book should be singled out for special mention:

●Worthington, B. S., Vermeersch, J., and Williams, S. R. *Nutrition in Pregnancy and Lactation*. St. Louis: Mosby, 1977 (paperback).

For the seeker of more technical information, the *American Journal of Clinical Nutrition* published a Supplement, April 1981, in which all of the articles were devoted to nutrition and nutrition assessment in pregnancy.

A superb audiovisual aid that all clinics and doctors' offices should show to mothers-to-be is *Inside My Mom*, described in Appendix C.

The person working with teenage pregnant girls should prepare by viewing this film:

●*Woman Child*, also from the March of Dimes.

Woman Child shows interviews with unmarried teenagers who have borne babies and makes unforgettably clear how they feel about themselves and their situations.

The entire issue of *Nutrition and the MD*, November 1980, was devoted to nutrition in pregnancy and contained many valuable pointers.

The American Council on Science and Health (ACSH) took the controversial stand in 1981 that pregnant women could drink alcohol, as long as they did so moderately. The editor of *Nutrition Today*, speaking for many authorities besides himself, angrily attacked their stand as irresponsible. His editorial, as well as the original ACSH paper, were both published in *Nutrition Today*, January/February 1982:

●Enloe, C. F., Jr. Thalidomide II, pp. 16-17.

●ACSH. Alcohol use during pregnancy, pp. 29-32.

Two other articles relevant to this debate are:

●Little, R. E. Moderate alcohol use during pregnancy and decreased infant birth weight. *American Journal of Public Health* 67 (1977):1154-1156.

●Even moderate drinking may be hazardous to maturing fetus (Medical News). *Journal of the American Medical Association* 237 (1977):2585-2587.

An excellent 10-minute film on fetal alcohol syndrome, *Born Drunk*, is available from ABC, 1330 Avenue of the Americas, New York, NY 10019.

An important film, *Nutritional Management of High Risk Pregnancy*, released in 1981, demonstrates the importance of nutrition in teenage pregnancies and shows how to manage the pregnancies of preeclamptic and diabetic women. The film is available from the Society for Nutrition Education, 1736 Franklin Street, Oakland, CA 94612.

The authoritative reference on nutrition assessment norms for pregnant women is the National Research Council's paperback:

●*Laboratory Indices of Nutritional Status in Pregnancy*. Washington, D.C.: National Academy of Sciences, 1978.

Many good references on breastfeeding are also available. We recommend:

● Jelliffe, D. B., and Jelliffe, E. F. P. "Breast is best": Modern meanings. *New England Journal of Medicine* 297 (1977):912-915.

This presents the reasons why, in the authors' opinion, breastfeeding is best even in developed countries such as the United States and Canada.

An outstanding, up-to-date reference for the health professional who is advising a breastfeeding mother is:

● Lawrence, R. A. *Breastfeeding: A Guide for the Medical Profession*. St. Louis: Mosby, 1980.

An international organization of women who believe in breastfeeding and who help each other with related concerns is the LaLeche League. The main office is at 9616 Minneapolis Avenue, Franklin Park, IL 60131; there are branches in many cities. Among the League's publications are a newsletter and a manual; it also highly endorses the manual listed last:

● *La Leche League News* (newsletter).

● *The Womanly Art of Breastfeeding* (manual).

● Brewster, P. B. *You Can Breastfeed Your Baby . . . Even in Special Situations* (500+ pages). Emmaus, Pa.: Rodale Press, 1979.

For more information on breast milk banking, contact the local LaLeche League office, or see:

● Human milk banking, *Nutrition and the MD*, March 1981.

● Williams, F. H., and Pittard, W. B., III. Human milk banking: Practical concerns for feeding premature infants. *Journal of the American Dietetic Association* 79 (1981):565-568.

FDA Consumer published an update on drugs excreted in breast milk:

● Hecht, A. Advice on breastfeeding and drugs. *FDA Consumer*, November 1979, pp. 21-22.

If you want to learn all there is to know about breastfeeding, you can get a giant head start by sending for the National Academy of Science's 58-page booklet prepared by the Committee on Nutrition of the Mother and Preschool Child:

● *A Selected Annotated Bibliography on Breast Feeding, 1970- 1977.*

Write to the Office of Publications, National Academy (address in Appendix J).

For patient education materials for pregnancy and lactation, turn to Appendix C.

Choosing Formulas and Milk Substitutes

Present formulas are not too bad for infants and for some may be beneficial or essential.

L. BARNESS

The how-to's of both breast and formula feeding were presented in Chapter 15, and a brief comparison of human milk with formula was made. For the person who needs to select a formula or milk substitute, further details are needed, and they are presented here.

For the first six months of a baby's life, mother's milk or formula is normally the only source of nutrients. The choice of formula must therefore be made carefully. At some time between six months and a year, when other foods have become responsible for supplying nutrients in significant quantities, formula can be replaced by milk or a milk substitute. Milk still plays a very important role in the diet, however, and if a substitute is selected, it must be chosen with care. This Highlight offers help with the questions:

1. Before six months: What formula is best?

2. Six months to one year: When should formula be replaced?

3. When formula is replaced: What milks or milk substitutes are best?

Selecting a Formula

Formula makers generally assume that human milk is the ideal milk for a young baby, and they duplicate it as closely as they reasonably can. Not all human milks are the same, however, and the standard ideally is "human milk taken from well-nourished mothers during the first or second month of lactation, when the infant's growth rate is high."[1]

Normally, the choice is a *starting formula*, that is, a formula designed to supply all the nutrient needs of a healthy infant for the first six months of life. Among starting formulas are *adapted* or *humanized formulas* and *medical formulas* (see the Miniglossary).

Fortunately for the person doing the choosing, national and international standards

[1]K. Brostrom, Human milk and infant formulas: Nutritional and immunological characteristics, in *Textbook of Pediatric Nutrition*, ed. R. M. Suskind (New York: Raven Press, 1981), pp. 41-64.

have been set for the nutrient contents of infant formulas. The standard referred to in this Highlight is the one developed by the American Academy of Pediatrics (AAP), which is widely used in the United States. The Infant Formula Act of 1980 requires that formulas meet nutrient standards based on the AAP recommendations, and in 1982 FDA adopted quality control procedures to be sure that they do. Formulas that meet the standard can be assumed to have about the same nutritional value; small differences in nutrient content are sometimes confusing but not usually important.

Table 1 shows characteristics of human, cow's, and goat's milk side by side, along with those of two starting formulas prepared from modified cow's milk. The animal milks clearly differ significantly from human milk in many respects; and you can see that the formulas are similar to the animal milks in some ways, and to human milk in others. The formulas resemble cow's milk in type and ratio of proteins, total fat, and calcium-to-phosphorus ratio; but they have been adjusted to approximate human milk in total protein, carbohydrate, linoleic acid, major minerals, and renal solute load. While obviously not identical to human milk, starting formulas present the same nu-

Table 1. Major Characteristics of Human Milk, Cow's Milk, Goat's Milk, and Infant Formula

Characteristic	Human milk	Cow's milk	Starting formula*	Goat's milk
Energy (kcal/100 ml)	74	67	68	76
Protein (g/100 ml)	1.1	3.5	1.5-1.6	3.3
Whey/casein ratio	80/20	20/80	20/80	18/82
Carbohydrate (g/100 ml)	7.2	5.0	7.0-7.2	4.7
Fat (g/100 ml)	2.7-4.6	3.5	3.6-3.7	4.1
Linoleic acid (% of total fatty acids)	10-15	4	13-23	-
Minerals				
Calcium (mg/l)	340	1,200	510-550	1,300
Phosphorus (mg/l)	140	955	390-460	1,060
Ca:P ratio	2.4	1.3	1.2-1.3	1.2
Iron (mg/l)	0.2-1.0	0.5	12 or 1.5†	0.5
Sodium (mEq/l)	7	25	11-12	18
Potassium (mEq/l)	13	35	18-20	46
Renal solute load (mOsm/l)	74	220	105-108	-
Vitamins (per 100 ml)				
Vitamin A (IU)	190-250	103 or 190‡	169-250	207
Thiamin (μg)	14-16	44	53-65	40
Riboflavin (μg)	36-37	175	63-100	184
Niacin (mg)	0.15-0.18	0.09	0.7-1.3	0.2
Vitamin B_6 (μg)	10-11	64	40	7
Pantothenic acid (mg)	0.18-0.23	0.4	0.3-0.32	0.3
Folacin (μg)	2-5	0.3	5-11	0.2
Vitamin B_{12} (μg)	0.03-0.05	0.4	0.15-0.21	0.06
Vitamin C (mg)	4.3-5.2	1.1	5.5	1.5
Vitamin D (IU)	2.2	1.3 or 38	40-42	2.4

Adapted from K. Brostrom, Human milk and infant formulas: Nutritional and immunological characteristics, in *Textbook of Pediatric Nutrition*, ed. R. M. Suskind (New York: Raven Press, 1981), and Milk-based and soy-based formulations used for feeding newborns in the hospital, January 1979, an information sheet from Ross Laboratories, Columbus, OH 43216. Data on goat's milk and on vitamins for all milk are adapted from S. J. Fomon, Milks and milk-based formulas, Chapter 11 in *Infant Nutrition* (Philadelphia: Saunders, 1967), Chapter 11, pp. 195-224.

*These numbers represent two formulas, Similac and Enfamil.

†These formulas are available unfortified or with iron fortification.

‡The higher value represents fortified milk, which should contain 2,000 IU vitamin A and 400 IU vitamin D per quart (1,900 and 375 IU per liter, respectively).

trients in roughly the same proportions for the most part.

Table 2 shows the AAP standard for the bulk ingredients of starting formulas and permits you to compare it with human milk and with typical starting formulas. As you can see, the AAP standard recommends higher protein than is in human milk; this is because the cow's milk protein does not present as perfect a balance of amino acids for the human infant. You can also see that the starting formulas meet the AAP standard for the nutrients listed. The rest of the AAP recommendations for vitamins and minerals are shown in Table 3 to facilitate comparison with

Table 2.   AAP Standard Compared with Human Milk and Infant Starting Formula

Content	Mature human milk	AAP standard	Starting formulas*
Energy (kcal/100 ml)	67-75	60-80	67
Protein (% of kcal)	5.2	7-18	9
Fat (% of kcal)	35-58	30-55	47-50
Carbohydrate (% of kcal)	35-44	35-50	41-43

Adapted from K. Brostrom, Human milk and infant formulas: Nutritional and immunological characteristics, in *Textbook of Pediatric Nutrition*, ed. R. M. Suskind (New York: Raven Press, 1981).

*Five formulas were used to generate these data: Similac (Ross), Similac 60/40 (Ross), Enfamil (Mead), SMA (Wyeth), Nan (Nestle).

any formula of your choice.

Table 4 compares other types of formulas with starting formulas and with human milk. You can see that adapted formulas are closer in composition than starting formulas to human milk (adjusted protein ratio, lower linoleic acid, lower sodium and other minerals). Either regular or adapted starting formula would be suitable for a full-term, healthy baby. (For premature babies, special premature formulas are available, but banked breast milk is preferable if it can be obtained, and the premature infant's very own mother's milk is best of all, as explained at the end of Chapter 15.) The medical formulas shown would be suitable for infants allergic to milk protein, because they are soy-based, or for infants with lactose intolerance, because the lactose has been replaced. For infants with other special needs, many other variations are available. Further details about the individual con-

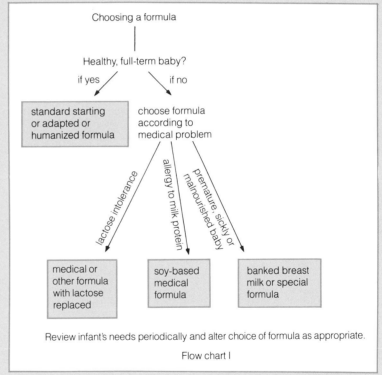

Flow chart I

stituents of milk and formulas can be found in technical references.[2] Flow Chart 1 shows the process of choosing a formula.

Replacing the Formula

As soon as the baby's nutrient needs are being met

[2]Brostrom, 1981.

mostly by solid food, at any time after six months, a less complete followup formula can be used. As long as formula is the baby's major food, however, it should not be replaced by milk — primarily because of the vitamin C and iron it provides.

Whole cow's milk in any form, fortified with vitamins

Table 3. AAP Recommendations for Nutrient Levels in Formulas

Nutrient	Recommended per 100 kcal	Recommended per 100 ml*
Protein (g)	1.8-4.5	1.3-3.2
Fat (g)	3.3-6.0	2.3-4.2
Essential fatty acids (linoleic acid) (mg)	300	210
Vitamins		
Vitamin A (IU)	250-750†	175-525
Vitamin D (IU)	40-100	28-70
Vitamin K (μg)	4	3
Vitamin E (IU)	0.3 (with 0.7 IU/g linoleic acid	2.1
Vitamin C (mg)	8	5.6
Thiamin (μg)	40	28
Riboflavin (μg)	60	42
Vitamin B_6 (μg)	35 (with 15 μg/g of protein in formula)	25
Vitamin B_{12} (μg)	0.15	0.11
Niacin (μg equiv)	250	175
Folacin (μg)	4	2.8
Pantothenic acid (μg)	300	210
Biotin (μg)	1.5	1.1
Choline (mg)	7.0	4.9
Inositol (mg)	4.0	2.8
Minerals		
Calcium (mg)	50	35
Phosphorus (mg)	25	18
Calcium/phosphorus ratio	1.1-2.0	1.1-2.0
Magnesium (mg)	6	4
Iron (mg)	0.15	0.11
Iodine (μg)	5	3.5
Zinc (mg)	0.5	0.4
Copper (μg)	60	40
Manganese (μg)	5.0	3.5
Sodium (mg)	20 (6 mEq‡)	(6 mEq‡)
Potassium (mg)	80 (14 mEq‡)	(14 mEq‡)
Chloride (mg)	55 (11 mEq‡)	(11 mEq‡)

Adapted from Committee on Nutrition, American Academy of Pediatrics, Commentary on breast feeding and infant formulas, including proposed standards for formulas, in *Pediatric Nutrition Handbook*, pp. 119-138. (Evanston, Ill.: American Academy of Pediatrics, 1979), Chapter 10.

*Assuming 70 kcal per 100 ml. If the formula contains 80 kcal/100 ml, multiply amount in "per 100 kcal" column by 0.8; if 60 kcal/100 ml, by 0.6; etc.

†250-750 IU would be 75-225 μg or RE (retinol equivalents).

‡Milliequivalents per liter of formula.

Table 4.   Comparison of Starting Formulas, Adapted (Humanized) Formulas, and Medical Formulas

Characteristic	Starting formulas*	Adapted formulas†	Medical formulas‡	Human milk
Energy (kcal/100 ml)	68	68	68	74
Protein (g/100 ml)	1.5-1.6	1.5-1.6	2.0-2.5	1.1
Whey:casein ratio	20/80	60/40	(No cow's milk protein)	80/20
Carbohydrate (g/100 ml)	7.0-7.2	6.9-7.2	6.8	7.2
Carbohydrate source	Lactose	Lactose	Sucrose, corn syrup, corn starch	Lactose
Fat (g/100 ml)	3.6-3.7	3.6-3.8	3.4-3.6	2.7-4.6
Polyunsaturated fatty acid (g/100 ml)	1.0-1.7	0.5-1.0	0.9-2.0	0.7-1.5
Minerals				
Calcium (mg/l)	510-550	400-440	700-790	340
Phosphorus (mg/l)	390-460	200-330	500-530	140
Ca:P ratio	1.2-1.3	1.4-2.0	1.4-1.5	2.3
Magnesium (mg/l)	41-47	42-53	50-74	40
Iron (mg/l)§	12 or 1.5	13 or 2.6	1.2-12.7	0.2-1.0
Zinc	4.2-5.0	3.7-4.0	5.0-5.3	1.6
Sodium (mEq/l)	11-12	6-7	13-16	7
Potassium (mEq/l)	18-20	14-15	18-19	13
Renal solute load (mOsm/l)	105-106	91-92	126-147	74
Vitamins				
Vitamin A (IU/100 ml)	169-250	250-264	169-250	190-250
Vitamin D (IU/100 ml)	40-42	40-42	40-42	2.2
Vitamin K (μg/100 ml)	3	3-6	-	2
Vitamin E (IU/100 ml)	1.3-1.5	1.0-1.5	1.5	0.2
Vitamin C (mg/100 ml)	5.5	5.5-5.8	5.5	4.3-5.2
Thiamin (μg/100 ml)	53-65	65-70	40-53	14-16
Riboflavin (μg/100 ml)	63-100	100-110	60-63	36-37
Vitamin B_6 (μg/100 ml)	40	33-40	40-42	10-11
Vitamin B_{11} (μg/100 ml)	0.15-0.21	0.11-0.15	0.21-3.0	0.03-0.05
Niacin (mg equiv/100 ml)	0.7-1.3	0.7-1.0	0.85-0.9	0.15-0.18
Folacin (μg/100 ml)	5-11	5.0-5.3	10.0-10.6	2-5
Pantothenic acid (μg/100 ml)	0.3-0.32	0.21-0.3	0.32-0.5	0.18-0.23

Adapted from Committee on Nutrition, American Academy of Pediatrics, Commentary on breast feeding and infant formulas, including proposed standards for formulas, in *Pediatric Nutrition Handbook* (Evanston, Ill.: American Academy of Pediatrics, 1979), Chapter 10, pp. 119-138.

*These numbers represent two formulas: Similac and Enfamil.
†These numbers represent two formulas: SMA and Similac 60/40.
‡These numbers represent two soy-isolate-based formulas: Isomil and Prosobee.
§Alternative numbers here are for standard and iron-fortified formulas.

A and D, is acceptable as a followup formula. The AAP recommends that it be introduced at one year, but it is safe to use it sooner and it may be desirable to do so in many instances, because it is less expensive than formula. (Don't offer plain, unmodified cow's milk before six months, though, because the infant's GI tract may be sensitive to its protein, and if so, may bleed.)

Cow's milk comes in many forms — pasteurized, homogenized, evaporated, powdered, and others. (The terms are defined in the Miniglossary.) Any pasteurized milk that has nutritional value equivalent to or superior to whole cow's milk is acceptable, but low-fat or skim milk should not be used routinely with infants under a year old; they need the fat of regular milk. Powdered milk is usually skimmed, but fat-containing varieties are available. Most people use either vitamin A and D-fortified whole or evaporated milk.

Milk Substitutes If a milk substitute must be used, the choice should be made carefully. Whatever substitute is chosen has an important role to play in supplying the nutrients other children get from milk. Among the possible substitutes are: boiled milk, goat's or other species' milk, enzyme-treated milk, soy milk, milk products such es plain yogurt and cheese,

nondairy foods containing the nutrients of milk, imitation milk, and supplements.

In theory, it should be easy to choose an appropriate milk substitute. If the child is allergic to milk, then the milk protein is the offending substance, and a substitute with altered or different proteins must be found. If the child is intolerant to lactose, then a lactose-free substitute is needed. It is often difficult, however, to determine why the child tolerates milk poorly (see To Explore Further). In practice, the selection of a substitute may have to proceed by trial and error.

Milk protein is denatured when milk is boiled. Some

cases of milk allergy can be solved by this simple means. Plain, boiled milk tastes strange to a person who is accustomed to drinking fresh milk but may be acceptable to an unprejudiced child. Alternatively, liquid or powdered milk can be cooked into foods such as custards, baked goods, and meat loaf.

Goat's milk proteins differ somewhat from cow's milk proteins and may be tolerated by the child who can't tolerate cow's milk. Table 1 permits comparison of cow's milk and goat's milk and shows that they are similar in most respects; both should be fortified with vitamins A and D, however, to be com-

Table 5. Lactose Contents of Dairy Products

Note that these are all fermented dairy products. A nonfermented milk product like ice cream has about the same amount of lactose per protein as milk (1 1/2 c has 93% of the lactose in 1 c milk).

Dairy product	Serving size to equal 1 c milk in protein	Amount of lactose as compared to that in 1 c milk
Yogurt	1 c	75%*
Strawberry yogurt	1 c	39%†
Pasteurized processed cheese food	3 T	33%†
Grated American cheese	3/4 oz	25%†
Cottage cheese	1/4 c	14%*
Aged cheddar cheese	2 cu in	6%*
Swiss cheese	1 oz	trace†
Extra sharp cheddar cheese	2 cu in	trace†

*Calculated from A. D. Newcomer, Lactase deficiency, *Contemporary Nutrition* (April, 1979).
†Calculated from D. E. Lee and C. B. Lillibridge, A method for qualitative identification of sugars and semiquantitative determination of lactose content suitable for a variety of foods, *American Journal of Clinical Nutrition* 29 (1976):428-440.

patible with the standard diet.

The treatment of milk with enzymes to digest its lactose offers a promising new solution to the problem of lactose intolerance. The enzyme preparation (Lact-Aid) can be purchased over the counter and mixed with the milk before the milk is served. A low-lactose milk may soon be available as an alternative.[3]

If lactose intolerance is the problem, the intolerance is usually not absolute. A child can handle small amounts of milk periodically throughout the day — up to half a glass each time. Fermented dairy products offer the same nutrients as milk but with a lower lactose content, because in fermenting the milk, bacteria use the lactose as an energy source to do their work. Fermented dairy products' lactose contents compare with the lactose in milk as shown in Table 5.

A product people sometimes wonder about is acidophilus milk. To give the end of the story first, it is *not* useful for lactose-intolerant

individuals. It was developed on the theory that *L. acidophilus* bacteria could be added to milk to compete against other bacteria that might otherwise grow there or that might grow in the intestines after the milk is ingested.[4] However, if *L. acidophilus* bacteria were allowed to grow in the milk and ferment the lactose, they would produce a sour by-product, lactic acid. (The human intestinal enzyme that digests lactose, in contrast, produces the monosaccharides it is made of, glucose and galactose.) Therefore, *L. acidophilus* bacteria are grown in another medium and then harvested and added to milk, where they are not allowed to act any further. Acidophilus milk tastes sweet because its sugars are sweet, but its composition is the same as that of milk.

Not only dairy products but also certain meats and vegetables can be used to help supply the nutrients of milk. If foods are to be chosen to help replace milk in the diet, their calcium and riboflavin contents should be the basis for making the choice, because milk and milk products normally supply about 75 percent of people's intake of calcium and about 40 percent of their riboflavin. In most foods, the

two nutrients occur together, so a selection made on the basis of calcium contents will serve both purposes. Foods to emphasize could be selected from Table 6. Many of these foods supply ample amounts of vitamin A as well, but their vitamin D contents are variable and unreliable. The growing child who is outdoors daily can make his or her own vitamin D from the sun (see page 555). A sick child needs a vitamin D fortified milk substitute or a vitamin supplement.

The alternatives offered for milk, so far, have been superior in the sense that they are whole dairy products or foods that offer many nutrients besides the ones listed in the tables. An inferior alternative is imitation milk. Imitation milk varies but typically consists of water, sugar, vegetable fat, a source of protein (casein or soy, usually), and flavoring agents and stabilizers. Whatever is listed first on the label is the predominant ingredient. Imitation milk may be lower in protein than milk (for example, 1 percent rather than 3.5 percent) and may not supply the nutrients typical of milk. A milk substitute is satisfactory only if it provides high-quality protein, calcium, phosphorus, riboflavin, and vitamins A and D in quantities comparable to those in fortified fresh milk. Use of imitation milks "in the diets of children and infants is generally undesir-

[3]LactAid was described in *Nutrition and the MD*, April 1982. Development of low-lactose milk was first reported in 1979. A. H. R. Cheng, O. Brunser, J. Espinoza, H. L. Fones, F. Monckeberg, C. O. Chichester, G. Rand, and A. G. Hourigan, Long-term acceptance of low-lactose milk, *American Journal of Clinical Nutrition* 32 (1979):1989-1993.

[4]New milk product was begun in OSU laboratory, *Journal of Milk and Food Technology* (June 1976), p. 431.

Miniglossary

acidophilus milk (acid-OFF-ih-lus): milk to which a culture of *Lactobacillus acidophilus* has been added. The theory is that the presence of these bacteria in the milk, and in the intestines after the milk is drunk, prevents the growth of other bacteria that might be harmful.

adapted (humanized) formula: a formula whose composition is closer to that of human milk than that of a starting formula. Adapted formula might be chosen under special circumstances such as low birth weight, immaturity, or illness.

casein or **sodium caseinate:** the principal protein of cow's milk. Other milk proteins, found in a higher percentage in human milk, are **whey** and **lactalbumin**.

condensed milk: evaporated milk to which sugar (sucrose) is added before processing, as a preservative. The percentages of kcalories from protein, fat, and carbohydrate in condensed milk are 10:24.5:65.5. Condensed milk contains 321 kcal/100 ml and is more than twice as concentrated as evaporated milk (146 kcal/100 ml). Accidental use of condensed milk in preparation of infant formula can cause dehydration.

evaporated milk: milk concentrated by evaporation. The milk is preheated (for example, at 120° C, or 248° F, for three minutes) and then run aseptically into cans. The ratio of fat to nonfat solids is the same as in the original milk. By adding water, you derive standard milk; the taste, however, is altered by this process. Whole or skim milk from any species can be evaporated.

evaporated milk formula: formula homemade from evaporated milk, sugar, and water — seldom used today.

filled milk: milk in which the butterfat has been replaced with vegetable fat or oil. The fat chosen may be anywhere from 3 percent to 30 percent polyunsaturated (coconut oil and partially hydrogenated soybean or cottonseed oil, respectively).

followup formula: a formula used as part of a baby's mixed diet after 6 months of age. Examples: vitamin A and D fortified whole cow's milk, evaporated milk.

fortified (with respect to milk): milk to which vitamins A and D have been added so that a quart contains 2,000 IU vitamin A and 400 IU vitamin D.

homogenized milk: milk treated to mix the fat evenly with the watery part (fat ordinarily floats to the top as cream). Heated milk is forced under high pressure through small openings to break up the fat into small particles, which then remain dispersed throughout the milk. Whole or partially skimmed milk from any species (cow, goat, or other) can be homogenized.

imitation milk: a substitute for milk, nutritionally inferior to milk in that it contains significantly less of one or more of the nutrients in milk. See *imitation* in Highlight 12.

medical (therapeutic) formula: a formula for use in special medical conditions such as PKU (Highlight 4) or cow's milk intolerance.

modified milk: cow's milk that is treated to denature the protein and thereby aid digestion.

pasteurized milk: milk that is heat treated to reduce its bacterial count to an acceptable level. Methods vary; a common one is to heat the milk to at least 72° C (161° F), hold it at or above this temperature for 15 seconds, then cool it rapidly to 50° C (148° F) or lower. Whole or skim milk from any species (cow, goat, or other) can be pasteurized.

powdered milk: completely dehydrated milk solids produced by a variety of processes. Some powdered milks are processed to rehydrate easily (instant milk); others require extensive blending. Both whole and skim milks can be powdered.

starting formula: a formula designed to meet all of an infant's nutrient needs in the first six months of life.

whole milk: cow's milk from which the fat has not been removed. The standard of identity for whole milk in most states requires that milk labeled whole must contain not less than 3.25 percent milk fat and not less than 8.25 percent nonfat milk solids.

Table 6. High-Calcium Foods

The total amount of calcium to aim for in a child's diet is 800 mg/day (1,200 mg for the over-11 crowd). If milk can't be used, the following foods will help supply calcium. Availability of calcium from greens is unsure; binders such as oxalic acid in the greens may appreciably reduce calcium absorption.

Foods providing

100+ mg calcium	150+ mg calcium	200+ mg calcium	250+ calcium
1 c cooked farina (quick type)	1 medium stalk broccoli	1 oz cheddar cheese	1 oz cheese (Swiss or Parmesan)
3 oz canned herring	1 c ice cream	1 c cottage cheese	1 c cooked collards
1 c cooked kale	1 c cooked mustard greens	1 c oysters	4 oz self-rising flour
1 tbsp blackstrap molasses	1 c cooked spinach	1 c cooked rhubarb	1 c milk
3 tbsp regular (light) molasses	3 oz pink, canned salmon		3 oz sardines
5 tbsp maple syrup			1 c cooked turnip greens

From G. B. Forbes, Calcium, phosphorus, and magnesium, in *Pediatric Nutrition Handbook* (Evanston, Ill.: American Academy of Pediatrics, 1979), Chapter 4, p. 38.

able and should be discouraged."[5]

Another product sometimes substituted for milk is filled milk, that is, milk in which the butterfat has been replaced by some other fat. Filled milk may be used in fat-modified diets, usually for adults.

Finally, the choice can be made to offer milk's nutrients in supplement form. Should the choice be made to deliver calcium that way, however, many disadvantages have to be overcome. A typical calcium supplement contains 100 mg of calcium per pill (in the salt, calcium lactate),

[5]Council on Foods and Nutrition, Substitutes for whole milk (a council statement), *Journal of the American Medical Association* 208 (1969), reprint.

and the recommended dose is nine pills a day. The calcium taken this way arrives in the body without benefit of all the nutrients that normally accompany it in milk and aid in its absorption (see page 417). Flow Chart 2 shows how to go about finding a milk substitute.

In a baby's first six months, the choice of formula is important, because whatever is chosen must supply the nutrients of human milk in similar forms and proportions. After the first year, the exact formulation of the milk selected is not so critical, but the choice is still important, because milk or its substitute occupies a place in the diet that no other type of food can fill. The health professional who takes the time and makes the

effort to learn what the key variables are will be able to offer substantial help to many people at an important time in life — the growing years.

To Explore Further

Nutrition and the MD, January 1980, provided information under the following titles:

● Milk allergy in infants.

● Lactose intolerance.

Nutrition and the MD, April 1982, provided information under the following titles:

● Dietary management of lactose intolerance.

● Milk vs. lactose intolerance.

● Evaluation of LactAid and acidophilus milk.

A book highly recommended by an American Dietetic As-

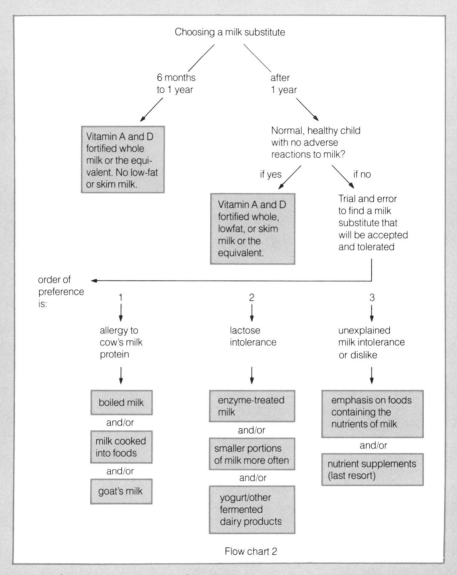

Choosing a milk substitute

6 months to 1 year

after 1 year

Vitamin A and D fortified whole milk or the equivalent. No low-fat or skim milk.

Normal, healthy child with no adverse reactions to milk?

if yes

if no

Vitamin A and D fortified whole, lowfat, or skim milk or the equivalent.

Trial and error to find a milk substitute that will be accepted and tolerated

order of preference is:

1
allergy to cow's milk protein

boiled milk
and/or
milk cooked into foods
and/or
goat's milk

2
lactose intolerance

enzyme-treated milk
and/or
smaller portions of milk more often
and/or
yogurt/other fermented dairy products

3
unexplained milk intolerance or dislike

emphasis on foods containing the nutrients of milk
and/or
nutrient supplements (last resort)

Flow chart 2

sociation reviewer that includes information on the selection of milk substitutes is:

● Bahna, S. L., and Heiner, D. C. *Allergies to Milk*. New York: Grune and Stratton, 1980.

Milk-free soy formulas are compared and critiqued in:

● Fomon, S. J. Milk-free formulas with comments on milk allergy. In *Infant Nutrition*, Chapter 12, pp. 225-244. Philadelphia:

Saunders, 1967.

Fomon's book is still one of the standard references on many aspects of infant nutrition. Look for the latest edition.

Another widely used reference is:

● Committee on Nutrition, American Academy of Pediatrics. Commentary on breast feeding and infant formulas, including proposed standards for for-

mulas. In *Pediatric Nutrition Handbook*, Chapter 10, pp. 119-138. Evanston, Ill.: American Academy of Pediatrics, 1979.

An up-to-date reference with more detail than this Highlight is:

● Anderson, S. A., Chinn, H. I., and Fisher, K. D. History and current status of infant formulas. *American Journal of Clinical Nutrition* 35 (1982): 381-397.

CHAPTER 16

CONTENTS

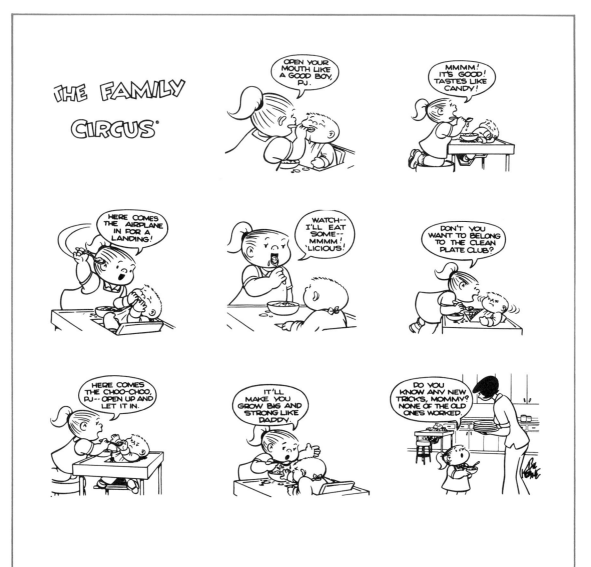

A one-year-old feels like eating less.

INFANT, CHILD, TEENAGER

Food habits are inextricably associated with the emotional and social development of a child from earliest infancy. The goal [is] not good nutrition, as such, but happy, satisfied, adjusted children.

ETHEL AUSTIN MARTIN

A single year of life was the subject of the last chapter; this chapter covers almost 20 years. The unequal emphasis is appropriate, because the first year, including the nine months of intrauterine life, is most critical to the individual's health and development through the following decades of life. Special relationships between nutrition and health exist in all the stages of life, however, and deserve their fair share of attention. This chapter relates nutrition and health in three life stages: infancy, childhood, and the teen years.

Nutrition of the Infant

The primary — indeed, the only — food needed by the infant for the first few months of life is milk, either breast milk or formula. The two modes of feeding milk were the subject of Chapter 15. This chapter begins at the point at which supplemental foods are introduced. The timing of these introductions is determined by the infant's need and developmental readiness for them.

Growth and Development   A baby grows faster during the first year than ever again, as Figure 1 shows. The birthweight doubles in four months, from 7 to 14 pounds, and another 7 pounds is added in the next eight months. (If a ten-year-old child were to do this, the child's weight would increase from 70 to 210 pounds in a single year.) By the end of the first year, the growth rate has slowed down, and the weight gained between the first and second birthdays amounts to only about 5 pounds. This tremendous growth is a composite of the differing growth patterns of all the internal organs. The generalization that many critical periods occur early still holds true.

The growth of infants and children directly reflects their nutritional well-being and is the most important parameter used in assessing their nutrition status. Chapter 18 tells how to measure height and weight of infants and children and how to use growth charts to follow their progress.

Figure 1 Weight gain of human infants (boys) in the first 5 years.

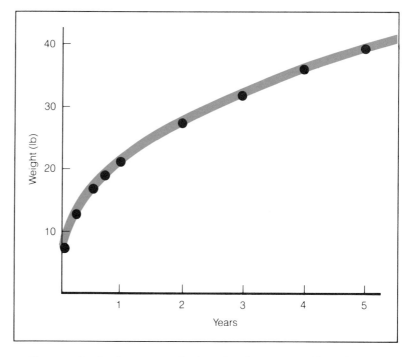

Changes in body organs during the first year affect the baby's readiness to accept solid foods. At first, all he can do is suck (and he can do that powerfully), but he can only swallow liquids that are well back in his throat. Later (at two months or so) he can move his tongue against his palate to swallow semisolid food. Still later, the first teeth erupt, but it is not until sometime during the second year that a baby can begin to handle chewy food. The stomach and intestines are immature at first; they can digest milk sugar (lactose) but can't manufacture significant quantities of the starch-digesting enzyme, amylase, until somewhat later and so cannot digest starch until perhaps three months.

The baby's kidneys are unable to concentrate waste efficiently, so a baby must excrete relatively more water than an adult to carry off a comparable amount of waste. This means that dehydration, which can be dangerous, can occur more easily in an infant than in an adult. Because infants can communicate their needs only by crying, it is important to remember that they may be crying for fluid. A baby's metabolism is fast, so his energy needs are high.

Baby's metabolism

  Heart rate: 120-140 beats/min
  Respiration rate: 20/min

Adult's metabolism
  Heart rate: 70-80 beats/min
  Respiration rate: 12-14/min

Nutrient Needs The rapid growth and metabolism of the infant demand ample supplies of the growth and energy nutrients. Babies, because they are small, need smaller total amounts of these nutrients than adults do; but as a percentage of body weight, babies need over twice as much of most nutrients. Figure 2 compares a three-month-old baby's needs with those of an adult man; as you can see, some of the differences are extraordinary. After three months, energy needs

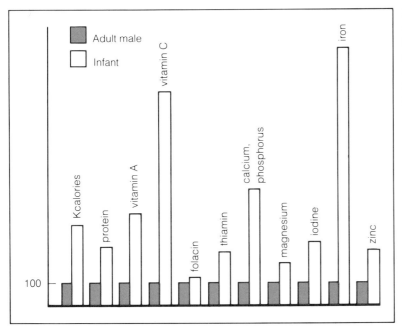

Figure 2 Comparison of the nutrient needs of a 3-month-old infant with those of an adult male (23 years or older) per unit of body weight. The adult male's needs are set at 100 percent (see RDA table, inside front cover).

continue to increase even though the growth rate slows down. As a baby nears the first birthday, the kcalories saved by slower growth are spent in greatly increased activity. (Babies are now known to require fewer kcalories in the middle of their first year than has been believed in the past, and new recommendations were being made as of 1981.[1])

Iron is the nutrient hardest to provide for infants, because it doesn't occur in adequate amounts in milk (except breast milk or iron-fortified formula). One U.S. survey showed in 1979 that by the end of the first year more than 70 percent of infants were receiving less than the RDA for iron, and almost half of them were receiving less than two-thirds of the RDA, a bottom line for adequacy. Iron was the nutrient most needing attention in infant nutrition.[2]

First Foods The baby's most important food is milk: breast milk or formula at first, cow's milk or a substitute after six months. Recommended transitions from one form of milk to another are shown in Table 1.

The timing for adding solid foods to a baby's diet depends on several factors. If the baby is breastfed, additions to the diet should probably

[1] Part of the significance of the infant's lower energy needs at six months is that breastfeeding will be seen to be more adequate when measured against them. R. G. Whitehead, A critical analysis of measured food energy intakes during infancy and early childhood in comparison with current international recommendations, *Journal of Human Nutrition* 35 (1981):339-348.

[2] G. H. Johnson, G. A. Purvis, and R. D. Wallace, What nutrients do our infants really get? *Nutrition Today*, July/August 1981, pp. 4-10, 23-26.

Table 1.   Transitions in Milk Feeding

Before 6 months

Breast-fed infant should receive:
    Breast milk.
    Vitamin D.
    Fluoride at pediatrician's discretion.

Formula-fed infant should receive:
    Vitamins A and D in formula separately.
    Vitamin C in formula or separately.
    Fluoride at pediatrician's discretion.

If weaning from breast milk before 6 months, wean to formula as above.

Wait to wean from formula until at least 6 months.

After 6 months

If weaning from breast milk after 6 months, wean to formula or whole cow's milk with supplementation.

Whole cow's milk (may be fresh or evaporated) should be supplemented with:
    Vitamins A and D if not fortified.
    Iron and/or iron-fortified cereals.
    Vitamin C and/or C-rich foods or juices.
    Fluoride at pediatrician's discretion.

After 1 year

When all four food groups are eaten daily, whole or low-fat cow's milk is acceptable.

Continue checking diet for vitamin C, iron, and all nutrients.

Continue fluoride supplements if necessary.

Adapted from recommendations made in *Pediatrics* 62 (1978):733 and *Nutrition and the MD*, March 1980.

A term used by many authorities to mean supplemental or weaning foods is **beikost** (BYE-cost).

wait until about six months, but not later. Babies not fed solid foods in the second half of the first year suffer delayed growth.[3] If the baby is formula-fed, a reasonable pattern for adding foods to the diet is as shown in Table 2. Solids should not be introduced too early, because infants are more likely to develop allergies to them in the early months.[4] But all babies are different, and the program of additions should depend on the individual baby, not on any rigid schedule.

The addition of foods to a baby's diet should be governed by three considerations: the baby's nutrient needs, the baby's physical readiness to handle different forms of foods, and the need to detect and control

[3] M. Winick, Infant nutrition: Formula or breast feeding? *Professional Nutritionist*, Spring 1980, pp. 1-3.

[4] L. A. Barness, Feeding children, *Journal of the Florida Medical Association*, April 1979, pp. 443-448.

Table 2.   First Foods for the Formula-Fed Baby

Age (months)	Addition
0-1	Supplement (depending on what's in formula)
1-2	Diluted orange juice (for vitamin C)
4-6	Iron-fortified rice cereal followed by other cereals (for iron; baby can swallow and can digest starch now)*
5-7	Strained vegetables and/or fruits and their juices, one by one
6-8	Protein foods (cheese, yogurt, cooked beans, meat, fish, chicken, egg yolk)
9	Finely chopped meat (baby can chew now)
10-12	Whole egg (allergies less likely now)
Later	Cottage cheese, toast, teething crackers (for emerging teeth)

*Later you can change cereals, but don't forget to keep on using the iron-fortified varieties. According to *Nutrition and the MD*, April 1981, the iron in cereal specially prepared for babies is so bioavailable that 3 level tablespoons a day is all they need.

Adapted from the 1979 *Recommendations for Infant Feeding Practices of the California Department of Health Services* as presented in *Current infant feeding practices, Nutrition and the MD*, January 1980.

allergic reactions. With respect to nutrient needs, a nutrient needed early, especially by the formula-fed baby, is vitamin C; and juices and fruits that contain vitamin C are usually among the first foods introduced. A nutrient needed later is iron. A baby's stored iron supply from before birth runs out after the birth weight doubles, so formula with iron; iron-fortified cereals; and later, meat are recommended.[5] Tables 1 and 2 show other examples of the ways nutrient needs dictate food choices for infants.

Physical readiness develops in many small steps. For example, the ability to swallow solid food develops around four to six months, and experience with solid food at that time helps to develop swallowing ability by desensitizing the gag reflex.[6] Later still, a baby can sit up, can handle finger foods, and is teething; then hard crackers and other hard finger foods should be introduced. These promote the development of manual dexterity and control of the jaw muscles. Table 2 gives more details.

Some parents want to feed solids at an earlier age, on the theory that "stuffing the baby" at bedtime will make him (or her) more likely to

[5]C. A. Finch, "Iron-Deficiency Anemia in the Pre-School Child," in *Pre-School Child Malnutrition, Primary Deterrent to Human Progress*. This publication reports the proceedings of publication 1282 (Washington, D.C.: NAS-NRC, 1966), pp. 93-95, an international conference on prevention of malnutrition in the pre-school child, Washington, D.C., December 1964.

[6]P. Pipes, When should semisolid foods be fed to infants? *Journal of Nutrition Education* 9 (1977):57-59.

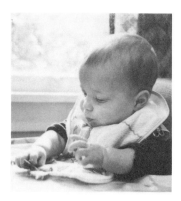

sleep through the night. There is no proof for this theory. On the average, babies start to sleep through the night at about the same age, regardless of when solid foods are introduced.[7]

New foods should be introduced singly so that allergies can be detected. For example, when cereals are introduced, try rice cereal first for several days; it causes allergy least often. Try wheat cereal last; it is the most common offender. If a cereal causes an allergic reaction (irritability, misery), discontinue its use before going on to the next food. About nine times out of ten, the allergy won't be evident immediately but will manifest itself in vague symptoms occurring up to five days after the offending food is eaten, so it isn't easy to detect.

About one out of every four people may have an allergy of one kind or another, and about half of these allergies are caused by foods — most commonly, milk, wheat, egg (whites), corn, and pork.[8] If a parent detects allergies in his infant's early life, he can spare the whole family much grief.

As for the choice of foods, baby foods commercially prepared in the United States and Canada are generally safe, nutritious, and of high quality. In response to consumer demand, baby food companies have removed much of the added salt and sugar their products contained in the past, and they also contain few or no additives.[9] They generally have high nutrient density, except for mixed dinners (which contain little meat) and desserts (which are heavily sweetened). An alternative for the parent who wants the baby to have family foods is to "blenderize" a small portion of the table food at each meal. This necessitates cooking without salt, though. Foods adults prepare for themselves often contain much more salt than even commercial baby foods. The adults can salt their own food after the baby's portion has been taken. And babies should never be fed canned vegetables; not only is the sodium content too high but also there is a risk of lead contamination.[10] It is also important to take precautions against food poisoning and to avoid the use of vegetables in which nitrites are likely to form — notably, home-prepared carrots, beets, and spinach.[11] Honey should never be fed to infants because of the risk of botulism.

[7]By three months, 74 percent are sleeping through the night whether or not they are receiving solid food. L. L. Clark and V. A. Beal, Age at introduction of solid foods to infants in Manitoba, *Journal of the Canadian Dietetic Association* 42 (1981):72-78.

[8]J. C. Breneman, Food allergy, *Contemporary Nutrition* 4 (March 1979).

[9]Gerber Products Company, Why we put what we put in Gerber baby foods (advertisement), *Nutrition Today*, September/October 1973, p. 24; and J. C. Suerth (chairman of the board, Gerber Products Company), Letter to the editor, *Nutrition Today*, May/June 1977, pp. 34-35. According to *Nutrition and the MD*, January 1980, there was no more sugar in Beechnut foods and much less in Heinz than formerly.

[10]C. M. Kerr, Jr., K. S. Reisinger, and F. W. Plankey, Sodium concentration of home-made baby foods, *Pediatrics* 62 (1978):331-335; Questions readers ask, *Nutrition and the MD*, May 1980.

[11]C. A. Thomson and I. S. Sheremate, Current issues in infant feeding, *Journal of the Canadian Dietetic Association* 39 (July 1978):189-194.

At a year of age, the obvious food to supply most of the nutrients the baby needs is still milk; 2 to 3 1/2 cups a day are now sufficient. More milk than this would displace foods necessary to provide iron and would cause the iron-deficiency anemia known as milk anemia. The other foods — meat, iron-fortified cereal, enriched or whole-grain bread, fruit, and vegetables — should be supplied in variety and in amounts sufficient to round out total kcalorie needs. A meal plan that meets these requirements for the one-year-old is shown in the margin.

Looking Ahead   The first year of a baby's life is the time to lay the foundation for future health. From the nutrition standpoint, the relevant problems most common in later years are obesity and dental disease. Prevention of obesity should also help prevent the development of the obesity-related diseases — atherosclerosis, diabetes, and cancer.

Infant obesity should be avoided. Probably the most important single measure to undertake during the first year is to encourage eating habits that will support continued normal weight as the child grows. Primarily, this means introducing nutritious foods in an inviting way; not forcing the baby to finish the bottle or the baby food jar; avoiding concentrated sweets and empty kcalorie foods; and encouraging vigorous physical activity. It has been suggested that the early introduction of sweet fruits to babies' diets might favor their developing a preference for sweets and lessen their liking for vegetables introduced later. To prevent this, the order should perhaps be changed: vegetables first, fruits later. This practice now has a wide following.

To discourage development of the behaviors and attitudes that plague the obese, parents should avoid teaching babies to seek food as a reward, to expect food as comfort for unhappiness, or to associate food deprivation with punishment. If they cry for thirst, they should be given water, not milk or juice. Babies have no internal "kcalorie counter"; and they stop eating when their stomachs are full, so low-kcalorie foods will satisfy as long as they provide bulk.

Beyond these recommendations, some thought is being given to the idea that infants should be started on a "prudent diet" like that recommended for heart patients: Restrict fat, increase the ratio of polyunsaturated to saturated fat, and reduce cholesterol intake. Such a diet has been tried with infants up to three years of age. It seems to have done them no harm, while lowering their serum cholesterol.[12] However, this kind of program is only experimental. Babies need the kcalories and fat of normal milk, and most experts agree that they should be fed whole or at least low-fat — not skim — milk until after they are a year old. The only exception might be the seriously obese baby, who should perhaps be started on a prudent diet as early as three months of age.[13] Tampering with the amount of protein in a baby's diet

milk anemia: iron-deficiency anemia caused by drinking so much milk that iron-rich foods are displaced in the diet.

Meal plan for a 1-year-old:

Breakfast
1 c milk
3 tbsp cereal
2-3 tbsp strained fruit
teething crackers

Lunch
1 c milk
2-3 tbsp vegetables
chopped meat
2-3 tbsp pudding

Snack
1/2 c milk
teething crackers

Supper
1 c milk
1 egg
2 tbsp cereal or potato
2-3 tbsp cooked fruit
teething crackers

Babies develop sensitivity to their own satiety (see page 269) at about 10 months, another example of developmental readiness.

For more about the prudent diet, turn to Chapter 26.

---

[12]G. Friedman and S. J. Goldberg, An evaluation of the safety of a low-saturated-fat, low-cholesterol diet beginning in infancy, *Pediatrics* 58 (1976):655-657.

[13]The prudent diet in pediatric practice, *Nutrition and the MD*, November 1979.

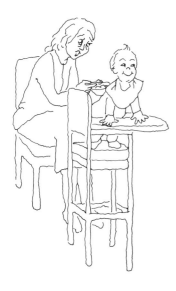

could be especially undesirable, because altered amounts of protein affect the baby's body composition, with unpredictable consequences.[14]

Normal dental development is promoted by the same strategies as those outlined above: supplying nutritious foods, avoiding sweets, and discouraging association of food with reward or comfort. In addition, the practice of giving a baby a bottle as a pacifier is strongly discouraged by dentists on the grounds that sucking for long periods of time pushes the normal jawline out of shape and causes the bucktooth profile: protruding upper and receding lower teeth. Further, prolonged sucking on a bottle of milk or juice bathes the upper teeth in a carbohydrate-rich fluid that favors the growth of decay-producing bacteria. Babies permitted to do this are sometimes seen with their upper teeth decayed all the way to the gum line. A photograph of this effect appears on page 458.

Mealtimes   The wise parent of a one-year-old offers nutrition and love together. Both promote growth. It is literally true that "feeding with love" produces better growth in both weight and height of children than feeding the same food in an emotionally negative climate.[15] It also promotes better brain development. The formation of nerve-to-nerve connections in the brain depends both on nutrients and on environmental stimulation.[16]

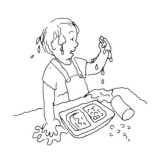

The person feeding a one-year-old has to be aware that this is a period in the child's life when exploring and experimenting are normal and desirable behaviors. The child is developing a sense of *autonomy* that, if allowed to flower, will provide the foundation for later confidence and effectiveness as an individual. The child's impulses, if consistently denied, can turn to shame and self-doubt.

In light of the developmental and nutritional needs of one-year-olds, and in the face of their often contrary and willful behavior, a few feeding guidelines may be helpful. Following are several problem situations with suggestions for handling them.

- He stands and plays at the table instead of eating. Don't let him. This is unacceptable behavior and should be firmly discouraged. Put him down and let him wait until the next feeding to eat again. Be consistent and firm, not punitive. If he is really hungry, he will soon learn to sit still while eating. A baby's appetite is less keen at a year than at eight months, and his kcalorie needs are relatively lower. A one-year-old will get enough to eat if he lets his own hunger be his guide.

[14]L. E. Holt, Jr., Protein economy in the growing child, *Postgraduate Medicine* 27 (1960):783-798.

[15]E. M. Widdowson, Mental contentment and physical growth, *Lancet* 1 (1951):1316-1318.

[16]J. Cravioto, Nutrition, stimulation, mental development and learning, *Nutrition Today*, September/October 1981, pp. 4-8, 10-15.

- She wants to poke her fingers into her food. Let her. She has much to learn from feeling the texture of her food. When she knows all about it, she'll naturally graduate to the use of a spoon.

- He wants to manage the spoon himself but can't handle it. Let him try. As he masters it, withdraw gradually until he is feeding himself competently. This is the age at which a baby can learn to feed himself and is most strongly motivated to do so. He will spill, of course, but he'll grow out of it soon enough.

- She refuses food that her mother knows is good for her. This way of demonstrating autonomy, one of the few available to the one-year-old, is most satisfying. Don't force. It is in the one- to two-year-old stage that most of the feeding problems develop that can last throughout life. As long as she is getting enough milk and is offered a variety of nutritious foods to choose from, she will gradually acquire a taste for different foods — provided that she feels she is making the choice. This year is the most important year of a child's life in establishing future food preferences. If a baby refuses milk, an alternative source of the bone- and muscle-building nutrients it supplies must be provided. Milk-based puddings, custards, and cheese are often successful substitutes. For the baby who is allergic to milk, soy milk and other formulas are available (see Highlight 15).

- He prefers sweets — candy and sugary confections — to foods containing more nutrients. Human beings of all races and cultures have a natural inborn preference for sweet-tasting foods. Limit them strictly. There is no room in a baby's daily 1,000 kcalories for the kcalories from sweets, except occasionally. The meal plan shown before provides more than 500 kcalories from milk; one or two servings of each of the other types of food provide the other 500. If a candy bar were substituted for any of these foods, the baby would lose out on valuable nutrients; if it were added daily, he would gradually become obese.

Infants Needing Special Attention   A baby with colic causes its parents much grief. Often the cause of colic is impossible to detect; but there are two known nutrition-related causes — overfeeding and underfeeding. Most often, it is *over*feeding that has made the baby so irritable. L. A. Barness, a pediatrician and authority on infant feeding, recommends that the parent's advisor (doctor, nurse, or nutritionist) obtain an accurate dietary history on a colicky infant and rule out these causes before recommending any change in food selections.[17]

Iron-deficiency anemia is too often a problem in infancy, as already mentioned, and can be difficult to manage.[18] All health professionals should be alert to the possibility that anemia may be contributing to an

colic: a syndrome seen in the young infant, usually not over 3 months. The infant cries as if feeling intense abdominal pain. The cause is unknown, but it helps to hug, pat, or rock the baby.

[17]Barness, 1979.

[18]Therapeutic trials in mild iron deficiency in infants, *Nutrition Reviews* 40 (1982):139-141.

To identify anemia in infants from hemoglobin, the line is often drawn at 11.5 g/100 ml.

Loose, watery stools are the identifying characteristic of **diarrhea.** A baby may have up to 8 normal movements a day and be fine. Treatment of diarrhea should be managed by the physician.

infant's abnormal behavior or development. Iron-fortified and iron-rich foods are an important part of therapy.

Diarrhea is a common symptom arising from many different kinds of infections and disturbances. It should never be taken lightly, especially in infants, because they can rapidly become seriously dehydrated. Diarrhea is the cause of more than half of all the deaths of children under four.

The most common cause of diarrhea is overfeeding, according to Barness.[19] Whatever its cause, maintaining fluid balance is the main part of treatment, even if this means feeding by tube or through a vein.

When diarrhea sets in, the intestine becomes irritated and inflamed; the enzyme lactase disappears from the intestinal wall; and the infant then cannot digest the lactose of milk. Instead, the intestinal bacteria attack the lactose and thrive on it, worsening the intestinal infection. If milk is given, it makes the irritation worse, and the intestine becomes abnormally permeable to food proteins. Some proteins may leak into the bloodstream and elicit an allergic reaction. Often, even after the episode of diarrhea has cleared up, the infant remains allergic to the offending food — often, milk itself. In counseling the parent of an infant with diarrhea not to offer protein-containing foods until a few days after the GI tract has settled down, you can be more persuasive if you explain this rationale.

There are many, many other diseases of infants, of course, that are not mentioned here. Part Four of this book is devoted to nutrition in disease states, and some diseases of infants are discussed there. Before leaving this subject, it should be said that illness, any illness, can quickly deplete an infant's nutrient stores. Half of the infants on the pediatric floor in any hospital are fighting malnutrition in addition to their other problems. Starvation worsens illness and hastens death. Whatever the disease or trauma, attention to nutrition is a crucial part of therapy.

One-year-old child and two-year-old child reduced to same height.

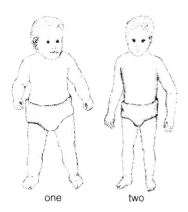

one   two

The Early Years

After the age of one, a child's growth rate slows, as shown in Figure 1. But during the next year, the body changes dramatically. At one, children have just learned to stand erect and toddle; by two, they can take long strides with solid confidence and are learning to run, jump, and climb. The internal change that makes these new accomplishments possible is the accumulation of a larger mass and greater density of bone and muscle tissue. The changes are obvious in the margin figure: Two-year-olds have lost much of their baby fat; their muscles (especially in the back, buttocks, and legs) have firmed and

[19]Barness, 1979.

strengthened, and the leg bones have lengthened and increased in density.

Thereafter, the same trend — lengthening of the long bones and an increase in musculature — continues, unevenly and more slowly, until adolescence. Growth comes in spurts; a six-year-old child may wear the same pair of shoes for a year, then need new shoes twice in the next four months.

A factor of importance is that there seems to be a period of rapid cell division in the fat tissue around the age of one or two. Like other critical periods, this one is limited in time; later, cell division slows down and the proportion of fat cells becomes fixed. If a baby is overfed during this time, the fat cell number may increase beyond the normal limit, leaving the child with too many fat cells. If the number of fat cells is involved in hunger regulation in the adult, this many mean that the fat baby is destined to be abnormally hungry for life and so to have a hard time fighting obesity.

The above hypothesis is not clearly established for human beings, but it is known that the obesity of childhood differs from adult-onset obesity in several respects. Excess weight in the early years places a demand on the skeletal and muscular tissues so that they, too, grow overly large. An obese child becomes an adult whose bones and muscles are denser than those of slimmer people. Excess weight is less often successfully and permanently lost in such an adult.

Just before adolescence, the growth patterns of girls and boys begin to become distinct. In girls, fat becomes a larger percentage of the total body weight, and in boys the lean body mass — muscle and bone — becomes much greater. Around this time, growth in height may seem to stop altogether for a while. This is the calm before the storm.

Nutritional Needs and Feeding   A one-year-old child needs perhaps 1,000 kcalories a day; a three-year-old needs only 300 to 500 kcalories more. Appetite decreases markedly around the age of one year, in line with the great reduction in growth rate. Thereafter, the appetite fluctuates; a child will need and demand much more food during periods of rapid growth than during periods of quiescence. The nutrients that need emphasis continue to be protein, calcium, and phosphorus, and the food best suited to supply them continues to be milk.

The preadolescent period is the last one in which parental food choices have much influence. As children gather their forces for the adolescent growth spurt, they are accumulating stores of nutrients that will be needed in the coming years. When they take off on that growth spurt, there will be a period during which their nutrient intakes, especially of calcium, cannot meet the demands of rapidly growing bones. Then they will draw on these nutrient stores. The denser their bones are before this occurs, the better prepared they will be.

The gradually increasing needs for all nutrients during the growing years are evident from the RDA table and the Canadian Dietary Standard, which list separate averages for each span of three years. To provide these nutrients, the Four Food Group Plan recommends the following:

- 3 servings of milk or milk products.
- 2 servings of meat or meat substitutes.
- 4 or more servings of fruits and vegetables.
- 4 or more servings of breads and cereals.

For meat, fruits, and vegetables, a serving is loosely defined as 1 tablespoon (T) per year. Thus at four years of age, a serving of any of these foods would be 4 T (1/4 c).

After the crucial first year, there is still much a parent can do to foster the development of healthy eating habits. The goal is to teach children to like nutritious foods in all four categories.

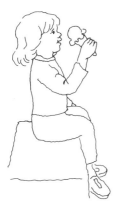

Calcium and riboflavin in a delicious form.

Experimentation with children's food patterns shows that candy, cola, and other concentrated sweets must be limited in a child's diet if the needed nutrients are to be supplied. If such foods are permitted in large quantities, there are only two possible outcomes: nutrient deficiencies or obesity. The child can't be trusted to choose nutritious foods on the basis of taste alone; the preference for sweets is innate.[20] On the other hand, an active child can enjoy the higher-kcalorie nutritious foods in each category; ice cream or pudding in the milk group, cake and cookies (whole-grain or enriched only, however) in the bread group. These foods, made from milk and grain, carry valuable nutrients and encourage a child to learn, appropriately, that eating is fun.

Children sometimes seem to lose their appetites for a while; this is nothing to worry about. The perfection of appetite regulation in children of normal weight guarantees that their kcalorie intakes will be right for each stage of growth. As long as the kcalories they do consume are from nutritious foods, they are well provided for. (One caution, however: Wandering school-age children may be spending pocket money at the nearby candy store.) An overzealous mother, unaware that her one-year-old is supposed to slow down, may begin a lifelong conflict over food by trying to force more food on the child than the child feels like eating.

Nutrition at School   While parents are doing what they can to establish favorable eating behavior during the transition from infancy to childhood, other factors are entering the picture. At five or so, the

[20]R. B. Choate, Selling cavities — U.S. style (address presented at the American Dental Association annual meeting, 11 October 1977, Council on Dental Health, American Dental Association). According to the speaker, the taste for sweetness already exists in the fetus, peaks at 14 years, and is more marked in blacks than in whites.

child goes to school and encounters foods prepared and served by outsiders. The U.S. government funds several programs to provide nutritious, high-quality meals for children at school. School lunches are designed to meet certain requirements: They must include specified servings of milk, protein-rich food (meat, cheese, eggs, legumes, or peanut butter), vegetables, fruits, bread or other grain foods, and butter or margarine. The design is intended to provide at least a third of the RDA for each of the nutrients. The School Lunch pattern was split into several patterns in 1980 to provide for the needs of different ages better than it had done in the past (see Table 3).

Parents rely on the school lunch program to meet a significant part of their children's nutrient needs on school days, but children don't always like what they are served. In response to children's differing needs and tastes, the school lunch program has been attempting to do better at feeding children both what they want and what will nourish them. The trend is:

● To increase the variety of offerings and allow children to choose what they are served.

● To vary portion sizes, so that little children may take little servings.

● To involve students (in secondary schools) in the planning of menus.

● To improve the scheduling of lunches so that children can eat when they are hungry and can have enough time to eat well.

A step toward making the lunches more consistent with today's ideals of healthful food has been to drop the requirement for whole milk and to offer low-fat or skim milk instead. Another alteration has been to eliminate the requirement that butter or margarine be served.

Television and Vending Machines   For the most part, children learn nutrition from parents or teachers who know very little about it. Meanwhile, they hear a great deal about foods from the television set. Many authorities are concerned that television commercials may have a less-than-desirable impact. It is estimated that the average child sees more than 10,000 commercials a year, of which many more than half are for sugary foods. Hundreds of millions of dollars are spent in the effort to sell these foods to children.[21] Most of the concern centers on the issue of sugar. You may recall that not all the public disapproval of sugar is based on scientific findings. However, there is widespread agreement on one point: Sticky, sugary foods left in the teeth provide an ideal environment for the growth of mouth bacteria and the formation of cavities. No regulations to prevent the promotion of sticky, sugary foods are in force, however.

Highlight 16 offers more about sugar and children.

[21]Choate, 1977.

It thus remains up to us to determine which food commercials we will believe and which we will not. Dentists, especially, have the obligation to educate their patients individually as long as misleading claims continue to appear on national television. A model eating plan that favors dental health is shown in Table 4.

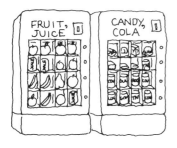

Television is not the only environmental force affecting children's food choices. Another is vending machines, especially in schools. The American Dental Association has established a National Task Force for the Prohibition of the Sale of Confections (sticky, sugary foods) in Schools and has resolved that the task force should seek changes in the School Lunch Act to eliminate the sale of confections as snacks in schools.[22] An experiment in six Canadian schools showed that children would choose more nutritious snacks if they were offered side by side with the sugary foods. When apples were made available in vending machines, there was a 27 percent reduction in the selection of chocolate bars. When milk was made available, soft-drink use dropped by 42 percent.[23]

Soft drinks contain not only sugar but also caffeine, which is a matter of some concern to pediatricians.[24] A cup of hot chocolate or a 12-oz cola beverage may contain as much as 50 mg caffeine; two or more such beverages are equivalent in the body of a 60-pound child to the caffeine in 8 cups of coffee for a 175-pound man.[25] Chocolate bars also contribute caffeine. Children and young adults who are troubled by irregular heartbeats or difficulty in sleeping may need to control their caffeine consumption.

Looking Ahead In children, as in infants, eating habits help determine whether development takes place in a positive or negative direction. To avoid obesity, the preschool child should be trained to "eat thin." Mealtimes should be relaxed and leisurely. Children should learn to eat slowly, pause and enjoy their table companions, and stop eating when they are full. The "clean your plate" dictum should be stamped out for all time. Parents who wish to avoid waste should learn to serve

[22]N. L. Shory, School confection sale bans: What can the dental profession do? (address presented at the American Dental Association annual meeting, 11 October 1977, Council on Dental Health, American Dental Association).

[23]L. Crawford, Junk food in our schools? A look at student spending in school vending machines and concessions, *Journal of the Canadian Dietetic Association* 38 (July 1977):193. Abstract cited in *Journal of the American Dietetic Association* 71 (1977):572. See also San Jose: Moving more nutritious lunches, *Institutions/Volume Feeding Magazine,* (1 August 1977), pp. 42-43; and E. Ott, Quieting our detractors' voices, *Food Management* 14 (1979):25-26.

[24]L. P. DiOrio, Improving nutrition: What should we eat? A dentist's perspective (address presented at the American Dental Association annual meeting, 11 October 1977, Council on Dental Health, American Dental Association); P. E. Stephenson, Physiological and psychotropic effects of caffeine on man, *Journal of the American Dietetic Association* 71 (1977):240-247.

[25]Some constructive ways to improve your diet, *Consumers' Research Magazine,* October 1976, p. 62.

Table 3. School Lunch Patterns for Different Ages

	Preschool ages 1-2	Preschool ages 3-4	Grades K-3	Grades 4-12	Grades 7-12
Meat or Meat Alternate one serving					
Lean meat, poultry, or fish	1 oz	1 1/2 oz	1 1/2 oz	2 oz	3 oz
Cheese	1 oz	1 1/2 oz	1 1/2 oz	2 oz	3 oz
Large egg(s)	1	1 1/2	1 1/2	2	3
Cooked dry beans or peas	1/2 c	3/4 c	3/4 c	1 c	1 1/2 c
Peanut butter	2 T	3 T	3 T	4 T	6 T
Vegetable and/or Fruit two or more servings					
both to total	1/2 c	1/2 c	1/2 c	3/4 c	3/4 c
Bread or Bread Alternate					
servings*	5 per week	8 per week	8 per week	8 per week	10 per week
Milk					
a serving of fluid milk	3/4 c	3/4 c	1 c	1 c	1 c

From School lunch patterns: Ready, set, go!, *School Food Service Journal* 34 (August 1980), p. 31.

*A serving is 1 slice of whole-grain or enriched bread; a whole-grain or enriched biscuit, roll, muffin, etc.; 1/2 c cooked pasta or other cereal grain such as bulgar or grits.

smaller portions or teach their children to serve themselves as much as they truly want to eat. Physical activity should be encouraged on a daily basis to promote strong skeletal and muscular development and to establish a habit that will undergird good health throughout life.

The child who has already become obese needs careful handling. As in pregnancy, weight loss may easily have a harmful effect on growth. J. L. Knittle, who has worked with obese children, recommends that they be fed so as to maintain a constant weight while they grow. The object is to restrict the multiplication of fat cells while promoting normal lean body development. Thus the child can "grow out of his obesity."[26]

Of all nutritional disorders other than obesity found in U.S. children, the most common is iron-deficiency anemia. It is most prevalent in low-birthweight infants, babies from six months to two years of age, and children and adolescents from low-income families.[27]

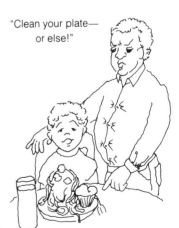

"Clean your plate— or else!"

[26]J. L. Knittle, Obesity in childhood: A problem in adipose tissue development, *Journal of Pediatrics* 81 (December 1972):1048-1059.

[27]S. J. Fomon, T. A. Anderson, H. Y. W. Stephen, and E. E. Ziegler, *Nutritional Disorders of Children: Prevention, Screening, and Followup*, DHEW publication no. (HSA) 76-5612 (Washington, D.C.: Government Printing Office, 1976), p. 100.

Table 4. Eating Habits to Favor Good Dental Health

Food group	Foods to eat	Foods to avoid
Milk and milk products	milk cheese plain yogurt	all dairy products with added sugar
Fruit	fresh fruit water-packed canned fruit	dried fruit sugar-packed canned fruit jams and jellies
Juice	unsweetened	sweetened
Vegetables	most vegetables	candied sweet potatoes glazed carrots
Grains	most grain products	grain products with added sugar

From L. P. DiOrio, What should we eat? A dentist's perspective (Address presented at the American Dental Association annual meeting, 11 October 1977, Council on Dental Health, American Dental Association).

Notice that granola bars are among the "bad guys" singled out by dentists. They are a grain food, but so sticky that dentists consider them akin to candy bars. Similarly, dentists see fruit yogurt as the equivalent of ice cream.

S. J. Fomon recommends supplementing the diet of infants to ensure an iron intake of 7 mg a day and modifying their food intakes as they grow older so that they will receive 5.5 mg of iron or more per 1,000 kcalories. To achieve this latter goal, milk must not be overemphasized in the diet, because it is a poor iron source. Too-high milk consumption causes a form of iron-deficiency anemia called milk anemia. If skim or low-fat milk is used instead of whole milk, there will be kcalories left for investment in such iron-rich foods as lean meats, fish, poultry, eggs, and legumes. Grain products should be whole-grain or enriched only, and children should be steered away from "dairy products (aside from the amount needed to ensure adequate calcium-riboflavin intakes), bakery goods unfortified with iron, candies and soft drinks."[28]

Cardiovascular disease is another condition to prevent, and many experts seem to agree that early childhood is the time to put practices into effect that until recently were recommended only for adults. Snacking on high-fat, high-sugar, and high-salt foods should be discouraged, because it sets a pattern that favors the development of atherosclerosis and hypertension. Instead, recommendations like those of the *Dietary Guidelines*, to emphasize foods with a high nutrient density, should be followed.

The *Guidelines* might also help to prevent or retard the onset of diabetes in children who have the genetic tendency toward it. Those who have been studying the effect of nutrition on cancer have suggested

[28]Fomon et al., 1976, p. 116.

that children should follow a "prudent diet," since evidence is
increasing that "appropriate biological control in terms of fat and
cholesterol may be set early in life."[29] The prudent diet was originally
developed for heart patients, but its outlines are the same as those
recommended by nutritionists interested in the prevention of cancer.

For more about prevention of
cancer, see Highlight 28.

Not everyone agrees that all children should be placed on diets
strictly limited in sugar, salt, and fat and high in fruits, vegetables, and
whole-grain cereals. However, even those who do not go this far
recommend that children be screened early with an eye to determining
what conditions each of them might be likely to develop and then
paying appropriate attention to diet in each special case. (Figure 3
outlines the screening process.[30]) Thus, the child of a parent with high
blood pressure should be raised on a diet relatively low in salt; the child
of a diabetic parent should avoid sugar and be encouraged to eat foods
high in complex carbohydrate; and the child of a parent with coronary
artery disease should eat foods low in fat, especially saturated fat, and
possibly cholesterol. In all these situations, the greatest success is likely
to be achieved if the whole family, and not just the child, follows the
recommended dietary guidelines.

Poor dental health is another preventable condition. The measures
recommended for its prevention center around two objectives. First,
adequate nutrition is needed to help so that the mouth and teeth
develop properly. This means providing an adequate diet, especially in
terms of protein; calcium; vitamins A, C, and D; and fluoride. Where
local water supplies are not fluoridated, direct application of fluoride to
the teeth may be necessary. Second, it is important to restrict the supply
of carbohydrate foods to the bacteria that cause tooth decay. This
means brushing the teeth or washing the mouth after meals (especially
meals high in carbohydrate), avoiding snacks that contain sticky
carbohydrate, and dislodging persistent particles with dental floss or
other devices.

Mealtimes   It is desirable for children to learn to like nutritious foods
in all of the food groups. With one exception, this liking usually
develops naturally. The exception is vegetables, which young children
frequently dislike and refuse. Even a tiny serving of spinach, cooked
carrots, or squash may elicit an expression that registers the utmost in
negative feelings (as well as great pride in the ability to make an ugly
face). Since most youngsters need to eat more vegetables, the next few
paragraphs are addressed to this problem.

Do you remember how you felt when first offered a cup of vegetable
soup, a serving of runny spinach, or a pile of peas and carrots? If the
soup burned your tongue, it may have been years before you were
willing to try it again. As for the spinach, it was suspiciously murky

[29]E. L. Wynder, The dietary environment and cancer, *Journal of the American Dietetic
Association* 71 (1977):385-392.

[30]Fomon et al., 1976, inside front cover.

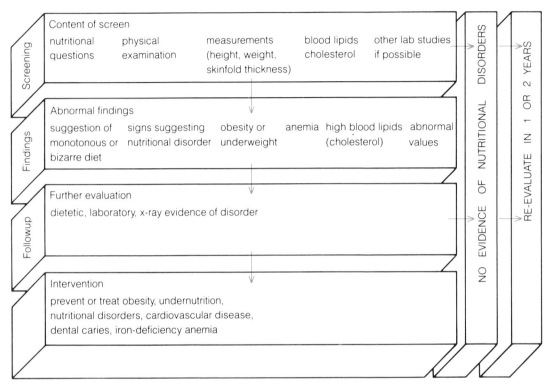

Figure 3 Nutritional screening of children.

From S. J. Fomon, T. A. Anderson, H. Y. W. Stephen, and E. E. Ziegler, *Nutritional Disorders of Children: Prevention, Screening, and Followup*, DHEW publication no. (HSA) 76-5612 (Washington, D.C.: Government Printing Office, 1976), inside front cover.

looking. (Who could tell what might be lurking in that dark, ugly liquid?) The peas and carrots troubled your sense of order. Before you could eat them, you felt compelled to sort the peas onto one side of the plate and the carrots onto the other. Then you had to separate, into a reject pile, all those that got mashed in the process or contaminated with gravy from the mashed potatoes. Only then might you be willing to eat the intact, clean peas and carrots one by one — perhaps with your fingers, since the peas, especially, kept rolling off the fork.

Why children respond in this way to foods that look "off" or "messy" to them is a matter for conjecture. Parents need only be aware that this is how many children feel and then honor those feelings. Children prefer vegetables that are slightly undercooked and crunchy, bright in color, served separately, and easy to eat. They should be warm, not hot, because a child's mouth is much more sensitive than an adult's. The flavor should be mild (a child has more taste buds), and smooth foods such as mashed potatoes or pea soup should have no lumps in them (a child wonders, with some disgust, what the lumps might be). Irrational as the fear of strangeness may seem, the parent must realize that it is practically universal among children and may even have a built-in biological basis.

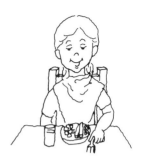

Little children like to eat at little tables and to be served little portions of food. They also love to eat with other children and have been observed to stay at the table longer and eat much more when in the company of their peers. A bright, unhurried atmosphere free of conflict is also conducive to good appetite. Parents who serve the food in a relaxed and casual manner, without anxiety, provide the emotional climate in which a child's negative emotions will be minimized.

Ideally, each meal is preceded, not followed, by the activity the child looks forward to the most. In a number of schools, it has been discovered that children eat a much better lunch if recess occurs before, rather than after, the meal. With recess after, they are likely to hurry out to play, leaving food on their plates that they were hungry for and would otherwise have eaten. Before sitting down to eat, small children should be helped to clean themselves thoroughly, washing their hands and faces so that they can enjoy their meal with "that clean feeling."[31]

Many little children, both boys and girls, enjoy helping in the kitchen. Their participation provides many opportunities to encourage good food habits. Vegetables are pretty, especially when fresh, and provide opportunities to learn about color, about growing things and their seeds, about shapes and textures — all of which are fascinating to young children. Measuring, stirring, decorating, cutting, and arranging vegetables are skills even a very small child can practice with enjoyment and pride.

When introducing new foods at the table, parents are advised to offer them one at a time — and only a small amount at first. Whenever possible, the new food should be presented at the beginning of the meal, when the child is hungry. If the child is cross, irritable, or feeling sick, don't insist but withdraw the new food and try it again a few days later. Remember, parents have inclinations and dislikes to which they feel entitled; children should be accorded the same privilege. Never make an issue of food acceptance; a power struggle almost invariably results in a confirmed pattern of resistance and a permanently closed mind on the child's part.

The key word (at one year) is *trust*; the parental behavior best suited to promote it is affectionate holding. At two years, the word is *autonomy*; parents should allow children to make their own choices, including giving them the right to say their favorite word (NO!) to offered foods — at the same time providing, of course, other nutritious foods to choose from. At four, when the development of *initiative* is their proudest achievement, children can be encouraged to participate in the planning and preparation of meals. At each age, food can be given and enjoyed in the context of growth in its largest, most inclusive

[31]We are indebted for many of these suggestions to Dr. Joyce Williams, coauthor (with M. Smith) of *Middle Childhood: Behavior and Development*, 2nd ed. (New York: Macmillan, 1980).

sense. If the beginnings are right, children will grow without the kind of conflict and confusion over food that can lead to nutritional problems.

At every age, there is a negative counterpart — distrust, shame, guilt, inferiority — to the desired development. These, too, can be promoted by unaware parents, even if they have the best of intentions. Mealtimes can be nightmarish for the child who is struggling with these issues. If, as she sits down to the table, she is confronted with a barrage of accusations — "Susie, your hands are filthy . . . your report card . . . and clean your plate! Your mother cooked that food" — mealtimes may be unbearable. Her stomach may recoil, because her body as well as her mind reacts to stress of this kind.

In the interest of promoting both a positive self-concept and a positive attitude toward good food, it is important for parents to help their children remember that they are good kids. What they *do* may sometimes be unacceptable; but what they *are*, on the inside, is normal, healthy, growing, fine human beings.

The Sick Child   A sick child who requires medical attention needs nutrition care just as much as, or more than, a well child. To deliver it, those who care for such children must be sensitive to their feelings and needs. Pointers from people experienced in working with children are:

- Notice the child's posture. Body language will tell you if a child is hurting or uncomfortable, when the child is unable or unwilling to speak.
- Touch the child often and lovingly. Your touch communicates more than your words.
- Let the child choose what to eat as much as possible. Choosing promotes acceptance.
- Make sure the child eats the food; notice if he doesn't. Putting it in front of him is not enough.
- Stay with the child or make sure a loved person is there during the meal. The child will eat and assimilate food better if her anxiety and loneliness are soothed.
- Encourage the child to eat what he needs most, first. Children live for now, not for the future. You watch out for the future.
- Let her eat with other children if possible. She'll enjoy mealtime more, accept more foods, and keep on eating longer.
- Avoid painful procedures near mealtimes. The stress of pain or fear shuts down digestion and turns off interest in food.

Not long ago, some researchers conducted a survey of 108 critically ill infants and children who had been in the hospital for over six months. Nutrition assessments showed that a third of them were at risk for growth retardation, while almost 20 percent were already growth retarded. A third of the children were suffering from mild to severe protein-kcalorie malnutrition, with the youngest being most affected.[32] In no way can infants and children with such serious malnutrition find an easy way back to good health.

Those who care for sick children may not be able to perform the dramatic medical and surgical miracles that save lives in a crisis, but they can provide steady, supportive love and nutrition care. In the long run, these factors contribute just as much to the miracle of recovery.

The Teen Years

Teenagers are not fed; they eat. For the first time in their lives, they assume responsibility for their own food intakes. At the same time, they are intensely involved in day-to-day life with their peers and preparation for their future lives as adults. Social pressures thrust choices at them: to drink or not to drink, to smoke or not to smoke, to develop their bodies to meet sometimes extreme ideals of slimness or athletic prowess. Few become interested in foods and nutrition except as part of a cult or fad such as vegetarianism or crash dieting. This section emphasizes the factors that affect their health for good or for ill and the information they need to develop and maintain food habits conducive to good health throughout adulthood.

Growth and Nutrient Needs   The adolescent growth spurt begins in girls at 10 or 11 and reaches its peak at 12, being completed at about 15. In boys, it begins at 12 or 13 and peaks at 14, ending at about 19. This intensive growth period brings not only a dramatic increase in height but hormonal changes that profoundly affect every organ of the body (including the brain) and that culminate in the emergence of physically mature adults within two or three years. The same nutrition principles apply to this period as to the growth periods previously discussed: The growth nutrients are needed in increased quantities, and there is an added need for iron, caused by the onset of menstruation in girls and by the great increase in lean body mass in boys. These changes, which are taking place in nearly adult-size people, may increase total nutrient needs at adolescence more than at any other time in life. A rapidly growing, active boy of 15 may need 4,000 kcalories or more a day just to maintain his weight. An inactive girl of the same age, whose growth is nearly at a standstill, may need fewer than 2,000 kcalories if she is to avoid becoming obese. Thus, there is tremendous variation in the nutrient needs of adolescents.

There is also tremendous variation in the rates and patterns of their growth. Growth charts used for children cannot be used any longer when the signs of puberty begin to appear. The only way to be sure a

[32] M. M. Pollack, J. S. Wiley, R. Kanter, and P. R. Holbrook, Malnutrition in critically ill infants and children, *Journal of Parenteral and Enteral Nutrition* 6 (1982):20-24.

Rule of thumb for teen girls:
For 5 feet, consider 100 lb a
reasonable weight.
For each inch over 5 feet, add 5
lb.
For each year under 25 (down
to 18), subtract 1 lb.

For men, see inside back cover.

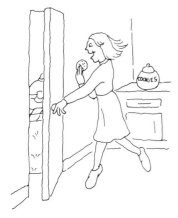

**Nutrients in a Hamburger,
Chocolate Shake, and Fries**

Nutrient	Percentage of need*
Protein	42
Calcium	47
Iron	21
Vitamin A	3
Thiamin	25
Riboflavin	57
Vitamin C	21

*Calculated from the RDA for a
teenage male.

teenager is growing normally is to compare his or her height and weight with previous measures taken at intervals and note whether reasonably smooth progress is being made. A teenager who wants to know what he or she should weigh should be reassured that any of a wide range of weights is considered normal at this time in life. The rule of thumb on the inside back cover can be modified for teenage girls down to age 18 (see margin) and considered a weight to aim at; but weights well in excess of these are normal, too. Teenage boys can be told that when they have finished growing, they should expect to weigh what the adult charts show, but that while they are growing it is not unusual for their weights to be quite different from the adult standards.

Teenagers as a group do have nutritional problems, however. Nearly every nutrient can be found lacking in one or another group: iron in girls, kcalories in young men (especially blacks), vitamin A in girls (especially Mexican- and Spanish-Americans), calcium, riboflavin, vitamin C, even protein. The insidious problem of obesity becomes more apparent, mostly in girls, especially in black girls. Serious nutritional deficiencies often arise in pregnant teenage girls.

Eating Patterns   Teenagers come and go as they choose and eat what they want when they have time. With a multitude of after-school, social, and job activities, they almost inevitably fall into irregular eating habits. The adult becomes a gatekeeper, controlling the availability but not the consumption of food in the teenager's environment. The adult can't nag, scold, or pressure teenagers into eating as they should, because they typically turn a deaf ear to coercion and often to persuasion. To "feed" effectively, the gatekeeper must make every effort to allow these young people independence while providing a physical environment that favors healthy development and an emotional climate that encourages adaptive choices.

In the home, a wise maneuver is to provide access to nutritious and economical energy foods low in sugar and fat and discouraging to tooth decay. The snacker — and a well-established characteristic of teenagers is that they are snackers — who finds only nutritious foods around the house is well provided for.

Inevitably, teenagers will do a lot of eating away from home. There, as well as at home, their nutritional welfare can be favored or hindered by the choices they make. A lunch of a hamburger, a chocolate shake, and french fries supplies nutrients in the amounts shown in the margin table, at a kcalorie cost of 780. Except for vitamin A, these are substantial percentages of recommended intakes at a kcalorie cost many teenagers can afford. Depending on how they adjust their breakfast and dinner choices, teenagers may serve their needs more than adequately with this sort of lunch. They need only supply fruits and vegetables (for vitamins A and C), a good fiber source, and more good iron sources.

On the average, about a fourth of teenagers' total daily kcalorie intake comes from snacks. Their irregular schedules may worry adults who think they are feeding themselves poorly, but at least one study shows that the kcalories they eat are far from empty. They receive substantial amounts of thiamin, protein, riboflavin, and vitamin C. The nutrients they often lack are calcium and iron and, to some extent, vitamin A and folacin. Protein usually need not be stressed, but some teenagers should be encouraged to recognize and consume more dairy products, for calcium, and more good vitamin A and folacin sources. (Wherever vitamin A is lacking, folacin is too, because both are found in green vegetables.)

The teenager's iron needs are a special problem, caused by several factors. Two already mentioned are the teenager's burgeoning iron need and the lack of iron in traditional snack foods. Other factors are the overemphasis on dairy products by some teenagers, vegetarianism, and the low contribution made by fast foods to iron intakes. A National Academy of Sciences committee, writing on this special problem, finds it doubtful that long-term administration of iron tablets is practical and advises against the measure of fortifying snacks and other foods with iron. Instead, the committee recommends that physicians and clinics screen all teenagers for low levels of iron in the blood. Their report stresses the fact that the best dietary source of absorbable iron is meats of all varieties, a point that should in turn be stressed in the nutritional education of teenagers.[33] A later section addresses the problem of teaching teens about nutrition.

Anorexia Nervosa and Bulimia A concern of teenagers, especially girls, is dieting to maintain a slim and beautiful figure. To accomplish this, many go on fad diets that are neither safe nor effective. The matters of obesity, overweight, and fad diets have been fully discussed elsewhere (see Chapters 7 and 8) but two special problems should be mentioned here: anorexia nervosa and bulimia. Anorexia nervosa is an extreme preoccupation with weight loss that seriously endangers the health and even the life of the dieter. Although no two persons with anorexia nervosa are alike, certain features are considered typical of the condition. The anorexic is almost always female and in her mid-teens. She is usually from an educated, middle-class, success-oriented, weight-conscious family that is proud of her and is surprised to see her develop a problem. She strives to achieve and chooses weight loss as one means of becoming successful herself. Being highly competitive and perfectionistic, she carries the weight-loss effort to an extreme: She will have the slimmest, most perfect body of anyone in her high school class.

For the nutritive value of selected fast foods, see Appendix N.

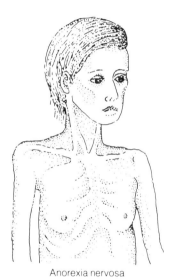

Anorexia nervosa

Copied from a woodcut accompanying Sir William Gull, Anorexia nervosa, *Lancet* 1 (1888).

anorexia nervosa: literally, "nervous lack of appetite," a disorder (usually seen in teenage girls) involving self-starvation to the extreme.

[33]Committee on Nutrition of the Mother and Preschool Child, Food and Nutrition Board, National Academy of Sciences, *Iron Nutriture in Adolescence*, DHEW publication no. (HSA) 77-5100 (Washington, D.C.: Government Printing Office, 1977).

So far this description probably fits many young women you know; but unlike most of them, this girl develops anorexia nervosa. When she has lost weight to well below the average for her height and is no longer slim but too slim, she still doesn't stop. Weight loss has become an obsession, she is afraid of losing control, and she allows her self-imposed starvation regimen to rule her life. At this point, according to Dr. Hilde Bruch, an authority who has studied and worked with anorexics, starvation has begun to affect her thinking patterns and personality, and physical symptoms are emerging. Although they are the symptoms of starvation, the girl sees them as desirable and prides herself on holding out against her extreme hunger.

Among the physical symptoms are:

- Wasting of the whole body, including muscle tissue.
- Arresting of sexual development and stopping of menstruation.
- Drying and yellowing of the skin, from an accumulation of stored carotene released from body fat.
- Loss of health and texture of hair.
- Pain on touch.
- Lowered blood pressure and metabolic rate.
- Anemia.
- Severe sleep disturbances.[34]

Right now I weigh 58 lbs., which isn't too bad for 5'2", though I want to lose a few more pounds — my hips are still fat. Lately I've got it down to no breakfast, a can of mushrooms for lunch, and a can of wax beans for dinner with lots of iced tea. I reward myself with a big, green apple at the end of the day, if I've stuck to The Plan.

— A. Ciseaux

Simultaneously, a set of bizarre mental symptoms develop in the anorexic, including an inability to see herself as others see her (she still sees herself as too fat), a preoccupation with death, a frantic pursuit of physical fitness by means of stringent exercise routines, and a manipulative way of dealing with her parents and family such that they make her the center of attention. Diet has become so all-engrossing, now, that she may be quite isolated socially except from friends who stick by her and worry about her without knowing how to help.

By this time, the anorexic has reached an absolute minimum body weight (65 to 70 pounds for a woman of average height) and is on the verge of incurring permanent brain damage and chronic invalidism or death.

Before 1950, the condition was very rare (1 in 2,000) and only 1 out of 4 such girls could be expected to recover. By 1970, the incidence was increasing and the success rate in treatment was closer to 3 out of 4. During the 1970s anorexia nervosa became still more widespread and familiar to doctors and therapists. Treatment was further improved to the point where success could be expected more often.

Dr. Bruch describes the treatment of the anorexic as a three-stage process. First, normal nutrition must be restored, by tube-feeding directly into the stomach if necessary. As she begins to return to normal weight, family interactions have to be dealt with. With progress in these

---

[34]H. Bruch, Anorexia nervosa, *Nutrition Today*, September/October 1978, pp. 14-18.

two areas, she can begin to be taught some new understanding and clear up some of her misconceptions about nutrition.[35]

Anorexia nervosa is a disease of the developed countries, and becomes more prevalent as wealth increases. Its victims seem to be reacting to the cultural values that emphasize fashion and material success over personal actualization and self esteem. Whatever its cause, it serves as but one of many possible examples of the ways teenagers feel pressured and the ways they react to those pressures.

Another reaction is bulimia, periodic binge-eating alternating with intervals of dieting or self-starvation. Bulimia was officially recognized only in 1980, although it had existed long before that. The binge eater typically ingests a large amount of food in an episode she or he feels is uncontrollable. The binge may last from minutes to hours and usually takes place in private. The foods chosen are usually sweet or starchy, require little chewing, and are high in kcalories. The binge ends when it would hurt to eat any more or when the person goes to sleep, induces vomiting, or is interrupted.[36]

Since 1980, bulimia has attracted much attention in the media, especially the variety in which the person binges and then vomits or takes laxatives to undo the "damage." A handful of professional articles have appeared on the subject, doubtless to be followed by many more.[37] It is not yet clear whether bulimic eaters are psychologically disturbed; they may simply be compensating for going to the extreme of self-imposed starvation by swinging to the other extreme of overeating. This is a not-surprising mode of behavior in a society that imposes an unrealistically thin ideal, especially on girls. As many as two or three out of every five women in some subgroups of society may be bulimic for some part of their lives (for example, dancers, who are often told they must weigh considerably less than the already-thin "ideal weight").

Although binge-eating is seldom life-threatening, at the extreme it can be physically damaging, causing lacerations of the stomach, irritation of the esophagus (in those who vomit frequently), and malnutrition (in the vomiters and laxative-takers). It is highly desirable that binge-eaters should learn to see food, and themselves, in a more positive light and should come to accept a realistic weight goal for themselves. Further thoughts on this problem are offered in Highlight 16.

The Pregnant Teenage Girl A special case of nutritional need is that of the pregnant teenage girl. Even if she were not pregnant, she would be hard put to meet her own nutrient needs at this time of maximal growth. Nourishing the baby doubles her burden. Figure 4

bulimia, bulimarexia: binge eating (literally, eating like an ox). Known popularly as "pigging out" or "blind munchies." When followed by self-induced vomiting or the taking of laxatives, this form of eating behavior has been called the **binge-purge syndrome.**

buli = ox
orex = mouth

[35] Bruch, 1978.

[36] R. L. Pyle, J. E. Mitchell, and E. D. Eckert, Bulimia: A report of 34 cases, *Journal of Clinical Psychiatry* 42 (1981):60-64.

[37] For example, Pyle, Mitchell, and Eckert, 1981; also J. Wardle and H. Beinart, Binge eating: A theoretical review, *British Journal of Clinical Psychology* 20 (1981):97-109.

Figure 4 Comparison of the nutrient needs of a 10-year-old girl with those of a pregnant 15-year-old girl. These values were calculated by adding the difference between the RDAs for a 10-year-old and a 14-year-old to the difference between the RDAs for a 14-year-old and a pregnant woman (see inside front cover).

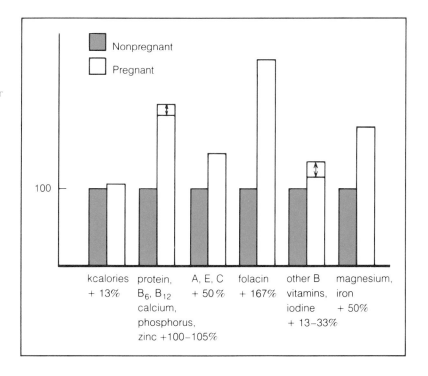

shows that her needs for many nutrients double, although her kcalorie allowance increases by only a few percent. In the case of a girl who begins pregnancy with inadequate nutrient stores or who lacks the education, resources, and support she needs, these problems are compounded.

The complications of pregnancy were discussed in Chapter 15, where it was shown that the consequences of poor nutrition are acute and long-lasting. Sickness is common in pregnant teenagers, with toxemia occurring in about one out of every five girls under the age of 15. If one pregnancy is followed by another, "the conditions are established for a rapid and irreversible slide from simple toxemia to renal [kidney] damage and hypertensive [heart] disease."[38]

Teenage pregnancy has become common. About one out of every five babies is born to a mother under 19 years of age, and more than a tenth of these mothers are 15 or younger.[39] The importance of preparing young girls for future pregnancy needs emphasis in public schools and public health programs. Faced with her parents' and classmates' often insensitive reactions, a pregnant girl is likely to wind up alone, with little or no money to buy food and no motivation to seek prenatal care. Programs addressed to all her problems are urgently needed, including

[38]B. S. Worthington, Nutritional needs of the pregnant adolescent, in *Nutrition in Pregnancy and Lactation*, ed. B. S. Worthington, J. Vermeersch, and S. R. Williams (St. Louis: Mosby, 1977), pp. 119-132.

[39]Worthington, 1977.

medical attention, nutritional guidance, emotional support, and continued schooling. A model program for giving nutritional help to teenage mothers, among others, is the WIC (Women's, Infants' and Children's) program.

Alcohol, Drugs, Caffeine   The teen years bring exposure to factors not encountered before. Some complicate the nutrition picture: use and abuse of alcohol, prolonged use of prescription medications, drug use (and abuse), caffeine, oral contraceptives, and many more. Because alcohol is by far the most widely used of all drugs in the United States, it receives the heaviest emphasis here.

In the mid-teens comes a choice point: whether to drink alcohol or to abstain. A 1975 study showed that more than half of all seventh graders nationwide had tried alcohol at least once within the previous year; nine-tenths of all high school seniors had had experience with alcohol.[40]

The year between the ages of 13 and 14 seems to mark the decision point for most white teenagers; and the year between 15 and 16 is critical for blacks. Another transitional stage occurs between the ages of 17 and 18, when infrequent drinkers apparently make a decision either to abstain or to drink more heavily. The highest proportion of heavy drinkers by ethnic group is found in Native American youth (16.5 percent), followed by Orientals (13.5) and Spanish (10.9). For whites, the proportion is 10.7 percent, and for blacks, 5.7 percent. Those receiving high grades in school are less likely to become alcohol drinkers; the heavy drinkers characteristically spend more time with peers who also drink.[41]

By the time students get to college, alcohol abuse is frequent and considered part of normal college life. About 90 percent of all college students use alcohol, and heavy drinking is common, with a third or more of all students getting drunk more than once a month.[42] Only a few college students are alcoholics, but 5 to 10 percent will experience serious complications as a result of drinking, and 1 in 12 will go on to become an adult problem drinker or an alcoholic.[43] Among adults in the United States, about 100 million drink, and 9 million are estimated to be alcoholics.

The nutrition implications of alcohol use and the consequences of its abuse were described in Highlight 9. To sum them all up, alcohol is an

[40]Young people and alcohol, *Alcohol Health and Research World*, DHEW publication no. (ADM) 75-157 (Washington, D.C.: Government Printing Office, Summer 1975), pp. 2-10.

[41]Drinking motivations: Habits of youth illuminated by national survey results, *NIAAA Information and Feature Service* 18, DHEW publication no. (ADM) 75-151 (Washington, D.C.: Government Printing Office, 26 November 1975).

[42]D. P. Kraft, College students and alcohol: The 50 + project, *Alcohol Health and Research World*, DHEW publication no. (ADM) 76-157 (Washington, D.C.: Government Printing Office, Summer 1976), pp. 10-14.

[43]G. Globetti, as quoted in *Alcohol Health and Research World*, Summer 1975.

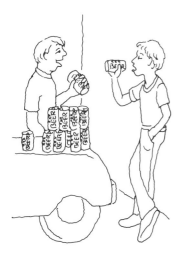

empty-kcalorie beverage and can displace needed nutrients from the diet while simultaneously increasing the demand for them. Those who are unable to use alcohol with moderation must abstain completely from its use if they are to maintain good health.

Many myths and misconceptions comprise the public's picture of alcohol use, and teenagers often cherish wrong beliefs that lead them to alcohol abuse and addiction if they are susceptible. Being susceptible to alcohol addiction, like being potentially diabetic, is probably an inherited trait and is therefore nothing to be ashamed of. The teenager, however, is apt to be exposed to peer pressure that favors everyone's drinking, and those who can't do so safely are in an unfortunate predicament. Chapter 24 offers some pointers useful in distinguishing safe from dangerous drinking and some strategies useful in the prevention and cure of addiction (alcoholism).

Among mistaken beliefs especially common among teenagers is the notion that a beer drinker can never become an addict. On the contrary, because beer contains alcohol, it is just as capable of contributing to alcoholism as is wine or "hard" liquor (whiskey, gin, vodka, and the like). It is not the beverage but the constitution of the consumer that determines whether he or she will become addicted to alcohol.

Some beer drinkers maintain that beer has some redeeming features. It makes people drunk less quickly, and it provides valuable nutrients. True, because the alcohol in beer is diluted, it will reach the bloodstream more slowly from the stomach than the same amount of alcohol taken straight. But the carbonation in beer stimulates the stomach, hastening the entry of alcohol into the intestine, where it will immediately be absorbed. As for the nutrient content of beer, an adult male would have to drink at least a six-pack of 12-oz cans to meet his niacin needs and nine six-packs to meet his protein needs.

Some young people choose to abstain from alcohol consumption because they know or suspect they are prone to an alcohol problem. Others make the same choice for other reasons. Such people have a hard time in some social settings, because drinking is often not only accepted but even demanded. It is hoped that this discussion will have shown why it is desirable not to pressure other persons to drink. Considerate hosts or social groups will welcome the nondrinker and provide nonalcoholic beverages for his or her enjoyment just as they would provide nonmeat food for a guest who is a vegetarian.

Not only alcohol but also many medicines affect the body's need for and use of nutrients. Prescription medications can affect nutritional status by:

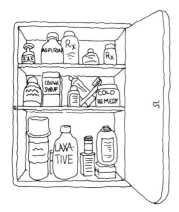

- Increasing or decreasing appetite.

- Causing nausea, vomiting, or an altered sense of taste.

- Inhibiting the synthesis of nutrients.

- Reducing the absorption or increasing the excretion of nutrients.

- Altering the transport, use, or storage of nutrients.

Foods and nutrients can also affect the drugs in the body. The interactions between drugs and nutrition status comprise such a big subject that a whole chapter of Part Four is devoted to them (Chapter 21).

The special case of the person taking oral contraceptives deserves a moment's attention. The Pill alters blood levels of several nutrients, raising some (vitamin A and iron) and lowering others (B vitamins and vitamin C). Women often wonder what vitamin supplements they should take while on the Pill. The answer seems to be "None. You are risking a nutritional deficiency only if your diet is grossly inadequate, especially in folacin. And if it is, you need diet counseling more than you need a vitamin pill."[44]

Like alcohol, marihuana also has characteristic effects on the body, and like alcohol, it has not been shown to have many pronounced harmful effects even with long-term use, unless the use is very heavy (five to six cigarettes a day for six months). The active ingredients are rapidly and completely (90 percent) absorbed from the lungs.[45] Then, being fat soluble, they are packaged in protein (possibly in lipoproteins[46]) before being transported by the blood to the various body tissues. They are processed by many tissues (not just by the liver), and they persist for several days in body fat, being excreted over a period of a week or more after the smoking of a single cigarette.[47]

marihuana: alternate spelling, **marijuana**

Smoking a marihuana cigarette has characteristic effects on hearing, touch, taste and smell and on perceptions of time, space, and the body; it also produces changes in mental sensations and alterations in the nature of sleep. Among the taste changes apparently induced is a great enjoyment of eating, especially of sweets ("the munchies"), but it is not known how this effect occurs.[48] The drug apparently does not change the blood glucose level.[49] Investigators speculate that the so-called hunger induced by marihuana is actually a social effect caused by the suggestibility of the group in which it is smoked.[50] Prolonged use of the drug does not seem to bring about a weight gain; in one small sample, regular users (30 smokers) have been observed to weigh less than

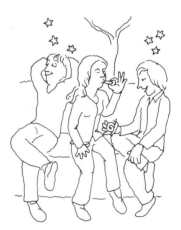

[44]D. A. Roe, Drugs, diet and nutrition, *Contemporary Nutrition* 3 (June 1978).

[45]L. J. King, J. D. Teale, and V. Marks, Biochemical aspects of cannabis, in *Cannabis and Health*, ed. J. D. Graham (New York : Academic Press, 1976).

[46]L. E. Hollister, Marihuana in man: Three years later, *Science* 172 (1971):21-29.

[47]King et al., 1976; Hollister, 1971.

[48]E. L. Abel, Effects of marihuana on the solution of anagrams, memory and appetite, *Nature* 231 (1971):260-261; C. T. Tart, Marijuana intoxication: Common experiences, *Nature* 226 (1970):701-704.

[49]L. E. Hollister, Hunger and appetite after single doses of marihuana, alcohol, and dextroamphetamine, *Clinical Pharmacology and Therapeutics* 12 (1971):44-49; J. D. P. Graham and D. M. F. Li, The pharmacology of cannabis and cannabinoids, in *Cannabis and Health*, 1976.

[50]Hollister, 1971.

comparable nonsmokers by about seven pounds.[51]

Many young people in the United States are turning to marihuana as an alternative to alcohol. The number of individuals using it at least once a day had grown from half a million in 1971 to over 3 million before 1980.[52] There is much disagreement about the desirability of this trend, and despite much current research, little is known about the possible risks of regular smoking.

It has become clear, however, that even in "socially acceptable" concentrations, the drug brings about a deterioration in some aspects of driving performance.[53] Another effect widely agreed on is that it causes alterations in heart action, including rapid and sometimes irregular heartbeat.[54] It also reduces the body's immune response and, in young men, reduces the sex hormone level and sperm count after a lag period of about six weeks. Reporting on this effect, the investigator points out that marihuana "is much like other drugs, such as tobacco and liquor, in that the greatest potential hazard exists for those who abuse it. . . . There is still no convincing evidence that casual, infrequent use of marihuana produces any ill effects."[55]

The potency of marihuana preparations reaching this country has been increasing. Before 1970, most marihuana used in the United States was a very weak domestic variety with an average THC content of about 0.2 percent. (THC is tetrahydrocannabinol, the primary active ingredient of marihuana.) During the 1970s, users shifted to a Mexican variety (about 1.5 percent THC), then to Jamaican and Colombian marihuana (3 to 4 percent). The present trend is toward even higher concentrations. Users looking for a greater "high" then sometimes shift to hashish oil, a much more concentrated form of the active drug (about 40 to 50 percent THC and up to 90 percent), at which point the risks probably increase dramatically.[56]

Most investigators agree that, with moderate use, the hazards of marihuana smoking are few and small. However, it should be remembered that, because possession and use of the drug is not legal, no controls are exerted by any agency, such as the FDA, on the content of preparations sold as marihuana. There is a significant hazard associated with the possibility that they may be contaminated with pesticides or that they may contain "hard" (addictive) drugs such as heroin, concealed in them by pushers to create a demand for a product they can sell for greater profits. Also, when marihuana use escalates into the use of other drugs, the nutrition and health effects become pronounced, as the next paragraph illustrates.

THC, or **tetrahydrocannabinol** (tet-ra-high-dro-can-NAB-in-ol): the primary active ingredient of marihuana.

[51]Marijuana: Truth on health problems, *Science News*, 22 February 1975, p. 117.

[52]T. H. Maugh, II, Marihuana: New support for immune and reproductive hazards, *Science* 190 (1975):865-867.

[53]Graham and Li, 1976; Pot update: Possible motor effects, *Science News*, 4 February 1978, p. 71.

[54]Graham and Li, 1976.

[55]Infrequent use might be defined as three cigarettes a week or less. Maugh, 1975.

[56]Maugh, 1975.

Alcohol and marihuana have received most of the attention here, but other drugs deserve a mention for their effects on nutrition. Among the drugs in most common use today are heroin, morphine, LSD, PCP, and cocaine. Users of these drugs face multiple nutrition problems:

- They spend their money for drugs rather than for food.

- They lose interest in food during "high" periods on drugs.

- Some drugs (for example, amphetamines) induce at least a temporary depression of appetite.

- Their lifestyle lacks the regularity and routine that would promote good eating habits.

- They often have hepatitis (a liver disease caused by the use of contaminated needles), which causes taste changes and loss of appetite.

- They often depend on alcohol, especially when withdrawing from drug use.

- They often become ill with infectious diseases which increase their need for nutrients.

During their withdrawal from drugs, one of the most important aspects of treatment is to identify and correct these nutritional problems while teaching and supporting adaptive eating habits.[57]

Like alcohol use, the use of caffeine-containing beverages — coffee, tea, and especially cola beverages — becomes common during the teens. Caffeine is less likely to be dangerously abused than alcohol, perhaps because its use neither dulls the senses nor impairs judgment. Caffeine is a true stimulant drug, increasing the respiration rate, heart rate, blood pressure, and the secretion of the stress and other hormones.[58] Its "wake-up" effect is maximal within an hour after the dose. In moderate amounts (50 to 200 mg a day), caffeine seems to be relatively harmless.

Caffeine is not addictive, but it is habit forming, and the body adapts to its use to some extent. A dose greater than what the body is adapted to causes jitteriness, nervousness, and intestinal discomfort. Sudden abstinence from the drug after long use, even if use has been moderate, causes a characteristic withdrawal reaction; the most frequently observed symptom is a headache. If a person has adapted to a much higher dose level than 50 to 200 mg caffeine, then dropping back to this level may cause the same withdrawal reaction.

hepatitis (hep-uh-TIGHT-us): a severe viral liver disease transmitted from person to person either through contaminated water or (as in the case of drug addicts) by way of contaminated needles.

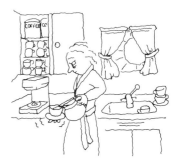

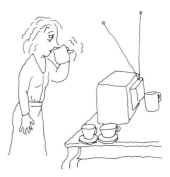

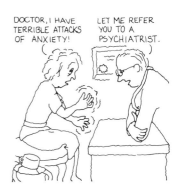

DOCTOR, I HAVE TERRIBLE ATTACKS OF ANXIETY!

LET ME REFER YOU TO A PSYCHIATRIST.

[57]R. T. Frankle and G. Christakis, eds., Some nutritional aspects of "hard" drug addiction, *Dietetic Currents, Ross Timesaver* 2 (July/August 1975).

[58]D. Robertson, J. C. Frolich, R. K. Carr, J. T. Watson, J. W. Hollifield, D. G. Shand, and J. A. Oates, Effects of caffeine on plasma renin activity, catecholamines, and blood pressure, *New England Journal of Medicine* 298 (1978):181-186; P. E. Stephenson, Physiologic and psychotropic effects of caffeine on man, *Journal of the American Dietetic Association* 71 (1977):240-247.

Caffeine Sources

Source	Caffeine (mg)
Brewed coffee (1 c)	85
Instant coffee (1 c)	60
Brewed black tea (1 c)	50
Brewed green tea (1 c)	30
Instant tea (1 c)	30
Decaffeinated coffee (1 c)	3
Cola beverage (12 oz)	32-65
Aspirin compound (pill containing aspirin, phenacetin, and caffeine)	32
Cope, Midol, etc.	32
Excedrin, Anacin (tablet)	60
Pre-Mens	66
Many cold preparations	30
Many stimulants	100
Cocoa (1 c)	6-42
No Doz (tablet) or Vivarin	100-200

Adapted from "Food allergy," *Nutrition and the MD*, July 1978; and P. E. Stephenson, Physiologic and psychotropic effects of caffeine on man, *Journal of the American Dietetic Association* 71 (1977):240-247.

An overdose of caffeine produces actions in the body that are indistinguishable from those of an anxiety attack.[59] People who drink between 8 and 15 cups of coffee a day, for example, have been known to seek help from doctors for complaints such as "dizziness, agitation, restlessness, recurring headaches, and sleep difficulties." Before prescribing a tranquilizer, the doctor would do well to inquire about the caffeine consumption of such patients.

A large dose of caffeine can also cause extra heartbeats and is believed to have caused heart attacks in people whose hearts were already damaged by degenerative disease.[60] However, neither caffeine nor its vehicle, coffee, can be considered a risk factor for the development of atherosclerosis.[61] Neither the Framingham Study nor a study of 7,705 Japanese showed any correlation between coffee drinking and heart attack risk.[62]

The Teenage Athlete Among the many interests some teens develop is a keen interest in athletics. Anyone who wants to have a beneficial impact on teenagers' food choices and health habits must be knowledgeable about factors affecting muscle size and strength, endurance, and body weight. Trainers often are not well versed in nutrition knowledge, but because they are expected to know the answers, they pick up and pass on whatever they can. Much of what athletes learn this way dates from centuries back and is a mixture of tradition, superstition, and fact. This section summarizes the minimum knowledge that a trainer or nutrition teacher who deals with athletes should have.

First, athletes often believe that their diets should be extremely high in protein. The bodies of athletes contain more protein than other tissues. Athletes do, in fact, use a little more protein in their activities than nonathletes, but only a little more — perhaps 10 percent. To protect muscle protein (to avoid losing more than they can easily replace), athletes need to be sure to eat enough protein-sparing kcalories to meet their energy needs, and they do spend significantly more energy than other people do. In short, what they need is extra kcalories, not extra protein. There is a margin of safety built into the protein recommendations for all people, and they are high enough for athletes.

To *build* muscle requires positive nitrogen balance (this was explained in Chapter 3), but even that doesn't mean eating more protein. Most young people's diets already contain about twice as much protein as they can possibly use, and they are actually wasting about half of the protein they eat, in the sense that they are using it not to

[59]"Food allergy," *Nutrition and the MD*, July 1978.

[60]Coffee: Downs and ups, *Nutrition and the MD*, April 1978.

[61]K. Yano, G. G. Rhoads, and A. Kagan, Coffee, alcohol, and risk of coronary heart disease in Japanese-Americans, *New England Journal of Medicine* 297 (1977):405-409.

[62]Coffee, 1978.

build body protein but rather for energy — a purpose any other energy nutrient could serve just as well, and less expensively.

There is no way to force extra protein into the muscles to make them grow just by eating more protein. Cells don't respond to what's given to them by helplessly accepting it — they work by responding to the demands put upon them and selecting from what is offered, what they need in order to perform. So the way to make muscle cells grow is to put a demand on them — that is, to make them work. They will respond by taking up nutrients, protein included, so that they can grow. In summary, don't *push* protein at them, but exercise them in order to demand that they *pull* protein in for themselves. Then make sure that protein is available by eating a diet that is adequate in protein. There's no need to make the diet "super-adequate" (whatever that might mean) and no advantage in doing so.

A technique some athletes have used to try to increase muscle mass is to take hormone preparations designed to duplicate the hormones of puberty (androgens or anabolic steroids), which favor muscle development in growing boys. The evidence on their effectiveness seems to show that they are ineffective when used alone.[63] They may seem effective when used in conjunction with hard physical conditioning and increased food intake, but the effects seen under these circumstances are more probably due just to the increased exercise and food.[64]

Hormones have profound and far-reaching effects on many target tissues, and these hormones are no exceptions. Hazards associated with their use include disturbed spermatogenesis and testicular degeneration in older athletes. Younger athletes may never reach their full potential height, because the bones of the lower back fuse to terminate growth early in response to the large dose of the hormones of puberty.[65]

Another issue athletes need to understand has to do with gaining and losing weight. An athlete who wants to gain weight in a hurry and doesn't care whether it is muscle or fat can add kcalories of any kind to the diet to achieve the desired gain. Because fat in foods is more kcalorie-dense than protein or carbohydrate, the athlete can most easily gain weight by eating a high-fat diet. This technique is said to be one of the most widespread nutrition-related abuses in sports; and it increases the risk of heart disease, to which athletes are not immune. The healthy way to gain weight is to build oneself up by patient and consistent training and at the same time to eat enough kcalories (of nutritious foods) to support the weight gain.

The athlete must remember to cut *down* on kcalories between and after training periods. Muscles respond to reduced demand by losing mass. It would be magical thinking to believe that that mass simply disappears. In fact, the cells slowly break down, and the materials they

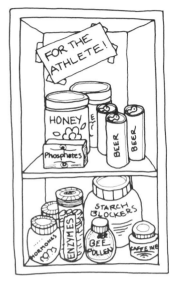

None of these foods or supplements is "ergogenic," no matter what the ads tell you.

ergogenic: a term referring to foods that are supposed to have unusual energy-producing power. Actually, no foods are ergogenic.

ergo = energy
genic = gives rise to

anabolic steroids: hormones, produced normally in males during puberty, that bring about maturation; dangerous when used by athletes to try to promote muscular development.

anabole = to build up

These hormones are also known as **androgens.**

andro = man
gen = gives rise to

spermatogenesis: the manufacture of sperm in the testicles.

---

[63]D. R. Lamb, Androgens and exercise, *Medicine and Science in Sports* 7 (1975):1-5.

[64]Lamb, 1975; N. J. Smith, Gaining and losing weight in athletics, *Journal of the American Medical Association* 236 (1976):149-151.

[65]Smith, 1976.

are made of (mostly carbohydrate, fat, and protein) become available as potential fuel for other body cells. Of course, this fuel will be stored as fat unless it is expended in activity. It should be no surprise, then, that a heavily muscled individual of twenty who stops working out but keeps on eating like a football player in training can become an oversized, flabby, and obese person at thirty. There's actually some truth in the notion that his muscle turned to fat, even though it's a slight oversimplification.

The athlete who wants to lose weight, like the one who wants to gain, can choose a wise or unwise course. To achieve ideal body composition — the optimum ratio of muscle strength to body mass — people must reduce only body fat, and they can't do this for more than a very few weeks at a rate faster than about two pounds a week. Hurry-up techniques, such as sauna bathing, exercising in a plastic suit (to sweat it off), using diuretics or cathartics, or inducing vomiting, achieve faster weight loss only by causing dehydration, and dehydration seriously impairs performance. The hazards of fasts and fad diets were described in Chapter 7, but a reminder should be repeated here: What is achieved by quick-weight-loss dieting is loss of lean tissue, glycogen, bone minerals, fluids — all materials vital to healthy body functioning. Abnormal heart rhythms have been seen in healthy adults after only ten days of fasting.[66]

Even if it is achieved by healthy methods, extreme weight loss can be hazardous to the athlete, as to any person. Occasionally one hears that an "elite runner" — in superb physical condition and at the peak of his career — has died suddenly at the end of an intensive exercise session. These deaths were a mystery until recently, but now a reason for them seems to be emerging. In each case, the person had been severely restricting kcalories and had reached a new, all-time low weight, while at the same time breaking his own previous records for distance or time. Exactly what causes the deaths is still not known, but severe kcalorie restriction and weight loss combined with hard training seem to be contributing factors.[67] Sometimes, however, an athlete obviously has heart disease, either hereditary or acquired. Diet can't always be blamed for sudden deaths in athletes.

Women athletes sometimes experience menstrual irregularity or even complete stoppage of the menstrual cycle. Athletic amenorrhea resembles the amenorrhea seen in women with anorexia nervosa or in the world's undernourished women and has been thought to be due to loss of body fat. The theory is that a certain minimum amount of body fat is necessary to support the making and using of the female hormones, which are fat-like compounds themselves. However, low body fat may not be the only cause; a change in the brain's regulation of sex hormone output may be responsible in the case of athletic

athletic amenorrhea (ay-men-or-REE-uh): the failure to menstruate in women athletes.

a = without
menor = menstrual cycle

[66]Nutrition and athletic performance, *Dairy Council Digest* 46 (1976).

[67]T. J. Bassler, Body build and mortality (letter to the editor), *Journal of the American Medical Association* 244 (1980):1437.

amenorrhea. In any case, the possibility serves as a reminder that all athletes should keep in mind the definition of ideal weight already mentioned: the optimum ratio of muscle strength to body mass. An optimum means having neither too much *nor too little* body mass.

Still another question has to do with the foods an athlete should eat to derive energy for training or competition. The fuel of muscle work is not protein but carbohydrate and fat. Muscles normally use a mixture of the two; but during intensive exercise they require glucose, and they store it as glycogen within their cells so that it will be available when needed. Two-thirds of the body's glycogen is in the muscles, and only one-third is in the liver to serve the rest of the body's needs for blood glucose. When a muscle uses glycogen, it first derives many glucose units from it, then breaks them down. The breakdown of glucose is a multistep process that releases energy at several of its steps, as Chapter 7 showed. (You may recall that the energy from glucose isn't used directly but goes to make other compounds, ATP and CP. The subsequent breakdown of these compounds provides the energy for the muscle to contract.) After glucose has released its energy, only carbon-dioxide gas and water are left — tiny waste products that can be excreted.

When you exert yourself extremely vigorously without relaxing for a moment, you experience muscle fatigue or even exhaustion and can't work your muscles at all. This effect results from the buildup of lactic acid — and knowing where it comes from can help an athlete to improve his (or her) endurance. The first few steps of glucose breakdown can be done without oxygen, until pyruvate (pyruvic acid) has been produced (see margin).

The next few steps require oxygen and end with the complete breakdown of pyruvic acid to carbon dioxide and water (margin). To break down glucose completely, then, and release the waste products, the muscle cells need abundant oxygen.

If the circulation can't bring them oxygen fast enough, the cells break glucose down as far as they can, to pyruvic acid, and then convert the pyruvic acid to the temporary waste product lactic acid. That is all they can do without oxygen. This acid accumulates, changes the acid balance in the muscle, and causes fatigue.

You can forestall the accumulation of lactic acid in two ways. Breathing is most important. The more oxygen you can bring to the muscle, the longer it can work aerobically, getting all of the available energy from its stored glucose. (This is why athletes, to get in the best possible shape, have to condition their cardiovascular and respiratory systems — that is, do aerobic exercise that requires speeded-up breathing and a rapid heartbeat, and not just weight-lifting or exercises that increase muscle strength only.) But during heavy physical exertion, the circulation can't keep up with the cells' need for oxygen, so lactic acid will accumulate. In this event, the strategy is to relax the muscles at every opportunity, so that the lactic acid and accumulated fluid can drain away. It can be relocated in the liver, if the circulation can carry it

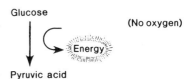

The anaerobic part of glucose breakdown.

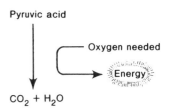

The aerobic part of glucose breakdown.

anaerobic: requiring no oxygen.

an = without
aer = oxygen

pyruvic acid (pie-ROO-vic): a breakdown product of glucose that can be produced anaerobically. To dispose of pyruvic acid without using oxygen, the cells convert it to lactic acid. See Highlight 7A.

aerobic: requiring oxygen.

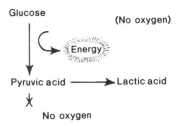

Pyruvic acid is shunted temporarily to lactic acid if oxygen isn't present to help oxidize it further.

lactic acid: an acid produced when oxygen is not available to oxidize pyruvic acid all the way to carbon dioxide and water. Lactic acid accumulates in hard-working muscles and makes them sore.

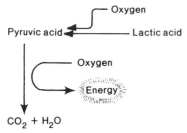

When oxygen is available again, lactic acid is reconverted to pyruvic acid and then completely oxidized.

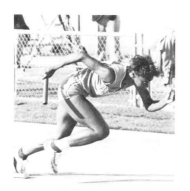

there, and disposed of later, when oxygen again becomes available. (At the end of the event, too, athletes shake and move their muscles to shift the fluid out of them so they won't become stiff.)

At the end of an event, the athlete continues to breathe fast, and the heart continues pounding for some time, because oxygen is still being circulated to the tissues to help break down the accumulated lactic acid. The carbon dioxide that results stimulates the brain to make the heart and lungs stay speeded up until the waste products have been disposed of.

This description has shown what provides fuel for intense muscular activity: glycogen, that is, carbohydrate. The message for the athlete is that meals high in protein not only don't help build muscle but also don't help fuel its activity. Many experiments have shown that extra protein in the diet confers no advantage on the athlete in terms of strength, endurance, or speed. [68]

Fat is also used for fuel by muscles but can be broken down only as long as oxygen is available. Fat deposits therefore supply energy only for moderate — not strenuous — muscular work. (That's why long, slow, moderately intense activity such as long walks can be very effective as an adjunct to a weight-loss effort.)

A great advantage to muscle conditioning is that it increases the muscles' ability to burn fat as fuel; they build up more fat-metabolizing machinery in response to demand. So people whose muscles are in good shape find it easier to keep off excess fat. Conditioned muscles will burn fat longer during activity, or at a higher-intensity exercise level, than poorly conditioned muscles. In competition, conditioned muscles will go much longer before starting to use glycogen. The point at which the body starts using glycogen is the beginning of the end, because glycogen stores are limited, whereas fat stores are (in effect) unlimited.

Athletes in training for an endurance activity such as long-distance running, cycling, or swimming may experience increasing fatigue as the days of training go on. One reason for this is that it takes 48 hours or more to restore muscle carbohydrate to its pre-exercise level after it has been completely exhausted. To replace the used-up carbohydrate, the athlete must eat a diet high in carbohydrate.[69] Two pointers for the athlete in training, then, are to take a periodic day's rest, if possible, during training, and to rest for a day or so before the event and eat a carbohydrate-rich diet.

Athletes who compete in long-distance endurance events naturally want to have as much stored energy in their muscles as they can. Glycogen loading is a technique of tricking the muscles into storing more glycogen than they normally have the capacity for. It involves first reducing carbohydrate intake for several days by eating meals high in protein and fat and simultaneously exercising heavily to deplete the

[68]Nutrition and athletic performance, 1976.

[69]F. I. Katch, W. D. McArdle, and B. R. Boylan, *Getting in Shape* (Boston: Houghton Mifflin, 1979), p. 109.

muscle glycogen stores. The second step is to reduce exercise intensity and switch abruptly to a diet high in carbohydrate. Muscle glycogen stores rebound to about two to four times the normal level and thus provide fuel that will last longer in an endurance event. Marathon racers can tell when they've run out of glycogen (they "hit the wall" and suddenly slow down); those who have "loaded" can keep going longer and so have the edge in the competition.[70]

Until the mid-1970s, the hazards of this practice were unknown. Now, unfortunately, it is clear that there are hazards (see margin).[71] Many top athletes feel that the side effects of tampering with their diets, muscle and cardiac pain from the "stuffing," and weight gain cancel the benefits conferred by loaded glycogen. It is also strongly suggested that this not be done more than about three times a year, due to the effects on heart function. However, some athletes feel they can get away with it without ill effects; it may be an individual matter.

To maximize endurance, the athlete pays attention not only to fuel reserves in the muscle (that is, glycogen) but also to the muscle's ability to use that fuel. That means maximizing all of the following:

- Aerobic capacity (by heart and lung conditioning).
- Hemoglobin levels (by optimal iron and protein nutrition).
- Metabolic regulators (by optimal vitamin and mineral nutrition).
- Muscular fat-using ability (by muscular conditioning).[72]

Athletes also want to know what food is best before an event. There seems to be no special food that should be eaten before an athletic contest. A meal of steak may boost morale, but a meal so high in fat may also stay on the stomach long enough to hinder performance. There's no need to avoid milk; the idea that it causes "cotton mouth" is pure superstition. Olympic training tables are laden with carbohydrate foods such as fruit, and this is the best choice, for the reasons described in the previous section.

A competitor who gets very excited before an event may be unable to digest any food very well. For this reason, many athletes tolerate liquid meals best. But there is no magic ingredient in a liquid meal, in spite of what advertisements may claim. Any meal should be finished a good two or even three or four hours before the event, because digestion requires routing the blood supply to the GI tract. By the time the contest begins, the circulating blood should be freed from the task of carrying newly arrived nutrients and available instead to carry oxygen and fuel to the muscles.[73]

The notion is widespread that it is smart to eat a candy bar or a few teaspoons of honey right before the event, for "quick energy." It may

Comment on glycogen loading:

The use of this dietary regime is . . . not without possible risks. Glycogen retains water and both may be deposited in the muscle to such an extent that a feeling of heaviness and stiffness is experienced. The resulting weight increase due to water retention may reduce the ability of the athlete to take up oxygen maximally. Carbohydrate loading designed to increase endurance has also been reported to produce cardiac pain and electrocardiographic abnormalities in an older marathon runner. The effect of this practice on heart function is worrisome enough to caution all athletes against its use.

Nutrition and athletic performance, 1976.

---

[70]P. Slovic, What helps the long distance runner run? *Nutrition Today* 10 (3) (1975):18-21.

[71]Nutrition and athletic performance, 1976.

[72]We are indebted to Dr. Sam Smith for suggesting this summary.

[73]Nutrition and athletic performance, 1976.

feel good to do this, but it probably confers a disadvantage physically, if it has any effect at all. The body's response is to secrete insulin, which retards fat use at a time when fat use should be maximal.

As to liquids, during heavy exertion, a person sweats, losing both water and salts. There is no question that this can disable the athlete more seriously than any other nutritional factor. Maintaining fluid balance is crucial to successful performance, because the first symptom of dehydration is fatigue. A rapid water loss equal to 5 percent of the body weight can reduce muscular work capacity by 20 to 30 percent.[74] According to the Food and Nutrition Board, a person should begin replacing salt as well as water after having drunk more than four quarts of water to replace that lost in heavy sweating; but according to recent research, the replacement need not be immediate and shouldn't be by way of salt tablets.[75] A person can sweat away as much as nine pounds of fluid and still perform well provided he or she drinks enough water, even without salt. When the event is over, eating regular food can make up the salt loss.[76] At that point, replacement of magnesium and potassium may be more important than replacement of sodium.

You may be wondering how this statement can be made when the makers of Gatorade and other "sweat replacers" claim that their mixtures of water with glucose, sodium, chloride, potassium, magnesium, and calcium enter the system "faster than water" and help football players win games. Actually, although such mixtures do resemble sweat in composition (except for the glucose) and do satisfy thirst, they are probably absorbed less rapidly, not more rapidly, than water, because the glucose in them holds them back.[77] Moreover, the body of a trained athlete stores extra amounts of the minerals in question and can replenish them perfectly well with ordinary food and fluids after the competition is over.[78] Furthermore, a person who sweats heavily (say, two liters) during competition *cannot* replace the lost fluid even by drinking that much, because the stomach can't absorb more than one liter in an hour's time. The best fluid for a marathon event is *diluted* juice (for example, one part orange juice plus four parts water) or plain water in small quantities. However, there is probably no great harm in the moderate use of sweat replacers. The sugar in them provides a boost; they taste good; and most importantly, they bolster morale.

Some athletes have anemia. It is not known whether this is always the result of nutritional deficiency, or whether in some cases it may be an adaptation to the athlete's way of life. It is possible that the athlete only appears to be anemic and in fact has a greater number of red

[74]J. Bergstrom and E. Hultman, Nutrition for maximal sports performance, *Journal of the American Medical Association* 221 (1972):999.

[75]S. Wintsch, Beading the heat, *Science '81* 2 (1981):80-82.

[76]Wintsch, 1981.

[77]Wintsch, 1981.

[78]Wintsch, 1981.

blood cells but an even greater plasma volume as a result of conditioning, so that the red blood cells are, in effect, diluted. This effect is enhanced when, during repeated days of heavy training, plasma volume may increase by almost a third because the kidney conserves sodium and water at these times.[79] Thus there may be two kinds of anemia in athletes — one, the adaptation just described, and the other, a true anemia that occurs especially in women athletes. For the latter, as for all persons with anemia, taking an iron supplement may be a good idea.

The case of athletes' anemia brings up a point that everyone should keep in mind. Not all apparent abnormalities are "bad." The body is a magnificent system that shows a remarkable ability to adapt to different lifestyles and situations. Athletes' anemia serves as a case in point. Don't take hasty action in cases like this; wait until the research is done and the proper course of action is known.

No doubt other differences between the bodies of athletes and nonathletes will be discovered in the future, and the finger will be pointed at nutrition again: "You wouldn't be that way if you would eat right." But the athlete being told this should keep in mind that the body may be wiser than the accuser and that the reason the body is different may be because of the different tasks it is called upon to perform.

This note is intended as a general note of caution. When new findings turn up in relation to nutrition and athletics, give them a chance to be responsibly investigated before jumping to conclusions and especially before going to any extremes in terms of food choices. In this field as in all fields of science, you can't find truth by a reasoning process, no matter how good the logic may be. Experimental testing must come first. Meanwhile, before the data are in and analyzed, be moderate in your nutritional practices.

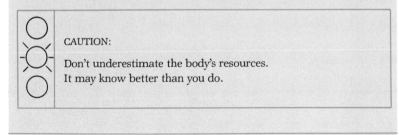

CAUTION:

Don't underestimate the body's resources.
It may know better than you do.

[79]D. L. Costill, A scientific approach to distance running, *Track and Field News* (Los Altos, Calif.: 1979), p. 22.

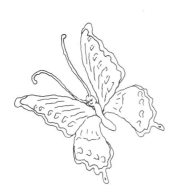

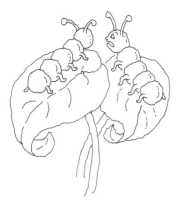

"You'll never get me up in one of those things."

The recommendations made here are simple, common-sense suggestions. To sum up, a normal varied diet is best for the athlete, as for anyone else. Athletes eat more food to get the extra kcalories they need, and if they choose their foods with reasonable good judgment, they will get the extra nutrients they need as well. An adequate fluid intake is indispensable to successful performance.

Teenagers' Food Choices   The teen years are well known as a time of rebellion. This rebellion extends to foods as well as to all other aspects of lifestyle. The choice of what to eat is up to teenagers themselves. Access points already mentioned include the refrigerator, the school lunch, and vending machines, but other than controlling the contents of these, adults can expect to have little impact on the nutrient intakes of adolescents — especially by such conventional means as education. Still, most young adults in this country are well fed, for reasons perceptively stated by R. M. Leverton: They get hungry; they like to eat; they want energy, vigor and the means to compete and excel in whatever they do; and they have many good habits, which are just as hard to break as the bad ones.[80]

Nutrition educators who wish to reach the teenager and young adult with nutrition information must find out and pay attention to two factors: why they sometimes are poorly nourished or develop poor food habits and what means of communicating turns them on.

The young person with poor food habits and a negative attitude toward food is likely to have at least one of the following characteristics:

- He thinks nutrition means eating what you don't like because it's good for you.
- She has been criticized for her eating pattern but feels fine and sees no ill effects.
- He is uninterested in food, and it plays a negligible role in his very busy life.
- The people she is most likely to listen to are not knowledgeable about nutrition.[81]

The parent or teacher concerned about a teenager's food habits should be aware of what teenagers feel about themselves (some reflection into your own past may recall painful memories in this connection). They crave acceptance, especially from their peers. They need to fit in. In many cases they are greatly dissatisfied with themselves. One of the most important aspects of their image is the body image. Young men want larger biceps, shoulders, chest, and

---

[80]R. M. Leverton, The paradox of teen-age nutrition, *Journal of the American Dietetic Association* 53 (1968):13-16.

[81]Leverton, 1968.

forearms; young women want smaller hips, thighs, and waists.[82] One study of U.S. teenagers revealed that 59 percent of the young men wanted to gain weight, although only 25 percent actually needed to do so. Similarly, 70 percent of the girls wanted to lose weight, but no more than about 15 percent were obese.[83] Words to the effect that "you look fine as you are" fall on deaf ears. (The same can be said of adults in some cases, up to the age of about 99.) To be effectively conveyed, nutrition information can be sold as part of a package that will bring about these desired changes. Fortunately, it happens to be true that nutrient-dense, low-kcalorie foods favor the development of strong biceps in men and a trim figure in women.

When the young person who is the target of your campaign possesses and cherishes nutrition misinformation, one of the first questions to ask is whether the practice is beneficial, neutral, or harmful. Opposing a loved ideal is more likely to polarize than to convert the opposition. A practice such as vegetarianism, dieting, or consuming a "muscle-building diet" can be encouraged — with modifications — rather than condemned. Only the most hazardous nutritional practices should be singled out for attention; silence is an option about the others.

One of the most effective ways to teach nutrition is by example. When nutrition teachers are moralists who fail to practice what they preach, their words fall on deaf ears. The coach and gym teacher, the friendly young French teacher, the admired city recreation director — those who enthusiastically maintain their own health — can have a great impact on teenagers. Remember, this is the period of identity formation, the time of seeking and emulating models.

When communicating nutrition information, above all be sure that you have it straight. We make fools of ourselves when we (for example) admonish our students to follow restrictive patterns when their own choices are already as good as ours or better. There may be no harm in using candy bars to meet part of the kcalorie allowance of an active young adult. It may not be necessary to drink milk if calcium, vitamin D, and riboflavin needs are being met by cheese or other food sources. Satisfactory diets can be designed on a great variety of foundations. It is the nutrient content and balance of foods, not the specific foods consumed, that make the difference between "good" and "bad" diets.

Much of the work of "teaching" nutrition can be delegated to teenagers themselves. Those who are interested and motivated can be guided to reliable sources and allowed to indulge their own desire to benefit their friends and classmates. Among the best materials prepared to teach teenagers the importance of good nutrition are those made by teenagers themselves.

Finally, remember that teenagers have the right to make their own decisions — even if they are ones you violently disagree with. You can

No other age group is as concerned about their bodies or as sensitive to or devastated by criticism and comparison as are adolescents. . . . It's not unusual to find these adolescents with distorted body images making inappropriate food choices and thus compromising optimal growth. — B. Lucas

[82]B. Lucas, Nutrition and the adolescent, in P. Pipes, *Nutrition in Infancy and Childhood,* 2nd ed. (St. Louis: Mosby, 1981), pp. 179-204.

[83]Lucas, 1981.

set up the environment so that the foods available are those you favor, and you can stand by with reliable nutrition information and advice, but you will have to leave the rest to them. Ultimately, they make the choices.

Summing Up

Additions to a baby's diet are selected according to the baby's readiness to handle them and its changing nutrient needs. Among the first nutrients needed in amounts beyond those provided by milk are iron and vitamin C. By a year of age, a baby can be eating foods from all four food groups. Normal weight gain, tooth development, and health can be promoted by feeding a balanced diet, avoiding empty-kcalorie foods, and encouraging infants to learn to like foods from all four food groups. The first year of life is the most important for setting future food habits.

After the age of one, a child's growth rate slows, and with it, the appetite. However, all essential nutrients, especially the growth nutrients, continue to be needed in adequate amounts from foods with a high nutrient density. Milk remains important but should not exceed three servings a day, because it is a poor source of iron and vitamin C.

When children go to school, their nutritional needs are partly met by school lunch programs. Another influential factor in the lives of children is television, with many advertisements for sugary foods; another is vending machines, which often limit choices to foods of low quality. Dentists and other health professionals are concerned that the advertisement and availability of sugary foods should be controlled; there may also be a need to control some children's caffeine consumption from cola beverages and cocoa products.

Sound nutritional practices may prevent future health problems to some extent. Obesity, iron-deficiency anemia, cardiovascular disease, and diabetes are conditions responsive to nutritional and other measures; screening for these conditions helps early detection. Good dental health can be promoted by avoiding sticky, sugary foods and adopting healthy eating habits as well as brushing teeth regularly.

It is desirable for children to learn to like nutritious foods in all the food groups. This liking seems to come naturally except, in some children, the liking for vegetables. The person who feeds the child must be aware of the child's psychological and emotional development. With wise handling, children can learn eating habits that will continue to promote their good health and well-being after they have become adults.

The teen years mark the transition from a time when children eat what they are fed to a time when they choose for themselves what to eat. Nutrition education becomes important as a means of encouraging healthy food habits. Teenagers' snacking patterns and lifestyles predispose them to certain nutritional inadequacies, notably a lack of iron, but teenagers vary so widely that generalizations are difficult. Screening for problems is one way to detect them early.

A special problem in the teen years is anorexia nervosa, self-imposed starvation. An anorexic may diet to only 65 to 70 lb and may need extremely careful treatment by knowledgeable professionals to recover. A related problem is bulimia, or binge-eating, which may be followed by self-induced vomiting or other "purging" strategies. Both anorexia nervosa and bulimia appear to be related to our society's overemphasis on extreme thinness as an ideal weight.

Special problems that may arise in the teen years and affect nutrition include pregnancy, alcohol, and drug use. The pregnant teenage girl, whose nutrient needs are higher than those of any other person, needs medical attention, nutritional guidance, and emotional support. Alcohol use is common among teenagers, and 90 percent of U.S. college students use alcohol. One out of 20 is likely to become an alcohol abuser. Beer, as well as hard liquor, can be abused and can lead to alcoholism.

Prolonged use of prescription drugs in the young adult and adult may affect appetite, nutrient synthesis, and other aspects of the body's handling of nutrients. Drugs also interact with one another and with alcohol, causing nutritional problems. Awareness of this and attention to diet planning provides safeguards against health hazards. Marihuana has characteristic effects on taste and appetite, but the long-term effects of heavy use are not well understood. Users of other drugs may suffer profound health damage, and an important part of the rehabilitation process is the identification and correction of nutritional problems.

Caffeine is a stimulant drug, habit-forming but not addictive, whose moderate use is not harmful. Excessive caffeine consumption may be the cause of anxiety symptoms and lack of sleep.

A major interest for many teenagers is athletics, and they are motivated to study nutrition to improve their performance. They need little or no extra protein, can utilize carbohydrate best as fuel, and need no special supplements but rather a balanced, varied diet. Fluid intake is important to athletic performance.

Teenagers and adults make their own choices. The nutrition educator is advised to be aware of the sources of their motivation and to convey important information in a way that honors their individuality.

To Explore Further

In relation to the profound effect that "feeding with love" can have on children, E. M. Widdowson described long ago how this variable "ruined" a nutritional experiment that some investigators tried to carry out. Love and attention had a bigger effect on the children's growth than the food:

- Widdowson, E. M. Mental contentment and physical growth. *Lancet* 1 (1951):1316-1317.

Conversely, the effect of lack of love and attention is now known to account for much of the growth and developmental failure wherever malnutrition of children is seen. A landmark article, reporting years of research, is:

● Cravioto, J. Nutrition, stimulation, mental development and learning. *Nutrition Today*, September/October 1981, pp. 4-15.

On nutrition in the first year of life, S. J. Fomon's book, *Infant Nutrition*, 2nd ed. (Philadelphia: Saunders, 1974), is an excellent comprehensive reference.

A tidy four-page statement on the nutritional needs of infants up to a year of age was published in the American Medical Association journal:

● Woodruff, C. W. The science of infant nutrition and the art of infant feeding. *Journal of the American Medical Association* 240 (1978):657-661.

The whole issue (all six pages) of *Nutrition and the MD*, May 1980, was also devoted to infant nutrition. This resource and the preceding one rely extensively on the authoritative word of the American Association of Pediatrics, whose Committee on Nutrition published the following recommendations:

● Commentary on breast-feeding and infant formulas, including proposed standards for formulas. *Pediatrics* 57 (1976):278-285.

According to a recent review, it is "irresponsible to make a dogmatic statement" about the timing or selection of additions of solid food to a baby's diet. This review gives details on what needs to be considered:

● Nutritional adequacy of breast feeding. *Nutrition Reviews* 38 (1980):145-147.

The USDA has published a manual giving the complete nutritional analysis of many baby foods:

● *Composition of Foods: Baby Foods — Raw, Processed, Prepared.* Agriculture Handbook no. 8-3. USDA Science and Education Administration, Washington, D.C.: 1978.

On the nutrition of children:

● Fomon, S. J. *Infant Nutrition*, 2nd ed. Philadelphia: Saunders, 1974.

● Pipes, P. L. *Nutrition in Infancy and Childhood.* St. Louis: Mosby, 1977 (paperback). This 205-page book is an authoritative, clear, understandable text, one of the best in the field.

On the prevention of adult health problems through good nutritional practices in childhood:

● Breslow, L., and Somers, A. R. Lifetime health monitoring: A practical approach to preventive medicine. *New England Journal of Medicine* 296 (1977):601-608. Breslow and Somers have studied the disorders most likely to appear at every age and have suggested an agenda for screening at intervals throughout life that would detect these disorders.

● Fomon, S. J., Anderson, T. A., Stephen, H. Y. W., and Ziegler, E. E. *Nutritional Disorders of Children: Prevention, Screening, and Followup.* DHEW publication no. (HSA) 76-5612. Washington, D.C.: Government Printing Office, 1976.

● Williams, C. L., and Wynder, E. L. A blind spot in preventive medicine. *Journal of the American Medical Association* 236 (1976):2196-2197.

● Blumenthal, S., and Jesse, M. J. Prevention of atherosclerosis: A pediatric problem. *Hospital Practice*, April 1973, pp. 81-90.

A review of the recent history of the nation's child nutrition programs is presented in:

- Vaden, A. G. Child nutrition programs: past, present, future. *Professional Nutritionist*, Winter 1981, pp. 7-10.

As the programs are being cut, data are also just beginning to be amassed, documenting the positive impacts of the child nutrition programs. There are fewer malnourished people in this country than there were 10 years ago.

The *School Lunch Journal* and the *School Foodservice Journal* are coming out monthly with creative new ideas. In addition:

- Frederick, L. *Fast Food Gets an "A" in School Lunch.* Boston: Cahner's Books, 1977. This book describes the fast-food style of serving school lunches, which has been proving successful in attracting children away from vending machines and off-campus eating places.

The entire issue of *Nutrition Reviews*, February 1981, was devoted to adolescent nutrition and included articles on all the topics discussed in this chapter.

Among the most thought-provoking and readable articles available on anorexia nervosa are three that appeared in the *American Journal of Nursing*, August 1980. The first is an account by an anorexic herself:

- Ciseaux, A. Anorexia nervosa: A view from the mirror. Pp. 1469-1470.

- Richardson, T. F. Anorexia nervosa: An overview. Pp. 1470- 1471.

- Claggett, M. S. Anorexia nervosa: A behavioral approach. Pp. 1471-1477.

Another excellent short article by the authority H. Bruch is:

- Anorexia nervosa. *Nutrition Today*, September/October 1978, pp. 14-18.

Bruch's book is still the authoritative reference on the subject:

- Bruch, H. *The Golden Cage: The Enigma of Anorexia Nervosa.* Cambridge, Mass.: Harvard University Press, 1978.

Two excellent films on the subject are also available: *Dieting: the Danger Point*, from McGraw-Hill, and *Diet unto Death*, from ABC Learning Corporation.

For the best readings and films on pregnancy, teenage and otherwise, see To Explore Further at the end of Chapter 15. For materials to recommend to clients, see Appendix C.

Infancy

Mrs. Trudeau is telephoning the nurse to ask what to do about her baby's constant crying. The nurse recalls the case: Tommy is a first baby and was a full-term, normal-weight infant delivered without complications and released from the hospital after four days without any unusual events. His mother was breastfeeding him.

Since then he has gained weight normally (he has had two checkups). His mother weaned him to formula at three weeks, fearing that her breast milk supply was inadequate because he was crying "all the time." He is now five weeks old and is still crying "all the time," especially after feedings.

The nurse checks the routine possibilities (do you burp him? does he have a fever? does he accept the formula?) and concludes that Tommy is probably colicky. She says this will pass in time, but when Mrs. Trudeau insists on having a suggestion what to do, she replies, "You might try a different formula. Sometimes a particular formula upsets the baby."

Study Question

1. Is there anything else the nurse should have said or done at this point?

At the three-month checkup, Tommy is normally alert and has gained approximately the expected amount of weight. The nurse has no time to talk with Mrs. Trudeau at this visit. Tommy misses his six-month appointment.

At nine months, Tommy has fallen behind in his growth, is listless, lacks appetite, and has some motor abnormalities indicative of anemia. His hemoglobin is below 11 g/100 ml.

A dietary interview now reveals that Mrs. Trudeau

tried a variety of formulas at the nurse's suggestion, without much success. Then she read somewhere that fortification iron can upset a person's stomach, so she switched to formula without iron. Later, when Tommy seemed cranky again, she switched to an iron-free, soy-based formula. She began introducing foods at four months, but whenever he seemed irritable (which was often), she withdrew them again. At nine months he was eating predominantly baby food fruits and teething crackers in addition to the formula.

Study Questions

2. Mrs. Trudeau got no nutrition advice from the nurse, and so she fended for herself. The nurse only heard Tommy's crying for a few minutes, but his mother listened to it in anguish for hours and could not live with it without trying everything she could think of to do. At what times and with what steps should the nurse have intervened?

3. What nutrition advice should she give now?

Sugar Abuse

Scene: Your place. Time of day: afternoon or evening. You are doing nothing in particular, when suddenly you feel like eating something sweet. You resist, but the feeling gnaws at you. With guilt fluttering in your conscience you head for the cookie jar, telling yourself, "Just one. Maybe two. Not more than three. Or four." But you already have calculated about how many cookies are in the jar and you know you may end up eating them all. . . . A jar of cookies, a piece of cheesecake, and two big bowls of ice cream later, you sit as if stunned. "Why did I do that?"

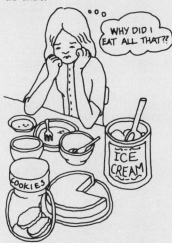

WHY DID I EAT ALL THAT??

You are full, uncomfortably full, maybe even in pain. You have eaten alone, and you hastily dispose of the evidence because you are ashamed of what you have done. You choose not to eat dinner, now, because you've eaten more than you intended to for the whole day. You resolve not to do it again.

There is no such thing as junk food. But there is such a thing as a junk diet.

H. A. GUTHRIE

Not all people see themselves in this description, but many more do than you might think — probably the majority of people in our society. Some are fat, some are at normal weight, and some are very thin. They are bingers — or, as they have variously been called, carboholics, hyperphagics, or bulimics. All of these people have a complex and intense relationship with their food that no one completely understands. Many factors are involved, from the body's purely chemical interaction with carbohydrate to the emotional involvement of the self with food and the consciousness of its social meaning. One factor is the tiny entity, the sugar molecule itself, which provides the sweet taste that started the binge.

This Highlight does not sort out all the factors in the tangled relationships of people with sweet foods, but it provides some help in understanding just what sugar has to do with this scenario. It is placed here after the chapter on children and teenagers, rather than after Chapter 1 (on Carbohydrates), because it seems particularly important for each parent to decide how to handle sugar in the diets of children. The one question we will try to answer (others will come up along the way) is whether sugar should be restricted in, or altogether eliminated from, the diets of children.

Arguments against Sugar We might as well begin with a sampling of the accusations made against sugar. It has been blamed for a host of ills in both children and adults. Most commonly, it is accused of causing hypoglycemia. One medical practitioner claims that "thousands of people . . . suffer from hypoglycemia," and describes the consequences:

Behavior and mood are affected, and the patient becomes depressed, restless, or anxious. Friends and relatives begin to notice signs of emotional instability. On the surface, the person appears to be neurotic rather than physically ill. . . . Some patients complain of itching, skin rashes, or numbness in certain areas. These symptoms can be traced to the effect that low blood-sugar levels have on nerve endings. . . . Often, hypoglycemia patients report an excessive craving for sweets.

He goes on to describe the "typical case" of an 18-year-old boy who was doing poorly in school and was unable to concentrate. He had emotional problems, felt worthless and depressed, and was unresponsive to friends. He complained of a craving for sweets and an acnelike rash. The practitioner diagnosed the case as hypoglycemia and recommended the standard treatment. "The results were gratifying. After a month the patient had new vigor [and] a return to normal health."[1]

Similarly, a probation officer who believes poor nutrition causes or worsens criminal behavior reports that of 106 prisoners on probation, many had symptoms of "hypoglycemia." The test used to identify hypoglycemia had respondents answer yes or no to such statements as: "I have cold sweats during the night; I feel well after eating candy, cakes, or soft drinks; I want revenge on society; I have crying spells; I have abdominal distress; I generally feel tired and weak; I feel very tense; I have trouble keeping jobs; I do not drink much water; my hands and legs feel cold."

The officer says that when the prisoners changed their diets, she saw remarkable changes in the way they felt and looked and how they behaved: "I've seen whole families change. One prisoner says, "Now I feel better than I ever have in my life.""[2]

The reader will recognize these descriptions as anecdotes and testimonials (Highlight 10) and will know that they do not constitute acceptable evidence that hypoglycemia was responsible for the subjects' feelings and behavior or that the change in diet accounted for the claimed dramatic cures. But they are typical of hundreds of cases that reveal how real the connection between behavior and diet is felt to be.

In cases of hypoglycemia, removal of pure, concentrated sugar from the diet is a necessary part of treatment. (The criteria for correct diagnosis and treatment are given in Chapter 25). If the diagnosis has been correct, then the change in diet brings about a welcome change in the experience of the client, who feels dramatically better and more energetic. The reason is that the dietary change has corrected the internal hormonal imbalance and so stabilized the blood glucose level. The

client may not understand how it works but will often report to friends, "I gave up sugar and I feel like a new person."

Chapter 1 showed that hypoglycemia is often wrongly diagnosed and is something of a fad. The cases described here may have suffered from true hypoglycemia, or they may have benefitted from the powerful placebo effect (Highlight 10) conferred by someone's taking a strong interest in their problems and presenting them with a cure that was guaranteed to be effective. The placebo effect is the more likely explanation, because it has been shown to account for more than half of all such cures. But the true cases of hypoglycemia, together with all these stories, are often taken to imply that sugar is a villain.

Sugar appears to be a villain, too, in other stories linking diet to behavior. For example, a physician describes a 4-year-old child whose favorite foods were sugar-coated cereals and other snack and junk foods. The physician noted:

Jim is the most active child I've seen in several months. He climbs on and off the table, he bounces around and gets into everything that isn't nailed down. His examination, otherwise, is essentially negative except for moderate pallor (even though a subsequent hemogram showed that he was not anemic) and circles under his eyes; his nasal mucosa appears pale and somewhat lavender; his

[1]The author was careful to point out that not all cases that present themselves this way turn out to be hypoglycemia. Another that appeared similar at first turned out to be multiple sclerosis. S. Walker, III, Sugar doctors push hypoglycemia, *Psychology Today*, July 1975, as quoted in L. Hofmann, *The Great American Nutrition Hassle* (Palo Alto, Calif.: Mayfield, 1978):259-262.

[2]B. Reed as quoted by C. Winter, Researchers look for link between diet and crime, *Miami Herald*, 13 October 1977.

teeth show several cavities which have been filled.

The diagnosis was "sugar allergy"; when sugar was eliminated from the diet, the mother reported:

> "Jim is a different child. He sleeps all night, he plays well and now listens to instructions." All foods had been re-added without reaction except for sugar. When the child ate sugar-containing foods, his symptoms reappeared within five minutes and lasted for some four hours.[3]

Other links between sugar and behavior (or should we say misbehavior?) are seen by such people as school principals and parents. A principal says: "Many of the children who ate a lot of this sugary food at the school site — these children were having problems with learning or with behavior."[4] A parents' group puts the case more strongly in the title of their booklet: "The Effects of Excessive Consumption of Refined Sugar on Learning Skills, Behavior Attitudes and/or Physical Condition in School-Aged Children — Some Consequences." They attribute all of the following problems in school children to overconsumption of refined sugar:

myopia . . . learning disabilities . . . fatigue . . . hyperactivity . . . behavior problems, mental disturbance and schizophrenia . . . violence . . . alcoholism . . . sugar addiction . . . auto accidents . . . cardiovascular disease . . . tooth decay . . . premature sexuality . . . arthritis.

They conclude their booklet, "If we do not respond by removing refined sugar from our children's diets, then we must all suffer the consequences of that inaction."[5]

It is hard to state the case any more strongly than this, but it has been done. An outraged pediatrician says sugar doesn't support higher brain function:

> So when a teacher is confronted with a child in her classroom who didn't eat a proper breakfast, she's just talking to a spinal cord or a gorilla. She should have the right to send the kid home.[6]

At this point, the case against sugar sounds like a crusade, with emotional and religious meaning for the participants. We will come back to the possible reasons for this ("Puritanism and Food," below), but first let us go on to see how strongly attractive sugar is in spite of all the negative effects attributed to it. Is it, as some people believe, an addictive substance?

The Case for Sugar as an Addictive Drug   A member of the board of Overeaters Anonymous who calls herself a "recovered sucroholic," says she is convinced that refined sugar can be as addictive as alcohol:

> Many of us use sugar like a drug. It is our lover, friend, comforter, and when stress comes into our lives we reach for it automatically. Giving it up is terribly difficult; many people go through withdrawal and get the shakes. For some of us, complete abstinence is the only way out. We cannot be social sugar eaters just the way other people cannot be social drinkers.[7]

Another person who calls himself an "addict" is William Dufty, the author of the bestseller *Sugar Blues*.[8] Dufty describes how he licked the sugar habit:

> I threw out everything that had sugar in it, cereals and canned fruit, soups and bread. . . . In about forty-eight hours, I was in total agony, overcome with nausea, with a crashing migraine. . . . I had it very rough for about twenty-four hours, but the morning after was a revelation. I went to sleep with exhaustion, sweating and tremors. I woke up feeling reborn.[9]

[3]W. G. Crook, An alternate method of managing the hyperactive child (letter to the editor), *Pediatrics* 54 (1974):656.

[4]G. Perry, school principal, as quoted in *The Sugar Film*, by Image Associates, P.O. Box 40106, 352 Conejo Road, Santa Barbara, CA 93103.

[5]J. F. Wallace and M. J. Wallace, *The Effects of Excessive Consumption of Refined Sugar on Learning Skills, Behavior Attitudes and/or Physical Condition in School-Aged Children* (Medford, Ore.: Parents for Better Nutrition, 1978).

[6]L. Smith, pediatrician and author of the national bestseller *Feed Your Kids Right*, as quoted in *The Sugar Film*, 1978.

[7]J. Pekkanen and M. Falco, Sweet and sour, *Atlantic Monthly*, July 1975, as quoted in Hofmann, 1978, pp. 252-259.

[8]W. Dufty, *Sugar Blues* (New York: Warner Books, 1975).

[9]Dufty, 1975, pp. 22-23.

According to *Sugar Blues*, if you allow yourself to get "hooked" on sugar, your addiction can lead to physical and mental ruin. The front cover describes sugar as "the killer in your diet," while the back cover states, "Like opium, morphine, and heroin, sugar is an addictive, destructive drug."

Is sugar a "killer"? Is it an addictive drug? Some intricate reasoning from experiments with animals sheds some needed light on the question. Figure 1 provides the details in case you are interested. The outcome was that animals can appear addicted to sugar under certain artificial circumstances; but when allowed access to normal food, they will not eat too much sugar. On a poor diet (low-protein), however, their reliance on sugar becomes excessive. *Addiction*, then, is too strong a term to use for their relationship to sugar.

Nevertheless, sugar's attractiveness shouldn't be underestimated. It does possess some of the characteristics of addictive drugs. "Sweetness is a supernormal, immediate reinforcer operating much like another supernormal, immediate reinforcer — opiates."[10] That means that when you taste it (behavior), you instantly feel pleasure (reward). You are inclined to taste it again. Furthermore, if you happen to be hungry, you quickly experience the reward of sugar's postingestive effects — the satisfaction of your hunger. So if you start eating a sugary food when you are very hungry, you are likely to overeat it until your appetite is sated and you are then too full for a nutritious meal. While *addiction* is too strong a word for what sugar elicits in people, *abuse* is not. And in a starving person, sugar's attractiveness can seem almost as powerful as drug addiction.

Furthermore, as has been mentioned in several previous chapters, sugar can displace from the diet foods

[10]Wallace and Wallace, 1978.

that contain needed nutrients — to the point where deficiencies of these nutrients arise. Nutrient deficiencies spell malnutrition. While the sugar doesn't cause the malnutrition directly in these cases, it certainly contributes indirectly.

Sugar Abuse and the Displacement of Needed Nutrients   Before going anywhere with this subject, let it be clear that any food can be abused in this sense. The overuse of milk, which causes depletion of iron in the diet and leads to milk anemia, could be called "milk abuse." Keeping this in mind, let us see what sorts of physical and behavioral abnormalities are caused not by the presence of sugar but by the simultaneous absence of other nutrients in a high-sugar diet.

The most common nutrient deficiency in children is iron deficiency. While its effects are hard to distinguish from the effects of other factors in children's lives, it is

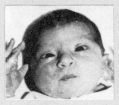 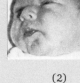 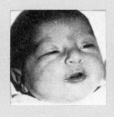 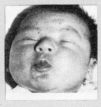 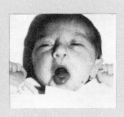

| (1) | (2) | (3) | (4) | (5) |

A newborn baby already likes sugar. This baby is resting (1), tasting distilled water (2), sugar (3), something sour (4), and something bitter (5).

Taste-induced facial expressions of neonate infants from the studies of J. E. Steiner in *Taste and Development*, ed. J. M. Weiffenbach, DHEW publication no. (NIH) 77-1068 (Bethesda, Md.: USDHEW, 1977), pp. 173-189.

likely that iron deficiency in children manifests itself in a lowering of the "motivation to persist in intellectually challenging tasks," a shortening of the attention span, and a reduction of overall intellectual performance. Anemic children perform less well on tests and have more conduct disturbances than their classmates.[11] This is very like a description of hyperactivity. Before blaming the presence of sugar for these problems, it makes sense to check for the absence of iron. Either way, the same kinds of diet changes may bring about improvement: substitution of nutritious foods for nutrient-poor foods.

Before blaming the presence of sugar ("junk foods") for any such problem, in fact, it makes sense to see if the diet is a nutrient-poor diet ("junk diet"). The two often go together, but the distinction is important because one accusation is just and the other is not.

Another nutrient that is easily lost from a "junk diet" is the trace mineral chromium. Diabetes is sometimes blamed on a high-sugar diet, but it is not seen in sugar-cane field workers. Their diet is high in sugar, but it is unrefined cane sugar, which hasn't been stripped of

its chromium. Diabetes is often seen where the diet is high in *refined* sugar, however. Refined sugar requires chromium for its utilization by the body, but does not provide it. (Whole grains do; see Chapter 13.)

A fascinating study that linked a "junk diet" to "neurotic behavior" traced the cause to still another displaced nutrient, thiamin. Unlike the testimonials quoted at the start, this study was published in a refereed journal (see Highlight 17). Twenty patients were identified who had a set of symptoms suggestive of thiamin deficiency, including pains in the chest and abdomen, sleep disturbances, personality changes (aggressiveness and hostility), fevers, GI upsets, chronic fatigue, and many more. Of the 20 patients, 12 were found to have a diet high in carbonated and other sweet beverages, candy, and common snack foods. All had abnormally low thiamin levels as identified by a blood test. Given thiamin supplements, all 20 "noticed marked symptomatic improvement or lost their symptoms completely after thiamin supplement":

> In all cases diet instruction was given. Some patients lost their craving for sweet tasting foods and beverages, although in some the process was extremely difficult and the temptation to succumb quite similar to that seen in people who express a wish to stop smoking.

In the ten who kept their re-

turn appointments, blood tests showed thiamin levels restored to normal.[12]

Thiamin is a nutrient that is easily displaced by nonnutritious foods. To be sure of getting enough vitamin A each day, you just have to eat a few carrots. To meet your vitamin C needs, an orange a day will do. But for thiamin, there is no single food you can eat daily that offers enough to meet the daily need. The only way to meet thiamin needs from food is to eat many servings of nutritious foods, relying on each to make a small contribution. Thus, a "junk diet" is especially likely to be low in thiamin.

People apparently cannot be trusted, then, to provide a nutritious diet for themselves by instinct alone. Given free access to poorly nourishing foods, they may make poor choices and so become malnourished.

> Kids see between 20 and 25 thousand TV commercials each year. Over $600,000,000 each year is spent advertising products to children, yet if kids were to eat only what they saw on television, they couldn't survive.
>
> Harry Snyder, legal advocate for Consumer's Union, as quoted in *The Sugar Film.*

[11] R. L. Leibel, Behavioral and biochemical correlates of iron deficiency: A review, *Journal of the American Dietetic Association* 71 (1977):399-404.

[12] D. Lonsdale and R. J. Shamberger, Red cell transketolase as an indicator of nutritional deficiency, *American Journal of Clinical Nutrition* 33 (1980):205-211.

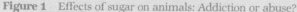

Figure 1   Effects of sugar on animals: Addiction or abuse?

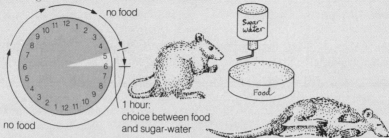

Figure 1a   There was an experiment which seemed to imply that rats could become addicted to sugar and could kill themselves eating it, even when good food was available to them. This kind of experiment has been widely misinterpreted to signify that if sugar is available to human beings, they will destroy themselves with it, as if it were a drug. What has been overlooked is the feeding schedule on which the rats were maintained. They were allowed access to food only for one hour a day, and starved the other 23 hours. During the one hour they were given a choice between nutritious food and pure sugar (in water). They chose the pure sugar every time, and starved themselves to death. Subsequent experiments showed that it wasn't just the sweet taste but also the "postingestive effects" of the sugar that reinforced the rats' choice. In other words, when they were starving, the rats consistently made the choice that most promptly gave them the feeling that their hunger was being relieved. Sugar is quickly absorbed and detected by the nervous system, so it wins the race.

From L. W. Hamilton, Starvation induced by sucrose ingestion in the rat, *Journal of Comparative and Physiological Psychology* 77 (1971):59-69.

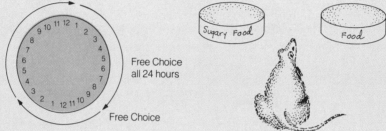

Figure 1b   Maintaining animals on such a schedule and allowing them to eat only when they are starving is different from allowing them free access at all times to a diet presenting a choice between sugary and more-nutritious foods. With free access and free choice between sugar and other foods, rats eat enough nutritious food to stay healthy and grow, although they also eat considerable sugar. Thus sugar alone doesn't kill rats. Rather, it is sugar administered on a weird schedule to starving rats.

From S. Muto, Dietary sweet: Exposure and preference among Japanese children and in laboratory rats, in *Taste and Development, the Genesis of Sweet Preference,* ed. J. M. Weiffenbach (Washington, D.C.: Government Printing Office, 1977), pp. 249-265.

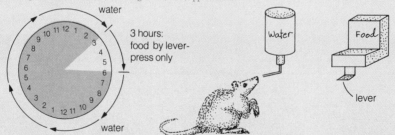

Figure 1c   An unnatural schedule can even induce a rat to over-use a harmless substance like water. An underfed rat, given access to food only 3 hours a day and made to press a lever for it, will drink about half his body weight in water during that 3-hour period, even though he has plenty of water for the other 21 hours as well. The experimenter who discovered this behavior in rats named it "water abuse." On returning to a normal schedule, the rats drank water normally again.

Alcohol abuse can be made to appear in rats by a similar manipulation of feeding time (rats normally refuse to become even interested in alcohol, much less abusers of it). After consuming large amounts of alcohol under these artificial conditions for many days, the rats are "hooked" (addicted). They react differently to alcohol now. Even when returned to a normal schedule they continue to drink alcohol as long as they have access to it.

A rat that is hooked on alcohol by the weird schedule technique and then given the choice between alcohol or a sugar solution (still on the weird schedule), will gradually shift his preference to the sugar solution. This experiment has been widely misinterpreted to mean that "sugar is even more addicting than alcohol," but sugar addiction is not what is seen here. It is sugar-preference-on-a-weird-schedule. Again in the words of the experimenter, "It takes unusual environmental arrangements for [water and sugar] to be abused and to become hazards to health, while ethanol and other agents with addiction liability produce their effects much more directly. . . . Further, addictive agents are viewed as instituting biochemical changes in the central nervous system which, functioning in a vicious circle, maintain a craving for the particular agent." Sugar preference in animals to the point of extreme self-harm does not persist when they are back on a normal schedule. Sweet abuse, then, is not addiction.

From J. L. Falk, Sweet abuse and the addiction model, in *Taste and Development*, 1977, pp. 374-386.

What about babies and children? Can they be trusted to select a nutritious diet for themselves without guidance? Years ago, an experiment was reported in which newly weaned babies were given free choice among a variety of foods. They chose a remarkably balanced diet, and this was taken to mean that their instincts could be relied on to choose the right foods. There was a catch though: No nonnutritious foods were offered to them.[13]

Puritanism and Food

From all the above, it is obvious that we need to "teach" children how to eat or to provide for them an environment in which they can't make the "wrong" choices. In our society, in which nonnutritious foods are occupying a larger and larger share of the marketplace, it has come about that we have had to adopt a puritanical attitude towards food: You must eat what you don't like; you must not eat what you do like. The famous anthropologist Margaret Mead described the development of this attitude with such insight that we have quoted her remarks at length on a nearby page.

A modern-day woman echoes Mead with a complaint about the guilt that accompanies eating for her:

Are we traumatized about food?

Myself, I am deathly afraid of eating too much. That fear is ridiculous since I am not "fat" — and yet every woman I know is similarly afraid. . . . Puritanism . . . is a vital force among women dieters in this country. It's not so much that fear of damnation actually prevents us from overeating: it's rebelling against imagined restrictions that blocks our true taste. When I eat something I don't want to eat, like a piece of cake, I don't taste it, just its forbidden-ness.[14]

By contrast, she says, the French have no such conflict over food. "When someone eats, she doesn't nourish just her body, but also her appetite, her heart, her memory."

Paradoxically, the puritanical commandment "Thou shalt not eat sweet foods" has given sweets a seductive attractiveness that adds to their natural reinforcing properties for people who feel like rebelling. What's forbidden is especially sweet. The coupling of guilt with pleasure may help to account for the kind of binge episode described at the start of this Highlight.

Binge Eating and Puritanism

The puritanically raised child who decides to break the rules is likely to think in these terms: "This is for you, mother (the spinach), and this is for me (ice cream)." Part of the pleasure comes from the sweet taste of the forbidden food, part from the feeling of getting away with it.

Turning from puritanism to physiology for a moment, there may be *additional* reinforcement in the binge episode. If a person is very hungry when she starts to binge, part of the pleasure soon starts coming from the postingestive effect, relief of the hunger pangs.[15] Thus the body as well as the mind falls victim to temptation.

No wonder sugar is seen as so all-powerful by those who hate and fear it. Precisely because they hate and fear it, it is especially powerful. Perhaps those who fear it less are less under its spell. How can we help ourselves and our children not to fear sugar but to put it in its proper place in the diet?

Sugar's Place in the Diet

Parents' and teachers' groups, as well as prison officers and others who are responsible for feeding groups of people, sometimes take vigorous action against sugar. In a school, for example, mothers may be told they may not send candy to school in their children's bag lunches; or children find that the vending machines offer-

[13]C. M. Davis, Self-selection of diet by newly weaned infants, *American Journal of Diseases of Children* 36 (1928):651- 679.

[14]E. Kendall, On food — and the American psyche, *Mademoiselle*, December 1974, pp. 40, 48, and 57, as quoted by Hofmann, 1978.

[15]There is also the possibility that the delivery of glucose to the body promotes the eating of *more* food, a positive feedback response (see Miniglossary). Eating is itself a trigger for the binge. Thus body and mind both fall victims to temptation.

ing cola beverages or candy have been replaced by others presenting milk and oranges.

Anyone who has read the preceding chapters will know that abundant information contained in

this book supports the notion that milk and oranges are a better choice for children's snacks than cola and candy. The evidence is perfectly clear on this point. Milk and oranges supply nutrients children need, cola and candy do

not. Adequately nourished children are healthier physically and mentally than poorly nourished children. Good health is no guarantee of good behavior, but poor health makes it hard for a child to behave well; unhealthy

Mead on Puritanism

People feel that they ought to eat correctly, or, less abstractly ("it's wrong to eat too much sweet stuff"), that, in fact, foods that are good for you are not good to eat, and foods that are good to eat are not good for you. So ingrained is this attitude that it may come as a surprise to learn that in many cultures there is no such contrast, that the foods which are thought to make people strong and well are also exclusively the foods which they like to eat, which they boast of eating, and without which they would be most unhappy. . . .

In the average home, the right food and the wrong food are both placed on the table; the child is rewarded for eating the "right" food and so taught that the right food is undesirable — for parents do not reward children for doing pleasant things. At the same time children are punished by having the "wrong" food taken away from them; here again the lesson is taught to the

child that that which is delicious is an indulgence — for which one is punished or with which one can be rewarded. A dichotomy is set up in the child's mind between those foods which are approved and regarded by adults as undelicious and those foods which are disapproved but recognized as delightful. A permanent conflict situation is established which will pursue that child through his life — each nutritionally desirable choice is made with a sigh or rejected with a sense of guilt; each choice made in terms of sheer pleasure is either accepted with guilt or rejected with a sense of puritanical self-righteousness. Every meal becomes an experience in which an individual must decide between doing right or enjoying himself. Furthermore, as doing right is closely associated with parental supervision, a secondary association is made linking autonomy, adulthood and masculinity with eating what one likes instead of what

mother approved of.

This situation is an eternally self-defeating one, for as long as materials for making the wrong food choice are as accessible as those for making the right, many individuals will make the wrong choice, fairly often. . . . we will never have a population which eats, gaily and unquestioningly, food based on the best nutritional science which we have. For each generation it has to be done all over again. The mother who has, with a great moral effort, learned to drink milk herself, does not merely place a pitcherful of milk on the table and let her children follow her example as she pours it out — although this is the simple method — but she, because of the conflict within her own personality, will argue, threaten, cajole, bribe and punish her children to make them "drink their milk."

children are likely to be listless, tired, inattentive, or irritable because they don't feel well.

The people promoting such changes have their hearts in the right place, but they sometimes have their facts wrong. They may, for example, promote the idea that sugar is "poison" or "an addictive drug." They would have their facts right if they said "our children need nutritious foods." Still, by eliminating sugar from the children's diets, they accomplish a desirable end. The diet of many of the children within the school becomes more nutrient-dense. Does it matter that the means were wrong in achieving this end?

To a student of nutrition science, it matters very much. To claim that sugar is a "poison," even if the intent is golden, is to broadcast a lie. Sugar is not a necessary substance in the diet, but it is not a poison. It can be life-sustaining in certain medical conditions.[16] In any case, it makes a harmless

and delightful addition to many diets that are superbly nourishing. Used artfully, it makes nutritious foods attractive to people who might not otherwise eat them. Many other points could be raised in its favor.

Why have sugar's opponents gone to such an extreme? Puritanism tends to be extreme anyway — but a spokesman for sugar may have hit upon another answer as well. Those making the judgments are not scientists trained in the impartial balancing of the evidence. Rather, they are consumer advocates or congressional committees who "often make it a practice to take an adversary position in order to prove a point. . . . Once the position is established, evidence is collected to back it with essential disregard for contrary evidence.[17]

In other words, they draw their conclusion first and then make the evidence fit. This is in direct contrast to the way a responsible reviewer of scientific evidence goes about evaluating the available data (as described in Highlight 10, for example).

The American Council on Science and Health has criticized the press for giv-

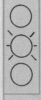

CAUTION:

When a statement about nutrition reads more like a witch hunt than a fair trial, ask yourself: Is the speaker biased to begin with? Is he or she reviewing all the evidence, or just the evidence that supports the bias?

ing uncritical coverage to scare stories about sugar:

It is essential that members of the media begin to help consumers sort myths from facts in the area of nutrition and health. A terrible disservice is performed in the name of news when [pure speculation] is presented to the public as accurate information."[18]

About Reinforcement

If Lenny and my parents wouldn't give me any attention, I would turn to someone who could love me back. Food loved me back.

R. Simmons

Deep inside there had always been a small child begging for my attention. . . . All I gave her was food. Now I give her love.

E. LeShan

[16]"Casual, though well meaning, recommendations that sugar be omitted from a child's diet can lead — in a case where sugar is medically required — to growth failure, weight loss, biochemical instability, or even be life threatening." D. E. M. Frances, *Journal of Human Nutrition* 33 (1979):146, abstract, *Journal of the American Dietetic Association* 75 (1979):197.

[17]G. M. Bollenbach, Sugar in health, *Cereal Foods World* 26 (1981):213-217.

[18]Health watch, *ACSH News and Views*, September/October 1980, p. 8

In contrast, some unbiased, although not perfect or final, reviews on sugar have concluded that it is innocent of some, but not all, of the charges leveled against it. For example, of eight substantial charges against sugar made in 1978 by the Federal Trade Commission (FTC), only one was upheld by that same agency and other review organizations in 1980. The 8 charges were:

1. Sugar has a causal relation to tooth decay.

2. Consumption of sugar robs the body of other nutrients.

3. Overconsumption of sugar leads to obesity.

4. Sugar consumption is related to cardiovascular disease.

5. Sugar intake increases blood lipid levels.

6. Some people are carbohydrate-sensitive.

7. Sugar may contribute to high blood pressure.

8. Sugar intake may contribute to diabetes.[19]

One charge was upheld: "The *only* demonstrated hazard that sugars pose to the public health . . . remains their contribution to dental decay." It was also agreed that sugar is safe at current levels of usage.[20]

Additional readings on sugar — pro and con —

are recommended in this Highlight's To Explore Further. Many more questions are raised and, to a great extent, answered in those readings. But it may be more important to remember the issues being discussed here than to have all the answers on the individual questions about sugar. When misinformation is promoted in the name of nutrition, a wrong is done. The credibility of all those who make statements about nutrition becomes suspect in the public view. Nutrition is a science, and as such, it helps us to make judgments about what to do from our perception of what is. Our statements about what is must be valid statements if they are to guide people accurately in deciding what to do.

If sugar is a poison, then what to do is to avoid it like — well, like poison. This notion may contribute to the beliefs that are so destructive to the binger, or bulimic.

The bulimic thinks, "If I touch this forbidden food, it will overwhelm me. Like alcohol to the alcoholic, sugar will cause me to lose control." Then he touches it — and loses control. The substance appears to have a magical power. Not only

that, the bulimic is also starving, having accepted society's thin standard. The hunger felt in starvation is real and powerful. It is no coincidence that many binge episodes in bulimics are preceded by strict dieting and that many unsuccessful dieters (bingers) believe that dieting involves severely limiting food intake.[21]

Sugar should be given less status. It should be demoted from a powerful, evil substance to a harmless but unneeded substance, one for which there is only a little room in a kcalorie-restricted diet. If binge eaters could see it this way, they might then bend their efforts towards figuring out where and how to use their restricted sugar allowance most effectively to enhance their eating pleasure. They could learn to think positively — not "I must never eat those foods," but rather "I must eat *these* (nutritious) foods and I may add a little sweetness where it pleases me the most." A cookie eaten at the end of a nourishing meal has considerably less power to precipitate a binge than a cookie eaten after 24 hours without food.

Both the binge eater and the child, in fact, need to

[19] Bollenbach, 1981.

[20] The FDA, USDA, and FTC all agree on this. Bollenbach, 1981.

[21] G. R. Leon, L. Roth, and M. I. Hewitt, Eating patterns, satiety and self-control behavior in obese persons during weight reduction, *Journal of Obesity and Bariatric Medicine* 6 (1977):172-181.

learn the same things to facilitate their developing healthful eating habits. In the following conversation, the person giving truthful answers (TA) is being much more helpful than the person giving puritanical answers (PA):

Q: Is sugar bad for me?
PA: Yes, it's a poison. You must never touch it.
TA: No, but it doesn't offer you the nutrients you need, either. You must learn to eat nutritious foods and use sugar in small amounts to increase your eating pleasure.

Q: Why do I like sugar so much?
PA: Because you're a bad, bad person and you have an addictive personality. It shows you can't trust yourself.
TA: Because you are a normal human being. Everybody likes sugar. It's delicious.

Q: I can't trust myself to choose foods that are good for me, can I?
PA: No, you will only like the foods that are bad for you.
TA: Yes, once you have learned how to eat well and have formed healthful eating *habits*. You will like nutritious foods very much, and then you can trust your habits.

One trainer of children put it this way: "Be sure they eat the foods they need first. Children live for the present. *You* protect their future." But this strategy by itself does nothing to prepare children for the time when they themselves will make the choices. It needs two words added: "Be sure they *learn to* eat the foods they need first." Our task as nutrition educators is not to teach children (or adults) *not* to eat. Our task is to teach them *how* to eat.

Miniglossary

addiction: a compulsive physiological need for a habit-forming drug such as alcohol or heroin.

bulimia, bulimarexia: binge eating (see Chapter 16).

carboholic: a popular term denoting a person "addicted" to carbohydrate.

hyperphagia: overeating.

positive feedback: a control system that responds to a signal by amplifying the signal. With reference to binge eating, the eating itself seems to trigger a binge, rather than turning off the binge as would be the case with *negative feedback* (see Highlight 2).

sucroholic: a popular term denoting a person "addicted" to sugar (sucrose).

To Explore Further

In another book, we examined more closely the relationship between diet and hyperactivity in children:

- Whitney, E. N., and Hamilton, E. M. N. Controversy 13, Hyperactivity. In *Nutrition: Concepts and Controversies*, 2nd ed. St. Paul, Minn.: West, 1982, pp. 449-454.

An important theory of what starts binges is that any kind of arousal — negative or positive emotional states — can be responsible. We didn't delve into it here because we had already overfilled our space:

- Stricker, E. M. Hyperphagia. *New England Journal of Medicine* 298 (1978):1010-1013.

Allergies to foods can be real and can cause apparent mis-

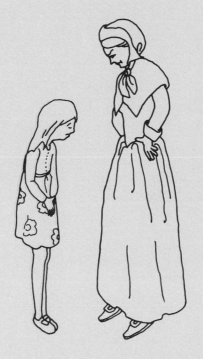

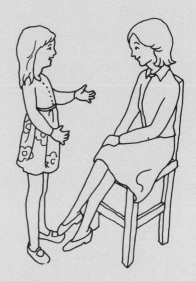

behavior. For the symptoms and an approach to diagnosis, see:

● May, C. D. Food allergy — material and ethereal. *New England Journal of Medicine* 302 (1980):1142-1143.

Chapter 23 also discusses food allergies.

The connections among malnutrition, learning, and behavior in children are clearly explained in a 33-page pamphlet from the National Institutes of Health:

● National Institute of Child Health and Human Development, Center for Research for Mothers and Children. *Malnutrition, Learning, and Behavior.* DHEW publication no. (NIH) 76-1036. Washington, D.C.: Government Printing Office, 1976.

A review of the recent research on malnutrition and behavior, including 173 references, is:

● Brocek, J. Malnutrition and behavior: A decade of conferences. *Journal of the American Dietetic Association* 72 (1978):17-23.

A colorful film that presents many viewpoints on sugar, although with a slight bias against it, makes an excellent basis for discussion: *The Sugar Film*, available from Image Associates, P.O. Box 40106, 352 Conejo Road, Santa Barbara, CA 93103. Telephone: (805) 962-6009.

CHAPTER 17

CONTENTS

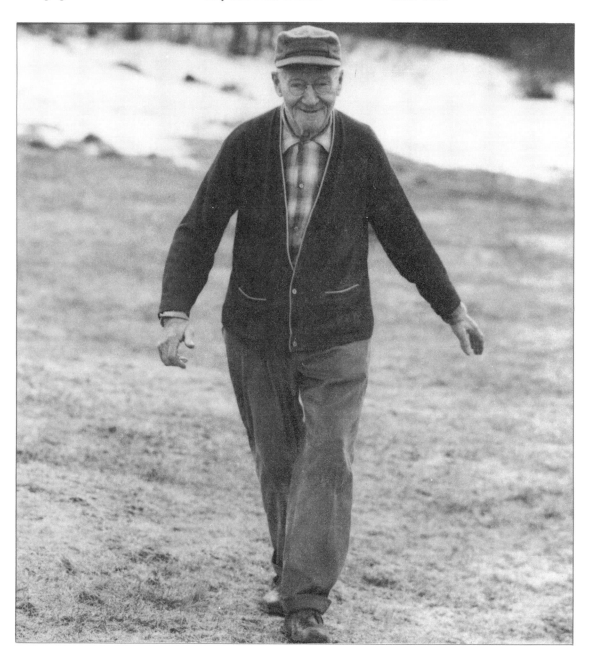

THE LATER YEARS

The increase in the number of aging is the most startling demographic characteristic of the 20th century. In 1900, one of every 25 persons was over 65. In 2030, it will be one of every 5.

UNKNOWN

One out of every nine citizens in the United States is above 65 years of age, and the percentage is increasing. This fact is evident everywhere. Retirement villages are springing up, especially in the warmer climates. Senior citizen centers are being established for congregate meals and leisure activities. Older adults can be heard on political matters at "silver-haired legislatures." The newspapers tell us the social security fund is nearing bankruptcy because many who were contributors are now retired and receiving from the fund. Civic and church organizations note that there is a preponderance of gray hair in their audiences. The data from recent census reports confirm these observations.

Older people cherish their independence. Contrary to the popular view, only 5 percent live in nursing homes.[1] Most live in the community, either alone or with nonrelatives, thus remaining independent. As we will see, this very independence fosters nutrition problems.

Of the 6 million elderly who live alone, 1.3 million are men and 4.7 million, women.[2] Most are in reasonably good health and have enough money to support themselves, if not in luxury, at least not in poverty. When we look around us and see the great needs of some people, we sometimes overlook those who are enjoying their later years. They have leisure to pursue some of their favorite activities and are unencumbered for the first time in their lives by family responsibilities. These facts contradict the popular belief that older people are all poor, lonely, and ill. They are not; they are as individual as all other age segments. Grouping them into a stereotype is a disservice to everyone, especially to young adults who might project into their futures a depressing view of old age. Just as only a few teenagers are reckless drivers, only a minority of older people have the "typical problems" attributed to them. Aunt Charlotte at 77 jets every winter to Europe to enjoy the social life of

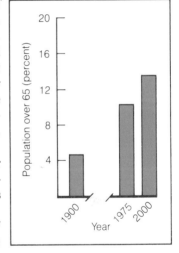

One out of every nine citizens in the United States is above 65. In 1900, 4% were over 65; 11% are over 65 today; 12.5% (30,500,000 people) will be over 65 in the year 2000.

[1] M. Chou, Selling to older Americans, *Cereal Foods World* 26 (1981): 633. Abstract, cited in *Journal of the American Dietetic Association* 80 (1982):277.

[2] U.S. Bureau of the Census, *Current Population Reports*, Series P-60, No. 101, "Money Income in 1975 of Families and Persons in the United States" (Washington, D.C.: Government Printing Office, 1976).

631

Paris; Uncle James at 84 is out early every morning in his vegetable garden hoeing his cabbages; and it is only Grandma Sadie who at 82 is lonely, withdrawn, ill, and forgetful, a problem to her family. Two-thirds of the elderly are relatively free of major problems.

However, the one-third who live at or below the poverty line deserve our attention. The average income of all older single people in the United States is $75 a week. Of aged black women, nearly half have a yearly income of under $1,000.[3] Clearly, these people need help in many areas, one of them being nutrition.

In exploring nutrition for the older adult, it will be necessary to remember statistics like these but also to recognize the wide range of individual situations represented in these statistics. It will be helpful to keep three questions in mind:

- What can I do now to prepare myself for the time when I will be an older adult?
- What can I do when I am older (or now that I am older) to keep myself healthy and vigorous so I will enjoy these years?
- How can I, as a relative or a health professional, help those who are in need?

Theories on Aging

The "increased life span" of people in the twentieth century is not a reality. Most people are not now living much beyond the limit of three-score years and ten mentioned in the Bible. In fact, in the last 25 years there has been no increase in life expectancy for people who are already 20 or older in spite of our miracle drugs and huge medical bills.[4] Since the beginning of the nineteenth century, as mortality from bacterial diseases has been brought under control by modern medicine, deaths from other causes have increased, so that the total life expectancy (for any individual) has remained at about 70 years. It is only the average length of life (for the population) that has increased. This has come about because more infants are surviving to adulthood, and so there are fewer infant deaths to bring the average down. Thus it seems that something built into the human organism (we call it aging) cuts off life at a rather fixed point in time.

Natural selection has not operated in favor of genes that promote longevity. However, the human race, with its superior brain, can collect and store information that helps keep individuals alive after they have reproduced. Longevity can be said to result from evolution only in the sense that the brain has evolved. In today's world, however, older people may contribute accumulated experience and wisdom to the

[3]U.S. Bureau of the Census, 1975.

[4]J. Mayer, Aging and nutrition, *Geriatrics* 29 (5) (1974):57-59.

benefit of society long after they have passed their reproductive years and the time when they would contribute genes.

We humans have not comprehended what is involved in the aging process, nor have we figured out how to prevent or postpone it. Even our definitions of the process are vague. One writer calls aging a certain kind of change in living systems due to the passage of time — the increased probability of death with increased chronological age.[5] Another calls it a decrease in viability and an increase in vulnerability.[6] However aging is defined, research into it has been scarce. Much is known about the growth, development, and nutrition needs of the human body from conception to maturity. But only in recent times has the scientific community become interested in the mechanism by which the human organism ceases to grow once it reaches maturity and then "runs down" and dies. Current interest is increasing, due in large part to the rising numbers of older people and the impact they are having on our social and governmental institutions, but answers are still few and far between.

Aging of Cells   Cells seem to undergo a built-in (genetic) aging process and also to age in response to outside (environmental) forces. Environmental stresses that promote aging include extremes of heat and cold, disease, lack of nutrients, the wear and tear of hard physical labor, and the lack of stimulation caused by disuse (for example, of the muscle cells in the legs of a cripple who can't exercise). But even in the most pleasant and supportive of environments, inevitable changes in the structure and function of the body's cells make them increasingly vulnerable to these environmental stresses.

All theories of aging have one element in common. They agree that at some point the cells become incapable of replenishing their constituents. In a complex organism such as the human body, the cells are interdependent. When some cells die and their function is lost, other cells dependent on the first ones suffer and also eventually die. A consequence of the gradual slowing down of cell function over the years is a reduction in the energy needs of older people.

A second common element seems to be that aging cells are programmed to stop reproducing once a certain stage of development has been reached.[7] Cells have different timetables for reproduction, but each type of cell seems to come to a natural end somehow. For example, red blood cells undergo division only as long as they are in the marrow of the long bones. When they are mature, they move out of the marrow to perform their function in the bloodstream. In the blood, they no longer reproduce; they work for three to six months and then die.

The brain cells are also programmed to stop reproducing, but they all stop within the first two years of life. Thus, at about 14 months of

[5]B. L. Strehler, *Time, Cells, and Aging,* 2nd ed. (New York: Academic Press, 1977).

[6]A. Comfort, *A Good Age* (New York: Crown, 1976).

[7]Strehler, 1977.

age, the human organism already has all the brain cells it will ever have. Many of them maintain themselves without further cell division, for about 70 years. Thousands die daily, but the daily loss is not noticeable. The accumulated loss over a lifetime is felt only in the slowing of reflexes and in garbled messages' going to other organs. It seems strange that the human species should have evolved such a magnificent instrument for receiving, storing, interpreting, and retrieving information and yet not have evolved a method of repairing it. Some scientists view this evolutionary mishap as a "self-destruct" mechanism for the human body.

Some cells seem never to die but only to reproduce. They take in nutrients from their environment and grow; profound changes take place in their internal structure; and the living material within them then divides itself equally between two poles while the cell splits down the middle. Each new daughter cell is an exact replica of the parent cell and contains the same material. Thus the parent cell still lives, in a sense, as two replicas of itself. However, even in optimal conditions, the cells of a multicellular organism seem unable to go on dividing in this manner forever. About 50 to 55 replications seems to be the maximum.

A third factor in the aging process seems to be that, with the passage of time, cells become cluttered with debris — partially completed proteins that are never totally dismantled. This intracellular "sludge" interferes with the efficiency of operations within the cells.[8] The material that accumulates in the cells is known as the pigment of old age.

The aging pigment is **lipofuscin** (lip-oh-FEW-sin).

Another factor may be that cells lose their ability to interpret the DNA genetic code words and so make their proteins incorrectly. As reduced amounts of protein or wrong proteins are produced, cell and organ functions that depend on those proteins also falter. Organs elsewhere in the body may also be adversely affected. A theory somewhat allied to this one is that through some environmental stress, such as the continuous bombardment of cosmic rays that penetrate the earth's atmosphere, the DNA code itself may become altered. This, too, would lead to the production of wrong proteins.

If wrong proteins are produced for any reason, another theory states, the body's immune system will react to them as if they were foreign proteins from outside and will produce antibodies to counteract them. Complexes then form between the antibodies and these proteins and accumulate in and among cells as useless debris. The autoimmune theory may account in part for the accumulation of deposits in joints, which causes arthritis.[9]

Finally, another theory of aging suggests that cosmic rays bombard molecules in the cells and split them into highly reactive compounds known as free radicals. These free radicals then bind rigidly to other

[8]M. Puner, *To the Good Long Life* (New York: Universe Books, 1974).

[9]Strehler, 1977.

cellular molecules by way of disulfide bridges. This disrupts the informational content of important molecules and so impairs their function. As in other cases, the cells in which this occurs, as well as others that depend on them, then die. (Some investigators have suggested that the formation of free radicals might be retarded by the taking of vitamin E supplements.)

Just as a chain is only as strong as its weakest link, so also is an organism only as long-lived as the least stable of its vital cells. The ability of cells to replenish the substances they need for life or to make fresh copies of themselves after they have reached maturity determines their life spans and ultimately the life span of the entire organism.

An analogy may help to show how all these processes work together to cause aging. A shipbuilding firm must have an office, where the plans and specifications for all the various boats are kept, and a warehouse, where the materials to carry out these orders are stored. There must also be a site where the actual construction takes place. When an order is received for a particular boat to be constructed, the plans on file are duplicated for a working copy, and messengers are sent to bring the materials to the construction site. Following the instructions, workers then build the boat.

If, through years of heavy use, the warehouse becomes cluttered and disorganized, then it will become increasingly difficult to fill the orders efficiently. (This parallels the theory that, with age, the cell fluid becomes cluttered with debris.) If some of the messengers take the wrong orders from the files or bring the wrong materials, this too will cause production to slow down or cease. (This parallels the cells' loss of ability to read the genetic code words.) With rain or fire damage to the files themselves, some of the specifications will become unavailable or illegible (like the cellular DNA's becoming altered by cosmic ray bombardment). Should one worker be instructed to burn the trash, he might lazily leave behind marred instructions or parts (as in the autoimmune theory). Vandalism (free radicals) might do further damage. With inefficient management of the warehouse, there might be delays in getting supplies. (For the cell, the nutrients might not be present in the blood because they were not taken in, or there might be a breakdown in the ability of the intestinal cells to absorb the nutrients.) Finally, the warehouse might have been set up for a limited order — its destruction, once it had produced a certain number of boats, might have been planned from the beginning. (This represents the idea that cells are programmed to self-destruct after a certain number of generations.)

None of the theories of cellular aging are more than theories, but some interesting work has been done in the attempt to solve the riddle of why cells age. One such experiment was conducted as early as the 1930s. Rats were fed a diet balanced in every respect except that it was severely restricted in kcalories. A control group was fed the same diet with ample kcalories. When the control group had reached maturity, the starved rats were still immature. They were then permitted to catch

For a picture of the disulfide bridges in insulin, a protein molecule, see p. 98.

There's more about vitamin E in Highlight 11.

up, by being fed ample kcalories. Surprisingly, the previously starved rats outlived the controls, averaging 1,465 days as compared with the controls' 969 days.[10] Similar experiments have since yielded similar results with many different species, and a tentative conclusion is that the key to success is keeping the animals in a juvenile state for longer than the normal period.

Obviously, such an experiment could not be carried out on human beings, but it suggested some interesting possibilities that were followed up in animals. It seems that their lives can be prolonged merely by reducing the protein content of the diet, and that some increased longevity will result even if the restriction doesn't begin until the animals are "middle-aged." Restriction of kcalories, protein, or fat also improves animals' resistance to age-related diseases such as cancer. Importantly, the diets that achieved these effects were not deficient in any nutrients; they represented "undernutrition, not malnutrition." It is impossible to know exactly what these findings mean for human beings, but it can be said that they lend added weight to the idea that being overnourished doesn't promote long life.[11]

Aging of Organs   The aging of cells is reflected by changes in the organs they are a part of. The most visible changes take place in the skin. As people age, wrinkles increase, partly because of a loss of the fat that underlies the skin and partly because of a loss of elasticity. The scars that have accumulated from many small cuts roughen the texture of the skin. Exposure to sun, wind, and cold hasten the drying process and contribute to wrinkling. The hair disappears also, particularly from the head and face of males.

Another obvious and traumatic change, in the digestive system, is painful deterioration of the gums and subsequent loss of teeth. According to the Ten State Survey, gum disease increases with age and exists in 90 percent of the population by age 65 to 74.[12] In addition, the senses of taste and smell diminish, which reduces the pleasure of eating.

In other parts of the digestive system, secretion by the stomach of hydrochloric acid and enzymes decreases with age, as does the secretion of digestive juices by the pancreas and small intestine. The GI tract muscles weaken with reduced use, so that pressure in the large intestine causes the outpocketings of diverticulosis.

The liver is somewhat different. Liver cells regenerate themselves throughout life, so with normal aging, the loss of liver cells is not a major problem. However, even with good nutrition, fat gradually

[10]Puner, 1974.

[11]J. E. Brody, Eating less may be the key to living beyond 100 years, *New York Times*, 8 June 1982.

[12]*Ten-State Nutrition Survey*, 1968-1970, DHEW publication no. (HSM) 72-8130-8133 (Atlanta, Ga.: Center for Disease Control, 1972).

infiltrates the liver, reducing its work output.[13] The response of the liver to moderate blood glucose levels is not appreciably altered with age, but the response to a large glucose load, as in the glucose tolerance test, is reduced. There may be two reasons for this: First, the blood may not be pushed strongly enough by the heart to reach the pancreas, so that it does not send its insulin message to the liver; second, there may be a reduction in the number of glucose-responsive cells in the pancreas.[14]

Glucose tolerance test: see Chapter 1.

As the heart and blood vessels age, the volume of blood that the heart can pump decreases. The arteries lose their elasticity. The amount of blood going into the networks of capillaries in the various organs decreases. Fat deposits form in the walls of the arteries, and calcium salts invade these deposits, making them hard and inflexible. Because all organs and tissues depend on the circulation of nutrients and oxygen, degenerative changes in this system critically affect all other systems.

The decrease in blood flow through the kidneys makes them gradually less efficient at their task of removing nitrogen and other wastes from the blood and maintaining the correct amounts of salts, sugar, and other valuable nutrients in the body fluids. As the heart pumps less blood into the capillary trees of the kidneys, the capillary trees diminish in size, causing some kidney cells to be deprived of their nutrient and oxygen supply. Cells formerly fed by these capillaries then die. Since both the heart rate and the volume of blood pumped into the kidneys depend on the muscular activity of the person, this degenerative process can be retarded by regular exercising.

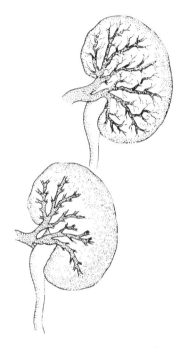

As the heart pumps less blood into an organ, the capillary trees within that organ recede, leaving some of the cells without nourishment. Exercise promotes maintenance and even growth of capillaries.

The ability of the brain to direct the activities of the body decreases during aging. However, the older adult compensates for this with a greater amount of stored information and wisdom. The nerve cells are not replaceable, so any damage by accident permanently diminishes mental ability. This is probably the greatest cause of unhappiness among older people and their relatives, because it decreases the ability to enjoy life. Visual impairment, hearing loss, loss of the senses of smell and taste, and loss of the sense of balance are all evidence of impaired nerve cell function.

Aging of the Skeleton   Like the body's other organ systems, the skeletal system is subject to change with the passage of time. Bone is a structure composed of salts of calcium, phosphorus, and other minerals. Bone-building and bone- dismantling cells are constantly working on this structure, remodeling it to adjust to the body's changing needs.

After 40, bone loss becomes more rapid than bone-building. Bone loss occurs in both sexes, although it is four times more prevalent in women than in men after 50, and no one knows for sure what the

For more about bones and osteoporosis, see Chapters 10 and 12.

[13] Mayer, 1974.

[14] Strehler, 1977.

causes are. The result, however, is osteoporosis — thinning and weakening of the bones so severe as to produce fractures in as many as one out of every three people over 65.[15] A hip fracture caused by osteoporosis may not be a clean break but a shattering of the bone into fragments that can't be readily reassembled. Repair can then only be accomplished by replacing the bone or joint with an artificial substitute.

Among the factors suspected of causing or contributing to osteoporosis are:

1. A too-low calcium intake.

2. Hormonal changes.

3. Reduced physical activity.

The person who wants to prevent or retard the process of bone loss should be aware of all these factors.

A too-low calcium intake is, of course, any intake that does not completely compensate for total calcium losses. But how much calcium is enough to ensure balance? Special populations have been known to maintain balance on as little as 200 mg calcium a day (the adult RDA is 800 mg), but for most men, the minimum intake appears to be above 400 mg, and for women after the menopause it is about 1,000 mg or even more.[16] In the light of several research findings confirming the high calcium need of older women, several authorities were by 1980 recommending a daily intake of 1 to 1 1/2 g calcium, the amount available from 5 c milk a day.[17]

The second factor named above is hormonal changes. The reduction of estrogen secretion in women after menopause is known to accelerate bone loss. Estrogen replacement therapy may help prevent bone loss but cannot strengthen bones already weakened. Other hormones are implicated in bone loss, and knowledge now being gathered may lead some day to effective therapy, but for the present the facts all point one way: It is better to prevent than to attempt to restore bone loss.[18]

The third factor, physical exercise, deserves strong emphasis. Bones lose material at a dramatic rate when they are inactive or immobilized. One prominent investigator considers it urgent to "educate middle-aged people to manage their lives to prevent . . . thinning of bone tissue" — meaning, primarily, to maintain regular physical activity.[19]

---

[15]L. Lutwak, Symposium on osteoporosis: Nutritional aspects of osteoporosis, *Journal of the American Geriatrics Society* 17 (1969):115-119.

[16]J. C. Gallagher and B. L. Riggs, Nutrition and bone disease, *New England Journal of Medicine* 298 (1978):193-195.

[17]Gallagher and Riggs, 1978; G. D. Whedon, Osteoporosis (editorial), *New England Journal of Medicine* 305 (1981):397-399; R. P. Heaney, Premenopausal prophylactic calcium supplementation: Questions and answers, *Journal of the American Medical Association* 245 (1981):1362.

[18]J. L. Marx, Osteoporosis: New help for thinning bones, Science 207 (1980):628-630.

[19]Marx, 1980.

Evidence is accumulating that bone loss can indeed be prevented by physical exercise.[20]

Another factor thought to increase the risk of bone loss is "thinness," and still another is "dieting."[21] There is also a concern that the person who drinks soft drinks rather than milk may be harming herself in two ways — first, by ingesting too little calcium, and second, by incurring greater calcium loss due to the high phosphorus content of soft drinks.[22] These factors blend readily into a picture of the figure-conscious older woman who has been "on a diet" for much of her lifetime and who drinks diet sodas rather than milk. This woman is a prime candidate for osteoporosis.

Perhaps the factors that promote or prevent the development of osteoporosis can be traced back to the growing years at the beginning of life. The higher the density of the bones at maturity, the later will be the development of osteoporosis. Heredity also plays some part. Men have denser bones than women, and Mediterranean, Latin American, and African populations have denser bones than Northern European and Asian peoples. Lifelong adequate intakes of both calcium and fluoride doubtless protect against osteoporosis; the condition is not usually seen in a person who has had a consistently high calcium intake.[23] In fact, people with osteoporosis give a lifelong history of exceptionally low calcium intakes.[24]

No one of middle age or over can, however, revisit her childhood, obtain the calcium and other nutrients she needs to build bone, and exercise them into place. Because "you can't learn younger," it is important for the person embarking on the later years to plan positively to obtain the needed nutrients and schedule physical workouts as part of a regular routine.

Arthritis, a painful swelling of the joints, is another problem that troubles many people as they grow older. During movement, the bones must rub against each other at the joints. The ends are protected from wear by cartilage and by small sacs of fluid that act as a lubricant. With age, the ends of the bone become pitted or eroded as a result of wear. The cause of arthritis is unknown, but it affects millions around the world and is a major problem of the elderly.

---

[20]J. F. Aloia, EXERCISE AND SKELETAL HEALTH, *Journal of the American Geriatrics Society* 29 (1981):104-107.

[21]B. A. Mosher, Letter, *American Journal of Public Health*, March 1981, as cited in *ACSH Media and Activity Update*, Spring 1981, p. 7; C. J. Lee, G. S. Lawler, and G. H. Johnson, Effects of supplementation of the diets with calcium and calcium-rich foods on bone density of elderly females with osteoporosis, *American Journal of Clinical Nutrition* 34 (1981):819-823.

[22]K. E. Wical and P. Brussee, Effects of a calcium and vitamin D supplement on alveolar ridge resorption in immediate denture patients, *Journal of Prosthetic Dentistry* 41 (1979):4-11.

[23]A. F. Morgan, Nutrition of the aging, *Gerontologist* 2 (1962):77-84.

[24]Lutwak, 1969.

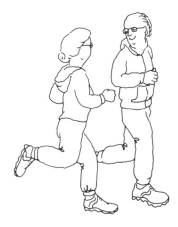

The aging of every body system is accelerated by a reduced flow of nutrients and oxygen to the system. To put this statement more positively, the process of aging can be retarded by maintaining a strong cardiovascular and respiratory system. Exercise, regular and active enough to increase the heartbeat and respiration rate, is one of the keys to good health in the later years. An added benefit of exercise, as you already know, is to prevent the atrophy of all muscles (not only the heart), which would take place with inactivity. A good flow of blood requires a strong heartbeat and strongly flexing muscles to press expelled lymph back into the bloodstream for recirculation. Many older persons believe that they can't participate in strenuous exercise, but studies have shown that they can do more than they think they can. Even modest endurance training can improve cardiovascular and respiratory function and promote good muscle tone while controlling the accumulation of body fat.[25] The older person who has never worked out hard before may be encouraged to learn that the trainability of older people does not depend on their physical prowess in their youth. Also, their increase in muscle strength during training is not due to the improvement in their muscles but to the improvement in the nervous system which results from the increased blood flow to the brain engendered by the exercise.[26]

Nutrition Implications of Aging

Good health habits, including good nutrition throughout life, are the best guarantee of healthy and enjoyable later years. Many of the nutrient needs of the elderly are the same as for younger persons, but some special considerations deserve emphasis.

kCalories   Energy needs decrease with advancing age. For one thing, the number of active cells in each organ decreases, bringing about a reduction in the body's overall metabolic rate. For another, older people are less active physically (although they need not be). In 1980, for the first time, the RDA tables presented recommended energy intakes for the older set; these recommendations reflect an estimated reduction of about 5 percent per decade in energy output. The variation is great, so the ranges are wide (see Appendix I), but average figures for people 75 and older are 2,050 kcal/day for the man and 1,600 for the woman. The margin table shows food patterns that would supply amounts of kcalories a little lower than the RDA tables show. Because overweight is

[25]K. H. Sidney, R. J. Shephard, and J. E. Harrison, Endurance training and body composition of the elderly, *American Journal of Clinical Nutrition* 30 (1977):326-333.

[26]H. A. DeVries, Physiological effects of an exercise training regimen upon men aged 52 to 88, *Journal of Gerontology* 25 (1970):325-336.

well recognized as a shortener of the life span, these seem to be life-sustaining recommendations.

Protein-kcalorie malnutrition is common in older people and often goes unnoticed. An observer, seeing the wasted muscle, weakness, and sometimes swelling of protein deficiency, may think, "That person looks old," when in fact he should recognize the symptoms of PCM. Older people who have been trying to lose weight or eating monotonous or bizarre diets are most likely to be affected.[27]

Protein foods should contribute about 20 to 25 percent of the kcalories in the older person's diet, fats no more than 20 percent, with the remainder coming from complex carbohydrates.[28] On such a limited kcalorie allowance, all foods must be nutrient dense. There is little leeway for such empty-kcalorie foods as sugar, sweets, fats, oils, or alcohol.

One side of the energy budget is for kcalories to be taken in, and the other side is for the expenditure of those kcalories. Increase in activity, as already mentioned, should be emphasized for any person interested in maintaining good health in the later years. People responsible for the care of older adults should encourage more activity of all kinds and shorter recuperation periods in bed following illnesses.

Protein   The need for essential amino acids is the same for older adults as it is for younger adults. However, the older person needs to get these essential nutrients from less food, so care should be taken that the protein is of high quality. The protein should also be protected from being used for energy by the inclusion of complex carbohydrates in the diet.

It has been shown that, for older persons living at home, milk or its equivalent in cheese is one of the foods most often omitted from the diet.[29] Another protein food, meat, is often omitted because it is difficult to chew; in one study, only those with excellent teeth had a high protein intake.[30] Both milk and meat may also be omitted because of difficulties with purchasing and storage. Low hemoglobin levels have been shown to correlate with protein (as well as iron) content of the diet,[31] and may be the cause of the fatigue and apathy so often mentioned as a problem by older persons. It has been recommended

Table 1   Eating Pattern Supplying the Recommended Proportions of Protein, Fat, and Carbohydrate for Older People

Food group	Number of exchanges	
	Woman (1,500 kcal)	Man (2,000 kcal)
Milk (skim)	3	3
Vegetable	2	3
Fruit	3	4
Bread	10	10
Meat (lean)	4	7
Fat	4	4

[27]S. R. Gambert and A. R. Guansing, Protein-calorie malnutrition in the elderly, *Journal of the American Geriatrics Society* 28 (1980):272-275.

[28]D. B. Rao, Problems of nutrition in the aged, *Journal of the American Geriatrics Society* 21(1973):362-367.

[29]J. S. Lyons and M. F. Trulson, Food practices of older people living at home, *Journal of Gerontology* 11 (1956):66-72.

[30]P. Swanson, Adequacy in old age, part II: Nutrition programs for the aging, *Journal of Home Economics* 56 (1964):728-734; C. S. Davidson, J. Livermore, P. Anderson, and S. Kaufman, The nutrition of a group of apparently healthy aging persons, *American Journal of Clinical Nutrition* 10 (1962):181-199.

[31]Morgan, 1962.

that the protein allowance for those over 65 be increased to 2 grams per kilogram ideal weight.[32]

Fat   For many reasons, fat should be limited in the older person's diet. Cutting fat helps cut kcalories (recall that fat delivers two and a half times as many kcalories as the other energy nutrients) and may also help retard the development of atherosclerosis. On the limited kcalorie allowance recommended for older adults, it would be difficult to obtain the many vitamins and minerals that come from protein-rich and complex carbohydrate foods if too high a percentage of the kcalories came from fat. Moreover, high fat intake interferes with calcium absorption, promoting osteoporosis.

On the other hand, if fat kcalories are restricted too greatly, the fat-soluble vitamins and linoleic acid may be deficient. Of the 20 percent of the kcalories to come from fat, about half should perhaps be from polyunsaturated fat to contribute linoleic acid, the essential fatty acid, and to displace the saturated fat thought to contribute to high levels of cholesterol in the blood.

Carbohydrate   Another emphasis in the older person's diet should be on securing a wide variety of complex carbohydrate foods to provide the vitamins and minerals contained in these foods. Older people often omit fruits and vegetables from their diets. It is not known whether this is due to earlier consumption patterns or to their finding fruits and vegetables too expensive or too difficult to store and prepare. Any educational campaign conducted to improve the diets of the elderly should emphasize the great amount of essential nutrients, minerals, and fiber contributed by complex carbohydrates. Programs such as congregate meals serving food to older people can furnish bags so that the participants can take home the fruit that was served for dessert, as a way of encouraging the use of fruit.

Vitamins   Many of the problems seen in the elderly may result from decreased vitamin intakes. Vitamin deficiency is likely unless great care is taken to include foods from each of the food groups. Studies have shown that the one food group omitted most often by the elderly is the vegetable group, which would contribute vitamin A.[33] About 18 percent of older people are reported to eat no vegetables at all. Fruit, a contributor of vitamin C, is lacking in many diets, and 34 percent in one study reported never eating fruit.[34] Some men and women do not eat whole-grain breads and cereals, which contribute the B vitamins; the mental confusion sometimes exhibited by the elderly may be caused not

Table 2   Vitamin C Intake of People 60 Years and Older (Ten-State Survey)

Category	Vitamin C intake (mg)
White males	30
White females	46
Black males	37
Black females	52
Spanish-American males	28
Spanish-American females	47

U.S. RDA for vitamin C: 60 mg

[32] Rao, 1973.

[33] Lyons and Trulson, 1956.

[34] J. Pelcovits, Nutrition to meet the human needs of older Americans, *Journal of the American Dietetic Association* 60 (1972):297-300.

by a loss of brain function but by a B-vitamin deficiency.[35] The destruction of vitamin E by heat processing and oxidation is well known, and the processed and convenience foods so often used by the elderly and by nursing homes are thought to contribute to a vitamin E deficiency if their use continues over several years.[36] These statistics have somber implications for the health of older persons.

Not only the omission of certain food groups but also other conditions contribute to vitamin deficiency in the elderly. Many are house- or hospital-bound and thus are deprived of the vitamin D they would get from sunshine on their skin. Many take laxatives regularly, and this causes such a rapid transit time through the intestine that many vitamins do not get absorbed. The use of mineral oil as a laxative especially robs the person of the fat-soluble vitamins. Some drugs regularly taken by older adults interact with vitamins. For example, some antibiotics kill bacteria in the intestine that produce vitamin K; and the anticonvulsant drugs used in the treatment of epilepsy produce a folacin deficiency.[37]

The recommended intakes for many of the vitamins are thought by some nutritionists to be too low for the over-65 group. They C, because toxicity from large amounts does not pose a great threat. However, other nutritionists feel that recommending vitamin supplements is a "cop-out" laying the elderly open to exploitation by quacks.[38] Money is better spent, they say, on food of higher quality. The older person would probably be wise to follow the rule of thumb that if the kcalorie intake is below about the 1,500 level, then a vitamin-mineral supplement is recommended — not a megavitamin, but just a once-daily type supplement. This means that many older persons, all except those who are so active that their kcalorie allowance has remained high, should take this precaution.

Chapter 21 provides more examples of the effects of drugs on nutrition status.

Minerals   Iron-deficiency anemia is common in older adults. Low blood hemoglobin can result from a diet low in protein, as already mentioned; but diets low in iron are also common. Heavy reliance on a "tea and toast" diet is cited as a double risk in this connection; what little iron the toast provides is poorly absorbable, while the tannins in tea inhibit iron absorption. But any diet that lacks color (and therefore lacks iron containing red meats and fruits and vegetables rich in vitamin C to aid in iron absorption) suggests risk of iron deficiency.

Aside from diet, other factors in many older people's lives increase the likelihood of iron deficiency:

[35]Mayer, 1974.

[36]H. H. Koehler, H. C. Lee, and M. Jacobson, Tocopherols in canned entrees and vended sandwiches, *Journal of the American Dietetic Association* 70 (1977):616-620.

[37]M. Balsley, M. F. Brink, and E. W. Speckman, Nutrition in disease and stress, *Geriatrics* 26 (1971):87-93.

[38]Mayer, 1974.

- chronic blood loss from ulcers, hemorrhoids, or other disease conditions.
- poor iron absorption due to reduced stomach acid secretion.
- antacid use, interfering with iron absorption.
- use of other medicines that cause blood loss, including arthritis medicines, anticoagulants, and aspirin.

The person counseling an older client on health and nutrition should not forget to ask about these possibilities.

Another mineral often lacking in older people's diets is calcium, the need for which increases with advancing age. Bone loss occurs insidiously, and may be alarmingly extensive and severe before a person realizes there is any problem at all. The recommendation that an older adult ingest the equivalent of 5 cups of milk a day is difficult to meet, especially for the person who is unaccustomed to using much milk at all. However, there are many alternative strategies for obtaining the needed calcium. If fresh milk causes flatulence (gas), as some older people report, then cheese should be included. Dry skim milk can be incorporated into many foods. Soup stock made from bones can be used daily. These and other strategies are offered in the next section ("Practical Pointers").

Salt, which contains the mineral sodium, should be curtailed in the older person's diet, not only by those with hypertension, congestive heart failure, or cirrhosis of the liver, but by all older people. Salt is conducive to the retention of fluid, which results in raised blood pressure. Convenience and processed foods are high in salt content and are widely used by older persons living alone, thus making it difficult for them to restrict their salt intake. Wherever possible, fresh foods should be eaten instead.

To obtain the needed minerals, the older person should follow the same recommendation as for vitamins. Every food group should be represented in the diet every day.

Fiber is discussed in more detail in Chapter 1.

Fiber The fiber recommendations for the general population should be stressed to older citizens as well: Increase the use of fruits, vegetables, and whole-grain cereals. The fiber content of these food groups is important to the health of the muscles of the intestinal tract. If there is bulk for these muscles to work against, it will be less necessary to resort to the use of laxatives. In addition, some fibers (except wheat bran) bind cholesterol and carry it out of the body.

Water The elderly need to be reminded to drink fluids because they are likely to be somewhat insensitive to their own thirst signals. They should drink six to eight glasses a day, enough to bring their urine output to about 1,500 ml (6 cups) per day. A large percentage of foster home operators note that one of the biggest problems with their elderly clients is getting them to use more water and fruit juices.[39]

Those older adults most at risk nutritionally are those who overemphasize one food group to the exclusion of another. Whenever one food group is excluded, the vitamins and minerals donated by that group become deficient in the diet. Even small amounts of food from each food group may protect from an overt deficiency. An example of such a skewed diet is that of a person who, for whatever reason, omits milk and dairy products. Calcium deficiencies would be expected and osteoporosis would be likely to develop if the omission had been continuing for most of the adult years. In the same manner, someone who excludes meat and cereals might be expected to develop an iron or zinc deficiency. The familiar maxim holds true throughout the life cycle: The best dietary guideline is to eat a balanced and varied selection of foods.

Practical Pointers

All of the above objectives may seem worthwhile, but they may be hard to achieve, especially for the person living alone who has difficulty buying groceries and preparing meals. Packages of meat and vegetables are often prewrapped in quantities suitable for a family of four or more, and even a head of lettuce will perish before one person can use it all. A large package of meat is often a good buy, but defrosting it enough to get a portion from it for dinner is time-consuming; furthermore, the rest tends to thaw, too. Small packages get "lost" in the freezer and ruined by freezer burn. For the person who has little or no freezer space, the problem of storage is further compounded. Following is a collection of ideas gathered from single people who are doing a good job of solving these problems and getting nourishing food:

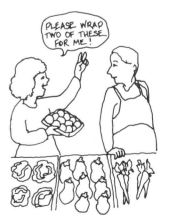

- Buy only three pieces of each kind of fresh fruit: a ripe one, a medium one, and a green one. Eat the first right away and the second soon, and let the last one ripen on your windowsill.

- Buy the small cans of vegetables even though they are more expensive. Remember, it is also expensive to buy a regular-size can and let the unused portion spoil in the refrigerator.

- Buy only what you will use. Don't be timid about asking the grocer to break open a package of wrapped meat or fresh vegetables.

- Think up a variety of ways to use a vegetable when you must buy it in a quantity larger than you can use. For example, you can divide a

[39]B. R. Bradshaw, W. P. Vonderhaar, V. T. Keeney, L. S. Tyler, and S. Harris, Community-based residential care for the minimally impaired elderly: A survival analysis, *Journal of the American Geriatrics Society* 24 (1976):423-429.

head of cauliflower into thirds. Cook one third and eat it as a hot vegetable. Put the other two thirds into a vinegar and oil marinade for use as an appetizer or in a salad. You can keep half a package of frozen vegetables with other vegetables to be used in soup or stew.

● Make mixtures, using what you have on hand. A thick stew prepared from leftover green beans, carrots, cauliflower, broccoli, and any meat, with some added onion, pepper, celery, and potatoes, makes a complete and balanced meal — except for milk. But see the uses of powdered milk that follow: You could add some to your stew.

● Buy fresh milk in the size best suited for you. If your grocer doesn't carry pints or half-pints, try a nearby service station or convenience store.

● Buy a half dozen eggs at a time. The carton of a dozen can usually be broken in half. However, eggs keep for long periods in the refrigerator and are such a good source of high-quality protein that you will probably use a dozen before they lose their freshness.

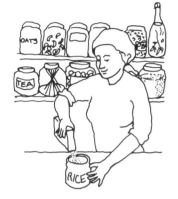

● Set aside a place in your kitchen for rows of glass jars containing shelf staple items that you can't buy in single-serving quantities. These could contain rice, tapioca, lentils or other dry beans, flour, cornmeal, dry skim milk, macaroni, cereal, or coconut, to name only a few possibilities. This will keep the bugs out of the foods indefinitely. They make an attractive display and will remind you of possibilities for variety in your menus. Cut the directions-for-use label from the package and store it in the jar.

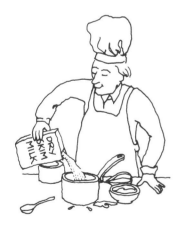

● Learn to use dry skim milk. It is the greatest convenience food there is. Not only does it offer much more calcium than any other food, it also is fortified with vitamins A and D. Dry milk can be stored on the shelf for several months at room temperature. It can be mixed with water to make fluid milk in as small a quantity as you like — but once it is mixed, it will sour just like fresh milk. One person says he keeps a jar of dry skim milk next to his stove and "dumps it into everything": hamburgers, gravies, soups, casseroles, sauces, even beverages such as iced coffee. The taste is negligible, but five "dumpings" of a heaping tablespoon each would be the equivalent of a cup of fresh milk. Ask a friend who is a member of Weight Watchers to give you some recipes for delicious milkshakes and ice cream using dry skim milk. Their recipes are for single servings.

● Make soup stock from leftover pork and chicken bones soaked in vinegar. The bones release their calcium into the acid medium, and the vinegar boils off when the stock is boiled. One *tablespoon* of such stock may contain over 100 mg of calcium.[40] Then cook something in this stock every day: vegetables, rice, stew — and of course, make soups with it.

[40] A Rosanoff and D. H. Calloway, Calcium source in Indochinese immigrants (correspondence), *New England Journal of Medicine* 306 (1982):239-240.

- Cook for several meals at a time. For example, boil three potatoes with skins. Eat one hot with margarine and chives. When the others have cooled, use one to make a potato-cheese casserole ready to be put into the oven for the next evening's meal. Slice the third one into a covered bowl and pour over it the juice from pickles. The pickled potato will keep several days in the refrigerator and can be used in a salad.

- Experiment with stir-fried foods. Use a frying pan if you don't have a wok. Ask your Chinese friends for some recipes. A variety of vegetables and meat can be enjoyed this way; inexpensive vegetables such as cabbage and celery are delicious when crisp-cooked in a little oil with soy or lemon added. Cooked, leftover vegetables can be dropped in at the last minute. There are frozen mixtures of Chinese or Polynesian vegetables available in the larger grocery stores. Bonus: Only one pan to wash.

- Depending on your freezer space, make double or even six times as much as you need of a dish that takes time to prepare: a casserole, vegetable pie, or meatloaf. Save the little aluminum trays from frozen foods and store the extra servings, labeled, in the trays in the freezer. Be sure to date these so you will use the oldest first. Somehow, the work seems worthwhile when you prepare several meals at once.

- Learn to connect food with socializing. Cook for yourself with the idea that you are also preparing for guests you might want to invite. Or turn this suggestion around: Invite guests and make enough food so that you will have some left for yourself at a later meal. These suggestions came from a young widow and an 86-year-old widow. The young widow, after her husband's death, purposely cooked generous amounts so she could make her own frozen dinners from the leftovers. With a wide variety of these on hand, she feels free to invite one or another of her single friends on the spur of the moment to "Come over and share my frozen dinners with me tonight." She says she devised this method of managing her food out of the need to manage her "five o'clock loneliness." The 86-year-old widow invites guests for dinner every Sunday, because "it is no fun to cook for one," and she, too, loves having the leftovers.

- Buy a loaf of bread and immediately store half, well wrapped, in the freezer. The freezer keeps it fresher than the refrigerator.

- If you have space in your freezing compartment, buy frozen vegetables in the very large bags rather than in the small cartons. You can take out the exact amount you need and close the bag tightly with a rubber band. If you return the package quickly to the freezer each time, the vegetables will stay fresh for a long time.

- If you have ample freezing space, you can buy large packages of meat such as pork chops, ground meat, or chicken when they are on special sale. Immediately divide the package into individual servings. Wrap in aluminum foil, not freezer paper: The foil can become the liner for the pan in which you bake or broil the meat, thus saving work over the sink. Don't label these individually, but put them all in a brown bag marked "hamburger" or "chicken thighs" or whatever the meat is, along with the date. The bag is easy to locate in the freezer, and you'll know when your supply is running low.

Although these suggestions will help you with the mechanics of food preparation and storage, they are only a part of what you can do for yourself. Loneliness, too, needs to be dealt with if single life in the later years is to be enjoyed. Even for nutrition's sake, it is important to attend to this problem.

Mealtimes Alone

The concept of old age as being a time of losses is a depressing one, certainly unpleasant to consider. But it is realistic and needs to be faced. Many people who arrive at this time of life don't comprehend the universality of the aging experience. They have made no mental preparations for it. Then, when faced with some of the normal experiences of later life — the children's wanting to be independent from the parents, for example — they turn inward for the explanation and conclude that there must be something wrong with them. Depression follows such reasoning and compounds the distress of the original problem.

Losses can occur in several areas. Old friends are lost whey they die or move away; offspring move away also and are too busy to write; there is loss of income on retirement and loss of status in the community. There is loss of control of the environment, such as finding that the home that was to be a haven in retirement now sits in the middle of a high-crime area so that one can no longer walk the streets or visit with neighbors. Familiar shops and fruit stands, where a person knows the owner and is known by them, may close. The aging person develops a feeling of deep loneliness as the familiar environment constantly shifts. But what place, you may well ask, does such a discussion have in a book on nutrition?

Many authorities believe that malnutrition among the elderly is most often due to loneliness.[41] For the 6 million adults over 65 who live alone, the pressing need seems to be for companionship first, then for food. Without companionship, appetite decreases. The association of food with human companionship is built into our genes, and our very first experience with food was combined with human body contact.

---

[41] Mayer, 1974; Rao, 1973; Pelcovits, 1972; J. Weinberg, Psychologic implications of the nutritional needs of the elderly, *Journal of the American Dietetic Association* 60 (1972):293-296; L. M. Williams, A concept of loneliness in the elderly, *Journal of the American Geriatrics Society* 26 (1978):182-187; J. Pelcovits, Nutrition for older Americans, *Journal of the American Dietetic Association* 58 (1971):17-21.

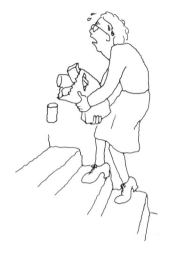

The social life of the adult is built around food. Most invitations into adults' homes are accompanied by an offer of food or drink. We must admit that feeding is, for human beings, as much a social and psychological event as a biological one.

Having spent a lifetime internalizing the concept of food as part of a social activity, the older adult, alone all day every day, must exert a wrenching effort to place enough importance on the nutrient content of food to prepare it and to eat it alone. The purchase, storage, and preparation of food and kitchen cleanup take a tremendous amount of energy. The lonely, depressed person, looking at the task, may forget about the body's needs and say, "What's the use?"

Dr. Jack Weinberg, professor of psychiatry at the University of Illinois, wrote perceptively of this problem:

> In our efforts to provide the aged with a proper diet, we often fail to perceive it is not *what* the older person eats but *with whom* that will be the deciding factor in proper care for him. The oft-repeated complaint of the older patient that he has little incentive to prepare food for only himself is not merely a statement of fact but also a rebuke to the questioner for failing to perceive his isolation and aloneness and to realize that food . . . for one's self lacks the condiment of another's presence which can transform the simplest fare to the ceremonial act with all its shared meaning.[42]

The lack of social interaction is no respecter of income. It is equally important in the lives of the financially secure and in the lives of the poverty-stricken. Newspapers occasionally carry stories of wealthy older persons' being discovered in their mansions, alone and without food. The stories are newsworthy because people wonder why such victims did not ask for help or make arrangements for someone to take care of them — after all, they had plenty of money. The reason is simple. Apathy evolves from loneliness; apathy is expressed in inaction. A victim may sit for long hours in a chair without the energy even to lift her arms. There is no energy to eat, even when food is just a phone call away. Without adequate food, nutrient deficiencies develop that increase the apathy and depression and eventually result in mental confusion. The downward spiral continues, unless interference of neighbors or friends breaks it at some point.

Let's look at what happens when a person receives too little food. In the first place, the body can't tell why it is receiving too few nutrients or kcalories. The situation is the same for a child dying in a famine in Bangladesh as for a wealthy solitary person who is depressed and refusing food. The B vitamins and vitamin C are quickly depleted because they are needed daily. The first organ to suffer from deprivation is the brain, since the B vitamins are necessary for the metabolism of the glucose energy that the brain requires. The brain responds by slowing down all muscular functions. This explains some of the apathy exhibited by the elderly who do not eat. If the carbohydrate kcalories and the B vitamins are not restored, mental confusion that resembles

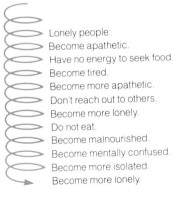

Lonely people:
Become apathetic.
Have no energy to seek food.
Become tired.
Become more apathetic.
Don't reach out to others.
Become more lonely.
Do not eat.
Become malnourished.
Become mentally confused.
Become more isolated.
Become more lonely.

---

[42]Weinberg, 1972.

The symptoms of B-vitamin deficiencies are listed in Chapter 9.

senility will be manifest and may even progress to hallucinations and insanity.

If protein foods, protected by complex carbohydrates, are insufficient, then enzymes to digest food and antibodies to protect against infection cannot be synthesized. When iron and vitamin C are absent, the protein hemoglobin cannot be made for the delivery of oxygen, so the feeling of weakness and tiredness grows. With tiredness from lack of food added to apathy from loneliness, there is even less energy with which to make the effort to secure nourishment. If the confusion of vitamin deficiency is diagnosed as senility, the elderly person may be wrongly confined to a nursing home.

The story is told of a woman who took her mother-in-law to live with her while the older woman waited for a place in a nursing home. The mother-in-law had exhibited the classic signs of senility — mental confusion, inability to make decisions, forgetting to perform important tasks such as turning off a stove burner — so the family had decided she needed institutional care. After several weeks in the daughter-in-law's home — eating good meals and enjoying social stimulation — she became her old self again and returned to her home. This story has been repeated with many variations and serves to remind us to seek a careful medical diagnosis before concluding that a person is senile and needs institutional care. What harm could there be in first trying good, balanced meals served with plenty of tender, loving care?

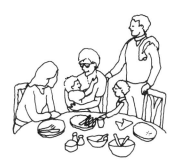

Money and Other Worries

To add anxiety to their problems, most retired persons have a loss of real income that occurs because the retirement check is fixed while all other expenses are increasing. This has a direct effect on the amount of money spent on food, because food (and clothing) purchases are among the few flexible items in the budget. Costs of shelter, utilities, and medical care must be paid and then the amount left over stretched to cover food and other needs.

Forced to practice economy, the older person usually first eliminates so-called "luxury" items such as fresh fruit, vegetables, and milk. In some cases, transportation to and from the market is both expensive and difficult, so that use is made of a nearby convenience store. The foods offered there are limited in variety and are, for the most part, more expensive than the same items in the larger markets. The amount of food that can be purchased is thus curtailed even further, and eating, one of the few pleasures left to the older person, becomes another reminder of reduced status.

Sometimes older persons fall prey to food fads and fallacies. Led by false claims to believe that health can be improved, aging forestalled, and illness cured by magical food and nutrient preparations, they spend money needlessly on fraudulent health-food products, thus depleting their already limited funds.

Two programs are helpful with older people's money problems, although they are not designed specifically for older people but for the poor of all ages. The Food Stamp program enables people who qualify to obtain stamps with which to "buy" food. The Supplemental Security Income (SSI) program is aimed at directly improving the financial plight of the very poor, by increasing a person's or family's income to the defined poverty level. This sometimes helps older people retain their independence.

A self-help effort aimed at enabling older people on limited incomes poverty level. This sometimes helps older people retain their independence.

A self-help effort aimed at enabling older people on limited incomes to buy good food for less money is the establishment of food banks in several areas. A food bank project buys industry's "irregulars" — products that have been mislabeled, underweighted, redesigned, or mispackaged and would ordinarily therefore be thrown away. Nothing is wrong with this food, the industry can credit it as a donation, and the buyer (often a food-preparing site) can buy the food for a small handling fee (10 cents a pound) and make it available for a greatly reduced price. A 1981 observation on this effort was "This kind of activity becomes even more important as we begin to realize that we're not going to get any additional federal money in the future. We have to find other ways to provide the same services."[43]

Besides loneliness, loss, and limited income, the older person faces an increased likelihood of illness and invalidism. Poor dental health, mental illness, and chronic alcoholism are other problems prevalent among the elderly. With all of these problems to live with, and with the increasing numbers of people in the older age group, it is not surprising that at least a few individuals and agencies are concerned enough to ask what can be done to help.

Assistance Programs

In recent years, we have come to recognize that the responsibility for support in old age cannot be left entirely to the individual. Two programs arising from this awareness have already been mentioned (the Food Stamp and Supplemental Security Income programs). The first venture into help for older persons grew out of the experiences of the depression years of the 1930s. The Social Security Act was put into effect in 1935. Under this act, employees and employers pay into a fund from which the employee collects benefits at retirement.

Social Security

A second major political move to benefit the elderly was the Older Americans Act of 1965. Title VII of this act is an amendment, Nutrition Program for the Elderly, which was signed into law by President Nixon in 1972. The major goals of this amendment are to provide:

Title VII of the Older Americans Act

[43]C. Schuster, Feeding at life's end, *Food Management* 16 (December 1981):41, 68-71, 76.

● Low-cost nutritious meals.

● Opportunity for social interaction.

● Auxiliary nutrition, homemaker education, and shopping assistance.

● Counseling and referral to other social and rehabilitative services.

● Transportation services.

Meals on Wheels

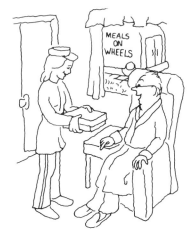

The nutrition program of Title VII was based on the belief that people living alone are apt to be poorly nourished. If their nutrition status could be improved, they might avoid medical problems, continue living in communities of their own choice, and stay out of institutions. The program was not designed as charity, but during its first years it was found that 80 percent of the participants had incomes less than $200 a month and 34 percent had incomes under $100 a month.[44]

Sites chosen for congregate meals under this program must be accessible to most of the target population. Church or school facilities are often used when they are conveniently located. Providing transportation increases the cost of meals by 20 to 30 percent, but it often is indispensable to the existence of a project. Some projects have been successful in recruiting volunteers to help with the transportation. Volunteers may also deliver meals to those who are homebound either permanently or temporarily: These efforts are known as Meals on Wheels. By 1980 there were several hundred such Meals on Wheels programs in the United States.

Every effort is made to persuade the elderly person to come to the congregate meal sites. The social atmosphere at the sites is as valuable as the nutrition. One participant was heard to remark, "It is better to come to the congregate meal and eat at a table with others, even if no one speaks to me, than it is to sit at home and stare at a wall while I eat."[45]

Independence is rated high by those over 65, and this is usually equated with staying in the home where they have lived many years. But this aloneness may not be a wise choice from a nutrition standpoint. There are alternatives that would enhance elderly people's health without threatening their independence. One alternative is covenant living, a lifestyle gaining in popularity. It is patterned after the communes of the young people of the 1960s, although the participants probably would deny this. A number of congenial people, wishing to live in a family group but having no family of their own, agree to live together. Sometimes they buy a house together or rent a house or, in some cases, rent the house of one of the members. The word *covenant* refers to the contractual agreements made among the parties before the arrangement begins. Sometimes it takes several months of talking to hammer out the details of problems that may arise.

[44]Pelcovits, 1972.

[45]Pelcovits, 1971.

The general work of running the house is shared. Either everyone shares equally in the work, taking turns at various jobs, or there is a division based on what each one likes to do or can do well. There are definite economic advantages, but the main advantage is in the sharing of meals and the abating of loneliness. One person described covenant living as coming out of "solitary confinement" into a warm family with the sound of laughter and people to touch.

Another way of gaining sociability while remaining independent is for several older persons to remain in their own homes but meet together regularly for meals, each one taking a turn at preparing the food. Socializing encourages a better food intake, and the one who prepares the food has leftovers to enjoy the next day. Some of the participants in the congregate meal programs have formed what they call a "diner's club" and go to restaurants in a group on the days when the congregate meal is not served. This kind of arrangement among friends helps improve the dietary intake of many older persons.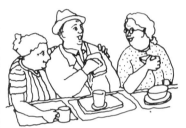

Another alternative is to move into a retirement community. Some are very expensive, but some have a rule that no one who has an income above a certain moderate amount is eligible. In these, a variety of living arrangements are available, from nursing home space to luxury apartments or separate homes on the grounds. In most, several services are maintained on the premises: an infirmary for slight illnesses, a restaurant, and barber shops and beauty salons. A daily check on persons who live alone is one of the valuable services.

Foster home care has proven to be an alternative for people who need some supportive care but do not need medical supervision. Foster homes have the advantage of being located within the community where the older person has lived, so that contact with friends and relatives can be maintained easily. The operators of such homes have no special qualifications and need help from nutritionists for some of their problems. One study of the problems of foster homes, involving 183 operators and 422 residents, showed the biggest problem they faced was the residents' lack of interest in food and other special diet needs. Guidance from nutritionists might help alert them to deterioration that, if allowed to continue, would necessitate more expensive medical care.[46]

Churches and synagogues are ideal organizations to help with the problems of the elderly for a number of reasons: (1) They have neighborhood facilities that lie idle a good portion of the week; (2) they are "caring" organizations; (3) they have a target population, either among their own members or in their neighborhood; and (4) they have a reservoir of volunteers to help cut down on labor costs. Many religious organizations have taken the lead in establishing retirement and nursing homes. However, these facilities are very expensive and usually

[46]Bradshaw et al., 1976.

necessitate the residents' leaving their own community, which means leaving behind the people who care about them. In addition, a nursing home is a medical solution to what, in many cases, is a social problem.[47]

A group of churches in Kansas City discovered the many needs of older people when they started plans to establish a retirement community.[48] Seven churches met together to build a nursing and retirement home and learned that what was really needed was a community service group capable of helping people remain in their own homes. The Shepherd's Center was the result of their planning. This center is now operated by 22 churches in the Kansas City area and has available eight home services, with new ones being made available as the need becomes apparent. The services are congregate meals in neighborhood churches; home delivery of hot meals; a shopping service by which people are taken to shop for groceries or purchases are made for them; a transportation service to take persons to medical appointments; a visitation program in which volunteers keep in personal touch with truly isolated persons; a handyman service to make minor repairs to the home; a crime assistance program; and a team that responds to emergencies at any hour.

In addition to these home services, the Shepherd's Center conducts classes on a wide range of topics taught by skilled or scholarly retired persons. The discovery that retired persons are eager to learn new skills and explore new areas of knowledge has been the experience of many other such groups as well. Health care is one topic of prime importance to older persons, and they are especially eager to study nutrition.[49]

For people who need constant medical care, nursing homes provide a less expensive facility than hospitals. Nursing homes are patterned after hospitals in their approach to their clients. Sometimes this is detrimental to clients' attitudes toward themselves and their future. However, for some, especially the crippled, paralyzed, or bedridden, the nursing home offers a valuable service. There has been a great deal of unfavorable publicity of some substandard homes, which makes many older people frightened at the prospect of having to enter one. But investigation by relatives can identify a home that provides the kind of service the individual needs.

The relative inquiring into nursing homes should ask the director or dietitian some questions about the food service. Is a choice given the resident in the selection of food? How often are the menus repeated (is the cycle monotonous)? How often are fresh fruits and vegetables served? Is the food fresh and tasty when served? Is a plate check

---

[47] R. L. Kane and R. A. Kane, Care of the aged: Old problems in need of new solutions, *Science* 200 (1978):913-919.

[48] E. C. Cole, An alternative to institutional care, *Interpreter*, March 1975.

[49] Cole, 1975; D. Boss, Reaching out: Diet and senior Americans, *Food Management* 12 (November 1977):70-73, 89, 91-93.

conducted regularly, at least once a week, to discover what the resident is consuming? Does the staff keep track of each person's weight? Is there good communication between the nursing staff and the dietitian so that the dietitian will know if someone is not eating? Is the resident encouraged and helped to go to the dining room to eat so that some socializing will occur? What is the environment like in which the residents eat? Does someone help those who can't manage feeding themselves? Are minced meats offered to those who have problems with their dentures? Are religious dietary restrictions honored? How high a proportion of the foods are prepackaged? (No guide can be given for what proportion is desirable, but it should be remembered that processed foods are low in vitamin content and high in salt.) Other questions that the investigator will want to ask have to do with the general atmosphere of the nursing home, in recognition of effect of social climate on a person's appetite. A nursing home that views residents as persons, not as patients, gets a mark in its favor.

In the nursing home, the dietitian, nutritionist, or nurse responsible for the residents' care should keep in mind the special needs associated with their time in life. The average age of a nursing home resident is 81, and many have problems that can affect nutrition status:

- At least one chronic disease.
- Constipation or incontinence.
- Confusion due to change in environment.
- Poor eyesight or hearing.
- Ill-fitting or missing dentures.
- Inability to feed self because of arthritis or stroke.
- Psychological problems, especially depression.
- Anorexia and loss of interest in eating.
- Lack of opportunity to socialize at mealtimes.
- Long-established food preferences.
- Slowed reactions (seeing, holding utensils, chewing, swallowing).[50]

On admission, their nutrition status should be assessed immediately, and the person responsible for their nutrition care should make every effort to rectify any problems promptly. Thereafter they should be reassessed at regular, frequent intervals and adjustments made as needed.

Opinions differ on the philosophy to adopt for nursing home menus. A multitude of different special diets is difficult and expensive to manage, and one authority recommends a "liberalized geriatric diet" for most cases, rather than modified diets. Based on the assumption

Chapter 18 presents all the instructions necessary to do a complete nutrition assessment.

[50]E. Luros, A rational approach to geriatric nutrition, *Dietetic Currents, Ross Timesaver* 8 (November-December 1981).

that older people "should have the right to choose the food they eat," this general, liberal approach provides in one package the key characteristics of several special diets:

- 1,500 to 2,000 kcal/day, mostly from nutrient-dense foods, with simple desserts not too high in kcal.
- Minimal salt used in preparation.
- 65 to 70 g protein per day from 2 c milk and 4 to 6 oz meat or alternate.
- At least 6 mg iron per day (the RDA for older people is 10 mg/day).
- Generous amounts of natural fiber and fluid intake of 64 oz/day.[51]

Nutrition needs incurred in disease are the subject of Part Five.

Further modifications can be made available for people with severe disease conditions.

Preparing for the Later Years

The programs just described can do much to help older people adjust to their changing circumstances, but the very best help we could give our elderly citizens would be a change of attitude. As a nation, we value the future more than the present, putting off enjoying today so that tomorrow we will have money or prestige or time to have fun. The elderly feel this loss of future. The present is their time for leisure and enjoyment, but they have no experience in the use of leisure time.

Our culture also values the doers, those concerned with action and achievement. The Spanish mother may enjoy her child because he is sitting in her lap and laughing in her face; however, the Anglo-American mother is more likely preoccupied with how well he is preparing for tomorrow. The elderly are aware of the status given those who are doing something and of the disrespect given those who lead a contemplative life in retirement.

It would take a near miracle to change the attitude of a nation, but there is a change in attitude that individual persons can make toward themselves as they age. Preparation for this period should of course include financial planning, but other lifelong habits should be developed as well. Each adult needs to learn to reach out to others, to forestall the loneliness that will otherwise ensue. Each needs to learn some skills or activities that can continue into the later years — volunteer work with organizations, reading, games, hobbies, or intellectual pursuits — which will give meaning to the activities of the days. Each needs to develop the habit of adjusting to change, especially when it comes without consent, so that it will not be seen as a loss of control over life. The goal is to arrive at maturity with as healthy a mind and body as it is possible to have, and this means cultivating good

[51]Luros, 1981.

nutrition status and maintaining a program of daily exercise.

Preparation for the later years begins early in life, both psychologically and nutritionally. Everyone knows older people who have gathered around themselves many contacts — through relatives, church, synagogue, or fraternal orders — and have not allowed themselves to drift into isolation. Upon analysis, you will see that their favorable environment came through a lifetime of effort. They spent their entire lives reaching out to others and practicing the art of weaving themselves into other people's lives. Likewise, a lifetime of effort is required for good nutrition status in the later years. A person who has eaten a wide variety of foods, has stayed trim, and has remained physically active will be most able to withstand the assaults of change.

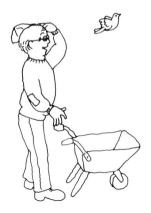

Summing Up

In the United States, 11 percent of the population is over 65, amounting to over 30 million people. Many live alone, and only a few are in nursing homes; their lifestyles are diverse, and fewer than half are poor.

Health of the elderly can be improved and prolonged by good nutrition, although aging is a natural process and in some ways cannot be prevented. Life still ends at about 70 for most people; the increase in the number of older people seen in U.S. census reports does not reflect an increase in life expectancy but an increase in the number of people surviving the early years and so living to about 70.

Aging of cells may occur for any of several reasons: They may accumulate debris; they may lose the ability to read the genetic code words that specify their functions; they may make wrong proteins, to which the body reacts by producing antibodies; or they may be programmed to divide a definite number of times before they die. Cellular aging is reflected in such familiar phenomena as the wrinkling of the skin, loss of digestive functions, loss of responsiveness to changes such as increased blood glucose, loss of elasticity of blood vessels, and loss of function of the kidneys. The brain and nervous system lose cells, and those that remain slow down in reaction time. To some extent these changes can be slowed by maintaining a strong cardiovascular and respiratory system by means of regular exercise. Adult bone loss (osteoporosis) is least likely in those whose bones were dense at maturity, thanks to good mineral and vitamin nutrition in the early years; some calcium loss does occur in aging, however. For many, arthritis makes movement difficult and painful.

Nutrition requirements of the older person are for fewer kcalories, increased protein, reduced fat, sufficient complex carbohydrates, sufficient vitamins and minerals (especially vitamin C, iron, and calcium), adequate water intake (six or seven glasses a day), and ample fiber (roughage) from fruits, vegetables, and whole grains. Meals should be regular and, as far as possible, prepared from fresh ingredients. The enjoyment of food is enhanced if loneliness — a major problem of older people living alone — can be alleviated. Eating with others often restores the appetite and health that may seem to be failing due to degenerative disease.

Having enough money is basic to coping with the nutrition problems of the later years. Government programs designed to help by providing money, either directly or for food, include Social Security, the Food Stamp program, and the Supplemental Security Income program. A government program that provides both food and settings in which to enjoy it is the Nutrition Program for the Elderly, which includes both congregate meals and Meals on Wheels. Alternatives to institutional care are desirable to preserve the older person's independence; among the possibilities are covenant living, diners' clubs, retirement communities, and foster home care. When a nursing home is chosen, its food service should be examined for characteristics that will facilitate good nutrition and appetite.

Old age need not be a time of despair, isolation, and ill health. Preparation for enjoyable later years should include financial planning, the establishment of lasting social contacts, the learning of skills and activities that can be pursued into later life, the maintenance of a program of regular physical activity, and the cultivation of healthy nutrition status throughout life.

To Explore Further

Recommended references on all nutrition topics are listed in Appendix J. In addition, we recommend highly the books by A. Comfort *(A Good Age)* and M. Puner *(To the Good Long Life)* listed in this chapter's notes.

A book that helps the reader understand the medical-social problems that develop with aging is:

● Field, M. *The Aged, the Family, and the Community.* New York: Columbia University Press, 1972.

Emphasized throughout is the need to preserve older individuals' feelings of worth and to safeguard their dignity.

The Journal of the American Geriatrics Society and *The Gerontologist* make good reading for the general reader.

A short article that takes a positive approach toward the nutrition problems of older people and presents up-to-date information on them is:

● Rowe, D. Aging — a jewel in the mosaic of life. *Journal of the American Dietetic Association* 72 (1978):478-486.

Among films and teaching aids that promote understanding of aging are:

● Pelcovits, J. Nutrition education for older Americans. *Cassette-a-Month*, February 1977. Available from the American Dietetic Association (address in Appendix J).

● *The String Bean*, a 15- to 20-minute long film, is a hauntingly poetic masterpiece portraying an old lady's devotion to life, love, and beauty. Available from McGraw-Hill Films, in care of Association Films, Inc., 600 Grand Avenue, Ridgefield, NJ 07657.

For the provider of nutrition for the elderly, we recommend one short and one long reference. The short reference is the one based on the philosophy that older people should be free to choose what to eat:

● Luros, E. A rational approach to geriatric nutrition. *Dietetic Currents, Ross Timesaver* 8 (November-December 1981). 6 pages, free from Ross Labs (address in Appendix J).

● Natow, A. B. *Geriatric Nutrition*. Boston: CBI Publishing, 1980. 332 pages, $15.95.

A chapter of Natow's book is devoted to nutrition education for the elderly, a topic not covered here. An important point she makes is that nutrition education materials need to be developed specifically for the elderly. Those prepared for younger people do not meet their needs. Indeed, the way is open for an abundance of literature and resources on nutrition for the elderly.

Mr. Acree, age 86, has recently become a widower. His sight is impaired to the extent that he is unable to care for himself at home, and his daughter and son-in-law have reluctantly decided to place him in a nursing home. Other than his near-blindness, he is in fair health and has no diagnosed chronic disease. On admission to the home his height and weight are found to be:

- Ht: 5′10″.
- Wt: 175 lb.

A month later, however, he is found to have lost 10 lb and is severely depressed.

Study Question

1. Itemize as many possible reasons for Mr. Acree's weight loss as you can. If corrective measures can be taken, indicate what they should be.

Chapter 18 presents the assessment procedures that might reveal additional, in-depth information about Mr. Acree's condition, and the chapters of Part Five present the nutrition implications of many different diseases. With that information, the nutrition provider can offer more sophisticated help, but even without it, the message here is important. An awareness of the person and of the circumstances and a simple monitoring of body weight are basic to adequate nutrition care.

Detecting Rip-offs

This is the last Highlight in the book directed to you, the consumer. From this point on, the Chapters and Highlights address you as a health professional who will be guiding others in their food choices. Before we leave you, we have a mission to complete, topping off your education in "How to be wise and wary in assessing nutrition information." This skill is especially important for older people who, because of their vulnerability to the diseases of advancing age, are often the targets of unscrupulous promoters of nutrition misinformation. It is not only old people, however, but all people who need this skill. No one is immune to the persuasions of the tricksters.

Each of the preceding chapters has contained words of caution to strengthen your ability to detect and avoid misinformation. Several themes have been introduced and developed along the way. These themes were always the subjects of digressions, incidental to the text; they were never quite in focus. Because they involve enjoyable subject matter and because they deserve direct attention in their own right, some of these themes have been gathered together here to be given a brief moment in the spotlight. There follows a last story with a moral.

The most widespread and expensive type of quackery in the United States today is the promotion of vitamin products, special dietary foods, and food supplements.

G. P. LARRICK

Review

One theme of our digressions has been the wisdom of the body. It is an ancient wisdom, arising from gradual evolution over eons of time. It signifies that the body has the equipment to handle the many variations its environment has presented in ages past and can be trusted to adjust beautifully to changing circumstances today. As a corollary, however, the body is *not* equipped to handle "new" things such as pure salt or sugar in large amounts, industrial pollutants in high concentrations, or man-made gimmicks it has never encountered before. False claims based on a misunderstanding or underestimation of the body's wisdom include these ideas:

- That you can second guess the body (Chapter 6) — for example, by eating foods singly to ease the body's work (Chapter 10).

- That you can improve the body's efficiency by offering it a drug used for illness (Chapters 4, 5).

- That you can meet vitamin or mineral needs better by taking pills or supplements than by eating foods (Chapter 9).

Another theme has been to warn you against self-diagnosis, for all kinds of reasons. Truckloads of worthless and dangerous medicines are unloaded on the gullible public by people using false suggestions such as:

- You probably have hypoglycemia (most people do) (Chapter 1).

- Anyway, you have symptom X, therefore you must have disease Y (Chapter 2).

- Therefore, you should buy and consume a certain food or nutrient preparation (Chapter 9).

Another theme has been the importance of reading food labels with an educated eye. You have been warned:

- About the use of the terms *organic*, *natural*, and *health food* (Introduction).

- About the implication that

honey or fructose in a product makes it superior to a product containing some other kind of sugar (Chapter 1).

- That the presence of a nutrient such as "protein" is not all you should look for on a label. You should also ask "*how much* protein" and "*what quality* protein (or fat or carbohydrate)" (Highlight 4) or "*which* fiber" (Chapter 6), and other such questions.

- That you should measure label amounts against a yardstick such as the RDA (Highlight 4, Chapter 12).

- That the boast "contains no X" (additives) may signify no advantage to the buyer (Highlight 13).

Highlight 12 offered all the basics about reading labels.

The differing significances of different *amounts* of substances were also pointed out in several other connections:

- Even an essential nutrient can be harmful at too high a dose level (Chapter 3). This is especially important with respect to fat-soluble vitamins and trace minerals (Chapters 11, 13).

- Even a deadly poison may be nothing to worry about at a low enough concentration (Chapter 13).

- Additive amounts are allowed in foods with a margin of safety such that they present no hazard under ordinary conditions of use (Highlight 13).

Miniglossary

refereed journal: a journal in which research reports are screened for acceptance by peers of the authors who are qualified to detect errors in method and invalid findings.

The most common tricks used by pushers of misinformation have also been exposed. To be on your guard against them, you should watch out for:

- Scare tactics (Chapter 13).

- Promises of easy, rapid weight loss — magical thinking (Chapter 8).

- Failure to distinguish between loss of fat and loss of weight (Chapter 7).

- The implication that what is safe or good for "nearly all people" is safe or good for you (Chapter 10).

- "New" treatments or products that have not yet been tested and are not proven to be effective and/or safe (Highlight 5).

- The use of logic rather than evidence (Chapter 5).

And to help you size up new weight-loss diets as they come along, a special rating scale was presented in the Self-Study for Highlight 14.

Another theme was developed around nutrition research and experiments and the caution needed in interpreting them. It was pointed out that:

- Correlation is not cause (Chapter 2).

- Human clinical studies involve many subtleties of experimental design and have to take into account the power of the placebo effect (Highlight 10).

- Animal research can't be applied uncritically to humans (Highlight 11).

Finally, Chapter 8 introduced the idea that you can't trust what you read, not only in newspapers but also in books, and recommended that you become acquainted with the scientific journals where the original research reports are located. Highlight 10 offered the cautious view that even a journal may report an invalid finding. Single research reports find their way into review articles, which draw a balanced picture of whole areas of research. The careful consumer of nutrition information learns to conduct such reviews or to rely on those carefully done by known, trusted authorities before arriving at any firm conclusions about what to believe.

All of these areas of awareness and strategies, taken together, provide the consumer with generally effective defenses against being taken in. This last story is told here, partly just because it is a good story, and partly because it puts the finishing touches on your sophistication as a consumer of nutrition information by introducing you to the *refereed journal*. It's the story of vitamin B_{15}.

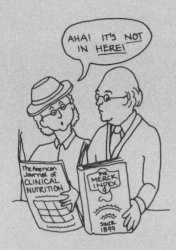

One Last Story   The story of vitamin B_{15} comes from a thoroughly researched review by Dr. Victor Herbert, professor of medicine at SUNY Downstate Medical Center in Brooklyn, New York, director of the Hematology and Nutrition Laboratory at the Bronx Veterans Administration Medical Center, and a highly respected, long-time scholar and researcher of vitamin facts and fallacies. The first episode occurred about 40 years ago, in 1943. Two researchers, Ernst Krebs, Sr., and Ernst Krebs, Jr., applied for a patent for a substance they claimed to have isolated from apricot kernels, which they called pangamic acid. They patented a trade name for it: vitamin B_{15}.[1]

Immediately, the first moral of this story can be

[1] Most of this story follows closely the excellent review of the history of pangamate: V. Herbert, Pangamic acid ("vitamin B_{15}"), *American Journal of Clinical Nutrition* 32 (1979):1534-1540.

drawn: Naming a compound a vitamin doesn't make it a vitamin. In the same way, Krebs, Jr., gave the name vitamin B_{17} to another chemical, laetrile, also isolated from apricot pits. Similarly, if you wished, you could name your next baby "Doctor" instead of Rachel or Nzingha or Cromwell, and the child could then be known by this name all its life without ever having earned an M.D. degree. As an adult, if the child decided to publish a diet, it could be called "Doctor So-and-So's diet". But to pursue this reasoning further would be to tell another story.

B_{15} into the 1980s   The *World Review of Nutrition and Dietetics* published in 1977 a review, "Pangamic Acid," which was "supported in part by a grant from the McNaughton Foundation" and which claimed that a similar review would soon be published in the *American Journal of Clinical Nutrition* with over 125 references, most of them clinical. The *Merck Index*, 9th edition, 1976, also published the structure of pangamic acid.

To the experienced reader of nutrition literature, these appear to be impressive evidence of legitimacy. But a closer look shatters the claims for pangamic acid based on them. First, the author of the review in the *World Review* is Krebs's stepson — not that a family relationship immediately proves a bias, but it does suggest the

possibility. Second, the "McNaughton Foundation" is a front name for Andrew McNaughton, the owner of a factory manufacturing laetrile. The "foundation's" previous publications were booklets promoting pangamic acid and laetrile as if they were vitamins. The review "to be published in the *American Journal of Clinical Nutrition*" was indeed submitted to the journal but was refused because it included:

- No quotation marks on the word "vitamin" as applied to pangamate, implying falsely that pangamate was already officially accepted as a vitamin.

- No mention of the Canadian and U.S. food and drug authorities' positions that evidence for pangamate as a vitamin was nonexistent and that its safety and benefit were not proven.

- No data on the chemical reactions in which pangamate might participate in the body.

- No data on absorption, blood levels, and other factors normally studied for vitamins.

- No foundation for the claims made or citation of conflicting evidence or claims.

In short, the review was not a scientific review and critique of all the available evidence but rather an uncritical collection of stories and uncontrolled studies from which no positive information could conclusively be drawn.[2] Hence, it was rejected for publication.

A second moral is now apparent in this tale. "To be published" does not mean "published"; it may be a statement of wishful thinking. And the fact that someone claims he or she has "clinical" evidence of a vitamin's effectiveness is not to say that such evidence actually exists. In other words, people sometimes lie.

One strong fact stands out in favor of the reality of pangamic acid as a substance, however: its publication in the *Merck Index*. Every chemist uses "the Merck" as a reference for the structure and properties of chemical compounds. The Merck is the standard for chemical identity; in short, the chemist's dictionary. So in spite of the lack of evidence and reliable publications on pangamate at present, the substance does exist and research in the future will show us exactly what it does. Right?

Wrong. Amazingly, the Merck slipped up — not once, but twice — when it came to pangamic acid. According to Dr. Herbert:

The *Merck Index*, 8th edition, 1968, notes pangamic acid [as one chemical, the 9th edition shows a

different structure]. The editor of the *Merck Index* indicated to this reviewer that "pangamic acid" and "vitamin B_{15}" will be deleted from the 10th edition, since they were deceived into listing it. Products marketed as B_{15} or pangamic acid, or calcium pangamate could contain any or all of the above materials, plus other materials, since there is no standard of identity for the product.[3]

Dr. Herbert, for all of the above and many more reasons, has concluded that vitamin B_{15} *alias* pangamic acid is "a label and not a substance." Its creator, he says, is a twice-convicted criminal who is a "doctor" only because he was given an honorary doctorate in science by a small Bible college in Oklahoma which had "no science department and no authority from Oklahoma to award the degree."[4] (That was another short story about "doctors.") The college itself no longer exists. (Here we could draw a moral about institutions of higher learning.)

When bottles labeled "pangamic acid" are bought and analyzed they are found to contain a variety of ingredients, not always the same but always identifiable as other compounds, not pangamic acid. One of these is a chemical which produces blood vessel dilation and a

drop in blood pressure so that the user experiences a "high" very shortly after taking it. The reaction of the uninformed: "Wow, this is really a powerful vitamin. I feel great already!" The promoters, who also sell laetrile, have become multimillionaires.[5] By now we have gleaned a multitude of morals, but there are still more to come.

The FDA and the *American Journal of Clinical Nutrition* have soundly condemned pangamic acid. *Nutrition and the MD* dubbed it the "quack nutrient of the year" in 1978. More recently it has been shown that one of the ingredients sometimes in the bottle is a compound that not only is not a vitamin but is a cancer-causing agent.[6] The sale of pangamate as a food, dietary supplement, or drug is illegal.[7] Canada has prohibited the sale of pangamate altogether since more than ten years ago.

Still, thousands of bottles of these compounds continue to be sold in health food stores, bearing the label "vitamin B_{15}" or "pangamic acid." The FDA has made a number of seizures of these products but has not stemmed the flow of them to the ever-believing public. No doctor can legally use or pre-

---

[2] Herbert, 1979.

[3] Herbert, 1979.

[4] V. Herbert, as quoted in: B_{15} blarney, *ACSH News and Views*, April 1980, pp. 4-5.

[5] B_{15} blarney, 1980.

[6] American Council on Science and Health, as quoted by ABC World News Tonight, April 1980.

[7] Herbert, 1979.

scribe the material without first securing permission from a committee composed of doctors authorized to make decisions about the ethics of experiments using human beings as subjects. Nor can a doctor proceed until after obtaining informed consent from the patient — *informed*, meaning that the patient reads a statement that the item has no known value in the treatment of any disease, is not known to be safe, and may be dangerous. However, doctors (and self-titled doctors) are as enthusiastic, impulsive, and ill-informed in many cases as the customers who hope to buy miraculous cures in pill form under this name.[8]

One Last Moral   This story illustrates many points that have been made before. The promoters of B_{15} were extraordinarily clever, and they broke through many barriers that should have held them back. Still, there were ways for the cautious consumer to tell this was a fraud. In this case the profit motive was clearly in evidence: Score one

against the sellers of B_{15}. Their credentials don't stand up to close examination, either: Score two. Their "evidence" was of the anecdotal, "case-history" kind which is never acceptable as sound scientific evidence of the safety or efficacy of a nutrient or drug in therapy for any condition. They had no controlled clinical studies of large samples of people with unbiased, double-blind scoring of results: Score three. But what this story illustrates, perhaps better than any other told so far, is that any authority, no matter how credible and reputable, can make an error on occasion, as the *Merck Index* did in this case. Seeing a statement on the pages of a book in black and white — no matter what the book — is no guarantee that it is a fact.

If you earnestly want to find out whether new nutrition information is valid, you have some effective strategies at your disposal, but you have to be willing to expend the time and energy to use them. To check on the credentials of a speaker, an inquiry by telephone to the institution where he or she claims to have gotten a degree is likely to be informative. To find out about the reality or reputation of an institution of higher learning, you can go to any good library and ask for a directory of colleges and universities or, in the case of organizations, for the *Encyclopedia of*

Associations.[9]

In reading published nutrition information, seekers after truth can glean much insight by simply asking themselves why it was published, as we have said before. In this case, it became easy to see that the object was promotion, not the presentation of evidence. Another question to ask, as we have also pointed out, is where it was published — or in this case, where it was *not* published. The trap that finally caught the rat was the *American Journal of Clinical Nutrition*, because it was a refereed journal. (You can find out from the *Encyclopedia of Associations* whether an association's journal is refereed.) This means that the articles submitted for publication are not automatically accepted. Each article is sent to at least two experts in the field who can judge the validity of each article and who are encouraged to be critical and careful in making their judgments. Only when these referees, or reviewers, have passed on an article is it allowed into print. That the

___

[8]Other names you may have read on labels or in literature making exaggerated claims are p-aminobenzoic acid (PABA), hesperidin, lipoic acid, and ubiquinone. These are not vitamins and are not needed by humans. V. Herbert, The vitamin craze, *Archives of Internal Medicine* 140 (1980):173-176.

[9]M. Fisk, ed., *Encyclopedia of Associations*, 11th ed. (Detroit: Gale Research Company, Book Tower, 1977). Or ask for W. A. Katz, *Magazines for Libraries*, 3rd ed. (New York: Bowker, 1978), which tells how to submit articles for publication in various journals. If the author is required to submit only one copy, then the article will not be refereed. Look for the latest editions of these reference books.

American Journal of Clinical Nutrition was alert enough to stop the misinformation about pangamic acid from going any further testifies to the critical judgment of its reviewers and shows how the screening of information for publication makes these journals far more trustworthy than most leaflets, pamphlets, and books you may pick up in the local food store or bookstore.

This section has perhaps told you more than you wanted to know about the publication of science facts. But there was an excuse, remember? Today's pangamic acid will disappear from the scene tomorrow, as surely as the snake-oil medicines of the 1920s have disappeared today. What you need to arm you against the next massive fraud of this kind is not the knowledge, specifically, of the history of pangamic acid, but the techniques to be able to determine — for *any* news — whether or not you should believe it.

PART FOUR

PRINCIPLES OF
NUTRITION SUPPORT

INTRODUCTION

NUTRITION IN HEALTH CARE

Nurse: *That which nourishes . . . (1529)*

Nutrition *(from the latin* nutrix, *nurse): Serving as, or supplying nourishment.*

OXFORD ENGLISH DICTIONARY

Throughout the earlier parts of this book you have developed an understanding of what nutrition is all about and how you can apply nutrition principles in your everyday life. You also saw how nutrient needs continue to change throughout life. Now the focus of the chapters shifts from you to your client.

The knowledge and skills you have gained from earlier chapters certainly can be applied to your clients. But you also need special information. Part Four provides some general guidelines for working with clients. The chapters help you identify your client's nutrient and nutrition education needs and show you how to communicate effectively with people, how hospitalized patients are fed, and how commonly used drugs interact with nutrients. What you learn in this section will help you work with all people. Nutrition for people with special disease conditions is the subject of Part Five.

As you shift your focus from yourself to others, keep in mind that clients have special needs. They are either sick or are preventing or controlling a disease. In many instances, they experience anxiety about their situation. Moreover, they are individuals with unique perceptions and varying knowledge about nutrition. For this reason, successful nutrition intervention must be tailored to the individual.

CHAPTER 18

CONTENTS

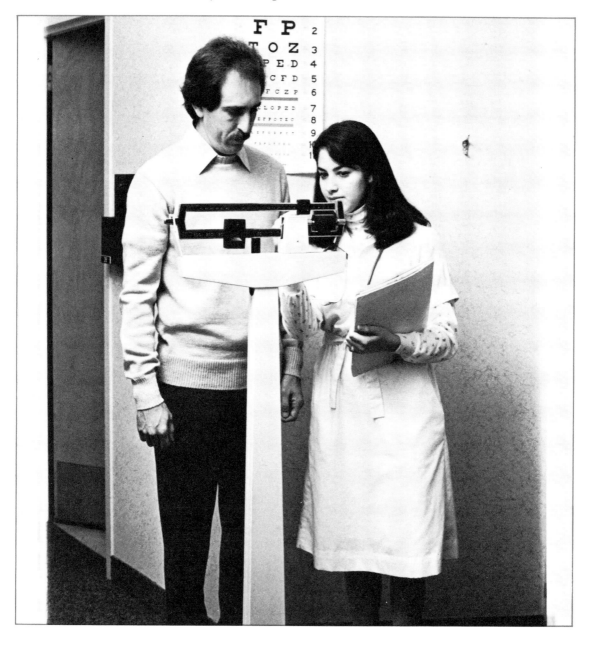

NUTRITION ASSESSMENT AND PLANNING

It is well known ... that malnutrition interferes with wound healing and increases susceptibility to infection. It thus becomes imperative to ensure that preventable malnutrition does not contribute to mortality, morbidity, and prolonged bed-occupancy rates of our hospital population.

CHARLES E. BUTTERWORTH, JR., M.D. (1974)

Patients in the hospital are in different states of health, have different nutrient needs, prefer different foods, and react differently to medical procedures and care. Supporting their health by way of diet is a complex and difficult task. Knowing the great difference that optimum nutrition makes, however, the health professional will make the maximum effort to deliver nutrition care tailored to the needs of each individual. To do so requires a systematic and logical approach.

The organized procedure through which nutrition needs are identified and possible solutions are implemented and evaluated is called the nutrition care process. This process includes several steps:

Nutrition care process

1. Assessing nutrition status.

2. Interpreting assessment data to determine nutrient requirements.

nutrition status: describes a person's nutrition health, i.e., how well the individual's nutrient needs are being met.

3. Developing a plan of action, including patient education, for meeting nutrition needs.

4. Implementing the care plan.

5. Evaluating the effectiveness of the care plan through ongoing assessment and making any appropriate changes.

Responsibility for developing and implementing nutrition care plans is shared by all health care providers, although the physician, nurse, and dietitian must assume the primary roles. The social worker, pharmacist, and physical therapist also can make valuable contributions to assessment and care (see Highlight 20B). Generally, the greater the participation of team members, the more realistic and attainable the care plan will be.

Throughout the next two chapters, we will be discussing the various steps which make up the nutrition care process. Although emphasis will be focused on hospitalized patients, the same principles apply to all people seen in outpatient clinics, community centers, nursing homes, private practice, or their own homes.

673

Overview of Nutrition Assessment

Nutrition assessment

Assessment, the first step in the nutrition care process, is an inventory of nutrition assets and liabilities. Nutrition assets are factors such as balanced eating habits, desirable body weight, and good skin tone which suggest that nutrient stores are adequate. On the other hand, loss of appetite, excessive weight gain, and anemia are liabilities, because they suggest nutrient imbalances. By comparing assets and liabilities, you can determine what actions will correct deficiencies or excesses or will maintain current status. A followup assessment helps determine if the actions you have taken are appropriate or if further action is required.

Appreciation for the important role of nutrition and nutrition assessment in patient care has developed only recently. This new interest has been sparked, in part, by the alarming discovery that from 30 to 65 percent of hospitalized patients surveyed in the 1970s suffered from a significant degree of malnutrition.[1]

Malnutrition   The word *malnutrition* generally evokes a picture of a hungry child in a Third World country. Malnutrition truly is a worldwide concern, and severe malnutrition is a very real and multidimensional problem (see Highlight 18).

undernutrition: inadequate intake of nutrients.

Simply defined, malnutrition describes a state of improper nutrition balance in the body. Malnutrition can be a problem of inappropriate ingestion, digestion, absorption, metabolism, or excretion of nutrients or a combination of several of these factors. Please note the use of the word *inappropriate* rather than *inadequate*. Malnutrition can be the result of nutrient excesses as well as deficiencies.

overnutrition: excessive intake of nutrients.

To illustrate the importance of this point, consider what can happen if people think of malnutrition only as undernutrition. They might notice an apparent nutrient deficiency, but in correcting it they might forget that a nutrient excess is also possible. Iodine is a case in point. In areas of the United States where the soil contained little iodine, goiter was a prevalent public health concern until iodized salt became widely used. Thereafter, iodine deficiency goiter was rarely seen, and iodine was all but forgotten.

Recently, however, there has been renewed interest in iodine. Data available from the Total Diet Study conducted by the FDA indicate

[1] B. Bistrian, G. Blackburn, J. Vitale, D. Cochran, and J. Naylor, Prevalence of malnutrition in general medical patients, *Journal of the American Medical Association* 235 (1976):1567-1570; J. Mullen, M. Gertner, G. Buzby, G. Goodhart, and E. Rosato, Implications of malnutrition in the surgical patient, *Archives of Surgery* 114 (1979):121-125; R. Weinsier, E. Hunker, C. Krumdieck, and C. Butterworth, Hospital malnutrition: A prospective evaluation of medical patients during the course of hospitalization, *American Journal of Clinical Nutrition* 32 (1979):418-426.

that iodine consumption in the typical American diet is now from four to thirteen times the RDA.[2] New processing technology and manufacturing practices have been cited as factors which may have increased the iodine content of the diet.[3]

There is generally a wide margin of safety when it comes to nutrient needs, so these findings do not necessarily imply a hazard. But certainly it will be important to monitor the situation closely.

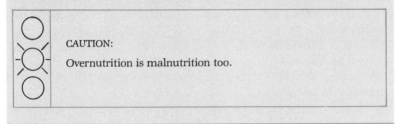

CAUTION:

Overnutrition is malnutrition too.

The classical nutrient deficiency diseases such as rickets, pellagra, and beriberi are seldom seen in the developed countries today. The word *classical* refers to severe deficiencies with clearly apparent signs and symptoms which can be attributed to a specific nutrient deficiency. Some examples include bowed legs in rickets or bleeding gums in scurvy. Chapters 9 to 14 discussed the roles of various nutrients and the consequences of deficient and excessive intakes. Classical nutrient deficiencies are apparent only after nutrient intake has been a problem over a long period of time.

Much more common today are subclinical nutrient deficiencies, which often go unnoticed. Detecting them is difficult and is complicated by the fact that many deficiencies generally occur simultaneously. One of the goals of nutrition assessment is to uncover early signs of malnutrition long before a classical deficiency disease develops.

The Ten State Nutrition Survey (also called the National Nutrition Survey) was conducted by the U.S. Department of Health, Education, and Welfare between 1968 and 1970 to explore allegations that hunger and malnutrition were widespread problems in the United States.[4] A cross-section of the population in each of ten states, representing different geographic, ethnic, economic, and other groups, was surveyed.

The results revealed that a significant number of people had energy intakes below the standards for their age, size, and weight. The groups

Subclinical deficiencies are those which are not yet obvious. They occur during the period of time when intake is deficient but before the outward symptoms have appeared.

[2] *Total Diet Study — Adults, Infants and Toddlers*, FDA Compliance Program 7305.002 (Washington, D.C.: Food and Drug Administration, 1979).

[3] Y. Park, B. Harland, J. Vanderveen, F. Shank, and L. Prosky, Estimation of dietary iodine intake of Americans in recent years, *Journal of the American Dietetic Association* 79 (1981):17-24.

[4] U.S. Department of Health, Education, and Welfare, *Ten-State Nutrition Survey*, 1968-1970, publication no. (HSM) 72-8130 (Atlanta: Center for Disease Control, 1972).

having the most nutrition problems included blacks, Spanish-Americans, adolescents, and low-income groups. The greatest numbers of people were deficient in iron, vitamin A, and riboflavin. Protein intake was a problem for pregnant and lactating women.

Nutrient excesses are also of major concern, because they are associated with chronic diseases in later life. A recent report from the Department of Health and Human Services identified several areas of national concern involving overnutrition.[5] These include excessive intakes of energy (obesity), sugar, sodium, cholesterol, total fat, and saturated fat.

Nutrition problems, then, are not confined to Third World countries or even to low-income or disadvantaged groups. Malnutrition is a problem for all of us. Of special interest here is the malnutrition that occurs in the hospital.

Protein-Calorie Malnutrition (PCM) in the Hospital Although the seriousness of PCM as a world health problem has been recognized for many years, only recently has attention been focused on its prevalence in the United States. The now classic article "The Skeleton in the Hospital Closet" sent shock waves through the health care community by exposing significant PCM in U.S. hospitals.[6] In response, several studies were conducted which confirmed the original findings.[7]

You may well wonder how something as basic as sound nutrition could be neglected in hospitals, where the latest technology abounds. Some of the causes are:

- Patients are often deprived of food for days at a time so that they can be given medical tests.
- Vitamin and mineral supplements are seldom given.
- Inadequate nutrient formulas (bottles of glucose and salts without protein, vitamins, or minerals) are given for long periods of time.
- Various health professionals fail to communicate accurately with each other.[8]

The parts of the body from which protein is lost are sometimes referred to as the **lean body mass**, which includes all body components except fat. A more accurate term is **fat-free body**.

Part of the reason nutrition care of the patient is neglected may be a basic failure of health care professionals, including physicians, to appreciate the role nutrition plays in the stress response. Ability to respond to stress depends, to a large extent, on energy reserves and protein, since the body's requirements for these nutrients increase in stress. When energy is not being supplied in adequate amounts from the diet for a period of time, the body uses protein to meet energy

[5]U.S. Department of Health and Human Services, *Promoting Health/Preventing Disease: Objectives for the Nation* (Washington, D.C.: Government Printing Office, Fall 1980), pp. 73-77.

[6]C. Butterworth, The skeleton in the hospital closet, *Nutrition Today*, March/April 1974, pp. 4-8.

[7]Bistrian et al., 1976; Mullen et al., 1979; Weinsier et al., 1979.

[8]Butterworth, 1974.

needs. When this adaptation occurs, functional protein is lost from skeletal muscle, from organs (liver, gut, lungs), and from circulating pools of protein (albumin, immune factors).

For the well-nourished patient, loss of *some* protein is not critical, since adequate protein remains to support vital functions. However, in prolonged stress or in malnutrition the protein loss can be serious. For example, it is not often appreciated that the malnourished patient is more likely to develop pneumonia following surgery. Loss of a critical number of functioning lung cells and decreased synthesis of immune factors lead to deterioration of lung function and depression of the immune system. The result: pneumonia.

Organs where cells are being replaced rapidly are among the first to be affected by PCM. One such organ system is the gastrointestinal (GI) tract. Once a patient develops PCM, the microvilli of the gut gradually shrink and become nonfunctional. Up to 90 percent of them can be lost. The patient then has grievous difficulty absorbing nutrients, and this makes the PCM worse.

Within the cell, PCM affects the synthesis of enzymes and other protein molecules which are necessary for proper metabolism and maintenance of the structure of the cells. These protein molecules usually are synthesized and degraded rapidly in our bodies to help us adapt promptly to changes in our environment. Losing this ability to adapt is critical.[9]

Protein and fat are used to meet energy requirements once glycogen stores are depleted. Thus, these body stores are of particular concern in nutrition assessment. When they are depleted, you know that the patient's defenses against disease are threatened.

While deficient intake can damage a person's nutrition status by causing primary deficiencies, disease also can affect nutrition status by altering the intake, utilization, or excretion of nutrients, causing secondary deficiencies. One or all of these factors may be operating to seriously interfere with a patient's ability to heal wounds, mount an immune response, and maintain the function of vital organs and skeletal muscle. Furthermore, malnutrition can cause longer hospital stays (which increase costs), higher morbidity and mortality rates, and a greater incidence of postoperative complications.[10]

Lack of understanding of the role of nutrition in recovery from disease may explain why weight loss often goes unnoticed, diets often are inadequate, and patients are allowed to reach an advanced state of depletion (which may be irreversible). Poor communication among various health care providers probably makes a major contribution to PCM. Because PCM is preventable and generally occurs while another disease is being treated, it is often referred to as *physician-induced malnutrition.*

When you first see the word *gut* it may seem out of place, but actually it's a shorthand way of referring to the GI tract.

primary deficiency: a nutrient deficiency caused by deficient intake of a nutrient.

secondary deficiency: a nutrient deficiency caused not by deficient intake but by impaired digestion, absorption, transport, metabolism, or excretion of a nutrient.

immune response: the body's system for defending against viruses, bacteria, and other foreign agents (see Highlight 22).

morbidity: unhealthiness; disease.

mortality: death.

Physician-induced malnutrition, technically, is **iatrogenic malnutrition** (ee-AT-ro-GEN-ic). This term includes malnutrition caused by prescription medication (see Highlight 17).

iatros = physician
genic = arising from

---

[9]W. Steffee, Malnutrition in hospitalized patients, *Journal of the American Medical Association* 244 (1980):2630-2635.

[10]Mullen et al., 1979; Weinsier et al., 1979.

The fact that a patient enters the hospital in good nutrition status is no guarantee that he or she will stay well nourished. Studies have shown that nutrition status often deteriorates during the course of hospitalization.[11] Therapy should be designed to maintain or improve nutrition status. Patients must be reassessed routinely to assure that the goals of nutrition therapy are being met.

Components of Nutrition Assessment

anthropometric: relating to measurement of the physical characteristics of the body, such as height and weight.

anthropos = human
metric = measuring

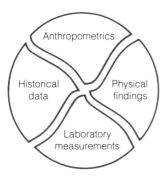

Figure 1 When you look at each parameter of nutrition assessment separately, the information you gather is difficult to interpret. But taken as a whole, the pieces fit together to form a complete picture of the person's nutrition status.

objective: based on facts.

subjective: influenced by judgment and perceptions rather than facts.

Many factors influence or reflect nutrition status. Consequently, information from many sources can help you make a nutrition assessment. These sources include anthropometric measurements, laboratory tests, physical examinations, and historical data. Although these sources make up a fairly extensive list, you can obtain most of this information routinely. For example, hospital admitting forms record such data as sex, age, height, weight, medical history, medications, diet, allergies, and complaints. Furthermore, some lab tests and a physical examination are routinely administered on admission to the hospital. These data can then be expanded and pulled together to describe an individual's nutrition status.

Anthropometric measurements and laboratory tests are relatively objective and are particularly valuable in assessing PCM. On the other hand, historical information is relatively subjective, because the information obtained is often dependent on the skills of the interviewer and the patient's cooperation, understanding, and memory. You can use historical information to determine food intake and factors (such as disease states and drugs) which may change your patient's nutrient needs. More importantly, historical information defines who a person is and what factors influence that person's eating habits. After all, intervention can only be successful if you tailor diet advice to the individual's needs.

Anthropometric and biochemical data are considered to be objective because they reflect measurable body compartments. But this type of data is not absolutely objective because the measurements are made by people, and the tools they use are also made by people.

As will be discussed, the accuracy of anthropometric measurements depends largely on the skills of the people who make them. The equipment used for such measurements isn't necessarily accurate. Additionally, the standards used for determining what is "normal" are adequate for populations but not for individuals. We do not know what measurements are "optimal" for each person.

[11] Mullen et al., 1979; Weinsier et al., 1979.

Similar problems are apparent with biochemical measurements. In the long run, then, none of these measurements are truly objective.

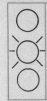

CAUTION:

Biochemical and anthropometric measurements are only "relatively" objective.

You have many resources available for obtaining the information needed for assessment. The patient's medical record is a good place to start. You can obtain additional information by talking with the patient, the family, and other health care providers; by using the drug record; and by observing what the patient eats.

An understanding of the community environment is also important in assessing nutrition status. For example, it is useful for you to know something about the food habits of the major ethnic groups within your locale, regional food preferences, and nutrition resources and programs available in the community. Local health departments and social agencies often can provide such information.

The more information you get about a person, the more accurate your assessment will be. But gathering information is a time-consuming process, and time is often a rare commodity in the health care setting. Recognizing that nutrition care is only one part of total care, you may not always find it practical or essential to collect detailed information on each person.

Later in the chapter, we will discuss which individuals need complete nutrition assessments. While you read through the following sections, keep in mind that, in the majority of hospitals, not all the parameters discussed are used routinely on each person. Furthermore, assessment data are more meaningful if interpreted by someone who has had extensive training and experience. A clinical dietitian is most likely to have those qualifications.

A **drug record** is a list of all medications a patient is to receive; the time each drug is given is recorded as well as the initials of the nurse administering the drug.

A **parameter** is one of a set of factors that characterize the whole (in this case, the whole is nutrition status).

Anthropometric Data

Anthropometrics are physical measurements which reflect growth and development. Anthropometrics taken on an individual are compared with standards specific for sex and age. These standards are derived from measurements taken on large numbers of people.

somatic: a term used to refer to the frame of the body as opposed to internal organs.

soma = body

somatic protein: skeletal muscle.

somatic fat: subcutaneous fat or fat found directly beneath the skin.

Height and weight are well-recognized anthropometrics. Others include the midarm circumference and various fatfold measurements. Anthropometrics provide an indirect assessment of skeletal muscle and body fat. Some are measured in specific situations, such as head circumference in infancy and abdominal girth in liver disease. Anthropometrics are particularly useful when you measure them periodically.

Anthropometric measurements are easy to take, and little equipment is required. However, their accuracy and value are limited by the skills of the measurer. Mastering the correct techniques takes time, and you need plenty of practice before you can use them reliably. Furthermore, significant changes in measurements are slow to occur in adults. When changes do occur in adults, they represent prolonged changes in nutrient intake.

Height-Weight   Growth retardation in infants and young children is an important sign of poor nutrition status. Once adult height has been reached, changes in body weight are useful in assessing overnutrition and undernutrition.

Although special equipment is available to measure an infant's length (see Figure 2), in many settings a less accurate method is used: With the infant lying on a flat surface, a measuring tape is run along the side of the baby from the top of the head to the heel of the foot. Regardless of the method used, care should be taken to insure that the infant's legs and body are straight. Since this is difficult to accomplish, it requires two people to obtain an accurate measurement.

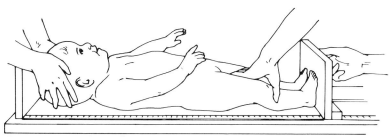

Illustration courtesy of Ross Laboratories.

Figure 2   An infant is measured lying down by use of a length measuring device with a fixed headboard and movable footboard. Note that two people are needed to measure the infant's length.

A child that can stand erect and cooperate can be measured in the same manner as an adult. The best way to measure height is to have the person being measured stand against a flat wall to which a measuring tape or stick has been affixed (see Figure 3). The person should not be wearing shoes and should stand erect with heels together. The person's line of sight should be horizontal, and the heels, buttocks, shoulders,

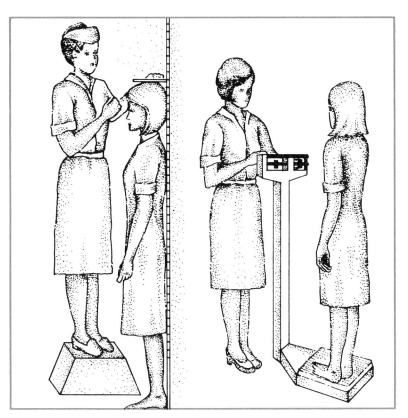

Figure 3   Height is measured most accurately when the person stands against a flat wall to which a measuring tape has been affixed. When the person is taller than the measurer, the measurer can stand on a stool to help insure that the proper height measurement is obtained.

Figure 4   Whenever possible, subjects are measured on beam balance scales to insure accuracy.

and head should be touching the wall. After carefully checking the height measurement, you should record the result immediately to avoid misplacing or forgetting the measurement. Height is recorded in either inches or centimeters, depending on the policy of the institution.

Although less desirable, the measuring rod of a scale can be used to measure height by using the same general procedure described above. The person should be facing away from the scale and extra care should be taken to insure that the person is standing as straight as possible.

Unfortunately, it is a common and inexcusable practice in many health care institutions to ask clients how tall they are, rather than measuring their height. A recent study of 1,610 men and 1,799 women found that men, particularly short men, tended to overestimate their

Inches (in)
$$= \text{centimeters (cm)} \times 2.54$$
$$\text{cm} = \frac{\text{in}}{2.54}$$

Checking the accuracy of an instrument is known as calibration. It's done by measuring a known quantity. For example, to calibrate a scale you weigh an item of known weight and then check to see if the scale measures the weight correctly. If not, you adjust the scale.

height while women tended to underestimate their height.[12] The height measurement may not be critical in itself, but it is used to estimate desirable weight and to interpret other assessment data. You should use self-reported height only as a last resort when measurement is not practical (in the case of an uncooperative patient, an emergency admission, or the like).

In adults, weight measurements should be taken on a beam balance which frequently is checked for accuracy (see Figure 4). By standardizing the conditions under which you weigh people, you increase the usability of repeated weight measurements. Whenever possible, a person should be weighed after voiding at the same time of day (preferably before breakfast), in the same amount of clothing (hospital gown, without shoes), and on the same scale. Bedridden patients can be measured with metabolic scales (see Figure 5). Bathroom scales are not accurate and should not be used. As with all measurements, you should record observed weight immediately.

You can compare weight measurements with desirable weight tables (see inside back cover), which are specific for height, sex, and frame size. The limitations of these tables have been discussed previously (p. 261).

A method of estimating frame size has been developed from a study

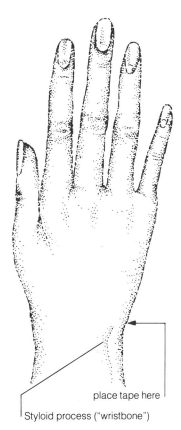

place tape here

Styloid process ("wristbone")

Figure 6 The wrist circumference is measured as shown above.

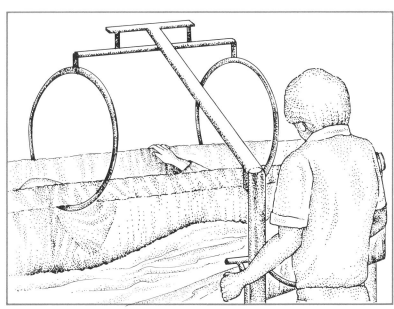

Figure 5 Metabolic bed scales are used to measure patients who cannot get out of bed.

[12] P. Pirie, D. Jacobs, R. Jeffery, and P. Hannon, Distortion in self-reported height and weight data, *Journal of the American Dietetic Association* 78 (1981):601-606.

of more than 100 males and 100 females.[13] The study compared the ratio (r) of height to wrist circumference and derived the expression for frame size shown in Table 1.

After you have determined frame size, you can easily locate the desirable or "ideal" weight range. Using a weight range, rather than pinpointing one weight, is a good reminder that we cannot determine a "perfect" weight for anyone.

By calculating the *percent ideal body weight* (%IBW) you can roughly estimate the degree of overnutrition or undernutrition. A %IBW greater than 115-120 is indicative of obesity. Undernutrition is evaluated as shown in Table 2.

A more valuable parameter for assessing weight measurements is the *percent usual body weight* (%UBW), which considers what is normal for a particular individual (see Table 3 and Highlight 8). You can easily overlook malnutrition in an obese subject when using %IBW rather than %UBW. The subject, family or friends, and older medical records are sources of information regarding usual weight.

You can determine any *recent weight change* by relating the %UBW to the time period over which a change, if any, has occurred. A 5 percent weight loss might be significant if it occurred within a month yet might not be significant if it occurred over five months. Always ask the patient about the weight change. Was the change intentional? Why does the patient feel his or her weight has changed? You may want to keep in mind that all weight measurements are difficult to evaluate in hospitalized patients. Diseases or therapy can cause fluid retention and mask significant weight loss. In fact, starvation itself is accompanied by an increase in extracellular fluid volume.[14]

$$\%IBW = \frac{\text{Actual weight}}{\text{Usual weight}^*} \times 100$$

$$\%UBW = \frac{\text{Actual weight}}{\text{Ideal weight}^*} \times 100$$

*Use the midpoint of the ideal weight range.

Recent weight change: remember to ask!

B.J. is a 45-year-old male of medium frame size with a height of 5′8″. He currently weighs 115 pounds. He has lost 15 pounds in the last month.

$$\%IBW = \frac{115 \text{ lbs} \times 100}{145 \text{ lbs}} = 79\%$$

Interpretation: Moderately depleted.

$$\%IBW = \frac{115 \text{ lbs} \times 100}{130 \text{ lbs}} = 89\%$$

Interpretation: Mildly depleted.

Recent weight change — weight loss is significant (almost 4 lb/week).

Table 1. Determining Frame Size from Height-Wrist Circumference Ratios (r)

	Male r values*	Female r values*
Small	>10.4	>11.0
Medium	9.6-10.4	10.1-11.0
Large	<9.6	<10.1

$$^*r = \frac{\text{Height (cm)}}{\text{Wrist circumference (cm)}\dagger}$$

†The wrist is measured where it bends (distal to the styloid process), on the right arm (see Figure 6).

[13]J. P. Grant, Patient selection, *Handbook of Total Parenteral Nutrition* (Philadelphia: Saunders, 1980), p. 15.

[14]H. M. Shizgal, A. H. Spanier, and R. S. Kurtz, Effect of parenteral nutrition on body composition in the critically ill patient, *American Journal of Surgery* 131 (1976):156-161; D. H. Elwyn, C. W. Bryan-Brown, and W. C. Shoemaker, Nutritional aspects of body water dislocations in postoperative and depleted patients, *Annals of Surgery* 182 (1975):76-84.

Figure 7   Examples of the use of growth charts. Growth charts are especially useful when a *sequence* of measurements can be made at intervals (for example, a year apart). Weights for age alone are not meaningful; they always have to be compared with heights. This figure gives you an idea of their usefulness; for actual interpretation see references on growth assessment.*

*An excellent reference is S. J. Fomon, *Nutritional Disorders of Children — Prevention, Screening and Followup*, DHEW publication no. (HSA) 77-5104 (Washington, D.C.: Government Printing Office, 1977), pp. 14-45.

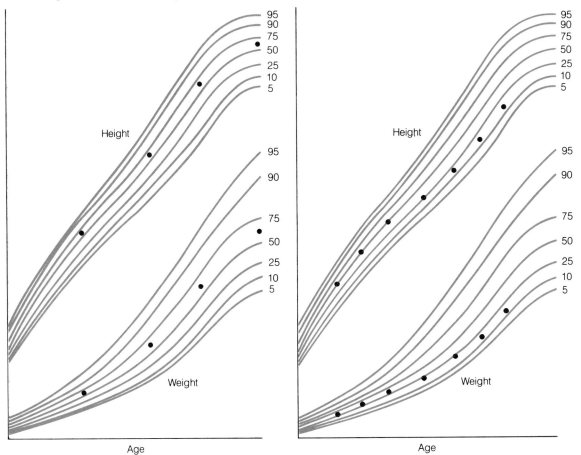

Figure 7a   Each percentile line divides the population into two segments. For example, the 25th percentile line divides the lower 25 percent of the population from the upper 75 percent. A child whose height is right on the 25th percentile line is taller than 25 percent of his age mates.

The points on this growth chart show how a normally growing child's height and weight might appear if graphed 4 times at 3-year intervals. Both height and weight fall between the 50th and 75th percentile lines each time they are plotted.

Figure 7b   This child's record suggests a failure of growth. He was graphed on the 50th percentile line on 3 successive visits, then fell to the 25th and then toward the 10th. Both height and weight were affected, a finding consistent with severe illness or malnutrition. Such a child should be further evaluated.

What makes the later points on this graph notable is the *comparison with the earlier points*. When a growth curve crosses a percentile line, it should be noticed. The last measurements taken, by themselves, would tell very little. Another child whose height and weight fell at the 15th percentile might turn out to be a perfectly normal child, just small — but you could only know this by noting that his previous measurements had all been at the 15th percentile.

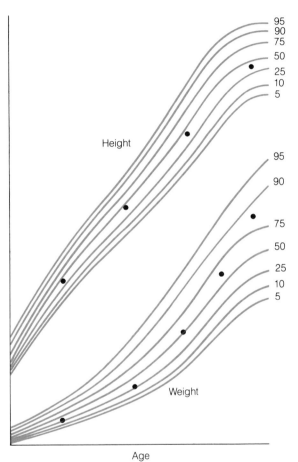

95
90
75
50
25
10
5

Height

95

90

75

50

25
10
5

Weight

Age

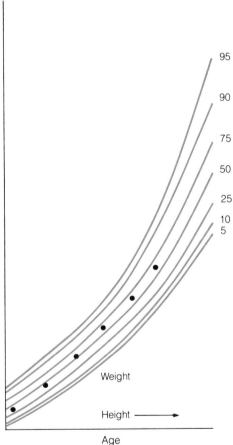

95

90

75

50

25

10
5

Weight

Height ⟶

Age

Figure 7c   This child has been gaining weight dispro-portionately fast relative to his gain in height. His weight has crossed two percentile lines while his growth in height is as expected. He should be evaluated further and may need nutrition consultation.

As in B, the weight and height measurements have to be assessed together to be interpreted correctly.

Figure 7d   Percentile data for height and weight can also be combined into a single set of weight-height curves. This graph shows that after 5 clinic visits in which this child's weight for height was right at the 50th percentile, his weight shot up to above the 95th percentile. The measurement should first be checked for error (perhaps it was misrecorded); if it is correct it suggests the onset of obesity and a need for further evaluation and consultation.

Generally, weights for height above the 95th percen-tile and below the 5th percentile are cause for concern.

Table 2. Relationship between Degree of Undernutrition and % IBW

% IBW	Degree of undernutrition
80-90%	Mildly depleted
70-79%	Moderately depleted
<70%	Severely depleted

Adapted from J. P. Grant, Patient selection, *Handbook of Total Parenteral Nutrition* (Philadelphia: Saunders, 1980), p. 11.

Table 3. Relationship between Degree of Undernutrition and % UBW

% UBW	Degree of undernutrition
85-95%	Mildly depleted
75-84%	Moderately depleted
<75%	Severely depleted

Adapted from J. P. Grant, Patient selection, *Handbook of Total Parenteral Nutrition* (Philadelphia: Saunders, 1980), p. 11.

We generally evaluate growth in infants and children by monitoring the rate of growth (height and weight) and comparing this rate to standard growth charts. (See Appendix E for growth charts.) Again, weight must be considered in relation to height — height and weight should be in approximately the same percentile. Although individual growth measurements may vary, in general, growth should be maintained along the same percentile throughout childhood (see Figure 7). In growth-retarded children, it is desirable that height and weight reach a higher percentile. In overweight children, weight should remain relatively stable as height increases, until weight becomes appropriate for height.

Because intrauterine growth proceeds at a faster rate than postpartum growth, special growth charts are available for use with premature infants. Weight gain grids also are available to assess weight gain in pregnant women (see Appendix E).

Midarm Circumference and Fatfolds   Midarm circumference is measured with a nonstretchable tape measure midway between the shoulder and the elbow (see Figure 8). The midarm circumference measures muscle mass and subcutaneous fat. This measurement decreases with both acute and chronic undernutrition and increases in obesity.

Approximately half the fat in our bodies is directly below the skin. In some parts of the body, this fat is more loosely attached, and you can pull it up between the thumb and forefinger. You can use these sites for measuring fatfold thickness (see Figure 9). By estimating subcutaneous fat, you get an idea of total body fat. Since fat stores decrease very slowly with inadequate energy intake, depletion of subcutaneous fat can reflect either long-term undernutrition or successful weight loss through dieting.

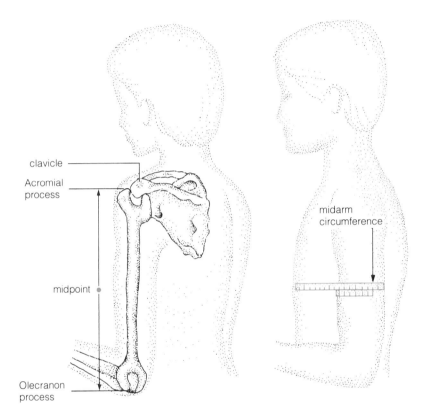

Figure 8   Finding the midpoint and midarm circumference.

1. Ask the subject to bend his arm at the elbow and lay his hand across his stomach. (If he is right-handed, measure the left arm, and vice versa.)

2. Feel the shoulder to locate the acromial process. It helps to slide your fingers along the clavicle to find the acromial process. The olecranon process is the tip of the elbow.

3. Place a measuring tape from the acromial process to the tip of the elbow. Divide this measurement by 2 and mark the midpoint of the arm with a pen.

4. Next, ask the subject to let his arm hang loosely at his side. Place the measuring tape horizontally around the arm at the midpoint mark. This measurement is the midarm circumference.

Figure 9 Measuring the triceps skinfold.

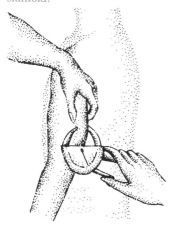

1. Find the midpoint of the arm.

2. Ask the subject to let his arm hang loosely at his side.

3. Grasp a fold of skin and subcutaneous fat between the thumb and forefinger slightly above the midpoint mark. Gently pull the skin away from the underlying muscle. (This step takes a lot of practice. If you want to be sure you don't have muscle as well as fat, ask the subject to contract and relax his muscle. You should be able to feel if you are pinching muscle.)

4. Place the calipers over the fatfold at the midpoint mark and read the measurement to the nearest 1.0 mm in 2 to 3 seconds. (If using plastic calipers, align pressure lines and read measurement to the nearest 1.0 mm in 2 to 3 seconds.)

5. Repeat steps 2 to 4 twice more. Add the 3 readings and then divide by 3 to find the average.

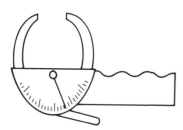

Precision skinfold calipers provide the most accurate tool for measuring skinfold thickness. A tool for calibrating the caliper is also available.

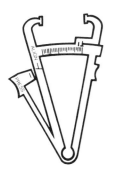

Plastic calipers are less expensive and easy to obtain. Although they are less accurate than standard calipers, they are an acceptable substitute.

Several types of calipers are available for making fatfold measurements. The most commonly used site for measuring fatfold thickness is the upper midarm, in the same area as the midarm circumference. This measurement, the triceps skinfold or triceps fatfold, is widely used because the upper midarm is easily accessible. Together with the midarm circumference, it can be used to calculate the derived midarm muscle circumference.

The midarm muscle circumference is derived indirectly, because it cannot be measured. Rather, it is obtained mathematically. Basically, you consider the arm to be circular and then subtract the fatfold circumference from the midarm circumference (Figure 10). The midarm muscle circumference is a measurement of muscle mass and, thus, is used as an indicator of protein nutriture.

Triceps skinfold, midarm circumference, and midarm muscle circumference measurements should be compared with percentile standards. The standards are shown in Appendix E.

Fatfold measurements, midarm circumference, and therefore, derived midarm muscle circumference are reproducible measurements if standard procedure is followed. Taking them according to standard procedure requires practice, however. Generally, the same person should measure the same subject routinely for best results.

Head Circumference Head circumference is generally measured in children under three years of age. Since the brain is rapidly growing during this time, it is believed that malnourished children will have fewer brain cells and a smaller head circumference. As with height and weight, you plot the measured head circumference on a percentile growth chart. Head circumference percentile should be similar to weight and height percentiles.

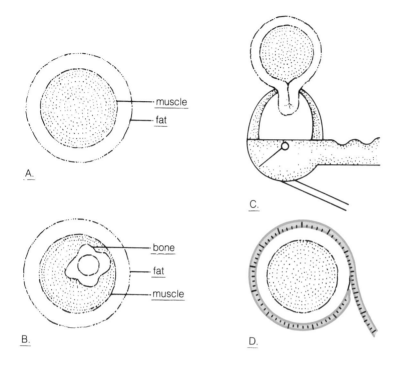

Midarm muscle
  circumference (cm)
    = Midarm circumference (cm)
    − [0.314* × Triceps
      skinfold (mm)]

*This factor converts the single skin-fold measurement to a *circumference* measurement and also converts the millimeters to centimeters.

B.J. has a midarm circumference of 24 cm (<5th percentile) and a triceps skinfold of 8 mm (about 25th percentile).

Midarm muscle circumference
  = 24 cm − (0.314 × 8 mm)

Midarm muscle circumference
  = 21.5 cm (<5th percentile)

Interpretation: All anthropomet-rics reveal significant depletion.

Figure 10 How the midarm muscle circumference is derived.

a The arm is visualized as an inner circle of muscle surrounded by an outer circle of fat.

b In reality, the arm is not circular, and there is some bone, but the simplified picture is approximately correct.

c This measurement (the fatfold) gives you two times the thickness of the fat.

d This measurement (the tape-measured outer circumference of the arm) defines the total area (muscle plus fat).

e The equation then subtracts the outer ring of fat from the total area, leaving the *area of the muscle*, an index of the body's total skeletal muscle mass.

In many facilities, arm an-thropometric measurements are compared with a single standard rather than percentile tables. These standards assume that one measurement is standard for every adult regardless of age or body frame. Furthermore, the single standards were developed for different purposes and on different population groups. Therefore, the use of percentile tables is recommended.

Laboratory Tests of Nutrition Status

While anthropometrics are used for measuring and assessing observable changes in the body, lab tests serve a different function — they help determine what's happening inside the body. Blood and urine samples are used to directly measure a nutrient or a metabolite (end product or enzyme) that is affected by that nutrient.

visceral protein: the protein contained in the blood and internal organs.

Biochemical measurements often can be used to detect subclinical malnutrition. The most common lab tests used in hospitals today for nutrition assessment help uncover PCM. These include albumin, transferrin, total lymphocyte count, nitrogen balance, and creatinine excretion tests. Although less commonly used, other lab tests are valuable in assessing vitamin, mineral, and trace element nutriture.

Blood tests often are ordered in packages which include several measurements. These packages are often referred to as SMAs followed by a number (e.g., SMA-l2 or SMA-l8). SMA means **simultaneous multiple analysis** and the number following SMA tells how many tests will be run.

Serum is the watery portion of the blood that remains after the cells and clot-forming material (fibrinogen) have been removed; **plasma** is unclotted blood. In most cases serum and plasma concentrations are similar to one another. The serum sample often is preferred because plasma samples occasionally clog the mechanical blood analyzers.

The word *laboratory* generally conjures up thoughts of precision and accuracy. Laboratory tests are generally performed with great care to assure accurate results. When a test result is obviously "way out of the normal range," the test is usually run again. But it is very important to recognize that many factors can influence lab test results and their subsequent interpretation.

One of the biggest problems is establishing "normal" values for test results. Individual values often differ from norms without apparent reason. The concentration of various blood constituents varies normally both within the individual and between individuals.[15] Considering how many lab tests are run daily in even one hospital, these variations are very significant. Some factors involved in normal variation include genetic influences, age, sex, environment, body build, diet, season, time of day, biological rhythm, posture when blood sample is drawn, immobilization, exercise, and administration of certain drugs.

Another consideration is that reference populations used to define "normal" and "deficient" ranges for lab tests may not be clearly defined, or they may be applied to hospitalized patients when they were established for "normal" subjects. All of this means that even lab test results must be interpreted with caution.

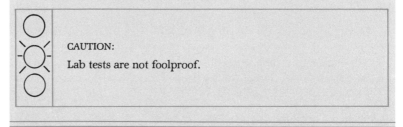

CAUTION:
Lab tests are not foolproof.

Laboratory tests and physical findings useful in assessing vitamin, mineral, and trace element status are listed in Table 4. Vitamin and mineral levels present in the blood and urine sometimes represent recent intake rather than long-term intake. This makes detecting a subclinical deficiency difficult. Furthermore, many nutrients interact; you should keep in mind that a lab value for one nutrient can be affected by the amounts of other nutrients in the body.

[15]S. Brown, F. Mitchell, and D. Young, eds., *Chemical Diagnosis of Disease* (Amsterdam: Elsevier/North-Holland Biomedical Press, 1979), p. 5.

Urinary Creatinine Excretion Creatinine excretion reflects skeletal muscle mass, because creatinine is a breakdown product of an energy source that is present specifically in skeletal muscle. Creatinine is excreted at a constant rate determined by the amount of skeletal muscle. As skeletal muscle atrophies during malnutrition, creatinine excretion decreases. Standards for creatinine excretion have been developed based on sex and height (see Appendix E). They are used along with the measured creatinine to derive the creatinine-height index (CHI):

$$\frac{\text{Measured urinary creatinine (24 hr sample)}}{\text{Standard creatinine for height}} \times 100$$

The measurement of urinary creatinine requires a 24-hour urine collection, which is often difficult to obtain. The test is invalid if the subject shows signs of kidney disease, since the disease might reduce the ability to excrete creatinine.

Albumin Albumin accounts for over 50 percent of the total serum proteins. It helps to maintain fluid and electrolyte balance and to transport bilirubin and many nutrients, hormones, and drugs. Albumin synthesis is dependent on the existence of functioning liver cells as well as on an appropriate supply of amino acids. Because there is so much albumin in the body and because it is not broken down by the body very quickly, albumin concentrations change slowly. Therefore, albumin is a useful indicator of prolonged protein depletion. Unlike creatinine, albumin levels can reflect the protein status of the blood and internal organs.

Many other conditions besides malnutrition can depress albumin concentration, including liver disease, nephrotic syndrome (advanced kidney disease), infection, cancer, and burns. Therefore, as is true for *all* parameters used in nutrition assessment, albumin cannot be used alone to determine protein status, but rather as one indicator among many.

Transferrin Transferrin is a protein that transports iron between the intestine and sites of hemoglobin synthesis and degradation. It is considered a more sensitive indicator of protein malnutrition than albumin, because it responds more promptly to changes in protein intake and has a smaller body pool.

Most transferrin is synthesized in the liver. Its concentration is inversely related to iron stores; transferrin levels are high in iron deficiency and low when iron storage is excessive. Therefore, the presence of abnormal iron nutriture makes interpretation of transferrin levels difficult. Liver disease, nephrotic syndrome, and burns also cause decreases in transferrin levels.

B.J.'s urinary creatinine excretion was 1,090 mg/24 hr.

$$\text{CHI} = \frac{1,090 \text{ mg} \times 100}{1,557 \text{ mg}} = 70\%$$

Interpretation: Based on the creatinine-height index, B.J.'s skeletal muscle mass is approximately 70% of that which would be expected in a man his size.

B.J. had a serum albumin of 2.4 g/100 ml.

Interpretation: B.J.'s serum albumin is moderately depleted (see Table 5).

Table 4. Selected Laboratory Tests and Physical Findings Useful for Assessing Some Vitamin and Mineral Deficiencies

	Laboratory test(s) used for assessment	Physical findings associated with deficiency
Vitamins		
Vitamin A	Serum vitamin A Serum carotene	Triangular, gray spots on eye; dryness of eye membranes and skin; softening of the cornea; plugging of hair follicles with keratin
Thiamin	Urinary thiamin Thiamin load test RBC transketolase	Loss of ankle and knee jerks; calf muscle pain; edema; wasting; mental confusion
Riboflavin	Urinary riboflavin RBC glutathione reductase Riboflavin load test	Dermatitis around lips and nostrils; cracking at corners of mouth; reddening of eyes; magenta-colored tongue
Niacin	Urinary N-methyl-nicotinamide Urinary 2-pyridone	Bilateral symmetrical dermatitis; swollen, edematous tongue; mental confusion
Vitamin B_6	Tryptophan load test Urinary B_6 Blood transaminase Blood B_6	Dermatitis; cracking of corners of mouth; smooth, red tongue
Folacin	RBC folate Urinary formiminoglu-tamic acid Serum folate	Smooth, swollen tongue with cracking
Vitamin B_{12}	Serum B_{12} B_{12} isotope methods Urinary methylmalonic acid Schilling test	Smooth, swollen tongue; heightened sensitivity of skin
Vitamin C	Serum vitamin C Urinary vitamin C Vitamin C load test	Swollen, spongy, bleeding gums; petechiae; poor wound healing

Table 4.   Selected Laboratory Tests and Physical Findings Useful for Assessing Some Vitamin and Mineral Deficiencies (continued)

	Laboratory test(s) used for assessment	Physical findings associated with deficiency
Vitamin D	Serum 25-hydroxy-cholecalciferol Serum alkaline phosphatase Serum calcium and phosphorus	Bowing of legs; beading of ribs; knock knees, wrist enlargement
Vitamin E	Hydrogen peroxide hemolysis test Plasma tocopherol	Edema in infants
Vitamin K	Prothrombin time	Bruising
Minerals		
Calcium	Serum calcium	Rickets; seizures
Magnesium	Serum magnesium	Tetany (extreme muscle contraction); muscle weakness
Iron	Hemoglobin Hematocrit Iron binding capacity	Pale nail beds, eye membranes, and palmar creases
Iodine	Serum protein-bound iodine Urinary iodine Radioiodine uptake	Enlarged thyroid
Zinc	Serum or plasma zinc Hair zinc concentration	Skin rash; hair loss; growth retardation

Table 5.   Relationship between Degree of Undernutrition and Serum Proteins

Degree of depletion	Indicator	
	Albumin (g/100 ml)	Transferrin (mg/100 ml)
Mild	2.8-3.4	150-200
Moderate	2.1-2.7	100-149
Severe	<2.1	<100

Total lymphocyte count (mm³)
   = WBC × % lymphocytes
   (mm³)

B.J.'s WBC count was 7,500 with 15% lymphocytes.

Total lymphocyte count (mm³)
   = 7,500 mm³ × 0.15
   = 1125 mm³

Interpretation: By this standard, too, B.J.'s nutrition status is moderately depleted.

induration: a raised, hardened area of skin.

   durus = hard

Some labs do not have the equipment necessary to determine transferrin levels directly. However, a reasonable estimate can be made by measuring total iron binding capacity (TIBC), a test which is widely available. The equation for converting TIBC to transferrin should be determined individually by each lab.[16]

Other serum proteins have been used to assess protein status, including thyroxin binding prealbumin[17] and retinol binding protein.[18] These tests are not in wide use at this time.

Measuring Immune Status   Various forms of PCM as well as individual nutrient deficiencies have been associated with depression of the immune system (see Highlight 22). The total number of lymphocytes appears to decrease as protein depletion occurs; so the total lymphocyte count is one index useful in nutrition assessment.

Another test of immune function is antigen skin testing. Organisms (usually three or four kinds) to which most people are immune are injected just under the skin. After 48 hours, the sites of the injections are inspected for raised, hardened areas (induration). Induration will be apparent in the well-nourished person, but in the malnourished person, hardened areas will not appear or will be very small.

Many factors other than nutrition can interfere with the immune response, and the value of skin testing as an index of nutrition status has recently been questioned.[19] No studies to date have considered all of the factors that might affect skin test results. Among these factors are age, certain allergies, and chemotherapy.

Nitrogen Balance   Nitrogen balance studies are useful in estimating the degree to which protein is being depleted or repleted in the body. A simple approach to measuring nitrogen is to measure urine urea nitrogen (UUN) on a 24-hour urine collection. During the same 24-hour period, an accurate record of the subject's protein (nitrogen) intake must be kept to complete the balance study.

Nitrogen intake is calculated by dividing protein intake (g) by 6.25 (g nitrogen/g protein). Nitrogen output equals the UUN plus a factor of 4 g to account for nitrogen lost through the lungs, hair, skin, and nails as well as nonurea nitrogen losses in the urine. The equation for nitrogen balance is:

$$\text{N balance} = \frac{\text{Protein (g)}}{6.25} - (\text{UUN g} + 4 \text{ g})$$

[16]J. P. Grant, P. C. Custer, and J. Thurlow, Current techniques of nutritional assessment, *Surgical Clinics of North America* 61 (1981):437-463.

[17]Y. Ingenbleek, M. DeVisscher, and P. DeNayer, Measurement of prealbumin as an index of protein-calorie malnutrition, *Lancet* 2 (1972):106-108.

[18]P. Peterson, Demonstration in serum of two physiologic forms of human retinal binding protein, *European Journal of Clinical Investigation* 1 (1971):437-444.

[19]P. Twomey, D. Ziegler, and J. Rombeau, Utility of skin testing in nutritional assessment: A critical review, *Journal of Parenteral and Enteral Nutrition* 6 (1982):50-58.

Table 6.   Summary of Body Compartments Assessed by Biochemical and Anthropometric Measurements

Assessment parameter	Body fat	Skeletal muscle	Visceral protein	Immune competence
Weight	X	X		
MAC	X	X		
MAMC		X		
TSF	X			
CHI		X		
Albumin			X	
Transferrin			X	
TLC			X	X
Skin testing				X

MAC: midarm circumference.
MAMC: midarm muscle circumference.
TSF: triceps skinfold.
CHI: creatinine height index.
TLC: total lymphocyte count.

Positive (N) balance
= N intake > N output

Nitrogen (N) balance
= N intake − N output

Negative (N) balance
= N intake < N output

B.J. had a protein intake of 45 g/24 hr and a urine urea nitrogen of 10 g/24 hr.

$$\text{N balance} = \frac{45g}{6.25} - (10g + 4g)$$
$$= 7.2g - 14g$$
$$= -6.8g$$

Interpretation: B.J. is in negative nitrogen balance; his intake of nitrogen is less than his body needs.

As with creatinine excretion, the kidneys must be functioning properly for measurement to be accurate. Additionally, abnormally high nitrogen losses (such as through burns) must be considered if this test is to be valid.

Nitrogen balance studies provide a prime example of the need for communication and cooperation between various health care providers and departments. A nitrogen balance study would be completely invalid if one urine specimen were thrown away or if food intake from one meal was not recorded. The whole procedure would have to be repeated. Consider the inconvenience to the patient as well as the waste of valuable staff time.

Laboratory tests add a dimension to nutrition assessment. However, as emphasized earlier, many factors influence lab tests; therefore, you cannot rely on a single test to assess nutrition status.

Physical Findings

Clues to a person's nutrition status can be identified by examining the person for clinical signs of malnutrition. However, many of these signs, too, are nonspecific; they can be associated with many nutrient deficiencies or can be unrelated to nutrition. So, again, physical findings can only be interpreted in light of other assessment findings.

Physical signs of malnutrition appear most rapidly in parts of the body where cells are being replaced at a high rate, such as in the hair, skin, and gastrointestinal tract. Table 7 lists some of the easily detectable signs of malnutrition and the nutrient deficiencies to which they are related.

Table 7. Physical Findings Associated with Various Nutrient Imbalances

Physical findings	Protein-kcalorie	Vitamin A	B vitamins	Vitamin C	Vitamin D	Iron	Other
Hair							
Dull, dry, sparse, readily plucked, lighter and darker bands (flag sign), depigmentation	X						
Face							
Swollen	X						
Dark areas of skin over eyes and under cheeks, flaky skin around nose		X					
Pale		X				X	
Eyes							
Triangular, shiny gray spots on exposed portion of conjunctiva (mucous membrane lining eyelid)		X					
Dull, opaque, or dry cornea		X					
Softening of cornea, inner eyelids		X					
Inner eyelids and whites dry and pigmented		X					
Cracked and red at corners			X				
Pale conjunctiva			X			X	
White ring around iris							Elevated blood-lipids
Raised yellow spots on eye							Elevated blood lipids
Lips							
Bilateral redness, cracking, scaling or scarring at corners of mouth			X				
Swollen, red lips with vertical cracks			X				
Tongue							
Swollen, magenta colored			X				
Smooth surface			X				
Atrophy of the surface structures			X				
Bright red, painful			X				

Table 7.   Physical Findings Associated with Various Nutrient Imbalances (continued)

	Protein-kcalorie	Vitamin A	B vitamins	Vitamin C	Vitamin D	Iron	Other
Teeth							
Caries							Excess sugar
Mottled enamel							Excess fluoride
Gums							
Bleeding, spongy, receding				X			
Glands							
Enlarged thyroid gland (located at front of neck)							Iodine
Enlarged parotid gland (located just below earlobes)	X						General undernutrition
Skin							
Depigmentation, patches of hyperpigmented skin which peels off (flaky-paint dermatosis)	X						
Dry, scaling, rough (skin may appear to have permanent goosebumps)		X					Essential fatty acids
Bilateral hyperpigmentation with redness and swelling on body areas exposed to sunlight; scrotal or vulval dermatosis			X				
Small red or purple skin hemorrhages				X			
Nails							
Spoon-shaped, brittle, ridged						X	
Pale nail beds						X	
Subcutaneous tissue							
Edematous (swollen)	X						
Decreased fat stores	X						
Excessive fat stores							Obesity

Table 7. Physical Findings Associated with
Various Nutrient Imbalances (continued)

	Protein-kcalorie	Vitamin A	B vitamins	Vitamin C	Vitamin D	Iron	Other
Musculoskeletal system							
Wasting of skeletal muscle	X						
Bleeding into muscles				X			
Enlarged wrists, knees, ankles				X	X		
Infants — softening of the back and sides of skull; bilateral enlargement at the front and sides of head; failure of soft spot to harden					X		
Beadlike lumps on sides of chest wall; bowed legs					X		Calcium
Bone fragility, chest deformities					X		
Nervous system							
Apathy	X						
Mental confusion; calf tenderness, loss of knee and ankle reflexes; sensory loss; loss of sense of balance and vibration; heightened sensitivity			X				
Other							
GI system: Enlarged liver and spleen	X						General undernutrition
Cardiovascular system: Enlarged heart, rapid heart rate			X				
High blood pressure							Excess sodium; obesity

Historical Data

Historical data are an extremely important part of nutrition assessment. Although such data are often subjective, they reveal many important facts about a person. Furthermore, through history taking you get a good sense of the whole person and really begin to understand him or her. An adept history taker uses the initial interview not only to gather facts but also to establish rapport.

In this section, we will only briefly review major points of significance in historical data, or the "whats" of history taking. The next chapter provides more detail on the "how" of history taking, and later chapters will further explain "why" certain factors are important in the nutrition assessment.

Medical History Most often, the medical record or chart contains the person's complete medical history. However, by conversing with the person, you can uncover valuable medical information which was not recorded because "no one asked" or because the patient was too upset on admission to think clearly.

The purpose of establishing a sound medical history when assessing nutrition status is to uncover any conditions which place a patient at risk for nutrient deficiencies. Table 8 lists important risk factors in the medical and diet histories. Remember that disease can have either long- or short-term effects on nutrition status by interfering with ingestion, digestion, absorption, metabolism, or excretion of nutrients.

Diet History A complete diet history includes general information about a person's intake, socioeconomic factors affecting intake, and specific food intake data. Food choices are a very important part of lifestyle and often represent an expression of personal philosophy. Questions you ask regarding food intake must always be nonjudgmental to elicit accurate information. As evidenced by the factors listed in Table 8, some questions are more delicate than others.

There are several methods for obtaining food intake data, including the 24-hour recall, food diary, and food frequency records. These methods will be discussed in detail in Chapter 19. Like anthropometrics and biochemical data, food intakes should be compared with "standards." In this case, the standards are recommended nutrient intakes. The question to be answered is how closely the person's diet meets the recommendations. Are any nutrients excessive or deficient?

A quick assessment can be made by comparing food intake with the Four Food Group Plan (see pp. 479-480). When you need detailed information about specific nutrients, the foods can be looked up in food composition tables and the final values compared with standards such as the RDAs. In some facilities, computer programs are available for easily determining nutrient intakes and comparing intakes with standards. Remember, though, that these standards were developed for

A quick method of calculating the kcalories needed to maintain the BMR was given on page 222. Another method, known as the **BEE (basal energy expenditure)**, which controls for the person's height, weight, and age as well as sex, is as follows:

$$66 + \left[13.7 \times \text{wt (kg)} \right] + \left[5 \times \text{ht (cm)} \right] - (6.8 \times \text{Age})$$

Females:
$$655 + \left[9.6 \times \text{wt (kg)} \right] + \left[1.7 \times \text{ht (cm)} \right] - (4.7 \times \text{Age})$$

To estimate the person's actual kcaloric needs, you multiply the BEE by the following factors:

Oral diet, weight maintenance: 1.20 × BEE

Oral diet, weight gain: 1.50 × BEE

Total parenteral nutrition: 1.75 × BEE

For the meaning of total parenteral nutrition (TPN), see Chapter 20.

The RDA or similar standards can be used to estimate protein requirements for maintaining the body's lean body mass. When lean body mass must be repleted, protein needs range from 1.2 to 1.5 g/day per kg of body weight.

Table 8.   Risk Factors for Poor Nutrition Status

Medical history

Recent major illness	Lung disease
Recent major surgery	Kidney disease
Surgery of the GI tract	Diabetes
Overweight	Heart disease
Underweight	Hormonal imbalance
Recent weight loss or gain	Hyperlipidemia
Anorexia	Hypertension
Nausea	Mental retardation
Vomiting	Multiple pregnancies
Diarrhea	Neurologic disorders
Alcoholism	Pancreatic insufficiency
Cancer	Paralysis
Circulatory problems	Radiation therapy
Liver disease	Teenage pregnancies

Diet history

Chewing or swallowing difficulties (including poorly fitted dentures, dental caries, and missing teeth)	Inadequate food budget
	Inadequate food preparation facilities
Inadequate food intake	Inadequate food storage facilities
Restricted or fad diets	Physical disabilities
Frequently eating out	Elderly
No intake for 10 or more days	Living (eating) alone
Intravenous fluids (other than total parenteral nutrition for 10 or more days	Cultural group
	Religious affiliation

Drug history*

Antibiotics	Catabolic steroids
Anticonvulsants	Oral contraceptives
Antihypertensive agents	Vitamin and other nutrient preparations
Antineoplastic agents	

*See Chapter 21 for specific interactions.

"healthy" people. Nutrient needs often change in disease, and these needs should be met by the diet (Chapters 22-27).

By gaining insight into what and how a person eats, you can pick up valuable clues as to how that person will accept diet changes, should they be necessary. You can use this information to provide realistic and attainable goals for your patient's nutrition care.

Drug History   The important interactions of foods and drugs have been increasingly recognized in recent years. Some general classifications of drugs which may influence nutrition status include antibiotics, anticonvulsants, antihypertensive agents, antineoplastic agents (used in chemotherapy), catabolic steroids, oral contraceptives, and vitamin and other nutrient preparations.

If a patient is taking any of these types of drugs, the amount and the length of time the drugs have been taken should be noted. Signs of any adverse effects also should be recorded. Nutrient-drug interactions are discussed in more detail in Chapter 21.

Classifying Nutrition Status

PCM is classified as either kwashiorkor, marasmus, or kwashiorkor-marasmus mix. In kwashiorkor, anthropometric measurements are normal or even above standard, while blood and organ proteins are depleted. A person with kwashiorkor will not have a positive skin test result. In the marasmic patient, blood and organ protein levels and immune function are adequate, while skeletal muscle and subcutaneous fat (as reflected in anthropometrics) are depleted. In people with kwashiorkor-marasmus mix, blood, organ, and skeletal protein, as well as subcutaneous fat, are depleted. The last-named type of malnutrition is the most serious. People with kwashiorkor-type malnutrition also may be at increased risk, but for a special reason: It is easy to assume they are "well-nourished," since they are often overweight, and so they may be overlooked.

Based on anthropometric, biochemical, and dietary information, B.J.'s malnutrition would be classified as kwashiorkor-marasmus mix.

Although assessment of hospital patients often concentrates on PCM, it is important to remember that other nutrient deficiencies also can occur. Determination of specific vitamin and mineral deficiencies is most often based on physical findings and laboratory confirmation.

The Nutrition Care Plan

A nutrition care plan translates assessment data into a strategy for meeting the client's nutrition and education needs. It concentrates on intervention and the client's response to intervention. For example, a care plan would not only document why a weight reduction diet was given but also how the client reacted to instruction on the diet.

The care process is continuous. As your client's needs change, you must adjust the care plan to meet them. Try a new approach when original plans fall short.

The nutrition assessment forms used as a part of the permanent medical record generally list only anthropometric, biochemical, and sometimes food intake data (see Form 1). Very little historical information is included. These forms are used to classify PCM, since this is the most common type of malnutrition seen in the hospital. You will need more information, however, to develop and implement a nutrition care plan.

Generally, dietitians or nurses keep the additional historical information in their respective care plans, rather than in the medical records. This system works well for several reasons. Much historical information is already recorded elsewhere in the chart, and thus duplication is avoided. Furthermore, historical information can be quite extensive, requiring a great deal of valuable chart space. Additionally, since the information is subjective, it may change considerably with time. Although it may be advantageous not to include historical data on a formal nutrition assessment form, this information should *always* be obtained. Furthermore, members of the health care team should communicate important historical information on a regular basis.

The initial care plan may change frequently during the hospitalization as new needs are identified. For example, a patient admitted on a medical floor for a diagnostic workup may later become a surgical patient and have different nutrient requirements.

Everyone seems to develop a personal system for nutrition assessment based on individual experience. Ideally, every hospital patient should receive a complete assessment shortly after admission. However, this is usually not possible. One easy way to determine who needs a complete assessment is to use the following steps:

1. Extract all relevant information from patient's medical record, including available lab data; height; weight; and drug, medical, and social history.

2. Visit patient, take diet history and food intake data. During this visit, observe patient for obvious physical signs of malnutrition.

3. Review information obtained in the first two steps to determine if the patient is at risk nutritionally. This process often is called *nutrition screening*. Generally, in-depth assessment is probably not necessary if a patient's weight for height is adequate but not excessive and if there has been no significant recent weight change, no prolonged use of drugs which interfere with nutrition status, no nutrition-related medical condition, and no bizarre eating habits. In this case, develop a care plan to maintain the patient's current status and reassess in one to two weeks if the patient still is in the hospital.

Form 1.   Nutrition Assessment Summary

Date _____   Admitting date _____

Patient _____   Room _____

Height _____   Admitting weight _____

Current weight _____   Usual body weight _____

Admitting diagnosis _____

Somatic protein and fat	Patient value	Degree of depletion			
		None	Mild	Moderate	Severe
Weight as % IBW*					
Weight as % UBW†					
Midarm circumference					
Triceps skinfold					
Midarm muscle circumference					
Urinary creatinine					
Creatinine-height index					

Visceral protein

Serum albumin					
Total iron binding capacity					
Transferrin (serum or calculated)					
Total lymphocyte count					
Cell mediated immunity					

Nitrogen balance: _____

Protein-kcalorie nutrition status

☐ Adequate

☐ Marasmus
  Somatic protein and fat depleted; visceral protein adequate

☐ Kwashiorkor
  Somatic protein and fat adequate; visceral proteins depleted

☐ Kwashiorkor-marasmus mix
  Somatic and visceral protein depleted

Other findings and comments

(Include pertinent food intake data, other laboratory tests and physical findings.)

_____

_____

_____
Signature of Assessor

*IBW: ideal body weight.

†UBW: usual body weight.

4. If patient is at risk, do a more complete assessment, including arm anthropometrics, and analysis of food intake for energy, protein, and other nutrients as appropriate; and recommend any additional necessary lab tests. Based on findings, develop a nutrition care plan which will maintain or improve the patient's nutrition status. Reassess regularly every one to two weeks.

You may well be frustrated with reading about nutrition assessment at this point. We have covered many general points without talking about specifics; and reading about general principles and putting them into practice are two different matters entirely! There are many "ifs" involved in nutrition assessment — no two patients have the same medical history, diet patterns, anthropometric findings, lab values, or physical appearance. So what do you do now?

Be patient. Reading subsequent chapters should help you develop a good grip on the nutrition implications of disease and medical therapy. Then you will have a basis for the real challenge — working with individuals! Pulling together facts and tying them together with the clinical judgment you develop with practice will make you a top-notch health care provider.

Summing Up

Nutrition assessment and nutrition care plans require continuous updating. Nutrition needs change as people change by aging, recovering from disease, developing complications, or leaving the hospital. When you develop nutrition care plans, consider each person's individual needs.

Many parameters are useful in assessing nutrition status, including anthropometric, laboratory, physical, and historical data. These assessment data form the foundation for interpreting nutrient needs and determining how these needs will best be met.

Anthropometric data mainly describe changes in skeletal muscle and subcutaneous fat, while lab tests are useful in assessing protein status of the blood and organs. Physical and historical findings provide information about possible nutrient deficiencies. Historical information also helps you understand clients so that their needs can be met. None of the parameters for assessing nutrition status stand alone in determining if malnutrition exists. Yet these pieces can be fitted together to define nutrition status.

To Explore Further

A comprehensive manual which discusses all aspects of nutrition assessment, including details of tests for vitamin-mineral status and an excellent section on food and drug interaction, is:

- Grant, A. *Nutritional Assessment Guidelines*, 1979. Available from Anne Grant, Box 25057, Northgate Station, Seattle, WA 98125.

More information on community assessment programs can be found in the booklet:

- Christakis, G. *Nutritional Assessment in Health Programs*, 1973. Available from American Public Health Association, Inc., 1015 Eighteenth Street, NW, Washington, DC 20036.

The original article exposing the prevalence of malnutrition in U.S. hospitals was:

- Butterworth, C. E. The skeleton in the hospital closet. *Nutrition Today*, March/April 1974, pp. 4-8.

An article, as well as teaching aid, entitled "Hospital Malnutrition and How to Assess the Nutritional Status of a Patient," by C. E. Butterworth and G. L. Blackburn, is available from *Nutrition Today*. The article appeared in the March/April 1975 issue, pp. 8-11.

Several useful free publications are available from drug companies:

- *A Guide to Nutritional Care*, 1981. Mead-Johnson, Nutritional Division, address in Appendix J.
- *Guidelines for Anthropometric Measurements*, 1978. Ross Laboratories, address in Appendix J.
- *Guidelines for Skin Testing*, 1979. Ross Laboratories, address in Appendix J.
- *Nutritional Assessment*, 1980. Cutter Medical, Cutter Laboratories, Berkeley, CA 94710.

A slide presentation entitled *A Nursing Role in Nutritional Assessment* is available through Ross Laboratories. This presentation is fairly comprehensive and is written at a more in-depth level. Ross Labs has also made an excellent film, *An Illusion of Nutritional Health*, demonstrating the importance of nutrition assessment in the care of hospital patients.

A very good book, invaluable in interpreting all types of lab tests, is:

- Wallach, J. *Interpretation of Diagnostic Tests*. Boston: Little, Brown and Company, 1978.

An excellent article which emphasizes how the nurse can uncover malnutrition while interviewing a client is:

- Swan, E., and Rohrback, C. Nutritional assessment — an investigative interview. *Nutritional Support Services*, May 1982, 12-15.

Mrs. Green, a 48-year-old homemaker, was admitted to the hospital for testing following a car accident. She was alert and her only obvious injury was a broken arm. After reviewing her chart, the health care team decided a complete nutrition assessment was necessary. The following significant information resulted:

Anthropometrics

- Height: 5'7".
- Weight: 150 lb.
- Midarm circumference: 29.3 cm.
- Triceps skinfold: 24 mm.
- Frame size: medium.

Physical findings

- Hair: dull, easily plucked.
- Others: negative.

Medical history

- No significant findings.

Laboratory findings

- Albumin: 3.0 g/dl.
- WBC: 9,000 mm^3.
- % lymphocytes: 10%.
- Urine urea nitrogen: 10 g/24 hr.

- Urinary creatinine excretion: 1,150 mg/24 hr.

Diet history

- Usual weight: 175 lb (6 weeks ago).
- Weight loss intentional.
- Protein intake: 45 g/24 hr.

Drug history

- 1 standard multivitamin tablet daily — no other.

Study Questions

1. Determine Mrs. Green's ideal body weight and calculate %IBW.

2. Calculate %UBW.

3. Consider Mrs. Green's recent weight change. What is a safe rate of weight loss (see Chapter 8)? How does Mrs. Green's weight loss rate compare with the safe rate?

4. Calculate Mrs. Green's derived midarm muscle circumference and compare all arm anthropometric measurements with the percentile tables in Appendix E. How would you classify her measurements (adequate, mildly depleted, moderately depleted, severely depleted)?

5. Calculate nitrogen balance and the creatinine-height index. What information do you get from these values?

6. What do Mrs. Green's lab values indicate with respect to her protein status?

7. Are there any other factors in Mrs. Green's medical and drug history or physical findings suggestive of malnutrition?

8. How would you classify Mrs. Green's nutrition status (adequate, kwashiorkor-type, marasmus-type, kwashiorkor-marasmus mix)?

9. What type of nutrition care would you recommend for Mrs. Green? What are her nutrition education needs?

The course of death from starvation is both tragic and terrible. An account of the Irish hunger strikers who refused all food in order to obtain political concessions from the British was recently detailed in a *Time* magazine article.[1] The hunger strikers lived only on water and salt. The course of starvation is known from observations of these strikers.

After the first two weeks, the overwhelming desire for food disappeared. Stomach cramps also ended. The hunger strikers spent a good deal of time in bed both to preserve strength and to stay warm. Their skin became parched and extremely dry, fillings dropped out of their teeth, and their throats became ulcerated.

After almost exactly 42 days of fasting, each striker experienced a gruesome ordeal. The strikers lost muscular control of their eyes — they rapidly jerked involuntarily up and down and from side to side. Efforts to look straight ahead were futile. These episodes were accompanied by constant spells of vomiting and dizziness. After about four or five days the ordeal ended, leaving the strikers in a more euphoric state.

[1] R. Ajemian, Ready to die in the Maze: What it is like to starve to death and why the I.R.A. men do it, *Time* 118 (7) (1981):46-48.

HIGHLIGHT 18

World Protein-kCalorie Malnutrition

If you give a man a fish, he will eat for a day. If you teach him to fish, he will eat for a lifetime.

UNKNOWN

As death approached, speech became slurred and the senses faded. Hearing became difficult, eyesight failed, and sense of smell diminished. The body progressively consumed itself until death became inevitable. Although intentional and total starvation is not typical of the protein-kcalorie malnutrition (PCM) seen in developing countries, it neverthless provides an example of what it is like to starve to death.

PCM in Developing Countries A more typical story of how PCM can occur in a developing country might go like this: A happy little one-year-old-girl lives in a shack with several brothers and sisters and her parents in Biafra (or Cambodia or some other developing country). A new baby has just arrived and is now nestled close to the mother, being fed from the

breast where once the little girl was held and fed. She has been banished. She must somehow learn to use a hard utensil to spoon a thin, tasteless cereal into her mouth. She pouts and cries with hunger, but no one listens. Finally she quits trying to acquire the new skill of eating from a bowl or spoon. She doesn't follow her brothers and sisters outside to play but wanders off into a corner and plays alone. The mother is disgusted with her withdrawal and doesn't try anymore to entice her to eat. "She will eat when she is hungry," thinks the mother. Sometimes the mother forgets about her altogether, the little girl is so quiet.

The little girl's body defends itself from destruction by adapting to the lower energy input with a lower energy output: She keeps still. She ingests few amino acids with which to build body tissue (hormones, enzymes, new cells). The amino acids she does receive and her entire body's resources are directed toward supplying energy to her brain, heart, and lungs. There is no energy left for the muscular activity of playing with her brothers and sisters or for smiling at her mother or even for crying for food. Apathy is the body's way of conserving energy. Its danger, in the case of an infant who depends on the mother to give it food, is that apathy can damage the mother-child

707

relationship to the point where the mother rejects the child. The downward spiral that is PCM has thus begun. If the little girl would eat the gruel, she might receive enough kcalories, but without a protein source she would probably develop kwashiorkor.

Textbooks usually describe marasmus and kwashiorkor as the two endpoints on a spectrum — lack of kcalories at one end and lack of protein at the other — with PCM occupying the central region. In clinical practice these distinctions are not so easily made. At all points between marasmus and kwashiorkor, protein deficiency produces symptoms, whether the underlying cause is lack of dietary protein or lack of kcalories to conserve the dietary protein. Furthermore, a diet deficient in protein and kcalories is invariably deficient in other nutrients as

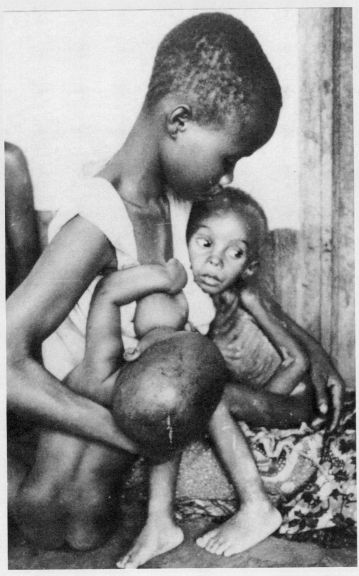

The sickness that invades the first child when the second child is born.

well. It seems to us that Cicely Williams had the right idea in urging that we quit worrying about the descriptions and the pathology of the disease and spend our energies instead on delivering the care that is needed and on correcting the underlying social, political, and economic causes.[2]

Protein-kcalorie malnutrition particularly affects vulnerable groups in the community, such as pregnant and lactating women, nursing infants, just-weaned children, and children in periods of rapid growth. These groups have a greater need for protein than the rest of the population because of the new tissues being formed in their bodies. They need ample kcalories to protect that protein from degradation, yet in many cultures they are the very ones who are denied protein.

Apathy like that of the little girl in our story is just one symptom of PCM. Other symptoms result from the disturbance of the water balance (edema), reduced synthesis of key hormones (lowered body temperature), lack of proteins to transport nutrients into and out of the circulatory system (anemia), lack of protein to carry oxygen to the cells (muscular weakness) or to carry away

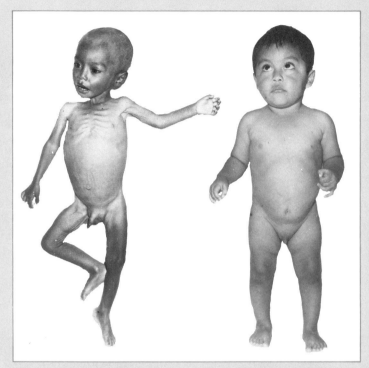

Courtesy of Dr. Robert S. Goodhart, M.D.

A child suffering from the extreme emaciation of marasmus.

The same child after nutritional therapy.

carbon dioxide (sleepiness), and lack of protein to build collagen for scar formation (poor healing of cuts) and for growth of bones and teeth (stunted growth).

Moreover, one of the most insidious and far-reaching effects of PCM is on learning ability. If the time of the insult occurs at a critical period of brain growth, children may never attain their intellectual potential — even if they are well nourished later. (It is difficult to determine, however, whether mental deficiencies observed in malnourished children are

due to PCM alone or to the social deprivation that goes with apathy.[3])

In order to study the effects of PCM on brain growth, Minick and his associates analyzed the brain tissue of young children who had died of severe marasmus as well as brain tissue from otherwise healthy accident victims (children of compar-

[2]C. D. Williams, On that fiasco, *Lancet* 1 (1975):793-794.

[3]J. Cravioto, Nutrition, stimulation, mental development and learning, *Nutrition Today*, September/October 1981, pp. 4-8, 10-15.

able ages).[4] They found that the number of brain cells of the marasmic children was significantly lower than the number in the well-fed children (See Figure 1). Since the number of brain cells does not increase significantly after about one year of age, this finding has serious implications for the intellectual development of the child who is deprived of protein and/or kcalories during gestation and the first year of life.

Factors Contributing to PCM   Figure 2 shows the areas of the world in which

[4]M. Winick, P. Rosso, and J. Waterlow, Cellular growth of cerebrum, cerebellum, and brain stem in normal and marasmic children, *Experimental Neurology* 26 (1970):393-400.

PCM is most severe. It is an extremely widespread problem, affecting almost every population of the world. The factors that contribute to its development are as varied and complex as the physical symptoms observed in people suffering from it. No one factor can be singled out as the only cause. Only a few are mentioned here to give an impression of its scope and complexity. Geography, education, traditions, economics, soil erosion, and birth rates are involved, and all are interdependent.

Geography   If the land is rocky or barren, it may require enormous effort to produce the minimum amount of food needed to support human life. Many of the developing countries are

in the subtropical or tropical regions. With their high temperatures and rainfall, they might be expected to produce an abundant harvest. However, their soils are poor. Furthermore, crop pests and bacteria also thrive in a warm humid climate, and they may substantially reduce the harvest. If the region is near the sea, fish may be plentiful, but again, in a warm climate spoilage will take its toll.

Education   The lack of education also contributes to PCM. Poorly nourished people are often caught in such a tangle of problems that, even when education is available, they can't take advantage of the opportunity. They may lack knowledge of birth control methods or may fail to understand that delaying the birth of the next child until the mother has replenished her body's supply of nutrients will be an advantage to the health of subsequent children. For these and other reasons, these people continue to produce children destined to die early or to live out their lives under great hardship.

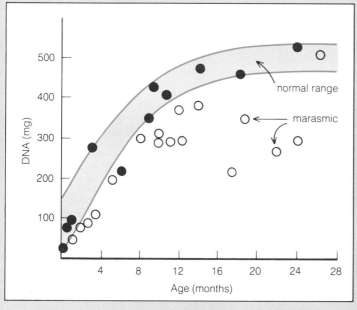
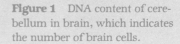

Figure 1   DNA content of cerebellum in brain, which indicates the number of brain cells.

From M. Winick, P. Rosso, and J. Waterlow, Cellular growth of cerebrum, cerebellum, and brain stem in normal and marasmic children, *Experimental Neurology* 26 (1970):393-400.

People in the regions of the world where PCM is rampant have no knowledge of efficient ways to plant, fertilize, and harvest crops and no capital with which to buy technology. Once the crops are harvested, the people do not know how to store them where insects and rodents will not destroy them or how to preserve them by drying or canning. These people suffer alternating periods of plenty and starvation, because one year's harvest, even if it is bountiful, cannot be made to stretch until the next harvest. Without knowledge of how to handle foods, they greatly reduce the nutrient levels of the food they do have.

Traditions Probably the saddest causes of PCM are human traditions. In many communities meat is for males; females are not allowed to eat meat during their reproductive years, the very years when they and their future offspring most need the complete spectrum of amino acids offered by meat.

Traditions within a group also produce food prejudices or beliefs that limit the use of valuable food. For example, some peoples of Southeast Asia view milk as belonging to the animal's offspring and thus as not rightfully theirs to take. If urged to drink it, they will admit that they think of it as an unclean body secretion.[5] Other groups have such a reverence for all life that they refuse to use pesticides. Thus a farmer's crop may support the lives of the crop insects while his own children die for lack of food.

[5] F. J. Simoons, The geographic approach to food prejudices, *Food Technology* 20 (1966):42-44.

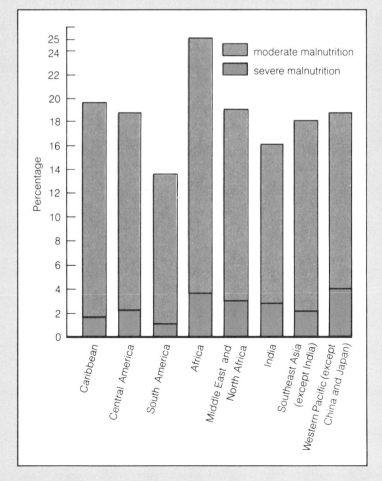

Figure 2 Prevalence of severe and moderate protein/kcalorie malnutrition, compiled from the results from 101 surveys in 59 countries, 1963-1973.

Adapted from J. M. Bengoa and G. Donoso, Prevalence of protein-calorie malnutrition 1963-1973, *PAG Bulletin* 4 (1) (1974):25-35.

Economic Systems   Countries need to have a marketable export item in order to produce a balance of payments with which to import other needed items. Sometimes to achieve this economic goal, they export food, even if it is badly needed by their own people. For instance, Africa imports high-carbohydrate foods, which its own land could produce, and exports pulses (peas or lentils), meat, and groundnuts, which its own people need. It has been estimated that a handful of groundnuts per person per day would solve India's protein problem,[6] yet India exports its groundnuts.

Birth Rates   As mortality from infectious diseases has decreased, more people have lived more years. But they have had to be fed from the same amount of land. The picture has been growing steadily worse. The world's grain stores are depleted, and since 1971 only three countries — the United States, Canada, and Australia — have had net exports of grain.[7] It is estimated that half of the world's people live in perpetual hunger.[8]

In spite of the introduction in the 1950s of improved contraceptive methods, which have achieved worldwide availability, populations have continued to increase faster than food production. Even the populations of the developed countries (including the United States) continue to increase. Figure 3 compares the size of the U.S. population in 2070 assuming a birth rate of three children per family to its size assuming a birth rate of two children per family. The figure shows that *even if the birth rate does decline, the population will still increase.* This difference can be likened to placing the population of seven more New York Cities into the United States between 1973 and 1998.

Visualize the problems connected with feeding seven new cities the size of New York. Land will be taken out of food production and covered with concrete; land will be taken away from forests and put into food production; the water needed for growing the food will run off into the ocean because of the loss of forests; more highways and trucks will be needed for transporting the food into the cities and the garbage out; additional energy will be required for this transportation network, as well as for cooking the food and for fertilizers. The problems seem severe even for a rich country. How, then,

[6] I. Palmer, UNRISD studies on the "green revolution," *Food and the New Agricultural Technology,* no. 5, Report no. 72.9 (Geneva: United Nations Research Institute for Social Development, 1972).

[7] F. H. Sanderson, The great food fumble, *Science* 188 (1975):503-509.

[8] F. H. Quimby and C. B. Chapman, in U.S. Senate, Select Committee on Nutrition and Human Needs, *National Nutrition Policy: Nutrition and the International Situation* (Washington, D.C.: Government Printing Office, 1974).

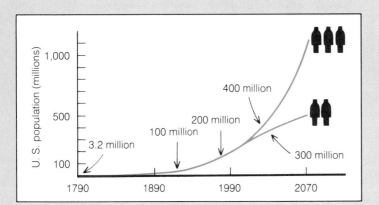

Figure 3 Comparison of U.S. population in 2070 with birth rate of 3 children per family and 2 children per family. Even if the birth rate declines, the population will still increase.

From F. H. Quimby and C. B. Chapman, in U.S. Senate, Select Committee on Nutrition and Human Needs, *National Nutrition Policy: Nutrition and the International Situation,* (Washington, D.C.: Government Printing Office, 1974).

can we hope to feed the exploding populations of the rest of the world?

Soil Erosion   Soil erosion is now accelerating on every continent, at a rate that threatens the world's ability to continue feeding itself. Erosion of soil has always occurred; it is a natural process — but in the past it has been counteracted by processes that build the soil up. Farmers should alternate soil-building crops with soil-destroying crops, a practice known as crop rotation. An acre of soil planted one year in corn, the next year in wheat, and the next in clover loses 2.7 tons of topsoil each year, but if it is planted only in corn it will lose 19.7 tons a year.[9] When a farmer must choose whether to make three times as much money planting corn year after year or rotate crops and go bankrupt, naturally he chooses the profits. Ruin will follow — but not immediately.[10]

Transportation   Then there is the problem of distributing food to the people that need it. The solution to this problem involves other areas. One is economics.

(Who is to bear the cost? Are the recipients able to pay?) Another is technology. (How are the roads to be built? How will the foods be kept from spoiling in transit? Who will pay for the trucks, planes, and other needed vehicles?) Another is energy. (Who will supply the petroleum for fertilizers, insecticides, farm machinery, and transport?)

How Can We Fight PCM?   Such is the maze of modern life that what started out as a discussion of protein and kcalorie deprivation has become a debate on questions of government policies, economics, and energy. But the problem *is* this complex, and all of these problems and more have to be dealt with. Our country's sending wheat to a starving population is analogous to giving a fish to a beggar at the door. Neither act helps to solve the underlying condition, even though both are well-meaning. What is needed is for policymakers to attack the problems of malnutrition on many fronts.

Hundreds of experts from different walks of life have become involved in and concerned about world hunger. Dozens of international conferences have been held, and policies have emerged from them that promise to benefit nations enlightened enough to adopt them.

There is no consensus regarding "the" solution to the

crisis or even about whether it can be solved. Many feel that it is too late and that it is only a matter of limited time before the human race enters a new Dark Age, beset by disease and starvation such as have never before been seen.[11] Others find cause for hope. The U.S. National Research Council has conducted a comprehensive study of the problem and has reached a conclusion of guarded optimism. The council recommends "a massive research and development effort to expand world food supply, reduce poverty, and curb soaring population growth."[12] In other words, we should go beyond feeding the hungry beggar at the door and help him solve his problems so that he can feed himself.

The National Research Council has outlined a means of combatting world PCM. Given a commitment by the U.S. government and parallel commitments from other government agencies, the council states that "it should be possible to overcome the worst aspects of widespread hunger and malnutrition within one generation."[13]

[9]National Agricultural Lands Study, *Soil Degradation: Effects on Agricultural Productivity, Interim Report No. 4* (Washington, D.C.: USDA, November 1980), as cited by L. R. Brown, World population growth, soil erosion, and food security, *Science* 214 (1981):995-1002.

[10]Brown, 1981.

[11]W. Paddock and P. Paddock, *Time of Famines* (Boston: Little, Brown, 1976).

[12]Steering Committee, National Research Council Study on Food and Nutrition, National Academy of Sciences, *World Food and Nutrition Study: The Potential Contributions of Research*, as cited in *Wilson Quarterly*, Autumn 1977, p. 55.

[13]National Research Council, 1977.

This seems to be an optimistic view, but what is needed most is the political will to take the initiative. So we must move from the scientific into the political arena.

On the personal level, if you are concerned about malnutrition, you can investigate the various movements that are attacking world hunger and can align yourself with the organization that best reflects your own philosophy. You can make your concerns known to political leaders, perhaps by joining a political action group. You also can implement ecologically sound conservation and nutritional programs in your own life. Don't be afraid to show your concern. The words of Benjamin Franklin, spoken in another context, apply to the world's PCM problem as well: "We must all hang together, or, assuredly, we will all hang separately."

To Explore Further

The world hunger problem is vast and severe, and no attempt has been made here to put its parts in perspective. For a readable and more in-depth treatment, see the paperbacks:

- Kirk, D., and Eliason, E. K. *Food and People* (second half). San Francisco: Boyd and Fraser, 1982.
- Gussow, J. D. *The Feeding Web*. Palo Alto, Calif.: Bull Publishing, 1978.

To study a single aspect of the problem more deeply, we suggest the article:

- Brown, L. R. World population growth, soil erosion, and food security. *Science* 214 (1981):995-1002.

CHAPTER 19

CONTENTS

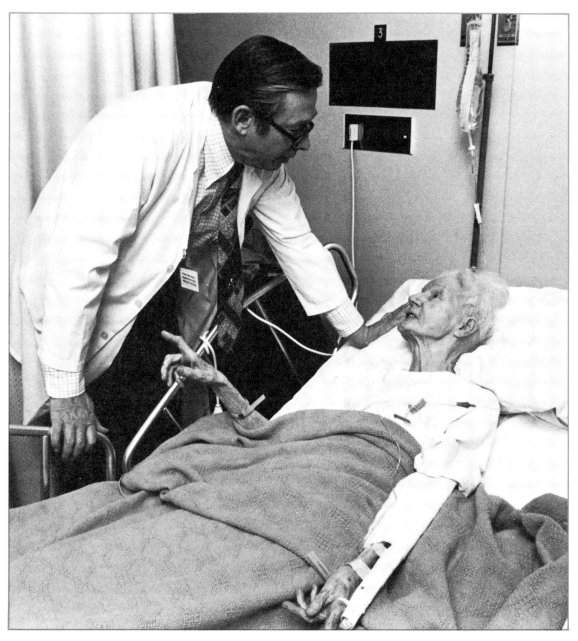

Communication makes the difference in patient care. Here, a patient airs her concerns with her physician.

NUTRITION COMMUNICATION NETWORKS

Half of what I say is meaningless, but I say it so that the other half may reach you.

KAHLIL GIBRAN

Close your eyes and for a moment, imagine that you are a hospitalized patient. You are frightened because you are not sure what's wrong with you or what will happen next. All of a sudden you have to depend on a lot of people to do things for you. You repeatedly have to ask someone to bring you the things you want or need. Even worse, you feel you have lost control of *yourself.* You must depend on someone else to find out what's happening inside your body and what the best treatment will be. How terrifying to be putting your health (your life) in someone else's hands (a stranger yet)! Your body is no longer private — everyone seems to be poking, sticking, and probing it. On top of that, you hurt, and many of the examinations, tests, and procedures you must undergo also hurt you. You need time to sort through your feelings, but how can you think when it seems that every few minutes someone is coming into your room to check vital signs, take blood, and ask endless questions that you feel you have already answered over and over.

Now open your eyes and remember to keep them open. You should be able to see how important communication becomes to the person reduced to a dependent state. Many fears and concerns felt by patients can be relieved when they feel satisfied that those they depend on listen, understand, and act on their needs. When the people around them respond in this way, patients retain some control over their environment, and therefore, themselves.

Furthermore, you will inevitably need to enlist your patients' cooperation to obtain accurate information or to motivate them to follow nutrition (or other) advice. If your patients do not feel they can talk to you, they certainly will be less willing to accept medical or nutrition advice. Therefore, a channel of two-way communication should always be operating.

Effective Communication

Communication involves the transfer of information from one person (sender) to another (receiver) for the purpose of eliciting a response. Information can be transferred verbally or nonverbally. Charting information in a patient's medical record is communication, as are touching, smiling, frowning, and the like. Regardless of the communication medium, to be an effective communicator you must formulate and express your ideas clearly, and the receiver must interpret what you say as you intended. As illustrated in Figure 1, the relationship is dynamic. The roles of sender and receiver are constantly switching between the parties involved in communication. When a person responds to your communication, you must correctly interpret that response.

Messages may not be perceived as intended if the words or actions used by the sender have a different meaning for the receiver. Values and ethnic and social influences affect everyone's perception of words and actions. For example, the way you say "How are you doing today" can have many meanings for the receiver, ranging from "What a dumb thing to say" to "He really cares about me." Smiling is generally an expression of friendliness, but a smile also can be inappropriate, for example, at a time of grief.

Effective communication

Active listening

Client-centered

Caring and trusting

Understandable terminology

Control the environment

When communication takes place between you and your client or patient, you must assume the role of helper. You can enhance communication by keeping in mind the following points:

- Give each person room to be himself. In other words, accept and value a person for who and what he is. If you react to what a person tells you with advice, criticism, or judgment, he will not feel free to relate important things about himself to you. He may not want to take the chance that you might belittle him either verbally or nonverbally.

- Become an active listener. The client should be the one doing most of the talking.

- Allow the client to control the direction of the discussion. Try not to follow a set form for asking important questions; rather, use such a form as a guide and ask questions based on what the patient is telling you. Effective communication in the health care setting is client-centered. After all, the client is the recipient of therapy.

- Establish a caring and trusting environment. Let the client know that you care about her as a person and that she can trust you.

- Avoid using medical terminology or abbreviations which may be confusing to a layperson. For example, a first-time surgical patient might be totally confused if told that after leaving the OR he would go to the RR and that he should expect to have an IV and an NG tube inserted before he awakens. Furthermore, always define the medical terms used to explain a patient's condition, diagnostic tests, or

Judgmental versus nonjudgmental responses:

Helper: Do you take any type of vitamin or mineral supplements?

Client: I take a vitamin E capsule and 2 grams of vitamin C every day.

Judgmental helper response: You know, of course, that there is no reason for taking these vitamin supplements.

Nonjudgmental helper response: Why do you take these vitamin supplements?

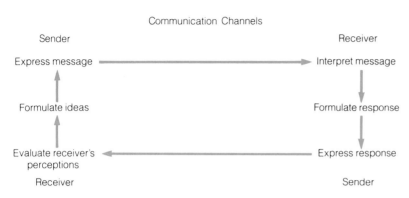

Figure 1 Communication channels.

therapy. The box, "That Latin's all Greek to me, doctor," written by Erma Bombeck, a syndicated columnist, illustrates the problem of miscommunication involving medical terminology.

That Latin's all Greek to me, doctor

Be honest now. Do any of you understand one word of what your doctor tells you?

Ever since I told a crowded room I had a Bavarian cyst and not only did no one laugh, but two others in the room had the same thing, I've been convinced doctor and patient do not speak the same language.

They speak Latin. We speak Reader's Digest.

I suspect I am like most people who are intimidated by anyone who wears white all winter and washes his hands 137 times a day.

It's not that I don't pay attention. It's just that I have a feeling something more important awaits him in the next treatment room.

Somehow, I cannot see me having this conversation with my doctor.

"You say this problem is my humorous bone? Humorous as in Woody Allen?"

"No, that's humerus."

"Would you spell that, please?"

"Of course. Give me a piece of scrap paper and I'll make a diagram and label it for you."

"Here, take the gown you gave me."

There is probably nothing more humiliating than to have a husband who always wants to know what the doctor said.

"It has something to do with my nose," I say.

"What part of your nose?" he asks.

"You know. The rectum."

"Try septum. What's wrong with it?"

"It's perverted."

"Deviated."

"Same thing."

I've talked with people who told me they had a Cather inserted in them for a week. (Not to be confused with novelist Willa Catheter who wrote "Death Comes for the Archbishop.")

Another friend I know could never remember his blood pressure numbers, but said if his diabolic reading was under his golf score, he was happy.

All of us who go to doctors suffer the same disease, timidity of the tongue. We don't open our mouths and ask questions. I don't know why. I only know a lot is lost in the translation.

When my grandmother once announced she had a prostate deficiency and was told it wasn't possible, she snapped, "The way I eat, anything is possible."

From "At Wit's End" by Erma Bombeck. 1981, Field Enterprises, Inc., courtesy of Field Newspaper Syndicate.

Before beginning any type of formal communication with a patient or client, be prepared! Check the chart to get an idea of the past and current history. Also, try to arrange for privacy and for the physical environment to be as comfortable as possible. It is difficult to communicate with anyone in a noisy, poorly lit, or stuffy-hot room.

Verbal Communication   The most appropriate verbal communication techniques are those which encourage the person to communicate openly and freely and to provide accurate information. Some of these techniques (in addition to those already discussed) include:

1. Introduction and statement of purpose. Always introduce yourself, verify the person's name, explain who you are, and define the purpose of your discussion. In so doing, you set the tone for the discussion and let the person know what is expected of him. At this time, it may be valuable to assure the person that all the information he gives you is confidential.

Open- vs closed-ended questions:

Open-ended: How do you feel about your new diet?

Closed-ended: You feel fine about your new diet, don't you?

2. Appropriate use of questions. Open-ended questions — broad questions which give the person a wide choice of answers — are particularly useful for initiating communication. On the other hand, closed-ended questions are very narrow, and they limit the person's responses.

Another kind of question that provides a limited choice of answers is sometimes called a double question. Avoid double questions.

Examples of double questions:

Do you drink orange or tomato juice with breakfast?

Have you followed a weight-reduction or low-cholesterol diet at home?

3. Continuous feedback. Providing the client or patient with continuous feedback lets her know that you are with her. Furthermore, you can use feedback to assure that you both understand each other correctly. Table 1 lists positive and negative feedback techniques.

4. Summary of the discussion. Prior to ending a discussion, be sure that you both agree on what has transpired. Misconceptions or misunderstandings can be clarified immediately. Furthermore, at this time you can arrange for whatever followup you may wish to make (I'll be back tomorrow; let's plan to talk again next week).

As you practice communicating with others, you will develop techniques which fit your individual style. However, while learning, try out all of the available techniques to discover which ones you use most comfortably and effectively.

Nonverbal Communication   The use of nonverbal communication techniques is extremely important to the communication process. Your body mannerisms often "speak" as much as your words do. Try to maintain eye contact during the communication process; sit at a close, yet comfortable, distance from the other person; and use appropriate facial expressions and gestures to clarify or emphasize important messages.

Table 1.   Providing Feedback: Do's and Don'ts

Do's	Examples
Encourage person (patient or client) to continue.	I see. MmHm. What else?
Repeat key phrases or ideas.	*Person:* I've been so distraught I've lost 10 pounds. *Helper:* You've lost 10 pounds?
Clarify what the person is saying.	I'm not sure I understand what you mean.
Validate person's responses.	*Person:* I get so nervous I begin eating like a horse. *Helper:* You eat when you're nervous?
Echo the person's feelings (sometimes called reflecting).	*Person:* After 4 weeks of dieting, I just can't believe that I only lost 2 pounds. *Helper:* You feel frustrated with how slowly you lose weight.
Remain silent, when appropriate, to let the person formulate ideas.	

Don'ts	Examples
Don't talk more than listen.	
Don't interrupt the person's thoughts.	*Person:* I could stay on my diet if . . . *Helper:* if you didn't live alone.
Don't judge or moralize	You have no excuse for not losing weight.
Don't use meaningless expressions.	I know you'll do fine.
Don't demean the person's situation or attitude.	You probably just don't understand how this diet works.
Don't put words into the person's mouth.	What did you have for breakfast today? (Assumes person eats or should eat breakfast.)
Don't give diet advice when seeking information.	You shouldn't eat candy on your diet. (The person may not tell you about other things he "shouldn't" be eating.)

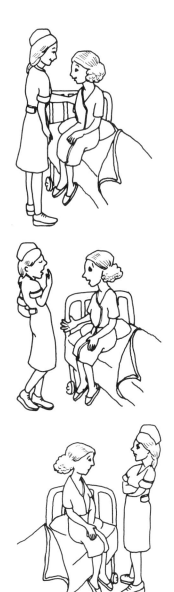

Body language tells people how you feel toward them.

"Tell me what kind of food you eat and I will tell you what kind of man you are."

Brillat-Savarin, *Gastronomy as a fine art*, in *Eating and Drinking — an Anthology for Epicures*, Peter Hunt, ed. (London: Edbury Press, 1976), p. 7.

One of the most powerful nonverbal communication techniques is silence. During a pause, the other person has a chance to formulate ideas and think. Occasionally, silence indicates that a thought is complete and provides a good time to move on to another topic or to end the discussion.

The Interview

The primary purpose of an interview is to gather information. Almost all health professionals conduct interviews to uncover important clues which affect their clients' or patients' health. Interviews also serve as a means of establishing a caring and trusting relationship that will enable the health professional to deliver health care effectively.

Why is developing a good relationship important to the diet interview? The information you seek to obtain in the interview generally represents a person's lifelong habits as influenced by complex social, cultural, psychological, religious, and economic factors. No one would share this much without trusting that the interviewer truly cared and would accept the information, whatever it might be. Otherwise, the interviewee might be worried that you would find her strange, think less of her, or be critical of her behavior.

The communication techniques discussed above provide the guidelines by which to conduct an effective diet interview. A checklist of important aspects of the interviewing process is provided in Table 2. Generally, the purpose of the initial interview is to obtain an account of the person's intake and factors which affect the intake (diet history). The information obtained is recorded on a diet history form (Form 1).

When recording information during an interview, let the person know what you are writing down. Furthermore, try not to write so much that listening becomes a problem. Remember that forms should be used only as a guide; let the person's responses determine the flow of the interview.

Diet History

Up to this point, we have been discussing the "how" of diet interviews. Now let's turn to the "what" of the interview. What information do we need to obtain, and why? Components of the diet history include food intake data, general data (such as age, sex, activity level), and food habits as influenced by socioeconomic, cultural, and psychological factors. Because the medical and drug histories may significantly affect nutrient intake and utilization, this information, too, is generally recorded on the diet history form (see Form 1).

Food Intake Data   There are several methods for obtaining food intake data. Some methods are more appropriate in certain settings

Table 2.   Interviewing Checklist

Preparation
- Obtain available background information from medical record and other team members.
- Arrange for privacy and improve physical environment, if necessary.

Initiating the interview
- Confirm person's identity.
- Introduce self.
- Explain purpose of interview.
- Establish rapport.

Conducting the interview
- Cover one thought at a time.
- Use language the person can easily understand.
- Remain objective.
- Look for verbal and nonverbal cues.
- LISTEN.
- Use open-ended questions.
- Provide appropriate feedback.
- Use nonverbal communication techniques.

Closing the interview
- A few minutes before closing the interview, let person know that time is almost over.
- Determine if person has questions.
- Answer any questions.
- Acknowledge person's cooperation during the interview.
- Explain the next step for followup, if needed.

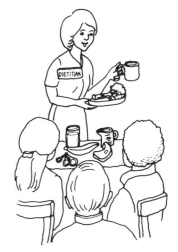

than in others. Obtaining food intake data is difficult and, at times, exasperating. You can make the process less tedious by helping the subject to visualize portion sizes using food models or measuring utensils. While you may think of a glass of milk as holding 8 oz, the subject's glass may hold 12 oz. By showing the patient what 8-, 10-, and 12-oz servings look like, you may be able to help her judge the serving size. Then, the information you obtain will be more accurate. You can use food containers such as empty cups, glasses, bowls, and spoons to help demonstrate portion sizes. Often, you must clarify information you receive by asking how foods were prepared and what might have been added to them, such as sugar, cream, sauces, butter, and margarine. People may also forget to include beverages when relating their intake.

Food models help people to report their intakes accurately.

Just the fact that you are asking about food patterns may cause people to respond with what they think you want to hear, rather than

Form 1. Diet History

Name _____ Birth date _____

Date _____ Sex _____ Height _____ Weight _____

Activity Level

Sleep _____ hrs/24 hrs

Physical activities (mostly ☐ sitting, ☐ standing, ☐ moving, ☐ active)

Food intake (past 24 hours or usual)

Time	Food	Amount

(If 24-hour recall is used, verify whether or not stated intake represents a typical day.)

General

Appetite _____ good _____ fair _____ poor

Alteration in taste/smell? _____

Difficulty in chewing/swallowing? _____

Food allergies? _____

Modified/restricted/fad diet? _____

If yes, reason _____

Members in household _____

Family member who shops _____ prepares meals _____

Food preparation/storage facilities? _____

Income adequate for food needs? _____

Food stamps? _____

Number of meals eaten away from home/week _____

Type (fast food, coffee shop, cafeteria, restaurant, bring from home, friend's home, other)

Food habits

Occupation _____ (hrs/day _____)

Religious dietary practices _____

Ethnic influences on diet _____

Regional influences on diet _____

Favorite foods _____

Food dislikes _____

Pertinent medical history

Current diagnosis:

Past history:

Drug history

Current medications (include dosage, length of time, prescription and nonprescription):

Significant medications in past (e.g., chemotherapy):

with facts. People may not be aware of their actual intakes, or they may be embarrassed about their eating habits. In the latter case, you must maintain an accepting and nonjudgmental attitude in order to encourage honest communication. Relating and emphasizing the purpose of the interview may be useful.

Several methods are used to determine food intake. The most commonly used method is the 24-hour recall. To use this method you ask the person to recount everything eaten or drunk in the past 24 hours or for the previous day (see Form 2). In order for the 24-hour recall to be a valid estimate of food intake, the day must be a typical one with respect to foods eaten.

Techniques for gathering food intake data:

(1) 24-hour recall

(2) Usual intake

(3) Food frequency

(4) Food diary

The major advantage of the 24-hour recall is that it is easy to obtain. Furthermore, it is less frustrating to elicit information from the past 24 hours than to require the person to approximate intake over a long period of time. The fact that the previous day's intake may not be usual, as well as the subject's inability to estimate amounts of foods eaten, are the disadvantages of this method.

A similar method is to obtain a usual intake pattern. Such an inquiry may begin with "What is the first thing you usually eat or drink during the day?" Similar questions follow until you have a typical intake pattern. This method is very similar to the 24-hour recall and can be

Form 2.   24-Hour Recall or Usual Intake

Name ———————————————   Interviewer ————————————————

Date ———————————————

Time	Food	Amount	Place eaten	Food group

Was this a typical day for you? ————

Form 3.   Food Frequency Record

Food item	Type	Amount	How often*
Meat			
Poultry			
Fish			
Eggs			
Cheese			
Legumes			
Peanut butter			
Nuts			
Citrus fruit			
Other fruit			
Leafy green vegetables			
Yellow vegetables			
Potatoes			
Other vegetables			
Milk			
Milk desserts			
Bread or cereal			
Rice or pasta			
Butter/margarine			
Oil/salad dressing			
Snack foods			
Sugar			
Sugar substitute			
Salt			
Salt substitute			
Soft drinks			
Alcoholic beverages			
Coffee/tea			
Other			

*Number of times consumed per week or month, seldom, or never.

recorded on the same form (Form 2). The method may be frustrating for a person whose intake varies widely from day to day. In such a case, the data obtained may be useless in estimating nutrient intake, which also may vary widely from day to day. However, this method is useful to verify food intake when the past 24 hours have been atypical.

Another approach is to use a food frequency record (Form 3). The purpose of this record is to ascertain how often an individual eats a specific type of food per day, week, month, or year. Subjects are asked to state how often they eat a certain food or food type, and this process is repeated for numerous food items. The information obtained can help pinpoint nutrients which may be excessive or deficient in the diet. Furthermore, when used in conjunction with the usual intake or 24-hour recall, the food frequency record enables you to double check the accuracy of the information obtained.

The food frequency record is generally the most frustrating for the interviewer as well as the interviewee and is extremely time consuming to obtain. Try completing a food frequency record on yourself to

Form 4.   Food Diary

Directions: Keep a complete 3-day record of the food you eat by writing down everything you put into your mouth (including liquids) and estimating the amount you have eaten. Be sure to include how the food was fixed (baked, boiled, fried, etc.) and what, if anything, you added to it (butter, margarine, salad dressing, etc.). Also, note the circumstances (birthday party, depressed, bored, etc.) at the time you ate.

Time and place	Food and preparation method	Amount	Circumstances

appreciate the difficulties involved. A typical response to this form of questioning includes "I don't know, sometimes I eat it once a day and then I won't eat it again for months!" You can encourage a person to cooperate if you patiently explain why the information is important to you.

Still another alternative is the food diary. Completion of a diary is often useful to determine food intake and the factors associated with intake (time of day, place eaten, mood, others present). The person keeping the diary is instructed to write down the required information immediately after eating. A food diary is generally useful in the outpatient setting but keeping one requires a good deal of cooperation and motivation (see Form 4).

The advantages of the food diary are many:

- The diary keeper must assume an active role.
- The person may for the first time begin to actually see and understand his own food habits.
- You get a good idea of the diary keeper's lifestyle and factors which affect his food intake.

For these reasons, food diaries are particularly useful in outpatient counseling for weight reduction. However, the diary also can be useful for many other situations, such as assessing a person's compliance to any diet or uncovering food allergies. The major disadvantages stem from poor compliance in recording data and conscious or unconscious changes in eating habits which may occur while the diary is being kept.

After food intake data has been collected, you can use it to determine if nutrient intake is appropriate. Comparison with standards such as the RDA or the Canadian Dietary Standard is the next step (see Chapter 18).

General Data   Age, sex, and activity level are important to note, because these factors affect nutrient requirements. To assess activity level you can ask people how many hours they sleep per 24 hours, what type of physical activity is associated with their job or daily routine (mostly sitting; mostly standing; heavy physical work), and what exercise they get after work. After considering these factors you can classify their activity level as either sedentary, light, moderate, or heavy (see Chapter 7 Self-Study).

It is extremely important to determine the presence of factors affecting food intake, such as appetite (poor, fair, good), alterations in taste or smell, difficulties in chewing or swallowing, food allergies, and any modified, restricted, or fad diet the patient may be following (see margin).

Consideration also should be given to several other factors. The number of people present in the household influences the total amount of money which must be spent on food. Important insight into current eating patterns and the number of people affected by such patterns also can be obtained. The family member responsible for food shopping and

---

anorexia (an-o-REX-ee-uh): lack of appetite.

an = without
orex = mouth

ageusia (uh-JYOOZE-ee-uh): partial or complete loss of the sense of taste.

a = without
geusia = taste

dysgeusia: impairment of the sense of taste; foods that normally taste one way have a completely different taste.

dys = distorted

anosmia: loss of the sense of smell.

osmia = smell

dysosmia: distortion of the sense of smell.

edentulous: without teeth.

e = without
dent = teeth

aphagia: inability to swallow.

phage = to eat

dysphagia: difficulty in swallowing.

preparation will have significant impact on food consumption patterns. Further, you need to know whom to include in any discussions you have with the patient or client concerning diet changes. The availability of facilities for food preparation (stove, hot plate) and storage (refrigerator) also affects food selection. Another consideration is the number of meals eaten away from home and the type of food eaten (fast food, lunch from home, cafeteria, restaurant).

Food Habits   As we have mentioned, the way you eat is influenced by many factors, including economic status, educational level, religious affiliation, and cultural background. Economic status influences the types and amounts of food available to an individual or family as well as the availability of food preparation and storage facilities. The individual's occupation also influences activity levels (and, therefore, energy requirements), as noted above.

Economic status

Information regarding a client's educational level may be useful in determining the best approach you can use for teaching. For example, the illiterate client will need written reinforcements in a pictorial form rather than a language form.

Educational level

Religious affiliation is often important in influencing eating patterns. Several religions define strict dietary patterns, including abstinence from certain foods (like all meats or beef) and specific methods for food preparation. As an example, the Jewish Dietary Laws are listed in Table 3. If you make recommendations for changing the diet without full consideration of religious food customs, your suggestions are doomed to fail.

Religious affiliation

Ethnic background is an important determinant of food selection and the timing and number of meals eaten per day. Ethnic food patterns are deep-seated and not readily changed, and you must work within them when giving diet advice. Figure 2 shows samples of typical meals of various ethnic groups.

Ethnic background

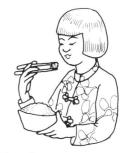

Psychological and personal attitudes also affect food intake. For example, a child forced to eat carrots may hate carrots as an adult. A food which represents security to a child, such as milk, may be used excessively to combat insecurity or depression in adulthood. The more you can learn about an individual's food habits and what these habits represent to that individual, the more likely your success in altering food habits.

What do you mean by a "serving" of rice?

The diet history is an important prerequisite for assessing people's nutrition status and understanding their food habits (see Chapter 18). Once you have such an understanding, you can work more effectively in reinforcing desired behavior and suggesting appropriate changes.

Psychological attitudes

Personal attitudes

Nutrition Counseling

Recently, there has been a tremendous explosion of knowledge regarding the effects of diet on health. However, this knowledge is all

Figure 2 The sample meals and the brief descriptions of the ethnic groups shown here are far from complete. They only serve to remind you that food means different things to different people. Also, the exact food patterns of ethnic groups must be determined on a local level. You would do well to learn

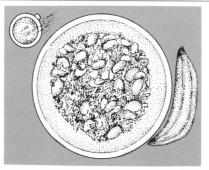

Puerto Rican

Rice and beans with a spicy sauce are served almost daily. Imported vegetables, like plantain (which look like large bananas) also are popular. Coffee con leche is a favorite beverage — each cup contains 2-5 oz milk.

Chinese

Popular Chinese dishes are often mixtures of vegetables (broccoli, pea pods, bamboo shoots, cabbage, mushrooms, and onions) quickly cooked at high temperatures. Fish, pork, or chicken is sometimes added. Rice is a staple, and tea is the favorite beverage.

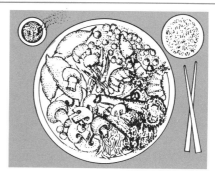

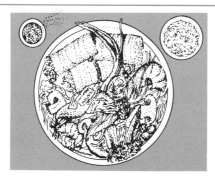

Vietnamese

As is true for other Asian cultures, rice and tea are frequently used items in the Vietnamese diet. Fish provides a popular protein source. Chao gio (rice paper rolls filled with meat, egg, and chopped vegetables and fish sauce) also are favorites.

Italian

Dishes made with pasta frequently grace the table, and bread is served at almost every meal. Favorite vegetables include greens, tomatoes, eggplant, zucchini, and artichokes. Cheese, too, is well liked.

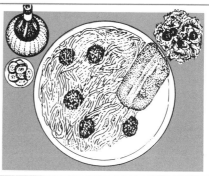

the habits of the predominant ethnic groups in your location. (References for food composition tables for foods used by various ethnic groups are given in Appendix H.)

Mexican

Dried beans are a fundamental part of the Mexican diet. Tortillas made from wheat, flour, or corn replace bread and are served as a part of other foods such as tacos, burritos, and enchiladas. Chili peppers are widely used; often as an ingredient in sauces.

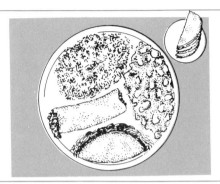

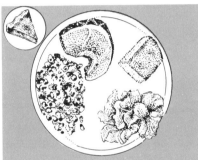

Southern black

The term *soul food* is used to describe traditional foods eaten by Southern blacks dating back to the days of slavery. Pork and chicken are still an important part of the diet. Vegetables, including dried peas and beans, squash, and greens, generally are cooked with salt pork or fatback.

Japanese

The Japanese diet is similar to the diets of other Asian cultures. Fish (especially raw fish) is served frequently, and vegetables are used abundantly. Soy sauce is often added to foods. Green tea is a favorite beverage.

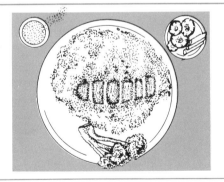

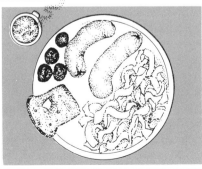

Polish

Polish favorites are often highly salted and seasoned. Sausages and smoked and cured meats are well liked, as are noodles, potatoes, dumplings, and breads. Coffee served with sugar and cream is a favorite beverage.

Table 3.   Example of Dietary Restrictions of Religious
Groups: Jewish Dietary Laws

Meat and meat alternates

- Meat is allowed from the forequarters of cattle, sheep, goats, and deer.
- Animals and poultry are slaughtered, soaked, and salted so as to remove as much blood as possible.
- Only fish that have scales and fins are permitted.
- Shellfish are forbidden.

Milk and dairy foods

- Dairy foods such as milk, cheese, and butter cannot be eaten with a meat meal. After a meat meal, six hours must pass before dairy foods are eaten. One half-hour after a dairy meal, meat can be eaten.
- Eggs can be served as either a meat or dairy meal.

Fruits and vegetables

- Vegetables and fruits can be eaten with either meat or dairy foods.

Fats and oils

- Animal fats are prohibited, unless they are specially certified. Vegetable fats are permitted with either meat or milk meals.

Meal preparation and food storage

- Homes which strictly follow the Jewish Dietary Laws have two complete sets of cooking utensils and dishes; one set for meat and one set for dairy foods. They are stored separately from each other.
- Dishes used for fish are not used for either dairy or meat foods.

but useless if the implications of nutrition research cannot be applied successfully by the individual. Nutrition counseling, therefore, must involve much more than simply giving information. As a counselor, you must integrate diet changes into your client's lifestyle and provide the motivation the client needs to follow through with your suggestions. In other words, counseling is only effective if it results in a change in the client's eating habits.

Nutrition counseling is no easy task. You will improve your counseling skills with practice, but always remember that even the best counselor has some failures. After all, it is not you, but your client, who must accept the responsibility for making the necessary diet changes.

You can enhance your counseling skills by following a logical and organized approach. This step-by-step procedure is referred to as the teaching-learning process: planning, implementing, and evaluating.

teaching-learning process: a logical and organized approach to teaching; consists of three major steps — planning, implementing, and evaluating.

The first step in the teaching-learning process is to adequately prepare for the counseling session. Only by thoroughly assessing a person's nutrition, educational, and emotional needs (Chapter 18) can you hope to make counseling relevant to and appropriate for that person.

Once you have identified a person's educational requirements, you must assess your own knowledge of the subject to be discussed. If you feel insecure regarding your knowledge of the diet, medical condition, future treatment plans, and so on, take the time to find out more before counseling begins. However, don't worry about being asked one or two questions you cannot answer. You can always check the information and get back to the person. This action is certainly preferable to giving incorrect advice or ignoring a question.

Following an assessment of the person's needs and your own knowledge level, you can move on to developing educational objectives. These objectives should be very specific and realistic. For example, when planning a low-cholesterol diet instruction, two objectives might be:

1. The person will be able to explain the rationale for the low-cholesterol diet.

2. The person will be able to plan a day's menu using the low-cholesterol diet booklet.

An unrealistic objective would be to expect the person to know the diet by memory at the end of the session. By defining objectives in terms of actions (behavior) that can be observed, you can better evaluate the effectiveness of nutrition counseling.

After developing specific objectives, you must consider the content of the session (the type and amount of information you will present) as well as the methods you will use (filmstrip, diet booklet, food models, practice menus, food diary). The person's motivational and educational level will guide your choice of methods and the content of the counseling session. For example, a diet instruction booklet in picture form would be useful for an illiterate adult or for a child. A highly educated and motivated person might benefit by knowing in-depth details about the diet, whereas the same information might overwhelm someone who is already confused.

The final consideration in the preparation step is to develop a tentative time frame for accomplishing objectives. Often (as in the hospital setting), you are limited to a certain number of counseling sessions, and you have to use each session optimally. Your time frame should be flexible and should finally be determined by the patient's or client's needs. Some people may move along much faster, and others slower, than originally anticipated.

As you can see, the preparation for a counseling session is as important as the session itself. In reality, these steps can be determined fairly rapidly as you gain experience and sharpen your assessment and planning skills.

The second step in the teaching-learning process is to implement your plan in the actual counseling session. The general communication techniques we discussed previously apply to the teaching-learning process (see Table 4). By the time you begin counseling, you will ideally

Assess needs.

Assess self-knowledge.

Develop objectives.

behavioral objectives: objectives written in such a way that the desired outcome can be either seen or heard.

Determine teaching method.

Implement the counseling session.

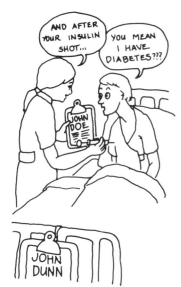

State objectives.

Stress personal responsibility.

Use relevant examples.

Let the patient/client actively participate.

Evaluate the counseling session.

have seen the person at least once and should have established some rapport. Nevertheless, be sure to confirm the person's identity and diagnosis, restate your identity, and take time to establish a trusting and caring atmosphere. Identify and communicate your objectives clearly. If a person knows, for example, that you will ask him to explain the rationale for his diet, he may listen more closely to your explanation. Furthermore, this gives him the opportunity to modify your expectations.

During counseling sessions, you should stress to clients that they are responsible for their health and for making the necessary diet changes. You will often hear statements such as "you need to talk to my wife, she does the cooking." It does help if the family member who prepares the food is present at the counseling session and understands the diet. However, the client *must* accept that it is he, not his wife and not the counselor, who needs the diet and that he is responsible for himself. He should be an active participant in the session.

When discussing recommendations for diet changes, be sure that the person can actually apply the changes. For example, the busy executive who frequently eats restaurant meals must know how to make appropriate food choices in restaurants. A person with a low-income may need help with incorporating lower-cost food items into the diet as well as tips on shopping economically. A person who follows a strictly kosher diet must know how to plan meals around the Jewish Dietary Laws.

You can make diet instructions more relevant to individuals by using many examples consistent with their own eating habits. This is more readily done if you are familiar with their diet histories. You can also have them plan personal menus or ask them to tell you what they would select in a restaurant. In some hospitals, patients select foods from the cafeteria line, and you also can use this experience to facilitate learning.

Always center diet counseling on patients or clients. Let them participate actively in the sessions and arrive at conclusions on their own. Stress the positives and successes rather than the negatives and failures in their current diets.

The third step in the teaching-learning process is evaluation. Ask yourself: Have the objectives of the counseling session been met? Is a change in the content or the methods of instruction required? Is more time needed for counseling? Have the person's nutrition needs changed? Furthermore, how effective was I as a counselor? What methods worked well and which were less effective? How can I improve my instructional techniques for further counseling sessions? The answers to these questions will direct your future actions.

The principles of the teaching-learning process can be applied in either an inpatient or outpatient setting. There are some special considerations with hospitalized patients. Unlike the outpatient, the hospitalized patient is a captive audience. It is not necessarily by choice that such a patient is discussing diet changes with you. Furthermore, the hospital environment is unlike the home environment. A person who has learned to make proper food selections from the hospital menu may still feel lost about what to eat when outside the hospital. Additionally, after the immediate danger of illness has passed, the person may soon give up following a special diet. For these reasons, it is advisable to follow up once the person is at home, through a phone call, home visit, or visit to you by the former patient. At the very least, the person should be referred to someone (either yourself or another agency) who can answer questions regarding the diet.

Follow up.

Table 4.   Nutrition Counseling Checklist

Preparation

- Assess person's needs.
- Develop objectives.
- Determine content of and methods to be used for counseling session.
- Establish tentative time frame for accomplishing objectives.
- Assess own knowledge of subject.
- Arrange for appropriate others to be present at session.

Implementation

- Establish identity and rapport.
- Improve physical environment.
- State objective of counseling session.
- Discuss rationale for diet changes.
- Center session around client or patient.
- Apply principles of diet to lifestyle.
- Reinforce all positive responses.
- Allow adequate time for counseling.
- Use familiar language.
- Use open-ended questions.
- LISTEN.
- Utilize nonverbal communication techniques.
- Use appropriate instructional aids.
- Provide accurate information.
- Answer questions.
- Acknowledge person's cooperation during session.
- Explain next step for followup, if needed.

Evaluation

- Determine if objectives have been met.
- Determine if content and methods have been suited to person's needs.
- Decide if additional counseling is required.
- Evaluate your effectiveness as a counselor.

The Hospital Patient's Perspective

From the patient's perspective, communication channels with health care providers may be very frustrating and confusing. Any one patient may be attended by a primary physician, several consulting physicians, residents, interns, three shifts of nurses that change daily, student nurses, nurses' aides, dietitians and dietary aides, and many other health team members (laboratory technicians, physical therapists, social workers, and so on). Many health care providers work only during the day and, generally, on weekends an entire hospital is covered by only a skeleton staff.

Consider for a moment just how many of these professionals a seriously ill patient encounters during the course of hospitalization. How exasperating for a patient to communicate a need or concern to one health care provider assuming that the information will be shared, only to have to repeat the request over and over again. In addition, miscommunication between professionals can result in inappropriate therapy, which ultimately lengthens the hospital stay and increases confusion for the patient.

As a health care provider, you have the responsibility to tie together the communication networks between patients and professionals. Closing communication gaps often is a very difficult job. You can help your patients most by following through with information or items you told them you would deliver, or explaining why compliance with some of their requests may be delayed or impossible. Often, requests must be forwarded to other departments (for example, requesting a certain food item from the dietary department).

Professional Communication Networks

There are many opportunities for discussion of patient concerns among professionals. Some of these opportunities will be discussed below. Keep in mind that maintaining strong professional communication networks is beneficial to both the patient and the health care team.

The Medical Record   The patient's chart, or medical record, is a compilation of the history, medical problems and therapy, and the expected outcome of treatment. The medical record is your way of sharing information with the health care team. Furthermore, reading the medical record gives you a continuous account of your patient's condition and response to therapy. From this information you can determine how to provide the best possible care for each patient.

You also should consider that the chart is a legal record of what the health care team has done or has failed to do for the patient. Therefore, the medical record is extremely important in malpractice suits and in evaluation of patient care. If you fail to document your actions, it may appear that they were never carried out.

medical record: a continuous written account of the patient's hospitalization.

diagnosis: the disease a person has or is thought to have.

gnosis = knowing

prognosis: the predicted course and outcome of a disease.

pro = ahead of time, before

A **patient care audit** is a thorough peer review of patient management, often conducted through review of documentation in medical records.

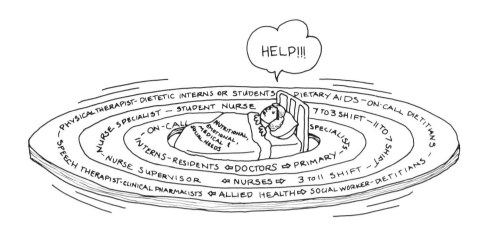

Patient in a sea
of confusion.

There are two basic types of medical records — source-oriented and problem-oriented. The traditional source-oriented medical record (SOMR) is organized according to the source of information. This type of record contains physicians' notes, nurses' notes, laboratory results, and so on, each filed separately in the chart. A major drawback of this system is the failure to focus on the whole patient.

Source-Oriented Medical Record (SOMR)

A new philosophy of organizing medical records involves use of the problem-oriented medical record (POMR), introduced by Lawrence Weed.[1] The POMR has been recommended as an improved method of documentation by all health professionals.[2] Under this system, a problem can be defined as "anything the patient presents with, that requires the health team to do one of three things about it: (a) obtain more information, (b) treat or (c) educate."[3] The physician writes the admission note and generates the initial problem list. Subsequently, each entry made in the chart specifically addresses diagnostic, therapeutic, and patient education actions as related to the problems identified. New problems are added to the problem list as they arise. All health care providers make entries in the same part of the chart. The two major advantages of the POMR are that:

Problem-Oriented Medical Record (POMR)

1. It places more emphasis on total patient care.

2. It recognizes the importance of the health team in patient care.

You will find a POMR easy to read, since it follows a logical flow of thought.

Regardless of the type of medical record used, you should always record important nutrition information in the patient's chart.

An entry made in a POMR is generally written in the form of a **SOAP note.** SOAP stands for Subjective, Objective, Assessment, and Plan.

[1]L. L. Weed, *Medical Records, Medical Education and Patient Care* (Chicago: Year Book Publishers, 1969).

[2]J. L. Ometer, Documentation of nutritional care, *Journal of the American Dietetic Association* 76 (1980):35-40.

[3]A. E. Voytovich, The dietitian/nutritionist and the problem-oriented medical record: I. A physician's viewpoint, *Journal of the American Dietetic Association* 63 (1973):639-641.

GOOD TIDINGS HOSPITAL

PATIENT: S. NICHOLAS

ADMISSION DATE: 12/26

DATA BASE

HEIGHT: 5'5" WEIGHT: 180% IBW

SEX: MALE AGE: OLD

CHEEKS: LIKE ROSES

NOSE: LIKE A CHERRY

GENERAL APPEARANCE: SOOTY

GOOD TIDINGS HOSPITAL

PATIENT: S. NICHOLAS

DATE	#	PROBLEM	INACTIVE DATE
12/26	1	OBESITY	
12/26	2	FROSTBITE	
12/26	3	STOMACHACHE	
12/26	4	EXHAUSTION	12/27
12/26	5	REINDEER BITE	
12/26	6	AMNESIA	
12/26	7	BACKACHE	

GOOD TIDINGS HOSPITAL

PATIENT: S. NICHOLAS

12/26 #3 STOMACHACHE

SUBJECTIVE: CLIENT REPORTS CRAMPS, PAIN, CRAVING FOR COOKIES & MILK, RECENT LARGE CANDY INTAKE.

OBJECTIVE: X-RAYS AND PHYSICAL—NO GI ABNOR- MALITIES. VITAL SIGNS— WITHIN NORMAL LIMITS.

ASSESSMENT: SUSPECT OVERINGESTION OF CONCEN- TRATED SWEETS CAUSING GASTRIC DISTRESS.

PLAN: DX—MONITOR VITAL SIGNS. RX—SUPPORTIVE CARE, LIQUIDS. ED—RE- QUEST DIETITIAN TO INFORM MR. NICHOLAS OF WISER FOOD CHOICES.

Examples of important information are:

- evaluation of patient's current diet
- nutrition assessment data
- recommended nutrition therapy
- patient's acceptance and tolerance of diet
- documentation of diet counseling
- any planned followup or referral to another person or agency
- patient response to nutrition care.

In addition to the formal medical record, various health care providers generally keep records of their own. For example, a nurse keeps a nursing care plan, and a dietitian keeps a nutrition care plan. These records contain some of the information contained in the formal medical record. However, they also include plans and notes which are more detailed and pertinent to the individual health team member. For example, a nutrition care plan may have more details regarding a patient's reaction to a diet, which will later be considered in preparation for diet counseling. Because nurses are involved with direct patient care more often than other team members are, it is wise to insure that the nursing care plan contains information regarding special nutrition needs.

Verbal Communication among Professionals   Generally, many opportunities exist for verbal communication among health team members. If one communication route fails, another can be used. When physicians are not in the hospital, they can be reached in the office, at home, or through an answering service. Health team members within the hospital can be phoned or paged.

Many physicians, particularly in teaching hospitals, conduct bedside rounds that all team members are welcome to attend. During rounds, patients are visited and examined as appropriate. A patient's case is discussed either prior to or following the visit. These discussions are prime opportunities for you to talk over the patient's nutrition problems and to exchange information about the patient's concerns and attitudes.

Nurses also report to one another at the end of each shift. This is a good time to pass along information regarding special nutrition needs required or requested by the patient.

Summing Up

To be effective, communication between health care providers and their patients or clients should be patient-centered, nonjudgmental, and based on trust and concern. Communication can be enhanced through active listening, adjustment of the physical environment, and the use of words that patients can understand.

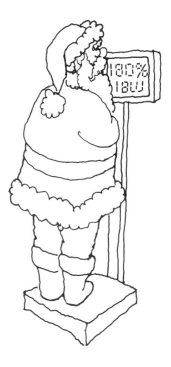

The primary purpose of interviewing is to gather information. During the diet interview, information regarding food intake and the factors affecting nutrient intake or utilization is obtained. Among the factors affecting nutrient intake and utilization are age, sex, activity level, appetite, alterations in taste or smell, difficulties in chewing or swallowing, food allergies, modified diet, religious affiliation, ethnic background, and psychological attitudes regarding food.

The teaching-learning process is a logical and organized approach to nutrition counseling. The three major steps in the teaching-learning process are planning, implementing, and evaluating. With the information you obtain through the assessment of nutrition status, which includes the diet history, you can determine a person's nutrition education needs.

Communication with other members of the health care team also is essential for optimal care of patients. A patient's chart is a legal document, a continuous record of the history, medical problems and therapy, and the expected outcome of the treatment. The medical record contains valuable input from all members of the health care team and is an appropriate place for sharing important information about each patient. Health team members should take advantage of opportunities to communicate nutrition needs.

To Explore Further

Numerous books that specifically deal with communication for nurses and allied health professionals can be found in university libraries. Some of these books are:

● Bernstein, L., Bernstein, R., and Dana, R. *Interviewing: A Guide for Health Professionals*, 3rd ed. New York: Appleton-Century-Crofts, 1980.

● Froelich, R., and Bishop, F. M. *Medical Interviewing: A Programmed Manual*, 2nd ed. St. Louis: Mosby, 1972.

● Edwards, B., and Brelhart, J. K. *Communication in Nursing Practice*. St. Louis: Mosby, 1981.

● Narrow, B. *Patient Teaching in Nursing Practice, a Patient and Family Centered Approach*. New York: Wiley, 1979.

A physician has written a very good book that profiles six patients with various diseases and includes actual dialogues in which the patients discuss how they cope with their diseases:

● Rosenberg, M. L. *Patients, the Experience of Illness*. Philadelphia: Saunders, 1980.

This book discusses many factors influencing food intake, including social, cultural, religious, and economic factors. The book is short and easy to read:

● Jenner, A. *Food: Fact or Folklore.* Toronto: McClelland and Stewart, 1973.

There are also excellent chapters on factors affecting food intake in the following books:

● Williams, S. R. *Nutrition and Diet Therapy,* 4th ed. St. Louis: Mosby, 1981, Chapter 13, pp. 266-290.

● Krause, M. V., and Mahan, L. K. *Food, Nutrition and Diet Therapy,* 6th ed. Philadelphia: Saunders, 1979, Chapter 17, pp. 355-366.

Several worthwhile articles on communicating, interviewing, and nutrition counseling include:

● Ling, L., Spragg, D., Stein, P., and Myers, M. L. Guidelines for diet counseling. *Journal of the American Dietetic Association* 66 (1975):571-575.

● Korsch, B. M. In search of doctor-patient rapport. *Therapaeia,* September 1981, pp. 64-65.

● Puckett, M. J., and Russell, M. The role of the allied health professional in improving patient adherence. *Journal of Allied Health,* Winter 1978, pp. 36-41.

● Jungman, L. B. When your feelings get in the way. *American Journal of Nursing,* June 1979, pp. 1074-1075.

● Almore, M. G. Dyadic communication. *American Journal of Nursing,* June 1979, pp. 1076-1078.

● Ramaekers, M. J. Communication blocks revisited. *American Journal of Nursing,* June 1979, pp. 1079-1081.

● Mahoney, M. J., and Caggiula, A. W. Applying behavioral methods to nutritional counseling. *Journal of the American Dietetic Association* 72 (1978):372-377.

● Ferguson, J. Dietitians as behavior-change agents. *Journal of the American Dietetic Association* 73 (1978):231-238.

Numerous references are available for obtaining information on problem-oriented medical records. Some that may be of interest to you are:

● Recording nutritional information in medical records. Chicago: American Hospital Association, 1976 (810 North Lake Shore Drive, Chicago, IL 60611).

● Voytovich, A., Walters, F. M., DeMarco, M., Chappelle, M., and Scholl, R. The dietitian/nutritionist and the problem-oriented medical record, Parts I-III. *Journal of the American Dietetic Association* 63 (1973):643-645.

● Rackel, R. E. The problem-oriented medical record (POMR). *American Family Physician* 10 (1974):100-111.

● Bernie, R., and Readley, H. *Problem-Oriented Medical Record Implementation,* 2nd ed. St. Louis: Mosby, 1978.

Rubber food models can be very expensive, but an inexpensive set of realistic cardboard models can be obtained from the National Dairy Council (address in Appendix J).

Identifying Nutrition Education Needs

Mr. Smith is a 68-year-old black male who lives with his 66-year-old wife in a rural community in South Georgia. Mr. Smith is 5′8″ tall and weighs 180 pounds. He has been seen irregularly in the health clinic for about three years for various and relatively minor complaints such as flu symptoms. During his last visit the physician noted that Mr. Smith had been gaining weight steadily and referred him to the nutritionist.

During the diet interview the nutritionist learned that Mr. Smith generally sleeps about six hours per day and usually enjoys working in his garden for about two to three hours per day, but that lately he has been spending less time gardening. Other types of activities are mainly sedentary, such as reading or watching TV. The nutritionist obtained a usual food intake pattern as follows:

Time	Food	Amount
8:00 a.m.	Grits	3/4 c
	Margarine	1 tsp
	Biscuits or cornbread (3-inch square)	2-3 pieces
	Margarine	2-3 tsp
	Bacon	2-3 slices
	Coffee	2 c
	Whole milk	2 tbsp
	Sugar	4 tsp
1:00 p.m.	Dried beans or peas (cooked with fatback)	1 c
	Collard, mustard, or turnip greens (cooked with fatback)	1 c
	Boiled potatoes or rice	1 c
	Cornbread (3-inch square)	2 pieces
	Margarine	2 tsp
	Iced tea	2 10-oz glasses
	Sugar	4 tsp
7:00 p.m.	Meat or poultry (usually pork or chicken)	2-3 oz
	Vegetables (cabbage, greens, or corn cooked with fatback or salt pork)	1 c
	Mashed sweet potatoes	1 c
	Cornbread (3-inch square)	2 pieces
	Margarine	2 tsp
	Iced tea	10 oz
	Sugar	2 tsp
	Pie or cobbler	3-inch wedge

Mr. Smith's appetite is good, but he wears poorly fitting dentures and has trouble chewing raw vegetables and many meats. His wife shops and prepares the food (she also is overweight). Mr. Smith is retired and he and his wife live on social security. Mr. Smith states that food prices have forced him and his wife into eating less meat.

Study Questions

1. Compare Mr. Smith's intake with the Four Food Group Plan. Are any food groups or food types omitted from the diet? Are any food groups or food types used excessively in the diet?

2. After reviewing the diet history, can you explain why Mr. Smith has been gaining weight steadily? Will Mr. Smith need nutrition counseling?

3. Compare Mr. Smith's eating habits with the food pattern for Southern blacks described in Chapter 19. Are Mr. Smith's eating habits typical of the region he lives in? Assume you have decided that nutrition counseling is appropriate for Mr. Smith. Prepare for the interview by considering the following:

4. What are Mr. Smith's nutrition and educational needs?

5. Should anyone other than Mr. Smith be present at the counseling sessions?

6. What dietary changes can you recommend consistent with Mr. Smith's cultural food preferences?

7. Will the changes you recommend be affordable to the Smiths?

8. What positive aspects of Mr. Smith's diet can you emphasize?

9. How can Mr. Smith's interest in gardening be used beneficially in his diet program?

10. What are your specific objectives for Mr. Smith and what methods would you use for accomplishing these objectives?

You have begun counseling Mr. Smith regarding his diet.

11. How will you evaluate whether or not your teaching objectives have been met?

12. How will you follow up with Mr. Smith to check his progress and to see if he understands his diet? Who could help you determine if Mr. Smith is eligible for any social services which might help reduce his personal food costs?

13. Write a SOAP note justifying your nutrition care plan for Mr. Smith.

Optional Extra

Take some time to complete a diet history form on yourself. What factors strongly influence your eating habits?

Saying More Than "Yes, Doctor"

Many people misunderstand the meaning of assertion on the job. They do not differentiate between assertion and aggression. But assertion does not signify ... punching a co-worker in the nose; it involves honest communication at the right moment to achieve mutual job goals.
HERBERT FENSTERHEIM, Ph.D., and JEAN BAUR

Dr. Block is an elderly surgeon who is extremely competent except for his lack of knowledge regarding nutrition. He is very difficult to talk to and he feels strongly that health care providers should "follow the doctor's orders" without making waves. Dr. Block's patient, Mrs. X, had extensive surgery three weeks ago and is still eating very poorly.

Miss Grey, the primary nurse, has done all she can to get Mrs. X to eat, with no results. The patient has lost 20 percent of her usual body weight and her surgical incisions are healing slowly. Miss Grey feels the patient should be fed by tube (see Chapter 20). Miss Grey's problem: How should she approach Dr. Block with her recommendations, get the results she wants, and not offend Dr. Block?

You may be thinking, what's the problem? Why can't Miss Grey just say "Mrs. X is malnourished, she is not eating, and she would probably benefit from a tube feeding"? Surely Dr. Block would realize that Miss Grey was only trying to help his patient. Unfortunately, this is not always the case.

Communication between Doctor and Health Care Provider   What happens to communication networks at the professional level? Although there are volumes of books that discuss communications between the various health care professionals and patients, very little has been written regarding how professionals communicate among themselves. Yet, only a few days of work in a health care setting will demonstrate that communication problems among professionals, particularly between physicians and other health care providers, are very common.

Physicians' complaints that other health care professionals fail to carry out their orders almost always stem from communication problems. Orders may be misinterpreted. Some orders may conflict with others. Some may be unrealistic or impossible to fulfill. For example, a diet instruction may be ordered for a patient leaving the hospital, and the dietitian may not be available to help with it. In one extreme case, an order was written for a 500 kcalorie weight reduction diet with milkshakes between meals!

On the other hand, nurses and other health care providers feel stuck when they cannot openly make recommendations for patient care without either being ignored or being reprimanded for "stepping out of line."

Rules of the Game   In 1967, Leonard I. Stein wrote an article in which he described communications between doctors and nurses as the doctor-nurse game.[1] Although the article specifically discusses communication between doctors and nurses, the general concepts also apply to other nonmedical professional groups.

Stein states that the object of the game is as follows: "The nurse is to be bold, have initiative, and be responsible for making significant recommendations, while at the same time she must appear passive. This must be done in such a manner as to make her recommendations appear to be initiated by the physician." Likewise, a physician who wants to hear a nurse's recommendations must ask for them without appearing to do so.

[1]Leonard I. Stein, The doctor-nurse game, *Archives of General Psychiatry* 16 (1967):699-703.

Let's go back to Dr. Block and Miss Grey and see how they could effectively play the game:

Miss Grey: Dr. Block, Mrs. X is still not eating and has lost a good bit of weight. Her family has expressed concern. Do you think a tube feeding might be helpful?

Dr. Block: Have the nurses tried everything else?

Miss Grey: Yes.

Dr. Block: Order a standard tube feeding. I will insert the tube this afternoon.

Miss Grey has made a recommendation without appearing to do so. Dr. Block has also asked for the nurse's recommendation by ordering a "standard tube feeding." The nurse then selects the formula from those available in the hospital or calls the dietitian to make the formula selection.

What happens when the game is not played according to the "rules?" Perhaps one of the most frustrating and counterproductive results is that the suggestion may be ignored. Furthermore, the nurse (or other health care provider) may be verbally berated. Doctors who fail to play the game (in other words, fail to pick up on subtle suggestions) are not treated to the courtesies extended to those who skillfully play the game.

Why Barriers Develop
What circumstances have allowed such a distorted communication system to develop? Stein identifies the training of both physicians and nurses as contributing to this system.[2] Early in medical training, physicians realize that if they make a mistake, the cost may be a patient's life. They understandably develop a fear of making mistakes, which they handle by assuming a posture of omnipotence.[3] Although the physician values the recommendations of others, overtly accepting advice from a nonphysician threatens this posture. So a system in which doctors appear to initiate all recommendations works well for them in some ways.

Nurses, on the other hand, are trained to treat physicians with utmost respect. Furthermore, they are taught that physicians are far more knowledgeable than they and, therefore, that physicians deserve special treatment. Sonja Herman believes that physicians and nurses perpetuate the nurses' subservient role.[4] "Behaviorally, nurses themselves perpetuate this by taking on other duties such as handing charts to physicians, or standing up and giving them their chair when they come into the nurse's station, referring patient questions to physicians, or remaining silent after the doctor criticizes them unjustly in front of patients."

A further consideration is the fact that most doctors are men and most nurses are women. Thus, patterns of male dominance and female subservience also come into play.

Communication among Other Health Care Providers   Unfortunately, communication problems do not involve only physicians. Communication blocks also are present within each health discipline and between the various health care professions. For example, day shift nurses may complain that night shift nurses do not follow through with nursing care plans. The dietitian may get disgusted with the nursing staff for failing to record a patient's intake. These problems are generally problems of miscommunication.

Breaking Communication Barriers   How can you overcome communication barriers in the health care setting? One positive step you can take is to get to know the people you work with as people. It is generally easier to communicate with people you know. And you also will feel better about your work situation.

Additionally, it is very important for you to understand and know the roles of the various health care pro-

[2]Stein, 1967.

[3]Stein, 1967.

[4]Sonja J. Herman, Barriers to nurses becoming assertive, in *Becoming Assertive: A Guide for Nurses* (New York: Van Nostrand, 1978), p. 127.

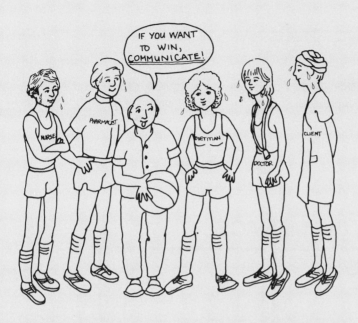

To be effective, health care teams must communicate openly with each other. Furthermore, by working with other team members each gains an appreciation for and an understanding of what other team members do. Hopefully, trends in education will continue to change, so that physicians will see their role in more realistic terms, and so that other health care providers will become more assertive.

Concluding Thoughts

A valuable resource is lost when "games" are the only method of communication. And that valuable resource is time. Furthermore, poor communications cause grumblings among physicians and other health care providers and end up hurting an innocent bystander — the patient. When optimal care (which must include effective communication) is not provided, the patient loses.

viders. If you fail to appreciate the part each health care discipline plays in therapy, you may feel some role is unimportant and create additional communication problems. The clinical dietitian provides a good example. Although these professionals receive intensive scientific training, they often are perceived by other health care providers (and patients) as "the ones who get the food."

The clinical dietitian, in trying to analyze a patient's intake, generally must rely on the nurse to record what the patient has eaten at each meal. The nurse who sees the dietitian as a "cook" may think the intake record is unimportant and may not comply with the dietitian's request. Worse yet, the nurse may not perceive nutrition as important to the patient's

care at all.

Communication can be made much more effective if you explain *what* you are doing and *why* you need another professional's help. Eventually, your role will be accepted.

Finally, when you do make recommendations, communicate clearly. Most importantly, know what you are talking about. Be ready to discuss the rationale for your recommendations.

Future Prospects   Are communications still where they were in 1967 when Stein wrote his article? Although actual research in this area is lacking, matters seem to be improving somewhat. Probably the most impressive change agent has been the development of the health care team (see Highlight 20B).

To Explore Further

An excellent reference for health care professionals who want to learn to become more effective in communicating is:

● Herman, S. J. *Becoming Assertive: A Guide for Nurses.* New York: Van Nostrand, 1978.

One of the most important messages in assertiveness training is to learn the difference between being *assertive*, which doesn't offend, and being *aggressive*, which does.

CHAPTER 20

CONTENTS

DENNIS the MENACE

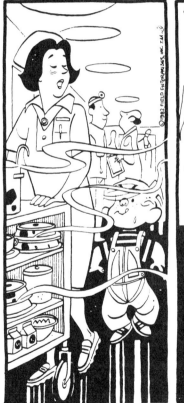
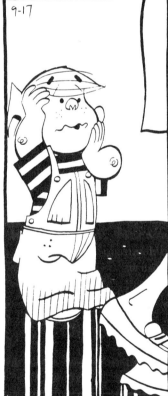

"SORRY, SONNY. THIS FOOD IS FOR **SICK** PEOPLE."

"I'M NOT FEELIN' SO HOT!"

"Dennis The Menace by permission of Hank Ketcham and by Field Enterprises, Inc."

SELECTION OF FEEDINGS AND FEEDING ROUTES

Whatsoever was the father of a disease, an ill diet was the mother.

GEORGE HERBERT

The general reaction to hospital food is negative. You may recall jokes you have heard about hospital food or the reaction of a person you know (maybe yourself) to hospital food.

Often, complaints about food are really the hospital patient's way of venting fear, frustration, anger, and physical pain. Eating, or refusing to eat, is one of the few experiences hospital patients can control. When they are worried about their health, upset over their progress or the way they are being treated, or in pain, they are likely to complain about food.

You also can consider that hospital food is not cooked as food is at home, which becomes a problem when the patient must eat three meals a day for many days in the hospital. Furthermore, hospital meals are served at times when many patients are not hungry. Unfortunately, the food may also be cold by the time it arrives in the room. The patient often must eat alone, in bed, which makes mealtimes more of a chore than a pleasurable experience.

Throughout Chapter 20, we will be discussing general concepts about diets served in the hospital. Alternative methods of feeding people who cannot eat table foods also will be explored.

Goals of Diet Therapy

The primary goal of diet therapy is to achieve or maintain optimal nutrition status. Optimal status is achieved when you provide appropriate amounts of energy, protein, carbohydrate, fat, vitamins, minerals, trace elements, and water to the cells. Furthermore, these nutrients must be provided in a form which is easy for the body to use and which will not stress the body physiologically. For example, if a patient's GI tract is not functioning, it will do no good to provide that patient with a standard diet.

In addition to the overall goal of diet therapy, each diet prescribed for someone has its own rationale and purpose. The rationale of a weight

When something is not produced by the body and must come from outside sources such as food, then that substance is said to be **exogenous** (ex-ODGE-uh-nus). A substance originating within the body cells or tissues is referred to as **endogenous** (end-ODGE-uh-nus).

A **modified,** or **therapeutic, diet** is a regular diet which has been adjusted to accommodate special nutrition needs. Such diets can be adjusted in consistency, in level of energy and nutrients, in amount of fluid, in number of meals, or by the elimination of certain foods.

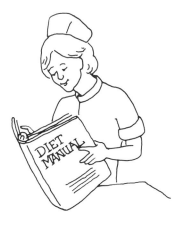

diet order: a physician's written statement in the medical record of what diet a patient should receive.

reduction diet is to provide less energy from food so that the person will use stored energy and lose weight. The purpose of weight reduction may vary from improving self-image to gaining better control of blood sugar levels.

In order for a person to benefit maximally from diet therapy, a thorough assessment of the person must be completed and nutrition needs must be correctly identified. The diet therapy selected must complement other medical therapy. For example, a diet planned for an insulin-dependent diabetic must be coordinated so that food is available during the times when the body will have insulin.

Standard and Modified Diets   A *regular* or *standard diet* is a diet which provides the recommended daily allowances of nutrients and includes all foods. On the other hand, a *modified diet* is a diet which differs from a regular diet in consistency, level of individual nutrients, energy or fluid, number of meals, or the elimination of certain foods. Table 1 lists examples of diets which have been modified in various ways.

The exact foods excluded or included on a specific modified diet differ among hospitals, generally in minor ways. These differences reflect different schools of thought regarding diet. The best way to familiarize yourself with a particular hospital's diet is by reading the diet manual.

In larger hospitals, diet manuals are compiled by the staff of dietitians and approved by the hospital administrator, several physicians, and representatives of the nursing service. Smaller hospitals may adopt the diet manual of another hospital or an organization such as the state dietetic association. The diet manual contains information regarding foods allowed and not allowed on each diet, the rationale and indications for use of the diet, sample menus, and information regarding the nutritional adequacy of the diet. The diets listed in the manual are those available through the dietary department. We will be discussing specific modified diets in later chapters as we look at nutrition in various disease states.

The physician is responsible for ordering the patient's diet, and the diet order is written in the medical record. The name given to the diet should be consistent with the name given in the hospital's diet manual. To avoid miscommunication the physician must describe exact modifications, when appropriate. For example, a 1,200 kcalorie diet, rather than a low kcalorie diet, should be specified. A diet required to be "low sodium" could be interpreted as containing anything from 500 to 4,000 mg of sodium.

What happens when a physician's order for a dietary modification is vague? In most cases, the responsibility for choosing the exact modification will fall to the dietitian or the nurse. The diet manual will generally give information as to what diet will be sent when vague orders are received by the dietary department. The dietitian, after seeing the patient and interpreting the physician's order, should chart the exact diet being sent in the patient's medical record. The dietitian or nurse often makes recommendations to physicians when diet orders are unclear or changes appear warranted. Whenever possible, the health team jointly recommends the most appropriate diet.

Because the physician is ultimately responsible for a patient's diet order, it is easy for others to follow the order without further consideration. But all health care providers are responsible for patient care.

Ideally, a dietitian should visit and review the chart of every patient admitted to the hospital. Generally, however, the dietitian is assigned to so many patients that this is virtually impossible. Therefore, most clinical dietitians see only patients on modified diets or patients they have been asked to see. In some smaller hospitals a clinical dietitian may not even be employed.

Typical examples of mistakes which occur daily because of inappropriate diet orders include the following:

● A grossly overweight patient is described as "well-nourished" and placed on a regular diet. Because the patient is not on a modified diet, the dietitian does not see him, and he receives an inappropriate diet and no nutrition advice.

● A patient is ordered N.P.O. by the physician, who wants a lab test to be run. Due to a miscommunication, the doctor thinks the order is changed after the test, but it isn't. The patient is needlessly "starved" for three or more days.

An order which reads "N.P.O." means that nothing is to be given to the patient orally (including food and medications). **N.P.O.** stands for *nil per os,* which means "nothing by mouth." On the other hand, **P.O.** stands for *per os,* which means "by mouth" or "orally."

● A patient routinely enjoys foods low in sugar and salt. Foods served on the regular diet are too salty for her. So she eats very little food. Furthermore, she feels the hospital has totally neglected its responsibility to provide nutritious foods to its patients.

Why isn't the diet ordered correctly in the first place? In cases where many doctors, interns, and residents are seeing a patient, miscommunication can easily occur. Furthermore, the patient may communicate needs more clearly and more often to the nurse or other health care provider than to the physician. Some doctors may not even consider nutrition to be a significant part of patient care.

CAUTION:

Written diet orders are not always appropriate.

Table 1. Examples of Modified Diets

Consistency modified diets	Nutrient modified diets	Diets excluding certain foods
Clear liquid diet	Reduced kcalorie diet	Allergy diet
Full liquid diet	High-kcalorie diet	Gluten restricted diet
Soft diet	Low-protein diet	Purine restricted diet
Low-residue diet	High-protein diet	Tyramine restricted diet
High-fiber diet	Low-fat diet	Lactose restricted diet
Tube feedings	Low-cholesterol diet	
	Low-potassium diet	
	High-potassium diet	
	Low-sodium diet	
	Fluid restricted diet	
	Force fluids	

In institutions which utilize a **centralized food service** system, meals are prepared and served from a central kitchen. In a **decentralized food service** system, food is generally prepared in a central kitchen but heated and distributed from smaller satellite kitchens located throughout the institution.

A **selective menu** is a menu from which patients can select the foods they will receive while hospitalized. **House diets** are preselected by the dietary department.

Oral Diets The majority of people in the hospital are given oral diets to provide for nutrient needs. Hospital diets should be as similar as possible to what they eat at home. The individual's history is of critical importance in determining what food is acceptable (see Chapter 19). Extra effort should be made to insure that foods are served at the correct temperature and that patients receive what they have ordered. These considerations are of special concern in the hospital patient whose illness, fears, and frustrations may significantly interfere with the desire to eat.

When someone's appetite is poor, individualizing the diet often helps correct the problem. When that step fails, supplementing the diet with appropriate foods or liquid formulas (see below) is tried. If the patient remains at risk nutritionally, alternative methods of feeding must be considered. These methods include tube feedings and intravenous nutrition, which we will be discussing in detail throughout the remainder of this chapter (see Figure 1).

Complete and Supplemental Liquid Nutrition As we have discussed previously, when someone cannot eat enough food, the first step is to try to supplement the diet. This can be accomplished by increasing the amount of food or by giving snacks between meals. Liquid supplementation often is useful, because food is easier to "drink" than to eat. Psychologically, liquids seem to be less filling, and they are much easier for debilitated patients to handle.

Liquid supplements can include common drinks like milk, milkshakes, or instant breakfast drinks. Commercially prepared liquid formulas also are available (some of these formulas are listed in Table 2). These liquids can be fortified with dry powdered milk to make them higher in protein. kCalories can be increased by adding a source of carbohydrate such as corn syrup or sugar. Commercial products (also listed in Table 2) can be used to increase the protein, fat, or carbohydrate content of any liquid supplement.

Even when a person enjoys a liquid supplement, palatability becomes a problem after long-term use. Sometimes you can relieve boredom by using more than one type of supplemental feeding. You can also add flavorings such as chocolate, decaffeinated instant coffee, and strawberry as well as other fruit flavorings. Commercially prepared flavor packets are available in a wide variety of flavors; these packets can conveniently be kept at the bedside for use as desired.

You can help a person accept liquid feedings more readily by serving them attractively. For example, a liquid feeding served from a can is far less appealing than one served in a glass. You can also help by serving the formula cold and providing an ice bath so that it can be kept cold and sipped as desired.

When a liquid formula supplies all the nutrients needed it is called a complete formula. A complete formula always should be used when the liquid formula is the sole source of nutrients. However, complete formulas also can be (and often are) used as supplemental feedings. When used in this way, they may not be given in quantities large enough to meet all nutrient needs. Table 2 lists some commercially available formulas.

Complete formulas can be made from table foods blenderized into a liquid form. Baby food meats, milk, iron-fortified baby cereals or potatoes, strained vegetables, and strained fruits are typical ingredients. The nutrient contents of these blenderized diets must be checked (usually by the dietitian) to assure that the recipient's nutrient requirements will be met. Of course, you can always add a liquid vitamin-mineral preparation to fortify the formula.

Blenderized diets made as described above are seldom used in institutional settings. Commercial formulas are far more convenient to use, their nutrient composition is constant, they flow through feeding tubes more readily, and far less risk of bacterial contamination is associated with their use. Commercially prepared formulas are available in a ready-to-use liquid form or in a powdered form which must be reconstituted with water.

As you can see from Table 2, many commercially prepared formulas are available. How do you know which one to select for your patient? What are those chemical ingredients and what do they mean?

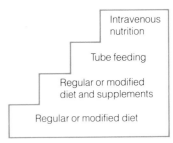

Figure 1 Selection of feeding method. Take one step at a time, starting from the bottom.

intravenous (IV): through a vein.

enteral nutrition: the delivery of nutrients utilizing the intestine. Oral diets and tube feedings are types of enteral nutrition.

enteron = intestine

parenteral nutrition: the delivery of nutrients through the veins (intravenously).

para = bypassing (the intestine)

blenderized diet: a liquid diet made from a combination of table foods. Blenderized diets usually contain pureed meat, vegetables, fruits, milk, and starches with vitamins and minerals added as necessary. They can be made in a blender or purchased commercially.

Table 2. Some Complete and Supplemental Formulas*

	Source of protein	kCalories per 100 ml	Protein (g) per 100 ml	Osmolality (mOsm)	Form
Hydrolyzed Formulas					
Criticare HN (Mead Johnson)	Small peptides, free amino acids	106	3.8	650	Ready to use
Travasorb STD (Travenol)	Oligopeptides	100	3.0	560	Powder
Travasorb HN (Travenol)	Oligopeptides	100	4.5	560	Powder
Vipep (Cutter)	Small peptides, free amino acids	100	2.5	520	Powder
Vital (Ross)	Peptides, oligopeptides, free amino acids	100	4.2	460	Powder
Vivonex STD (Norwich-Eaton)	Free amino acids	100	2.2	550	Powder
Vivonex HN (Norwich-Eaton)	Free amino acids	100	4.4	810	Powder
Intact formulas					
Blenderized formulas					
Compleat-B (Doyle)	Meat, milk	107	4.0	405	Ready to use; contains lactose
Compleat-Modified (Doyle)	Meat, calcium caseinate	107	4.3	300	Ready to use
Formula II (Cutter)	Wheat, meat, egg, milk	100	3.8	435-510	Ready to use; contains lactose
Vitaneed (Organon)	Meat, calcium caseinate, vegetables	102	3.5	375	Ready to use
Isolate formulas:					
Ensure (Ross)	Caseinates, soy protein isolate	106	3.7	450	Ready to use
Ensure Plus (Ross)	Caseinates, soy protein isolate	150	5.5	600	Ready to use
Isocal (Mead Johnson)	Caseinates, soy protein isolate	106	3.4	300	Ready to use
Isocal HCN (Mead Johnson)	Caseinates	200	7.5	690	Ready to use
Magnacal (Organon)	Caseinates	200	7.0	590	Ready to use
Meritene liquid (Doyle)	Milk	100	5.8	505-570	Ready to use; contains lactose

Osmolite (Ross)	Caseinates, soy protein isolate	106	3.7	300	Ready to use
Precision Isotonic (Doyle)	Egg white solids	96	2.9	300	Powder
Precision LR (Doyle)	Egg white solids	110	2.6	480	Powder
Precision HN (Doyle)	Egg white solids	105	4.4	557	Powder
Renu (Organon)	Caseinates	100	3.5	300	Ready to use
Sustacal liquid (Mead Johnson)	Caseinates, soy protein isolate	100	6.1	625	Ready to use
Sustacal HC (Mead Johnson)	Caseinates	150	6.1	650	Ready to use

Supplemental formulas	Use	Description	Form
Casec (Mead Johnson)	Protein supplement	Protein source is caseinate; 4 g protein and 17 kcal per tbsp	Powder
Citrotein (Doyle)	Protein and kcalorie supplement	Protein source is egg white solids; 7.7 g protein and 127 kcal per serving	Powder
Pro-Mix (NAVACO)	Protein supplement	Protein source is whey; 5 g protein and 22 kcal per tbsp	Powder
Propac (Organon)	Protein supplement	Protein source is whey; 3 g protein and 16 kcal per tbsp	Powder
Controlyte (Doyle)	Carbohydrate (kcalorie) supplement	35 kcal per tbsp	Powder
Moducal (Mead Johnson)	Carbohydrate (kcalorie) supplement	30 kcal per tbsp powder; 2 kcal per ml liquid	Powder, liquid
Polycose (Ross)	Carbohydrate (kcalorie) supplement	32 kcal per tbsp powder; 2 kcal per ml liquid	Powder, liquid
Sumacal (Organon)	Carbohydrate (kcalorie) supplement	2 kcal per ml	Liquid
Sumacal Plus (Organon)	Carbohydrate (kcalorie) supplement	2.5 kcal per ml	Liquid
MCT Oil (Mead Johnson)	Fat supplement	7.7 kcal per ml in the form of medium-chain triglycerides	Liquid
Microlipid (Organon)	Fat supplement	4.5 kcal per ml; contains essential fatty acids	Liquid

*This table is not intended as a complete listing of all available formulas. The amounts of nutrients were accurate at the time the list was compiled. The osmolality of some formulas varies depending on the flavor.

Formula Characteristics

The ideal formula for an individual is one that meets nutrient needs with the least risk of complications and at the least cost. When a formula is given orally, it also must taste good. Other factors important in selecting a formula include osmolality, residue, and individual tolerance.

intact protein formula: a liquid diet that contains a complete protein that has not been altered.

protein isolate: a type of intact protein; a protein with high biological value that has been separated from a source containing a variety of proteins. A **protein isolate formula** contains a protein isolate as the source of protein.

hydrolyzed protein: an intact protein treated with acids or enzymes to yield a combination of free amino acids and short peptide chains.

The term **monomeric** (MON-oh-MERR-ic) is sometimes used to describe formulas which have hydrolyzed protein or free amino acids as the source of protein. **Polymeric** (POLL-ee-MERR-ic) formulas contain an intact protein source.

Some hydrolyzed formulas are called **elemental** or **defined formula diets** because the nutrients are present in the most elemental or simple form. The term *defined formula diet* is preferable to the term *elemental diet.*

Meeting Nutrient Needs   A person can only benefit from a diet which meets energy, protein, fat, vitamin, and mineral needs. This is of particular importance for patients receiving liquid formulas, because they often have altered nutrient needs due to illness. Furthermore, you are depending on one food source to meet all of these needs.

Providing a person with appropriate amounts of nutrients will do no good if the nutrients cannot be digested and absorbed. Patients who do not have a functioning GI tract are not candidates for oral or tube feedings. However, patients with minimal GI function may be able to benefit from certain formulas. Therefore, the chemical composition of the protein, fat, and carbohydrate in the formula must be considered.

There are two major types of formulas. Those that contain protein, carbohydrates, and fats of higher molecular weights are called intact formulas. The patient must be able to digest and absorb nutrients without difficulty to use this type of formula. Intact formulas can be blenderized diets or protein isolate formulas. (A protein isolate formula contains a purified protein.)

The second type of formula is hydrolyzed formula. These formulas contain smaller molecules of protein (including dipeptides and tripeptides), fat, and carbohydrate. They are, in a sense, "predigested," and therefore only minimal further digestion is needed. Patients who lack digestive capabilities or who have a smaller than normal area for absorbing nutrients may benefit from these formulas.

Defined formula diets are the simplest of the hydrolyzed protein formulas. They contain free amino acids, simple carbohydrate, and very little fat. Several recent studies suggest that the dipeptides and tripeptides available from hydrolyzed formulas may actually be better absorbed than free amino acids, however.

A small number of formulas are termed modular feedings. Some are intact, and some are hydrolyzed. They serve only to add certain nutrients or energy to the diet, rather than being complete in themselves.

Osmolality   Osmolality is a measurement of the concentration of molecular and ionic particles in a solution. The greater the number of particles in a solution, the greater the osmolality. The important thing to know about osmolality is that water flows from an area of low osmolality to one of higher osmolality (see also Chapter 14, pp. 488-489).

The osmolality of normal blood serum is about 300 milliosmoles per liter (mOsm). The osmolality of formulas ranges from about 250 mOsm to over 800 mOsm. A formula that approximates the osmolality of the serum is referred to as an isotonic formula. A hypertonic formula has a higher osmolality than serum.

When a hypertonic formula moves into the intestine, water from in and around the body cells eventually also moves out into the intestine. If the patient's body has had time to adapt to the hypertonic solution, this is usually not a problem. However, if adaptation has not occurred, diarrhea, vomiting, cramps, or nausea can result.[1] Therefore, the most desirable formulas are those as near isotonic as possible.

A hydrolyzed formula may contain exactly the same amount of protein as an intact formula, but it contains many more particles. Hydrolyzed formulas are therefore higher in osmolality than most intact protein formulas and so are more likely to cause the GI symptoms discussed above.

Residue   Residue is a combination of undigested and unabsorbed food in the colon. Intestinal secretions, bacteria, and the turnover of intestinal cells also produce residue. The residue content of the diet is largely responsible for fecal bulk. As we will be discussing in Chapter 23, people with certain gastrointestinal disorders need diets that are very low in residue. Higher-residue diets may help stimulate normal bowel function in people who do not need low-residue diets.

Since hydrolyzed formulas are almost completely absorbed, they leave very little residue in the gut. Protein isolate formulas have a low to moderate residue content. Blenderized formulas are the highest in residue of the types discussed earlier.

Individual Tolerances   Many individual tolerances must be considered in formula selection. If the patient has any allergies or food intolerances, then the formula selected must not contain the offending substances.

osmolality: the number of molecular and ionic particles (osmoles) per kilogram of water in a solution.

isotonic formula: a formula with an osmolality similar to that of blood serum (300 mOsm).

iso = the same
ton = tension

hypertonic formula: a formula with an osmolality higher than that of blood serum.

hyper = greater, more

Figure 2   Advantages and disadvantages of formula types.

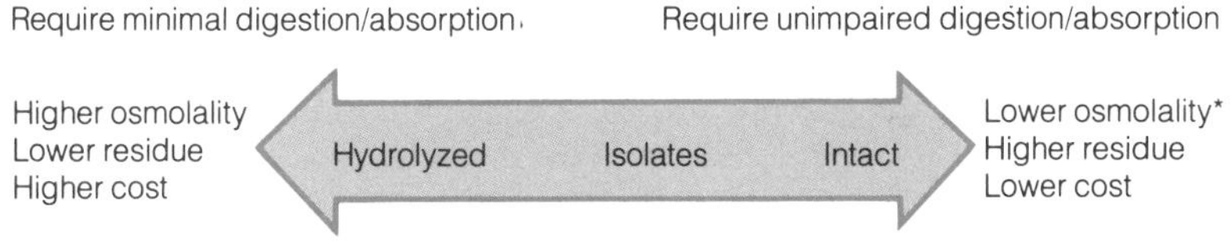

Require minimal digestion/absorption.   Require unimpaired digestion/absorption

Higher osmolality
Lower residue
Higher cost

Hydrolyzed   Isolates   Intact

Lower osmolality*
Higher residue
Lower cost

*Except for the isotonic formulas which are, for the most part, made from protein isolates, the osmolality of protein isolate formulas and intact formulas are similar.

[1]S. B. Heymsfield, J. Horowitz, and D. Lawson, Enteral hyperalimentation, in *Developments in Digestive Diseases*, ed. J. E. Birk (Philadelphia: Lea and Febiger, 1980), pp. 59-83.

Many adults who normally tolerate milk become temporarily lactose intolerant following GI surgery or during radiation therapy or chemotherapy. When they are given a formula with lactose, they become bloated and develop cramps and diarrhea. The nurse or dietitian who is alert to this possibility can save such a person much misery and pain.

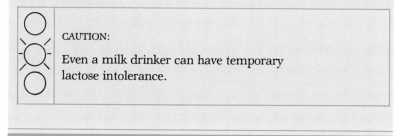

CAUTION:

Even a milk drinker can have temporary lactose intolerance.

When a patient is taking a formula orally, palatability is a major concern. You can generally keep in mind that the more hydrolyzed a formula and the lower its fat content, the less tasty it will be. However, people's likes and dislikes vary greatly, and what might seem quite unpalatable to you or me might be perfectly acceptable to someone else.

Cost   A final but important consideration in selecting a formula is cost. Costs vary greatly for individual products in different parts of the country and for different hospitals. However, as a general rule, hydrolyzed formulas are far more costly than intact formulas because they require more commercial modification.

No formula is perfect. The more digestible the formula, the higher its cost and osmolality and the lower its palatability. Since hydrolyzed formulas have many disadvantages and are more likely than other formulas to cause complications, they should be used only for patients who cannot digest and absorb nutrients adequately. Figure 2 diagrams the chief advantages and disadvantages of various formula choices.

Tube Feedings

A patient who has a functioning GI tract but who is unable to orally ingest enough nutrients to meet present needs is a candidate for a tube feeding. Such a patient may have physical problems that make chewing and swallowing difficult, may have no appetite, may be in a coma, or may have very high nutrient requirements. Tube feedings are generally not used for patients who have severe vomiting, upper gastrointestinal bleeding, or complete intestinal obstructions.[2]

Feeding Tube Placement   You may be wondering just how someone is fed by tube. The thought of being "force fed" may seem terrible to you. You may feel better knowing that the administration of tube feedings has improved dramatically in recent years. In this section, we will discuss how tubes are placed and what the implications are for each type of placement.

Feeding tubes are most commonly inserted through the nose and passed into the stomach or intestine. This is called transnasal placement (see Figure 3). When patients are fully alert during the procedure they help pass the tube by swallowing. When the correct size and type of tube are used and the person is emotionally prepared for the procedure, feeding tubes can be passed transnasally with minimal discomfort.[3] The major disadvantage of transnasal tube placement is that the disoriented or uncooperative patient can easily pull the tube out. Furthermore, if an inappropriate tube is selected the nasal passages and the esophagus can become irritated.

When a feeding tube cannot be passed through the nose, esophagus, or stomach due to an obstruction, a feeding ostomy may be created (see Figure 4). A feeding ostomy is a surgically-made opening into the

transnasal: through the nose. A *transnasal feeding tube* is one that is passed through the nose.

   naso = nose

nasogastric (NG): from the nose to the stomach.

nasoduodenal (ND): from the nose to the duodenum.

nasojejunal (NJ): from the nose to the jejunum.

nasoenteric: from the nose to the intestine. *Nasoenteric feedings* include both nasoduodenal and nasojejunal feedings.

feeding ostomy: a surgically made opening through which a feeding tube is passed. An ostomy can be made in various parts of the GI tract.

   ostomy = a surgically formed opening

esophagostomy (eh-SOFF-uh-GOSS-toh-mee): a surgically made opening in the esophagus through which a feeding tube can be passed.

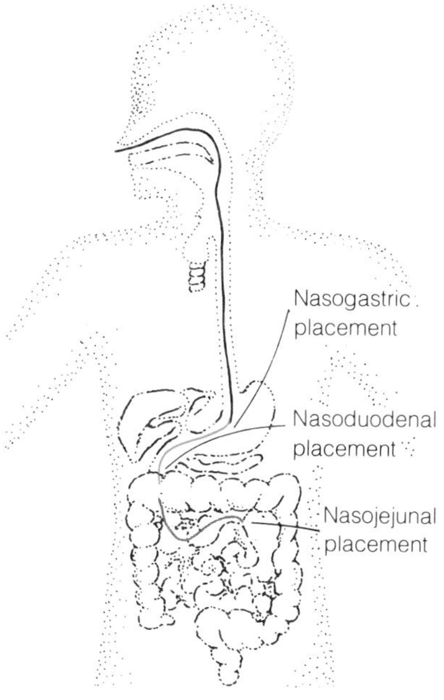

Figure 3   Transnasal tube placement. 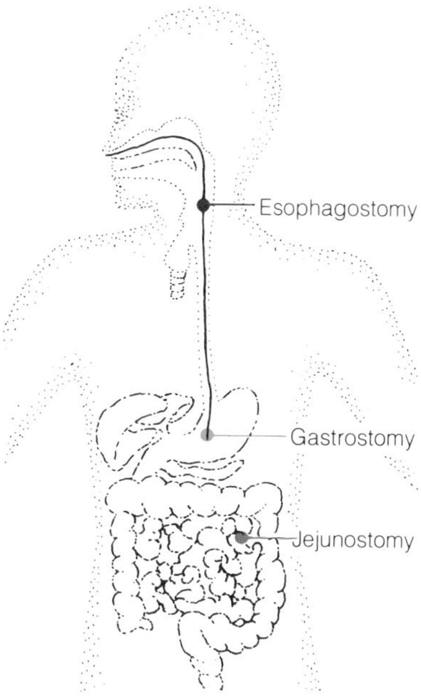   **Figure 4**   Feeding ostomy sites.

[2]Heymsfield, Horowitz, and Lawson, 1980.

[3]R. Chernoff, Nutritional support: Formulas and delivery of enteral feeding, Part II, *Journal of the American Dietetic Association* 79 (1981):430-432.

gastrostomy (gas-TROSS-toh-mee): a surgically made opening in the stomach through which a feeding tube can be passed.

jejunostomy (jee-june-OSS-toh-mee): a surgically made opening in the jejunum through which a feeding tube can be passed.

A **duodenostomy** (doo-oh-deen-OSS-toh-mee) is not used for tube feedings because the duodenum swings toward the back of the body and is not easily accessible (see Figure 5).

An infection of the lung caused by inhaling fluids regurgitated from the stomach is called **aspiration pneumonia.** Aspiration pneumonia can be a fatal complication of tube feeding.

esophagus, stomach, or jejunum through which a feeding tube is passed. Feeding ostomies also are useful for patients on long-term tube feedings, because they are invisible under clothing. Additionally, they eliminate feeding tube irritation. The most obvious disadvantage of the feeding ostomy is that it involves surgery.

When you administer a feeding by either the NG (nasogastric), esophagostomy, or gastrostomy route, the digestive process begins in the stomach. The stomach empties its contents at a controlled rate, giving the intestine time for adequate digestion and absorption. The disadvantage of these feedings is that people sometimes tend to regurgitate them. If the regurgitated fluids are inhaled and reach the lungs, a fatal infection may develop.[4]

Intestinal feedings into the duodenum or jejunum are less likely to cause regurgitation of fluids, because the fluid has to travel further to come back up. More importantly, two sphincters are working to keep the fluid down: the pylorus and the cardiac sphincter (see p. 151). The disadvantage of intestinal feedings is that the controlled emptying action of the stomach is lost. Formulas must be more carefully selected and tube feedings must be given at a slower rate to avoid diarrhea and dehydration.

The skin surrounding a gastrostomy or jejunostomy site sometimes becomes irritated from the gastric and intestinal secretions that may leak around the ostomies. Infection can result. Skin care is usually effective in treating this problem.

Table 3 lists the features of the various feeding tube placement sites. As you can see, each is useful in a different set of circumstances.

Figure 5   Anatomy of the GI tract.

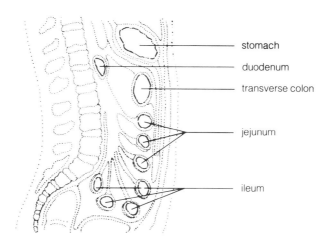

stomach

duodenum

transverse colon

jejunum

ileum

[4]B. A. Griggs and M. C. Hoppe, Update: Nasogastric tube feeding, *American Journal of Nursing* 79 (1979):481-485; B. A. Griggs, R. Chernoff, M. C. Hoppe, and J. F. Wade, Enteral nutrition for hospitalized patients, *ASPEN Monograph* (Rockville, Md.: American Society for Parenteral and Enteral Nutrition, 1980).

Table 3.   **Features of Various Tube Feeding Sites**

	Insertion	Potential irritations	Risk of regurgitation*	Long-term tolerance	Chance of removal by uncooperative patient
Nasogastric	Nonsurgical	Nasal passages, esophagus	High	Fair†	Likely
Nasoduodenal	Nonsurgical	Nasal passages, esophagus	Low	Fair†	Likely
Nasojejunal	Nonsurgical	Nasal passages, esophagus	Low	Fair†	Likely
Esophagostomy	Surgery required	—	High	Good	Unlikely
Gastrostomy	Surgery required	Skin irritation	Moderate	Good	Unlikely
Jejunostomy	Surgery required	Skin irritation	Low	Good	Unlikely

*Relative to the other feeding sites. The absolute risk of regurgitation is small.

†When the appropriate type and size of tube are used.

Feeding Tubes   The safety and comfort of tube feedings have been enhanced greatly through the development of soft, flexible, small-diameter feeding tubes. Traditional feeding tubes, made from stiffer materials (rubber or polyvinyl chloride), were sometimes referred to as "garden hoses." They became even stiffer when exposed to digestive juices and were extremely irritating to patients. Further, large-diameter tubes cause the cardiac sphincter to open more, increasing the likelihood of regurgitation.

The newer feeding tubes, which are gaining wide acceptance, are much smaller in diameter and are made from pliable materials which cause less irritation.[5] They do not stiffen when exposed to gastric juice. Indeed, the patient generally becomes unaware of the tube's presence within several hours after it has been inserted.[6]

Many newer tubes are designed for placement in the intestine. These tubes are longer and are weighted at one end, to help them pass spontaneously from the stomach into the intestine during peristalsis.

Generally, the physician assumes responsibility for ordering the feeding tube; but occasionally, the nurse or dietitian orders it. The most important points to keep in mind about feeding tubes are:

● The use of polyvinyl chloride or rubber tubes is seldom appropriate.

● The tube size ordered should be the smallest through which the feeding will flow.

A weighted feeding tube passes spontaneously from the stomach to the intestine during peristalsis. See p. 151.

[5]Heymsfield, Horowitz, and Lawson, 1980.

[6]M. H. Torosian and J. L. Rombeau, Feeding by tube enterostomy, *Surgery, Gynecology and Obstetrics* 150 (1980):918-927.

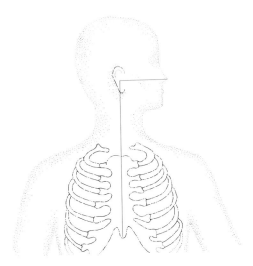

Figure 6 Measuring for the correct feeding tube length. The correct length of tubing to be passed for an NG feeding is estimated by measuring the combined distance from the nose to the earlobe to the xiphoid process.

Table 4.   Guide to Feeding Tube Sizes by Formula Types

Formula	Tube sizes (French)*
Intact protein formulas (excluding protein isolates)	8-12 F
Protein isolates	7-10 F
Protein hydrolysates	5-6 F

*The smaller sizes can be used when the feeding is delivered by pump.

Table 4 gives some general guidelines regarding the proper tube sizes for various types of formulas.

Steps in Formula Selection

As we have said earlier, you must thoroughly assess a patient's nutrition status before starting a tube feeding. Once you have a thorough understanding of the patient's needs, you can follow a few simple steps to select the right formula (see Figure 7).[7]

[7]C. B. Cataldo and C. L. Smith, *Tube Feedings: Clinical Applications* (Columbus, Ohio: Ross Laboratories, 1980), pp. 10-12.

Digestive and Absorptive Function   You can narrow down the choice of formulas considerably just by determining if the patient's GI tract is functioning. Throughout the next several chapters, we will be discussing what diseases cause problems with digestion and absorption. Don't worry about that for now. Just remember that any patient with impaired digestive or absorptive function may need a hydrolyzed formula. If, however, the patient's GI tract is functional, intact formulas are a better choice, since they are lower in osmolality and are less likely to cause complications.

Placement of the Tube   You have to be careful in selecting a formula that is to be delivered directly into the intestine. Although the formula must be easily digested, it does not have to be hydrolyzed when the GI tract is functional. However, the small intestine is more sensitive than the stomach to hypertonic solutions; so the feedings should be as near isotonic as possible. When a hydrolyzed formula is not required, isotonic protein isolate formulas work very well for intestinal feedings.

Nutrient Requirements   The selection of formulas is narrowed even further by the patient's energy, protein, vitamin, mineral, and trace element requirements. These nutrient needs often are altered considerably in various diseases.

A patient (J.K.) needs a total of 3,000 ml of a formula per 24 hours to meet her nutrient needs. Therefore, she eventually will need 125 ml every hour to get 3,000 ml for the day.

Another nutrient to consider is water. As a general guideline, most adults require from 1,500 to 2,000 ml of pure water a day. A patient with a high fever may require an additional 500 to 1,500 ml a day.[8] Other conditions, such as heavy sweating and some types of kidney disease, may increase water requirements. In other types of kidney disease, as well as in liver and heart disease, the total water may need to be restricted.

The formula itself already contains some water. In general, you can figure that formulas which contain 1 kcal/ml contain about 850 ml of water per liter of formula. (Table 2 shows the kcal/ml in various formulas.) Any additional water needed can be given between feedings or to rinse out the feeding tube.

If a formula contains 850 ml water per liter of formula, and a patient is given 2.5 liters of the formula, then he will be getting 2,125 ml water in the feeding solution.

$$\frac{850 \text{ ml}}{1 \text{ L}} \text{ as } \frac{X \text{ ml}}{2.5 \text{ L}}$$

$$(2.5 \text{L} \times 850 \text{ ml}) \div 1\text{L} = 2{,}125 \text{ ml}$$

Other Considerations   The final considerations deal with individual tolerances. Often, lactose-free formulas are less likely to lead to complications. Food allergies must also be considered.

You really can only make an educated or informed guess when selecting a formula. Therefore, it becomes critical to monitor each patient's nutrition status and tolerance to the formula to insure that individual needs are being met. Table 5 lists the major steps in monitoring patients on tube feedings.

[8]E. Goldberger, Water loss syndromes, in *A Primer of Water, Electrolyte and Acid-Base Syndromes* (Philadelphia: Lea and Febiger, 1980), p. 43.

Figure 7 Narrowing the choice of tube feeding formulas.

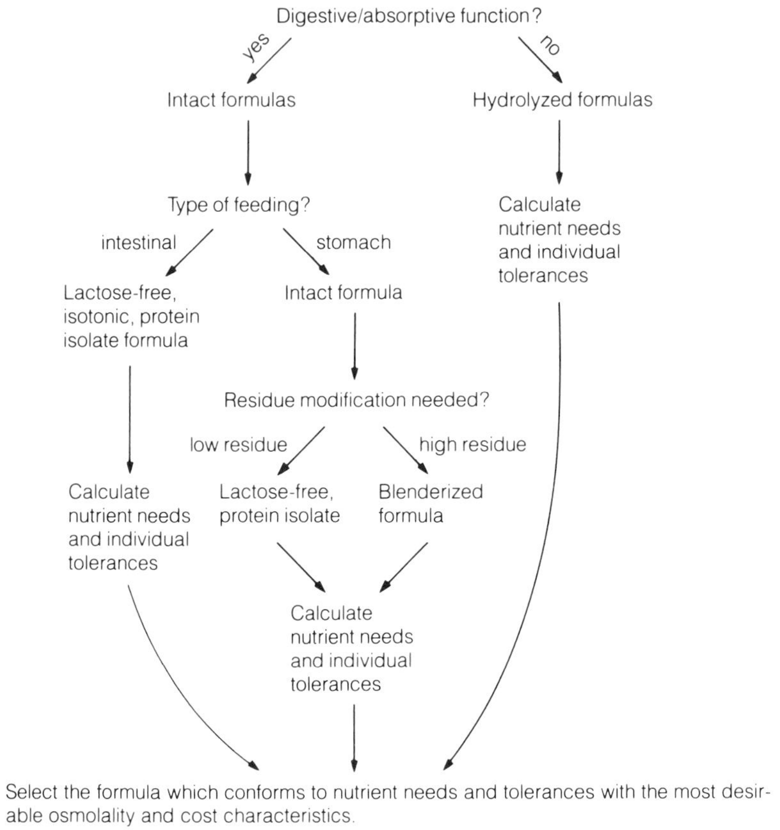

Digestive/absorptive function?

yes / no

Intact formulas — Hydrolyzed formulas

Type of feeding? — Calculate nutrient needs and individual tolerances

intestinal / stomach

Lactose-free, isotonic, protein isolate formula — Intact formula

Residue modification needed?

low residue / high residue

Calculate nutrient needs and individual tolerances — Lactose-free, protein isolate — Blenderized formula

Calculate nutrient needs and individual tolerances

Select the formula which conforms to nutrient needs and tolerances with the most desirable osmolality and cost characteristics.

Figure 8 Diluting a formula to desired strength.

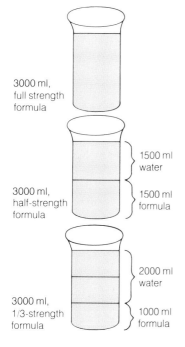

3000 ml, full strength formula

3000 ml, half-strength formula
{ 1500 ml water
1500 ml formula }

3000 ml, 1/3-strength formula
{ 2000 ml water
1000 ml formula }

Administering a Tube Feeding

Patients who go on tube feedings often have had surgery or have not eaten for several weeks. When a tube feeding is initiated, they cannot tolerate large volumes or highly concentrated nutrients.

When a tube feeding is first started, water is usually added to the formula to dilute it to one-half or one-third strength (see Figure 8). The formula is given slowly at first, at about 50 ml/hour. If the patient tolerates the formula, the rate of feeding can be increased by 25 ml/hr every eight to twelve hours. Once the final desired rate has been reached, the strength is increased. If a new rate or strength is not tolerated, you can back up and try increasing it more slowly, giving the patient more time to adapt.

There are many ways to give a volume of a formula. For example, a patient can be fed four to six times daily. In such a case, the total

Table 5.   Checklist for Monitoring the Tube-Fed Patient

Before starting a new or in-termittent feeding:	Complete a nutrition assessment. Check the tube placement. Check amount of re-sidual (if 150 ml, consider possible reasons for delayed gastric emptying).	The nurse started the feeding at 50 ml per hour at 1/2 strength and then progressed the feeding as follows:
Every half-hour:	Check gravity drip rate when applicable.	After 8 hours
Every hour:	Check pump drip rate when applicable.	75 ml/hour at 1/2 strength
Every 2 to 4 hours of continu-ous feeding:	Check residual.	After 16 hours 100 ml/hour at 1/2 strength After 24 hours
Every 4 hours:	Check vital signs, including blood pressure, temperature, pulse, and respiration.	125 ml/hour at 1/2 strength After 36 hours
	Check sugar and acetone in urine; in non-diabetic patient can be discontinued after 48 hours if consistently negative.	125 ml/hour at full strength
	Refill feeding container.	The patient tolerated the feeding well. The formula met her nu-trient needs by the second day of administration.
Every 8 hours:	Check intake and output.	
	Check specific gravity of urine.	
	Chart patient's acceptance of and tolerance to tube feeding.	
Every day:	Weigh patient.	If our patient, J.K., received her formula intermittently 6 times a day, at each feeding she would need 500 ml of formula.
	Change feeding bag and tubing.	
	Check electrolytes, blood urea nitrogen, and blood glucose daily until stabilized.	3,000 ml ÷ 6 = 500 ml
Every 7 to 10 days:	Check all laboratory findings.	If she received the formula only 4 times a day, she would need 750 ml of formula at each feed-ing.
	Reassess nutrition status.	
As needed:	Observe patient for any undesirable re-sponses to tube feeding, e.g., nausea, vomit-ing, diarrhea.	3,000 ml ÷ 4 = 750 ml
	Check tube placement (for NG placement only).	She would probably tolerate this volume of solution very poorly if it was given to her within a few minutes at each meal.
	Check nitrogen balance.	
	Check laboratory data.	
	Clean feeding equipment.	
	Chart significant details.	

volume of formula needed for the day is divided by four or six, respectively. If this amount of fluid is given within a few minutes, it is called a bolus feeding. Feedings given by this method are poorly tolerated — they lead to more complaints of abdominal discomfort,

bolus delivery: giving a 4 to 6 hour volume of feeding solution within a few minutes.

intermittent feeding by slow drip: giving a 4 to 6 hour volume of feeding solution over 20 to 30 minutes.

continuous drip administration: giving a feeding solution continuously over a 16 to 24 hour period.

If J.K. received continuous drip feedings over 24 hours, she would receive 125 ml/hr.

3,000 ml ÷ 24 hr = 125 ml/hr.

If she received the total volume of solution continuous drip for 16 hours she would receive 187.5 ml/hr.

3,000 ml ÷ 16 hr = 187.5 ml/hr

nausea, fullness, and cramping. Thus, bolus feeding should be discouraged.[9]

When feedings are delivered intermittently (four to six times a day) but allowed to infuse over a longer period (20 to 30 minutes), the patient generally tolerates the feeding much better. This makes sense. After all, you would not gobble down a meal in just a few minutes, especially if you were not feeling well anyway. Further, when feedings are given intermittently, the patient has greater freedom of movement between meals.

Feedings also can be delivered over a 16- to 24-hour period. This feeding method is called continuous drip. Sometimes pumps (similar to those used for delivering intravenous solutions) are used to insure that the formula is given slowly. Continuous drip administration is useful for patients who have poor tolerance to large volumes of formula. Generally, intestinal feedings (particularly jejunal feedings) should be delivered by continuous drip.

Regardless of the method used to deliver a formula, the patient's head should be elevated to at least a 30 degree angle during the feeding and for 30 minutes following an intermittent feeding. This measure minimizes the possibility of regurgitation.

Complications Associated with Tube Feedings

The complications most frequently seen with tube feedings often can be prevented. Patients who receive the proper formula, administered correctly, seldom have problems. Tube feedings should always be carefully monitored, however, to prevent major complications from arising.

Diarrhea   Diarrhea is the most frequently cited complication of tube feedings. Diarrhea can result from a number of causes, including bacterial contamination of the formula, lactose intolerance, hypertonic formulas, low serum albumin, and drug therapy.

Some people may find it appalling to think that a formula could actually become contaminated in the hospital. However, contamination can and does occur. To prevent contamination, formulas are generally made fresh every 24 hours under very clean conditions. Unopened cans of formula can be stored unrefrigerated; but once a can is opened or a powder mixed with water, the container should be dated and refrigerated. Opened containers of formula should be discarded if not used within 24 hours. New formula should not be added to formula still in the feeding container. The feeding bag and tubing (not including the transnasal tube) should be changed every 12 to 24 hours to reduce the risk of bacterial overgrowth.

[9]M. E. Heitkemper, D. L. Martin, B. C. Hansen, R. Hanson, and V. Vanderburg, Rate and volume of intermittent enteral feeding, *Journal of Parenteral and Enteral Nutrition* 5 (1981):125-129; Griggs, Chernoff, Hoppe, and Wade, 1980.

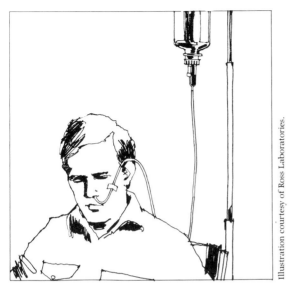

A patient being tube fed. The feeding is being delivered by gravity drip.

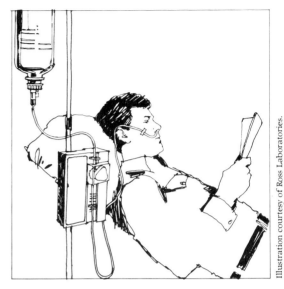

Tube feedings can also be delivered by a pump. A typical setup is shown here.

Lactose-free formulas should be used whenever a patient is lactose intolerant or when the possibility of lactose intolerance is high. Lactose intolerance is fairly common in any adult population;[10] in adult blacks, Indians, Mexican Americans, Jews, and Oriental populations, the incidence approaches 60 to 95 percent.[11] Temporary lactose intolerance also can occur following surgery, radiation therapy, and chemotherapy.

Inappropriate delivery of hypertonic solutions into the intestine also can cause diarrhea. Remember that water flows from an area of low osmolality to one of high osmolality. When a concentrated solution reaches the lumen of the intestine, water from the intestinal capillaries moves into the lumen to equalize the osmolality of the solution. Diarrhea results. The initial dilution of hypertonic formulas with a gradual increase in concentration helps eliminate the problem. Feeding the patient by continuous drip also allows the gut to adapt to a hypertonic formula.

The patient who has low serum albumin due to malnutrition or other causes may have problems with diarrhea.[12] The actual problem is very similar to what was described above. Albumin helps keep water inside the body's blood vessels. If the albumin concentration is low, even a normal osmolar load is like a hyperosmolar load. Water flows from

To find more information on lactose intolerance, see Highlight 15 and Chapter 23.

lumen: the inner open space of a tubular organ like the intestine.

[10]R. Chernoff, Nutritional support: Formulas and delivery of enteral feeding, Part I, *Journal of the American Dietetic Association* 79 (1981):426-429.

[11]J. D. Welsh, Diet therapy in adult lactose malabsorption: Present practices, *American Journal of Clinical Nutrition* 31 (1978):592-596.

[12]M. V. Kaminski, Jr., Enteral hyperalimentation, *Surgery, Gynecology and Obstetrics* 143 (1976):12-16.

Compounds which prevent diarrhea are known as **antidiarrheal agents.** Opiates, kaolin, and pectin are some types of antidiarrheal agents.

The rapid loss of water which is excreted with sugar in the urine is called **osmotic diuresis** (dye-you-REES-iss). It occurs when blood sugar levels get too high.

hypernatremia (high-per-nay-TREE-me-uh): excessive levels of sodium in the blood.

hyperchloremia (high-per-clor-EE-me-uh): excessive levels of chloride in the blood.

azotemia (ay-zoh-TEE-me-uh): the presence of urea and other nitrogen-containing compounds in increased amounts in the blood.

   azo = containing N in a special configuration

The term **tube-feeding syndrome** is used to refer to the dehydration, hypernatremia, hyperchloremia, and azotemia which results from excessive protein intake with inadequate fluid intake in tube-fed patients. The symptoms include mental confusion and decreasing levels of consciousness.

the blood and body fluids into the intestine, and diarrhea can result. Sometimes albumin is given by vein to help bring up serum albumin levels. The feedings given are diluted until the patient can tolerate them.

Patients also may develop diarrhea which is unrelated to the tube feeding. Drug therapy is frequently the culprit. In this case, they can often be given other drugs which correct the problem of diarrhea.

Dehydration   Dehydration can occur in people with excessive diarrhea, in those who cannot handle a high carbohydrate load, and in those receiving excessive protein intakes. In most alert people, water intake is regulated by thirst.[13] But in the unconscious or confused person, dehydration can be a real problem.

People with excessive diarrhea lose a large amount of fluid in the stool and become dehydrated unless the fluid they lose is replaced. For some patients, especially diabetics, the carbohydrate content of the tube feeding may be hard to handle. Their blood sugar gets very high and they begin to "spill" sugar in their urine. As the sugar is excreted in the urine, it carries water with it. Severe dehydration and eventually coma can result. To prevent this type of dehydration, the patient should be monitored for sugar levels in the blood and urine. The problem can be managed by the administration of insulin, administration of tube feeding by continuous drip, or both. Continuous drip prevents the delivery of large amounts of carbohydrate at any one time.

When high protein diets are fed to patients not receiving adequate fluid, dehydration, mental confusion, and decreasing levels of consciousness can result.[14] In addition, serum sodium, chloride, and urea levels become high. Monitoring serum electrolytes and urea levels can prevent this problem.

Aspiration Pneumonia   We have previously discussed the problem of a formula's being regurgitated and then inhaled into the lungs. This may cause an infection — aspiration pneumonia. There is a high risk of aspiration in patients who are unconscious or comatose, severely debilitated, or restrained. In these patients, the placement of the feeding tube should be nasoenteric, or a gastrostomy or jejunostomy should be considered. If a transnasal tube is used, it should have a small diameter. Elevating the head of the bed to at least 30 degrees during feeding and for at least 30 minutes following intermittent feeding reduces the likelihood of aspiration. Using the continuous drip method of delivery also helps minimize the possibility of regurgitation. Because aspiration pneumonia is potentially fatal, precautions must be taken to guard against its occurrence.

[13]E. Pearson and H. S. Soroff, Burns, in *Nutritional Support of Medical Practice*, ed. H. A. Schneider, C. E. Anderson, and D. B. Coursin (Hagerstown, Md.: Harper & Row, 1977), p. 234.

[14]B. C. Walike, Nasogastric tube feeding: The nursing perspective, in *Dietetic Currents* (Columbus, Ohio: Ross Laboratories, 1975).

Other Gastrointestinal Problems Problems with vomiting, nausea, cramps, and distention have been mentioned earlier. If the patient vomits, the tube feeding should be stopped immediately.[15] Generally, you can prevent other GI problems by selecting the appropriate formula and giving it slowly at first. Warming the feeding to room temperature before giving it also may be helpful.

The source of nausea in a patient must be investigated. Sometimes it indicates that the feeding is not moving through the intestinal tract. The presence of a large volume of formula in the stomach increases the likelihood of vomiting and aspiration. If there is some sort of blockage, continuous feeding can lead to a gastric rupture, another potentially lethal complication.[16] To prevent this problem, the amount of formula left in the stomach prior to the next feeding can be measured, and a decision can be made to stop feeding, if necessary. When a feeding is being given continuously, the amount of formula left in the stomach can be checked every two to four hours.[17]

The amount of formula left in the stomach after a feeding is measured by **checking the gastric residual.** A syringe is used to gently withdraw fluid which may be left in the stomach through the tube. The gastric residual is checked before each feeding. With continuous drip, residual is checked every 2 to 4 hours. Residual of greater than 150 ml indicates delayed gastric emptying, and the feeding must be temporarily stopped.

Table 6 summarizes the major complications of tube feedings and their causes. Familiarity with the preventive measures listed there can enable you to ease the problems of tube feeding patients.

A typical nurse's reaction to the news that a patient will be tube fed is "Oh, no!" In her mind's eye she sees a picture of endless trips to the patient's room to check tolerance, refill formula bags and, worse, handle messy complications like diarrhea. But tube feeding doesn't have to be that way. The few simple measures taken to eliminate tube feeding problems not only help the patient, but also save the nurse's valuable time. When handled skillfully, tube feeding is simple and gives the nurse the satisfaction of knowing that the patient's nutrient needs are being met.

Psychological Implications of Tube Feedings In Chapter 19, we discussed the many factors that contribute to the way we eat. When someone is tube fed, all these associations are lost. The feeding is merely "nourishment" rather than an expression of religious, social, cultural, and psychological beliefs. Furthermore, the person may experience physical and emotional discomforts from the tube, tube feeding, illness itself, or hospitalization.

The person may feel self-conscious about how the tube looks and may feel tied down by the feeding equipment. You can encourage tube-fed patients to walk about and socialize whenever possible.

[15]Chernoff, 1981.

[16]Griggs and Hoppe, 1979.

[17]Griggs and Hoppe, 1979.

Walking around will help them realize that movement is not impossible, and socializing may help them forget about the tube.

There are some other steps you can take to make the tube feeding experience more tolerable. When the person is allowed to eat or drink other foods, you can give the food he or she prefers. Sometimes a person can "drink" a favorite beverage or food (blenderized) through a tube for psychological satisfaction.

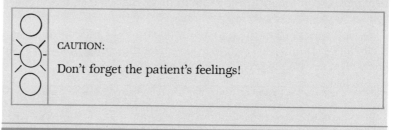

The more complex the procedure that a helper is responsible for, the more likely the helper is to focus on the procedure and forget the patient's feelings. Remember, no matter how many technicalities you have to keep in mind, you must never forget the person who is the object of your care.

CAUTION:

Don't forget the patient's feelings!

What to Chart   We have previously discussed the medical record and its importance as a communication tool. Information about tube feeding that should be documented includes:

- Type of feeding tube.
- Tube placement.
- Patient's response to tube insertion.
- Administration schedule (concentration and rate).
- Method of delivery (intermittent or continuous).
- Patient's tolerance to tube feeding (note any complications and any corrective actions taken).
- Patient's response to tube feeding.
- Education about feeding received by patient.

Appropriate charting helps all members of the health care team to maintain an optimal level of patient care.

Intravenous Nutrition

Many types of nutrient solutions can be administered by vein in patients unable to eat or drink. These intravenous, or parenteral, solutions consist of water, glucose, electrolytes, amino acids, fat, vitamins, trace elements, and combinations of the above.

Table 6.   Causes and Prevention of Tube Feeding Complications

Complications	Cause	Prevention
Diarrhea	Bacterial contamination	Take care in preparation, storage, and administration of formula.
	Lactose intolerance	Use lactose-free formula in high-risk groups.
	Hypertonic formula	Dilute formula and increase concentration gradually; use continuous drip administration of formula.
	Low serum albumin	Dilute formula and increase concentration gradually; consider giving albumin by vein.
	Drug therapy	Use antidiarrheal agents; change drug therapy, if possible.
Dehydration	Excessive diarrhea	See above 5 items.
	Inadequate fluid intake	Give water.
	Carbohydrate intolerance	Use continuous drip administration of formula; monitor sugar levels in blood and urine; consider administering insulin.
	Excessive protein intake	Monitor blood electrolyte levels.
Aspiration pneumonia	Regurgitation of formula, which is subsequently inhaled into lungs	Use nasoenteric, gastrostomy, or jejunostomy feedings in high-risk patients; use small-diameter transnasal tube; elevate head of bed during feeding; use continuous drip method of delivery.
Vomiting	Obstruction, stomach emptying slowly	Check gastric residual; use continuous drip method of administration.
Nausea, cramps, distention	Obstruction, stomach emptying slowly; intolerance to concentration or volume of formula	Check gastric residual; use continuous drip method of administration; dilute formula, increasing gradually.

peripheral veins: the smaller-diameter veins which bring blood to the extremities (arms, legs).

central veins: the larger-diameter veins located close to the heart (see Figure 9).

TPN (total parenteral nutrition): a method of meeting all nutrient requirements by vein.

IVH (intravenous hyperalimentation): same as TPN. Hyperalimentation means feeding higher-than-normal amounts of nutrients either orally, enterally, or parenterally.

hyper = greater than normal
alimentation = the process of providing nutrients to the body

dextrose: a form of glucose that is very soluble in water and is therefore used in IV solutions. Dextrose already contains a little water; therefore, while glucose provides 4 kcal/g, dextrose provides only 3.4 kcal/g.

As early as 1831, a Scottish physician named Latta successfully injected a salt solution into the bloodstream of his patients.[18] Later, glucose and hydrolyzed protein and many other substances were successfully infused. While these solutions were important for providing the water, electrolytes, and the minimal amount of kcalories essential to support life, they were far from complete. People who couldn't eat for long periods of time and those who had high nutrient requirements simply withered away. If they did not starve to death, they became too weak to withstand the treatment they needed and died of their diseases or of infections they could not fight.

Gradually, the techniques of infusing nutrients by vein improved. Interest in the importance of nutrition in recovery from disease heightened, and researchers began to look for ways of giving patients all the nutrients they needed by vein. The big problem was that the small-diameter peripheral veins became irritated and eventually collapsed when highly concentrated nutrient solutions were infused. However, if the patient received less concentrated solutions, it would take 12 to 15 liters of solution a day to deliver all the needed nutrients. This volume is far more than the body can safely handle.

The answer to the problem seemed to lie in using a very large-diameter central vein. Almost a gallon of blood rushes through one such vein, the superior vena cava (see Figure 9), each minute.[19] Here, highly concentrated solutions could be quickly diluted. By the time the solutions reached the peripheral veins, they would not be irritating.

Studies of total parenteral nutrition (TPN) were initiated in 1949, at first with adult dogs. In 1965, Dr. Stanley Dudrick demonstrated that puppies fed entirely by vein could achieve full adulthood. This study showed that TPN could be used safely. In 1967, Dr. Dudrick successfully fed a newborn infant entirely by vein for 45 days.[20]

You can see how recent the use of TPN really is. Although someone who cannot eat need not starve to death today, much more research still must be done to improve the use of TPN.

Peripheral Intravenous Solutions

The routine use of simple parenteral solutions given by peripheral vein is widespread in the hospital. Simple IV solutions contain water and combinations of dextrose, electrolytes, and occasionally other nutrients. These solutions are used to maintain fluid and electrolyte as well as acid-base balance. For the well-nourished postsurgical patient who is expected to eat within a few days, simple IV solutions are very useful.

[18]J. P. Grant, History of parenteral nutrition, in *Handbook of Total Parenteral Nutrition* (Philadelphia: Saunders, 1980), pp. 1-3.

[19]D. Ingber, People who never need to eat, *Science Digest*, January, 1982, pp. 34-35.

[20]S. J. Dudrick, A clinical review of nutritional support of the patient, *American Journal of Clinical Nutrition* 34 (supplement, June 1981):1191-1198.

Figure 9   The central veins used for TPN. The superior vena cava is one of the largest-diameter veins and is usually used for giving TPN solutions. When it cannot be used, the internal jugular vein is the next choice, followed by the external jugular vein. Can you see why?

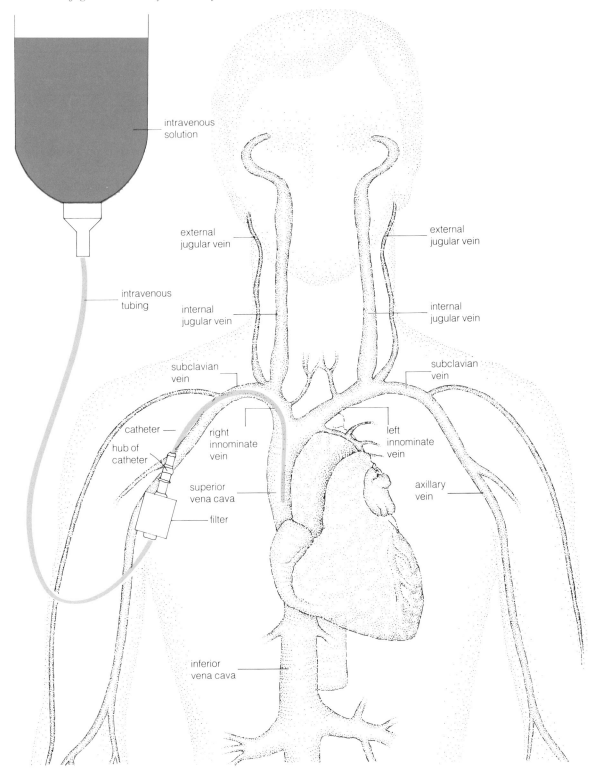

Several abbreviations are used to name IV solutions, including:

D: dextrose
W: water
NS: normal saline (0.9% sodium chloride solution)

These abbreviations are combined to specify the IV solution as follows:

D_5W

Read as: 5% dextrose in water (the subscript following the D tells you the percentage of dextrose required)

$D_{10}W$

Read as: 10% dextrose in water

$D_5 1/2NS$

Read as: 5% dextrose in a 1/2 normal saline solution (0.45% sodium chloride)

How would you read $D_{50}W$?

Generally, adult patients with normally functioning kidneys receive from 2 1/2 to 3 1/2 liters of a 5 percent dextrose solution following a major trauma or surgery. Electrolytes are replaced as necessary. Three liters of a 5 percent dextrose solution give the patient about 150 g glucose or about 510 kcal/day (see box, "How to Calculate the Nutrient Content of IV Solutions"). The protein-sparing effect of glucose is minimal at this level; so these solutions are not appropriate for long-term use or for malnourished patients.

How to Calculate the Nutrient Content of IV Solutions

You will feel less apprehensive about IV solutions if you know what's in them. The basic thing to remember is that the percentage of a substance in solution tells you how many grams of that substance are present in 100 ml. For example, in a 5% dextrose solution, there are 5 g of dextrose per 100 ml. A 3.5% amino acid solution contains 3.5 g of amino acids (protein equivalents) per 100 ml. A 0.9% normal saline solution contains 0.9 g of sodium chloride per 100 ml.

A patient receiving 1,500 ml of 50% dextrose and 1,500 ml of 7% amino acid solution would get:

$$\frac{50 \text{ g dextrose}}{100 \text{ ml}} \quad \text{as} \quad \frac{x \text{ g dextrose}}{1,500 \text{ ml}}$$

$$(50 \text{ g} \times 1,500 \text{ ml}) \div 100 \text{ ml} = 750 \text{ g dextrose}$$

$$\frac{7 \text{ g amino acids}}{100 \text{ ml}} \quad \text{as} \quad \frac{x \text{ g amino acids}}{1,500 \text{ ml}}$$

$$(7 \text{ g} \times 1,500 \text{ ml}) \div 100 \text{ ml} = 105 \text{ g amino acids}$$

To calculate the total kcalories in the mixture simply multiply by kcalories per gram:

$$750 \text{ g dextrose} \times 3.4 \text{ kcal/g} = 2,550 \text{ kcal}$$
$$105 \text{ g protein} \times 4.0 \text{ kcal/g} = \underline{420 \text{ kcal}}$$
$$2,970 \text{ kcal}$$

Protein-Sparing Therapy with Amino Acids   Dextrose solutions have been used as the traditional method of protein sparing for many years. More recently, however, it has been suggested that giving glucose without protein could lead to a kwashiorkor-type of malnutrition (blood and organ proteins become depleted).[21] Studies on stressed patients and on normal subjects show that amino acid solutions alone are more effective in promoting nitrogen balance than are glucose

---

[21]J. P. Flatt, Panel report on nutrient-hormone interaction, *American Journal of Clinical Nutrition* 34 (supplement, June 1981):1255-1257.

solutions.[22] The effect on nitrogen balance of adding glucose to the amino acid solutions has been variable. In one study, nitrogen balance responded equally well to amino acids alone and to amino acids with glucose.[23] Others have observed that nitrogen balance improves when glucose is added to the amino acid solution.[24]

No one knows exactly why amino acids produce a superior nitrogen-sparing effect in the stressed patient. One theory is that the high level of insulin elicited by glucose causes several undesirable effects. The insulin causes the uptake of amino acids and glucose into skeletal muscle cells. You may recall that insulin also inhibits the breakdown of fat to meet the energy requirement. So the rest of the body cells must rely on the breakdown of vital visceral (organ and blood) protein to meet energy needs. When amino acids are infused, insulin levels don't rise as high. Fat can be freely used to help meet energy needs and to spare the amino acids for visceral protein synthesis.

The use of amino acid solutions for protein sparing is controversial. The body still requires glucose, which cannot be made from fat. Therefore, some of the amino acids will be used for making glucose — and amino acids are a very expensive source of glucose. Furthermore, the breakdown of fat causes the formation of ketones (pp. 56 and 212). The long-term effects of ketosis are not clear; however, ketosis does suppress the appetite, which may make it more difficult for patients to return to an adequate oral diet.

IV Fat and Peripheral TPN   Just as protein and carbohydrate can be provided intravenously, so can fat. The use of IV fat serves two general purposes. First, it prevents essential fatty acid deficiency in patients who will be fed only intravenously for long periods of time. This type of intravenous feeding will be discussed later. IV fat can safely be used to provide up to 60 percent of the total daily energy requirement.

The second purpose that IV fat can serve is to supplement kcalories. When IV fat is given in addition to amino acids, the patient can receive approximately 2,000 kcalories per day by peripheral vein. (You can

Nitrogen balance reflects the body's use of protein. If it is negative, the body is losing protein. See p. 106.

Technically, **protein sparing** refers to any type of nutrient solution given orally or intravenously which decreases the use of protein for energy; more commonly, the term is used to refer to amino acid solutions given by peripheral veins. Oral protein sparing also has been used in the treatment of obesity (pp. 215-216).

Technically, **peripheral parenteral nutrition** refers to the provision of any nutrient solution through a peripheral vein; however, it most commonly refers to a system of meeting all maintenance nutrition requirements by peripheral vein. Dextrose, amino acids, fat, vitamins, electrolytes, and trace elements may be provided. The preferred term for this type of therapy is **peripheral TPN**.

[22]H. N. Munro, Energy intake and nitrogen metabolism, in *Assessment of Energy Metabolism in Health and Disease, Report of the First Ross Conference on Medical Research,* ed. J. Kinney (Columbus, Ohio: Ross Laboratories, 1980), p. 108.

[23]A. R. Greenberg, E. B. Marliss, G. H. Anderson, B. Langer, W. Spence, E. B. Tovee, and K. N. Jeejeebhoy, Protein-sparing therapy in post-operative patients: Effects of added hypocaloric glucose or lipid, *New England Journal of Medicine* 294 (1976):1411-1416.

[24]D. H. Elwyn, F. E. Gump, M. Iles, C. L. Long, and J. M. Kinney, Protein and energy sparing of glucose added in hypocaloric amounts to peripheral infusions of amino acids, *Metabolism* 27 (1978):325-331; A. J. W. Sim, B. M. Wolfe, V. R. Young, D. Clark, and F. D. Moore, Glucose promotes whole-body protein synthesis from infused amino acids in fasting man, *Lancet* 1 (1979):68-71; L. Howard, A. Dobs, R. Chodos, R. Chu, and T. Loludice, A comparison of administering protein alone and protein plus glucose on nitrogen balance, *American Journal of Clinical Nutrition* 31 (1978):226-229.

provide more kcalories in a smaller volume of a fat emulsion.) This form of nutrition can supply all nutrient needs for some patients, and therefore it can be called peripheral TPN. IV fat is also isotonic to blood and does not irritate the veins.

IV fat is available in either a 10 percent or 20 percent concentration (Intralipid 10 percent, 20 percent; Liposyn 10 percent, 20 percent). The 10 percent fat emulsion contains 1.1 kcal/ml, and the 20 percent fat emulsion contains 2.0 kcal/ml. The actual fatty acid compositions of the two brands differ, but each has been shown to be effective in preventing essential fatty acid deficiency.

When IV fat is used as a kcalorie supplement and given by peripheral vein, generally two bottles or 1,000 ml of 10 percent IV fat are given daily. Patients who are candidates for peripheral TPN include those who need only short-term nutrition support (about 7 to 14 days), patients with normal renal function who do not have excessive energy requirements, patients in whom inserting a central line might be difficult, and patients on tube feedings who may need additional nutrients.

An **infusion pump** is a mechanical device that accurately controls the rate at which a solution is delivered. A **controller** has a sensing device that controls the number of drops of a solution; no pressure is exerted by a controller. A **volumetric pump** measures a volume of solution and then supplies pressure to deliver the solution.

Fat emulsions are never mixed in the same container with glucose and amino acids, because the fat emulsion would break down. Rather, they are given from separate containers and through separate tubing (see Figure 10). A Y-connector joins the tubing just before it enters the vein, so that the solutions only mix for a very short time. The flow rate of each solution is controlled separately by infusion pumps.

Initially, IV fat is given at 1 ml/min for 15 to 20 minutes. If the patient tolerates the infusion, the rate is increased so that 500 ml is infused within four hours. Generally, only one bottle is infused the first day.

Some patients react adversely to IV fat emulsions. Immediate reactions may include fever, warmth, chills, backache, chest pain, allergic reactions, dizziness, blurred vision, and lymphocytosis (excess number of lymph cells). Irritation and inflammation of the vein also have been reported. After long-term administration the most commonly observed adverse effect is the deposition of a brown pigment in certain liver cells. These pigments disappear after parenteral therapy is stopped, and their effect on liver function is unknown. Other effects of long-term administration may include enlarged liver and spleen and decreased number of blood platelets and white blood cells.

Before IV fat is administered, the patient's liver function, blood count, and plasma lipids are evaluated. Once the infusion has begun, weight, electrolytes, blood urea nitrogen, serum triglycerides, cholesterol, and blood count should be assessed regularly. The use of IV fat is contraindicated in patients with disturbances of normal fat metabolism.

TPN by Central Vein

The previous section discussed peripheral TPN. When the term TPN is

Figure 10   Peripheral infusion of IV fat, amino acids, and dextrose solutions.

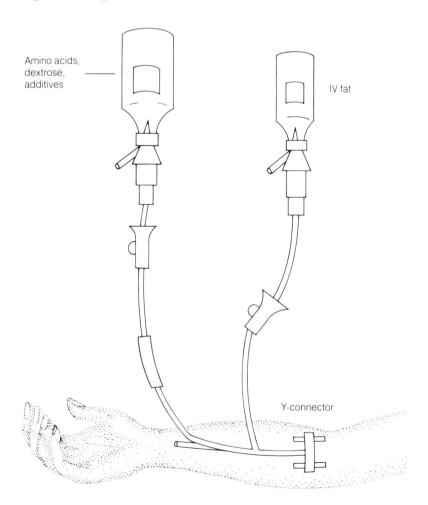

Amino acids, dextrose, additives

IV fat

Y-connector

used alone, it usually refers to TPN by central vein. People who cannot or should not be fed through the GI tract are candidates for TPN; usually it is indicated whenever long-term parenteral nutrition will be required. Also, when nutrition support is urgent in a malnourished patient whose GI function is questionable, TPN should be considered. Some specific conditions which may necessitate its use are listed in Table 7. The actual need for TPN must be determined by the individual patient's medical and nutrition needs. Ideally, the patient should not reach a severely depleted state before TPN is initiated. It is much easier to maintain nutrition status than to try to replenish lost nutrient stores.

The TPN Solution   The actual concentrations of amino acids and dextrose which compose the final TPN solution are determined by the patient's nutrient needs. Patients who are extremely malnourished or who are highly stressed (by burns or infection) require higher levels of

Table 7. Possible Indications for TPN by Central Vein*

Severe protein-kcalorie malnutrition
Nutritional repletion necessary to improve response to surgical or medical therapy
Prolonged vomiting
Prolonged diarrhea
Anorexia nervosa
GI tract obstruction
Prolonged absence of intestinal peristalsis (ileus)
Enterocutaneous fistulas
Short bowel syndrome
Inflammatory bowel disease
Cancer
Burns
Trauma
Pancreatitis

*Please note that these indications are not absolute. Occasionally patients with these indications can be fed orally or by tube successfully.

TPN catheter: the thin tube inserted into a central vein through which the TPN nutrient solution is given.

protein and kcalories than moderately malnourished or mildly stressed patients. A typical standard TPN solution contains 25 percent dextrose and 3.5 percent amino acids. Three liters of such a solution provide about 3,000 kcalories and 105 g protein daily.

In addition to dextrose and amino acids, electrolytes and vitamins are added to the TPN solution. The normal ranges of requirements for these nutrients are listed in Table 8. Trace elements should also be added to the solution, since trace element deficiencies can otherwise arise (such deficiencies have been reported in patients maintained on TPN). Although exact trace element requirements are unknown, Table 9 lists suggested trace element additions to the TPN solution. Essential fatty acid requirements can be met by giving IV fat periodically (about 500 ml of fat emulsion two times a week) or by applying corn or safflower oil (10 to 15 ml) to the skin three times a day.[25] Other additions to the TPN solution include:

- Albumin to increase serum albumin concentration.
- Heparin to prevent clots from forming on the IV catheter which might obstruct the flow of the TPN solution.
- Insulin to help regulate blood sugar levels.

Adding albumin, heparin, and insulin directly to the TPN solution is a controversial practice. Not all institutions consider these substances TPN additives.

[25]J. P. Grant, Septic and metabolic complications: Recognition and management, in *Handbook of Total Parenteral Nutrition* (Philadelphia: Saunders, 1980), p. 138.

Table 8.   Normal Range of Daily Vitamin and Mineral Requirements during TPN

Vitamins*	Recommended amounts
Vitamin A (IU)	3,300
Vitamin D (IU)	200
Vitamin E (IU)	10
Vitamin C (mg)	45
Folacin (μg)	400
Niacin (mg)	40
Riboflavin (mg)	3.6
Thiamin (mg)	3.0
Vitamin B_6 (mg)	4.0
Vitamin B_{12} (μg)	5.0
Pantothenic acid (mg)	15
Biotin (μg)	60

Minerals†	Normal ranges
Sodium (mEq)	60-150
Potassium (mEq)	70-150
Chloride (mEq)	Equal to sodium
Calcium (mEq)	0.2-0.3/kg
Magnesium (mEq)	0.35-0.45/kg
Phosphorus (mmoles)	7-10/1,000 kcal

*Data from American Medical Association, Department of Foods and Nutrition, Multivitamin preparations for parenteral use: A statement by the Nutrition Advisory Group, *Journal of Parenteral and Enteral Nutrition* 3 (1979):258-262.

†Data from J. P. Grant, Administration of parenteral nutrition solutions, in *Handbook of Total Parenteral Nutrition* (Philadelphia: Saunders, 1980), p. 98.

Table 9.   Guidelines for Trace Element Use in Parenteral Nutrition

Trace elements	Suggested IV intake	Comments
Zinc	2.5-4.0 mg	Add 2.0 mg for adult in acute catabolic state; add 12.2 mg per liter of small bowel fluid lost; add 17.1 mg per kg of stool or ileostomy output
Copper	0.5-1.5 mg	
Chromium	10-15 μg	Add 20 μg for stable adult with intestinal losses
Manganese	0.15-0.8 mg	

Data from American Medical Association, Department of Foods and Nutrition, Guidelines for essential trace element preparations for parenteral use, a statement by an expert panel, *Journal of the American Medical Association* 241 (1979):2051-2054.

The term used to describe the presence of disease-causing bacteria in the blood is **sepsis.** Sepsis is a major complication of TPN.

Insertion and Care of the TPN Catheter   The TPN catheter is the tube that is inserted into the patient's central vein (generally the subclavian). The TPN solution is delivered through the catheter directly into the vein (see Figure 9). Because of the proximity of the catheter insertion site to the heart, the danger that disease-causing microorganisms will enter the bloodstream and heart is very great. The nurse must be very careful to keep the catheter site clean.

A catheter insertion is a surgical procedure performed by a physician. However, the catheter often is inserted at bedside rather than in an operating room. The patient generally is awake but is given a local anesthetic. The patient should understand the procedure to avoid unnecessary apprehension and should be told to expect some pain.

Physician, assistants, and patient all are masked to reduce the risk of bacterial contamination. The physician wears sterile gloves and often a sterile gown. The patient's skin is shaved and thoroughly cleansed around the catheter insertion site. Once the catheter has been inserted, its correct placement must be confirmed by x-ray before the TPN solution can be infused.

The dressing around the catheter site is generally changed about three times a week, or more often if necessary. During the dressing change, the catheter site is examined for redness and edema and the catheter itself is examined for position, leaks, and obstructions. The skin is thoroughly cleansed before a new dressing is applied.

The tubing that leads to the catheter is changed daily. To guard against bacterial contamination, the TPN catheter generally is not used to draw blood or to administer any other medications.

Administering the TPN Solution

Like a tube feeding, a TPN feeding is started slowly to give the patient time to adapt to the high glucose concentration and osmolality of the TPN solution. During the first 24 hours, the patient receives 1 or 2 liters of TPN solution by continuous drip. Usually, an infusion pump is used to insure a slow rate of delivery. The patient is monitored for electrolytes and blood and urine glucose. If the blood glucose is unacceptably high (greater than 200 mg/100 ml) with a high urine glucose (4+), the cause must be investigated and treated.[26] After the first 24 hours the infusion rate is increased by a liter a day until the desired volume of solution is given within 24 hours. Changes in the infusion rate can cause significant hypoglycemia or hyperglycemia,

[26]Grant, 1980, pp. 129-131.

Table 10. Complications Associated with TPN

Complications related to catheter insertion or care

Fluid in the chest (hydrothorax)

Air or gas in the chest (pneumothorax)

Blood in the chest (hemothorax)

Catheter tip breaks off, obstructing blood flow (catheter embolism)

Air leaks into catheter, obstructing blood flow (air embolism)

Hole or tear made in heart by catheter tip (myocardial perforation)

Catheter inadvertently placed in subclavian artery (arterial puncture)

Improperly positioned catheter tip

Sepsis

Blood clots (thrombosis)

Metabolic complications

Elevated blood glucose (hyperglycemia)

Low blood glucose (hypoglycemia)

Dehydration

Coma from excessive glucose load (hyperosmolar, hyperglycemic, nonketotic coma)

Low blood magnesium (hypomagnesemia)

Low blood calcium (hypocalcemia)

High blood phosphorus (hyperphosphatemia)

Low blood phosphorus (hypophosphatemia)

Low blood potassium (hypokalemia)

Essential fatty acid deficiency

Trace element deficiencies

High blood ammonia levels (hyperammonemia)

Acid-base imbalances

Elevated liver enzymes

which can lead to coma, convulsions, and even death,[27] so all changes should be made gradually and with caution. When the administration of solution gets behind or ahead of schedule, the drip rate should be adjusted to the correct hourly infusion rate, but no attempt should be made to speed up or slow down the drip rate to meet the originally ordered volume. Table 10 lists the many types of complications

[27]J. P. Grant, Administration of parenteral nutrition solutions, in *Handbook of Total Parenteral Nutrition*, p. 108.

associated with TPN, and Table 11 summarizes how patients on TPN are monitored.

When a patient is being taken off TPN, the infusion rate of the solution must be gradually tapered; otherwise hypoglycemia might occur. The infusion rate of patients who have been on 3 liters of solution per day may be decreased to 2 liters for a day, then to 1 liter for a day, then discontinued.

cyclic parenteral nutrition: the periodic administration of standard TPN solutions.

Another way of administering TPN is called cyclic parenteral nutrition; this method of administration may help prevent a problem that has been observed when TPN is given continuously. When a patient receives a TPN solution by continuous drip, insulin levels stay high. In turn, the patient cannot mobilize fat stores for energy, and eventually, fat may be deposited in the liver. Studies are currently being conducted to determine if cyclic infusion of TPN might correct this problem.

A patient on cyclic parenteral nutrition receives a standard TPN solution for 14 to 16 hours a day, and then only amino acids and fat for 8 to 10 hours a day. Cyclic administration more closely approximates a normal diet, since during sleep there usually is no nutrient intake. Liver function returns to normal when this form of TPN is used. Additionally, it seems that fewer kcalories are necessary for maintaining nitrogen balance, probably because the patient uses body fat for energy.

Transitional/Combination Feedings

Whenever a patient has been on some form of special nutrition support, care must be taken to insure that his or her nutrient needs will continue to be met after the special support is discontinued. For example, a patient on a tube feeding should be taking adequate food by mouth before the tube feeding is discontinued. The patient should be allowed to eat "around the tube," and meanwhile, the volume of the tube feeding is gradually tapered off. In many cases, the patient is able to take by mouth the same formula that was earlier delivered by tube.

The transition from parenteral to enteral nutrition can be accomplished in more than one way. One method is to place the patient on a tube feeding. The volume of the parenteral nutrition solution is decreased as increases in the tube feeding volume are tolerated. If the tube feeding is not tolerated, the patient can still rely on TPN to meet nutrient needs, since the catheter is still in place. The patient also can be weaned from the TPN solution while oral intake is increased, avoiding the use of a tube. The decision whether or not to tube feed depends on the patient's medical condition, appetite, and attitude.

Occasionally, patients must continue tube feedings or TPN long after their medical conditions have stabilized. These patients can continue to receive specialized nutrition support at home. Highlight 20 discusses the techniques and ideas behind home nutrition support programs.

Table 11.   Guidelines for Monitoring Patients on TPN

Frequency of monitoring	Clinical or biochemical parameter
Every 4 to 6 hours:	Urinary glucose Vital signs (respiration, pulse, temperature)
Daily:	Weight Strict intake and output Urine specific gravity
Daily until stable and then 2 to 3 times weekly:	Serum glucose Serum electrolytes Blood urea nitrogen
Weekly:	Nutrition assessment Serum protein Serum calcium Serum phosphorus Serum ammonia levels Complete blood count

Summing Up

The major goal of diet therapy is to achieve or maintain optimal nutrition status. Therefore, the diet must provide all nutrients the patient needs in a form the body can handle. The most appropriate diet and feeding method cannot be determined without a complete assessment of the patient's nutrition status.

Whenever possible, the patient should be fed a standard or modified diet orally. When intake is inadequate, liquid nutrition supplements given by mouth may increase the patient's intake considerably. If the patient is at risk nutritionally and is still unable to ingest adequate nutrients, tube feeding is the next alternative. However, if the GI tract is not functioning, parenteral nutrition should be considered. Figure 11 summarizes steps in deciding how to feed a patient.

Many types of formulas are available for tube and supplemental feedings, generally classed by the chemical characteristics of the nutrients they contain. Intact formulas require the patient to have normal digestive and absorptive capabilities. Hydrolyzed formulas require minimal digestion and are more readily absorbed.

Tube feedings can be delivered by many routes, and can be used to provide for all of a patient's nutrient requirements. The rate, concentration, formula selection, and method of delivery should be individualized in the way that allows each patient to best tolerate the tube feeding.

Figure 11   Selecting the feeding route.

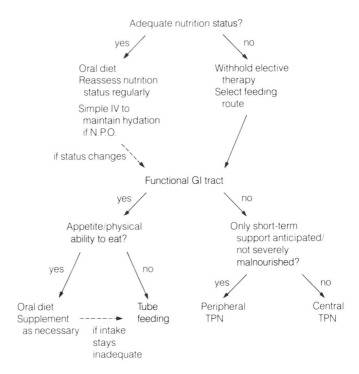

Simple intravenous solutions are often given to patients simply to prevent dehydration or to maintain acid-base balance when oral intake is inadequate. Intravenous protein-sparing therapy with dextrose or amino acids helps maintain nitrogen balance but falls short of meeting all the patient's nutrient needs.

Peripheral TPN can provide all needed nutrients to support a patient who does not have high kcalorie needs. When a patient is severely malnourished or in a hypermetabolic state, central TPN can provide all nutrient needs. TPN is only used when the GI tract cannot be used, because it is associated with far more complications, the patient must undergo a surgical procedure, and the cost is very high. On the other hand, when indicated, TPN can be used safely and should be started before the patient becomes severely depleted.

To Explore Further

Many publications give useful information on parenteral and enteral nutrition. *The Journal of Parenteral and Enteral Nutrition* (428 E. Preston Street, Baltimore, MD 21202) is the publication of the American Society for Parenteral and Enteral Nutrition (A.S.P.E.N.). The journal presents research findings and discusses technical areas related to special nutrition support. *Nutritional Support Services* (12849 Magnolia Boulevard, North Hollywood, CA 91607) is a new publication which focuses on the practical application of clinical nutrition concepts.

Excellent review articles and manuals on tube feedings are also available. They include:

● Cataldo, C. B., and Smith, C. L. *Tube Feedings: Clinical Applications.* Columbus, Ohio: Ross Laboratories, 1980. Available free of charge through Ross Laboratories (address in Appendix J).

● Rombeau, J. L., and Miller, R. A. *Nasoenteric Tube Feeding: Practical Aspects.* Mountain View: Health Development Corporation, 1979. Available free of charge from HEDECO Corp., 2551 Casey Avenue, Mountain View, CA 94043.

● Chernoff, R. Nutritional support: Formulas and delivery of enteral feedings, Part I and II. *Journal of the American Dietetic Association* 79 (1981):426-432.

● Griggs, B. A., and Hoppe, M. C. Update: Nasogastric tube feeding. *American Journal of Nursing* 79, (1979):481-485.

● Hemysfield, S. B., Bethel, R. A., Ansley, J. D., Dixon, D. W., and Rudman, D. Enteral hyperalimentation: An alternative to central venous hyperalimentation. *Annals of Internal Medicine* 90 (1979):63-71.

A good article which reviews the many types of equipment used with tube feedings is:

● Hoppe, M. The new tube feeding sets: A Nursing 80 product survey. *Nursing*, March 1980, pp. 79-85.

A slide series entitled *Nutritional Principles of Nasogastric Tube Feeding* is available through Ross Laboratories (address in Appendix J).

Two articles dealing with tube insertion are:

● Valden, C., Grinde, J., and Carl, D. Taking the trauma out of nasogastric intubation. *Nursing*, September 1980, pp. 64-67.

● McConnell, E. A. 10 problems with nasogastric tubes . . . and how to solve them. *Nursing*, April 1979, pp. 78-81.

In the area of parenteral nutrition, this book is an excellent reference:

● Grant, J. P. *Handbook of Total Parenteral Nutrition.* Philadelphia: Saunders, 1980.

Dr. Grant discusses central TPN in detail in an easy-to-follow way.

A good chapter on parenteral nutrition can be found in the following book:

● Schneider, H. A., Anderson, C. E., and Coursin, D., eds. *Nutritional Support of Medical Practice.* Hagerstown, Md.: Harper & Row, 1977.

The chapter entitled "Parenteral Nutrition: Principles, Nutrient Requirements, Techniques, and Clinical Applications" was written by H. C. Meng.

A useful 1977 manual entitled *Clinical Parenteral Nutrition* (S. J. Dudrick, guest editor) is available free of charge from McGaw Laboratories, Irvine, CA 92714.

The Role of Fat in Parenteral Nutrition (1979), by K. M. Jeejeebhoy, is available free of charge through Abbott Laboratories, North Chicago, IL 60064. Also available from Abbott Laboratories is *Parenteral Nutrition in the Neonate* (1980), by W. C. Jacobs, A. Lazzara, and D. J. Martin.

Highlight 21 provides references on home enteral and parenteral nutrition.

CASE-STUDY

Total Parenteral Nutrition

Mr. Small has been admitted to the hospital for a diagnostic workup. He has been steadily losing weight. He appears emaciated and states that he cannot swallow and has lost his appetite. He was frightened of coming to the hospital and has waited a long time before admitting himself. After a thorough examination, Mr. Small has been found to have an obstruction in his esophagus. The nutrition assessment reveals severe PCM. Surgery will be required as soon as possible. Mr. Small is placed on central TPN prior to surgery. He progresses well, gains weight, and undergoes surgery about two weeks after admission. During surgery, a feeding jejunostomy is made.

About two days after surgery, Mr. Small begins to receive feedings through the jejunostomy. His digestive and absorptive capacity are intact.

4. Specifically, what type of formula would you recommend for Mr. Small's tube feedings?

5. How does the feeding route influence your selection of formula?

6. How would you begin the tube feeding? How would you progress it? How would you deliver it?

7. When should Mr. Small be taken off central TPN? How should this be accomplished?

8. After several weeks, Mr. Small is ready to take some foods by mouth. How does this affect his tube feeding?

Study Questions

1. What factors in Mr. Small's history indicate the need for central TPN?

2. How would you explain the catheter insertion procedure and the need for TPN to Mr. Small?

3. Is the placement of a feeding jejunostomy during surgery a good idea? Why or why not?

Mrs. Reed has been hospitalized for over 14 months. She suffers from Crohn's disease (Chapter 23) and has had repeated operations to remove parts of her small intestine. An abnormal opening, or fistula, has formed between her small intestine and skin. Drainage which leaks through the opening can cause serious fluid and electrolyte disturbances. The patient was admitted to the hospital severely malnourished, and the repeated operations have put a great stress on her body. Because food taken by mouth increases the drainage from the fistula and also leaks through the opening, Mrs. Reed has been on central TPN. She has steadily improved. At various times during the course of hospitalization, oral intake has been tried unsuccessfully. From a medical standpoint, Mrs. Reed is stable and could probably manage well at home. She is in the hospital primarily to receive TPN. Mrs. Reed is becoming very depressed about staying in the hospital. The nutrition support team (see Highlight 20B) has been asked to evaluate her for a home TPN (HPN) program.

Goals and Objectives of HPN The actual goals of HPN must be individualized to meet each person's unique requirements. For example, some patients will only be on

HIGHLIGHT 20A

Special Nutrition Support at Home

The best treatment of any chronic illness is one which minimizes dependence and fosters a restoration of normal, purposeful behavior.

ALBERT R. JONSEN

HPN temporarily, while others may require HPN permanently.

One objective of HPN, as with TPN in the hospital, is to maintain or achieve adequate nutrition status. However, HPN has an added dimension: Patients can go home to familiar surroundings and gain more control over their situation. They can resume many activities they gave up while hospitalized and can begin leading more normal lives. Additionally, hospital care is extremely expensive. Care is less costly when patients and their families take over responsibilities formerly left up to the professional hospital staff.

Selecting Patients for HPN The input of all members of

the nutrition support team is very important in deciding which patients are candidates for HPN. In addition to medical considerations, the person's psychological profile and financial resources must also be considered. The hospital must be able to provide appropriate training for the patient. Finally, the patient must have access to the equipment and supplies that will be necessary for HPN.

From a medical standpoint, Mrs. Reed is a candidate for HPN. She is unable to maintain adequate nutrition by mouth, and resting her GI tract is appropriate therapy. Generally, patients with untreatable terminal diseases are not considered candidates for HPN.

Psychologically, the person on HPN must have a stable personality. (Just think of the severe consequences that could result if a patient mixed his formula incorrectly or improperly cared for the catheter site!) The patient must be able to rationally handle problems as they arise.

The HPN candidate must be intellectually capable of learning the techniques of HPN and also must understand possible complications which might arise. Several authors also have identified the need for a partner who is firmly committed, stable, and highly motivated to assist the patient in the HPN program.[1]

Although home care may be less costly than hospital care, HPN is expensive. A recent article estimated the cost of HPN (when provided on a non-profit basis) to range from $25,000 to $30,000 per person per year.[2] Most people could not afford such a program without help from private insurance, Medicare, or Medicaid. Even with such support, the patient will most likely still have to pick up many expenses. Occasionally, volunteer groups or private donations can help supplement the patient's resources.

Not all hospitals, even those with nutrition support teams, are capable of training patients for HPN. Most HPN training programs are provided through academic medical centers.[3] The quality and safe use of HPN depend on the patient's complete understanding of the HPN program. Patients must be taught how to mix and administer the HPN solution as well as how to care for the catheter. They also must be made aware of catheter-related and metabolic complications and know what actions to take if they occur.

Patients are trained while they are in the hospital. They must be able to assume responsibility for their care before they are discharged. Practicing in the hospital gives the patient a chance to try the system out, with help nearby, if needed.

Once the person is at home, he or she must be able to return to the training center or the physician for followup and be visited by a qualified nurse regularly. Also, a qualified nurse or physician must be available 24 hours a day to answer questions and to deal with emergencies.

The patient must have access to the supplies necessary to maintain a HPN program. Generally, supplies are obtained through the hospital or through an outside pharmacy. Recently, commercial supply services have been developed which send all products and equipment the patient needs directly to the home. When the patient is traveling, the supplies can be sent to other locations.

How HPN Works There are different types of HPN programs. Generally, patients are given as much responsibility as they can handle. A special type of catheter often is inserted for HPN; it enters the subclavian vein but is tunnelled under the skin and eventually exits near the middle of the chest (see Figure 1). This way patients can

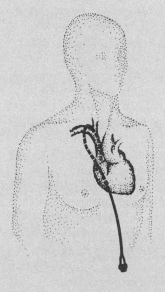

Figure 1 Placement of an HPN catheter. In this case, the catheter is tunnelled under the skin before going into the subclavian vein; in other cases, the catheter may enter the subclavian directly. The catheter has a dacron cuff; connective tissue from the person's skin grows into this cuff and helps hold it in place.

[1] I. L. Mackenzie, Evaluation of the patient for home parenteral nutrition, *Nutritional Support Services*, February 1982, pp. 16-19; S. J. Dudrick, D. M. Englert, A. O. Barroso, T. G. Jensen, C. Pacinda-Ortiz, P. A. Lee, and B. J. Rowlands, Update on ambulatory home hyperalimentation, *Nutritional Support Services*, April 1981, pp. 18-21; M. Perl, R. C. W. Hall, S. J. Dudrick, D. M. Englert, S. K. Stickney, and E. R. Gardner, Psychological aspects of long-term home hyperalimentation, *Journal of Parenteral and Enteral Nutrition* 4 (1980):554-560.

[2] Mackenzie, 1982.

[3] J. L. Mullen, Home parenteral nutrition, in *Clinical Nutrition Newsletter* (Philadelphia: University of Pennsylvania, February 1982), p. 1.

more easily look down and see the catheter and can do their own dressing changes.

The most common method of administration is for the patient to use an infusion pump set at a rate to insure that the total solution is delivered within 12 to 14 hours. The patient can infuse the solution while sleeping or at any other convenient time to allow freedom of movement during a good part of the day. The patient starts the solution slowly to avoid hyperglycemia and tapers it at the end of the feeding to avoid hypoglycemia. Then the patient disconnects the IV tubing and injects heparin into the catheter to prevent clotting.

Using another system, nutrients are infused over 24 hours. A small pump and IV bags fit neatly into a lightweight vest, allowing the patient to move around freely with little inconvenience (see Figure 2).

Some people prepare their own HPN solutions from bottles of IV dextrose and amino acids. Others receive their bottles premixed. Of course, the premixed bottles are more costly, but they are advantageous when the patient's (or family member's) ability to correctly mix the solution is questionable.

How Do HPN Patients Cope? Several articles are available which discuss the social and psychological problems which have accompanied the use of HPN.[4] These problems must be adequately recognized and considered in working with HPN patients. Many such patients suffer depression which is most apparent in the first months of treatment. Depression seems to be related to whether or not they expect to regain eating function.[5]

However, HPN also allows patients to resume many activities, including employment, sexual activity, recreation, social activity, and travel. Oftentimes, restrictions on activities are related more to the patient's illness than to HPN.[6]

[4]Perl and co-authors, 1980; A. E. Robinovitch, Home total parenteral nutrition: A psycho-social viewpoint, *Journal of Parenteral and Enteral Nutrition* 5 (1981):522-525; B. S. Price and E. L. Levine, Permanent total parenteral nutrition: Psychological and social responses of the early stages, *Journal of Parenteral and Enteral Nutrition* 3 (1979):48-52.

[5]Perl and co-authors, 1980.

[6]Perl and co-authors, 1980.

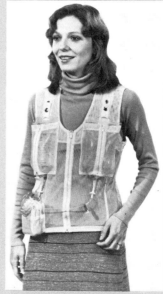

Photograph courtesy of Cormed, Inc.

Figure 2 This lightweight vest contains a small pump and bags of nutrient solution so the patient is free from machines.

One person on HPN has been quoted as saying "Do I miss the taste of real food? Sure. But you get used to it. Look at the alternative. Ten years ago I would have been dead of starvation."[7]

HPN does offer a great deal of potential for people like Mrs. Reed. HPN is monitored nationally; data collected through the registry in 1978 showed that at that time there were already about 1,000 HPN patients. For people who can be supported at home by use of tube feedings, the alternative of HEN is available.

[7]D. Ingber, People who never need to eat, *Science Digest*, January 1982, pp. 34-35.

Home Enteral Nutrition (HEN)   HEN is managed in much the same way as HPN. Patients who require long-term tube feeding are thoroughly trained in administering and mixing the feedings and managing complications.

Feeding ostomies often are placed for long-term tube feedings. Some people learn to use a transnasal tube, which they insert at each feeding. When possible, an intermittent feeding schedule is arranged so that the person is free to move about between meals. Generally, infusion pumps are used only if necessary, because they are expensive to purchase or rent. Patients who must receive a continuous drip feeding can be trained to use the pump. One system available for HEN is similar to the vest used for HPN patients[8] (see Figure 3).

[8]C. L. Kien, Employment of a mobile infusion system for continuous ambulatory tube feeding, *Journal of Parenteral and Enteral Nutrition* 5 (1981):526-527.

The patient may be able to make a tube feeding from blenderized table food, if it is tolerated. However, most patients prefer to purchase a premixed formula, which is far more convenient to prepare. A premixed formula should be used whenever the patient's ability to mix the formula is questionable.

Generally, a nurse visits the patient at home, and the patient sees his physician at regular intervals. A qualified nurse, dietitian, or physician must be available to answer

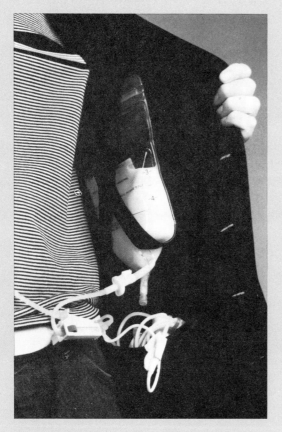
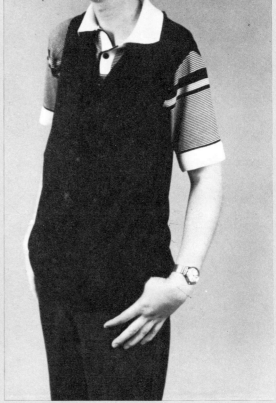

Figure 3   For home enteral nutrition, this outfit is available.

From C. Lawrence Kien, M.D., Ph.D., Associate Professor of Pediatrics and Biochemistry (Medical College of Wisconsin), Director of Nutrition and Metabolism (Milwaukee Children's Hospital), *Journal of Parenteral and Enteral Nutrition* 5 (1981):527.

questions which arise, often shortly after the patient leaves the hospital.

HEN or HPN: What Works Best?   Whenever possible HEN is selected over HPN. A recent study showed that both HPN and HEN can successfully be used to maintain or restore optimal nutrition status in patients.[9] But the techniques of HEN are easier for the patient to learn, and fewer complications are associated with its use. Further, an HEN program costs from 10 to 20 times less than an HPN program.

[9] S. A. Chrysomilides and M. V. Kaminski, Home enteral and parenteral nutritional support: A comparison, *American Journal of Clinical Nutrition* 34 (1981):2271-2275.

The Team Approach to Nutrition Support

The metabolic consequences of severe illness oblige us to employ diet therapy with maximum leverage to reduce morbidity and mortality. . . . The multidisciplinary approach of the nutrition support service . . . can lead to . . . optimal nutritional care for the hospitalized patient.
GEORGE L. BLACKBURN and BRUCE R. BISTRIAN

Eight o-clock Wednesday morning nutrition support rounds. Each patient receiving a tube feeding, peripheral TPN, or central TPN is being discussed. The core members of the nutrition support team include a physician, a dietitian, a nurse, a pharmacist, and, of course, the patient, who is the center of the team. Efforts made by the team are made on behalf of the patient. Furthermore, the patient's cooperation is an important ingredient for the successful use of nutrition support.

Each professional health team member possesses specialized knowledge. When this specialized knowledge is shared, the patient receives the benefits of combined expertise. A nutrition support team helps assure the safe and appropriate use of special nutrition support by the entire hospital staff.

Functions of a Nutrition Support Team

The nutrition support team performs many important functions. One is to identify patients who may be at risk nutritionally. Once malnourished or potentially malnourished patients have been identified, the team is available to consult on any patient as requested by the patient's physician. Furthermore, each team member serves as a resource person to the hospital staff to answer nutrition-related

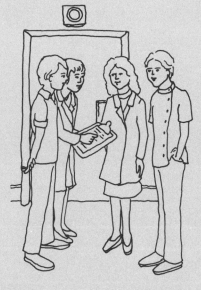

questions and solve technical problems if they arise.

The nutrition support team also monitors all patients on special nutrition support and maintains records of benefits and complications which arise as a result of such support. The team analyzes new products and techniques to help ensure cost and quality control. It is essential that all team members keep abreast of new developments which affect special nutrition support.

Team Roles

The Physician   The director of the nutrition support team is generally a physician. The physician's functions include: supervising the activities of other team members and developing guidelines for the safe use of nutrition support techniques; monitoring the rate of complications and, when possible, correcting problems that arise; and conducting in-hospital educational and training programs for the professional staff.

Additionally, other physicians may consult with the nutrition support physician, in which case the physician becomes involved with direct patient management. During nutrition support rounds the physician reviews the progress of each patient receiving special support and makes recommendations as appropriate.

The Dietitian[1] The dietitian has an obvious role on the nutrition support team as the nutrition "expert." The dietitian is invaluable in determining nutrient requirements and in translating the physician's diet orders into food or feedings.

Generally, the dietitian is directly responsible for assessing the patient's nutrition status. The dietitian may measure, calculate, record, and evaluate nutrition status parameters or may supervise the gathering of data necessary to complete the assessment.

The dietitian must have a complete and thorough knowledge of liquid formulas in order to determine which products will best meet the needs of patients using these products. For tube fed patients, the dietitian should be able to recommend not only the correct formula and feeding tube but also an appropriate administration schedule. The dietitian should be familiar with all enteral feeding equipment so that questions can be answered as they arise. The dietitian also should be able to recommend alternative

formulas and administration schedules when the patient does not tolerate the original formula.

The dietitian plays an important role in helping patients understand and cope with special nutrition support. Visiting the patient daily, continuously assessing nutrient intake, and effecting the transition from parenteral nutrition or tube feeding to oral intake are other responsibilities of the dietitian. The dietitian also assists in selecting and training patients for home parenteral and enteral nutrition programs. Whenever possible, the dietitian should make home visits to all special nutrition support patients receiving tube feedings or special formulas orally.

The Nurse[2] The nurse on a nutrition support team plays a central role in patient care management and patient relationships. The nurse is generally responsible for explaining nutrition support techniques to patients and their families. This includes explaining the need for special nutrition support as well as describing catheter or trans-

nasal tube insertion. When patients go home on special nutrition support, the nurse assumes the primary responsibility for teaching them how to follow their programs. The nurse also coordinates discharge from the hospital, being sure the patient has all the supplies and equipment needed. The nurse is usually the person available 24 hours a day to answer the home patient's questions.

For patients on parenteral nutrition, the nurse is responsible for assuring that the proper techniques of catheter insertion and care are followed. In some hospitals, the nutrition support nurse is responsible for inserting transnasal tubes for patients on enteral support. In other facilities, the nurse supervises the staff nurses to be sure that no problems arise.

Like other members of the nutrition support team, the nurse contributes to carefully monitoring patients, looking out for mechanical or metabolic complications. The nurse also administers skin tests and assesses reactions to them (see Chapter 18).

An important function of the nutrition support nurse is to act as a liaison between the nursing staff and the team. The nurse teaches the staff nurses, on a group and individual basis about the techniques of and the rationale for special nutrition support. The nurse also as-

[1] R. Chernoff, The team concept: The dietitian's responsibility, *Journal of Parenteral and Enteral Nutrition* 3 (1979):89-90; S. N. Aker, C. Cheney, S. DeHoog, M. McFadden, R. Miller, and K. Moore, *Role of the Clinical Dietitian on a Nutrition Care Team*, A.S.P.E.N. Monograph (Rockville, Md.: A.S.P.E.N., 1980).

[2] M. C. Hoppe, Grow professionally in a growing field as a nutritional support nurse, *Nursing*, May 1981, pp. 108-110; P. Rowan-Page, S. L. Turnamian, P. B. Hawkes, and M. J. Lambert, Nutritional support: The role of the nurse-clinician, *Nutritional Support Services*, April 1981, pp. 36-37.

sists in training physicians and other concerned health care professionals.

The Pharmacist[3] The pharmacist on the nutrition support team is responsible for assuring that intravenous fluids are prepared correctly and for providing training for the hospital staff who will be handling these fluids. The pharmacist must develop a knowledge of available nutrient solutions and should be able to assist in writing IV fluid orders, formulate nutrient infusions that are not commercially available, and detect any stability problems in IV solutions.

The pharmacist plays a key role in pointing out possible nutrient-drug interactions. This team member also shares in the responsibility of monitoring patients, training patients for HPN, and teaching concerned health care professionals about nutrition support techniques.

[3]R. J. Hopkins, Expanding the pharmacist's role in nutritional support service, *Nutritional Support Services*, December 1981, pp. 20-23; The role of personnel, in *Establishing a Nutritional Support Service* (Chicago: Abbott Laboratories, 1980), pp. 41-44.

Other Team Members
Other health care professionals can be an important part of the nutrition support team. The physical therapist can provide an individualized exercise program to enhance skeletal muscle protein synthesis or mineral uptake by bone and can help the patient gain independence by developing muscular strength. The social worker is extremely important, particularly for patients on home nutrition support programs. The social worker is helpful in finding funding and social services for individuals who need financial assistance. Staff, IV, and infection control nurses may wish to participate in nutrition support rounds to discuss problems they have encountered or suggestions they have regarding nutrition support.

How the Team Approach Works

The actual members of the nutrition support team and their duties may vary considerably in different hospitals. Many times, duties overlap. For example, the dietitian and nurse may both do nutrition assessments, insert nasogastric tubes, or administer skin tests. As pointed out, all team members share in monitoring and

visiting patients.

A recent study has demonstrated the benefits of the team approach to nutrition support. The study showed a decreased risk of complications from TPN when a team was used to implement and monitor appropriate TPN techniques.[4] This decrease in complications means that patients can be maintained more safely and that hospital costs will be reduced.

Nutrition support rounds are just about over. The physician reports that Mrs. A is to go home tomorrow after the successful use of TPN. Thanks to the dietitian, Mr. B is off tube feedings and eating a regular diet. The nurse was able to provide important information about Ms. C's problem with an infusion pump and so may have prevented a case of hyperglycemia. The pharmacist pointed out an easily correctable problem the pharmacy was having with fluid orders. Once the problem was solved, valuable time was saved, and more time was available for patient care. Teamwork works!

[4]A. E. Nehme, Nutritional support of the hospitalized patient: The team concept, *Journal of the American Medical Association* 243 (1980):1906-1908.

CHAPTER 21

CONTENTS

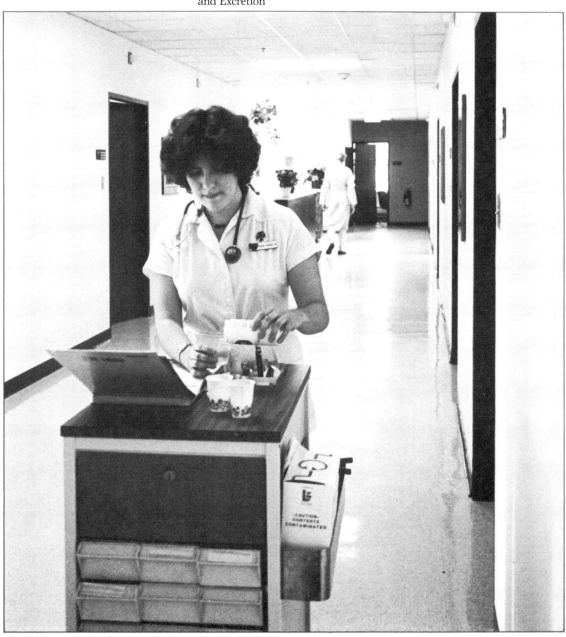

NUTRITION AND DRUG THERAPY

The more subtle manifestations of drug toxicity, particularly those which are not associated with specific symptoms or signs, or those which occur only after extremely prolonged periods of drug administration, may escape notice.

DAPHNE A. ROE, M.D.

For many years, the possibility that food and drugs might interact was largely ignored. However, in recent years we have begun to know more and more about how drugs affect nutrition status and how nutrition status affects drug metabolism. The body of information regarding food and drug interactions changes rapidly as we gain experience with the use of newer drugs.

Not all the drug-nutrient interactions we will be discussing are significant for every person. Many factors influence the risk of adverse drug-nutrient interactions. Drug-induced nutrient deficiencies are more likely to occur in people who must take drugs over a long period of time. The more drugs someone is taking, the greater the risk that deficiencies will occur. Furthermore, the person whose nutrition status is poor when drug treatment begins is more likely to develop nutrient deficiencies. Therefore, the elderly and people who have higher nutrient requirements are more likely to develop problems.

Nutrients and drugs may interact in many ways, producing one or more of the following effects:

- Alteration of food intake.

- Changes in the absorption of the nutrient or the drug.

- Interference with the intended action of the drug.

- Alteration of the metabolism and excretion of the nutrient or the drug, which changes nutrient or drug requirements.

Nutrients themselves also can be classified as drugs when they are given in amounts far in excess of physiologic needs.

Although some drug-nutrient interactions are produced intentionally, more often than not these interactions are unintentional. To protect against undesirable interactions, health care professionals must be alert to the effects of drugs and nutrients on one another.

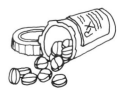

Drugs and Food Intake

Drugs can affect food intake in several ways. A drug may stimulate or depress the appetite, alter perceptions of taste and smell, cause sores or inflammation of the mouth, or induce nausea and vomiting.

Occasionally some such effects are desirable, but often they are not. For example, amphetamines often are prescribed in the treatment of obesity specifically because they depress the appetite. But amphetamines also are used to treat hyperactive children, and in this instance, the appetite-depressing effects are undesirable. Table 1 lists drugs which have been shown to interfere with food intake.

Antineoplastic agents used in the treatment of cancer patients may cause many undesirable effects on food intake. In addition to depressing the appetite, they can cause taste alterations, mouth sores, nausea, and vomiting (see also Chapter 28). The use of marihuana in alleviating nausea and vomiting in patients receiving chemotherapy is discussed in Highlight 21.

Many drugs can cause nausea. Sometimes giving these drugs with meals helps alleviate the nausea; drugs which should be given with foods are listed in Table 2.

Absorption and Drug-Nutrient Interactions

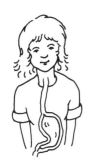

The absorption of drugs can be positively or negatively affected by the presence of food or particular nutrients in the GI tract, and the reverse is also true. Like foods, drugs taken by mouth are often absorbed in the intestine. When you consider how many processes are operating during digestion and absorption, you can see that nutrients and drugs have many opportunities to interact.

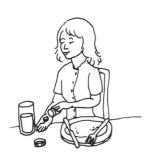

Effects of Food on Drug Digestion and Absorption Food can affect a drug by enhancing, delaying, or decreasing its absorption. When a drug is given by mouth, it may be given in tablet, capsule, or liquid form. Tablets and capsules must dissolve before they can be absorbed, and the pH of the stomach affects the way in which they dissolve. The presence of food in the stomach causes the secretion of gastric acid, which lowers the pH of the stomach. Therefore, drugs which are negatively affected by increased acidity should be taken on an empty stomach. For example, some antibiotics are degraded by a low pH. Conversely, some capsules are coated so that they dissolve in the higher pH of the small intestine. If they are given with milk (which raises the stomach's pH) they dissolve in the stomach — an undesirable effect.

The presence of food in the stomach also stimulates the secretion of bile acids into the intestine, which enhances fat digestion and absorption. Some medications dissolve in and are better absorbed along with fat. These drugs should be given with food. Griseofulvin, for

Table 1. Examples of Drugs Affecting Food Intake*

Depress appetite

    Amphetamines
    Antineoplastic drugs
    Alcohol (chronic use)
    Laxatives (methyl cullulose, guar gum)
    Cardiac glycosides

Stimulate appetite

    Antihistamines
    Tranquilizers
    Antidepressants (chloropromazine, chlordiazepoxide, diazepam)
    Hypoglycemic agents (insulin, tolbutamide, chlorpropamide)
    Corticosteroids

Induce nausea and/or vomiting

    Analgesics
    Antibiotics
    Anticonvulsants
    Antineoplastic drugs
    Anti-inflammatory drugs
    Chelating agents
    Cardiac glycosides
    Mineral preparations

Alter taste sensitivity

    Antineoplastic agents
    Amphetamines
    Anesthetics
    Penicillamine
    Levodopa
    Clofibrate

*This list is not all-inclusive. Furthermore, not every drug within each major classification causes the effect (e.g., not all antibiotics cause nausea and vomiting).

Data from D. A. Roe, Interactions between drugs and nutrients. *Medical Clinics of North America* 63 (1979):985-1007; A. O. Moore and D. E. Powers, *Food-Medication Interactions*, ed. C. H. Smith (Tempe, Ariz.: A. O. Moore and D. E. Powers, 1981); J. A. S. Carson and A. Gormican, Disease-medication relationships in altered taste sensitivity, *Journal of the American Dietetic Association* 68 (1976):550-553; C. J. Maslakowski, Drug-nutrient interactions/interrelationships, *Nutritional Support Services*, November 1981, pp. 14-17.

example, is an antifungal drug which is better absorbed with fat.

    Food delays the rate at which the stomach empties. Therefore, when you want a drug to work rapidly, you should give it on an empty stomach. For example, an aspirin given on an empty stomach works faster than one given on a full stomach. However, aspirin also can be

Table 2. Recommended Timing of Drug Administration with Meals

Drug	Give on empty stomach (1 hour before or 2-3 hours after meals)	Give 1/2 hour before meals	Give with food or milk	Don't give with milk or dairy products	Don't give with fruit juices	Can give with or without meals
Allopurinol			X			
Aminophylline			X			
Amoxicillin						X
Ampicillin	X				X	
Aspirin			X			
Atropine sulfate		X				
Belladonna		X				
Bisacodyl				X		
Cephalexin						X
Chlorodiazepoxide		X				
Chlorothiazide			X			
Chlorpromazine			X			
Chlorpropamide			X			
Cimetidine			X			
Cloxacillin sodium	X				X	
Demeclocycline	X			X		
Dicloxacillin sodium	X					
Doxycycline hyclate				X		X
Erythromycin						X
Erythromycin, enteric coated			X			
Erythromycin estolate						X
Erythromycin, succinate or stearate	X					
Ferrous sulfate, fumarate, lactate, or gluconate			X			
Glycopyrrolate		X				
Griseofulvin			X			
Hydrocortisone			X			
Indomethacin			X			
Isoniazid			X			
Levodopa			X			
Lincomycin	X					

Table 2. Recommended Timing of Drug Administration with Meals (continued)

Drug	Give on empty stomach (1 hour before or 2-3 hours after meals)	Give 1/2 hour before meals	Give with food or milk	Don't give with milk or dairy products	Don't give with fruit juices	Can give with or without meals
Methylsergide maleate			X			
Metronidazole			X			
Minocycline						X
Nalidixic acid			X			
Nitrofurantoin			X			
Oxacillin sodium	X					
Oxyphenbutazone			X			
Oxytetracycline	X			X		
Penicillin, G	X					
Penicillin, K						X
Phenformin			X			
Phenylbutazone			X			
Potassium salts			X			
Prednisolone			X			
Prednisone			X			
Procainamide						X
Propantheline bromide		X				
Rauwolfia serpentina			X			
Reserpine			X			
Rifampin	X					
Sulfinpyrazone			X			
Tetracycline	X			X		
Theophylline			X			
Tolbutamide			X			
Triamterene			X			
Trihexyphemidyl			X			
Trimeprazine			X			
Zinc sulfate			X			

Data from C. Giovannetti and T. Schwinghammer, Food and drugs, managing the right mix for your patient, *Nursing*, July 1981, pp. 26-31; M. L. Lambert, Drug and Diet Interactions, *American Journal of Nursing* 75 (1975):402-406; J. A. Visconti, Ed., Drug-food interaction, in *Nutrition in Disease*, ed. R. A. Dell (Columbus, Ohio: Ross Laboratories, 1977).

Miniglossary of Drug Actions

amphetamines: stimulate the central nervous system; used in the treatment of obesity and of hyperactivity in children.

analgesics: relieve pain.

anesthetics: block sensations of pain or touch.

antacids: neutralize the acidity of the stomach.

antibiotics: kill microorganisms or interfere with their growth.

anticoagulants: prevent or slow down blood clotting.

anticonvulsants: prevent or reduce the occurrence of seizures.

antidepressants: help alleviate severe depression.

antidiabetic agents: reduce blood sugar levels.

antifungal agents: kill fungus or prevent its growth.

antihistamines: counteract inflammation; also used to treat allergies.

antihypertensive agents: reduce blood pressure.

anti-infective agents: kill microorganisms or interfere with their growth.

anti-inflammatory agents: reduce tissue inflammation.

antilipemics: counteract or prevent accumulation of fats in the blood; cholesterol-lowering agents are antilipemics.

antimicrobials: kill microorganisms or interfere with their growth.

antineoplastic agents: prevent or inhibit the growth of malignant tumor cells.

antitubercular agents: inhibit growth of the bacteria that cause tuberculosis.

cardiac glycosides: increase the force of heart muscle contractions.

cathartics: cause rapid expulsion of intestinal contents, usually in semiliquid form; very strong laxatives.

chelating agents: bind to toxic heavy metals (lead, arsenic, gold, mercury) to promote their excretion.

corticosteroids: can be used as antiflammatory agents, to suppress undesirable immune responses, or as replacement therapy for people who cannot synthesize corticosteroids.

diuretics: increase the excretion of urine.

hypocholesterolemics: reduce blood cholesterol levels.

hypoglycemic agents: reduce blood sugar levels; same as *antidiabetic agents*.

laxatives: cause intestinal contents to be rapidly expelled.

oral contraceptives: prevent pregnancy.

irritating to the GI tract. The presence of food can act as a buffer and reduce this irritation. So when rapid action is not essential, giving aspirin (or other drugs) with food can help reduce nausea, GI distress, and possible damage to the intestinal mucosa.

Additionally, there are instances in which the desired action of a drug must be timed with food intake. For example, some drugs used to treat ulcer patients decrease gastric acid secretion and gastric motility. The patient should take the drug just before a meal so that it will be effective while the meal is stimulating gastric acid secretion.

Specific nutrients in food also can have a negative effect on drug absorption. A classical example is the interaction of tetracycline and dairy products. The calcium from a dairy product can bind to tetracycline, thereby reducing the amount of tetracycline which is absorbed. Antacids that contain calcium carbonate (such as Tums) also can reduce the absorption of tetracycline.

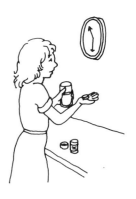

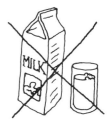

Many people believe that drugs available without a prescription (over-the-counter, or OTC, drugs) are harmless. Such is not the case. For example, simple aspirin (probably the most common OTC drug) can lead to anemia and possibly hemorrhage when it is used over long periods of time.

A further danger in using OTC drugs is that they can allow a serious problem to be masked by covering up the symptoms. For example, a person who repeatedly takes antacids for stomach discomfort may be ignoring the signs of an ulcer. Furthermore, some antacids contribute significant amounts of sodium (Alka-Seltzer — 521 mg/tablet) or calcium (Tums — 500 mg calcium/tablet), or can lead to a depletion of phosphorus (drugs containing aluminum hydroxide). Although these effects may be insignificant in healthy individuals, they can aggravate some medical conditions.

ac: *ante cibes*; before meals.
bid: *bis in die*; twice daily.
c: *cum*; with.
hs: *hora somni*; at bedtime.
pc: *post cibum*; after meals.
qid: *quater in die*; four times daily.
tid: *ter in die*; three times daily.

Over-the-counter (OTC) drugs: drugs that can be purchased without a prescription.

A FLAG SIGN OF A SPURIOUS CLAIM
IS THE ASSERTION THAT:

Nonprescription drugs are harmless.

Effects of Drugs on Food Digestion and Absorption   Drugs can act very similarly to food in altering pH, digestive secretions, and gastrointestinal motility. These drug effects influence the digestion and absorption of nutrients. Some drugs can inactivate enzyme systems necessary for the absorption of some nutrients, and some can actually damage the mucosal cells that absorb nutrients. Still other drugs bind to specific nutrients so that they cannot be absorbed (see Table 3).

Table 3. Selected Drug-Nutrient Interactions

Drug	Effect on nutrients	
Alcohol	Energy	⇓ intake
	Protein	⇓ intake
	Fat	⇑ buildup in liver
		⇓ absorption
	Thiamin	⇓ absorption ⇓ storage
	Vitamin B$_6$	⇓ activation
	Folacin	⇓ absorption, utilization
	Vitamin B$_{12}$	⇓ absorption
	Magnesium	⇑ urinary excretion
	Zinc	⇑ urinary excretion
Analgesics		
Aspirin	Folacin	⇓ serum levels; altered transport
	Vitamin C	⇑ urinary excretion
	Thiamin	⇑ urinary excretion
	Vitamin K	⇑ urinary excretion
	Iron	may cause blood loss
Amphetamines	⇓ Intake	causes anorexia, dry mouth, metallic taste, nausea, vomiting
Antacids		
Aluminum hydroxide	Phosphorus	⇓ absorption
Other types	Thiamin	⇑ destruction
Anticoagulants	Vitamin K	⇓ conversion to active form
Anticonvulsants	Folacin	⇓ serum levels
	Vitamin B$_6$	⇓ serum levels
	Vitamin B$_{12}$	⇓ serum levels
	Vitamin D	⇓ conversion to active forms
	Vitamin K	⇑ requirement
Antimicrobials		
Chloramphenicol	Riboflavin	⇑ requirement (?)
	Vitamin B$_6$	⇑ requirement (?)
	Vitamin B$_{12}$	⇑ requirement (?)
Penicillin	Potassium	⇑ urinary excretion
Neomycin	Fats	⇓ absorption
	Nitrogen	⇓ absorption
	Carbohydrates	⇓ absorption
	Folacin	⇓ absorption
	Vitamin B$_{12}$	⇓ absorption
	Fat-soluble vitamins	⇓ absorption
	Calcium	⇓ absorption
	Iron	⇓ absorption
	Potassium	⇓ absorption

Table 3.   Selected Drug-Nutrient Interactions (continued)

Drug		Effect on nutrients
	Vitamin K	$\Downarrow$ intestinal synthesis
Tetracycline	Fat	$\Downarrow$ absorption
	Amino acids	$\Downarrow$ absorption
	Calcium	$\Downarrow$ absorption
	Iron	$\Downarrow$ absorption
	Magnesium	$\Downarrow$ absorption
	Zinc	$\Downarrow$ absorption
	Niacin	$\Uparrow$ urinary excretion
	Riboflavin	$\Uparrow$ urinary excretion
	Folacin	$\Uparrow$ urinary excretion
	Vitamin C	$\Uparrow$ urinary excretion
Antineoplastic agents		
Methotrexate and pyrimethamine	Folacin	folacin antagonist
	Vitamin B_{12}	$\Downarrow$ absorption
	Fat	$\Downarrow$ absorption
	$\Downarrow$ Intake and general malabsorption	anorexia, nausea, vomiting, mouth sores
5-Fluorouracil	Protein	$\Downarrow$ absorption and synthesis
Antitubercular drugs		
Cycloserine	Vitamin B_6	vitamin B_6 antagonist
	Protein	$\Downarrow$ synthesis
	Calcium	$\Downarrow$ absorption (?)
	Magnesium	$\Downarrow$ absorption (?)
	Vitamin B_6	$\Downarrow$ serum levels (?)
	Folacin	$\Downarrow$ serum levels (?)
	Vitamin B_{12}	$\Downarrow$ serum levels (?)
Isonicotinic acid hydrazide (INH)	Vitamin B_6	vitamin B_6 antagonist $\Uparrow$ urinary excretion causes deficiency
	Niacin	causes deficiency
	Vitamin B_{12}	$\Downarrow$ absorption, $\Downarrow$ serum levels
Para-aminosalicylic acid	Folacin	$\Downarrow$ absorption
	Vitamin B_{12}	$\Downarrow$ absorption
	Fat	$\Downarrow$ absorption
	Iron	$\Downarrow$ absorption
Chelating agents		
Penicillamine	Vitamin B_6	$\Uparrow$ requirement $\Uparrow$ urinary excretion
	Zinc	$\Uparrow$ urinary excretion
	Iron	$\Uparrow$ urinary excretion

Table 3. Selected Drug-Nutrient Interactions (continued)

Drug		Effect on nutrients
	Copper	⇑ urinary excretion
	⇓ Intake	alters taste; causes anorexia; nausea, vomiting
Cholesterol-lowering agents		
Cholestyramine	Fat and cholesterol	⇓ absorption
	Fat-soluble vitamins	⇓ absorption
	Folacin	⇓ absorption
	Iron	⇓ absorption
	Vitamin B$_{12}$	⇓ absorption
		⇓ blood levels
	Calcium	⇑ urinary excretion,
		⇓ blood levels
Clofibrate	Vitamin B$_{12}$	⇓ absorption
	Iron	⇓ absorption
	⇓ Intake	alters taste; causes nausea and GI irritation
Colchicine	Fat	⇓ absorption
	Nitrogen	⇓ absorption
	Folacin	⇓ absorption
	Vitamin B$_{12}$	⇓ absorption
	Sodium	⇓ absorption
	Potassium	⇓ absorption
Corticosteroids	Vitamin D	⇑ metabolism,
		⇑ requirement
	Vitamin B$_6$	⇑ requirement
	Vitamin C	⇑ requirement,
		⇑ urinary excretion
	Calcium	⇓ absorption,
		⇑ urinary excretion
	Phosphorus	⇓ absorption
	Zinc	⇑ urinary excretion,
		⇓ serum levels
	Glucose	⇑ serum levels
	Triglycerides	⇑ serum levels
	Cholesterol	⇑ serum levels
	Potassium	⇑ urinary excretion
	Nitrogen	⇑ urinary excretion
Diuretics		
Furosemide	Calcium	⇑ urinary excretion
	Sodium	⇑ urinary excretion
	Potassium	⇓ serum levels
	Chloride	⇓ serum levels
	Magnesium	⇓ serum levels
	Zinc	⇑ serum levels,
		⇓ storage in liver

Table 3.   Selected Drug-Nutrient Interactions (continued)

Drug	Effect on nutrients	
Mercurials	Thiamin	⇑ urinary excretion
	Calcium	⇑ urinary excretion
	Sodium	⇑ urinary excretion
	Potassium	⇑ urinary excretion
	Chloride	⇑ urinary excretion
	Magnesium	⇑ urinary excretion
Thiazides	Sodium	⇑ urinary excretion
	Potassium	⇓ blood levels
	Chloride	⇓ blood levels
	Calcium	⇑ urinary excretion, ⇑ blood levels
	Magnesium	⇑ urinary excretion
	Phosphorus	⇓ blood levels
	Glucose	⇑ blood levels (?)
Triamterene	Sodium	⇑ urinary excretion
	Folacin	⇓ serum levels
	Vitamin B$_{12}$	⇓ serum levels
Glutethimide	Vitamin D	⇑ metabolism
Hypoglycemics		
Phenformin and metaformin	Vitamin B$_{12}$	⇓ absorption
Hydralazine	Vitamin B$_6$	⇑ urinary excretion
Laxatives		
Cathartics	Fat	⇓ absorption
	Glucose	⇓ absorption
	Vitamin D	⇓ absorption
	Calcium	⇓ absorption
	Potassium	⇓ absorption
Mineral oil	Fat-soluble vitamins	⇓ absorption
	Calcium	⇓ absorption
	Phosphates	⇓ absorption
Levodopa	Amino acids	⇑ requirement
	Vitamin B$_6$	⇑ requirement
	Vitamin C	⇑ requirement
	Sodium	⇓ urinary excretion
	Potassium	⇓ urinary excretion
Oral contraceptives	Vitamin B$_6$	⇑ requirement, ⇓ blood levels
	Riboflavin	⇑ requirement, ⇓ blood levels
	Folacin	⇓ absorption, ⇓ blood levels
	Vitamin B$_{12}$	⇓ blood levels
	Vitamin C	⇓ blood levels

Table 3.   Selected Drug-Nutrient Interactions (continued)

Drug	Effect on nutrients	
	Vitamin A	⇈ blood levels
	Calcium	⇈ absorption
	Iron	⇈ serum levels
	Copper	⇈ serum levels
	Magnesium	⇊ blood levels (?)
	Zinc	⇊ blood levels (?)
Potassium salts	Vitamin B_{12}	⇊ absorption
Sulfonamides		
Salicylazosulfapyridine	Folacin	⇊ absorption,
		⇊ blood levels
	Iron	⇊ blood levels
Others	Folacin	⇊ intestinal synthesis
	Vitamin K	⇊ intestinal synthesis
	B vitamins	⇊ intestinal synthesis

⇈   increases

⇊   decreases

(?) possible effect

Data from R. E. Hodges, Drug-nutrient interactions, in *Nutrition in Medical Practice* (Philadelphia: Saunders, 1980), pp. 323-331; R. C. Theuer and J. J. Vitale, Drug and nutrient interactions, in *Nutritional Support of Medical Practice*, ed. H. A. Schneider, C. E. Anderson, and D. B. Coursin (Hagerstown, Md.: Harper & Row, 1977) pp. 297-305; A. O. Moore and D. E. Powers, *Food-Medication Interactions*, ed. C. H. Smith (Tempe, Ariz.: A. O. Moore and D. E. Powers, 1981); A. Grant, *Nutritional Assessment Guidelines* (Seattle: A. Grant, 1979), pp. 63-96; D. C. March, *Handbook: Interactions of Selected Drugs with Nutritional Status in Man* (Chicago: American Dietetic Association, 1978).

When drugs cause a change in the intestinal environment (by changing motility, altering pH, or interfering with bile acids) the change is called a **luminal effect**.

lumen = the inside (of a tube)

Drugs that interfere with a nutrient's ability to be absorbed across the intestinal mucosa are said to exert a **mucosal effect**. Mucosal effects include actual damage to the mucosal cells and inactivation of enzyme systems.

Antacids change the pH of the stomach and can decrease iron absorption. A lower pH enhances the formation of ferrous iron, which is the absorbable (+2) form of iron. Potassium chloride (used as a potassium supplement) decreases the pH of the small intestine, interfering with the absorption of vitamin B_{12}.

Several drugs increase the absorption of nutrients. For example, cimetidine, a drug commonly used to prevent the secretion of gastric acid, has been shown to be effective in reducing malabsorption of fat and improving the absorption of protein and carbohydrate in people with short bowel syndrome.[1] In addition to reducing gastric acid secretion, it also reduces gastric output to help improve absorption.

[1] D. A. Roe, Interactions between drugs and nutrients, *Medical Clinics of North America* 63 (1979):985-1007.

When malabsorption is due to lack of pancreatic enzymes, drugs known as enzyme replacements aid in the digestion and absorption of various nutrients. Additionally, lactase enzyme replacements are available to aid in the digestion of lactose in people with a lactase deficiency.

Laxatives, drugs which cause the gastrointestinal contents to be rapidly expelled, may give nutrients little time for absorption. Taking laxatives regularly can lead to decreased absorption of fat-soluble vitamins, protein, calcium, and glucose. Chronic use of some laxatives damages the structural integrity of the intestinal cells. Mineral oil, another laxative, interferes with the formation of micelles, particles formed in an early step of fat digestion. The fat-soluble vitamins (A, D, E, and K) dissolve in the oil and are lost in the feces rather than absorbed. Calcium and phosphorus also are malabsorbed.[2]

Drugs which help reduce cholesterol levels (hypocholesterolemics) can decrease the absorption of many nutrients, including fat-soluble vitamins, vitamin B_{12}, glucose, iron, and fat. Vitamin K deficiency has been reported in people receiving therapeutic doses of cholestyramine, one hypocholesterolemic agent.[3]

Neomycin, an anti-infective agent, also binds bile salts and has been reported to reduce absorption of fat, fat-soluble vitamins, amino acids, vitamin B_{12}, lactose, potassium, calcium, and iron. In addition to binding bile salts, neomycin appears to decrease the activity of pancreatic lipase; it also damages mucosal cells.[4] Furthermore, by destroying the intestinal bacteria which synthesize vitamin K, it may induce a vitamin K deficiency with long-term use. Other antibiotics may cause similar malabsorption problems.

Metabolic Food-Drug Interactions

We have been discussing examples of ways in which foods and drugs interact to cause changes in food intake and nutrient and drug absorption. Food and drugs can also interact to alter metabolism and excretion.

Effects of Nutrients and Foods on Drug Metabolism   Two basic types of food-drug interactions affect the way a drug works:

● The presence of certain nutrients can change the way the body uses a drug.

[2]D. C. March, *Handbook: Interactions of Selected Drugs with Nutritional Status in Man* (Chicago: American Dietetic Association, 1978).

[3]L. Gross and M. Brotman, Hypoprothrombinemia and hemorrhage associated with cholestyramine therapy, *Annals of Internal Medicine* 72 (1970):95-96.

[4]D. A. Roe, Drug-induced malabsorption, in *Drug-Induced Nutritional Deficiencies* (Westport, Conn.: AVI, 1976), p. 133.

Table 4.   Nutrients That May Be Affected by Drugs

Nutrients	Drugs that affect nutrient status
Protein	5-fluorouracil; neomycin
Carbohydrates	metformin; phenformin; corticosteroids ; chlorothiazide
Fats and fatty acids	neomycin; cholestyramine; clofibrate
Thiamin	antacids; ethanol; carbohydrates
Riboflavin	boric acid; oral contraceptive steroids
Niacin	isoniazid; 6-mercaptopurine; 5-fluorouracil
Vitamin B_6	isoniazid; ethanol; oral contraceptive steroids; penicillamine; hydralazine; cycloserine; L-dopa
Folates	diphenylhydantoin; methotrexate; pyrimethamine; ethanol; oral contraceptive steroids; phenylbutazone
Vitamin B_{12}	para-aminosalicylic acid; barbiturates; colchicine; cholestyramine; phenformin; oral contraceptive steroids
Vitamin C	aminopyrine; cigarettes; diphenylhydantoin; oral contraceptive steroids; paraldehyde; salicylates
Vitamin A	mineral oil (disputed); cholestyramine; oral contraceptive steroids
Vitamin D	phenobarbital; diphenylhydantoin; cholestyramine; mineral oil
Vitamin E	mineral oil; iron; polyunsaturated fatty acids; cholestyramine
Vitamin K	sodium warfarin (Coumadin); barbiturates; ascorbic acid; mineral oil
Essential fatty acids	continuous infusions of glucose
Sodium	thiazides; ethacrynic acid; Aldactone
Potassium	thiazides; cathartics

Table 4.   Nutrients That May Be Affected by Drugs (continued)

Nutrients	Drugs that affect nutrient status
Calcium	oxalates; fatty acids; phytates; phosphates
Phosphorus	aluminum hydroxide; total parenteral nutrition
Magnesium	ethanol; ethacrynic acid
Iron	phytic acid; oxalates; phosphates; ascorbic acid
Zinc	ethanol; penicillamine; oral contraceptive steroids
Copper	ethanol; penicillamine; phytates; corticosteroids

From R. E. Hodges, *Nutrition in Medical Practice* (Philadelphia: Saunders, 1980), p. 328. Reprinted with permission.

● Certain substances in foods can interact with drugs to alter the drug's action (see Table 3).

When vitamins are given in pharmacologic doses they can lower blood levels of some drugs and thereby reduce the drugs' effectiveness. For example, high doses of vitamin B_6 or folacin can reduce blood levels of diphenylhydantoin and phenobarbitol (drugs used to treat seizure disorders). Very high doses of vitamin K can reduce the effectiveness of some drugs (dicoumarol and warfarin) which prevent blood from clotting. Green leafy vegetables such as spinach, turnip greens, and brussels sprouts are foods high in vitamin K.

Occasionally, people with severe depression are treated with drugs called monoamine oxidase (MAO) inhibitors, which block the action of the enzyme monoamine oxidase. Tyramine, a substance found in some foods, normally undergoes conversion in the body to an inactive form through the action of monoamine oxidase. When MAO inhibitors are given, tyramine remains active and causes the release of norepinephrine. As a result, the patient can develop severe hypertension and headaches. Blood pressure can rise high enough to be fatal. Table 5 lists foods that are major sources of tyramine.

People taking certain types of diuretics which cause loss of potassium may need to be cautioned about eating genuine licorice, which can cause more potassium loss and more retention of water and salt. Most American-made licorice uses synthetic licorice flavoring, which is not a problem. However, imported licorice may contain the natural extract.

Effects of Drugs on Nutrient Metabolism   Some drugs have a chemical structure similar to that of a vitamin or of a metabolite. Such

pharmacologic dose: a dose of a nutrient which exceeds normal requirements and can produce a drug-like effect. The amount of a nutrient the body needs and can use is termed a **physiologic dose**.

pharmaco = drug

Table 5.   Food Sources of Tyramine*

Foods very high in tyramine	Cheeses, aged
	Boursalt
	Camembert
	Cheddar
	Stilton
	Yeast extracts
Foods high in tyramine	Bologna
	Dried, salted, or pickled herring
	Dried, salted, or pickled cod
	Pepperoni
	Salami
Foods moderately high in tyramine	Cheeses
	Blue
	Brick, natural
	Brie
	Gruyere
	Mozzarella
	Parmesan
	Romano
	Roquefort
	Chianti wine
	Meat tenderizers
Foods moderate in tyramine	Broad beans (fava, Chinese pea pods)
	Caffeine (in large amounts)
	Chocolate (in large amounts)
	Liver, chicken, and beef
	Pineapple
	Plums
	Raisins
	Soy sauce
Foods low in tyramine	Ale
	Avocados
	Bananas
	Beer
	Cheeses
	American, processed
	Cottage
	Cream
	Ricotta
	Figs
	Sherry
	Sour cream
	White wine

*The tyramine content of each type of food varies. Data on tyramine content may be based on small sample sizes.

a drug can displace the vitamin or metabolite from an enzyme and block a normal metabolic pathway. Many types of drugs used to treat cancer are of this type. Cancer cells, like normal cells, need the real vitamin to grow. When the vitamin is not available, they die. Unfortunately, other growing cells in the body also need the vitamin, and vitamin deficiency results. Methotrexate and pyrimethamine, which are structurally similar to folacin, are examples of this type of drug (see Figure 1).

Anticonvulsants interfere with vitamin metabolism in a different way. You may recall that once vitamin D has been absorbed it is converted to 25-hydroxy vitamin D in the liver and then to its more active form, 1,25-dihydroxy vitamin D, in the kidney. Anticonvulsants interfere with the conversion of vitamin D in the liver. Less 25-hydroxy vitamin D reaches the kidney, so that less of the dihydroxy vitamin is formed.

A drug can also bind to a nutrient, thereby making it unavailable to the body. An example is a drug called isonicotinic acid hydrazide (INH), used to treat tuberculosis. INH binds with vitamin B_6 and both are excreted in the urine.

An **antivitamin**, or **vitamin antagonist**, is a substance structurally similar to a vitamin which interferes with the normal activity of the vitamin.

anti = against

An **antimetabolite** is similar to an antivitamin, but it affects the activity of a metabolite. (A **metabolite** is any compound produced during metabolism.) An example is 5-fluorouracil, an antimetabolite of uracil, a base necessary for RNA synthesis.

Food-Drug Interactions and Excretion

When some foods (breads and protein-rich foods) are metabolized, their end products can potentially produce an acid urine. Other foods (fruits, vegetables, and milk) potentially produce an alkaline urine (see also Table 2, Chapter 14). The pH of the urine affects the degree to

Figure 1 Because methotrexate and pyrimethamine are structurally similar to folacin, they compete for the enzyme which normally activates folacin.

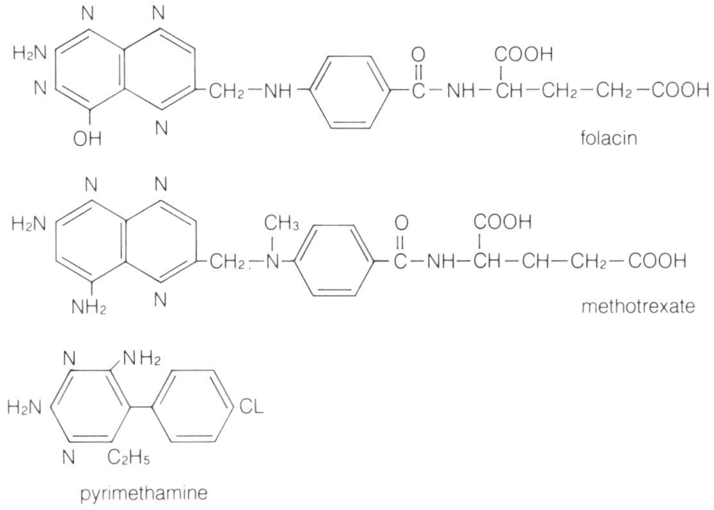

which some drugs are reabsorbed from the renal tubules back into the blood. A low urinary pH decreases the excretion of acidic drugs like aspirin and phenobarbitol. Thus, these drugs remain in the blood for longer periods of time when the urine is acidic. Since bacterial growth is inhibited in a low-pH urine, it is often desirable to decrease the urinary pH when antibiotics are given for urinary tract infections. Vitamin C is sometimes given in large doses to acidify the urine.

Drugs can increase or decrease the excretion of nutrients in the urine. For example, some diuretics can increase the excretion of calcium, potassium, magnesium, and zinc. Birth control pills, on the other hand, may decrease the urinary excretion of calcium, phosphorus, magnesium, and zinc.

The excretion of a nutrient may be increased when a drug causes it to be displaced from the plasma protein that normally transports it. When attached to the larger protein, some nutrients would not be filtered by the kidney; however, the much smaller unbound nutrient is readily excreted. An example is aspirin, which may increase folacin excretion by displacing folacin from its carrier protein.[5]

A Word about Alcohol

The interactions between alcohol and nutrition status are so numerous that they deserve special emphasis here (see also Highlight 9), especially since alcohol is a widely used and abused drug. Alcohol affects the intake, absorption, metabolism, and excretion of nutrients.

The severe thiamin deficiency frequently seen in alcohol abusers is believed to cause **Wernicke's encephalopathy**, a syndrome characterized by mental disturbances and an inability to coordinate muscular movements.

encephalo = brain
path = disease

Chronic use of alcohol suppresses the appetite and thus interferes with the ingestion of nutrients. Alcohol is directly toxic to the pancreas, liver, and GI tract.[6] Damage to the pancreas leads to insufficient production of digestive enzymes, which may explain why amino acids and fats are malabsorbed in alcoholics.[7] (Alcohol also reduces the absorption of thiamin, folacin, and vitamin B_{12}.) The damaged liver may be unable to adequately store nutrients or activate enzyme systems necessary for nutrient metabolism. The metabolism of thiamin, folacin, vitamin A, and vitamin D are affected by liver disease. Zinc, magnesium, and potassium are excreted in increased amounts in the urine. In addition, iron may be stored excessively in the liver, increasing liver damage.

[5]H. J. Alter, M. J. Zvaifler, and C. E. Rath, Interrelationship of rheumatoid arthritis, folic acid and aspirin, *Blood* 38 (1971):405-416.

[6]Roe, 1976, p. 203.

[7]Roe, 1976, p. 205.

Alcohol not only affects nutrients but also interacts with other drugs. Highlight 7 presents some of the reasons why.

Drugs and Modified Diets

A relationship between foods and drugs that often goes unnoticed is the contribution of nutrients from drug sources. For example, many drugs contain considerable sodium, sugar, potassium, and other electrolytes. This must be kept in mind for people who are following diets restricted in sodium, electrolytes, or sugar. Many liquid preparations have sugar added to make them taste better. Antibiotics often contain considerable amounts of sodium. Intravenously administered medications may provide sodium or dextrose.

People being fed by tube often are given medications through the tube. Generally, medicines in tablet form should be finely crushed to prevent clogging of the tube. However, some types of tablets and capsules are intended to slowly release their contents, and they should not be crushed, or the patient might be exposed to an excessive dosage of the drug at one time. The place where the feeding is delivered is also of considerable importance. A drug that dissolves in the acidic environment of the stomach may not be as readily absorbed if delivered directly to the duodenum or jejunum. Similarly, a drug that is absorbed optimally in the duodenum may be poorly absorbed in the jejunum.

Unpleasant-tasting drugs are sometimes mixed with a food or beverage to make them more palatable. This practice should be used cautiously since, as previously discussed, pH can have an effect on the absorption and stability of the drug. The same cautions should be exercised when medications are given with tube feedings, which, like foods, vary in pH.

Summing Up

Many interactions between drugs and nutrients can affect nutrition status. Also, nutrients or foods can affect the usability and availability of a drug. The likelihood of developing nutrient deficiencies from drugs increases with the length of time, dosage, and number of drugs a person is taking. People whose nutrition status is poor or whose nutrient requirements are high are more likely to develop nutrient deficiencies. Table 6 summarizes the ways in which drugs and nutrients can interact.

Table 6.   Mechanisms of Food-Drug Interactions

Drugs can change food intake by:
> Altering the appetite
> Interfering with taste or smell
> Inducing nausea or vomiting
> Causing sores or inflammation of the mouth

Foods can change drug absorption by:
> Changing the pH of the GI tract
> Stimulating secretion of digestive juices
> Altering GI motility
> Binding to drugs

Drugs can change food absorption by:
> Changing the pH of the GI tract
> Altering digestive juices
> Altering GI motility
> Inactivating enzyme systems
> Damaging mucosal cells

Foods can change drug metabolism by:
> Interfering with a drug's action
> Contributing pharmacologically active substances (example: tyramine)

Drugs can change food metabolism by:
> Acting as structural analogs
> Interfering with metabolic enzyme systems
> Binding to nutrients

Foods can change drug excretion by:
> Changing the pH of the urine

Drugs can change nutrient excretion by:
> Altering reabsorption in the kidneys
> Displacing nutrients from their plasma protein carriers

To Explore Further

Information about food and drug interactions changes rapidly. When you need specific information about how best to give a drug, how it acts, how it is metabolized, or what exactly it contains (electrolytes, glucose, and so on), you can always consult the manufacturer or the hospital pharmacist. Several good general drug references include:

- American Medical Association. *AMA Drug Evaluations*. New York: Wiley, 1980.

- Bressler, R., Bogdonoff, M. D., and Subak-Sharpe, G. J., eds. *The Physician's Drug Manual: Prescription and Nonprescription Drugs*. Garden City, N.Y.: Doubleday, 1981.

- *The Physician's Desk Reference*. Oradell, N.J.: Medical Economics Company.

The *PDR* is updated annually. The same publisher currently produces *The Physician's Desk Reference for Nonprescription Drugs*.

General drug references often do not give specific information on drug-nutrient interactions; the following books can give you more information. A handy pocket-size reference on food-drug interactions has been developed:

- Moore, A. O., and Powers, D. E. *Food-Medication Interactions*, 3rd ed., 1981. Available in single copies for about $7.00 each from Food-Medication Interactions, P.O. Box 26464, Tempe, AZ 85282.

There also are two excellent books written by Dr. D. A. Roe, who has done much of the work in this area. Her books are among the best:

- Roe, D. A. *Drug-Induced Nutritional Deficiencies*. Westport, Conn.: AVI, 1976.

- Roe, D. A. *Handbook: Interactions of Selected Drugs with Nutrients in Patients*. Chicago: American Dietetic Association, 1982 (address in Appendix J).

Another good reference is:

- Hathcock, J. N., and Coon, J., eds. *Nutrition and Drug Interrelationships*. New York: Academic Press, 1978.

A monograph is available free of charge through Ross Laboratories (see Appendix J for address):

- Visconti, J. A., Ed. Drug-food interaction, in *Nutrition in Disease*, ed. R. A. Dell. Columbus, Ohio: Ross Laboratories, 1977.

A useful and well-referenced table on food and drug interactions can be found in:

- Grant, A. *Nutritional Assessment Guidelines*. This book can be obtained for about $10 from the author at Box 25057 Northgate Station, Seattle, WA 98125.

Food and Drug Interactions

Mrs. O'Connor visited her physician after she began noticing pain on urination and a general run-down feeling. The results of blood tests and urinalysis confirmed a diagnosis of a urinary tract infection and iron-deficiency anemia. The doctor prescribed tetracycline (250 mg four times a day) for the urinary tract infection and 300 mg of ferrous sulfate (an iron supplement) three times a day. On her return visit two weeks later, the physician discovered that both her urinary tract infection and her anemia persisted. The doctor checked her drug and meal history and found that she has been taking her medications as follows:

> 7:00 a.m. Tetracycline
> Iron tablet

(Soon after Mrs. O'Connor takes these medications, she often feels nauseated, so she takes two antacids containing calcium carbonate.)

> 8:00 a.m. Breakfast
> 12:00 p.m. Tetracycline
> Iron tablet

(Feels nauseated — takes two more antacids.)

> 1:00 p.m. .Lunch
> 5:00 p.m. Tetracycline
> 6:00 p.m. Supper
> 10:00 p.m. Tetracycline
> Iron tablet

(Feels nauseated — takes two more antacids.)

> 11:00 p.m. Bed

Study Questions

1. Can you spot any possible drug-nutrient interactions in Mrs. O'Connor's drug and diet history?

2. What could be causing Mrs. O'Connor's nausea? Can anything be done to correct the problem?

The doctor told Mrs. O'Connor to stop taking the tetracycline and iron at the same time and to discontinue the antacids altogether. He recommended that she eat a small amount of food (no dairy products or foods high in calcium) when she took her medications.

3. Was the doctor's advice sound? Why or why not?

4. Try working out a new schedule for Mrs. O'Connor so that the iron is given either three hours before or two hours after the tetracycline. Remember that the tetracycline should preferably be given one hour before or two hours after meals.

Medical Uses of Marihuana

Nothing is intrinsically good or evil, but its manner of usage makes it so.

ST. THOMAS AQUINAS

Since the mid-sixties the illegal use of marihuana as a "social" drug has been on the increase. An article written in 1980 reported that 43 million Americans (about 30 percent of the adult population) have tried marihuana at least once, while 16 million use it regularly. Even more significantly, 4 million regular users are under the age of 17.[1] These facts are particularly important because the regular use of marihuana is associated with a variety of health hazards affecting behavior, performance, and function of various organs (see Chapter 16).

Ironically, while reports confirm the harms associated with the social use of marihuana, new research on the medical uses of marihuana is showing promise. It is the medical uses of marihuana that we will be discussing in this Highlight.

The Metabolism of Marijuana   The active substance in marihuana is tetrahydrocannabinol, or THC. When marihuana is smoked, approximately 50 percent of the THC is absorbed into the bloodstream. When taken by mouth, only about 5 to 10 percent is absorbed. The availability of THC from smoking, then, is five to ten times greater than from ingestion of the drug.[2]

Once in the blood, a single dose of THC takes about 30 days to be completely eliminated. Therefore, when marihuana is taken regularly, high levels eventually accumulate in the blood. About 15 percent of the THC is eventually excreted as urinary metabolites, and 40 to 50 percent is excreted in the feces.

Marihuana has been used medically for centuries in remote Asian and African communities. Texts from ancient China, Persia, and India record the use of marihuana in infusions, vapors, ointments, and suppositories.[3]

Some medical uses for marihuana were also reported in the late nineteenth century, but such reports dwindled by the twentieth century with the increased use of marihuana as a social drug. Today, renewed interest in marihuana as therapy has stimulated research that has yielded some hopeful findings.

Marihuana and Chemotherapy   The most promising medical use of marihuana and THC is in the treatment of nausea and vomiting associated with chemotherapy, which is widely used to control or cure many types of cancer. Unfortunately, chemotherapy affects all cells in the body (see Chapter 21) and causes many side effects; nausea and vomiting are among the most common. Some anti-cancer drugs produce such severe vomiting that people refuse further treatment even though the therapy is effective. For this reason, vomiting has been called a lethal side effect of chemotherapy.[4]

In 1975, a group of researchers at the Sidney Farber Cancer Institute in Boston reported the results of

[1]J. Elliott, Many questions, fewer answers, about pot, *Journal of the American Medical Association* 243 (1980):15, 18.

[2]G. G. Nahas, Current status of marijuana research, *Journal of the American Medical Association* 242 (1979):2775-2778.

[3]S. Cohen, Marijuana as medicine, *Psychology Today* 11 (1978):60-64, 73.

[4]J. S. MacDonald, Associate Director of the Cancer Therapy Evaluation Program, National Cancer Institute, Statement to the Select Committee on Narcotics Abuse and Control Substances, U.S. House of Representatives, May 20, 1980.

a well-designed study in which the antiemetic properties of THC were compared with those of a placebo (an inactive substance) in people undergoing chemotherapy.[5] The antiemetic effect of THC was seen in 14 of 20 THC treatments and none of 22 placebo treatments. Since then, other studies have confirmed THC's antiemetic properties.[6] However, one of these studies, conducted at the Mayo Clinic, found that THC was associated with undesirable side effects and that it was no more effective in preventing vomiting than a standard, widely used antiemetic.[7] These results conflicted with those of a later study which found a relatively good response to THC, especially among younger subjects.[8] Still other studies have reported that THC is effective in people who do not respond favorably to standard antiemetics.[9]

In a recent statement, the American Medical Association's Council on Scientific Affairs has suggested that additional research is needed to determine who will best respond to THC without side effects. In the older age groups, response to THC is poorer and side effects such as drowsiness, hallucinations, anxiety, and rapid heartbeat are more frequent complaints.[10]

Further research into the effectiveness of marihuana cigarettes, as opposed to THC capsules, also is needed. Currently, some evidence suggests that inhaling THC is more effective than taking it orally. Inhaled THC, you recall, is more rapidly and completely absorbed. Furthermore, smoking a marihuana cigarette may offer the smoker more control over the amount of THC reaching the bloodsteam and, thus, reduce the risk of side effects. To understand how this works, consider a person smoking a marihuana cigarette to control nausea. Inhaled THC is quickly absorbed. As THC levels rise in the bloodstream, nausea promptly subsides. The person can quit smoking as soon as the nausea is relieved. By contrast, a THC capsule must be digested and absorbed before the blood level rises; so it will be some time before the nausea is relieved. Furthermore, less THC is absorbed by the gut, so higher doses must be taken. It may be harder to determine the exact dose that is right for an individual. Too much THC might lead to undesirable side effects. Another concern is that some people cannot swallow capsules because of retching and vomiting. However, because it is difficult to standardize the content of marihuana cigarettes, research using cigarettes is far more difficult to carry out and interpret, and THC capsules are therefore the form studied.

[5]S. E. Sallan, N. E. Zinberg, and E. Frei, III, Antiemetic effect of delta-9-tetrahydrocannabinol in patients receiving cancer chemotherapy, *New England Journal of Medicine* 293 (1975):795-797.

[6]S. Frytak, C. G. Moertel, J. R. O'Fallon, J. Rubin, E. T. Creagen, M. J. O'Connell, A. J. Schutt, and N. E. Schwartau, Delta-9-tetrahydrocannabinol as an antiemetic for patients receiving cancer chemotherapy, *Annals of Internal Medicine* 91 (1979):825-830; S. E. Sallan, C. Cronin, M. Zellen, and N. E. Zinberg, Antiemetics in patients receiving chemotherapy for cancer, *New England Journal of Medicine* 302 (1980):135-138; A. E. Chang, D. J. Shiling, R. C. Stillman, N. H. Goldberg, C. A. Seipp, I. Barofsky, R. M. Simon, and S. A. Rosenberg, Delta-9-tetrahydrocannabinol as an antiemetic in cancer patients receiving high-dose methotrexate, *Annals of Internal Medicine* 91 (1979):819-824.

[7]Frytak and co-authors, 1979.

[8]Sallan and co-authors, 1980.

[9]V. S. Lucas, Jr., and J. Laszlo, Delta-9-tetrahydrocannabinol for refractory vomiting induced by cancer chemotherapy, *Journal of the American Medical Association* 243 (1980):1241-1243; L. E. Orr, J. F. McKernan, and B. Bloome, Antiemetic effect of tetrahydrocannabinol, *Archives of Internal Medicine* 140 (1980):1431-1433.

[10]Council on Scientific Affairs, Marijuana: Its health hazards and therapeutic potentials, *Journal of the American Medical Association* 246 (1981):1823-1827.

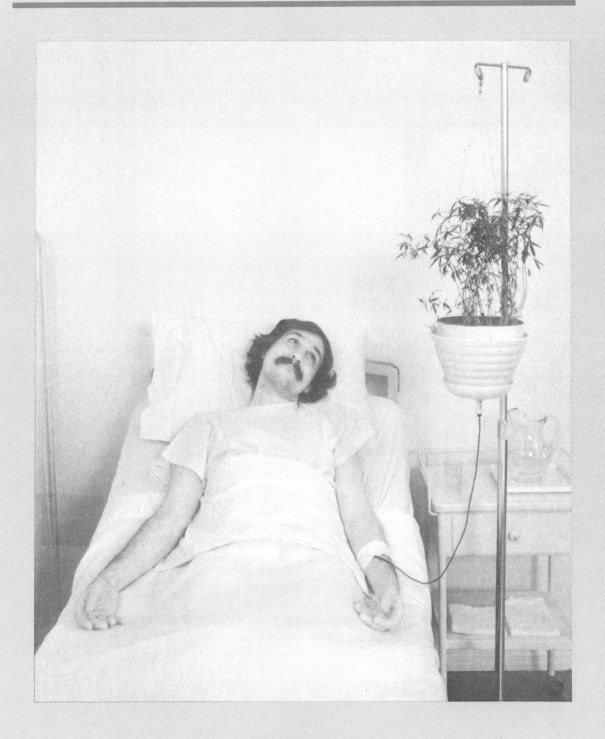

Photo reprinted from S. Cohen, Marijuana as medicine, *Psychology Today* 11 (April 1978):61, courtesy of the author and publisher.

Research on the value of THC in the control of nausea and vomiting for people undergoing chemotherapy is far from complete. However, there is a general consensus that THC is at least as effective as currently available antiemetic drugs and that it may be beneficial for people who don't get relief from standard antiemetics.

THC and Glaucoma
Glaucoma is a disease of the eye in which pressure builds up within the eyeball, causing poor vision and possibly blindness. THC capsules and marihuana cigarettes appear to be effective in reducing this pressure. Studies in this area continue and more investigations will be needed in the future to know what dosages are effective, what side effects are produced, and what mode of administration is best.

Other Medical Uses The most widely researched medical uses of marihuana and THC are for people with cancer and glaucoma. Other scattered reports have suggested that THC can be used as a bronchodilator for people with asthma, as a decongestant for the relief of flu symptoms, and as an antispasmodic agent in paraplegia.[11]

The Legal Picture Since 1978, well over 20 states have approved the medical use of marihuana for people with cancer and glaucoma. However, there is a catch. Since marihuana is considered to be an investigational drug that has a high potential for abuse, only the federal government can grow and distribute marihuana (and THC) legally. In order for a state to be able to legally distribute marihuana for medical use, the state must submit a research plan to the Food and Drug Administration (FDA). Once the plan has been approved, only physicians who can comply with the research guidelines can prescribe THC.

The intent of such a procedure is to gather more reliable information, so that the drug can be legally marketed if it is effective. In reality, the value of the information obtained may be questionable, because the guidelines are so general that high quality research is not assured.[12] In the meantime, while this procedure allows some practicing physicians to prescribe THC, many people who could benefit from using it cannot legally obtain it. Some of these people will do without. Others will obtain unpurified marihuana illegally, a choice for which they could theoretically be jailed for up to a year and fined $5,000 under federal law. (It is doubtful, though, that such a case would be prosecuted.)

It is likely that THC capsules or a synthetic derivative will be legally marketed before marihuana cigarettes become available. As previously mentioned, there are many problems in standardizing the THC content of marihuana. Even adjacent leaves of the same plant picked at different times of the same day yield different amounts of THC by unit weight.[13] In the meantime, several drug companies are studying synthetic derivatives in the hope that these derivatives will maximize THC's effectiveness while eliminating undesirable side effects. Preliminary data on the synthetic derivatives are promising,

[11] Council on Scientific Affairs, Marihuana reexamined: Pulmonary risks and therapeutic potentials, *Connecticut Medicine* 44 (1980):521-523.

[12] R. W. Rhein, Jr., Marijuana therapy, *Medical World News*, April 1980, pp. 39-44.

[13] Council on Scientific Affairs, 1980.

but further testing will be required before any of these drugs can be marketed. It is hoped that the legal and medical issues surrounding the use of marihuana and THC for people with cancer and glaucoma can be resolved in the near future. Only then can everyone who needs treatment have access to this potentially beneficial drug.

To Explore Further

All the references listed in the Highlight notes are very informative. A particularly good article is the one in *Medical World News* (note 12). A patient-oriented book is also available:

● Roffman, R. *Using Marijuana in the Reduction of Nausea Associated with Chemotherapy.* Seattle: Murray Publishing, 1979.

This book contains information on the physiological effects of marihuana, its medical uses, and advice on obtaining and preparing it (including recipes). The appendixes list researchers studying THC as well as general references. The book can be obtained from the Murray Publishing Company, 2312 Third Avenue, Seattle, WA 98121, for about $3.00.

PART FIVE

NUTRITIONAL IMPLICATIONS OF DISEASE

INTRODUCTION

THE DIET AS THERAPY

Let thy food be thy medicine.

HIPPOCRATES

In Part Four, we began to look at how nutrition is applied to patients in the health care setting. Emphasis on the patient continues in Part Five. Now, though, we will look more closely at the role of nutrition in different diseases.

Nutrition can play a part in preventing or treating some disorders. For some of these disorders, the part that nutrition plays in treatment is crucial. In other disorders, nutrition has a smaller place in the treatment plan. Still other disorders require no special diet therapy other than a well-balanced diet.

Part Five focuses on those disorders in which nutrition plays a significant role in treatment. For this purpose, each chapter involves a particular organ system and diseases that affect it.

Diet therapy is constantly changing. As more and more research on different disorders becomes available, some dietary treatments have become controversial. We have tried to point out current areas of controversy to alert you to the fact that dietary recommendations do change with time.

A final note before you read on: Keep in mind that physicians are responsible for prescribing diets. We have approached diet therapy as if the doctor has given this responsibility to you, in the hope that you will, indeed, assume an active role in the nutrition care of patients. In any case, you should feel confident enough to discuss your dietary recommendations with the physician.

CHAPTER 22

CONTENTS

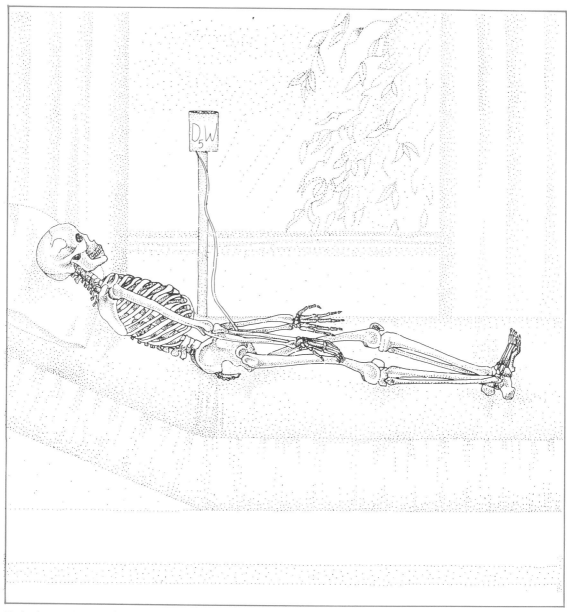

Neglecting nutrition can have serious consequences for the stressed patient.

NUTRITION AND STRESS: Surgery, Infection, and Burns

Almost no germ is unconditionally dangerous to man; its disease-producing ability depends upon the body's resistance.

HANS SELYE, M.D.

You can think of stress as an influence which interferes with the body's normal balance. The complex changes the body undergoes when confronted with stress are collectively referred to as the stress response. Stress can be mild or severe. It can be caused by normal states such as growth or pregnancy. In this chapter, however, we will be discussing the more severe stresses imposed by illness or injury to the body. Some of these stresses are surgery, broken bones, infection, and fever.

The Metabolic Response to Starvation

Fasting and starvation represent one type of stress. It will help to understand the metabolic changes that occur with starvation because this condition presents a fairly uncomplicated picture. If you can visualize this picture, then you can see how added stresses such as illness or injury further tax the body. Starvation is often superimposed on illness and injury because they lead to poor intake.

After a short period of starvation the body must draw on stored carbohydrate, fat, and protein to meet energy needs. Liver glycogen, which represents the available stored form of carbohydrate, breaks down to maintain blood glucose levels. Fatty acids, which can provide fuel for many cells in the body are also mobilized. However, the brain must have glucose for fuel, and fatty acids cannot be converted into glucose.

Glycogen stores become depleted fairly soon after starvation begins. The body must have another source of glucose, and so protein tissues begin to break down to supply those amino acids which can be used to make glucose. Glycerol from fat also can be used to make new glucose, but this process is inefficient. Generally, in the first few days of starvation, amino acids provide about 90 percent of the needed glucose, and glycerol about 10 percent.

homeostasis: a state of balance, or equilibrium, within the body. (See also p. 47).

physiologic stress: stress that occurs as part of the body's normal and healthy functioning. Growth and pregnancy are physiologic stresses. **Pathologic stress** represents stress imposed by disease or an abnormal bodily insult such as surgery, burns, fever, or infection.

One type of stress is **trauma** — a physical injury to the body such as a broken bone, a gunshot wound, or surgery.

Metabolically, **fasting** and **starvation** have the same consequences in the body. In fasting, food intake is voluntarily discontinued, whereas in starvation, lack of food intake is involuntary.

The adaptation that occurs when the body tissues and brain begin using ketones to supply energy needs is called **ketoadaptation**.

Thereafter, the body adapts to a different energy source and so conserves vital protein. As fat continues to break down, the liver begins to synthesize ketones (see pp. 211-212), and the brain and other tissues begin to use the ketones as an energy source, reducing the need for glucose. (The brain still needs some glucose, though.) At the same time, the body reduces its energy needs by slowing its metabolic rate. The net effect is that the body conserves its fat and lean tissue. However, this also means that the starved person is less able to perform work and that the functioning of vital organs (including the GI tract, heart, and lungs) is compromised. It has been estimated that a weight loss of 40 to 50 percent, which represents losses of about one-quarter to one-third of body protein mass, is fatal.[1]

When additional stress such as an infection or surgery is placed on a starving person, body tissues break down to a greater degree, increasing the loss of vital protein. Multiple stresses can very easily occur in one person — for example, a patient may not be eating following surgery and may develop an infection with a fever.

The Response to Severe Stress

The way the body responds to stress depends on the type of stress and its severity. A well-nourished person undergoing minor elective surgery is only mildly stressed, whereas a person with extensive burns suffers the most severe type of stress. However, in general, the metabolic responses to various types of stress are similar (see Table 1). Table 2 describes the relative severity of several types of stress.

hypermetabolism: accelerated metabolic activity.

catabolism: metabolic breakdown of body energy reserves.

The **acute**, or **flow**, phase of the stress response is the catabolic period immediately following the onset of stress. During the **adaptive phase**, the body adjusts to the stress to minimize losses. If adaptation fails, **exhaustion** follows.

The stress response is mediated by hormonal changes and is characterized by an increase in metabolic activity (hypermetabolism) and an accelerated breakdown of body energy reserves (catabolism). Table 3 lists changes in hormone levels during stress and their effects on metabolism. In the period following injury, the stressed patient has elevated blood glucose levels (hyperglycemia), negative nitrogen balance, increased retention of fluid and sodium, and increased excretion of potassium.

The metabolic changes that occur during the initial stress response are believed to be positive changes that help support the immune system, repair damaged tissues, and maintain vital organ function.[2] These changes constitute an adaptation that is sustained for as long as possible. Then the rate of catabolism decreases, blood sugar levels fall, and nitrogen balance is slowly restored. The amount of time it takes for the body to return to normal depends on the degree of stress. A well-nourished person can tolerate a short period of severe stress

[1] D. W. Wilmore and J. M. Kinney, Panel report on nutritional support of patients with trauma and infection, *American Journal of Clinical Nutrition* 34 (1981):1213-1222.

[2] P. Benotti and G. L. Blackburn, Protein and caloric or macronutrient metabolic management of the critically ill patient, *Critical Care Medicine* 7 (1979):520-525.

Table 1.   Summary of Metabolic Events in Early versus Late Starvation

	Early starvation	**Late starvation**
Brain	Relies on glucose for fuel	Adapts to using ketones and some glucose for fuel
Liver glycogen	Breaks down to supply glucose	Stores exhausted
Amino acids, glycerol	High demand for making glucose	Significantly reduced demand for making glucose
Fatty acids	Supply energy directly for most tissues	Increasingly converted to ketones
Metabolic rate	Normal	Reduced
Net effect	High use of protein to supply glucose for brain and of fat to supply energy to other tissues	Less need for glucose, conservation of protein and fat reserves

Table 2.   Changes in Metabolic Activity in Stress

Stress	Percent change in metabolic activity*
Mild starvation	-15-0%
Uncomplicated surgery	0-5
Peritonitis	5-25
Long bone fracture	15-30
Severe infection	30-55
Multiple trauma	30-55
Multiple trauma patient requiring ventilator	50-75
Burns (by percent of body surface area burned)	
10%	25
20%	50
30%	70
40%	85
50%	100
60%	105
70%	115

*The percentages represent ranges within which most people's metabolic activities will fall. Extremes outside these ranges are possible.

Data adapted from D. W. Wilmore, *The Metabolic Management of the Critically Ill* (New York: Plenum Medical Book Company, 1977).

Table 3. Major Hormonal Changes That Occur During Severe Stress

Hormone	Alteration	Metabolic effect
Catecholamines	Increase	Glucagon release ⇑
		Insulin/glucagon ratio* ⇓
		Glycogen breakdown ⇑
		Glucose production from amino acids ⇑
		Mobilization of free fatty acids ⇑
Cortisol	Increases	Mobilization of free fatty acids ⇑
		Glucose production from amino acids ⇑
		Utilization of glucose by many cells except brain ⇓
Glucagon	Increases	Glucose production from amino acids ⇑
		Glycogen breakdown ⇑
Insulin	Decreases	Storage of glucose, amino acids and fatty acids ⇓
Antidiuretic hormone	Increases	Retention of water ⇑
Aldosterone	Increases	Retention of sodium ⇑

*Whenever the ratio of insulin to glucagon decreases, the net effect is that catabolism predominates.

without adverse effects. However, a severely malnourished person does not have the protein reserves necessary to continue meeting the **increased metabolic demands of severe injury. The result is exhaustion and other complications, such as infection or organ failure, which can be fatal.**

Nutrition and the Surgical Patient

Nutrition plays an important role in a person's ability to recover from surgery. Studies have shown that malnourished patients undergoing surgery have a higher incidence of postoperative mortality, complications, infections, and delayed wound healing.[3] Furthermore, the surgical procedure itself may directly influence intake, digestion, and absorption of nutrients, which may lead to malnutrition. A patient who develops complications following surgery is even more likely to become malnourished because of the additional stress placed on the body. The

[3]J. L. Mullen, Consequences of malnutrition in the surgical patient, *Surgical Clinics of North America* 61 (1981):465-487.

following discussion will concentrate on the nutrition needs of general surgical patients. The next chapter will discuss specific nutrition needs associated with various surgeries of the GI tract.

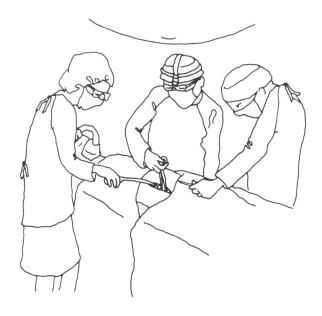

Nutrition before Surgery   Whenever possible, a person's nutrition status should be optimal prior to surgery. Optimal status may be difficult to achieve, however, since the illness which necessitates the surgery may interfere with food intake or nutrient utilization, increasing the likelihood of malnutrition. Additionally, many diagnostic and laboratory tests can be given only after the person to be tested has fasted or has followed a nutritionally inadequate liquid diet, which further taxes nutrition status. On the other hand, obesity also is a risk factor, and weight should be reduced before surgery whenever possible.

A regular diet is generally adequate for well-nourished people who are expected to have uncomplicated surgery. They can withstand short-term starvation and some degree of protein catabolism without serious consequences. Regular hospital diets provide ample kcalories and generally exceed the RDA for protein.

For malnourished patients, diets higher in kcalories and protein are often given prior to surgery. In most hospitals these patients receive high-kcalorie and high-protein supplements and snacks between meals. Such diets generally provide about 1,000 kcal more than a regular diet and 125 g of protein daily. For people who cannot consume an adequate intake orally, tube feeding may be indicated. Furthermore, TPN may be initiated before surgery if use of the GI tract is contraindicated (see Chapter 20). However, the value of vigorous

Remember to check the hospital's diet manual to determine what exactly a "regular" and a "high-kcalorie, high-protein" diet contain.

nutrition support for short periods of time before surgery remains controversial.[4]

Vitamins, minerals, and trace elements should be provided to meet individual needs. A person with iron deficiency anemia will be given iron supplementation before elective surgery or a blood transfusion when surgery must be performed immediately. The need for B-complex vitamins increases when kcalorie and protein intakes increase. However, diets higher in kcalories and protein normally also will contain increased amounts of these nutrients; thus the person who is accepting the variety of foods offered needs no supplements.

All food and fluids are generally withheld for at least eight hours before surgery. This step helps prevent regurgitation and aspiration, which can occur during anesthesia or recovery. Usually, food and fluid are withheld from the midnight prior to surgery. For people undergoing GI surgery, liquids or foods low in residue are given for two or three days before surgery to minimize the amount of fecal material in the gut and help prevent distention after surgery. Low-residue and residue-free liquid supplements are available to meet all the nutrient needs of patients on liquid diets. These supplements can be given either orally or by tube to patients who are malnourished or who will be unable to eat for some time after surgery.

Nutrition after Surgery   The immediate nutrition-related concern following surgery is the maintenance of fluid and electrolyte balance. The loss of blood, fluid, and electrolytes from the body during surgery can lead to dehydration and shock. Additional fluids may be lost after surgery from draining wounds, vomiting, and diarrhea. Following surgery, fluids and electrolytes are replaced by IV infusion because, in the immediate postoperative period, peristalsis in the GI tract has stopped. Absence of peristalsis (ileus) is most common following GI surgery. Until peristalsis returns, food and fluids cannot be given orally. (See box, "How to Check for Normal Bowel Activity").

The exact diet prescribed after surgery depends on the type of surgery and on the patient's nutrition status. People on TPN prior to surgery will most likely be kept on TPN until their oral intake is adequate. The surgeon who anticipates that a patient may have difficulties in resuming oral intake may construct a feeding jejunostomy during surgery. Jejunostomies are well-tolerated because peristalsis and absorption in the small intestine return within several hours of surgery. Motility in the stomach, on the other hand, is impaired for about 24 to 48 hours.[5]

shock: a sudden drop in the blood volume, which disrupts the supply of oxygen to the tissues and the return of blood to the heart. There are many causes of shock, including bleeding, trauma, and dehydration.

ileus (ILL-ee-us): absence of normal gastrointestinal activity.

[4]R. V. Heatley, R. H. Williams, and M. H. Lewis, Pre-operative intravenous feeding — a controlled trial, *Postgraduate Medical Journal* 55 (1979):541-545.

[5]L. Hultén, H. Andersson, I. Bosaeus, S. Fasth, R. Hellberg, B. Isaksson, O. Magnusson, and I. Warnold, Enteral alimentation in the early postoperative course, *Journal of Parenteral and Enteral Nutrition* 4 (1980):455-459.

How to Check for Normal Bowel Activity

Before a patient can be fed after surgery, a check must be made to insure that normal peristalsis has returned. While the patient is lying down, a stethoscope is placed over his or her intestine. An active intestine makes bubbling or soft gurgling noises irregularly every 5 to 15 seconds. The abdomen should be soft and flat. Additionally, the patient is asked if he or she has passed gas (flatus), another sign that bowel activity has returned.

The objective of postsurgical nutrition support is to prevent weight loss and the depletion of nutrients. Generally, the diets of people who are not receiving special nutrition support (IV or tube feedings) progress from clear liquids to full liquids and on to a regular diet as tolerated. A clear liquid diet consists of foods that are clear and liquid or that liquefy at room temperature. A full liquid diet includes both

Take a close look at the foods allowed on a clear liquid diet. You can imagine why someone just recovering from surgery would find these foods unappetizing. Even more disturbing, consider the nutritional quality of the diet. It is deficient in kcalories and most nutrients for the normal person. A stressed person has even greater requirements. Therefore, care must be taken to insure that no one is kept on a standard clear liquid diet for any great length of time.

CAUTION:

Standard clear liquid diets
are nutritionally deficient.

Often the postsurgical diet order simply says "diet as tolerated." The nursing personnel consult with the patient and use their discretion in advancing the diet from liquids to regular. Many times someone forgets to advance the diet. Other times a patient truly cannot tolerate foods other than clear liquids; in these cases, further steps must be taken. Clear liquid nutrition formulas can be fed either orally or by tube as needed to meet nutrient needs. Occasionally, total or supplemental intravenous nutrition may be necessary.

clear and opaque liquid foods and those which liquefy at room temperature. Table 4 lists foods allowed on clear and full liquid diets.

A well-nourished person who is tolerating regular foods after uncomplicated surgery will do well on a standard hospital diet that is adequate in all required nutrients. People with depleted nutrient stores and people with complications need high-kcalorie, high-protein diets. No less than 1.5 g protein per kg of ideal body weight should be supplied. To increase energy intake, the fats and carbohydrates in the diet also are increased. The nutrition status of people with inadequate protein intakes can become seriously depleted, especially if complications arise after surgery. These people are weak and vulnerable to infection and have delayed wound healing.

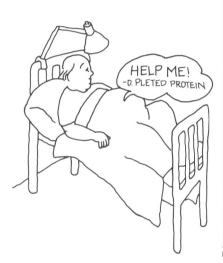

When you think of nutrient-depleted people, don't forget that overweight people can be depleted, too. It is very easy to overlook malnutrition in these individuals. Although overweight persons may have adequate fat stores, their bodies may have lost vital protein. The period immediately following a major injury or surgery is not the time for a weight reduction diet.

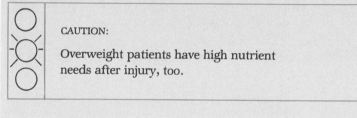

CAUTION:

Overweight patients have high nutrient needs after injury, too.

He may look as if he has adequate nutrient stores, but looks can be deceiving!

As mentioned previously, the need for B-complex vitamins increases when energy and protein intakes must be increased. Special attention also must be paid to vitamin C; it helps form collagen, which plays an important role in wound healing. Vitamin K is important in postsurgical patients because it functions in blood clotting. Like vitamin C, zinc plays a role in wound healing. Depending on the type of surgery and the quality of the diet, supplements of these nutrients may be necessary.

Malnutrition in the postsurgical patient may be further complicated by anorexia and immobilization. Lack of appetite can be improved by serving foods the patient likes, at the correct temperature, in an attractive manner. Some patients tolerate more frequent, smaller meals or snacks while others prefer larger meals served less often. Individualizing the diet is very important. Exercise is important too: Patients are encouraged to get out of bed and begin minimal exercise (such as walking) as soon as medically safe.

Table 4. Foods Included in Liquid Diets

Clear liquid diets

Bouillon
Broth, fat-free
Carbonated beverages
Coffee, regular and decaffeinated
Fruit juices, strained
Gelatin
Popsicles
Tea

Full liquid diets

All clear liquids
Cooked cereals, strained
Custard
Flavorings
Fruit ices
Ice cream, plain
Honey
Potatoes, mashed and diluted in cream soups
Pudding
Sherbet
Soups, strained vegetable, meat, or cream
Syrup
Vegetable juices
Vegetable purees, diluted in cream soups

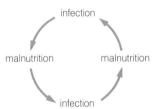

Malnutrition and infection: a vicious cycle.

Nutrition and the Infected Patient

In areas of the world where people suffer from malnutrition, the incidence of infection is high. The discovery of this association has sparked great interest in how nutrition affects the immune system. In recent years, research in this area has increased tremendously. The role of nutrition in immunology will be discussed in Highlight 22.

Once an infection has developed, the metabolic events that follow greatly influence nutrient needs. The response to infection is for the most part similar to the response that occurs with surgery or other injury. However, the body takes longer to adapt to using ketones for energy, so the early protein losses are more severe. Infection often develops in people who have already been stressed by surgery or some other injury. The anorexia, nausea, vomiting, diarrhea, and immobilization which may occur in infected persons place further demands on nutrient stores.

immunology: the study of how people are protected from diseases, particularly infections.

During an **infection**, the body is invaded by a disease-causing microorganism or virus which grows and causes illness. **Sepsis** results from the presence of microorganisms or their poisonous products directly in the bloodstream. **Septicemia** is a synonym for sepsis.

The **incubation period** of an infection is the interval between exposure to the infection and development of related symptoms.

A **fever** is an increase of temperature of more than 1° F above normal (98.6° F).

A patient who is **febrile** (FEE-brile) has a fever; **afebrile** (AY-fee-brile) means without fever.

The **convalescent period** of an infection describes the period of recovery from illness, during which the body develops positive body balances.

A.J. is a 22-year-old male who is 5′9″ tall, weighs 160 lb, and has a temperature of 103° F. To calculate the impact of fever on his energy needs we first determine his BMR. (For males: 1 kcal/kg/hr; for females: 0.9 kcal/kg/hr.)

$1 \text{ kcal} \times \dfrac{160 \text{ lb}}{2.2}$

(to convert lb to kg)

$\times 24 \text{ hr}$

$= 1{,}746 \text{ kcal/day}$

A.J.'s temperature is 4.4° F above normal. His BMR increases by:

$4.4° \text{F} \times 7\% = 31\%$

His energy needs increase by:

$1{,}746 \text{ kcal} \times 31\% = 541 \text{ kcal}$

His total energy needs are:

$1{,}746 \text{ kcal} + 541 \text{ kcal} = 2{,}287 \text{ kcal}$

Fever has added more than 500 kcal daily to A.J.'s energy needs. If he is still active or is very restless, he may need an additional 500 to 1,000 kcal.

The course of an infection goes something like this: Following exposure to an infective agent, a period of time (generally a few days) passes before the first symptoms of the infection appear. Shortly after this period, most infections cause a fever to develop. After the onset of fever, the catabolic changes which characterize the stress response begin. Hyperglycemia develops. The body's losses of nitrogen (from protein catabolism) and intracellular electrolytes (potassium, magnesium, phosphorus, zinc, and sulfur) exceed intake, and negative body balances develop. These negative balances are aggravated by decreased intake of food. If diarrhea and vomiting also occur, the body loses even more nutrients. Because of hormonal changes, the infected individual retains water and sodium.

When an infection lasts for a long time, the person gradually begins to conserve nitrogen. However, this occurs after he or she has already suffered marked weight loss and muscle wasting. Once the illness has ended, the person generally develops positive balances which restore the body to its normal composition. The time it takes for the body to reach a positive balance and the duration of the positive balance depend on the extent of nutrient deficiencies as well as the quality and quantity of food intake. During this time, a good diet is essential to restore vital nutrient reserves. A good diet may also help guard against the development of additional infections.

The major concern in the infected person is to identify and eliminate the invading organism. Often, antibiotics are prescribed.

Nutrient Needs Fever is a major factor in determining the energy needs of the infected person. The basal metabolic rate (BMR) increases approximately 13 percent for each 1° C (7 percent for each 1° F) the temperature rises above normal (98.6° F; 37° C). Additional kcalories should be given for activity, particularly for the restless patient. Patients should be weighed daily to monitor changes in body weight. When body weight is assessed, it is important to remember patients may retain sodium and water or be dehydrated. Therefore, their scale weight may not always reflect tissue weight changes.

The immune system functions best when protein status is optimal. The actual protein requirements of the infected patient depend largely on the total kcalories the patient is receiving. However, at a minimum, the protein intake should be consistent with the RDA for age, weight, and sex. These allowances should be increased by 10 percent per 1° C (5.5 percent per 1° F) of fever.

An infected patient must be monitored to insure that fluid needs are being met. In some infectious diseases, particularly those which involve vomiting, diarrhea, or considerable sweating, fluid needs may be as high as 3 to 4 liters per day. On the other hand, the infected patient may be retaining water because of hormonal changes which accompany fever. Excessive fluid in these patients can cause fluid overload. Usually, for patients with generalized infections which are not accompanied by diarrhea, vomiting, or excessive sweating, dehydration is not a problem.[6]

Little information is available regarding increased requirements for specific vitamins and minerals during infection. As mentioned, the need for B-complex vitamins increases with increased intake of kcalories and protein but remains consistent with the RDA. Vitamins should be given in their normal doses throughout the course of illness or, at most, given in amounts not more than two times the RDA to cover the possibility that vitamins may be metabolized or excreted in increased amounts during hypermetabolic states.[7] Likewise, losses of intracellular electrolytes (which are also in negative balance during an infection) can generally be covered through foods. Sodium may have to be restricted in patients who are retaining this electrolyte. The general guidelines for feeding surgical patients also apply to patients with infections (see p. 834).

A.J.'s protein needs can be calculated from his RDA for protein:

0.8 g (RDA for protein)

$\times \dfrac{160 \text{ lb}}{2.2}$ (to convert lb to kg)

= 58 g protein

The fever increases his protein needs as follows:

$4.4° \times 5.5\% = 24\%$
$58 \text{ g} \times 24\% = 14 \text{ g}$

His total protein needs are:

$58 \text{ g} + 14 \text{ g} = 72 \text{ g}$

Anemia of Infection   People with infections often develop a type of anemia (anemia of infection) that does not respond to iron, folacin, or vitamin B_{12} therapy. At the onset of an infectious illness, blood levels of iron rapidly decline as iron moves into the liver cells for storage. The iron, then, is not available to make new hemoglobin, and anemia results. However, this shift of iron from the blood to the liver helps fight the infection. Once in storage, the iron is unavailable to bacteria, which need it to carry out metabolic functions. Therefore, supplemental iron is not given for this type of anemia.

Nutrition and the Patient with Burns

An extensive burn represents the most extreme state of stress that a person can experience. The metabolic response to a burn results in tissue catabolism and a very rapid loss of body mass. The burned patient quickly uses up the energy and protein reserves necessary for survival.

Nutrition needs of the person with extensive burns are very high. Moreover, most burned patients experience anorexia, which compromises their ability to meet nutrient demands. The burn injury itself may make eating difficult because of the pain associated with it or because of its physical location (for example, the hands). Immobilization and lack of exercise further aggravate the situation.

A burn is sometimes called a **thermal injury.**

[6]W. R. Beisel, Infectious diseases, in *Nutritional Support of Medical Practice*, ed. H. A. Schneider, C. E. Anderson, and D. B. Coursin (Hagerstown, Md.: Harper & Row, 1977), pp. 350-366.

[7]Beisel, 1977.

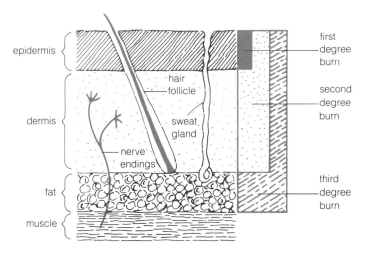

Figure 1 Depth of burn wounds.

Not all people with burns require aggressive nutrition support. People who are well nourished and whose burns cover less than 20 percent of their body surface area (BSA) can do well on regular diets. A panel of medical experts recently reached a general consensus regarding persons that would require nutrition replacement.[8] These persons have the following characteristics:

1. Greater than 20 percent BSA burn.

2. Poor nutrition status prior to injury.

3. Preinjury illness or disease.

4. Morbid obesity.

5. Patterns of alcohol or drug abuse.

6. Other injuries associated with the burn, such as fractures, infections, and the like.

7. Complications such as infection, lung failure, or hormonal imbalance which may follow a burn injury.

8. Weight loss of greater than 10 percent from preburn body weight during hospitalization.

In the discussion on burns, we will focus on the nutrient needs of this group.

---

[8]W. Schumer, Supportive therapy in burn care: Consensus summary on metabolism, *Journal of Trauma* 19 (Supplement 1979):910-911.

Nutrient Needs   Immediately after a person is burned, dramatic changes take place in the circulatory system. Plasma proteins (mainly albumin) and electrolytes leak through the capillaries into the interstitial space and into the burned area. The collection of fluid in the interstitial space causes considerable edema. Plasma volume can be decreased by as much as 75 percent in patients with 40 percent BSA burns.[9] During this time, then, the primary consideration of therapy is providing enough fluid and electrolytes to maintain circulatory volume and prevent shock. Fluids are given to maintain urinary output (the amount of urine excreted) at about 50 ml per hour. Isotonic fluids are given intravenously because the severely burned patient experiences a temporary absence of peristalsis (ileus) and cannot take fluids by mouth. On an average, 3 to 5 liters are needed to replace fluid losses daily. However, in some cases over 10 liters of fluid may be required.

Normal bowel activity usually returns in the period following fluid replacement, and attention to adequate nutrition becomes essential. Hypermetabolism reaches a peak at about the end of the first postburn week and then gradually becomes normal over a period of several weeks. The duration of the hypermetabolic state depends on the severity of the burn. Hypermetabolism is associated with extreme protein catabolism and weight loss. The rate of hypermetabolism also is related to the severity of the burn, reaching a maximum with a 50 percent BSA burn.

An estimate of the patient's kcalorie needs can be made by using the following formulas.[10]

Adults:

25 kcal × Preburn body weight (kg) + $\left[\right.$ 40 kcal × % BSA burned $\left.\right]$

Children:

30-100 kcal (use RDA for age) × Preburn body weight (kg)
+ $\left[\right.$ 40 kcal × % BSA burned $\left.\right]$

Adjustments in kcalorie intake can be made as indicated by body weight changes or complications (such as infection) which may change energy needs.

Nitrogen balance can generally be achieved by giving 2 to 3 grams of protein per kilogram of body weight per day in adults. Children may need from two to four times the RDA for protein (as appropriate for age) per day.

The fluid containing plasma proteins and electrolytes which leaks out through the capillaries is called the **exudate.**

B.T. is a 39-year-old female who weighs 130 lb. She recently sustained a 60% BSA burn. Her energy needs can be calculated as follows:

25 kcal
× Preburn body weight (kg)
+ 40 kcal × % BSA burned
25 kcal × $\dfrac{130 \text{ lb}}{2.2 \text{ kg}}$
(to convert lb to kg)
+ $\left[\right.$ 40 kcal × 60 $\left.\right]$
= 3,877 kcal

An approximation of B.T.'s protein needs is:

$2 \times \dfrac{130 \text{ lb}}{2.2} = 118\text{g}$

$3 \times \dfrac{130 \text{ lb}}{2.2} = 177\text{g}$

B.T. needs from 118 to 177 g protein daily.

D.Z., an 11-month-old baby who weighs 20 lb, recently suffered a 30% BSA burn. His energy needs can be calculated as follows:

$\left[\right.$ 108 kcal/kg (RDA for age)
× $\dfrac{20 \text{ lb}}{2.2}$ (to convert lb to kg) $\left.\right]$
+ $\left[\right.$ 40 kcal × 30 $\left.\right]$
= 2,182 kcal

D.Z.'s protein needs range from 26 to 38 g daily:

2×1.4 g/kg (RDA for age)
× $\dfrac{20 \text{ lb}}{2.2} = 26$ g
3×1.4 g/kg
× $\dfrac{20 \text{ lb}}{2.2} = 38$ g

[9] P. R. Rogenes and J. A. Moylan, Restoring fluid balance in the patient with severe burns, *American Journal of Nursing* 76 (1976):1953-1957.

[10] P. W. Curreri, Nutritional replacement modalities, *Journal of Trauma* 19, Supplement 1979, pp. 906-908.

My Child Never Cried

My child never cried. He was a 6-year-old black boy. You couldn't really tell how beautiful he was because he was burned over 50% of his body, including part of his face, but you sensed it anyway. His life was sustained by intravenous feedings, and, because of his age, the extent of skin loss secondary to burn, and the size of his veins, he required a "cutdown" for their administration.

This minor surgical procedure, in which a vein is located under local anesthesia through a small incision and a cannula is inserted therein, had to be repeated frequently because either the cannula would pull out of the vein or it would clog up because his fragile tissues could not support the apparatus. Cutdowns were performed at the bedside by the intern assigned to the Children's Burn Service. That was me.

It was the fourth cutdown I was doing on him, and he never cried. It was unnerving. He didn't make a sound. He lay there immobile, his flesh stinking with burn, and stared at me with hot eyes, black as smoke, from behind his heavily bandaged body, his tiny lips firmly closed, paling in clenched tension. It was a frustrating job. To change a cutdown at 3 a.m. after a 12-hour day on the wards was a drag of the first order. It was the middle of July, and the County Hospital wasn't air-conditioned. It was muggy; sweat dripped into my eyes, and I was having a hard time finding the vein. My mouth tasted sleep. A small lamp lit the bedside area at which I was working. The rest of the stuffy room was dark. I had been at the job for over ten minutes, and as I probed through the bleeding tissues, seeking the tiny vessel, I could hear turnings and whimperings from the other 30-odd restless children in the ward, moving painfully through their burned-out dreams. But my child never cried.

I injected more novocaine. I could never tell whether or not he really needed it. He never talked. He just stared at me with an awful mixture of trust and hate. And he never cried. So I injected more novocaine. I kept searching for the vein. I would find it if it took all night. The wound was like a mouth. A blistered mouth that mocked me as I struggled to find the vein. I would find the vein and place the cannula, and then I would again pour life into him. We all knew he would die, as indeed he must have also known. Children with 50% body burns seldom live. And as I bent over his tiny, charred body in the middle of that hot, dark night, alone on that restless ward in that lonely building, I realized I was not searching only for his vein, but also for something within myself. I was trying not only to save his life, but something in my own as well.

My child never cried. Later perhaps I would. For both of us.

Irwin M. Siegel, A piece of my mind: My child never cried, *Journal of the American Medical Association*, August 7, 1981, Vol. 246, p. 617. Copyright 1981, American Medical Association.

Specific vitamin and mineral requirements for patients with burns have not been established. However, in consideration of the high energy and protein requirements, as well as nutrients needed for tissue repair and blood and skin losses, additional vitamins are generally given. Adults can be given two standard multivitamins per day with an additional 1 to 2 grams of vitamin C.[11] Children may be given from 500 to 700 mg of vitamin C in addition to one to two doses of a pediatric multivitamin preparation. Many liquid vitamin preparations (commonly used for children) do not contain vitamin K and folacin, and these vitamins may require additional supplementation. Generally, mineral requirements are met with a diet adequate in protein and kcalories, although some studies suggest that supplemental zinc may help burn wounds heal more quickly. If iron deficiency anemia is present, iron supplementation should be given.

Goals for Meeting Nutrient Needs   As soon as the bowel becomes active, feeding should begin. At the latest, nutrition support should begin by the fourth postburn day. If bowel activity has not resumed by this time, then peripheral or central parenteral nutrition should be started. By the seventh postburn day, kcalorie intake should approximate energy demands. If a patient has active bowel motility but cannot eat enough food, then tube feeding should be initiated.

When encouraging the burned patient to eat, you must remember to keep the total person in mind. Emotional support is very important. Understandably, food may seem unimportant to the patient who faces a lengthy hospital stay, a great deal of pain, and fear of permanent disfigurement. Burn therapy, which generally includes whirlpool baths and the cutting away of dead skin and tissue, is extremely painful. If possible, these treatments should be scheduled so as not to interfere with mealtimes.

Patients may feel awkward about eating when the location of a burn interferes with self-feeding. Sometimes this problem can be worked out with the aid of an occupational therapist, who may be able to adapt feeding utensils for the patient. Patients also should be encouraged to get up and walk around and begin physical therapy as soon as possible. This measure helps prevent further catabolism associated with injury, improves morale, and also may help to increase appetite.

Skin Grafting   Gradually, as the dead skin separates from the wound, an extensive burn wound becomes ready for grafting. Skin can be taken from another part of the patient's body, from another human body, or from an animal, usually a pig (the latter two types of grafts are only temporary). Adequate nutrition is necessary to help heal the grafted area as well as the donor site.

[11] E. Pearson and H. S. Soroff, Burns, in *Nutritional Support of Medical Practice*, ed. H. A. Schneider, C. E. Anderson, and D. B. Coursin (Hagerstown, Md.: Harper & Row, 1977) pp. 222-235.

A significant number of people with extensive burns develop deep ulcers (usually in the duodenum) called **Curling's ulcers**, which can cause major bleeding. When bleeding is profuse, the patient cannot be fed orally. For these patients, TPN may be indicated. (See Chapter 20.)

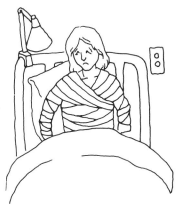

Psychological and emotional concerns of the burn patient outweigh interest in food.

Dead, burned skin is called **eschar** (es-CAR). As the eschar becomes loose, it is removed so that the burn wound can close as soon as possible. The removal of the eschar is called **debridement.**

Hydrotherapy, sometimes called **tanking**, is used to cleanse the burn wound and help loosen the eschar. The patient is placed in a large tub where the wounds are gently cleansed with a special soap that helps prevent infections.

Nutrition and Other Trauma

Physical therapy for burned patients is very important for preventing **contractures**, or loss of joint function. As the burn wound heals, the new skin is very tight, and it may pull the area surrounding a joint into a nonfunctional position.

Three types of skin are used for grafts. In an **autograft**, the patient's own skin is taken from an unburned area and used to cover the burn wound. In a **homograft**, skin is taken from another human (usually a cadaver); and in a **heterograft**, skin is taken from an animal (usually a pig). Autografts grow and become a permanent part of the person's skin. Homografts and heterografts are used only temporarily to cover a burn wound.

Bedsores caused by constant pressure exerted on the skin are called **decubitus** (dee-KYOO-bi-tus) **ulcers.**

decumbere = to lie down

Although there are some differences in the nutrition care of patients with various types of stress and trauma, for the most part the care is very similar. Diets high in kcalories, protein, vitamins, and minerals, with close attention to fluids, are the general rule. The same is true for other types of mechanical trauma such as bone fractures.

Immobilization, which commonly occurs during periods of other stress and trauma, is itself an additional stress on the body. During immobilization the body losses nitrogen and calcium. Calcium is lost from bone when the weight bearing and muscle tension produced by normal activity do not occur. In prolonged immobilization, blood and urine levels of calcium may increase, causing calcium stones to form in the kidney and bladder. Restricting dietary calcium does not alleviate the problem. The best treatment is for the patient to become actively mobile as soon as possible. A high-protein diet helps minimize negative nitrogen balance.

Bedsores occur when constant pressure is exerted on the skin, causing it eventually to break down and die. The tissues and muscles under the skin, as well as bone, may also be involved in the breakdown. Preventing or minimizing negative nitrogen balance helps avert the development of bedsores. Turning and repositioning the patient regularly also alleviate pressure and death of tissue. Once a bedsore has developed, an adequate diet is essential to speed up the healing process.

Hospitalized or injured people often are afraid and anxious. These feelings increase the activity of the stress hormones (see Highlight 6) and so intensify stress. In addition, they can interfere with food intake by causing anorexia or nausea. Therefore, whenever you can relieve someone's anxiety, you help his or her physical recovery as well.

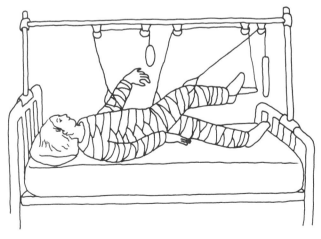

The injury itself can interfere with food intake.

Nutrition Assessment in Stress

Of course, all of the parameters of nutrition assessment discussed in Chapter 18 are applicable to the stressed or injured patient. However, some very important aspects of the assessment should be emphasized here:

1. An accurate assessment of the patient's *preinjury nutrition status* is vital for determining nutrient needs.

2. Careful and continuous monitoring of nutrition status is critical to insure that nutrient needs are being met by the diet. Patients' nutrient stores can become depleted rapidly.

3. For patients on oral diets, a careful history of food likes and dislikes will be invaluable in encouraging adequate oral intake.

4. Anthropometrics must be interpreted cautiously in the period immediately following the injury, because patients may be retaining or losing water. Also, the location of wounds may make arm anthropometrics impossible.

5. In burn patients, low serum albumin and transferrin levels are due to the loss of plasma proteins through the burn wound and into the interstitial fluid. Low values are to be expected and are difficult to interpret as an index of nutrition status.

6. In all stressed patients, serum albumin concentrations may decrease for awhile. Levels which remain depressed for more than seven days following the insult can be evaluated as an indicator of poor protein status.[12]

Summing Up

When the body's normal state is challenged by illness or injury, the stress response, mediated by hormonal changes, follows. The result is rapid depletion of energy reserves, elevated blood glucose levels, negative nitrogen balance, and weight loss. A well-nourished person can withstand short periods of stress without adverse effects. People whose nutrient stores have been depleted, though, do not have the reserves necessary to meet the metabolic changes imposed by injury.

Stressed patients need more kcalories, protein, vitamins, and minerals to meet nutrient needs. They may retain fluids or become dehydrated, so fluid intake must be carefully monitored. Increasing food intake is often difficult because of the anorexia, immobility, and pain which may occur along with stress.

---

[12] J. P. Grant, P. B. Custer, and J. Thurlow, Current techniques of nutritional assessment, *Surgical Clinics of North America* 61 (1981):437-463.

To Explore Further

In addition to the references cited in the footnotes, many other sources of information about nutrition and stress are available.

A teaching aid and syllabus entitled *Stress*, by H. Selye, is available from the Nutrition Today Society (address in Appendix J).

An excellent book that is easy to read and understand is:

● Wilmore, D. W. *The Metabolic Management of the Critically Ill*. New York: Plenum Medical Book Company, 1977.

The book uses a question-and-answer format, contains practical guides to calculating nutrient needs, and also includes case studies.

Two excellent chapters pertaining to stress and injury can be found in the book *Nutritional Support of Medical Practice*, edited by H. A. Schneider, C. E. Anderson, and D. B. Coursin (Hagerstown, Md.: Harper & Row, 1977). The chapters are:

● Pearson, E., and Soroff, H. S. Burns. Pp. 222-235.

● Beisel, W. R. Infectious Diseases. Pp. 350-366.

A well-illustrated reference is:

● Abston, S. Burns in children. *Clinical Symposia* 28 (1976):1-36.

Address correspondence to: Medical Education Division, CIBA Pharmaceutical Company, Summit, NJ 07901.

The June 1981 issue of *Surgical Clinics of North America* was devoted to nutrition for surgical patients. More detailed information, particularly on metabolism, can be found in this reference. It also contains chapters on nutrition in trauma and infection, enteral and parenteral nutrition, and nutrition assessment.

A shorter summary of nutrition and stress is:

● Wilmore, D. W., and Kinney, J. M. Panel report on nutritional support of patients with trauma or infection. *American Journal of Clinical Nutrition* 34, Supplement, 1981, pp. 1213-1222.

More detailed and advanced information on hormonal and metabolic consequences of stress can be found in *Journal of Parenteral and Enteral Nutrition* 4 (March-April 1980), which reported on the "Symposium on the Metabolic Response to Surgery and Injury."

A *Journal of Trauma* supplement (November 1979) included several articles on metabolism and nutrition therapy in burn patients (pp. 898-911).

Articles which provide more specific information on selected topics include:

● Bruner, V. Nutritional support of the trauma patient: Nursing considerations. *Nutritional Support Services*, February 1982, pp. 41-42.

● Cerra, F. B. Sepsis, metabolic failure and total parenteral nutrition. *Nutritional Support Services*, April 1981, pp. 26-28, 50.

● Elwyn, D. H. Nutritional requirements of adult surgical patients. *Critical Care Medicine* 8 (1980):9-20.

● Wieman, T. J. Nutritional requirements of the trauma patient. *Heart and Lung* 7 (1978):278-285.

● Wilmore, D. W. Nutrition and metabolism following thermal injury. *Clinics in Plastic Surgery*, October 1974, pp. 603-619.

● Curreri, P. W., Richmond, D., Marvin, J., and Baxter, C. R. Dietary requirements of patients with major burns. *Journal of the American Dietetic Association* 65 (1974):415-417.

● Kirkpatrick, J. R., and Nelson, R. Preoperative nutritional support: Indications and strategies. *Nutritional Support Services*, June, 1981, pp. 28-34.

● Faintuch, J., Waitzberg, D. L., Azevedo, S. A., Gama-Rodrigues, J. J., and Gama, A. H. Influence of malnutrition on the length of hospitalization after moderate and severe surgical injury. *Nutritional Support Services*, September 1981, pp. 29-30.

● Choctaw, W. T., Fujita, C., and Zawacki, B. E. Prevention of upper gastrointestinal bleeding in burn patients. *Archives of Surgery* 115 (1980):1073-1076.

Several publications are available free of charge from pharmaceutical companies. See Appendix J for addresses.

● Progressive hospital diets. In *Dietary Modifications in Disease*. Columbus, Ohio: Ross Laboratories, 1976.

● Major body burns. In *Dietary Modifications in Disease* Columbus, Ohio: Ross Laboratories, 1977.

● Gastineau, C. F., ed. Nutrition in trauma and burns. *Dialogues in Nutrition* 2 (March 1977). Available from Mead Johnson laboratories.

Severe Stress

Mrs. Sampson, a 48-year-old homemaker, has been admitted to the emergency room. She has been in a car accident. The emergency room physician has found that she has a fractured leg; multiple bruises and cuts on her head, arms, and legs; and a third-degree, 40 percent BSA burn. Other information:

- Ht: 5'5".
- Wt: 125 lb.
- Serum albumin: 2.8 g/dl.

Study Questions

1. Identify Mrs. Sampson's immediate postinjury needs. Should she be fed orally during this time? Why or why not?

2. How will you determine when Mrs. Sampson can begin eating foods orally?

3. Do you have enough information to determine Mrs. Sampson's preinjury, preburn nutrition status? If not, what do you need? How would you assess her serum albumin level?

4. Calculate Mrs. Sampson's kcalorie and protein needs for burn healing. Discuss what other nutrients must be considered.

5. How do the other injuries affect Mrs. Sampson's nutrient needs?

6. Discuss some general guidelines for providing all of Mrs. Sampson's nutrient needs. What physical and emotional factors must be considered?

7. If Mrs. Sampson cannot get adequate nutrients orally by the fourth to seventh postburn day, how should she be fed? If she developed major GI bleeding, how could she be fed?

8. Discuss the role of physical therapy and exercise in Mrs. Sampson's treatment.

HIGHLIGHT 22

AN OPTIONAL CHAPTER
Nutrition and Immunity

In the broadest terms, the development of immunity is a process by which the body learns from experience of past infections to deal more efficiently with subsequent ones.

SIR MACFARLANE BURNETT

The remarkable capacity of people to survive in an environment teeming with disease-causing organisms is a tribute to the human immune system. The immune system is composed of various organs whose function is to defend the body against foreign materials such as microorganisms like bacteria and viruses or damaged body cells that must be eliminated. Immunity, then, depends on the ability to recognize foreign materials and destroy or otherwise neutralize them.

The "First Line of Defense" The body's first line of defense against foreign materials is found in body surfaces exposed to the outside environment. The skin itself is a formidable barrier. Additionally, secretions of glands associated with the skin (sweat, tears, and the oily secretions of the sebaceous glands) contain chemicals toxic to some types of bacteria. The mucus produced by mucous membranes also contains antimicrobial chemicals, and more important, it is sticky; it "catches" foreign materials, which can then be disposed of. Mucus from the lungs is eliminated through the cough reflex or swallowed. If it is swallowed, the acid environment of the stomach together with digestive enzymes can destroy many microorganisms. If the invader does gain entry into the body, a second line of defense is called into action.

The "Second Line of Defense" The cells that participate in the immune function can be found throughout the body, but they are primarily housed in lymph tissue — the thymus, lymph nodes, spleen, bone marrow, and areas lining the GI tract (see Figure 1). Most important among these cells are the three types of white blood cells, the granulocytes, monocytes, and lymphocytes.

immune system: the body's system of defense against foreign materials.

immunity: the body's ability to recognize and eliminate foreign materials.

immunology: the study of the immune system.

sebaceous glands: glands generally associated with hair follicles which secrete fat droplets that lubricate the skin.

Table 1.   Major Components of the Immune System

First line of defense

> Skin
> Mucus
> Tears, sweat, secretions of sebaceous glands
> Digestive enzymes

Second line of defense

> Granulocytes
> Macrophages

Third line of defense

> Sensitized T-lymphocytes
> Antibodies

White blood cells **(leukocytes)**:

granulocytes
  (polymorphonuclear
  leukocytes, or PMNL)
monocytes
lymphocytes

phagocytosis: the process by which some cells engulf and destroy foreign materials.

One chemical released by one type of granulocyte is histamine; one of its effects is increased blood flow to an invaded area.

The white blood cells are the mobile components of the immune system. When the body is wounded or invaded by a microorganism, white blood cells transported to that area by way of the circulatory system provide a rapid and potent defense against infection. As mentioned, there are three types of white blood cells, the granulocytes, monocytes, and lymphocytes, and all three are formed from the same precursor cells (see Figure 2).

The first type of white blood cell, the granulocytes, function in two ways. Some granulocytes are capable of engulfing (ingesting) and digesting foreign particles in a process called phagocytosis (see Figure 3). Other granulocytes release chemicals which play a role in the immune response.

The second type of white blood cells, the monocytes, reach the invaded or wounded area and mature into macrophages. Macrophages also participate in phagocytosis.

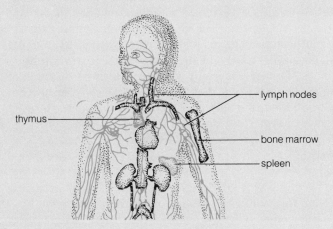

Figure 1 The lymph tissues and bone marrow. The bone marrow is not lymph tissue, but it is the site of production of cells important to the immune response. Not shown: the patches of lymph tissues in the GI tract.

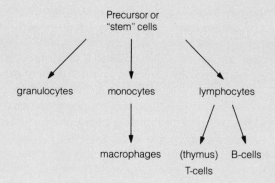

Figure 2 The various types of white blood cells are derived from the same precursor cells.

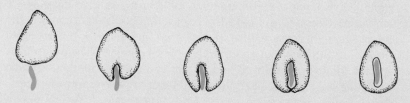

Figure 3 During phagocytosis, a foreign substance is engulfed by a white blood cell and eventually surrounded and digested.

The process of phagocytosis must be selective to insure survival of the body. Macrophages and granulocytes must be able to distinguish foreign or damaged cells from functional cells so that the body does not digest itself. Still, phagocytosis is a general process; many types of foreign particles can be handled in this way.

The "Third Line of Defense" The lymphocytes, a third type of white blood cells, serve a different function in the immune system. All lymphocytes originate from precursors in the bone marrow but are released from the bone marrow and mature into two distinct types of lymphocytes — T-cells and B-cells. T-cells travel to the thymus and are then housed in the lymph tissues. The thymus produces a hormone which influences the activity of these cells.

The B-cells do not travel to the thymus after release from the bone marrow. Indeed, we are not certain where these cells go. They are called B-cells because, in the chicken, they travel to the bursa of Fabricus.

Unlike the macrophages and granulocytes, the lymphocytes are important in the body's defense against specific invading organisms. This more specific immune response depends on prior exposure to the invading organism, recognition of it when exposed again, and reaction to it.

Immunity directed at foreign organisms in general is called **nonspecific**, or **innate**, immunity. The skin, mucous membranes, granulocytes, and macrophages are a part of nonspecific immunity.

lymphocytes:
 T-cells
 B-cells

Immunity directed at specific organisms is called **specific**, or **acquired, immunity.** The lymphocytes mediate this type of immunity, which depends on prior exposure, recognition,and reaction to invading organisms. Two types are cell-mediated immunity and humoral immunity.

cell-mediated immunity: immunity conferred by the actual reaction of cells (sensitized T-cells) to an invading organism.

The T-cells participate in cell-mediated immunity. T-cells travel directly to the invasion site, where they become "sensitized" to the particular invading organism. Although the mechanism is unknown, a sensitized T-cell is then capable of releasing powerful chemicals when the invading organism is encountered again. The chemicals kill foreign cells and also stimulate other immune functions, including phagocytosis. Some of the sensitized lymphocytes serve as memory cells; if a person is exposed to the same invading organism again, the immune system remembers how to produce the right type of T-cell and so can respond much more quickly. T-cells are especially active in defending the body against fungi, viruses, parasites, and a few types of bacteria; they can also destroy cancer cells. T-cells are involved in the rejection of newly transplanted tissues.

humoral immunity: immunity conferred by antibodies secreted by B-cells and carried to the invaded area by way of the body fluids. Antibodies: see p. 128.

A substance foreign to the body that causes the formation of antibodies is an **antigen.**

B-cells are important in humoral immunity. When a foreign substance reaches the lymph tissues containing the B-cells, these B-cells rapidly divide, and then differentiate into plasma cells which produce antibodies (see p. 128). Unlike the T-cells, the B-cells don't travel to the invasion site themselves. Instead, they send their secreted antibodies to the site. Antibodies, like sensitized lymphocytes, react selectively with a specific foreign organism. The body remembers how to make specific antibodies, so that the next time the foreign organism is encountered, the immune response can occur with greater speed. B-cells play a bigger role in resistance to infection than do T-cells.

In summary, the body's first line of defense against foreign materials is provided by the skin, the mucous membranes, and various body secretions. Should a microorganism gain entrance into the body, the second line of defense, which includes the macrophages and granulocytes, is called into play. At the same time, antibodies and sensitized lymphocytes are produced. They play a vital role as a third line of defense if the general immune responses are unsuccessful or if the organism has been previously encountered.

The preceding discussion of the immune system is an oversimplification of a very complex subject. The three systems discussed here as separate entities are really interdependent and synergistic; furthermore, much information has not been included. However, our intent is merely to provide some general background so that you can appreciate the role that nutrition plays in immunology.

The Role of Nutrition

For some time it has been recognized that people who suffer from malnutrition in developing countries also develop more infections. A vicious cycle develops in which malnutrition decreases resistance to infection, and infection further aggravates malnutrition. Exactly how this happens isn't clear yet. But researchers have been uncovering information which is helping to solve the puzzle (see Table 2).

Table 2.   Effects of Malnutrition on the Immune System

Immune system components	Effect of malnutrition
Skin	Thinner with less connective tissue and collagen
Mucous membranes	Microvilli flattened; secretory immunoglobulin A reduced
Lymph tissues	Thymus gland atrophied; lymph nodes and spleen smaller; T-cell areas depleted of lymphocytes
Phagocytosis	Kill time delayed
Cell-mediated immunity	Circulating T-cells decreased
Humoral immunity	Circulating immunoglobulin levels normal; antibody response may be impaired

The first barriers a foreign material encounters when trying to enter the body are the skin and the mucous membranes. Malnutrition causes changes in these tissues which compromise their function. During malnutrition the skin becomes thinner, with less connective tissue and collagen. The microvilli of the mucous membranes become flattened.[1] Also, one type of antibody present in mucous membrane secretions is depressed in malnutrition.[2] This may help explain why malnourished children have repeated lung and GI tract infections.[3]

The antibody of mucus that is depressed in malnutrition is **secretory immunoglobulin A.**

Malnutrition does not appear to interfere with phagocytosis by granulocytes once an organism has entered the body.[4] However, some investigators have found that malnutrition delays phagocytosis by macrophages. Therefore, bacteria stay in the body longer, although eventually, malnourished cells will kill as many bacteria as control cells.[5]

Cell-mediated immunity, which is a function of the T-lymphocytes, appears to be significantly affected by malnutrition. In children with severe protein-kcalorie malnutrition, the thymus gland atrophies, and

[1]L. Vasantha, S. G. Srikantia, and C. Gopalan, Biochemical changes in the skin in kwashiorkor, *American Journal of Clinical Nutrition* 23 (1970):78-82.

[2]S. Sirisinha, R. Suskind, R. Edelman, C. Asvapaka, and R. E. Olson, Secretory and serum IgA in children with protein-calorie malnutrition, *Pediatrics* 55 (1975):166-170.

[3]R. E. Hodges, Nutrition in relation to infection, *Medical Clinics of North America* 48 (1964):1153-1167.

[4]R. M. Suskind, Malnutrition and the immune response, in *Nutrition in Clinical Care* (New York: McGraw-Hill, 1982), pp. 403-417.

[5]W. P. Faulk and J. J. Vitale, Immunology, in *Nutritional Support of Medical Practice*, ed. H. A. Schneider, C. E. Anderson and D. B. Coursin (Hagerstown, Md.: Harper & Row, 1977), pp. 341-346.

the lymph nodes and spleen are smaller in size.[6] The areas of the lymph tissues which house the T-cells are depleted of lymphocytes.[7] The number of T-cells circulating in the blood are also reduced in children with malnutrition, and their number increases when the poor nutrition status is improved.[8] The skin testing procedure discussed in Chapter 18 is one measurement of cell-mediated immunity. Several studies have shown that malnourished people do not react to skin testing (indicating that cell-mediated immunity is impaired) and that vigorous nutrition support can reverse the situation.[9]

Malnutrition seems to affect T-cell function more than B-cell function. Antibodies secreted from B-cells belong to a family of proteins commonly called immunoglobulins. In malnourished people, the blood levels of immunoglobulins are not decreased.[10] Furthermore, the total numbers of B-cells in blood samples have been found to be normal in malnutrition.[11] However, as already noted, one type of immunoglobulin found in mucous secretions is depressed as a result of malnutrition. Some investigators have found that the antibodies are less effective in malnutrition, but the studies are difficult to interpret because different antigens produce different responses.[12]

The Role of Individual Nutrients

Just as generalized malnutrition has an effect on the immune system, so can deficiencies or excesses of individual nutrients. A workshop sponsored by the American Medical Association on single-nutrient effects on immunologic functions was useful in tying together available information on the subject.[13] Still, the currently available data are far from complete.

Changes in immune function in humans have been associated with deficiencies of folacin, iron, and zinc and with excesses of vitamin E

[6]Suskind, 1982.

[7]Faulk and Vitale, 1977.

[8]A. C. Ferguson, G. J. Lawlor, C. G. Neumann, W. Oh, and E. R. Stiehm, Decreased rosette-forming lymphocytes in malnutrition and intrauterine growth retardation, *Journal of Pediatrics* 85 (1974):717-723.

[9]D. K. Law, S. J. Dudrick, and N. I. Abdou, Immunocompetence of patients with protein-calorie malnutrition: The effects of nutritional repletion, *Annals of Internal Medicine* 79 (1973):545-550, H. D. Willcutts, D. Linderme, D. Chlastawa, and H. S. Willcutts, Anergy: Is nutritional reversal possible/outcome significant, *Journal of Parenteral and Enteral Nutrition* 3 (1979):292.

[10]W. P. Faulk, E. M. Denmaeyer, and A. J. S. Davies, Some effects of malnutrition on the immune response in man, *American Journal of Clinical Nutrition* 27 (1974):638-646.

[11]Faulk and Vitale, 1977.

[12]R. Dionigi, F. Gnes, A. Bonera, and L. Dominioni, Nutrition and infection, *Journal of Parenteral and Enteral Nutrition* 3 (1979):62-68.

[13]W. R. Beisel, R. Edelman, K. Nauss, and R. M. Suskind, Single-nutrient effects on immunologic functions, *Journal of the American Medical Association* 245 (1981):53-58.

and essential fatty acids. Furthermore, a few clinical reports suggest that changes in immune function accompany deficiencies of vitamins A, B_6, B_{12}, and pantothenic acid and elevated blood cholesterol levels. Studies in animals link the levels of many vitamins, minerals, trace elements, amino acids, fatty acids, and cholesterol with immunologic changes in animals. Table 3 lists nutrients known to influence immune function. (See Highlight 10 for a discussion of vitamin C in infections.)

As you can see, nutrition plays an important role in our ability to defend ourselves against disease-producing organisms. You may recall from Chapter 22 that the stress of injuries such as surgery and burns often makes a person vulnerable to infection. Now you can see why attention to nutrient needs becomes even more important in stress.

Table 3.   Effects of Selected Nutrient Deficiencies on the Immune System

Nutrient deficiency	Effect
Vitamin A	Depletion of T-lymphocytes;* increased frequency and severity of some infections;* increased incidence of infections (humans)†
Vitamin B_6	Depressed cell-mediated and humoral immunity;* reduced antibody responses to vaccines (humans)
Folacin	Impaired response to skin tests; lymph tissue atrophy;* decreased numbers of white blood cells;* impaired cell-mediated and humoral immunity*
Pantothenic acid	Depressed antibody responses (humans)
Vitamin B_{12}	Some reduction of phagocytosis by granulocytes (humans)
Vitamin E§	Depressed antibody responses;* impaired response to skin tests*
Iron	Atrophy of lymph tissue; impaired response to skin tests; defective phagocytosis (humans)
Zinc	Atrophy of lymph tissues; abnormalities in cell-mediated and humoral immunity (humans)
Individual amino acids	Impaired humoral immunity*

*Information is from animal studies.

†Some reports support this finding, but more information is needed.

§Vitamin E excess can cause inhibition of multiple immune functions in humans.

To Explore Further

In addition to the references already cited, a very clear and informative discussion of immunology can be found in:

● Vander, A. J., Sherman, J. H., and Luciano, D. S. Defense mechanisms of the body. In *Human Physiology — The Mechanisms of Body Function*. New York: McGraw-Hill, 1975, pp. 476-499.

Two publications are available through pharmaceutical companies:

● Vitale, J. J. Impact of nutrition on immune function. In *Nutrition in Disease*. Columbus, Ohio: Ross Laboratories, 1979.

● Ruggiero, R. P., Mills, C. B., and Kaminski, M. V. *Cell Mediated Immunity and Nutrition*, physicians monograph. Berkeley, Calif.: Cutter Laboratories.

A thorough review of the effects of individual nutrients and immunity is available in:

● Beisel, W. R. Single nutrients and immunity. *American Journal of Clinical Nutrition* 35 (Supplement 1982) pp. 417-468.

CHAPTER 23

CONTENTS

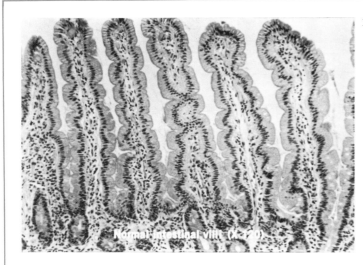

Normal intestinal villi

Villi affected by celiac disease

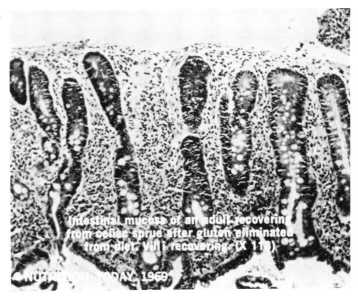

Disease of the GI tract can severely disturb absorbing surfaces, causing malnutrition

Reproduced with permission of Nutrition Today magazine, P.O. Box 1829, Annapolis, Maryland 21404, September 1968.

GASTROINTESTINAL DISORDERS

Between the actual consumption of good food and the nourishment of all the cells and tissues of the body, there must be digestion, assimilation, and delivery of nutritional elements to the cells. The requirements of our cells are the basis for our need to eat.

ROGER J. WILLIAMS

You would be a very rare individual if you went through life without experiencing some type of gastrointestinal upset. Many common complaints can be minor, such as indigestion, nausea, or a temporary bout of diarrhea. Other GI problems can be more severe, such as the intense cramping and vomiting that accompany severe food poisoning. Little wonder that a great deal of attention has been focused on how the diet can prevent or alleviate symptoms of GI disorders. After all, anything that causes a change in GI function can alter the intake, digestion, and absorption of food and nutrients. Furthermore, food itself may contain components which are either irritating or easy for the GI tract to handle.

Problems of the Upper GI Tract

The upper GI tract includes the mouth, throat, and esophagus. Problems with any of these areas have dietary implications.

Difficulties in Chewing and Swallowing   The mouth and teeth play an important part in reducing the size of food particles so that they can be swallowed and digested. When teeth are missing or decayed, when the gums and mouth are sensitive, or when the mouth is dry or ulcerated, food must be provided in a form that minimizes the discomfort of swallowing. If the diet of a person with any of these problems is not adjusted, you will probably see the person eating less and losing weight. Nutrition status will deteriorate. Table 1 lists some conditions which may interfere with ability to chew.

The diet used to reduce the discomfort of chewing and swallowing is a highly individualized modification of a regular diet called a mechanical soft diet. It merely eliminates those foods the person cannot easily chew or swallow. The permitted foods may be liquid, chopped, or pureed foods, or regular foods with a soft consistency.

The process of chewing is sometimes called **mastication.**

masticare = to chew

mechanical soft diet: a diet that excludes all foods that are difficult to chew or swallow; also called a **dental soft diet.**

857

People vary in the consistency of foods they can tolerate, so you must always obtain a complete diet history. The foods provided to a patient should be as similar to those of a regular diet as possible. These foods will offer the most variety, increasing the patient's acceptance of them and reducing the likelihood of nutrient deficiencies. For example, although a patient with a newly broken jaw may only be able to handle liquids, an edentulous patient may be able to eat baked chicken or fish, ground beef, casseroles, canned fruits, and many soft cooked vegetables.

All seasonings and types of foods are allowed on a mechanical soft diet. However, highly seasoned or acidic foods (citrus fruits, tomatoes) may cause pain to someone with mouth ulcers. Also, foods that contain nuts or seeds such as breads with sesame or poppy seeds are generally avoided because they can easily get trapped in the ulcer and cause discomfort.

Stop and think about a pureed diet for a moment. A typical dinner on a regular diet that consists of baked chicken, boiled potatoes, and diced green beans is now white mush, more white mush, and one green blob added for color. Pureed foods are even replaced by baby foods in many hospitals. Although baby foods are nutritious, they are often very bland tasting, since they are prepared without salt and extra spices. Furthermore, whether pureed or baby food, the consistency of the food is a psychological block to the patient's intake. Malnutrition can result.

Is there any way you can help improve the situation? The answer is yes! First of all, be sure your patient actually needs pureed rather than chopped foods. Second, try to help your patient select meals that will provide for a variety of colors. For example, consider substituting mashed sweet potatoes for white potatoes in the meal above. Such a change can add appetizing color to a meal. The food can be served attractively and at the right temperature. Lastly, be sure the patient understands that unless the physician has ordered otherwise, salt, pepper, and other spices can be added to the food to improve the taste. Many patients do not think they are allowed to have additional seasonings.

CAUTION:

Pureed diets can look and taste unappealing, causing decreased intake.

Table 1. Conditions That Interfere with Chewing and Swallowing

Dental caries	Dryness of the mouth
Missing teeth	Periodontal disease
No teeth	Ulceration of mouth or gums
Ill-fitting dentures	Oral surgery
Sensitivity to hot or cold	Broken jaw

Dysphagia   The esophagus, which transports food from the mouth to the stomach, is important in swallowing. It makes sense that disorders of the esophagus can cause dysphagia. Dysphagia can be the result of psychological problems as well as physiological ones; in this section we will discuss only those causes of dysphagia which can be helped by diet.

One such disorder is achalasia. In achalasia the nerves which control the motility of the esophagus are not functioning properly, and the muscles of the esophagus do not propel the food bolus downward toward the stomach. Additionally, the cardiac sphincter (see p. 151) does not relax and open during swallowing to allow the food to pass into the stomach. When the person with achalasia eats or drinks, foods and fluids accumulate in the esophagus. The person generally describes a sensation of food sticking in the throat in addition to dysphagia. Gradually, either the pressure of the food causes the cardiac sphincter to open, or the person must regurgitate to expel the food.

At first, the person with achalasia may experience only temporary and mild dysphagia. As the condition worsens, the symptoms become more painful. The esophagus widens as achalasia progresses (see Figure 1). The person becomes fearful of eating, gradually reducing food intake. Marked weight loss and other nutrient deficiencies are likely to be present by the time the person sees a doctor. There is a danger that the person will aspirate the food into the lungs, and this may lead to serious lung infections.

The treatment for achalasia is either to stretch or partially slit the cardiac sphincter so that it is no longer functional. This will make the person more comfortable, but it will not restore motility to the esophageal muscles. Because the cardiac sphincter remains open, another problem, reflux esophagitis, is a common complication (see below).

Before the cardiac sphincter is opened, the patient will need to consume only liquid or semiliquid foods, and avoid large servings at any one time. The use of liquid supplements which meet all nutrient needs should be considered. Tube feedings and parenteral nutrition may be indicated, particularly if the patient is severely malnourished or is unable to consume adequate nutrients orally.

dysphagia (dis-FAGE-ee-uh): difficulty in swallowing.
dys = bad, difficult
phagein = eating

achalasia (ack-uh-LAY-zee-uh): dysfunction of the esophagus. Achalasia is sometimes called **esophageal dyssynergia** (es-ahf-uh-GEE-ul dis-sin-ERJ-ee-uh) or **cardiospasm.**
a = without
chalasis = relaxation
synergia = cooperation

The cardiac sphincter is often called the **lower esophageal sphincter (LES)** or the **gastroesophageal sphincter.** (For sphincter muscles in general, see p. 150.)

The fear of eating is called **sitophobia** (SIGH-toh-FOE-bee-uh).
sitos = food

When an organ, such as the esophagus, becomes enlarged beyond normal dimensions it is said to be **dilated**. Making an organ or vessel larger is called *dilation* or *dilatation*.

The backflow or regurgitation of gastric contents from the stomach into the esophagus is called **reflux**.
re = backwards
flux = flow

Stretching the cardiac sphincter is accomplished by inserting an instrument through the mouth and esophagus. The end of the device has a balloon-like attachment which is inflated under pressure, stretching the sphincter. The procedure is called **pneumatic** (noo-MAT-ic) or **forceful dilation**.

pneuma = air, respiration

Partially slitting the cardiac sphincter requires a major surgical procedure. Surgery is generally not used unless the sphincter does not respond to forceful dilation.

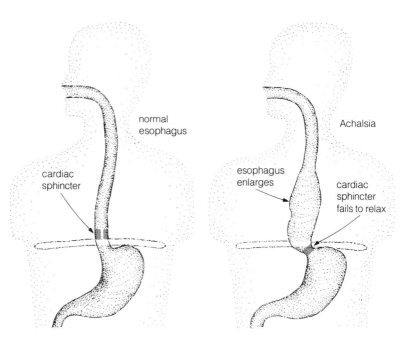

Figure 1 In achalasia the muscles of the esophagus lose their tone, and the esophagus gradually becomes enlarged.

The continuous reflux of gastric juices may cause scarring of the esophageal mucosa. As scar tissue forms, the diameter of the esophagus narrows. This condition is referred to as an **esophageal stricture**.

strictura = to bind tight

heartburn: a burning pain felt behind the sternum which may spread into the neck and throat.

Reflux Esophagitis Reflux esophagitis is an irritation in the lower esophagus. It occurs when the cardiac sphincter does not close tightly enough and highly acidic gastric contents splash backwards into the esophagus, irritating the esophageal mucosa. You can see why people being treated for achalasia often develop esophagitis. However, reflux esophagitis can occur at any time if the pressure of the cardiac sphincter is not great enough to keep it closed. When esophagitis becomes chronic, the inner diameter of the esophagus may become narrowed by inflammation and scarring, causing dysphagia and the same problems seen in achalasia. Chronic esophagitis also can cause ulcers to form in the esophagus. Table 2 lists some foods and substances which affect cardiac sphincter pressure.

A burning pain called heartburn occurs when the gastric juices reflux into the esophagus. Heartburn usually hurts behind the sternum, often spreading into the neck and back of the throat in waves, and may cause enough pain to awaken a sleeping person. Heartburn is especially likely when presure in the stomach exceeds pressure in the esophagus; so it occurs more frequently when a person lies down or bends over. bends over.

The treatment of reflux esophagitis centers around three principles:

● Prevention of esophageal reflux.

● Reduction of gastric acidity to prevent irritation.

● Use of foods which are least likely to irritate an already inflamed esophagus.

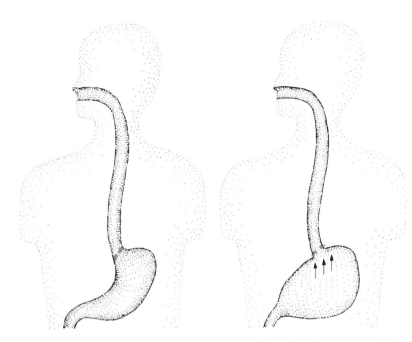

Figure 2 Whenever the stomach becomes overdistended, the pressure in the stomach is greater than the pressure in the esophagus, increasing the chance of reflux. Overeating or drinking large amounts of liquids can cause the stomach to become overdistended.

Food and drugs that lower cardiac sphincter pressure are avoided. For example, fatty meals trigger the release of cholestokinin from the small intestine, and cholecystokinin decreases cardiac sphincter pressure. Therefore, fatty foods are avoided. Protein foods, on the other hand, stimulate the release of gastrin, which helps increase cardiac sphincter pressure. Caffeine-containing beverages (see p. 602) and foods are also avoided because caffeine decreases cardiac sphincter pressure. The same is true for alcohol, peppermint and spearmint oils (found in some liqueurs), and cigarette smoking. Decaffeinated coffee must also be eliminated from the diet because, even without the caffeine, it stimulates gastric acid secretion. Red pepper must be avoided for the same reason.

Acidic juices such as orange, grapefruit, and tomato juice may be irritating to the esophagus; they should be avoided by a person experiencing the symptoms of reflux esophagitis. This person should eat should avoid drinking liquids for one hour before and after meals (see Figure 2). You can remind such a person to avoid lying down and bending over for about three hours after eating and to refrain from wearing tight-fitting garments, particularly after eating. The head of the person's bed should be elevated so that the chest is higher than the stomach to help prevent reflux (see Figure 3). Weight loss is important for the obese person with esophagitis.

In addition to changes in diet, the frequent use of antacids is recommended to neutralize the acidity of the gastric juices. Other drugs

Principles of nutrition care for people with reflux esophagitis:

Limit fat in diet; fat decreases sphincter pressure.

Eat high-protein foods; protein increases sphincter pressure.

Avoid alcohol, caffeine-containing beverages, decaffeinated coffee, red peppers, and peppermint and spearmint oils; these foods either decrease sphincter pressure or stimulate gastric acid secretion.

Eat smaller, more frequent meals; large meals cause distention of the stomach.

Avoid liquids for one hour before and one hour after meals; large amounts of liquids can distend the stomach.

Do not lie down, bend over, or exercise vigorously after eating; these actions can cause pressure in the stomach to increase.

Do not wear tight-fitting garments; tight garments can increase pressure in the stomach.

Lose weight, if necessary; excessive fat around the abdomen can increase pressure in the stomach.

Two drugs which increase cardiac sphincter pressure and the rate at which the stomach empties are bethanechol (beh-THAN-uh-call) and metoclopropamide (MET-uh-cloh-PROH-puh-mide). They are sometimes useful for people with reflux esophagitis.

Table 2.   Action of Some Foods and Other Substances on Cardiac Sphincter Pressure

Increase Pressure	Decrease Pressure
Protein	Alcohol
Bethanechol	Caffeine-containing beverages
Metoclopropamide	Chocolate
	Fat
	Peppermint and spearmint oils
	Cigarette smoking
	Atropine
	Anticholinergic agents

also may be prescribed. Generally, esophagitis can be controlled through diet and drugs. However, in some instances surgery is attempted when medical management fails.

> People with reflux esophagitis tend to become chronic users of antacids. You may recall from Chapter 21 that nutrient imbalances are likely to develop in people using drugs for long periods of time. It is important to remember that some antacids contain high amounts of sodium (those containing sodium bicarbonate) and calcium (those containing calcium bicarbonate). The chronic use of a particular antacid may be contraindicated for people with other medical problems.

esophageal hiatus (high-AY-tus): the opening in the diaphragm through which the esophagus passes.

hiatal hernia: an outpouching of a portion of the stomach through the esophageal hiatus of the diaphragm. There are several types: sliding, rolling, or short-esophagus (see Figure 4).

hiatus = to yawn

Hiatal Hernia   Normally, the stomach lies completely below the diaphragm. The esophagus passes through the diaphragm by way of an opening, the esophageal hiatus. A hiatal hernia results when the opening in the diaphragm weakens, allowing a portion of the stomach to protrude above the diaphragm (see Figure 4). The symptoms of hiatal hernia result from esophagitis caused by the reflux of the acidic gastric juices into the esophagus. The goals of nutrition care for hiatal hernia are the same as those given earlier for esophagitis: that is, to prevent reflux, to neutralize gastric acidity, and to eliminate foods that irritate the esophagus.

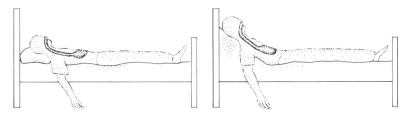

Figure 3   Elevating the head of the bed reduces the likelihood that food will back up from the stomach to the esophagus.

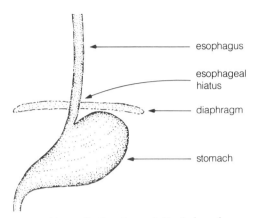

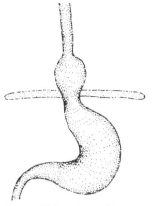

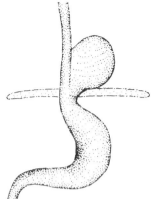

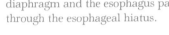

a. Normally the stomach lies below the diaphragm and the esophagus passes through the esophageal hiatus.

b. A **sliding hiatal hernia** is the most common type of hiatal hernia.

c. A **paraesophageal hernia** is relatively rare; reflux is not a problem in this type of hiatal hernia because the lower end of the esophagus and its closing mechanism lie below the diaphragm.

Figure 4

Diseases of the Stomach

Whenever you turn on the television set you are likely to see at least a few advertisements touting cures for indigestion, heartburn, and gas. These terms have become so ingrained in the minds of the public that any GI discomfort may be incorrectly described as one of these disorders.

Indigestion or dyspepsia is a vague term used to describe any discomfort in the GI tract. Indigestion can be a symptom of many disorders, either in the GI tract or in other organs. Oftentimes, indigestion is caused by emotional tension. You may hear people making comments such as "I have a nervous stomach," or "I got so mad my stomach felt like it was in a knot." In addition to emotional factors or underlying medical conditions, indigestion can be caused by eating too much or too rapidly or chewing poorly.

Generally, no diet modifications are necessaary for a temporary bout of indigestion. When indigestion occurs frequently, the cause (whether it be physical, emotional, or dietary) should be identified. You can give some dietary advice that may help. Eating slowly, at regular times, and in a relaxed atmosphere is often helpful. Avoiding excessive amounts of fats, highly spiced or seasoned foods, alcohol, and caffeine-containing beverages also can help. And, of course, people should avoid any food that they know gives them indigestion.

When indigestion is persistent, the person may decrease intake of food. Therefore, you should take a careful diet history to determine if the diet has been adequate. Persistent indigestion may be a symptom of two disorders we will be discussing later in this section: gastritis and peptic ulcers.

dyspepsia: a vague term used to describe abdominal discomfort. Dyspepsia is a symptom, not a disease.

dys = bad, difficult
peptein = to digest

When a disease or a symptom has a rapid onset and lasts only for a short time, it is described as **acute; chronic** conditions, on the other hand, develop slowly and are of long duration.

Vomiting is another symptom which can occur in several types of disorders. When a person vomits, the waves of peristalsis have reversed direction, and the contents of the stomach are propelled up through the esophagus and mouth. If vomiting continues long enough or is severe enough, the reverse peristalsis will carry the contents of the duodenum, with its green bile salts, into the stomach and then up the esophagus. Simple vomiting is certainly unpleasant and wearying for the nauseated person, but it is no cause for alarm. Vomiting is one of the body's adaptive mechanisms to rid itself of something irritating.

But vomiting can be a symptom of a more serious disorder. Furthermore, vomiting itself can be serious enough to require a doctor's care. When large quantities of fluid are lost from the GI tract, fluid leaves the interstitial spaces to replace it. This interstitial water must be replaced from somewhere. The nearest supply is in the capillaries of the circulatory system. To resupply the circulatory system, fluid is drawn from the cells. The danger in prolonged vomiting is that eventually fluid is taken from every cell of the body. Leaving the cells with the fluid are electrolytes — particularly sodium, potassium, chloride, and bicarbonate — which are absolutely essential to the life of the cells. These electrolytes and fluid must be replaced, which is difficult while the vomiting continues. Intravenous feedings of saline and glucose with electrolytes added are frequently necessary while the doctor is diagnosing the cause of the vomiting and instituting corrective therapy.

In an infant, vomiting is especially serious; a doctor should be contacted soon after onset. Babies have a higher proportion of fluid in the interstitial space, so it is much easier for their body water to be depleted and their electrolyte balance upset than it is for adults to suffer these consequences.

Projectile vomiting is another kind of vomiting that is not the simple type associated with nausea. In this type, the contents of the stomach are expelled with such force that they leave the mouth in a wide arc, arching far out from the body like a bullet leaving a gun. There are a number of causes for this type of vomiting, and all of them require immediate medical care.

To identify specific GI disorders, the physician correlates biochemical and clinical data. One tool often used to help diagnose disorders of the esophagus and stomach is the gastroscope, a long tube equipped with a special optical device that allows the physician to see and photograph (if desired) the physical appearance of the esophagus, stomach, and upper portion of the duodenum.

A word that describes the region of the body just over the stomach is **epigastric**.

epi = above

Gastritis   Gastritis is a common disorder, characterized by inflammation of the mucosal lining of the stomach. The person with gastritis may complain of anorexia, nausea, vomiting, belching (see below), a feeling of fullness, and epigastric pain.

Acute gastritis is most often caused by ingesting aspirin or other drugs which irritate the gastric mucosa. Alcohol abuse, food irritants, food allergies, food poisoning, radiation, stress, and infections also can cause gastritis. There are two principles to keep in mind for the dietary management of acute gastritis:

- Eliminate irritating foods.
- Reduce gastric acidity.

If the person with gastritis cannot eat because of nausea or vomiting, food is generally withheld for one or two days. The diet is then progressed from liquids to a bland diet as tolerated. A bland diet eliminates foods that are irritating to the gastric mucosa, such as those named in Table 3.

When the gastric juices secreted in the stomach contain no hydrochloric acid, the condition is called **achlorhydria** (ay-clor-HIGH-dree-uh). In **hypochlorhydria** (HIGH-po-clor-HIGH-dree-uh), there is some hydrochloric acid in the gastric juice, but less than normal.

a = without
chlorhydria = hydrochloric acid
hypo = too little

In Chapter 6 you saw how the use of logic rather than evidence can be misleading. A good example demonstrating this point is the bland diet. For many years, bland diets that eliminated many spices, raw fruits and vegetables, and other foods high in fiber were widely prescribed. In 1971, the American Dietetic Association (ADA) developed a position paper on bland diets.[1] The ADA reviewed the literature and found that the rationale for many restrictions on the bland diet was not supported by scientific evidence. For example, traditional bland diets frequently recommended milk to neutralize gastric acidity. However, milk has actually been shown to *increase* gastric acid secretion.[2]

Despite the fact that a more liberal diet approach has been adopted by the ADA and gastroenterologists, traditional bland diets continue to be widely used without proven benefit.

This discussion should help to reinforce a happy thought: that in at least some instances the diet that is best for your client's health may be the one he likes. To promote the health of the digestive tract, your client should indulge in eating as a pleasant experience that contributes to a tranquil state of mind.

Chronic gastritis has the same symptoms as acute gastritis, but persists for longer periods of time. As the disease progresses, the gastric cells atrophy and gastric secretions decrease. Unlike acute gastritis,

[1] American Dietetic Association, Position paper on bland diet in the treatment of chronic duodenal ulcer disease, *Journal of the American Dietetic Association* 59 (1971):244-245.

[2] A. F. Ippoliti, V. Maxwell, and J. I. Isenberg, The effect of various forms of milk on gastric-acid secretion: Studies in patients with duodenal ulcer and normal subjects, *Annals of Internal Medicine* 84 (1976):286-289; J. Behar, M. Hitchings, and R. D. Smyth, Calcium stimulation of gastrin and gastric acid secretion: Effect of small doses of calcium carbonate. *Gut* 18 (1977):442-448; M. J. Brodie, P. C. Ganguli, A. Fine, and T. J. Thomson, Effects of oral calcium gluconate on gastric acid secretion and serum gastrin concentration in man, *Gut* 18 (1977):111-114.

Table 3. **Liberal Bland Diet**

1. Eliminate foods irritating to the individual.
2. Avoid pepper, chili powder, and cocoa.
3. Avoid caffeine, cola beverages, coffee (both caffeinated and decaffeinated), and tea.
4. Avoid alcohol.

peptic ulcer: an eroded mucosal lesion in the esophagus, stomach, or duodenum.

lesion: an abnormal change in structure.

pepsin: a gastric protease. It circulates as a precursor, pepsinogen, and is converted to pepsin by the action of stomach acid.

The word that describes how a disease starts and then develops is **pathogenesis**.

  patho = disease
  genesis = beginning

A condition in which a person develops tumors of the pancreas which secrete excessive amounts of gastrin is called the **Zollinger-Ellison syndrome.** The gastrin triggers the release of excessive gastric acid and pepsin, leading to ulceration of the stomach and small intestines.

Ulcers that develop following severe physiologic stress (surgery, burns, shock, or infection) are called **stress ulcers**. Generally, once they have healed they do not recur.

chronic gastritis has no known cause. Overeating; eating too rapidly; eating when emotionally upset; eating certain foods; using alcohol, tobacco and coffee; and having infections and nutrient deficiencies all have been implicated as possible causes, but conclusive evidence is lacking. Because so little is known about chronic gastritis, it is not clear what the most appropriate diet therapy may be. However, a bland diet may help relieve gastrointestinal symptoms in some cases. In some people, vitamin B_{12} deficiency may develop because of decreased availability of intrinsic factor (see pp. 332-333). Therefore, it is important to assess vitamin B_{12} status. This assessment should be repeated at regular intervals, because it may take two to three years before the body's stores of vitamin B_{12} become depleted.

Peptic Ulcers Ulcers can occur in many places outside and inside the body. However, used alone, the term *ulcer* generally refers to an ulcer in the stomach (gastric ulcer) or duodenum (duodenal ulcer). The term *peptic ulcer* includes both of these. An ulcer is an erosion of the top layer of cells from the wall of the stomach or intestine, leaving the second and succeeding underlying layers of cells exposed to gastric juices. The erosion may proceed until the capillaries that feed the area become exposed. Bleeding results and can eventually be fatal. If the erosion penetrates all the way through the stomach or duodenum, a major infection (peritonitis) can rapidly develop and can be fatal.

Normally, the stomach lining in a healthy person is well protected from gastric acid and pepsin by its mucous coat. Why, then, do ulcers form? Two factors are required: a weakness in the mucosal lining of the stomach and the presence of gastric acid and pepsin to erode the weak spot (see Chapter 5). The exact cause of the initial weakness is unknown. Some factors that are believed to predispose the individual to ulcers include smoking, poor nutrition, lack of rest, drug ingestion (aspirin, glucocorticoids), stress (both physiological and psychological), and genetic factors. Once the mucosal barriers have weakened, the secretion of gastric acid and pepsin makes the ulcer worse. A person with an ulcer may experience a gnawing, burning pain which lasts up to several weeks. Although symptoms generally disappear for periods of time, they usually recur eventually.

The origin and development of a gastric ulcer is different from that of a duodenal ulcer. A commonly accepted theory to explain how a gastric ulcer starts postulates that the gastric mucosa are damaged by the reflux of duodenal contents (bile) into the stomach. The bile then breaks the mucosal barrier, and acid and pepsin facilitate ulcer formation. This theory also explains why people with gastric ulcers almost always have chronic gastritis.

Duodenal ulcers are more common than gastric ulcers. It appears that most people with duodenal ulcers have higher than normal levels of acid in gastric secretions. The duodenum is less well protected against acid than the stomach. Stress may play a role in duodenal ulcer development. You may recall that the secretion of digestive juices is regulated by hormones and nerves. Both hormonal and neural activity are influenced by mental state. Excessive anxiety and worry may be a cause of the initial ulcer lesion; they are clearly related to the excessive acid secretion that makes an ulcer worse.

Currently there is no cure for ulcers. Instead, treatment is aimed at relieving pain, healing the ulcer, and reducing the likelihood of recurrence. The treatment for both gastric and duodenal ulcers is the same.

The objectives of peptic ulcer therapy are to neutralize gastric acidity and to decrease gastric acid secretion. These measures help protect the stomach and duodenum wall from the eroding effect of gastric acid and pepsin. You or the physician may tell the patient to:

● Use antacids. Take them one hour after meals to prolong their effect.

● Eliminate any food that routinely causes indigestion or pain. In addition, eliminate any food known to irritate the gastric mucosa or increase acid secretion (see liberal bland diet — Table 3).

● Use drug therapy, which may include anticholinergics or cimetidine (see Figure 5).

● Reduce stress. Learn how to handle stress without overreacting or becoming upset; learn how to relax, to get enough sleep, and to enjoy life.

● Eliminate drugs that irritate the stomach (aspirin).

● Reduce or eliminate cigarette smoking.

At one time, the ulcer patient was advised to eat smaller, more frequent meals. However, food stimulates gastric acid secretion, and therefore, three regular meals a day are indicated for people with healed ulcers.

Most patients and nutritionists agree that strict bland diets are unnecessary during periods when the patient is symptom-free. There is less agreement over what to do when the ulcer is active. When the traditional approach is used, the diet is progressed in stages. In the first stage, the patient is served 3 to 4 oz milk every one to two hours during the day and, if he or she awakens, during the night. Antacids are also given. As the pain subsides (usually in about three or four days) the patient advances to the second stage. Here, small feedings of very soft-fiber foods are added to the diet, and the interval between feedings

Principles of nutrition care for people with peptic ulcers:

Eliminate foods that cause discomfort.

Avoid caffeine, cola beverages, coffee, tea, alcohol, pepper, chili powder, and cocoa.

Eat frequently.

Relax during and between meals.

anticholinergics: drugs that decrease gastric acid secretion and gastric motility. They produce many undesirable side effects, including blurred vision and dry mouth.

cholinergic = working in the same way as acetylcholine (neurotransmitter)

erg = work

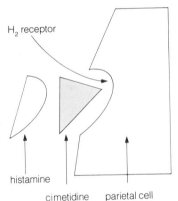

Figure 5 When cells that are located near the parietal cells of the gastric glands are stimulated by nerve impulses, they secrete histamine. There is a receptor for histamine on the parietal cell called an H_2 receptor. When histamine acts on the H_2 receptor hydrochoric acid (HCl) is produced. The drug *cimetidine* acts by blocking the H_2 receptor so that the production of HCl is inhibited.

A new drug used overseas to heal ulcers is carbenoxolone (car-ben-OX-uh-lone) sodium. It has not been approved for use in the U.S. The drug is derived from glycyrrhitinic (GLY-si-ri-TIN-ic) acid, which is extracted from licorice, and it can cause sodium and fluid retention and possibly renal damage (see also Chapter 21).

asymptomatic: free of symptoms.

The first stage of the restrictive bland diet is sometimes called the **Sippy diet.** It consists of milk or cream given in small amounts every one to two hours.

People who drink significant amounts of milk in conjunction with some types of antacids can develop hypercalcemia and alkalosis. Permanent kidney damage can result. This condition is called the **milk-alkali syndrome.**

is increased until a six-feeding-per-day schedule is established. The patient who remains symptom-free reaches the third stage. The third-stage diet eliminates all foods eliminated on the liberal bland diet (see Table 3) as well as highly seasoned foods, most raw fruits and vegetables, whole grain breads and cereals, fried foods, and foods containing seeds, nuts, or coconut.

The exact foods included and excluded on a traditional bland diet vary widely among institutions. The facility's diet manual can be consulted to determine what foods are served when a traditional bland diet is given.

Many physicians recommend that the third-stage diet be continued even when the patient is asymptomatic. However, as we have already said, this recommendation is not supported scientifically and is unnecessarily restrictive.

People on bland diets may be either underweight (when pain or tension stops them from eating) or overweight (from eating too much, too frequently). All efforts should be made to encourage these people to achieve and maintain ideal body weight and to include enough protein in the diet to speed healing of the ulcer. Usually, ulcer patients can be managed medically. However, surgery may be necessary for those who do not respond to medical treatment or for those who develop complications such as bleeding, perforation, or obstruction.

Sample bland diet menu (stage 3)

Breakfast
½ c grapefruit juice
1 soft cooked egg
1 slice toast with butter
½ c milk

Midmorning Snack
½ c corn flakes
½ c milk
2 tsp sugar
½ banana

Lunch
Roast beef sandwich
(2 slices white bread,
2 oz meat)
1 tsp mayonnaise
½ c green beans
½ c milk

Midafternoon Snack
½ c pudding
2 sugar cookies
1 c decaffeinated tea
with sugar

Supper
2-3 oz broiled fish
½ c rice
½ c carrots
Ginger ale

Evening Snack
½ c cottage cheese
in a peach half
2 saltine crackers
4 oz milk

Gastric Surgery

Many different types of gastric surgery can be employed in the management of peptic ulcers, gastric cancer, and damage following trauma (gunshot wound, auto accident). Figure 6 shows several types

Some interesting observations by two doctors, named Wolf and Wolff, set in motion the line of inquiry that was to culminate in today's agreement that stress is the primary factor that aggravates an ulcer. Wolf and Wolff were doctors at a hospital that admitted a most unusual patient one day in 1939. This patient, remembered in scientific circles only as "Tom," had had since childhood an opening from the outside of his body through the abdominal wall into his stomach. Through this fistula he had learned to feed himself and, keeping his condition secret, had grown to manhood and had lived a near-normal life.

At the age of 53, while performing hard manual labor, he tore the edge of the opening of the fistula and was taken to the hospital where Wolf and Wolff were on the staff. The two doctors managed to gain Tom's confidence. He cooperated with them by allowing them to make observations of his stomach lining through the fistula. As a result, they learned that emotions called forth unique responses from the stomach. Aggressive emotions, such as anger and hostility, made the capillaries in the stomach lining flush with blood and caused the gastric juices to pour forth as if food had been introduced. However, when Tom was sad and depressed, there was no secretion of gastric juices, and the capillaries were pale pink instead of red. These emotional states and the stomach's responses to them were entirely independent of Tom's feelings of hunger.

The discovery was exceedingly important and was duly reported in the journals. Probably the most important result of these observations was that they stimulated other doctors to experiment with their patients who had fistulas. Thus researchers began to learn exactly which foods were irritating to the lining of the stomach and which foods neutralized the acidity, instead of relying on tradition and logical thinking for this knowledge. For instance, they found that the majority of the foods that had been classified as irritating to the stomach actually had more effect when applied to the skin of the arm! This story should remind you once again that caution must be applied when decisions are made on the basis of logic (see p. 157).

CAUTION WHEN YOU READ!

A logical conclusion cannot be accepted as true
until it is supported by experimentation.

of commonly used gastric surgery procedures, and the accompanying Miniglossary defines some types of gastric surgery. The general nutrition care described in Chapter 22 for all surgical patients applies to those who undergo gastric surgery. However, there are additional nutrition concerns following gastric surgery.

After undergoing gastric surgery, many people lose a significant amount of weight. Some have trouble regaining their preoperative weight. Others develop specific nutrient deficiencies. Weight loss can be the result of decreased food intake, malabsorption, increased metabolic requirements, or a combination of these.

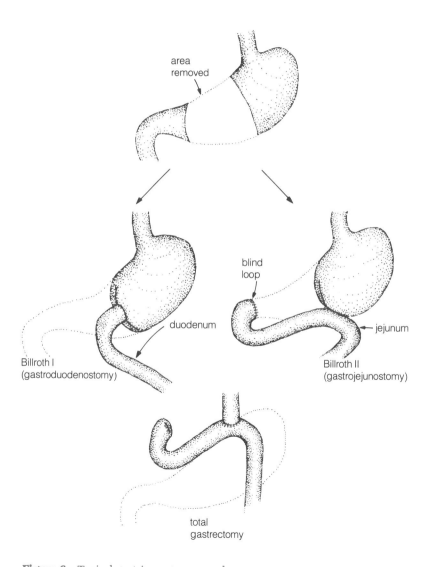

Figure 6   Typical gastric surgery procedures.

Miniglossary of Gastric Surgery Terms

anastomosis (an-ASS-to-MOCE-is): the site where two distinct spaces or organs are surgically joined together.

ana = upward
stoma = opening

blind loop: the section of intestine that is bypassed but not removed after gastric surgery (see Figure 6).

esophagoenterostomy (e-SOFF-uh-go-ent-er-OSS-to-me): a surgical procedure in which the esophagus is connected to the intestine after the stomach is removed. In an **esophagoduodenostomy** (e-SOFF-uh-go-doo-oh-den-OSS-to-me), the esophagus is connected to the jejunum.

gastrectomy: a surgical procedure in which part (partial gastrectomy) or all (total gastrectomy) of the stomach is removed. A gastrectomy may also be called a **gastric resection.**

gastroenterostomy (GAS-troh-en-ter-OSS-to-me): a surgical procedure in which a portion of the stomach is removed and a new connection is made between the stomach and intestine. When the new connection is made with the duodenum, a **gastroduodenostomy** (GAS-troh-duo-oh-den-OSS-to-me) has been performed. In a **gastrojejunostomy** (GAS-troh-jee-joon-OSS-to-me), the stomach is connected to the jejunum.

pyloroplasty (pie-LO-ro-plasty): a surgical procedure used to increase the diameter of the pyloric channel.

vagotomy (vay-GOT-oh-me): a surgical procedure often performed along with other gastric surgery to sever the vagus nerve either totally or partially. (The vagus nerve supplies nerves to the stomach, among other organs.) A vagotomy helps to reduce HCl production and to delay gastric emptying.

Dumping Syndrome   One problem that may occur in the person who has had significant portions of the stomach removed is called dumping syndrome. A typical scenario goes something like this: Patient X had a fairly extensive gastric resection about a week ago, and has just begun eating solid foods. He swallows the food and about 15 minutes later he begins to feel weak and dizzy. He looks pale, his heartbeat is rapid, and he breaks out into a sweat. Shortly thereafter he develops diarrhea. What causes this sequence of events?

Because of the surgery, the patient has lost an important function of his stomach. Food no longer empties at a controlled rate into his intestine. Instead it gets "dumped" rapidly into the jejunum. (even if the duodenum was not bypassed during surgery, it is so short that food

dumping syndrome: the physiological events that result from the presence of undigested food in the jejunum.

The hypoglycemia sometimes seen in patients following gastric surgery is called **alimentary** (al-i-MENT-ary) or **postgastrectomy hypoglycemia**.

aliment = food

postgastrectomy diet: a diet given to prevent the dumping syndrome and hypoglycemia that sometimes follow gastric surgery.

Postgastrectomy diet guidelines:
   Maintain fluid and electrolyte balance.
   Restrict total carbohydrate; eliminate concentrated sweets.
   Eat small meals, frequently.
   Drink liquids 30 to 60 min after meals.
   Lie down after eating.
   Tailor diet to individual needs.

passes quickly into the jejunum.) As the food is digested, the intestinal contents become hypertonic (see Chapter 20). Water from the intestinal capillaries move into the lumen of the jejunum to equalize the osmolar load. The volume of the circulating blood decreases rapidly, causing **weakness, dizziness, and rapid heartbeat. The large fluid load in the jejunum causes hyperperistalsis, and diarrhea results. Figure 7 outlines the sequence of events that occur in dumping syndrome.**

After about two to three hours, Patient X develops many of the same symptoms again: dizziness, fainting, nausea, and sweating. This time the cause is different. Carbohydrates from the meal were rapidly **hydrolyzed and then absorbed, causing blood glucose levels to rise quickly. The pancreas responded by overproducing insulin. The symptoms of hypoglycemia are now occurring as blood glucose levels fall rapidly. It has been postulated that intestinal hormones, blood hormones, and the hydrogen ion content of the stomach may play a role in mediating the dumping syndrome response.**[3]

Not all patients who have had gastrectomies develop dumping syndrome. Even fewer develop hypoglycemia. Many people who initially experience dumping syndrome gradually adapt to a fairly normal diet. However, a special diet is available for the period immediately following surgery or for prolonged or severe cases.

The postgastrectomy diet is used to control the symptoms of dumping syndrome and hypoglycemia. Fluid and electrolyte balance should be monitored carefully and any imbalance should be corrected. To help people follow the diet, encourage them to eat more foods containing protein and fat, because these nutrients are hydrolyzed more slowly than carbohydrate in the intestine and so do not increase the osmolar load as rapidly as carbohydrates do. Advise patients to be especially careful not to eat concentrated sweets (sugar, cookies, cakes, pies, soft drinks), because they are the most rapidly hydrolyzed carbohydrates. Recommend that patients eat smaller, more frequent meals to fit the reduced storage capacity of the stomach. Tell them to wait until about 45 minutes after eating before drinking liquids; this helps decrease the rate at which food passes from the stomach to the intestine. You can also try having patients lie down immediately after eating to help slow down the transit of food to the intestine and help prevent the symptoms of dumping. Table 4 lists foods included and excluded on the postgastrectomy diet, and a sample menu is illustrated in the text.

[3]K. T. Shultz, F. A. Neelon, L. B. Nilsen, and H. E. Lebovitz, Mechanism of postgastrectomy hypoglycemia, *Archives of Internal Medicine* 128 (1971):240-246; A. Cushieri and O. A. Onabanjo, Kinin release after gastric surgery, *British Medical Journal* 3 (1971):565-569; S. R. Bloom, C. M. S. Royston, and J. P. S. Thomson, Enteroglucagon release in the dumping syndrome, *Lancet* 2 (1972):789-791; N. R. Thomford, K. R. Sirinek, S. E. Crockett, E. L. Mazzaferri, and S. Cataland, Gastric inhibitory polypepide: Response to oral glucose after vagotomy and pyloroplasty, *Archives of Surgery* 109 (1974):177-182; J. P. S. Thomson, R. C. G. Russell, M. Hobsley, and L. P. LeQuesne, The dumping syndrome and the hydrogen ion concentration of the gastric contents, *Gut* 15 (1974):200-206.

Sample postgastrectomy menu

Breakfast
  1 fried egg
  1 slice toast
  1 tsp butter
  ½ c whole milk
    (take 30-60 min after meal)

Midmorning Snack
  ¼ c cottage cheese
  1 graham cracker

Lunch
  2 oz hamburger patty
  ¼ c mashed potatoes
  1 tsp margarine
  ¼ small cantaloupe
  ½ c whole milk
    (take 30-60 min after meal)

Midafternoon Snack
  2 T peanut butter
  3 saltine crackers

Supper
  2 oz boiled ham
  ¼ c rice
  ½ c carrots
  2 tsp butter
  ¼ c unsweetened peach slices
  ½ c whole milk
    (take 30-60 min after eating)

Evening Snack
  ¼ c tuna
  1 tsp mayonnaise
  1 slice bread

The diet must be carefully tailored to meet each person's individual needs. Initially, visit the patient after each meal to determine food tolerances and intolerances. Gradually, many patients will be able to tolerate small amounts of concentrated sweets, larger quantities of food, and some liquids with meals. Some patients develop lactose intolerance and cannot tolerate milk at all (see below). Diet is not successful in correcting the symptoms of dumping syndrome for everyone. A study by one group of researchers suggests that adding pectin (a type of dietary fiber) to the diet may be useful in preventing the symptoms of dumping syndrome.[4] When all dietary measures fail, additional surgery is sometimes necessary to correct the problem.

Other nutrition concerns arise in gastrectomy patients. Anemia is commonly seen. Iron-deficiency anemia can result from the initial blood loss accompanied by poor nutrition and poor iron absorption. Fifty percent of iron absorption normally takes place in the duodenum, but following gastric surgery, the transit time through the duodenum may be rapid or the duodenum may be bypassed altogether. An iron supplement can be given to correct iron-deficiency anemia.

Anemia also can be caused by a deficiency of vitamin B_{12} or folacin. You may recall that vitamin B_{12} cannot be absorbed without intrinsic factor (IF), which is synthesized in the stomach. Depending on the location and extent of the gastric resection, IF production may be reduced or absent and vitamin B_{12} absorption correspondingly impaired. Vitamin B_{12} must then be given by injection to correct the deficiency.

[4]D. J. A. Jenkins, M. A. Gassull, A. R. Leeds, G. Metz, J. D. Dilawari, B. Slavin, M. R. C. Path, and L. M. Blendis, Effect of dietary fiber on complications of gastric surgery: Prevention of postprandial hypoglycemia by pectin, *Gastroenterology* 73 (1977):215-217.

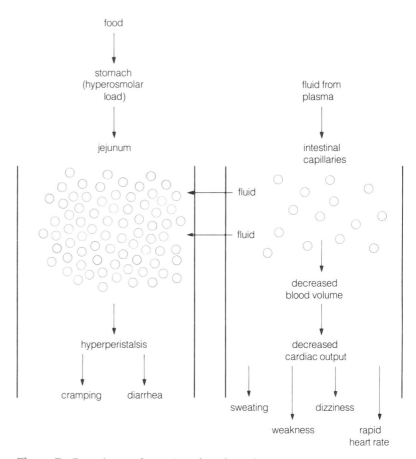

Figure 7 Dumping syndrome is a physiological reaction to the presence of a hyperosmolar load in the jejunum.

steatorrhea (stee-AT-or-REE-uh): fatty diarrhea. The stools are foamy, greasy, and odorous, reflecting fat malabsorption.

The problems of fat malabsorption and vitamin B$_{12}$ and folacin depletion that can result from the overgrowth of bacteria in a bypassed segment of the intestine are collectively called the **blind loop syndrome**. Synonymous terms: **small intestinal stasis** (STAY-sis) **syndrome, contaminated small bowel syndrome,** and **stagnant loop syndrome.**

stasis = standing still

Absorption of both vitamin B$_{12}$ and folacin can be impaired because of an overgrowth of bacteria in the portion of the intestine that has been bypassed. The bacteria compete with the host for the vitamin B$_{12}$ and folacin, decreasing the available supply. The bacteria also partly dismantle bile salts so that they become ineffective in fat digestion and absorption or even inhibit these processes. Fat may be malabsorbed as a result. To help correct the problem, parenteral vitamin B$_{12}$ and/or oral folacin supplements are given along with antibiotics to inhibit the bacterial growth. Fat may be restricted to prevent steatorrhea. Sometimes the bypassed intestinal segment must be removed surgically.

General malabsorption is a problem in a person who has had a total gastrectomy or in a person whose stomach has been surgically connected directly to the jejunum. Normally, when food enters the duodenum the hormones secretin and cholecystokinin are released. In turn, these hormones mediate the release of digestive enzymes and bile, which are then secreted into the duodenum. When the duodenum is bypassed, these normal digestive processes also are bypassed. Additionally, malabsorption can result from the rapid passage of food through the GI tract, a problem when the stomach no longer controls the rate of gastric emptying.

Common GI Problems

Several GI problems are occasionally experienced by practically all of us. In some cases, these problems are symptoms of an underlying disease process. However, they can occur as isolated incidents and, often, they present no cause for alarm.

Gas   Many people complain of problems that they attribute to excessive gas. For some, belching is the complaint. Others blame intestinal gas for abdominal discomforts such as cramping or distention. Almost all these people feel that the problems occur after they eat certain foods.

Excessive gas in the stomach or the intestines is sometimes called **flatulence** (FLAT-you-lence) or **flatus** (FLAY-tus). Flatus also describes the expulsion of gas through the mouth (belching) or through the rectum.

flatus = blowing

Another word for belching is **eructation** (ee-ruck-TAY-shun).

eructatio = to belch

Reprinted by permission of Tribune Company Syndicate, Inc.

Contrary to popular belief, belching is not caused by gas formed from certain foods in the stomach. Rather, belching results when air that has been swallowed or sucked in is expelled. People who complain of excessive belching have acquired a bad habit, usually unconsciously. They suck in or swallow air, often as a result of tension. Occasionally, belching can be a sign of a more serious disorder. People with gallbladder pain, colonic distress, or an impending obstruction of a coronary blood vessel may belch frequently.[5]

Very little is known about the production of intestinal gas. It appears that some gas is derived from swallowed air. Other gases appear to be formed by bacteria in the gut. This happens because humans lack the enzymes necessary to digest and absorb certain types of carbohydrate that are found in some vegetable products, such as beans. The gut bacteria do have the necessary enzymes, and so they metabolize the

[5]F. J. Inglefinger, How to swallow, and belch and cope with heartburn, *Nutrition Today*, January/February 1973, pp. 4-13.

Table 4. **Postgastrectomy Diet**

Food item	Allowed	Excluded	Comments
Meats/meat alternatives	X		Any type
Breads/cereals/starchy vegetables			
Plain breads, crackers, rolls, unsweetened cereal, rice, pasta, corn, lima beans, parsnips, peas, white potatoes, sweet potatoes, peas, pumpkin, yams, winter squash	X		Limit to 5 servings daily
Sweetened cereal; cereal containing dates, raisins, or brown sugar		X	
Nonstarchy vegetables			
Chicory, Chinese cabbage, endive, escarole, lettuce, parsley, radishes, watercress	X		As desired
Asparagus, bean sprouts, beets, broccoli, brussels sprouts, cabbage, carrots, cauliflower, celery, cucumbers, eggplant, green pepper, greens, mushrooms, okra, onions, rhubarb, sauerkraut, string beans, summer squash, tomatoes, turnips, zucchini	X		Limit to two 1/2-c servings daily; individual tolerances will vary
Vegetables prepared with sugar		X	
Fruits			
Unsweetened fruits and fruit juices	X		Limit to three servings daily
Sweetened fruits and fruit juices		X	
Fats	X		Any type
Beverages			
Milk (whole or skim milk or buttermilk)	X		If tolerated
Coffee, tea, dietetic carbonated beverages	X		
Alcohol, carbonated beverages, sweetened milk, cocoa, fruit drinks		X	
Desserts			
Cakes, cookies, ice cream, sherbet		X	
Other			
Honey, jam, jelly, syrup, sugar		X	

undigested carbohydrate, producing gas. (One type of gas, methane, is produced in only a third of the population.) It's easy to see why people who absorb carbohydrates poorly (such as those with a lactase deficiency) are likely to complain of excessive gas.

People whose excess gas production results from malabsorption can be treated accordingly. For people who are methane producers, however, diet has little effect. Foods that produce gas usually must be determined individually. You can have your client test foods suspected of forming gas by omitting them individually for a trial period and seeing if there is any improvement. Some foods that have been accused of causing gas are listed in Table 5.

Diarrhea Diarrhea occurs when bowel movements become more liquid or more frequent than usual. This sort of stool indicates that the intestinal contents have moved too quickly through the intestines for fluid absorption to have taken place or that water has been drawn from cells lining the intestinal tract and added to the food residue.

Emotional stress, nervous tension, and overeating can trigger diarrhea, as can some drugs, foods, and spices that irritate the GI tract. Spoiled food and bacterial overgrowth in the gut can also be causes. Many times an acute case of diarrhea develops and remits in 24 to 48 hours. Unless it is very severe, this type of diarrhea seldom requires medical treatment. Eliminating food irritants or drinking clear liquids can sometimes be helpful.

On the other hand, chronic diarrhea is a cause for concern. Chronic diarrhea can result from other disorders (malabsorption, protein-kcalorie malnutrition) or medical treatments (radiation therapy, drugs). The person with chronic diarrhea loses large amounts of water and electrolytes and can become dehydrated. Zinc is also lost.

Oftentimes, the GI tract is rested in cases of severe diarrhea. All foods and beverages may be withheld for 24 to 48 hours. During this time, fluids and electrolytes are replaced intravenously. The patient is then placed on a clear liquid diet and progressed to a full liquid diet and, finally, a regular diet as tolerated. If the diarrhea increases as the diet is progressed, then the patient can be given nothing by mouth, and intravenous nutrition must be supplied. Depending on the cause of the diarrhea, the patient may suffer from weight loss and multiple nutrient deficiencies. Care should be taken to prevent or correct these problems.

Once the patient is on an oral diet, applesauce or scraped raw apples are sometimes given every two to four hours. These foods contain pectin, a carbohydrate that attracts water and improves the consistency of the stools. Of course, if a food is known to have irritated the intestine, it should be eliminated. The exact treatment plan depends on what is causing the diarrhea.

When identifiable injury to the GI mucosa results in diarrhea, the diarrhea is called **organic**. On the other hand, in **functional** diarrhea, no such cause is observable.

When diarrhea results from an increased movement of fluids and electrolytes from the intestinal capillaries into the lumen of the intestine, then **secretory diarrhea** is present. When unabsorbed water and electrolytes cause diarrhea by increasing the osmolar load in the intestine, **osmotic** diarrhea exists. When fat is not absorbed but excreted in the stools, the resulting diarrhea is steatorrhea, already mentioned. Severe, chronic diarrhea is often called **intractable diarrhea**.

stear = hard fat

Table 5. **Foods That May Increase Intestinal Gas Production**

Apples	Carrots	Pastry
Apricots	Celery	Potatoes
Bagels	Citrus fruits	Pretzels
Bananas	Eggplant	Prune juice
Beans	Milk	Raisins
Bread	Milk products	Wheat germ
Brussels sprouts	Onions	

Adapted from information in L. O. Sutalf and M. D. Levitt, Follow-up of a flatulent patient, *Digestive Diseases and Sciences* 24 (1979):652-654.

constipation: the condition of having painful or difficult bowel movements (elapsed time between movements is not relevant).

defecate (DEF-uh-cate): to move the bowels, eliminate wastes.

defaecare = to remove dregs

irritable bowel syndrome: a common GI tract disorder characterized by spasms of the colon. It is also called spastic colon, spastic constipation, spastic diarrhea, and mucomembranous colitis.

Constipation You may joke about or be irritated by the laxative commercials that frequently seem to appear on the TV screen during the dinner hour, but most persons believe the message the advertisements are sending — that Mrs. X must have a daily bowel movement or else she will be headachy and irritable and lose all her marvelous personality. The screen then shows Mrs. X the next day feeling her old jovial self because her pharmacist has persuaded her to take a laxative.

Each person's GI tract responds to food in its own way, with its own rhythm, so that the fecal matter arrives at the rectal area in a fairly constant number of hours. Each GI tract thus has its own cycle, which depends on its "owner's" physical makeup and such environmental considerations as the type of food eaten, when it was eaten, and when the person's schedule allows time to defecate. If several days pass between movements but these movements take place without discomfort, then the person is not constipated, nor did she absorb any "toxins" that would cause irritable behavior. Nor does anyone need to worry about an inability to have daily movements — TV commercials nothwithstanding.

What then is constipation? When a person receives the signal that says to defecate and ignores it, the signal may not return for quite a few hours. In the meantime, water will continue to be withdrawn from the fecal matter, so that when a person does decide to defecate the movement will be drier and harder. If the bowel movement is hard and is passed with difficulty, discomfort, or pain, then it can be said that the person is constipated. (Note that in this definition of constipation no mention has been made of the amount of time that has elapsed since the previous bowel movement; that is irrelevant.) Constipation occurs when the muscles of the colon are loose and fail to push the intestinal contents along.

Constipation also can occur as a result of irregular and excessive contractions of the colon. This disorder, the irritable bowel syndrome, seems to be associated with emotional stress. Because of the spasms, intestinal contents move irregularly along the colon and can result in either diarrhea or constipation or both in an alternating sequence.

What can be done about constipation? If discomfort is associated with passing fecal matter, a doctor's help should be sought in order to rule out the presence of organic disease. For example, constipation can be a sign of an intestinal obstruction or tumor or diverticulitis (discussed later). If the constipation is found to be functional rather than organic, dietary or other measures for correction can be considered.

Careful review of daily habits may reveal the causes of the constipation. Being too busy to respond to the defecation signal is a common complaint. The patient's daily regimen may need to be reexamined with the idea of instituting regular eating and sleeping times that will allow time in the day's schedule, at the dictate of the person's body, to have a bowel movement.

Another cause of constipation that requires some rearrangement of lifestyle is the lack of physical activity. In modern society many people drive cars or ride buses to work, stand at assembly lines, or sit behind desks, then sit in front of a television set in the evening. People who do not have the time or money to work out at a spa are finding that they can park their cars a distance from the office and walk the extra blocks, or they can walk up several flights of stairs rather than take the elevator. The muscles that are responsible for peristalsis are improved by any activity that increases muscle tone of the entire body.

Increasing the fiber and fluid content of the diet may help to relieve constipation. Fiber absorbs a lot of water and so softens stools. Because fiber is not digested, it also adds bulk to the stool. Fiber can be added to the diet by increasing the use of whole grain breads and cereals and raw fruits and vegetables. Cereal fiber is more effective than fruit and vegetable fiber for increasing stool weight.[6] (See Appendix K for the fiber contents of selected foods.) The average daily diet should ideally contain about 12 to 15 grams of crude fiber.[7] (Most Americans consume about 4 to 5 grams of crude fiber daily.) Bran can be used to significantly increase the fiber content of the diet. A rounded teaspoon of unprocessed bran contains 2.4 grams of fiber. Bran can be sprinkled on cereal, salads, applesauce and many other food items or added to beverages. Many breakfast cereals contain a considerable amount of crude fiber. It has been suggested that drinking liquids also promotes peristalsis by providing the physical stimulation of increased bulk. Fluids help augment stool weight and softness.

Two terms, *fiber* and *residue*, are used to describe the contents of the colon. People often use these terms interchangeably, although it is incorrect to do so. *Fiber* describes the portion of food that is found in the colon because we don't have the right enzymes to digest it. *Residue* refers to the total amount of material in the colon; it includes undigested food, intestinal secretions, bacteria, and the turnover of intestinal cells. High-fiber foods are also high-residue foods with one exception: Milk is a fiber-free food that leaves residue in the gut following digestion.

There is a scarcity of laboratory research into the laxative quality of foods. It has been determined, however, that prunes contain a laxative.[8] If a morning defecation is desired, prunes or prune juice can

[6]J. Scala, Fiber, the forgotten nutrient, *Food Technology* 28 (1974):34-36.

[7]B. J. Dolin and H. W. Boyce, Jr., Dietary management of gastrointestinal disorders, *Journal of the Florida Medical Association* 66 (1979):395-401.

[8]This substance is dihydroxyphenyl isatin.

be taken at bedtime; if the evening is preferred, prunes or prune juice at breakfast may be useful.

Some constipation may be relieved by the addition of fat to the diet. It was previously thought that the success of this regimen was due to the lubricating effect of the fat, but it now appears to be due instead to its stimulation of cholecystokinin, which causes bile to be secreted into the duodenum. The bile acts in the same way that a saline laxative does; that is, its high salt content draws an abundance of water from the intestinal wall, which stimulates peristalsis and softens the fecal matter.

cholecystokinin: see p. 161.

These suggested changes in diet or lifestyle should correct chronic constipation without the use of laxatives. Occasionally, laxatives may be indicated, but they should only be used after a doctor has been consulted.

Hospitalized or institutionalized patients often suffer from constipation. Stress from disease, nervous tension, and inactivity are all contributing factors.

Ironically, frequent use of laxatives can actually lead to chronic constipation. Laxatives are generally safe when they are used on occasion, but when you use them for too long, the colon loses its ability to respond to natural stimulation. The lining of the intestine becomes irritated and muscular reflexes diminish. Thus, a temporary problem can become permanent. Furthermore, as you may recall from Chapter 21, nutrient deficiencies can develop when laxatives are used.

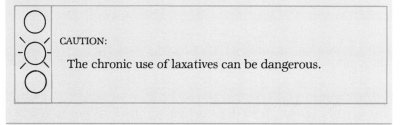

CAUTION:

The chronic use of laxatives can be dangerous.

Painful clusters of dilated and twisted veins in the lower rectum and anus are called **hemorrhoids** (HEM-or-oids).

haimo = blood
rhein = to flow

Most cases of constipation are harmless, although some may be accompanied by abdominal discomfort. Chronic constipation, on the other hand, is believed to be associated with other problems. The constant pressure of straining to defecate may result in hemorrhoids or the formation of diverticula (see below).

Disorders of the Intestine

In some diseases of the intestine, diet can play a significant role in preventing uncomfortable symptoms and injury. In some cases, diet may influence the incidence of certain diseases.

The malabsorption of nutrients is of primary concern in many disorders that involve the intestine. Malabsorption can occur when food is improperly digested, when the surface area of the bowel is reduced, or when normal mechanisms for absorbing nutrients are impaired. Many disorders can result in malabsorption; we will be discussing some of them throughout the remainder of this chapter. The effect of inadequate digestive enzymes is discussed in Chapter 24. Table 6 highlights the risk factors for poor nutrition status that may occur in patients with malabsorption.

Table 6. Risk Factors for Poor Nutrition Status in Malabsorption Syndromes

Decreased Intake	Increased Nutrient Losses	Increased Nutrient Needs
Emotional stress	Diarrhea	Surgery
Abdominal pain	Steatorrhea	Drug therapy
Bowel rest	General malabsorption	
	Short-bowel syndrome	
	Blind loop syndrome	

Whenever fat is malabsorbed, it is lost in excessive amounts in the stool, and steatorrhea exists. The loss of fat represents lost kcalories. Furthermore, when fat is malabsorbed, fat-soluble vitamins also are lost, since the two are absorbed together. Loss of vitamin D can result in calcium depletion. Calcium (and magnesium) are also lost in the feces with fat because they form soaps with unabsorbed fatty acids.

The loss of calcium with fatty acids can cause another problem, enteric hyperoxaluria. Oxalate, present in some foods, normally binds with calcium in the gut and both are excreted. But when calcium binds instead to fatty acids, the oxalate is left unbound and can be absorbed. Because oxalate is not metabolized by the body, this increased absorption leads to increased excretion of oxalate in the urine. High urinary oxalate favors the formation of kidney stones (see Chapter 27).

The primary treatment of steatorrhea is to treat the underlying disorder. To go with this treatment, fat is restricted and fat-soluble vitamins are supplemented in a water-miscible form that is easier to absorb. Medium-chain triglycerides (MCT) can be used to increase kcalories (see box "How MCTs are Digested and Absorbed"). Therapy for enteric hyperoxaluria involves treating the steatorrhea, restricting dietary oxalate, and supplementing the diet with calcium to bind the oxalate. Oxalates are present in tea, cocoa, leafy green vegetables, and products made with unbleached flour.

enteric hyperoxaluria (en-TERR-ic HY-per-ox-al-YOOR-ee-uh): a condition of excess oxalate absorption that comes about because calcium is unable to bind oxalate in the gut; leads to kidney stone formation.

enteric = intestinal

**How Medium-Chain Triglycerides (MCT) are
Digested and Absorbed**

You may recall from Chapter 2 that triglycerides contain a molecule of glycerol to which three fatty acids are attached. Most naturally occurring triglycerides have fatty acids that contain at least 14 carbon atoms. But some fats (such as coconut oil) contain fatty acids with only 6 to 12 carbon atoms. This type of triglyceride is called a **medium-chain triglyceride (MCT).** Unlike long-chain triglycerides (LCT), MCT do not require pancreatic lipase or bile for digestion and absorption. MCT do not form micelles and are absorbed into the portal vein (like amino acids and simple sugars) rather than into the lymphatic system. Thus, MCT can be digested and absorbed very easily by people who can't digest and absorb LCT. MCT can be used as a source of extra kcalories but not as a source of essential fatty acids.

---

diverticulosis (DYE-ver-tic-you-LOH-sis): a condition in which pouches of intestinal lining balloon out through the muscles of the intestinal wall. The pouches are called **diverticula** (DYE-ver-TIC-you-luh; the singular is **diverticulum**); they can become inflamed, a condition called **diverticulitis** (DYE-ver-tic-you-LIGH-tus).

fistula (FIST-you-luh): an abnormal opening between two organs or from an organ to the skin.

fistula = pipe

Diverticular Disease Sometimes pouches, or diverticula, form along the intestine in weak areas of the intestinal muscles, often at points where blood vessels enter the muscle. Evidence suggests that the pouches result from very high pressures in the intestinal lumen. The high pressures are the result of excessive intestinal contractions which cause segments of the intestine to be pinched off. Since the pressure cannot escape completely from the segment, it forces the membrane of the intestine through the weakened intestinal muscle layer (see Figure 8). Diverticulosis is the condition in which diverticula have formed in the intestine.

The person with diverticulosis is symptom-free and may not know the disorder exists. But in some people, fecal material gets trapped in the diverticula, causing inflammation and infection; this condition is called diverticulitis. People with diverticulitis may complain of cramps, alternating periods of diarrhea and constipation, dyspepsia, flatus, and abdominal distention. Occasionally a diverticulum may rupture; this is life-threatening. If the diverticula become inflamed repeatedly, the intestinal wall can thicken, narrowing the intestinal lumen and resulting in an obstruction. An inflamed bowel segment can also stick to other pelvic organs, which can result in fistula formation and obstruction of the intestine — serious medical problems that can be fatal.

For many years, people with diverticulosis have been advised to adopt low-fiber diets. It was believed that fiber could become trapped in the diverticula and cause irritation. However, this advice has changed dramatically in recent years. Many studies suggest that a high-fiber diet is more beneficial than a low-fiber one. One author has suggested that the large fecal mass produced by a high-fiber diet prevents the opposite walls of the intestine from contacting each other

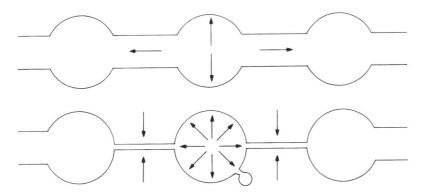

Figure 8 Pressures inside the intestine normally can be dissipated along the length of the bowel. But if contractions are excessive and they pinch off a segment of bowel the pressure cannot escape by the normal route and pouches can form.

(see Figure 9).[9] It is widely believed that a high-fiber diet may reduce the incidence of diverticulosis.[10] Furthermore, many people with established diverticular disease remain symptom-free while following a high-fiber diet.[11]

You can help a client adjust to a high-fiber diet by advising him to increase fiber gradually. During the first few weeks on the diet, the person may feel bloated, pass gas more frequently, or experience heartburn. If the person is forewarned about these symptoms, compliance with the diet will be better.

Many people with diverticulosis, particularly older people, have been following a low-fiber diet for many years. They may be apprehensive about switching to a high-fiber diet. After all, they had been told that the low-fiber diet would prevent symptoms and they may be fearful of trying once-forbidden foods. They may be skeptical about any diet after having received such contradictory advice. What can you do? In addition to following the advice given above, you can acknowledge their concerns and try to stress the value of the diet. Also, try gaining their involvement and cooperation during the teaching process.

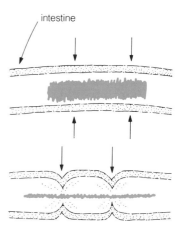
intestine

Figure 9 Rationale for the use of a high-fiber diet in diverticulosis. A large fecal mass physically prevents the opposite walls of the intestine from contacting to meet each other. This reduces the likelihood of segmentation and resulting high intralumenal pressures which predispose the individual to diverticulosis.

[9]S. A. Broitman and N. Zamcheck, Nutrition in diseases of the intestine, in *Modern Nutrition in Health and Disease*, ed. R. S. Goodhart and M. E. Shils (Philadelphia: Lea & Febiger, 1980), p. 943.

[10]N. S. Painter, A. Z. Almeida, and K. W. Colebourne, Unprocessed bran in treatment of diverticular disease of the colon, *British Medical Journal* 2 (1972):137-140; A. J. M. Brodribb, Treatment of symptomatic diverticular disease with a high-fibre diet, *Lancet* 1 (1977):664-666; J. M. P. Hyland and I. Taylor, Does a high fibre diet prevent the complications of diverticular disease? *British Journal of Surgery* 67 (1980):77-79.

[11]Hyland and Taylor, 1980.

Crohn's disease: inflammation and ulceration along the length of the GI tract, often with granulomas.

ulcerative colitis: inflammation and ulceration of the colon.

granuloma (gran-you-LOH-muh): a granular tumor or growth.

  oma = a growth

Inflammatory Bowel Disease Several conditions can cause inflammation of the bowel and can result in malabsorption. In this section we will be discussing two such disorders, Crohn's disease and ulcerative colitis, which frequently are accompanied by malnutrition.

Crohn's disease and ulcerative colitis are two distinct disorders that show similar clinical, pathologic, and biologic features. Their cause or causes remain unknown. In Crohn's disease inflammation of the bowel is accompanied by cracklike ulcers and many granulomas. The incidence of Crohn's disease has been increasing worldwide, and it has become a problem of major concern.[12] Symptoms can occur anywhere in the GI tract but most often are found in the ileum and colon. The person with Crohn's disease often reports weight loss, fever, diarrhea, and cramping abdominal pain. The disease may be self-limited and eventually be cured, but it often recurs. Inflammation and scarring may narrow the intestinal lumen, sometimes causing obstruction.

Antibacterial drugs (most commonly sulfasalazine) and corticosteroids are given to treat the disease. Oftentimes, the diseased portion of the bowel must be removed surgically. Even after surgery, the disease often flares up in other areas of the bowel and surgery may have to be performed several times.

The person with Crohn's disease is at high risk for developing nutrient deficiencies for many reasons. For one, malabsorption limits the availability of nutrients. Diarrhea can upset fluid, electrolyte, and zinc balances. The person usually has lost weight, and during periods when the disease is active, abdominal pain and emotional stress may cause food intake to be reduced considerably. Also, many times oral intake is withheld so that the bowel can rest, particularly when the person has developed an obstruction or when a fistula has formed. Furthermore, the drug therapy used to treat the disease can also affect nutrition status (see Chapter 21). Sulfasalazine appears to interfere with the absorption and utilization of folacin, and corticosteroids interfere with the absorption of calcium.[13] If surgery is required, nutrient needs become even greater. Because a portion of the bowel is removed during surgery, the surgery itself can contribute to malabsorption.

As you can see, restoring and maintaining nutrition status for the person with Crohn's disease can be an extremely difficult task. Multiple nutrient deficiencies can develop, and they may reduce the effectiveness of drug therapy and threaten immune function.[14] Deficiencies of calcium, magnesium, zinc, iron, vitamin B_{12}, folacin, vitamin C, and

[12]J. B. Kirsner and R. G. Shorter, Recent developments in "nonspecific" inflammatory bowel disease, part I. *New England Journal of Medicine* 306 (1982):775-785.

[13]M. D. Sitrin, I. H. Rosenberg, K. Chawla, S. Meredith, J. Sellin, J. M. Rabb, F. Coe, J. B. Kirsner, and S. C. Kraft, Nutritional and metabolic complications in a patient with Crohn's disease and ileal resection, *Gastroenterology* 78 (1980):1069-1079.

[14]Kirsner and Shorter, 1982.

fat-soluble vitamins are commonly reported.[15]

As mentioned earlier, during the acute stages of the disease, bowel rest is sometimes desirable. This may be true when any food intake increases diarrhea significantly, when the bowel is obstructed, or when resting the bowel might help a fistula to close. When complete bowel rest is desired, the patient can be given all nutrients intravenously by means of TPN (see Chapter 20). In some cases, complete bowel rest can eliminate the need for surgery.[16]

Hydrolyzed and elemental diets have been used successfully during acute periods of Crohn's disease to provide nutrition without the need for TPN. Since hydrolyzed formulas are easily absorbed in the upper small intestine, they also allow the bowel to rest. The person may accept the formula by mouth if you experiment with different flavors and serving techniques. However, a tube feeding can be used if the person can't drink the formula. A word of caution: Hydrolyzed formulas are hypertonic. They can worsen diarrhea if they are not administered properly (see Chapter 20).

During periods of remission, people with Crohn's disease often are advised to follow low-fiber diets. This suggestion is based on the belief that roughage may increase the chance that an intestinal obstruction will form. However, the value of this suggestion has been questioned.[17] You can help patients most by encouraging them to eat a nutrient-rich, well-balanced diet and by reassessing their nutrition status frequently to assure that their nutrient needs are being met.

> The person with Crohn's disease often needs a lot of emotional support. The typical patient is young (the incidence is highest in teenagers) and often depressed. After all, the disease is highly unpredictable. Just when a person feels well, a relapse may occur, necessitating another round of surgery. The person may feel that food itself causes the disease, and may react by eating very little.

Unlike Crohn's disease, which can occur anywhere along the GI tract, ulcerative colitis occurs only in the large intestine. It is characterized by severe diarrhea, rectal bleeding, cramping, abdominal pain, anorexia, and weight loss. The diarrhea can be almost continuous, resulting in poor absorption of nutrients and great losses of fluids and electrolytes. Anemia may be present because of blood loss from rectal bleeding. The

---

[15]Nutrient deficiences of inflammatory bowel disease. *Nutrition and the MD*, June 1981; Nutritional support in Crohn's disease, *Nutrition and the MD*, March 1977.

[16]C. O. Elson, T. J. Layden, B. A. Nemchausky, J. L. Rosenberg, and I. H. Rosenberg, An evaluation of total parenteral nutrition in the management of inflammatory bowel disease, *Digestive Diseases and Sciences* 25 (1980):42-48.

[17]K. W. Heaton, J. R. Thornton, and P. M. Emmett, Treatment of Crohn's disease with an unrefined-carbohydrate, fibre-rich diet, *British Medical Journal* 2 (1979):764-766.

same dietary principles discussed for Crohn's disease apply to the person with ulcerative colitis. However, complete bowel rest with the use of TPN has been less successful for ulcerative colitis than for Crohn's disease.[18]

Intestinal Surgery   Surgery of the intestine may be necessary for some people with inflammatory bowel diseases, cancer of the intestine, obstruction, diverticulitis, or impaired blood supply to the intestine. In an intestinal resection a segment of intestine is cut out. Generally, up to 50 percent of the small bowel can be resected without serious consequences. The actual absorption of nutrients after a small bowel resection depends on three factors:

- The extent and location of the resection.
- The presence or absence of the ileocecal valve (p. 151).
- The adaptive ability of the remaining bowel.

When a large segment of the small intestine must be resected, the absorptive surface of the small intestine is reduced considerably. The person may experience diarrhea, weight loss, muscle wasting, protein and fat malabsorption, hypocalcemia, hypomagnesemia, and anemia. When several of these conditions occur at the same time they are collectively called the *short-bowel* or *short-gut syndrome.*

People with short-bowel syndrome generally absorb carbohydrates and most water-soluble vitamins without difficulty. When more than 8 feet of the proximal jejunum have been resected, however, the absorption of fat, protein, fat-soluble vitamins, calcium, and magnesium can be impaired. When the ileum has been resected, vitamin B_{12} must be supplemented parenterally, since the ileum is the site of vitamin B_{12} absorption. Also, bile salts are normally reabsorbed in the ileum. If they are not reabsorbed there will be a decreased body pool of bile salts available for recycling and repeated fat absorption.

The ileocecal valve plays an important role in controlling the rate at which the intestinal contents move from the small to the large bowel. When the valve is absent, transit time through the small intestine is rapid, decreasing the time available for the absorption of nutrients.

Following a resection of the small intestine, a remarkable adaptive mechanism occurs provided that adequate nutrients have been given. The portion of the bowel that remains intact gets bigger, thus expanding its ability to absorb nutrients. The presence of nutrients in the remaining gut appears to stimulate this adaptive process. However, it is important to note that if too much bowel has been resected, even this adaptation will be inadequate. People who become malnourished despite all other efforts at prevention may require permanent support by parenteral means.

Immediately after surgery, the primary nutrition concern is the replacement of fluids and electrolytes. Parenteral feedings are given in

short-bowel syndrome: a complex of symptoms, which may include diarrhea, weight loss, malabsorption, hypocalcemia, hypomagnesemia, and anemia, that can occur whenever the absorptive surface of the small bowel is reduced.

proximal: the first part or the part that is closest to the point of attachment.

creatorrhea (cree-AT-or-REE-uh): excretion of excessive amounts of amino acids and peptides in the stool.

   creato = creatinine, a nitrogen-containing substance

---

[18]Elson and co-authors, 1980.

the period immediately after surgery. Oral feeding, tube feeding, or TPN should be initiated as soon as possible to insure that kcaloric and protein needs are met. The diet is gradually progressed to a high-protein, low-fat, oral diet. The recommendation to restrict fat is based on the finding that reducing fat intake reduces steatorrhea and, thus, helps minimize the loss of fat, fat-soluble vitamins, calcium, and magnesium (see also steatorrhea, p. 881). MCT can be used to provide additional kcalories. It is important to note, however, that a high-fat diet has also been found successful in managing short-bowel syndrome.[19] Although steatorrhea increased when fat intake increased, the total amount of fat absorbed also increased, and weight gain was possible. Further studies will be required to clarify which therapy is best.

When the large intestine is resected, individual nutrient deficiencies are less likely to occur, because absorption has already taken place before the intestinal contents reach the colon. Still, losses of fluids and electrolytes can become a problem, since they are normally reabsorbed in the colon.

An ileostomy involves the removal of the entire colon and rectum; a stoma, or opening, is made from the ileum and brought out through the abdomen to allow for defecation (See Figure 10). In a colostomy only the rectum and anus are removed and the stoma is formed from the remaining part of the colon. A watery stool will result from an ileostomy, while a more formed stool is produced by a colostomy.

Figure 10

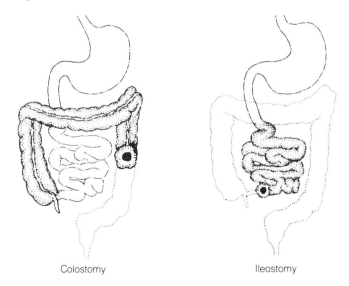

Colostomy   Ileostomy

[19]V. Simko, A. M. McCarroll, S. Goodman, R. E. Weesner, and R. E. Kelley, High-fat diet in a short bowel syndrome, *Digestive Diseases and Sciences* 25 (1980):333-339; V. Simko and W. G. Linscheer, Absorption of different elemental diets in a short-bowel syndrome lasting 15 years, *American Journal of Digestive Diseases* 21 (1976):419-425.

ostomate (OSS-toh-mate): a person who has a surgically formed opening from the bowel to the outside of the body, bypassing the anus. An **ileostomate** (ill-ee-OSS-toh-mate) has an **ileostomy**; a **colostomate** (co-LOSS-toh-mate) has a **colostomy**.

stoma = window

A health care professional specially trained to work with ostomates is the **enterostomal** (en-ter-oh-STOME-al) **therapist (E.T.)**.

celiac disease (SEEL-ee-ac): a sensitivity to gliaden that causes flattening of the intestinal villi and generalized malabsorption. Also called **gluten sensitive enteropathy** (en-ter-OP-uh-thee) or celiac sprue.

gluten (GLOOT-en): a protein found in wheat, oats, rye, and barley.

gliaden (GLEE-uh-den): a fraction of the gluten protein.

atrophy: shrinking.
a = without
trophy = growth

disaccharidase: see p. 99.

protein losing enteropathy: excessive loss of protein into the bowel; can result from numerous disorders.

After oral intake is initiated following surgery, ileostomy and colostomy patients are generally placed on a bland, low-fiber diet to help promote healing of the stoma and prevent irritation. However, as soon as possible each patient should be encouraged to resume a normal diet. Foods should be added individually and in small amounts so that their effects can be assessed. If a new food causes problems, it can be tried again a few months later.

Ostomy patients are often concerned about gas, odor, and loose and watery stools. Foods that cause excessively watery stools must be determined individually for each patient. Some raw fruits and vegetables and highly spiced foods cause problems for some ileostomates. Beer and other alcoholic beverages may cause diarrhea and gas. Gas and odors can be caused by such foods as beans, onions, green pepper, cabbage, turnips, and beets.

You must stress the importance of drinking plenty of fluids to the ostomate. Such patients may be inclined not to drink fluids, in hopes of controlling their diarrhea. But since they are not absorbing water in the colon, dehydration can result if fluids are not adequately replaced. Reassure patients that excess fluid, taken above and beyond the amount lost via the ostomy, will be absorbed and excreted by the kidneys and will not worsen the diarrhea.

New ostomates have many adjustments to make after surgery. They may feel they have lost control over a very basic and private function. The retraining required to care for the ostomy and maintain bowel function may be difficult. Ostomates may also be worried that loved ones, particularly spouses, may find them unattractive. The health care team must work closely with each patient and family to help them make the necessary adjustments and resume normal activities.

Celiac Disease   Adult celiac disease provides an example of how changes in intestinal mucosal cells can cause malabsorption. The incidence of celiac disease is about 1 in every 2,000 to 3,000 births. The individual with celiac disease is sensitive to gluten, a protein found in wheat, oats, rye, and barley. A fraction of the gluten protein, gliadin, acts as a toxic substance. It causes the intestinal villi to atrophy, seriously reducing the absorptive surface of the intestinal tract. The disaccharidases and carrier molecules normally found on the villi become deficient. Malabsorption of many nutrients, including fat, protein, carbohydrate, fat-soluble vitamins, iron, calcium, magnesium, zinc, and some water-soluble vitamins, results.

The person with celiac disease often experiences steatorrhea, diarrhea, weight loss, and malnutrition. Anemia may occur as a result of iron, folacin, or vitamin B_{12} deficiency. Because protein is malabsorbed, serum protein levels can fall dramatically and edema and swelling result. The celiac patient may bleed easily because of clotting abnormalities precipitated by a vitamin K deficiency. Furthermore, calcium deficiency can result in tetany (p. 414) and bone pain.

Fortunately, the intestinal changes can gradually return to near normal when gluten is removed from the diet. Generally, improvement can be expected within a few weeks if the diet is strictly followed. However, lactase deficiency and lactose intolerance may be permanent. If the patient does not follow the diet, symptoms return.

The treatment for celiac disease sounds deceptively simple: eliminate gluten. Unfortunately, gluten is found in many common foods. As you can see from Table 7, many foods contain wheat, oats, rye, or barley in some form. Wheat flour is used as an extender in many processed foods (ice cream, salad dressings, canned foods). The patient must understand how to read labels and must appreciate the importance of avoiding offending substances.

You can help the celiac patient not only by helping her to understand what foods to avoid but also by helping her make palatable dietary substitutions. Arrowroot, corn, potato, rice, and soybean flours can be used to replace wheat flour in some recipes. A low-gluten wheat starch flour is also available for use as a substitute (see Appendix C for some references for people with allergies and intolerances).

Disaccharidase Deficiencies The disaccharidases are the enzymes that split disaccharides (lactose, sucrose, and maltose) to monosaccharides (glucose, galactose, and fructose) so that they can be absorbed. The disaccharidases are normally found along the intestinal villi. When there is a deficiency of any disaccharidase, carbohydrate malabsorption results. The unhydrolyzed disaccharide remains unabsorbed in the intestine, causing the intestinal contents to become hyperosmolar. Large volumes of water are drawn into the gut to equalize the osmolarity, and this results in cramps, distention, and diarrhea. Bacteria present in the intestine metabolize the undigested sugars to irritating acids that further contribute to cramping and diarrhea.

Lactase deficiency is the most frequently seen disaccharidase deficiency. In rare cases a person is simply born with a deficiency of lactase. More often, lactase deficiency develops as a consequence of another disease, or lactase levels decrease as the person ages.

The intestinal cells that produce lactase are located on the delicate fringe of microvilli that form the brush border of the intestinal villi (see p. 173). Any condition that changes the brush border can lead to lactose intolerance. We have already discussed some disorders and conditions that can result in either temporary or permanent lactose intolerance: inflammatory bowel disease, celiac disease, protein-kcalorie malnutrition, GI tract surgery, and radiation therapy.

Some people are born with normal lactase levels that gradually decrease to low levels as they become adults. This type of lactose intolerance is more prevalent among blacks, native Americans, and Orientals than among Caucasians.

The amount of lactose that can be tolerated varies greatly among individuals. Many can include moderate amounts of lactose-containing

Principles of dietary management of celiac disease:

Eliminate wheat, oats, rye, and barley. (How to remember: WORB.)

Read labels carefully.

Substitute arrowroot, potato, corn, rice, and soybean flours for wheat flour.

lactose intolerance: malabsorption of lactose because of a lactase deficiency. A person born with little or no lactase activity has **primary lactose intolerance. Secondary lactose intolerance** is caused by another disease. **Developmental lactose intolerance** describes a lactase deficiency that develops as a person ages. More on lactose intolerance appears in Highlight 15, with a table of the lactose contents of foods.

Table 7.   Gluten-Restricted, Gliadin-Free Diet

Foods allowed

Beverages

Carbonated drinks, cocoa (no wheat flour added), coffee, decaffeinated coffee to which no wheat flour has been added, fruit juices and drinks, milk (at least 2 cups a day), tea

Breads and flour products

Bread products made only from arrowroot, buckwheat, cornmeal, wheat starch, soybean flour, or gluten free wheat starch; cornbread, muffins, and pone with no wheat flour; cornstarch; gluten free macaroni products; gluten free porridge; rice wafers; soybean wafers, pure; rice, sago, and tapioca

Foods excluded

Beverages

Ale, beer, cereal beverages such as Postum and Ovaltine, commercial chocolate milk with cereal additive, instant coffee containing wheat, root beer

Breads and flour products

Breaded foods, breads, rolls, crackers, etc., made from wheat, rye, oats, or barley; commercial gluten bread; commercially prepared mixes for biscuits, cornbread, muffins, pancakes, buckwheat pancakes, waffles, etc.

The following list of foods to be avoided is not all-inclusive (read labels):

All-purpose flour
Baking powder biscuits
Barley flour
Bran
Bread crumbs
Bread flour
Cake mixes
Cookie mixes
Cracker meal
Graham flour
Macaroni
Malt
Matzoth
Noodles
Pancakes
Pastry flour
Pretzels
Rye flour
Rye krisp
Spaghetti flour
Self-rising flour
Vermicelli
Waffles
Wheat, cracked wheat, and whole wheat flours
Wheat germ
Zwieback

Table 7.   Gluten-Restricted, Gliadin-Free Diet (continued)

Foods allowed

Cereals

Corn or rice cereals such as (read labels):

Cornmeal
Cornflakes
Cream of Rice
Hominy
Puffed rice
Rice flakes

Foods excluded

Cereals

All cereals containing malt, bran, or wheat germ or made of rye, wheat, oats, or barley.

The following is not an all-inclusive list:

All Bran
Barley
Branflakes
Cream of Wheat
Farina
Grapenuts
Grapenuts Flakes
Instant Cream of Wheat
Kaska
Krumbles
Oatmeal
Pablum
Pep
Pettijohns
Puffed wheat
Ralston
Ralston Bits
Shredded Ralston
Shredded wheat
Super farina
Wheatena
Wheat flakes
Wheaties
Wheat Oata
Whole Bran

Desserts

Cakes, cookies, pastries, etc., prepared with permitted low gluten flours or instant potato granules; custard; gelatin desserts; homemade cornstarch and rice puddings; ice cream and sherbet if they do not contain gluten stabilizers; tapioca pudding

Desserts

Cakes, cookies, commercial ice cream with gluten stabilizers, doughnuts, ice cream cones, pie, prepared mixes, prepared pudding thickened with wheat flour

Fats

Butter; corn oil; French dressing, pure; margarine, fortified; mayonnaise, pure; olive oil, other animal and vegetable fats and oils

Fats

Commercial salad dressings that contain gluten stabilizers, homemade cooked salad dressings if thickened with flour

Miscellaneous

Pepper, pickles, popcorn, potato chips, sugars and syrups, vinegar, molasses

Soups

Broth, bouillon, clear meat and vegetable soups, cream soups thickened with cream or allowed starches or flours

Soups

All soups thickened with wheat products or containing barley, noodles, or other wheat, rye and oat products in any form

Source: American Dietetic Association, *Handbook of Clinical Dietetics* (New Haven, Conn.: Yale University Press), 1981.

foods with no ill effects. Others may be hypersensitive to as little as a few grams of lactose such as might be found in a capsule of medicine. Highlight 15 contains information on the lactose content of foods.

Food Allergies and Sensitivities

People can have many adverse reactions to food. Food allergy mediated by the immune system is one such reaction. Others, not mediated through the immune system, have been variously called food sensitivities, food intolerances, and (incorrectly) food allergies; authorities differ as to the definitions of these terms. For our purposes, it seems prudent to avoid use of all these terms except food allergy and to group these poorly understood conditions under the term *adverse reactions to food.*

A true food allergy can arise in more than one way. Sometimes a protein from food is absorbed whole into the bloodstream instead of being digested and then absorbed as amino acids in the normal way. Once inside the body, the protein acts as an antigen (Highlight 22), eliciting the formation of antibodies. Thereafter, the body "remembers" to react to this particular protein and the person is allergic to the food. Even if its proteins don't get into the bloodstream again, the presence of this food in the GI tract triggers an allergic reaction. Symptoms vary, but can include bloating, belching, nausea, diarrhea, or constipation, as well as skin rashes, nasal congestion, bronchitis, and asthma.

Common food allergies include allergies to milk, wheat, eggs, nuts, fish, and seeds. They tend to be most prevalent early in life, with the incidence declining later in childhood. Oftentimes, an allergy to one food is associated with allergies to other foods in the same biological family. Sometimes allergic reactions occur shortly after a food has been ingested, but in other cases hours or even days may lapse before symptoms appear.

elimination diet: a diet used to detect food allergies. At first, all common food allergens are omitted; then new foods are introduced gradually, one by one.

allergen: a substance that causes an allergic reaction.

Food allergies are difficult to diagnose and may go undetected. If an allergy is suspected, it can be identified by means of systematic detective work including clinical history, diet diaries, elimination diets, food challenges, and laboratory tests.

The simplest type of elimination diet requires that the person avoid all suspected foods for a period of time. If the symptoms abate, then suspected foods are added back individually or in small groups to see if the symptoms reappear. Another, better controlled approach is to present the person with suspected substances in a vehicle such as cookies, applesauce, or large capsules. Repeated allergic responses to a particular food, together with non-responses to placebos presented in the same fashion can pin down an allergy quite accurately.

When the offending food or foods have been identified, they are eliminated from the diet. In young children the food can be reintroduced 6 to 12 months later to determine if they have developed a tolerance for it.

It is generally believed that the likelihood of food allergies is reduced if potent food allergens such as unmodified milk, eggs, and wheat are withheld for the first 9 months of life. During early life these allergens may be more readily absorbed through the immature GI tract. In any case, foods should be introduced into the infant's diet one at a time so that possible allergens can be identified.

Not all adverse reactions to food are true allergies. For example, celiac disease, already discussed, involves an adverse reaction to a protein in wheat, but this reaction does not seem to be mediated by the immune system. Another adverse reaction previously mentioned is lactose intolerance, caused by the lack of an enzyme and the resulting bacterial fermentation of milk sugar. It is important to identify conditions like this so that the offending foods can be avoided.

Careful testing will sometimes show, however, that there is no allergy or other physical response to the food at all. The person reacts only if he knows he is eating the foods — but then the reaction can be dramatic. People have strong feelings about food, including intense fears and food aversions. Highlight 16 sorts out some of the feelings people can have about "guilt trip" foods like sugar, and Chapter 28 describes the way in which food aversions develop.

Nutrition Assessment of Patients with GI Disorders

As we have seen, diseases of the GI tract can affect nutrition status by interfering with food intake, affecting the absorption of nutrients, or increasing nutrient needs. Some important points to remember in interpreting nutrition assessment data follow:

1. It is of utmost importance to get a very detailed history of weight fluctuations, food tolerances, and chronic drug use. Weight loss commonly occurs in GI tract disorders, and the GI patient is at risk for protein-kcalorie malnutrition. Likewise, the chronic drug use often prescribed for people with GI tract disorders can contribute to malnutrition. A history of food tolerances is extremely important in planning a diet that will cause the least discomfort.

2. Anthropometric measurements will be affected by the state of hydration. Keep in mind that anthropometric measurements, including weight, may be deceptive in people who have edema. Remember that people with low serum albumin levels (malabsorption, weight loss) often have edema.

3. Biochemical measurements may falsely appear to be high in dehydration. You should consider dehydration a possibility in anyone who is is experiencing severe diarrhea or vomiting.

4. Individual nutrient deficiencies can be present in people with long-standing GI tract disorders. You must assess not only their intake but also note any possible interferences with absorption (short gut, dumping syndrome).

Summing Up

Disorders of the GI tract often have an impact on nutrition status because they affect intake, absorption, and nutrient needs. The intake of food can be difficult for people with disorders that alter normal chewing and swallowing. Intake can also be affected when nausea, vomiting, or other abdominal disorders are present.

Many disorders can cause the malabsorption of nutrients: decreased availability of digestive enzymes or bile salts, decreased surface area for absorption, or changes in the intestinal villi that reduce ability to absorb nutrients. Steatorrhea is commonly seen in malabsorption. When fat is lost in the stool, weight loss is likely to occur. Fat-soluble vitamins, calcium, and magnesium are lost along with the fat, increasing the likelihood that deficiencies will be present.

In actuality very little is known about the effects of different nutrients on the GI tract. There is controversy over what the best diet is for almost every GI tract disorder. For the present, the best policy is to work closely with the individual, tailoring the diet to his or her personal tolerances.

To Explore Further

The number of references devoted to diseases of the GI tract and their interactions with nutrition is overwhelming. It would be impossible to list more than a few here.

Excellent reviews that discuss several GI tract disorders with emphasis on nutrition include:

- Heizer, W. D. Nutritional problems in gastrointestinal diseases. *Gastrointestinal Diseases* 7 (1981):59-64.

- Dolin, B. J., and Boyce, H. W. Dietary management of gastrointestinal disorders. *Journal of the Florida Medical Association* 66 (1979):395-401.

- Leslie, J. Nutrition and diet, part 8: Care of the patient with gastro-intestinal disease. *Nursing Mirror*, September 1977, pp. 28-30.

- Gastrointestinal diseases. *Dietary Modifications in Disease*. Columbus, Ohio: Ross Laboratories, 1978 (address in Appendix J).

- Council on Foods and Nutrition. Diet as related to gastrointestinal function. *Journal of the American Medical Association* 176 (1961):935-941.

- Holt, P. R. Malabsorption. *Nutrition in Disease*. Columbus, Ohio: Ross Laboratories, 1977 (address in Appendix J).

The entire issue of *Nutrition and the MD*, August 1982, discussed nutrition care in common disorders involving the GI tract.

Reviews and research articles on specific disorders include:

- Lee, K. A. *Dysphagia and Its Dietary Management: A Review for Dietitians.* New York: K. A. Lee, 1981. Available for about $2 from K. A. Lee, 112 Circle Road, Staten Island, NY 10304.

- Pope, C. E. Pathophysiology and diagnosis of reflux esophagitis. *Gastroenterology* 70 (1976):445-454.

- Pops, M. A. Peptic ulcer disease: Should you prescribe a diet? *Nutrition and the MD*, May 1978.

- Spiro, H. M. Is milk all that bad for the ulcer patient? *Journal of Clinical Gastroenterology* 3 (1981):219-220. This article takes a positive view of the traditional ulcer diet.

- Samborsky, V. Drug therapy for peptic ulcer. *American Journal of Nursing* 78 (1978):2064-2066.

- Levine, A. S. The relationship of diet to intestinal gas. *Contemporary Nutrition* 4 (1979).

- Battle, E. H., and Hanna, C. E. Evaluation of a dietary regimen for chronic constipation. *Journal of Gerontological Nursing* 6 (1980):527-532.

- Eshchar, J., and Cohen, L. Re-education of constipated patients — a non-medicinal treatment. *American Journal of Proctology, Gastroenterology and Colon and Rectal Surgery*, September 1981, pp. 16-24.

- Hyland, J. M. P., and Taylor, I. Does a high fibre diet prevent the complications of diverticular disease? *British Journal of Surgery* 67 (1980):77-79.

- Ornstein, M. H., Littlewood, E. R., Baird, I. M., Fowler, J., North, W. R. S., and Cox, A. G. Are fibre supplements really necessary in diverticular disease of the colon? A controlled clinical trial. *British Medical Journal* 282 (1981):1353-1356. This article touched off a lot of controversy, as it concluded that bran does not help diverticular disease except in that it reduces constipation.

- Fielding, J. F., and Melvin, K. Dietary fibre and irritable bowel syndrome. *Journal of Human Nutrition* 33 (1979):243-247.

- Kirsner, J. B., and Shorter, R. G. Recent developments in "nonspecific" inflammatory bowel disease, parts 1 & 2. *New England Journal of Medicine* 306 (1982):775-785, 837-848. This excellent review contains almost 400 references on Crohn's disease and ulcerative colitis.

- Janowitz, H. D. Crohn's disease — 50 years later. *New England Journal of Medicine* 304 (1981):1600-1602.

- Heaton, K. W., Thornton, J. R., and Emmett, P. M. Treatment of Crohn's disease with an unrefined-carbohydrate, fibre-rich diet. *British Medical Journal* 2 (1979):764-766.

- Logan, R. F. A., Gillon, J., Ferrington, C., and Ferguson, A. Reduction of gastrointestinal protein loss by elemental diet in Crohn's disease of the small bowel. *Gut* 22 (1981):383-387.

- Nutrient deficiencies of inflammatory bowel disease. *Nutrition and the MD*, June 1981.

- Nutritional support in Crohn's disease. *Nutrition and the MD*, October 1977.

- Nutritional considerations in ulcerative colitis. *Nutrition and the MD*, February 1978.

- Klish, W. J., and Putnam, T. C. The short gut. *American Journal of Diseases in Children* 135 (1981):1056-1061.

- Dietary management of ostomy patients. *Nutrition and the MD*, May 1978.

- Behm, V., Murchie, G., and King, D. R. Nutritional care of the patient following gastric surgery. *Dietetic Currents*, March-April 1974. Available from Ross Laboratories (address in Appendix J).

- Curreri, P. W., and Richmond, D. Nutritional management following massive small bowel resection. *Dietetic Currents*, July-August 1974. Available from Ross Laboratories (address in Appendix J).

- Treatment of lactose intolerance. *Medical Letter* 23 (1981):67-68.

- Welsh, J. D. Diet therapy in adult lactose malabsorption: Present practices. *American Journal of Clinical Nutrition* 31 (1978):592-596.

Several booklets for people with allergies are listed in Appendix C.

- Corman, M. L., Veidenheimer, M. C., and Collier, J. A. Cathartics. *American Journal of Nursing* 75 (1975):273-279. It lists about 90 over-the-counter laxatives by brand name with classification and site of action.

Crohn's Disease

Tim was first diagnosed with Crohn's disease when he was 21 years old. At that time he weighed 155 lb and was 6 ft 2 in tall. His normal weight had been about 180 lb until he began having the symptoms that eventually were found to be caused by Crohn's disease. Since that time he has been hospitalized several times and has undergone surgery twice to resect portions of his bowel. He has had an ileostomy. He is now 24, his weight has slipped down to 130 lb and he is in the hospital again with a suspected intestinal obstruction. As anticipated from his weight loss and history, Tim's nutrition assessment reveals that he is suffering from protein-kcalorie malnutrition. Tim's doctor has decided to begin TPN, with strict orders that Tim have nothing by mouth. The doctor hopes that further surgery can be avoided.

Study Questions

1. Review Tim's weight history. What is his ideal weight? What is his %IBW? What is his %UBW? What does his weight history suggest about his food in-take? What measures could have been taken to avoid the 50-lb weight loss that Tim has experienced over the past three years? Can this rate of weight loss continue?

2. Do you agree with the doctor's decision to place Tim on TPN? Why or why not? If Tim were allowed to take food by mouth what type of diet should probably be prescribed?

3. Assume that Tim does well on TPN and is able to avoid surgery. What type of diet should he be placed on? Are any food precautions made necessary by his ileostomy? What individual nutrients should be considered?

4. Consider Tim's long-term dietary management. What goals for weight gain would you establish? How would you monitor results?

Optional Extra

Try placing yourself on a traditional bland diet for a day. Plan your day's food in advance taking into account your nutrient needs, schedule, and budget. Make your diet adequate. If you are on duty in the hospital at lunchtime, take along a lunch that is permitted. If you have to shop for special items, notice how this affects your pocketbook.

Remember to eliminate all coffee, alcohol, pepper, highly spiced foods, raw fruits, raw vegetables, fried meats, and luncheon meats for the day. How does all this planning and changing of your habitual routine affect you physically? Psychologically? Carry a writing pad with you and jot down notes about every two hours on what you ate/are eating and how you feel.

This exercise should give you insight into what we are really demanding of clients when we "put" them on special diets. Share your experiences with other class members in a class discussion.

Surgery: Last Hope for Weight Loss

Physicians recommending and surgeons carrying out jejunoileostomy for morbid obesity must understand they are creating one disease to alleviate another. A careful risk-benefit evaluation must be done to justify the induction of potentially fatal malnutrition of the lean body and skeleton as the price for the mobilization of unwanted lipid in adipocytes.

NUTRITION REVIEWS

At 25 years old, Mary is desperate. She has been grossly obese since childhood. Now she finds herself, at 5 feet 4 inches tall, weighing 315 pounds. Over the years she has developed high blood pressure, and recently she has been diagnosed with diabetes. She is at high risk for developing heart disease. Mary has reached the point in her life when she realizes how many things have passed her by because of her weight. She thinks about the job she wanted but couldn't get, friends and boyfriends she never had, and the endless jokes and advice she has heard about her weight. Worst of all, she lives with the feeling that it is "all her fault" — that she is a failure.

Mary's doctor also is alarmed. Mary's mounting health problems and her mental state are major concerns. Mary and her doctor have tried everything they could think of to help her lose weight: low-kcalorie diets, supervised fasting, exercise programs, behavior modification techniques, and even diet pills. It came as no surprise to the doctor when Mary asked him about her last hope: surgery.

Mary's doctor, who wasn't experienced with surgery for morbid obesity, told Mary he had some questions he wanted answered before he could advise her about the surgery. Here are some of the things he learned before he saw Mary again.

Who is a Candidate for Surgery?

One thing is clear: surgical procedures for weight loss present significant danger and should be used only when all else fails. Major and sometimes fatal complications can occur.

Although the exact standards used to determine whether an obese person is a candidate for surgery vary, some typical considerations include the following:

● The person must be morbidly obese. Some surgeons take this to mean that the person must be at least 100 lb overweight. For others, morbid obesity means a body weight twice or more the average desirable weight as given in life insurance tables.

● The person with a chronic disease such as diabetes, high blood pressure, or heart disease or the person whose life is otherwise in danger because of obesity may be considered for surgery.

● The candidate must have tried seriously and repeatedly to lose weight, by such means as dieting in several different ways, exercising, and taking medications, if approved.

● The candidate must be willing to return for followup for a number of years.

● People with liver disease or alcoholism, kidney disease, or gastrointestinal disease (except gallstones) are *not* candidates for surgery.

Prior to surgery the candidate must understand that there are many potential complications from the surgery; she may have to live with some of them, such as diarrhea, for the rest of her life. Furthermore, the candidate should know that she may need surgery again either to reverse or revise the original procedure.

Types of Surgery for Obesity

There are two basic approaches to surgery for obesity — gastric and intestinal — and each approach includes several types of operations. Figure 1 shows some of these operations, and the Miniglossary defines some relevant terms.

The first surgical approach used to treat obesity was the intestinal approach, also called the jejunoileal (JI) bypass. The idea behind the JI bypass is that shortening the intestine leaves less area for absorption of nutrients. The duodenum is left intact. A short length of the jejunum (about 12 inches) is left intact and connected to the last portion of the ileum (about 4 inches). About 90 percent of the small intestine is bypassed.

Another, more recent, surgical approach is the gastric bypass. With this procedure a small pouch is created in the first part of the stomach with an opening to allow food to pass into the rest of the intestine. In effect, the surgeon makes the stomach so small that it cannot hold very much at a time. The pouch is made to hold only about 60 ml (about 1-1/2 oz), and the diameter of the outlet is only 12 mm (about 1/2 in).

The Jejunoileal Bypass
It was originally thought that weight loss would result

> **Miniglossary**
>
> **gastric bypass:** surgical procedure in which a small pouch is created in the upper part of the stomach to reduce its storage capacity. In the **Roux-Y** (ROO-WYE) **procedure**, a loop of jejunum is attached to the stomach and an opening created (see Figure 1). In **gastroplasty** or **gastric plication** (GAS-troh-plasty, pligh-CAY-shun), the stomach is partitioned with surgical staples. A small opening is left for gastric emptying.
>
> **Jejunoileal (JI) bypass:** surgical procedure in which a short segment of jejunum is attached directly to the terminal ileum, bypassing about 90 percent of the small intestine. In an **end-to-end** procedure, the bypassed bowel is closed off at the jejunal end, while the ileal end is attached to the transverse colon. If an **end-to-side** procedure is used, only the jejunal end of the bypassed bowel needs to be closed (see Figure 1).
>
> **morbid obesity:** twice or more the average desirable weight given in life insurance tables or 100 lb more than the desirable weight.
>
> **take-down:** the surgery to reverse a JI bypass.

from malabsorption in people with a JI bypass, but this turned out to be only partly true. Studies have shown that food intake is decreased in JI bypass patients and that this contributes to

their weight loss.[1] Weight loss is rapid right after surgery, but it levels off after about 12 to 24 months. After this time weight actually increases somewhat in most patients. The typical patient loses about two-thirds of the excess weight after JI bypass surgery. The leveling off of weight loss occurs when the remaining functional intestine has increased in size so that it can absorb more nutrients.

Although the JI bypass is an effective way for the morbidly obese person to lose weight, the big question is, at what price? Serious and numerous complications have been associated with the procedure. Fluid and electrolyte imbalances are commonly reported, particularly if too much of the bowel has been resected. All JI bypass patients suffer from diarrhea, although its severity varies widely. The diarrhea can precipitate fluid and electrolyte imbalances, rectal irritation, severe itching, and anal sores and abrasions.

[1]W. W. Faloon, A. Rubulis, J. Knipp, C. D. Sherman, and M. S. Flood, Fecal fat, bile acid, and sterol excretion and biliary lipid changes in jejunoileostomy patients, *American Journal of Clinical Nutrition* 30 (1977):21-31.

Figure 1

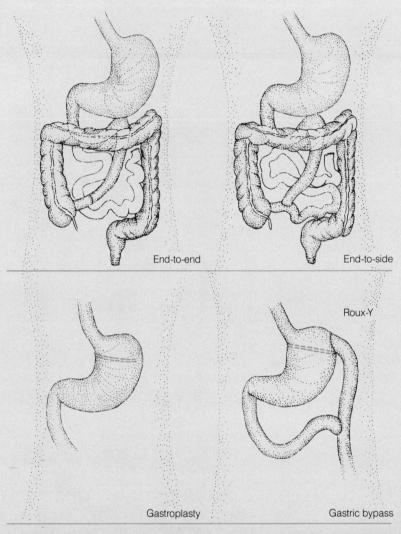

Jejunoileal bypass

End-to-end

End-to-side

Roux-Y

Gastroplasty

Gastric bypass

People who have undergone JI bypass have a very high incidence of hyperoxaluria (see Chapter 23) and are prone to developing kidney stones. Renal failure has been reported in about 3 percent of all JI bypass patients. Liver failure, seen in about 2 to 4 percent, is fatal for more than half of the patients in whom it occurs. Although the cause of the liver failure is unknown, it has been suggested that bacterial overgrowth in the bypassed bowel segment may be responsible. The liver changes are similar to those seen in kwashiorkor; so it has also been suggested that protein malnutrition and essential fatty acid deficiency play a role.

Understandably, nutrient deficiencies can occur; protein, trace element, fat-soluble vitamin, potassium, calcium, and magnesium deficiencies have been reported. Hair loss, dermatitis, muscle wasting, bone pain, kidney disease, gallstone formation, arthritis, abdominal distention, vomiting, and chronic flatulence also may be present. Table 1 lists some of the complications that have been reported in JI bypass patients.

If serious complications arise, the JI bypass must be either reversed or revised. People who have had the surgery reversed have regained and sometimes even exceeded their original weight.

The myriad serious complications associated with the JI bypass have led many physicians to stop performing the operation. Instead, many surgeons have turned to the gastric bypass. In some cases, people have had a JI bypass reversed and replaced with a gastric bypass.

Gastric Bypass Gastric bypass surgery is a relatively new development in the treatment of morbid obesity. In one type of gastric bypass (gastroplasty), a row of surgical staples is placed across the upper stomach to form a pouch, and no resection of tissue is necessary.

Since long-term followup information on gastric bypass patients is scant, it is impossible to know exactly what the consequences of this surgery will be. Patients lose about 60 percent of their excess weight by about two years after surgery, and so far, they seem to experience fewer complications than JI bypass patients.

Table 1. Complications Reported in JI Bypass Patients

Abdominal distention	Hair loss
Anorectal disorders	Hyperoxaluria
Arthritis	Liver failure
Chronic flatulence	Muscle wasting
Dermatitis	Nutrient deficiencies
Diarrhea	Renal failure
Fluid and electrolyte imbalances	Surgical complications
Gallstone formation	Vomiting

On the negative side, some serious early postoperative complications have been reported. Patients may develop severe and unrelenting nausea and vomiting, dumping syndrome, or blind loop syndrome (see Chapter 23). Narrowing or ulceration of the small opening from the pouch can develop. Bile acids may reflux into the stomach, causing gastritis. Sometimes the staples come loose, widening the gastric reservoir and thus defeating the purpose of the procedure. Perforation and bleeding can also occur.

Some patients begin eating frequently to compensate for the small volume they can accommodate, and some start drinking high-kcalorie liquids. These people, of course, fail to lose weight. Other patients develop nutrient deficiencies; for example,

thiamin deficiency is suspected of resulting from gastric bypass surgery.[2] Table 2 summarizes the complications now known to be associated with gastric bypass.

How Successful Are Bypass Operations?

The success of bypass operations can only be measured by weighing the risks of obesity against the risks of the procedures. Table 3 summarizes the many disorders that are associated with obesity. The reader is also referred to Chapter 8 and Highlight 8 for more discussion of obesity and its risks.

[2]R. W. Haid, L. Gutmann, and T. W. Crosby, Wernicke-Korsakoff encephalopathy after gastric plication, *Journal of the American Medical Association* 247 (1982):2566-2567.

Table 2. Complications Reported in Gastric Bypass Patients

Bile acid reflux	Outlet narrowing
Blind loop syndrome	Perforation
Dumping syndrome	Staple disruption
Gastritis	Ulceration
Inadequate weight loss	Vomiting
Nausea	

The majority (about 85 percent) of both JI and gastric bypass operations are considered to be successful based on weight loss. Weight loss should be significant enough to reduce the risk of death and illness from obesity and improve the quality of life. It is interesting to note that sometimes people express satisfaction with the results of surgeries that their physicians consider medically unsatisfactory.[3]

Concluding Thoughts

Mary's doctor talked to her

[3]T. B. Van Itallie and J. B. Kral, The dilemma of morbid obesity, *Journal of the American Medical Association* 246 (1981):999-1003.

Table 3.   Disorders Associated with Morbid Obesity

Cardiorespiratory dysfunction	Kidney disease
Diabetes mellitus	Liver/gallbladder disease
Edema of ankles and legs	Osteoarthritis
Heart disease	Psychosocial disorders
High blood pressure	Thromboembolic disease
Increased operative risk	Uterine fibroid and
Increased susceptibility to infection	endometrial cancer

about what he had found out about surgery for obesity. He advised her to try dieting again and when that was unsuccessful, he gave her the name of a surgeon.

The surgeon, Dr. Smith, agreed that Mary was a candidate for surgery. Dr. Smith told Mary that she no longer did JI bypasses and then made sure Mary understood the risks and side effects of the gastric bypass. She gave Mary three months to think about her decision. Is weight loss worth the risks? Only Mary can decide what is best for her. And as a health care provider, you have the responsibility of supporting her decision.

CHAPTER 24

CONTENTS

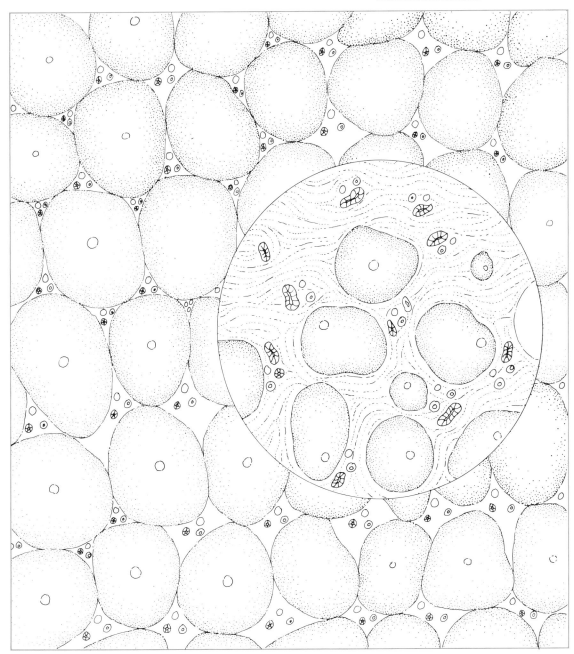

DISORDERS OF THE LIVER, EXOCRINE PANCREAS, AND GALLBLADDER

If you drink alcohol, do so in moderation.

DIETARY GUIDELINES FOR AMERICANS

The GI tract, liver, pancreas, and gallbladder are all part of the digestive system. The liver is like a processing plant; nutrients and other metabolites arriving there may be metabolized, stored, or detoxified. Furthermore, the liver is the place where bile salts (necessary for fat digestion and absorption) are made. The bile salts are then stored in the gallbladder until they are released into the small intestine.

The pancreas has both endocrine and exocrine functions. In this chapter we will be talking about its exocrine function (see Chapter 25 for diabetes, related to endocrine function). The pancreas secretes many digestive enzymes along with a bicarbonate-rich digestive juice that raises the intestinal pH for optimal activity of the enzymes.

biliary tract: the gallbladder and the duct system that conveys bile from the liver to the intestine (see p. 156).

exocrine: see p. 82.

Alcoholism

In 1977, more than 30,000 people in the United States died from cirrhosis of the liver, and 95 percent of the deaths were alcohol-related. Alcohol contributes to several other leading causes of death in young adults and adults, and is directly responsible for certain cancers of the liver. It is also a risk factor in various other cancers and sometimes in diabetes, and it is an indirect cause in many of the 150,000 annual deaths from accidents, homicides, and suicides. This book does not have a chapter on alcoholism in and of itself, but this chapter begins with alcoholism because of the major contribution it makes to liver disease.

Alcoholism is a serious and debilitating disease. About 10 million adults in the United States (7 percent of the adult population) are problem drinkers.[1] In addition, among 14- to 17-year-olds there are an estimated 3.3 million problem drinkers (19 percent of that age group). The cost of alcoholism in the United States is estimated at $43 billion, almost $13 billion of which is spent directly on medical and health care costs. Thus alcoholism is a major public health problem.

People sometimes think that alcoholism only overtakes "the other guy" or "people I don't know," but in fact alcoholism is so prevalent that practically everyone must know several people who are or will become alcoholics. The trick to discovering who they are, a necessary first step before obtaining help for them, is to realize that they do not fit the popular image of a falling-down, raggedy drunk. Contrary to prevailing myths, alcoholism is:

- Not related to what is drunk (for example, a beer drinker can just as easily be an alcoholic as a whiskey drinker).

- Not related to how much is drunk (a person who does not drink at all for many days at a time can still be an alcoholic; a person who drinks too much and passes out at a party may not be an alcoholic).

- Not related to social class or station (alcoholics come in all garbs — rich, poor, male, female, black, white).

- Not always obvious (your best friend can successfully hide an alcohol problem for years if you are not tuned in to it).

alcoholism: a disease characterized by a pathological dependence on alcohol.

disease: a definite morbid process having a characteristic train of symptoms.

Alcoholism: A Disease   What alcoholism is (since it is not all these things), is a disease: a definite morbid process having a characteristic train of symptoms. A disease may affect the whole body or any of its parts; in the case of alcoholism, many parts are affected. A disease may be of known or unknown cause; in the case of alcoholism, the cause is unknown.

The criteria for diagnosis of alcoholism are very complete. A person can make an informal self-diagnosis by answering a quiz (see box: "Self-Quiz on Alcohol"). For greater precision, the diagnostician uses a 93-item inventory of symptoms and behaviors.[2] But you need neither of these to recognize an alcoholic pattern developing. A description of the typical course of events in the life of an alcoholic diagnosed far into the progression of the disease reveals an average 30-year sequence of stages:

- 17 — first drink.
- 21 — regular drinking.
- 30 — excessive drinking.
- 35 — first blackout.
- 37 — uncontrolled drinking.
- 39 — first DTs.

[1]U.S. Department of Health, Education, and Welfare, *Third Special Report of the U.S. Congress on Alcohol and Health from the Secretary of Health, Education, and Welfare* (Washington, D.C.: Government Printing Office, 1978).

[2]National Council on Alcoholism, Criteria Committee, Criteria for the diagnosis of alcoholism, *American Journal of Psychiatry* 129 (August 1972):127-135.

● 42 — first treatment for alcoholism.

● 45 — arrival at a residential treatment center.[3]

By the time the person has checked in for a month-long, $1,000-5,000 rehabilitation effort, the disease is full blown and every body organ is affected. Social and financial consequences may by this time be severe and irreversible. But the disease has been under way for almost 30 years. Meanwhile, of every 10 or 15 young people who drink, one is already headed in the same direction. By age 25 or 30, an alcoholic has enough signs of the disease so that any alert individual (including the drinker himself) can identify it and take steps to arrest its progress.

DTs (delirium tremens) (de-LEER-ee-um TREM-unz): a violent delirium with tremors that occurs during withdrawal from alcohol after long use; a dangerous, life-threatening state that requires emergency medical treatment.

This book is about *diet* and disease, but space is given here to the identification of alcohol addiction because, like the hospital malnutrition of a decade ago, it is going unrecognized right under the nose of many a health professional who deals with it. Prevention is far preferable to after-the-fact attempts at cure, but can't take place unless professionals train themselves to "see" this insidious disease, which masquerades in so many different guises. Nor can any efforts at nutrition rehabilitation take place if an alcohol problem is not dealt with.

Alcoholism goes unrecognized inside and outside the hospital for many reasons. For one thing, people with alcohol problems do not want to admit to them; most are unaware that alcoholism is a disease and believe instead that it is a reflection on their character, something they should be ashamed of. For another, family members subscribe to the same belief and help their relatives to hide the problem. Finally, health professionals join the conspiracy of silence because they know too little about alcoholism, are afraid to confront it, and don't know how to deal with it. Instead, they ignore it and deny its existence, treating their clients for side-effects instead of bringing the problem into the open and meeting it head on.

In some hospitals, diagnosed alcoholism accounts for about a third of all the people being treated, but in only one hospital has the question been asked how prevalent it really is. In that hospital, 50 percent of the patients were found to be alcohol abusers, although the word *alcohol* did not appear on a single chart.[4] In some VA hospitals, alcohol abuse probably contributes to the illnesses of 95 percent of the patients. Alcoholism is estimated to cost half a million hospital days each year in the United States alone.

---

[3]J. H. Williams, Characteristics of an alcoholic sample (Mimeographed paper available from the Bureau of Alcoholic Rehabilitation, Division of Mental Health, Florida Department of Health and Rehabilitative Services, P.O. Box 1147, Avon Park, FL 33825).

[4]*Preventive Medicine, USA: Health Promotion and Consumer Health Education* (New York: Neale Watson Academic Publications, 1976), p. 6.

Self-Quiz on Alcohol

The following is a typical short quiz anyone can use to get a first clue as to the seriousness of his or her possible alcohol problem. There are dozens of versions. In this one, a "yes" answer to any question indicates a symptom of alcoholism. Several "yes" answers to questions 1-8 indicate the early stage; to questions 9-21, the middle stage; and to questions 22-26, the beginning of the final stage. Several "yes" answers to any part indicate a need for further information and advice.

Yes No

☐ ☐ **1.** Do you occasionally drink heavily after a disappointment, a quarrel, or when the boss gives you a hard time?

☐ ☐ **2.** When you have trouble or feel under pressure, do you always drink more heavily than usual?

☐ ☐ **3.** Have you noticed that you are able to handle more liquor than you did when you were first drinking?

☐ ☐ **4.** Did you ever wake up on the "morning after" and discover that you could not remember part of the evening before, even though your friends tell you that you did not "pass out"?

☐ ☐ **5.** When drinking with other people, do you try to have a few extra drinks when others will not know it?

☐ ☐ **6.** Are there certain occasions when you feel uncomfortable if alcohol is not available?

☐ ☐ **7.** Have you recently noticed that when you begin drinking you are in more of a hurry to get the first drink than you used to be?

☐ ☐ **8.** Do you sometimes feel a little guilty about your drinking?

☐ ☐ **9.** Are you secretly irritated when your family or friends discuss your drinking?

☐ ☐ **10.** Have you recently noticed an increase in the frequency of your memory "blackouts"?

☐ ☐ **11.** Do you often find that you wish to continue drinking after your friends say they have had enough?

☐ ☐ **12.** Do you usually have a reason for the occasions when you drink heavily?

Yes No

☐ ☐ **13.** When you are sober, do you often regret things you have done or said while drinking?

☐ ☐ **14.** Have you tried switching brands or following different plans for controlling your drinking?

☐ ☐ **15.** Have you often failed to keep the promises you have made to yourself about controlling or cutting down on your drinking?

☐ ☐ **16.** Have you ever tried to control your drinking by making a change in jobs, or moving to a new location?

☐ ☐ **17.** Do you try to avoid family or close friends while you are drinking?

☐ ☐ **18.** Are you having an increasing number of financial and work problems?

☐ ☐ **19.** Do more people seem to be treating you unfairly without good reason?

☐ ☐ **20.** Do you eat very little or irregularly when you are drinking?

☐ ☐ **21.** Do you sometimes have the "shakes" in the morning and find that it helps to have a little drink?

☐ ☐ **22.** Have you recently noticed that you cannot drink as much as you once did?

☐ ☐ **23.** Do you sometimes stay drunk for several days at a time?

☐ ☐ **24.** Do you sometimes feel very depressed and wonder whether life is worth living?

☐ ☐ **25.** Sometimes after periods of drinking, do you see or hear things that aren't there?

☐ ☐ **26.** Do you get terribly frightened after you have been drinking heavily?

From *What Are the Signs of Alcoholism?* a leaflet published by the National Council on Alcoholism. A 35-item quiz for the same use was published by R. D. Hurt, R. M. Morse, and W. M. Swenson, Diagnosis of alcoholism with a self-administered screening test, *Mayo Clinic Proceedings* 55 (1980):365-370.

If thousands of people are in hospitals because of alcohol abuse and almost no one's chart says "alcoholism," what do the charts say? Where are all these people being treated for? They are on every floor of the hospital, under a multitude of other diagnoses. Among them:

● Accidents (cuts, bruises, fractures from automobile accidents, falls, fights).

● Anemia, other blood disorders.

● Cardiomyopathy.

● Cystitis.

● Flu and other respiratory disorders.

● Gastritis and other GI disorders.

● Liver disease (the only alcohol-related disease that is often recognized as such).

● Pancreatitis.

● Prostatitis/impotence.

● Psychiatric disorders (depression, aberrant behavior, family violence including child abuse and spouse abuse, other).

● Skin infections.

● Many, many other.

The first person to recognize the root cause of the problem being treated may be you in your role as diet advisor — not because others have not had the opportunity to see it but because it has been invisible to them. If you suspect an alcohol problem, remind yourself that it is seldom a kind act to allow a disease to proceed unchecked. If the problem is not dealt with, the illness will recur. Therefore, assert yourself, and alert the health care team. Say, "Alcohol abuse often contributes to this problem," or "Let's find out if this person is a problem drinker." Not to say something is to refuse to be an effective health care provider — and didn't you get into the business originally in order to really benefit people's health?

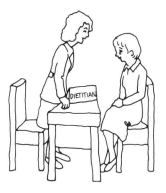

CAUTION:

Many illnesses reflect an invisible alcohol problem. Put on your educated eyeglasses, see it, and take action.

To identify an alcoholic, keep four points in mind. First, the concept of addiction helps make alcoholism understandable. An addictive substance is one that is needed to relieve the symptoms caused by its

addiction: a pathological dependence on a substance such that a craving develops when the substance is withdrawn; only the substance itself can relieve the pain associated with its withdrawal.

tolerance: with respect to alcohol, an ability to metabolize increasing quantities with repeated exposure so that more has to be taken before the effects are felt.

blackout: a time-limited, retrospective amnesia that develops after a drinking episode and makes the person unable to remember what happened while he or she was drinking; considered by some authorities to be a distinguishing feature of alcoholism.

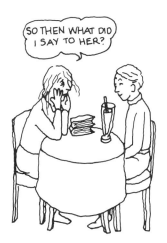

own withdrawal. Most people feel about alcohol that they can "take it or leave it," but about one in every ten drinkers, for unknown reasons, becomes an addict and develops a risky relationship with alcohol. Although these people may be able to drink moderately on several occasions, on others they drink far more than they intended to, exhibiting loss of control. These occasions occur unpredictably, so that the first drink becomes a gamble: The addict may or may not be able to stop. Episodes of uncontrolled drinking become more frequent with time. The addict's craving for alcohol becomes marked by several features. He or she thinks about alcohol a lot (obsession), takes it in spite of resolving not to (broken promises), and then suffers remorse. When someone exhibits feelings that strong about a substance, you should suspect addiction. Note, too, that these feelings do not reflect moral degeneracy. The person is simply someone whose internal makeup makes the body react in a special way to alcohol.

Second, the alcohol addict develops a tolerance to alcohol and requires larger and larger doses to achieve the same effect. Anyone can learn to handle more alcohol with practice than at first, but the alcoholic becomes so "good" at metabolizing alcohol that he or she ceases to get any pleasure out of drinking.

Tolerance reflects an adaptation of the alcohol-metabolizing enzymes in the liver, as described in Highlight 7. The alcoholic's liver may be able to metabolize two or three times as much alcohol per unit of time as the nonalcoholic's liver. When liver disease sets in, however, tolerance rapidly declines until it is poorer than at first. One drink can then make the person drunk.

A third key to recognizing alcoholism is the blackout. A blackout is a peculiar kind of event. What happens is that a person, while drinking, may behave perfectly normally — talking, moving around, acting as usual until the end of the evening. But then, the next day, the person can't remember anything at all that happened beyond a certain time the day before. The blackout, then, is a kind of amnesia — but it happens after the fact. You conduct yourself normally at the time, but later, you can't remember what you did. A blackout is not at all the same as "passing out," although one may pass out during a blackout. Most people who drink do not experience blackouts (their memory of the previous evening may be hazy, but the evening's events are not totally beyond recall). Some alcohol counselors consider blackouts to be the single most characteristic diagnostic feature of alcoholism.

Fourth and finally, because alcoholism is a disease, it can be diagnosed and brought to a halt at any time during its course — early as well as late. (One brings alcoholism to a halt by stopping drinking altogether: simple to say, although sometimes very hard to do.) Theoretically, alcoholism begins before the first drink is ever taken, because it is characteristic of the person, not of the behavior. Therefore early detection and intervention can have literally life-transforming effects.

Often, the health care provider can and should do no more than recognize and speak up about an alcohol problem. It is not the province of a dietitian, for example, to offer psychologic counseling to addicts or their families. But all health care providers should know where, in the local community, such help is available and how to make referrals to the appropriate agencies. (Additional information about alcoholism is available in the references listed at the end of this chapter.)

With all of this by way of introduction, it is time to turn to the physical consequences of alcohol abuse. The chronic use of ethanol has damaging effects on virtually every organ system, including the liver, pancreas, GI tract, brain, heart, muscles, and gonads. The liver is the site of ethanol metabolism and is particularly susceptible to alcohol-related injury. The pancreas is another organ sensitive to alcohol abuse, and chronic pancreatitis often develops. Table 1 summarizes some effects of alcohol on the body.

Alcohol and Nutrition   Liver disease requires one kind of nutrition care; pancreatitis, another. The specifics of diet for each of these diseases are given later in this chapter. No matter what organ is first affected, however, all alcohol abusers tend to have certain nutrition problems in common.

Highlight 9 offered insight into many of the interrelationships between alcohol abuse and nutrition and showed why alcohol abusers tend to have multiple nutrient deficiencies, especially of protein, B vitamins, and minerals. At the peak of the disease, alcohol abusers typically ingest as many as half their kcalories in the form of alcoholic beverages, therefore losing out on some 900 kcalories of nutrient-bearing foods. Nutrition rehabilitation of these people requires that they give up alcohol and replace its kcalories with nutritious foods, especially foods rich in protein and B vitamins (folacin, vitamin B_6, thiamin, and vitamin B_{12}). In addition, the alcohol abuser is likely to have some special nutrition problems.[5]

All of the fat-soluble vitamins can be affected by alcohol abuse. Vitamin A is affected because, in adapting to metabolize great quantities of alcohol, the addict's liver synthesizes supernormal amounts of the enzyme alcohol dehydrogenase (ADH). This enzyme happens to degrade not only alcohol (ethanol) but also retinol. (The *ol* ending signifies that both are alcohols.) Instead of being converted to retinal and then used to maintain functions of the eye and testes, retinol is degraded; hence the eyes' adaptation to darkness and the making of sperm are both impaired in the alcoholic. The remedy is not to take extra vitamin A, which is toxic, but to stop drinking and thereby stop inducing the destructive enzyme.

[5]Many of the statements that follow are based on the detailed review provided in S. Shaw and C. S. Lieber, Nutrition and alcoholism, in *Modern Nutrition in Health and Disease*, 6th ed., ed. R. S. Goodhart and M. E. Shils (Philadelphia: Lea & Febiger, 1980), pp. 1220-1243.

Table 1.   Adverse Effects of Alcohol on the Body

GI tract

Esophageal lesions
Tears at the gastroesophageal junction
Motor dysfunction of the esophagus
Esophageal varices
Gastritis
Peptic ulcers
Diarrhea
Malabsorption
Increased risk of cancer of the tongue, mouth,
   pharynx, esophagus, and larynx

Liver

Fatty liver
Hepatitis
Cirrhosis
Increased risk of cancer of the liver

Pancreas

Pancreatitis
Pancreatic damage

Nervous system

Wernicke-Korsakoff syndrome
Structural brain changes
Impaired sensorimotor performance
Impaired perceptual capacity
Impaired visual-spacing ability
Impaired memory function
Peripheral neuropathy

Endocrine system

Increased cortisol
Increased aldosterone
Inhibition of oxytocin release
Inhibition of antidiuretic hormone release
Increased insulin
Reduced testosterone in males

Muscles

Muscle weakness and breakdown

Blood

Anemia
Abnormal platelet production
Decreased WBCs

Cardiovascular system

High blood pressure
ECG abnormalities
Enlarged heart
Biventricular heart failure

Table 1.   Adverse Effects of Alcohol on the Body (continued)

Lungs

    Tuberculosis

    Airway obstruction

Reproductive system

    Impotency

    Early postmenopausal amenorrhea

    Fetal alcohol syndrome (see Chapter 15)

Other

    Interference with drug metabolism (see Chapter 21)

    Malnutrition

Vitamin D is also affected in alcohol abuse. Normally, the liver performs a step in the making of active vitamin D (Chapter 11), and the defect in alcoholism may be caused by liver damage; but this is not certain. Alcohol also affects the kidney, the liver's vitamin-D degrading system, and the adrenal and parathyroid glands, so the defect may be caused by these. In any case, alcoholics tend to develop bone disease, which can be halted only by discontinuing alcohol abuse. Alcohol also directly inhibits the absorption of calcium as well as promoting its excretion, worsening this problem.

Iron status is of great concern in the alcohol abuser, but not because of iron deficiency. Alcohol excess increases iron absorption, making overload likely, and iron overload injures the liver. Certain wines contain large amounts of iron, adding to the risk. While anemias (from deficiencies of vitamin A, vitamin B_6, vitamin B_{12}, folacin, and vitamin C) often occur in alcohol abusers, iron-deficiency anemia is not one of them. Furthermore, many of the other side effects of alcohol abuse make iron absorption greater: pancreatic insufficiency, folacin deficiency, cirrhosis, and others. Also, alcohol abusers sometimes try to protect themselves against nutrient deficiencies by taking supplements, and these supplements sometimes contain iron. Vitamin C megadoses taken with the iron can greatly increase its absorption, making the problem worse. A rule of thumb for the diet counselor is that alcoholics are not likely to be iron deficient unless they have been bleeding extensively. Transfusions and iron therapy should be used with caution, and supplements containing iron should not be given.

Another nutrition problem common in alcohol abusers is hypoglycemia. Ironically, this may prompt a person to drink, because a dose of alcohol "fools" the body into thinking it has received sugar. Actually, alcohol sensitizes the pancreas to glucose so that it tends to oversecrete insulin, causing hypoglycemia. At the same time, alcohol depletes the liver's glycogen and damages its glucose-making system so that it becomes harder to recover from hypoglycemia. Add to these the fact that the drinker often doesn't eat, and you can see why he or she is often admitted to the hospital in a severely hypoglycemic state. After emergency treatment, the tendency towards hypoglycemia tends to persist for many days before the liver and pancreas regain normalcy. The diet advisor rightly counsels the person recovering from a bout of heavy drinking by recommending frequent small, protein-containing meals to stabilize blood glucose level. Recovering alcoholics counsel each other to eat lots of protein, especially peanut butter, which they know to be high in B vitamins, and to "reach for a sweet instead of a drink" if they feel "down."

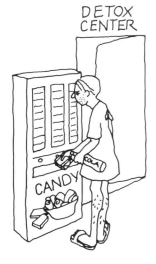

Nutrition management principles for clients recovering from alcoholism:

Stress abstinence from alcohol above all other measures.

Replenish depleted nutrients.

Emphasize protein, kcalories, nutrient-dense foods.

Correct anemia with caution. Consider B vitamins first; assume no iron deficiency except in severe bleeding.

Offer frequent meals to avert hypoglycemia.

The early stage of recovery from alcohol abuse is often characterized by a behavior you might be tempted to call sweet abuse. An alcoholic rehabilitation center is likely to have several vending machines selling candy, cola beverages, coffee with cream and sugar, and the like. They are heavily used.

Don't be tempted to judge this behavior negatively. You might not want to see such heavy consumption of sweets in a child, but a child is choosing sweets over fruits and juices, a negative choice. The recovering alcoholic, in contrast, is using sweets to satisfy the craving for a drink, a positive choice. Encourage this behavior enthusiastically. Keep it in mind (but in the back of your mind) that when sobriety is firmly established and there is little risk that the client will resume drinking, *then* you can encourage gradual improvement of eating habits.

 CAUTION:

Use of sweets may be a positive choice.
Ask yourself: What is the alternative?

For the same reasons, an ex-alcoholic's weight may change rapidly in the early stages of recovery. This may be a matter of concern (for example, in a hypertensive client who is already overweight), but if at all possible, the concern should be deferred a while. Top priority is for the client to stop drinking. Other agenda items should wait.

The principles of nutrition therapy for the recovering alcoholic are shown in the margin. The diet advisor can best get through to the recovering alcoholic by offering abundant support for the decision not to drink and a few simple diet guidelines tailored to the client's particular concerns.

Many alcohol abusers end up in the hospital with liver disease or pancreatitis. Besides the guidelines given here, additional concerns become relevant in these diseases. The next sections give attention to these concerns.

Disorders of the Liver

At one time it was widely believed that malnutrition in the alcoholic was due solely to poor food intake. Now we know that in addition to having poor intake, alcoholics also digest, absorb, and utilize nutrients poorly. It has been suggested that alcohol abuse is the most common cause of vitamin and trace element deficiencies in the United States.[6]

In the past it was also believed that malnutrition, rather than alcohol per se, was the factor leading to liver disease in alcoholics. However, studies have shown that cirrhosis can develop in baboons that ingest large amounts of alcohol, even when their diets are nutritionally adequate.[7] This suggests that alcohol is directly toxic to the liver, although the way in which alcohol affects the liver is unknown.

Liver disease can, of course, result from many causes besides alcoholism; the rest of this section describes several types of liver disease. The diet advice you give depends to a large extent on the type and severity of the disease.

Considering how many functions the liver performs, there is little wonder that diseases of the liver can affect nutrition status or that malnutrition can adversely affect liver function. Table 2 summarizes important functions of the liver.

Fatty Liver   Fatty liver can occur when triglycerides are being synthesized excessively, when triglycerides aren't being oxidized to fatty acids, when the liver takes up excessive triglycerides from the blood, when the liver can't release the triglycerides into the blood, or when a combination of these factors is present. Highlight 9 discusses the development of fatty liver in the alcoholic.

fatty liver: the accumulation of triglycerides in the liver. Also called **hepatic steatosis** (stee-uh-TOE-sis).

stea = fat

When triglycerides accumulate in the liver, the liver enlarges. Fatty liver itself is usually not harmful and often can be reversed. However, the accumulation of fat suggests the presence of an underlying disease that can be serious. Aside from alcohol abuse, fatty liver can be associated with the use of some drugs (corticosteroids, tetracycline), kwashiorkor, obesity, mismanaged TPN, and small bowel bypass surgery. Fatty liver associated with small bowel bypass surgery can rapidly progress to more serious liver disease and death.

In cases of fatty liver caused by malnutrition, the liver changes can be reversed by correction of nutrition deficits. In alcoholism, abstinence

---

[6]M. J. Eckardt, T. C. Harford, C. T. Kaelber, E. S. Parker, L. S. Rosenthal, R. S. Ryback, G. C. Salmoiraghi, E. Vanderveen, and K. R. Warren, Health hazards associated with alcohol consumption, *Journal of the American Medical Association* 246 (1981):648-666.

[7]C. S. Lieber, L. DeCarli, and E. Rubin, Sequential production of fatty liver, hepatitis, and cirrhosis in sub-human primates fed ethanol with adequate diets, *Proceedings of the National Academy of Sciences USA* 72 (1975):437-441.

from alcohol in addition to a good diet is necessary. If drug ingestion is responsible, the drug is stopped. Otherwise, there is no specific therapy for fatty liver.

hepatitis: inflammation of the liver.

jaundice: yellowing of the skin, whites of the eye, mucous membranes, and body fluids caused by an accumulation of bile pigments in the blood.

Hepatitis   Hepatitis is a more serious liver disease in which liver tissue becomes inflamed. The most common causes are virus infections (types A, B, and C), alcohol, and drugs. The type A virus is spread through contaminated water, food, or sewage. The type B virus is transmitted parenterally (through blood transfusions, dialysis, use of contaminated needles by drug addicts) and results in a more serious type of hepatitis. (Type C, at present, is little understood, but the name should alert you to the fact that there may be other causes of hepatitis.) Hepatitis is sometimes a minor illness but it can be fatal.

In the early stages, the person with hepatitis may suddenly develop anorexia, nausea, vomiting, and fever. Later, as bile pigments spill from the diseased liver into the blood, the person develops jaundice (yellowing of the skin, whites of the eyes, mucous membranes, and body fluids) and a dark urine. The liver also may be enlarged.

A normal, well-balanced diet is given to the person with hepatitis. Adequate amounts of nutrients are important in helping liver cells to regenerate. When anorexia is severe, IV glucose solution may be given temporarily. Giving small, frequent meals may help. Liquid supplements may be easier for some anorectic people to accept. Tube feedings should be considered if nausea or anorexia is severe, and intravenous feedings may be necessary if vomiting becomes a problem. Occasionally, a person with hepatitis develops liver failure and hepatic coma, which will be discussed below.

cirrhosis (seer-OH-sis): a disease of the liver characterized by scarring. **Laennec's cirrhosis** is the type associated with alcohol abuse and malnutrition.

The **portal vein** is the vein carrying nutrients from the digestive organs to the liver; the **hepatic artery** is the artery bringing oxgyen-rich blood from the heart to the liver.

portal hypertension: increased blood pressure in the portal vein caused by obstructed blood flow through the liver.

Cirrhosis   Either fatty liver or alcoholic hepatitis may progress to cirrhosis. Cirrhosis can also result from congenital causes, chemicals, infections, biliary obstructions, heart disease, or unknown causes. In cirrhosis, liver cells filled with fat or damaged by inflammation die and scar tissue invades the liver. The liver is remarkable in that even after many cells have died, those that remain alive can multiply and regenerate healthy tissue. Still, cirrhosis is the most serious and irreversible type of liver injury.

In the United States, chronic alcohol abuse is the most common cause of cirrhosis. Not all alcoholics develop cirrhosis, however; its incidence among alcoholics is about 10 to 12 percent. Still, in 1975, cirrhosis was the sixth most common cause of death.[8]

Because the liver is so vital in maintaining the body's homeostasis, you can expect that severe liver damage will result in many harmful effects. Normal liver tissue is soft and flexible, but scars are unyielding. Normally, the portal vein and the hepatic artery carry 1 1/2 quarts every

[8]D. H. Van Thiel, H. D. Lipsitz, L. E. Porter, R. E. Schade, G. P. Gottlieb, and T. O. Graham, Gastrointestinal and hepatic manifestations of chronic alcoholism, *Gastroenterology* 81 (1981):594-615.

Table 2.   Functions of the Liver

Protein metabolism

> Conversion of amino acids to energy sources
>   (oxidative deamination)
> Synthesis of nonessential amino acids (transamination)
> Synthesis of nitrogen-containing compounds from
>   amino acids (purines, pyrimidines)
> Urea synthesis
> Plasma protein synthesis

Carbohydrate metabolism

> Maintenance of normal blood sugar levels
> Glycogen storage
> Conversion of monosaccharides to glucose

Fat metabolism

> Synthesis of cholesterol, phospholipids, and lipoproteins
> Production of ketone bodies
> Oxidation of fatty acids
> Synthesis of triglycerides

Other

> Synthesis of bile salts
> Synthesis of blood coagulation factors
> Detoxification of alcohol, drugs, wastes, and other
>   foreign substances

minute through the miles of intermeshed capillaries in the liver. This huge volume of blood cannot pulse easily through the mass of scar tissue in the cirrhotic liver, and so it backs up into the portal vein. Blood pressure in the vein increases sharply in consequence, causing portal hypertension.

As pressure rises, plasma is forced out of the liver's blood vessels into the abdominal cavity, and the belly swells up. The accumulation of fluid in the abdominal cavity is the kind of edema called *ascites*, a self-aggravating condition. Because the volume of blood in the circulatory system is now reduced, less blood reaches the kidneys, and they respond by calling for more aldosterone. As a result, the body retains sodium, and edema now spreads to all body compartments. To make matters worse, the diseased liver cannot dispose of aldosterone as it normally does, so aldosterone levels remain high.

Normal blood flow through the liver is blocked, so some of the blood takes a detour through smaller vessels around the liver and out to the rest of the body. These shunts, or collaterals, often develop in the area of the esophagus. Frequently, the raised pressure enlarges them so that they bulge into the lumen of the esophagus, like varicose veins in the legs, creating esophageal varices. The lining of the esophagus on top of the varices eventually erodes. Many times the erosion penetrates into

ascites (uh-SIGHT-eez): accumulation of fluid in the abdominal cavity.

collaterals: small blood vessels developed to divert blood flow away from an obstructed organ. These blood vessels are also called **shunts**.

esophageal varices (uh-SOFF-uh-GEE-ul VAIR-ih-seez): protruding tangles of distended blood vessels into the esophagus.

A high blood level of ammonia is called **hyperammonemia**.

the varices themselves and massive bleeding follows. A person who has bled from esophageal varices will very likely bleed again, and there is a 50-50 chance that death will occur during any bleeding episode.[9]

Under normal circumstances the liver removes ammonia from the circulation and converts it to urea (see p. 206). A seriously diseased liver can't synthesize urea and so can't clean up the ammonia from the blood. The problem is further aggravated by the fact that some blood carrying ammonia is not even reaching the liver; instead, it is bypassing the liver by way of the collaterals. High blood ammonia levels insult the central nervous system, increasing the risk of hepatic coma, which will be discussed later (see also the accompanying box entitled "Production of Ammonia").

[9]S. S. Hanna, W. D. Warren, J. T. Galambos, and W. J. Millikan, Bleeding varices: 2. Elective management, *Canadian Medical Association Journal* 124 (1981):42-47.

Production of Ammonia

Blood ammonia comes from several sources, but principally from the GI tract. In the GI tract, protein digestion by enzymes and bacteria yields ammonia as one of its products. Therapy to reduce blood ammonia therefore has to be aimed at reducing the amount of protein present in the GI tract. An obvious way to do this is to limit food protein, but even if no protein is given in the diet, the GI tract will contain protein available for digestion, because it constantly sheds cells into its lumen, and they then can be digested. Moreover, the person with liver disease is likely to be bleeding in the GI tract from gastritis, ulcers, or esophageal varices; the blood serves as an additional source of protein. These three main protein sources in the GI tract — food, shed mucosal cells, and blood — account for about two thirds of the ammonia found in the blood. Another source of ammonia in the GI tract is urea (see Figure 1). Most of the blood urea is filtered into the urine for excretion, but about 25 percent of the body's urea finds its way into the GI tract instead, where gut bacteria metabolize it to ammonia. Another small, but significant ammonia source is metabolic processes carried on by cells all over the body.

The ammonia produced in the GI tract enters the body by way of the portal vein. In liver disease, the many narrowed and blocked blood vessels of the liver offer resistance; some ammonia-laden blood therefore bypasses the liver and enters the peripheral circulation, raising the body's total ammonia content.

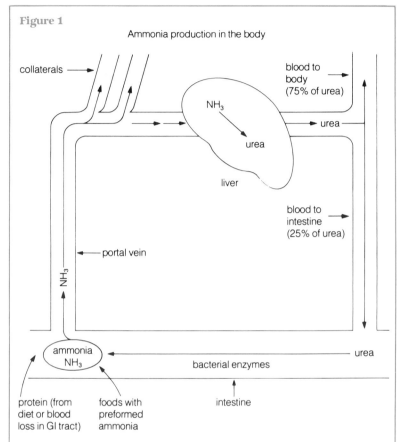

Figure 1

Ammonia production in the body

Diagrams on p. 206 show how the liver and kidneys normally cooperate to remove excess nitrogen from the body. The liver performs the first step (converting ammonia to urea); the kidneys, the second (filtering urea into the urine). A diseased liver fails to do its job for two reasons — first because, as already mentioned, the ammonia isn't flowing into the liver as it should; and second because the liver's dead and dying cells can't efficiently convert the ammonia they receive. In fact, the ammonia is directly toxic to them, as it is to all cells of the body.

You can see how the vicious cycle feeds itself: more ammonia is produced, the body gets sicker, and less can be detoxified. (You can also see why, in liver disease, blood ammonia is high, while in kidney disease blood urea is high).

Many drugs used in the treatment of liver disease work on the intestine to disrupt this vicious cycle. At the same time, diet, by supplying just enough but not too much protein (nitrogen), helps relieve the metabolic load of the liver.

Specific guidelines:

Protein: 0.5-1.0 g/kg ideal body weight.

Energy: 35-50 kcal/kg ideal body weight.

D.K., a 125 lb, 5 ft 7 in male alcoholic undergoing a detoxification program, is ready to begin oral intake. His energy needs can be calculated as follows:

$\dfrac{125 \text{ lb}}{2.2 \text{ kg}}$ (to convert lb to kg)

$\times$ 35 kcal $= 1{,}988$ kcal

$\dfrac{125 \text{ lb}}{2.2 \text{ kg}} \times 50$ kcal

$= 2{,}840$ kcal

Since he is underweight, you will try to give him the upper range of kcalories. His protein needs are:

$\dfrac{125 \text{ lb}}{2.2 \text{ kg}} \times 0.5$ g $= 28.4$ g

$\dfrac{125 \text{ lb}}{2.2 \text{ kg}} \times 1.0$ g $= 56.8$ g

The time it takes for clotting to occur is measured by a test called **prothrombin time;** both vitamin K deficiency and liver disease can prolong the time it takes for the blood to clot.

Diet therapy in cirrhosis involves the tricky business of providing just the right amount of protein so that liver cells can regenerate. Enough carbohydrate and fat must accompany the protein so that none is degraded for energy. Providing too much protein can precipitate hepatic coma. Too much protein necessitates deamination of excess amino acids (and ammonia results); too little halts repair of the liver. The guideline is that the diet should be adequate in kcalories and should meet the RDA for protein (0.5-1.0 g/kg) in the absence of hepatic coma. Total abstinence from alcohol is necessary to protect the liver from further injury. Indeed, the cirrhotic person should never drink again.

To accompany the protein, a daily intake of 35-50 kcal/kg body weight (about 2,000 to 3,000 kcal) is recommended to maintain the person in positive nitrogen balance. A few studies have suggested that higher protein intakes may be desirable,[10] but if coma is likely, the excess protein makes it even more likely (by generating ammonia). Therefore, it seems wise that protein intake should be moderate. Of course, the protein given should be of high quality.

Fat helps make foods attractive to a person whose appetite is poor. In addition, fat delivers kcalories efficiently. It has been thought that the cirrhotic liver could not handle fat, and indeed, such a liver exposed to the continued onslaught of alcohol can't manufacture the transport proteins to make lipoproteins and rid itself of accumulated lipids. But without alcohol, and with enough protein as new raw material, the cirrhotic liver seems to manage well enough. Therefore, fat is not restricted unless the cirrhotic person develops steatorrhea, a clear sign that fat absorption has failed.[11] Even then, the diet should probably supply fat, but as MCT (see p. 882).

The diet is usually supplemented with large amounts of water-soluble vitamins (up to five times the RDA). Remember that the B vitamins, in particular, are coenzymes necessary for the liver's many enzymes to do their metabolic and repair work, and that in malnutrition the water-soluble vitamins are among the first to be depleted. A person with a prolonged prothrombin time should be offered vitamin K supplements. Otherwise, fat-soluble vitamins are generally not deficient, and RDA amounts of these vitamins should be adequate.

For people with ascites, fluids and sodium are also restricted. The level of the restriction varies with the severity of the ascites. Sodium amounts may range from 250 to 2,000 mg a day; fluids, from 1,500 to 2,000 ml a day. The person is weighed *daily* to assess changes in fluid

[10]J. Smith, J. Horowitz, J. M. Henderson, and S. Heymsfield, Enteral hyperalimentation in undernourished patients with cirrhosis and ascites, *American Journal of Clinical Nutrition* 35 (1982):56-72.

[11]S. Shaw and C. S. Lieber, Alcoholism, in *Nutritional Support of Medical Practice*, ed. H. A. Schneider, C. E. Anderson, and D. B. Coursin (Hagerstown, Md.: Harper & Row, 1977), pp. 202-221.

balance. If weight gain is rapid, the person is gaining fluid. Weight loss, on the other hand, indicates that the person is losing water weight. Table 3 shows patterns used for various sodium-restricted diets.

It is difficult to provide a diet very low in sodium, stimulate the appetite, and still keep protein intake adequate, since many high-protein foods (eggs, meat, milk) also contain significant amounts of sodium. Special low-sodium supplements and milk products are available to help deal with this problem. When sodium intake must be severely restricted, it is important to note even the sodium content of medications.

The person who has bleeding esophageal varices will be unable to take food by mouth. When there is no bleeding, the person with esophageal varices should avoid foods that are irritating to the mucosa, such as caffeine and pepper, and should chew food thoroughly before swallowing it, to be sure that no particles get caught in or around the varices.

Sample low-sodium menu (1,000 mg)

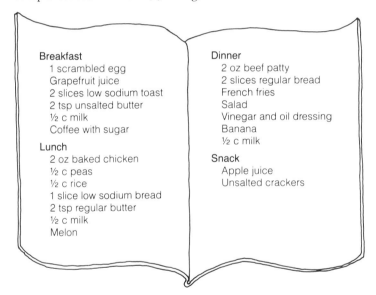

Breakfast
1 scrambled egg
Grapefruit juice
2 slices low sodium toast
2 tsp unsalted butter
½ c milk
Coffee with sugar

Lunch
2 oz baked chicken
½ c peas
½ c rice
1 slice low sodium bread
2 tsp regular butter
½ c milk
Melon

Dinner
2 oz beef patty
2 slices regular bread
French fries
Salad
Vinegar and oil dressing
Banana
½ c milk

Snack
Apple juice
Unsalted crackers

The person with cirrhosis has anorexia, and may accept food more willingly in small, frequent meals than in a few large ones. Diet is so vital to recovery from cirrhosis that it is very important to do everything possible to insure its acceptance. Work closely with the cirrhotic patient and family and do what you can to individualize the diet as well as to serve the food attractively. These tactics will be a big help in encouraging the person to eat.

If the person with cirrhosis cannot take adequate foods by mouth, little time should be wasted in beginning a tube feeding or parenteral nutrition, if necessary. Both types of special nutrition support have been used successfully in people with cirrhosis.

Table 3. Low-Sodium Diets

| Foods | Number of Servings Allowed on Various Levels of Sodium Restriction | | | | | |
	250 mg	500 mg	1,000 mg	2,000 mg	Serving size	Sodium per serving (mg)
Skim, whole, and evaporated milk	0	2	2	2	8 oz	120
Low-sodium milk	2				8 oz	7
Meat, fish, poultry, and unsalted cheese	4	4	4	6	1 oz	25
Egg	1	1	1	1	1	60
Bread and allowed ready-to-eat cereal	0	0	2	5	1 slice or 3/4 oz	200
Low-sodium bread, cereal, and cereal products	7	7	7	4 or more	varies	5
Fresh, frozen, or canned without salt: asparagus, bean sprouts, broccoli, brussels sprouts, cabbage, cauliflower, cucumbers, egglant, endive, escarole, green pepper, collard and turnip greens, lettuce, mushrooms, okra, onions, radishes, rhubarb, rutabaga, string beans, summer squash, tomatoes, watercress, zucchini, and low-sodium tomato and vegetable juices	2	2	2	not restricted	1/2 c	9
Fresh, frozen, or canned without salt: corn, lima beans, parsnips, peas, potatoes, pumpkin, winter squash, yam, and sweet potato	1	1	1	not restricted	1/2 c	5
Canned vegetables and vegetables frozen with salt	0	0	0	1	1/2 c	200
Salted butter, margarine, regular mayonnaise	0	0	2	6	1 tsp 1-1/2 tsp	50 50

General diet guidelines:

The foods listed below cannot be used unless they have been calculated into the diet. However, allowances can be made, particularly when the higher levels of sodium are allowed. For example, if a person on a 2 g sodium diet does not drink milk, you can allow 240 mg of sodium from any other food source (see Appendix I for the sodium content of foods). With this in mind, avoid the following foods:

1. Salt in cooking or on the table.
2. Highly salted snacks such as potato chips, corn chips, tortilla chips, salted popcorn, and pretzels.
3. Barbeque sauce; bouillon cubes (except low sodium); catsup; celery salt, seeds, or leaves; chili sauce; garlic salt; horseradish made with salt; meat extracts, sauces and tenderizers; monosodium glutamate; prepared mustard; olives; onion salt; pickles; relishes; saccharin; soy sauce; and Worcestershire sauce.
4. Commercial foods made with milk; ice cream; sherbet; malted milk; milk mixes; and milkshakes.
5. Artichokes, Chinese or red cabbage, greens (except those listed with vegetables in table above), sauerkraut, spinach, beets, and carrots.

6. Maraschino cherries, crystallized or glazed fruits, and dried fruit with sodium sulfite added.

7. Brains; kidneys; canned salted, or smoked meats; bacon; luncheon meats; chopped or corned beef; kosher meats; shellfish; regular cheeses; egg substitutes; and regular peanut butter.

8. Salted butter or margarine, salt pork, commercial salad dressing (except low sodium), and salted nuts.

9. Leavening agents such as baking powder, baking soda, rennet tablets, pudding mixes, and molasses.

10. Fountain beverages; instant cocoa mixes; prepared beverage mixes (including fruit-flavored powders); and commercial candy, cakes, cookies, sweetened gelatin mixes, pastries, puddings, cakes, and biscuit mixes.

11. Most commercial dry cereals or instant hot cereals. Puffed wheat, puffed rice, and shredded wheat are allowed.

Adapted from American Dietetic Association, *Handbook of Clinical Dietetics* (New Haven, Conn.: Yale University Press), 1981.

Hepatic Coma   Hepatic coma is a dangerous complication of liver disease. Typically, the person with impending hepatic coma exhibits mental disturbances such as changes in judgment, personality, or mood. Sometimes sleep patterns change. Furthermore, such a person may be unable to reproduce a simple shape, such as a star. A sweet, musty, or pungent odor may develop on the breath. Flapping tremor is also seen in the pre-coma state. Just before passing into coma, the person becomes very difficult to arouse.

The exact mechanisms causing hepatic coma are unknown, but rising blood ammonia levels play an important role. Protein is therefore restricted when coma is impending. Other nitrogen-containing compounds that appear to be produced from the metabolism of methionine by bacteria in the colon may also be involved. It has been found that the blood amino acid pattern changes in hepatic coma. This change may cause the production of unusually high levels of certain substances that act like neurotransmitters (see Highlight 5), and these substances contribute to hepatic coma. The nature of the change and its implications for nutrition treatment of hepatic coma are the subjects of Highlight 24.

When a person shows signs of impending coma, the physician prescribes additional dietary modifications. Protein intake must be restricted to 20 to 35 g (or less) high-quality protein per day. Once coma has set in, the person may be given no protein. If improvement becomes evident, protein can gradually be increased in 10- to 15-g increments per day five to seven days until the RDA for protein is reached. People should not be kept on zero-protein diets for more than a few days, because this causes breakdown of body proteins, which can make matters worse. (More information on low-protein diets will be given in Chapter 27.)

Some other foods also should be restricted because they contain preformed ammonia or contain amino acids that readily form ammonia in the body. These foods include cheeses (American, beer, cheddar, domestic blue, tilsit), some poultry and meat (chicken, ground beef, ham, salami), buttermilk, gelatin, Idaho potatoes, onions, and peanut butter.[12]

hepatic coma: a state of unconsciousness that results from liver disease. Also called **portal systemic encephalopathy**.

flapping tremor: uncontrolled movement of the hand that occurs when a person puts his arms out in front of him, bends his wrists upward, and separates the fingers.

Guidelines for diet in liver disease:
1. 35-50 kcal/kg body weight.
2. Protein:
   Liver disease: 0.5-1.0 g/kg body weight.
   Impending coma: Drop back protein to 20-35 g/day; increase in increments of 10-15 g/day for 5 to 7 days until individual tolerance or 1.0 g/kg body weight (whichever is lower) is reached.
   Coma: Give no protein. Gradually increase as above as client improves.
3. If ascites is present, restrict sodium to 250-2,000 mg/day and fluid to 1,500-2,000 ml/day. Increase sodium and fluid intake as tolerated as liver function improves.

[12] D. Rudman, R. B. Smith, A. A. Salam, W. D. Warren, J. T. Galambos, and J. Wenger, Ammonia content of foods, *American Journal of Clinical Nutrition* 26 (1973):487-490.

Limited data suggest that vegetable protein may be better tolerated than meat protein,[13] perhaps because vegetable protein has fewer amino acids that readily form ammonia. Another reason why diets high in plant foods may be beneficial is that the fiber contained in such diets prevents constipation, decreasing the time available for the production and absorption of ammonia in the gut.

In our discussion of these diets, try to picture what the diet really consists of. Consider, for example, what the person on a 30 g protein diet is actually getting. On such a diet the total protein allowance would be spent on just 1 egg, 2 oz meat, 1/2 c milk, and 1 serving each of vegetables and bread. You can probably already see some problems. The amounts of foods allowed from the major food groups are very small. The kcalorie content of the foods is also low. You may be able to see why fat is not restricted unless necessary — adding fat wherever possible can help boost kcalorie intake a lot. Other foods that do not contain protein, such as some candy, jelly, and sugar, can also help. But this diet is obviously difficult to plan and follow.

Adding a sodium restriction, especially a strict one, is like adding insult to injury. A person offered such a diet may not want to eat at all. He or she will need all the encouragement you can offer.

Drugs can also be used to help reduce blood ammonia levels. Two drugs commonly used for this purpose are neomycin and lactulose. Neomycin kills the intestinal bacteria that produce ammonia. The mechanism of action of lactulose is unknown, but it has been suggested that it works by causing diarrhea (thus loss of ammonia) and by converting ammonia to a form that can't be reabsorbed into the body.

Disorders of the Exocrine Pancreas

The pancreas normally produces many enzymes necessary for the digestion of protein, fat, and carbohydrate. Additionally, it secretes a bicarbonate-rich juice that provides an optimal pH for activation of the enzymes. Therefore, diseases of the pancreas can have significant impact on absorption and, consequently, nutrition status.

Fat malabsorption is the biggest problem in pancreatic disorders, because only the pancreas makes lipase, which is necessary for fat digestion. In contrast, the intestine can help somewhat with the

[13]N. J. Greenberger, J. Carley, S. Schenker, I. Bettinger, C. Stammes, and P. Beyer, Effect of vegetable and animal protein diets in chronic hepatic encephalopathy, *American Journal of Digestive Diseases* 22 (1977): 845-855.

digestion of protein and carbohydrate by secreting its own amylase, disaccharidases, and proteases.

Pancreatitis   Pancreatitis is an inflammation of the pancreas that is most often caused by biliary tract disease, surgery (often of the stomach or biliary tract), or alcoholism. Exactly how these disorders cause pancreatitis is unknown. Blood vessels supplying the pancreas increase in permeability, allowing fluid and plasma proteins to leak into the space between the pancreas cells and cause localized edema. The damage to the pancreas causes retention of pancreatic secretions, including enzymes. The enzymes become activated and begin to digest the pancreas itself. Some of these enzymes are picked up by the blood. This is why serum amylase and lipase levels rise and can be used as indicators of pancreatitis. If the edema compresses blood vessels, the oxygen supply to the cells can be cut off, resulting in cell death. If the enzymes destroy blood vessels, bleeding can occur. Fat tissue near the pancreas can also die.

The typical person with pancreatitis has high serum amylase levels, severe abdominal pain, and oftentimes, nausea and vomiting. The goal of therapy in pancreatitis is to reduce the stimulation of pancreatic secretions. No food is given by mouth, since food stimulates bicarbonate and enzyme secretions from the pancreas. An NG tube is inserted, but not for feeding. Instead, the tube acts like a straw to suction out the stomach's contents; this further reduces stimulation of the pancreas.

IV fluids are given to correct fluid and electrolyte imbalance, which can be caused by the edema and also by loss through NG suction. If pancreatitis is severe or if the person is severely malnourished, TPN should be started; it does not stimulate pancreatic secretions as food does.

When the person is free of abdominal pain and has active bowel sounds and normal or near-normal serum amylase levels, he or she can have food by mouth again: first clear liquids, then a low-fat diet (see Table 4), and finally a regular diet as tolerated. At the first sign of pain, or if serum amylase levels rise, food is withheld, and when these signs and symptoms subside, food can be reintroduced. Six small meals may be better tolerated than larger, less frequent meals.

People with milder forms of pancreatitis may benefit from tube feedings of hydrolyzed formulas. Pancreatic secretions may actually be decreased by the administration of a defined formula diet (see Chapter 20).[14] The feeding tube should be passed into the jejunum to minimize stimulation. Once the person improves, he or she can take food by mouth again.

Sometimes an acute attack of pancreatitis doesn't subside, or acute attacks occur at frequent intervals. This is chronic pancreatitis, most

pancreatitis: inflammation of the pancreas caused by invasion of its tissue by its digestive enzymes.

amylase: the pancreas's starch-digesting enzyme.

Guidelines for diet in acute pancreatitis:

1. Initial treatment:
   If severe, use TPN and NG suction.
   If mild, use hydrolyzed tube feeding formula delivered into jejunum.
2. After pain stops and serum amylase falls, progress to a low-fat oral diet, then a regular oral diet.

[14]R. G. Keith, Effect of a low fat elemental diet on pancreatic secretion during pancreatitis, *Surgery, Gynecology, and Obstetrics* 151 (1980):337-343.

commonly caused by repeated alcohol abuse. Pancreatic tissue is destroyed and, like nerve tissue, cannot regenerate.

Maldigestion and consequent malabsorption of nutrients doesn't occur until a good bit of pancreatic tissue has been destroyed. The pancreas normally excretes enzymes far in excess of needs, so even after extensive damage has occurred, digestion may still proceed normally. Therapy of chronic pancreatitis during active attacks is the same as given above. Between attacks, the client should follow a bland, low-fat diet.

The goals of diet therapy in chronic pancreatitis are to:

● Maintain optimal nutrition status.

● Reduce steatorrhea.

● Miminize pain.

● Avoid subsequent attacks of active pancreatitis.

The diet eliminates all foods that stimulate gastric acid secretion (caffeinated and decaffeinated coffee, tea, and pepper). Offering small meals may be helpful. The person with chronic pancreatitis usually tolerates about 50 to 70 g fat per day; restricting fat to less than this amount is unnecessary. (Table 4 lists foods excluded on a low-fat diet.) The person takes enzyme replacements with meals to aid the digestion and absorption of protein and fat. When the person needs extra kcalories, they are given as MCT so as not to cause steatorrhea. Always make sure the person understands that absolutely no alcohol is permitted. If steatorrhea persists, fat-soluble vitamins are given in supplement form. Vitamin B_{12} absorption may be reduced, and so injections of vitamin B_{12} may be required.

Enzyme replacements are extracts of hog or beef pancreatic enzymes. They help with digestion but are not as effective as human enzymes.

Sample low-fat menu

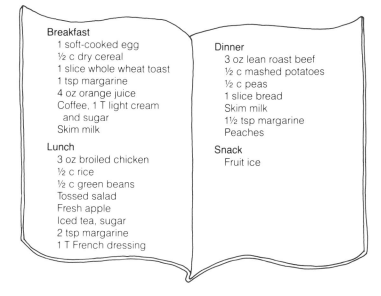

Breakfast
    1 soft-cooked egg
    ½ c dry cereal
    1 slice whole wheat toast
    1 tsp margarine
    4 oz orange juice
    Coffee, 1 T light cream
        and sugar
    Skim milk

Lunch
    3 oz broiled chicken
    ½ c rice
    ½ c green beans
    Tossed salad
    Fresh apple
    Iced tea, sugar
    2 tsp margarine
    1 T French dressing

Dinner
    3 oz lean roast beef
    ½ c mashed potatoes
    ½ c peas
    1 slice bread
    Skim milk
    1½ tsp margarine
    Peaches

Snack
    Fruit ice

Table 4.   Low-Fat Diet (50 g fat)

Do not use:

1. Whole milk, chocolate milk, whole-milk cheese, and ice cream.

2. Pastries, cake, pie, sweet rolls, and breads made with fat.

3. More than one egg a day, fried or fatty meats (sausage, luncheon meats, spare ribs, frankfurters), duck, goose, and tuna packed in oil (unless well drained).

4. More than six servings of fat. One serving is as follows:

   1 t butter, margarine, shortening, oil, or mayonnaise.
   1 strip crisp bacon.
   1 T heavy cream or Italian or French dressing.
   1/8 avocado.
   2 T light cream.
   6 small nuts.
   5 small olives.
   If fat is used to cook or season food, it must be taken from this allowance.

5. Desserts, candy, and anything made from chocolate or nuts.

6. Creamed soups made with whole milk.

Use:

1. Skim milk, skim-milk cheeses, yogurt made from skim milk, sherbet, and fruit ices.

2. Angel food cake and fruit whips made with gelatin, sugar, and egg-white meringues.

3. Up to 6 oz of lean meats and poultry, low-fat egg substitutes, up to 3 regular eggs per week, and chicken without skin.

4. Plain white or whole grain bread, nonfat cereals, pasta, rice, noodles, and macaroni.

5. Clear soups and cream soups made with skim milk.

6. All vegetables prepared without fat.

7. Jelly, jam, honey, sugar, gumdrops, jelly beans, and marshmallows.

Suggestions:

1. To make the diet still lower in fat, reduce the fat and meat (and egg) servings.

2. To increase the fat content, give additional fat or meat servings.

3. To increase acceptance of the diet, check the fat content of a well-liked food and allow that food if possible.

Pancreatitis damages not only the cells that produce digestive enzymes for the GI tract but also, sometimes, the cells that produce insulin. The individual with pancreatitis then becomes glucose intolerant like a diabetic and must follow a diabetic diet in addition to the restrictions stated above (see Chapter 25).

People with acute pancreatitis are often in pain, one of the most severe kinds of pain known in any illness. The worst of it usually subsides in about two to three days. You should try to do everything you can to ease your client through this difficult time. Obviously it will help not to discuss food and diet, even though you want to be sure nutrition needs are met, until the patient feels better.

cystic fibrosis (CF): a hereditary disorder that affects many organs, including the pancreas, lungs, liver, heart, gallbladder, and small intestine.

Cystic Fibrosis   Cystic fibrosis (CF) is a hereditary disease that may affect many organs, including the pancreas, lungs, liver, heart, gallbladder, and small intestine. It is the most common cause of pancreatic insufficiency in children and young adults.[15] People with CF often have three major symptoms: pancreatic insufficiency, chronic lung disease, and abnormal electrolyte levels in the sweat. The pancreas is affected in 80 to 85 percent of people with CF.

CF is characterized by production of a very thick mucus by glands throughout the body. The mucus obstructs the small pancreatic ducts and interferes with the secretion of digestive enzymes and pancreatic juices. Eventually, the enzyme and bicarbonate-secreting cells are surrounded by the mucus and are gradually replaced by fibrous tissues.

fibrous: composed of fibers.

pulmonary: of the lungs.

The airways of the lungs also become plugged with mucus, making it difficult for the person to breathe. Lung infections become likely and are the usual cause of death in CF.

People with CF frequently are malnourished. A common misconception is that they regularly eat large amounts of food. Although this may be true when they are well, it is not true during periods of illness. Furthermore, they do not eat enough during well periods to make up for what they lose while ill. As a result, many young people with CF experience growth failure and are short and very thin for their age. Furthermore, they malabsorb fats, protein, fat-soluble vitamins, and vitamin B_{12}, becoming malnourished.

You may be asked about selenium in the treatment of CF. "I have heard that selenium can cure CF. Can you tell me how much I should take?"

An article in a national lay magazine of fairly wide circulation suggested that selenium supplementation in CF might reverse the disorder. The article was based on a report of a child who had been taking selenium supplements. The child was admitted to the hospital with very low blood chloride levels that may have been a

[15]P. A. DiSant' Agnese and P. B. Davis, Cystic fibrosis in adults: 75 cases and a review of 232 cases in the literature, *American Journal of Medicine* 66 (1979):121-132.

complication caused by selenium overdose. Usually people with CF have high levels of chloride in their sweat (indeed, this is one way they are diagnosed). However, in this child sweat chloride was normal, probably because her blood chloride was so low. When she was given IV therapy to correct the electrolyte imbalance, the sweat chloride was again elevated. The child, who had many problems, died.

The article picked up on the fact that the child's sweat chloride had reverted to normal, without reporting the abnormally low blood chloride or the subsequent tragic outcome. The opinion of most participants at a conference held at the National Institute of Health in September of 1979 was that "there was no direct evidence to support the concept that selenium is a causative factor in CF or plays a beneficial role in the routine treatment."[16] Still, unfortunately, many people with CF are now experimenting with selenium supplements, which will probably do harm rather than good and whose long-term effects are still largely unknown. As we have pointed out before, supplements of any nutrient, but especially of trace elements (Chapter 13), can have dangerous, unforeseen consequences.

The misuse of selemiun supplements in cystic fibrosis is merely another example of wishful thinking based on unfounded rumors. We have offered many previous cautions to help you protect your clients against hurting themselves this way — cautions against self-diagnosis (p. 21), against magical thinking (p. 264), and against believing what you read in unrefereed publications (Highlight 17). If you care, keep alert.

The energy needs of people with CF are about 150 percent of the RDA for their sex and age. This is because they lose energy nutrients through malabsorption and have frequent infections. Furthermore, they need extra energy just to breathe, since breathing is so laborious.

Aside from providing adequate energy, the diet should be nutritionally balanced and tailored to the individual's tolerance.[17] In the past, diets for people with CF were often severely restricted in fat. However, individuals generally know how much fat they can take before uncomfortable GI symptoms occur. Furthermore, fat is an important source of kcalories and essential fatty acids. For patients who cannot tolerate fat, MCT oil can be used to provide additional kcalories.

An important part of therapy is the use of enzyme replacements. Enzyme replacements help decrease malabsorption considerably, but they do not correct it completely. People who have persistent

---

[16]V. S. Hubbard, G. Barbero, and H. P. Chase, Selenium and cystic fibrosis (editorial), *Journal of Pediatrics* 96 (1980):421-422.

[17]V. S. Hubbard and P. J. Mangrum, Energy intake and nutrition counseling in cystic fibrosis, *Journal of the American Dietetic Association* 80 (1982):127-131.

steatorrhea (frequent, foul-smelling stools), gas, flatulence, and abdominal distention may need to have their dosage of enzyme replacements adjusted.[18]

The best way to insure that people with CF are eating enough is to assess their nutrition status regularly, with particular attention to monitoring height and weight. Nutrition care plans can then be revised as necessary.

Vitamin supplements (two tablets daily) are usually given. The fat-soluble vitamins should preferably be given in a water-miscible form which can be absorbed without fat. (Table 5 lists appropriate amounts of fat-soluble vitamins.) Zinc supplements may also be needed.

Another nutrition concern in CF is possible depletion of electrolytes (sodium and chloride). This can happen as a result of a fever, high environmental temperature, or diarrhea. During such times, the person needs extra salt.

Fat-soluble vitamins that readily mix with water and can be absorbed without fat are **water-miscible** vitamins.

You may recall from Chapter 18 that when iodine was added to the food supply as iodized salt, the iodine content of the typical American diet increased considerably. A reverse situation may have considerable impact on infants with CF.

Since 1977 manufacturers have stopped adding salt to baby foods. Also, more people use baby formula instead of whole cow's milk to supplement or replace breast milk in the early months of life. Formula is lower in salt than cow's milk. Consequently, the sodium intake of infants has decreased substantially.[19] This is probably a desirable change for normal, healthy infants. For infants with CF, however, it is not.

In a recent report, one hospital admitted five CF infants with a total of eight episodes of electrolyte depletion.[20] Six episodes were not related to high temperatures, fever, or significant GI symptoms. The authors suggest that infants with CF who are fed primarily breast milk or infant formula and commercial baby foods should receive salt supplementation.

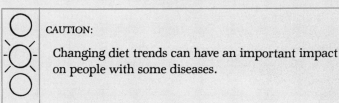

CAUTION:

Changing diet trends can have an important impact on people with some diseases.

---

[18]Hubbard and Mangrum, 1982.

[19]J. J. Laughlin, M. S. Brady, and H. Eigen, Changing feeding trends as a cause of electrolyte depletion in infants with cystic fibrosis, *Pediatrics* 68 (1981):203-207.

[20]Laughlin, Brady, and Eigen, 1981.

Table 5. Recommended Fat-Soluble Vitamin Supplementation in Cystic Fibrosis

Vitamin	Amount per day
A	5,000-10,000 IU
D	400-800 IU
E	200 IU*
K	50-100 μg

*In preschool or older children.

From H. P. Chase, M. A. Long, and M. H. Lavin, Cystic fibrosis and malnutrition, *Journal of Pediatrics* 95 (1979):337-347.

Disorders of the Gallbladder

The gallbladder stores and concentrates the bile produced in the liver. Sometimes it can become inflamed (cholecystitis), most commonly because of a bacterial infection. Sometimes, stones form in the gallbladder (cholelithiasis). If a stone obstructs the outlet of the gallbladder, choledocholithiasis can result.

The symptoms associated with cholecystitis vary. Pain in the area of the gallbladder may occur gradually or suddenly and can be quite severe. Frequently, nausea, vomiting, and flatulence are present.

Many factors are involved in gallstone formation. Hereditary factors, gender (being female), obesity, and some drugs may predispose the individual toward developing gallstones. Diabetes, ileal disease or resection, and diet may also be implicated. Women are more likely to develop gallstones than men, but gallstones do occur in men, and the incidence increases in both sexes with aging.

Gallstones are of two general types: cholesterol gallstones and pigment gallstones. About 85 percent are of the cholesterol type, which form when the cholesterol in the bile gets too concentrated, either from excessive cholesterol synthesis or a decreased bile pool. The cholesterol becomes insoluble in the bile and precipitates; and as more and more cholesterol precipitates, stones form. Restricting cholesterol in the diet does not alter the course of cholesterol stone formation.

Low-fat diets have traditionally been prescribed for people with gallbladder diseases. The rationale was that fat in the intestine causes the gallbladder to contract, which can cause pain. However, the symptoms of cholecystitis may not be related to fat intake.[21] Some clinicians report that people with gallbladder disease have no more problems with fat than other people do.[22] A psychological factor seems to be involved: if people *think* they are receiving less fat, they may feel

cholecystitis (coal-ee-sis-TYE-tis): inflammation of the gallbladder.

chole = bile

A person with gallstones has **cholelithiasis** (COAL-ee-lith-EYE-uh- sis). If the stones obstruct the duct leading to the intestine, **choledocholithiasis** (coal-ee-DOCO-lith-EYE-uh-sis) is present.

litho = stone

[21]J. W. Manier, Diet and cholelithiasis, in *Nutrition and Metabolism in Medical Practice*, ed. S. Halpern, A. L. Lukby, and G. Berensen (New York: Futura, 1973).

[22]W. H. Price, Gall-bladder dyspepsia, *British Medical Journal* 2 (1963):138-141.

cholecystectomy (coal-ee-sis-TECK-to-me): surgical removal of the gallbladder.

cyst = bladder
ectomy = removal

Two drugs used to treat gallstones are *chenodeoxycholic* (KEEN-oh-dee-OXY-COAL-ic) *acid* and its derivative *ursodeoxycholic* (ERR-so-dee-OXY-COAL-ic) acid. Both are bile acids.

less GI discomfort, even though they actually are being given fat that they don't recognize as such.[23]

The best advice for your clients with gallbladder ailments seems to be to consume a well-balanced diet with careful attention to individual tolerances. Some people are truly intolerant to fat or to particular foods, and their diets should be adjusted accordingly. Obese patients should be encouraged to lose weight. It has been suggested that a high-fiber diet helps prevent gallstone formation.[24] However, more research will need to be done before this can be confirmed.

Oftentimes, people with gallstones must have their gallbladders removed (cholecystectomy). Following surgery, the same care is given as outlined in Chapter 22 for other surgical patients. After surgery, fat need not be restricted.

Efforts are being made to dissolve gallstones with drugs. The results have been variable but encouraging.

Nutrition Assessment Parameters of Concern

When you assess the nutrition status of people with disorders of the liver, pancreas, and gallbladder, you should keep several points in mind:

1. People with diseases of the liver and pancreas (especially alcoholics) are often malnourished. It is very important to obtain an accurate diet history for calculating nutrient requirements.

2. When the pancreas or gallbladder is diseased, the diet history also offers the opportunity to estimate the person's tolerance for fat.

3. The cirrhotic may be retaining considerable amounts of fluids. This will affect weight measurements and, if generalized edema is present, also arm anthropometrics. Under these circumstances, weight is not useful to keep track of body tissue gains and losses but can be monitored to see if the patient is mobilizing fluids. Weight loss, then, is a good sign that indicates that some liver function is returning.

4. Another strategy useful in people with ascites is to measure abdominal girth. Place a tape measure around the back and over the person's abdomen directly over the umbilicus. Repeat the measurement periodically. A decreasing abdominal girth indicates that fluid is being mobilized. If girth increases, the ascites is becoming worse.

5. In people with extensive liver disease, serum albumin levels will be low. Supplying extra amino acids will not help if the liver doesn't function well enough to synthesize albumin. Serum albumin levels may also be low in people with pancreatitis. Usually, people with CF have normal albumin levels.

[23]R. M. Donaldson, Diet and gastrointestinal disorders (editorial), *Gastroenterology* 52 (1967):897-900.

[24]D. A. Smith and M. I. Gee, A dietary survey to determine the relationship between diet and cholelithiasis, *American Journal of Clinical Nutrition* 32 (1979):1519-1526.

Summing Up

Diseases of the liver can be expected to have a major impact on the processing of nutrients. The liver synthesizes bile salts, which are necessary for the absorption of fat and fat-soluble vitamins. The metabolism of virtually all nutrients is affected by liver disease.

Alcoholism is a major cause of liver disease. The alcoholic is at risk of poor nutrition status because of poor food intake, malabsorption, and often liver disease. Alcoholism is a major health problem with many adverse consequences.

The goal of diet therapy for people with severe liver disease is to provide adequate energy and protein for liver cell regeneration without increasing the risk of hepatic coma. The person with ascites must restrict intake of both sodium and fluids. Protein restriction is necessary in the person who shows signs of impending hepatic coma.

People with pancreatitis run the risk of malnutrition caused by malabsorption of nutrients. Nutrition problems may be compounded for alcoholics with pancreatitis. A low-fat diet may be needed in chronic pancreatitis, along with fat-soluble vitamin and vitamin B_{12} supplements.

People with cystic fibrosis can follow a normal diet restricted only in those foods to which they are intolerant. Enzyme replacements are used to decrease fat losses in the stool. A high-kcalorie diet and daily vitamin supplements are usually a part of diet therapy. Nutrition status should be assessed regularly.

People with gallbladder disease should avoid only foods that cause pain or excessive gas. Obese clients should be instructed to lose weight and maintain ideal weight to reduce their risk of gallstone formation. Adding fiber to the diet may be helpful.

To Explore Further

Two articles on nutrition and liver disease are of interest (see also chapter footnotes):

- Tomaiolo, P. P. Nutritional problems in the alcoholic. *Comprehensive Therapy*, July 1981, pp. 24-27.

- Morgan, M. Y. Alcohol and the liver. *Journal of Human Nutrition* 33 (1979):350-356.

A symposium on alcoholism and malnutrition was published in:

- *American Journal of Clinical Nutrition* 33, December 1980.

A series of articles providing an in-depth look at how vitamins are affected by alcoholism appeared in the following issues of *International Journal for Vitamin and Nutrition Research*:

- Ascorbic acid. 49 (1979):434-441.

- Folate and vitamin B_{12}. 50 (1980):96-121.

- Vitamin B_6. 50 (1980):215-230.

- Thiamin. 50 (1980):321-338.
- Riboflavin; Niacin; Pantothenic acid; Biotin. 50 (1980):425-440.
- Vitamin A. 51 (1981):166-177.
- Vitamin D; Vitamin E; Vitamin K. 51 (1981):307-318.

A publication by S. Shaw and C. S. Lieber entitled Nutrition and alcoholic liver disease, *Nutrition in Disease* (Columbus, Ohio: Ross Laboratories, 1978) is available from Ross Laboratories (address in Appendix J).

Two excellent articles on hepatic coma are:

- Steigmann, F. Preventing portal systemic encephalopathy in the patient with cirrhosis. *Postgraduate Medicine*, February 1979, pp. 118-126.
- Hoyumpa, A. M., Desmond, P. V., Avant, G. R., Roberts, R. K., and Schenker, S. Hepatic encephalopathy. *Gastroenterology* 76 (1979):184-195.

Some worthwhile references on cystic fibrosis include:

- Chase, H. P., Long, M. A., and Lavin, M. H. Cystic fibrosis and malnutrition. *Journal of Pediatrics* 95 (1979):337-347.
- Hubbard, V. S., and Mangrum, P. J. Energy intake and nutrition counseling in cystic fibrosis. *Journal of the American Dietetic Association* 80 (1982):127-131.
- Hubbard, V. S., Barbero, G., and Chase, H. P. Selenium and cystic fibrosis. *Journal of Pediatrics* 96 (1980):421-422.

Two good articles about gallbladder disease are:

- Redinger, R. N. Cholelithiasis: Review of advances in research. *Postgraduate Medicine*, June 1979, pp. 56-71.
- Facts and fallacies about gall stones. *British Medical Journal* 283 (1981):171.

Cirrhosis

T.J. was a busy executive. The first time he was admitted to the hospital (after an auto accident) no one even considered that he might be an alcoholic. Somehow most of us have the misconception that most alcoholics are skid-row bums. T.J. was socially respected. And since neither the health team nor T.J. realized that his drinking was excessive, he went undiagnosed for some time.

Many hospitalizations and years later, T.J. is in the hospital again. This time a diagnosis of alcoholic cirrhosis has been confirmed. At 5 ft 7 in tall, T.J., who once weighed 150 lb, now weighs 120 lb. He looks thin, although his abdomen is quite large, and his skin is yellow. He is no longer a busy executive — he started missing so much work that he was fired. His wife and children tried for years to get him the help he needed but nothing worked.

They eventually left him. His liver disease is advanced, and he is showing signs of impending hepatic coma.

Study Questions

1. From the limited information available, what can you say about T.J.'s nutrition status? What are his %IBW and %UBW? Do you expect his blood albumin levels to be normal? If not, why not? What specific nutrient deficiencies would you look for in T.J.?

2. Discuss factors that lead to nutrient deficiencies in the alcoholic. Explain the interrelationships among malnutrition, alcoholism, and liver disease.

3. What dietary changes would you have recommended to T.J. if he had been diagnosed to have alcoholism on his first hospital admission? How would these recommendations have changed when he was diagnosed with liver disease? How will his diet be altered now that he is in a pre-coma state? If he is able to avert coma or as he recovers from coma, how should his diet be altered?

4. Why is T.J.'s abdomen distended? Explain the development of ascites in liver disease. How is the diet adjusted for people with ascites?

5. Would you expect T.J.'s blood ammonia levels to be high? Why or why not? Explain why blood ammonia can increase in liver disease.

6. Define portal hypertension and jaundice.

Nutrition in Hepatic Coma: A Look at What's New

Scientic progress is not a series of revelations of new truths but a set of successive approximations of a picture of reality that fits the observed facts.

E. N. WHITNEY

The purpose of this Highlight is to provide the interested reader with a review of some newer concepts about hepatic coma that involve nutrition. These ideas remain controversial, both because they have not been completely tested and because results of the few studies so far undertaken have been variable.

An important thing to keep in mind as you read is that the ideas presented here are by no means all-inclusive. We will only be looking at some areas where nutrition might play a big role in correcting hepatic coma.

The Case

Imagine that you are sitting on a jury. The case of Neurotransmitters versus Ammonia will begin. The judge is about to address the jury.

"Ladies and gentlemen of the jury, today we are hearing the case of two theories regarding the cause of hepatic coma. As you listen to the testimony keep in mind that to be a causative factor in hepatic coma, a substance should fulfill at least three criteria:

1. It should be present in abnormal amounts when hepatic coma is present.
2. When the abnormality is created, coma should be induced.
3. Coma should be reversed when the abnormality is corrected.[1]

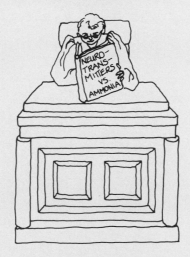

With these instructions in mind, we will begin hearing the evidence against the defendent, Ammonia."

Arguments for the Prosecution

The prosecution attorney will now address the jury:

"Ladies and gentlemen of the jury, I am sure you will agree that ammonia causes hepatic coma. Indeed, as you know, the usual treatment of hepatic coma aims at controlling ammonia production through diet (protein restriction) and drugs (lactulose, and neomycin). Will our first witness take the stand, please? . . . Dr. X, please answer the following question for the jury. Is ammonia present in abnormal amounts when hepatic coma is present?"

"Well (with slight hesitation), yes, in most people in hepatic coma, ammonia levels in the blood and cerebral spinal fluid are elevated. But ammonia levels do not correlate with the severity of hepatic coma. For example, you can't say that everyone with a certain degree of hyperammonemia will be in coma. However, one must keep in mind that blood ammonia levels do not reflect the concentration of ammonia in the brain, and most routine hospital determinations of blood ammonia are inaccurate.[2] The best correlation between the severity of hepatic coma and lab tests are with spinal fluid glutamine and ketoglutarate. These two substances accumulate in the brain in the presence of excess brain ammonia."

[1] L. Zieve, The mechanism of hepatic coma, *Hepatology* 1 (1981):360-365.

[2] P. Misra, Hepatic encephalopathy, *Medical Clinics of North America* 65 (1981)209-226.

"Thank you, Dr. X. Now can you tell the jury if coma can be created by giving excess ammonia?"

"Of course, we cannot purposely give excess ammonia to humans to try to induce coma, so animal models must be used. When animals are given high doses of ammonia there is an increase in the size and number of certain nerve cells which have also been seen in the brains of people who died with coma.[3]

"There is also another bit of evidence to suggest that hepatic coma is induced by excess ammonia levels. Children who have certain congenital enzyme defects have high blood ammonia levels. They also may lapse into a type of coma similar to hepatic coma.[4] This suggests that ammonia is causal."

"One last question, Dr. X. Can hepatic coma be reversed by lowering blood ammonia levels?"

"Well, as you stated in your opening remarks, reducing blood ammonia levels is the cornerstone of conventional therapy for hepatic coma. Ridding the intestine

---

Miniglossary

aromatic amino acids (AAAs): amino acids with aromatic rings as part of their structures (see p. 96) — phenylalanine, tyrosine, and tryptophan.

branched-chain amino acids (BCAAs): amino acids containing branched carbon chains as part of their structures — leucine, isoleucine, and valine.

cerebral spinal fluid: the fluid bathing the brain and spinal cord.

dopamine: a neurotransmitter derived from tyrosine which increases blood pressure.

F080: an intravenous solution of amino acids high in BCAAs and low in AAAs. The enteral counterpart to this product is Hepatic Acid (McGraw Laboratories).

neurological: pertaining to the nervous system.

neurotransmitters: see Highlight 5.

norepinephrine: a neurotransmitter derived from tyrosine that causes (among many effects) constriction of blood vessels (see also p. 85).

---

[3]M. D. Norenberg, A light and electron microscopic study of experimental portal-systemic (ammonia) encephalopathy, *Laboratory Investigation* 36 (1977):618-627.

[4]V. E. Shih, Hereditary urea-cycle disorders, in *The Urea Cycle*, ed. S. Grisolia, R. Báguena, and F. Mayor (New York: Wiley, 1976), pp. 367-414.

---

of substances that produce ammonia (bacteria, and protein) has been successful in reversing coma."

"Thank you, Dr. X, that will be all."

Arguments for the Defense

The defense attorney will now present her case:

"Ladies and gentlemen of the jury, I submit for your consideration, that excess ammonia does not induce hepatic coma. Rather, high blood ammonia levels are one of several side effects of the deranged metabolism of amino acids. This deranged metabolism also results in changes in various neurotransmitters — and it is these changes that eventually lead to hepatic coma. Our next witness will explain this theory in more detail.

"Dr. Y, can you explain why you think that altered amino acid metabolism causes hepatic coma?"

"Well, yes. First of all, in people with liver failure, the ratio of glucagon to insulin is increased. This hormonal imbalance results in a state of catabolism. Since there is less production of glucose and ketone bodies from the liver, the effect is compounded. Anyway, what happens is that skeletal muscle stores are broken down to provide energy. The muscle itself retains the branched-chain amino acids (or BCAAs) leucine, isoleucine, and valine to make energy for its own use. The aromatic amino acids (or AAAs), namely phenylalanine, tyrosine, and tryptophan, are normally metabolized in the liver, so when the liver is damaged those amino acids accumulate in the blood.

"So what you have is an altered pattern of amino acids in the blood. The AAAs are elevated and the BCAAs are low. When this abnormal mixture of amino acids reaches the brain, the amino acids compete with each other for transport into the brain on a limited number of carriers. Because there are more AAAs, more AAAs will come in contact with the carriers, and consequently more of them will be transported into the brain.

"Tryptophan (one of the AAAs) is a precursor of the neurotransmitter serotonin. Since more tryptophan gets into the brain, more serotonin is produced. In animals (rats and cats), increased serotonin is associated with drowsiness and sleep and decreased serotonin is associated with arousal.[5] The altered amino acid pattern may also deplete the levels of some true neurotransmitters (like dopamine and norepinephrine) and increase the levels of other compounds that, in this circumstance act as neurotransmitters, too — false neurotransmitters. The false transmitters may replace the true ones and thus alter neurological responses."

"Thank you very much, Dr. Y. Now can you tell the jury if this altered amino acid pattern is present when people are in hepatic coma?"

"Yes, in people with the type of hepatic coma seen in chronic liver disease levels of AAAs are increased, and levels of BCAAs are decreased."

"Dr. Y., if altered amino acid levels were responsible for hepatic coma, you would expect that giving feeding solutions high in BCAAs and low in AAAs would normalize the amino acid pattern and reverse coma. Does this happen?"

"Well, yes and no. The use of intravenous solutions high in BCAAs and low in AAAs has had mixed results. Some researchers report that people in coma tolerate higher levels of protein when these mixtures are used and that they awaken sooner.[6] However, other studies have been less promising."[7]

The Cross-Examination

The prosecution attorney will now cross-examine the witness.

"Dr. Y, if altered amino acid patterns were responsible for hepatic coma, you would expect that amino acid patterns would have to normalize before the person would awaken. Does this happen?"

"Not always. Some people in hepatic coma improve even though changes in most amino acids do not appear.[8] Furthermore, unpublished observations suggest that people successfully treated with conventional therapy for hepatic coma have reduced blood ammonia levels not associated with changes in amino acid levels."[9]

"Thank you, Dr. Y. I would like to call one more witness to the stand. Dr. Z, an expert on neurotransmitters, will share some additional comments about neurotransmitters in hepatic coma. Dr. Z?"

[5]G. Curson and P. J. Knott, Environmental, toxicological, and related aspects of tryptophan metabolism with particular reference to the central nervous system, *CRC Critical Reviews in Toxicology*, September 1977, pp. 145-187.

[6]J. E. Fischer and R. H. Bower, Nutritional support in liver disease, *Surgical Clinics of North America* 61 (1981):653- 660.

[7]H. Michel, G. Pomier-Layrargues, O. Duhamel, B. Lacombe, G. Cuilleret, and H. Bellet, Intravenous infusion of ordinary and modified amino-acid solutions in the management of hepatic encephalopathy, *Gastroenterology* 79 (1980):1038.

[8]A. Cascino, C. Cangiano, V. Calcaterra, F. Rossi-Fanelli, and L. Capocaccia, Plasma amino acids imbalance in patients with liver disease, *American Journal of Digestive Diseases* 23 (1978):591-598; M. Y. Morgan, J. P. Milsom, and S. Sherlock, Plasma ratio of valine, leucine, and isoleucine to phenylalanine and tyrosine in liver disease, *Gut* 19 (1978): 1068-1073.

[9]F. L. Weber, Therapy of portal-systemic encephalopathy: The practical and the promising, *Gastroenterology* 81 (1981): 174-181.

"Yes. In hepatic coma, plasma and urine levels of false neurotransmitters are elevated. This tends to support the neurotransmitter theory. However, shortly after people in hepatic coma have died, the levels of tryptophan in their blood are elevated, but brain serotonin is not increased.[10]

"Furthermore, the changes in neurotransmitters have not been shown to induce hepatic coma. Studies in rats have shown that infusing high levels of one false neurotransmitter did cause dopamine and norepinephrine levels to be reduced by more than 90 percent, but the rats still remained alert.[11] Additionally, some people under psychiatric treatment take large doses of tryptophan. Their plasma levels of tryptophan may increase approximately a hundredfold without any apparent toxic effect."[12]

[10]Zieve, 1981.

[11]L. Zieve, Hepatic encephalopathy: Summary of present knowledge with an elaboration on recent developments, in *Progress in Liver Diseases*, vol. 6, ed. I. H. Popper and F. Schaffner (New York: Grune and Stratton, 1979), pp. 327-341.

[12]Curson and Knott, 1977.

The Verdict

The jury is hung on the cause of hepatic coma. More evidence will have to be collected to determine whether one of the alterations just described will be found to be the cause of coma or if some new alteration will be found responsible. When more is known, the case will be retried.

To Explore Further

A brief and clear review that calls itself a unifying hypothesis to explain the roles of ammonia and BCAAs in hepatic coma is:

● Hepatic encephalopathy: a unifying hypothesis. *Nutrition Reviews* 38 (1980):371-373.

CHAPTER 25

CONTENTS

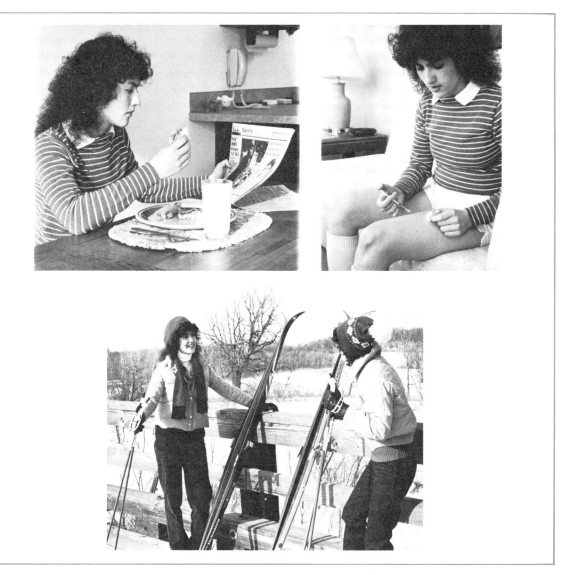

The three major factors in diabetes care: diet, insulin, and exercise.

DIABETES MELLITUS AND HYPOGLYCEMIA

Acute and chronic complications of diabetes are to a large degree controllable if the client understands and follows adequate treatment.

RITA NEMCHIK

Diabetes mellitus and hypoglycemia are two metabolic disorders that result in an imbalance of blood glucose homeostasis. Recognizing the importance of blood glucose in providing fuel for the brain and other tissues, you can imagine why these disorders can have a wide range of effects.

It has been estimated that nearly 10 million people in the United States have diabetes, although fewer than half know they have it.[1] The frequency of diabetes is increasing. Indeed, this disorder is one of the four major causes of death in the United States.

Hypoglycemia is a widely misdiagnosed disorder. People often diagnose themselves as hypoglycemic, and it is fashionable to attribute many ill effects to low blood glucose.

Diabetes Mellitus

The problem in people with diabetes is that their blood glucose is too high. In the diabetic, energy metabolism is altered by either an absolute or relative deficiency of insulin.

Diabetes mellitus is not a single disease. Rather, it is a group of disorders with different causes, clinical features, and outcomes. The two major types of diabetes are insulin dependent diabetes (IDDM or type I diabetes) and non-insulin dependent diabetes (NIDDM or type II diabetes). Some features of the major types of diabetes are summarized in Table 1.

Genetic factors appear to predispose the individual to both types of diabetes. Fewer than 15 percent of diabetics have IDDM; this type of diabetes frequently occurs in childhood and often follows a viral infection. The cells of the pancreas that produce insulin are destroyed and insulin must be replaced.

diabetes mellitus (dye-uh-BEET-eez-MELL-uh-tus): a metabolic disorder of energy metabolism caused by an absolute or relative deficiency of insulin.

mellitus = honey sweet (from sugar in the urine)

Another type of diabetes, which is caused by inadequate secretion of antidiuretic hormone, is called **diabetes insipidus** (in-SIP-id-us). It is treated by giving antidiuretic hormone.

insipid = without taste (no sugar in the urine)

[1]A. Drash, Nutrition vs. diabetes, in *The Medicine Called Nutrition*, ed. D. T. Mason and H. Guthrie (Westport, Conn.: CPC International, 1979), pp. 54-60.

Table 1.   Features of IDDM and NIDDM

	IDDM	NIDDM
Other names	Type I diabetes	Type II diabetes
	Juvenile-onset diabetes	Adult-onset diabetes
	Ketosis-prone diabetes	Ketosis-resistant diabetes
	Brittle diabetes	Lipoplethoric diabetes
		Stable diabetes
Age of onset	< 40 (mean age, 12)	> 40 (about 80% over 50)
Associated conditions	Viral infection	Obesity
Insulin requirement	Yes	Sometimes
Insulin receptors	Normal	Low or normal

A type of NIDDM that develops during the teen years has been termed **maturity-onset diabetes in the young** (MODY).

NIDDM usually develops later in life and is often associated with obesity. Here, insulin secretion is not the major problem. Rather, the cells of the peripheral tissues (muscle, fat) become insensitive to insulin. Obesity makes the insulin resistance worse. Even though the body may make enough insulin, it can't be used. About 85 percent of diabetics have type II diabetes; it is usually milder and it progresses more slowly than type I diabetes.

There are other, less common, classifications of diabetes mellitus. Some people have hyperglycemia without any symptoms of diabetes. In the past this condition was called *chemical diabetes* but now it is classified as *impaired glucose tolerance*. Additionally, some women develop hyperglycemia while pregnant but revert to normal when not pregnant. This is called *gestational diabetes mellitus*. People who develop diabetes during stress (for example, after surgery or infection or during pregnancy) but who are normal at other times are classified as having a *previous abnormality of glucose tolerance*. These people should be followed closely to insure that they do not develop diabetes later in life. *Potential abnormality of glucose tolerance* is another classification of diabetes; it includes people who have a higher-than-average chance of developing diabetes. This group includes people who have close relatives with diabetes and women who have given birth to babies weighing over nine pounds. These people also should be followed closely. Finally, diabetes can develop secondary to other disorders such as pancreatitis and cystic fibrosis or through exposure to some drugs or other chemicals.

The symptoms of diabetes:

Hyperglycemia
Glycosuria (gligh-cose-YOO-ree-uh)

What Happens in Diabetes?   The basic problem in diabetes is that glucose has a lot of trouble getting into cells. Instead, it builds up to very high levels in the blood, causing hyperglycemia. Normally, the kidneys retain glucose rather than excreting it. But when blood levels get too high the excess glucose "spills" into the urine (glycosuria). Glycosuria generally occurs when blood glucose levels exceed 180 mg/ml (see Figure 1).

Figure 1 Overview of diabetes.

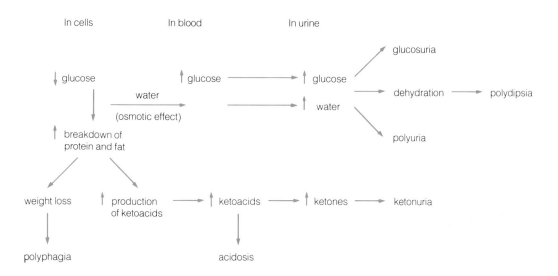

People with uncontrolled diabetes also can become severely dehydrated. The blood glucose concentration rises and creates an osmotic effect, causing water to move from the cells into the blood. (Remember that water moves from a less concentrated to a more concentrated solution.) Furthermore, as glucose spills into the urine, it takes water with it (also an osmotic effect). Thus, both the intracellular fluid and the extracellular fluid become depleted. The diabetic produces excessive urine (polyuria) and, being dehydrated, also may become excessively thirsty (polydipsia). Polyuria and polydipsia are often early symptoms of diabetes.

Dehydration

Polyuria (polly-YOU-ree-uh)
Polydipsia (polly-DIP-see-uh)

Normally, the presence of insulin signals the body that it has been fed and directs cellular activities that favor the storage of protein, carbohydrate, and fat. Insulin enhances the uptake of amino acids into cells and increases protein synthesis. It also enhances the uptake of glucose into cells, increases glycogen synthesis in the liver and muscle, and increases the synthesis of fat. The net effect is to reduce blood glucose levels. When we are fasting, the continued presence of some insulin prevents our bodies' energy stores from being mobilized excessively.

When not enough insulin is produced, or when the cells cannot respond to insulin, they are deprived of the substrates they need for energy. Amino acids and glucose may abound in the cells' fluid environment but the cells have limited access to them and therefore must mobilize their own protein and fats as energy sources. Because of the large amounts of fat being broken down, the liver begins making ketone bodies, and these also accumulate in the blood, compounding the problem of dehydration. The losses of both glucose and ketone bodies (both energy substrates) in the urine and the breakdown of

Biochemical Tests for Diabetes

The diagnosis of diabetes mellitus can be made based on a person's plasma glucose level after an overnight fast. If the person has a plasma glucose concentration of greater than 140 mg/100 ml on two separate occasions, the diagnosis is positive.[2]

Another method of diagnosing diabetes is the glucose tolerance test. The person should follow a high carbohydrate diet for at least three days before the test and should not be taking medication, smoking, or exercising during the test. Furthermore, the person should not be emotionally or physiologically stressed if the test is to be valid.

A glucose tolerance test works like this: The person is given a set amount of glucose to take by mouth in the form of a flavored drink. Blood is drawn before the glucose is given (after an overnight fast) and then at 30, 60, 90, and 120 minutes after the glucose is given. Table 2 lists the upper limits considered normal and the values suggestive of diabetes for each time interval. At least two of the glucose levels should exceed the latter values in order for diabetes to be diagnosed. A person whose glucose levels fall between the upper limits of normal and the values suggestive of diabetes is diagnosed as having impaired glucose tolerance.

Urine tests often provide the first suggestion that a person may be diabetic. Urine tests for sugar and ketones are often performed during routine physicals. Although positive tests for these substances do not always mean diabetes (for example, ketones may be present in people who are following low-carbohydrate diets or fasting), they suggest the need for blood tests. Urine is tested by dipping indicator paper or a paper stick into the urine sample. The color that results is then compared with a color chart to determine the approximate concentration of glucose. The results are read as 0, 1+, 2+, 3+, or 4+, depending on how much glucose is present.

Another method of urine testing involves adding a tablet to the urine sample; the color that results is then compared with a color chart. People are generally advised to check their urine at home using the methods they have learned in the hospital or clinic to be sure their insulin and diet are appropriate, and to keep careful records to review at their next appointment. The urine is checked before meals and at bedtime. The *double-void* method of urine collection is recommended. The person voids once, voids again one-half hour later, and tests the second sample. This method insures that the glucose concentration does not reflect the concentration of urine stored in the bladder for a long period of time.

[2]J. M. Moss, New diagnostic classification of diabetes mellitus, *American Family Physician* 23 (1981):179-181.

Table 2.   Interpretation of Glucose Tolerance Test Results*

Time (min)	Upper limits of normal (mg/100 ml)	Values suggestive of diabetes (mg/100 ml)
0	115	140
60	200	> 200
120	140	200

*This is one of many variations of the glucose tolerance test.

Urine testing is gradually being replaced by direct monitoring of blood glucose levels at home. Blood testing is more sensitive because blood glucose levels must exceed 180 mg/100 ml before glucose spills into the urine. When used properly, home monitoring of blood glucose can help maintain blood glucose levels between 60 and 140 mg/100 ml. To use this method, the diabetic makes a finger stick to get a blood sample (the same method as used to determine hematocrit). Paper strips (as with urine samples) can be used to determine blood glucose concentrations. Meters that give a read-out of the actual glucose concentration and are more accurate than paper strips are also available. However, they are more expensive as well. One author suggests the following schedule for home glucose monitoring:

- Test blood during fasting, two hours after breakfast and lunch, and two hours before and after supper for several days.

- Then test blood at the same times one or two days a week.[3]

A new test used to monitor control of blood glucose levels is the measurement of *glycosylated hemoglobin* (or hemoglobin A$_{1c}$). As blood glucose levels rise, a small glucose molecule attaches to an amino acid on hemoglobin. The altered hemoglobin no longer releases oxygen properly, and it remains in circulation for the life of the red blood cell (120 days). For most of us, only 4 to 8 percent of our hemoglobin is glycosylated. But when blood glucose levels are high for a period of time, this percentage can go up to 16 percent. Measurement of glycosylated hemoglobin allows the physician to determine how successful diabetes control has been over the past two to four months. The test has another advantage. Urine and blood glucose tests are a reflection of diabetes control just prior to the test. A person who has been in poor control can have a normal urine and blood test just by starving or using more insulin the day before going to the doctor. But glycosylated hemoglobin reflects control over several months, so you can't "cheat" on the test.

[3]P. H. Forsham, Diabetes mellitus: A rational plan for management, *Postgraduate Medicine*, March 1982, pp. 139-154.

Weight loss
Polyphagia (polly-FAY-gee-uh)

protein lead to weight loss. This is why the insulin dependent diabetic is likely to be thin. It is also why the diabetic may eat excessively (polyphagia). (Type II diabetics, as mentioned earlier, tend to be obese, rather than thin as type I diabetics are. They overeat because their cells, lacking energy fuels, are hungry; but then the insulin they do have slowly takes effect, and they end up storing as fat the excess energy they have consumed.)

Acetone breath
Ketosis
Ketonuria

If type I diabetes goes uncontrolled, excessive levels of ketones persist in the blood (ketosis). The presence of one ketone (acetone) can be detected by a fruity odor in the breath of the uncontrolled diabetic. The ketones are acidic; when they build up in the blood they cause the pH of the blood to decrease. Ketones begin to appear in the urine (ketonuria), and sodium and potassium become depleted because they are excreted along with the ketones. The loss of sodium and potassium, both base-formers, worsens the acidosis. When acidosis becomes severe enough, the diabetic can lapse into a potentially fatal coma.

Diabetic coma
Hyperosmolar hyperglycemic
  nonketotic coma

People with type II diabetes generally are not prone to ketosis, since they have enough insulin to prevent the excessive buildup of ketoacids. However, they can develop another kind of coma, hyperosmolar hyperglycemic nonketotic coma. As the name implies, this occurs when blood glucose levels become excessive, resulting in osmotic diuresis and dehydration. Acidosis is not present.

The metabolic aberrations seen in diabetes can be used in the clinical setting to help test people for the presence of diabetes. These tests are described in the box "Biochemical Tests for Diabetes."

pruritus vulvae (proo-RIGH-tus VULL-vye): severe itching of the external female genitalia.

pruritus = to itch
vulva = external female
          genitalia

gangrene: death of tissue that usually occurs when the blood supply is cut off.

microangiopathies (MY-cro-AN-gee-OP-uh-these): disorders of the capillaries often seen in diabetes; **retinopathy** is a type of microangiopathy affecting the capillaries of the eye; **neph-ropathy** affects the kidney.

micro = tiny
angio = blood vessel
pathy = disease
retino = of the retina
nephro = of the kidney

Other Complications of Diabetes The person with diabetes often suffers from related complications. The diabetic is more likely to develop infections because of the high levels of glucose in the blood and urine. Urinary tract infections and pruritus vulvae are fairly common. For this reason, the diabetic must pay special attention to hygiene.

Diabetics also are prone to many diseases involving the vascular system. These vascular diseases are of two types: those of the large blood vessels and those of the smaller vessels. Atherosclerosis tends to develop early in diabetics (see Chapter 26) and is the major cause of death in NIDDM. The arteries become blocked by the formation of plaques. When blood flow to the limbs (often the legs) is blocked, the cells die and the limbs must be amputated. Diabetics have a fiftyfold higher incidence of gangrene than the nondiabetic population.[4]

Diabetics frequently develop disorders of the small blood vessels (capillaries), called microangiopathies. The eyes, kidneys, and nervous system may be involved. About 85 percent of diabetics have either retinopathy (involvement of the capillaries of the eye) or nephropathy (involvement of the capillaries of the kidney). Diabetes is a leading cause of both blindness and renal disease.

[4]Forsham, 1982.

Nerve tissues also can deteriorate, a condition called neuropathy which can be quite painful. Loss of sensation in the hands and feet can occur, causing the diabetic to be unaware of injuries to these areas. An infection, once started, can then progress rapidly, because the bacteria thrive on the high blood glucose available to them. This is another chain of events leading to amputation of a limb and again points to the need for good hygiene, especially care of the feet.

The treatment of the person with diabetes depends on the type of diabetes. However, for all diabetics the goals of therapy are to:

- Maintain blood glucose levels in an acceptable range.
- Prevent or delay the onset or progression of the associated complications.
- Encourage people to resume normal activities.

Diet therapy for all diabetics encompasses these goals. Additionally, diet therapy should be designed to:

- Help people achieve and maintain optimal nutrition status.

The diabetic has the same nutrient requirements as a nondiabetic of the same age, stature, and activity level. The diet is designed to minimize changes in blood glucose levels and is modified when complications of diabetes make such a change necessary.

No one knows if maintaining blood glucose levels within a fairly normal range can prevent the complications of diabetes. However, evidence is accumulating that control of blood glucose levels does produce this benefit, and it surely does no harm.

Treating the Insulin Dependent Diabetic

A diagnosis of insulin dependent diabetes can be devastating. It may seem like the end of the world to a child just about ready to pass into adolescence, a time when peer pressure dictates that no one should be "different." The fear of having to inject insulin daily and of possible complications may be difficult to come to terms with for a person of any age. Then there is the diet to be followed. And, finally, there is the impressive task of coordinating diet, insulin, and exercise. Overwhelming as they may seem at first, these difficulties can be overcome. The insulin dependent diabetic today can lead a normal and full life and should be encouraged to think positively.

We have already mentioned the three basic components that must be coordinated in the diabetic's treatment — insulin, diet, and exercise. Let's start by taking a closer look at insulin.

Insulin   Since type I diabetics can't make insulin, their insulin must come from another source. Commercially made insulin is commonly extracted from the pancreas of cattle. There are different types of

Insulin was first used successfully in diabetic dogs by F. G. Banting and C. H. Best in 1922. Shortly after its discovery, insulin became available to thousands of persons with diabetes.

Some people become allergic to a particular kind of insulin (beef or pork) or to the type of alcohol that is used to clean or sterilize a particular kind of insulin. This is called **insulin allergy.** In this case, the diabetic must switch to another kind of insulin.

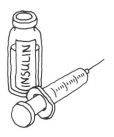

An example of insulin dosage is as follows:

45 minutes before breakfast — an injection of 60% rapid-acting and 40% intermediate-acting insulin.

30 minutes before supper — an injection of 40% rapid-acting and 60% intermediate-acting insulin.

Rapid-acting insulin peaks within 4 hours; intermediate at about 8 to 10 hours.

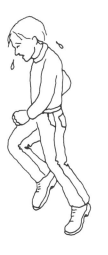

insulin; they are grouped as fast acting, intermediate acting, or long acting, depending on how quickly they begin to work and how long they remain active. Table 3 lists examples of the various types of insulin and their actions.

Normally, we secrete insulin after a meal and therefore have it available to enable us to store energy nutrients when they are plentiful. But the type I diabetic has to take insulin at a prescribed time, and so has to make sure to have nutrients from food available when the insulin is present. The exact type, dosage, and administration schedule of insulin is prescribed by the physician based on the individual's needs. Stage of growth, activity patterns, eating habits, and individual responses must all be considered. If the diabetic gets too little insulin or doesn't get insulin when glucose from foods is available, hyperglycemia and diabetic ketoacidosis can result. If the diabetic gets too much insulin or has too little glucose available when insulin is high, severe hypoglycemia may follow (see further discussion below). Even though the discovery of insulin has been invaluable, insulin therapy cannot achieve the same degree of blood glucose control as the body can.

Insulin needs change as growth occurs. As a rule of thumb, about 0.5 to 1.0 unit of insulin is given per kilogram of body weight. (It is important for children with diabetes and their parents to understand this, so that they will know that increased insulin needs do not necessarily mean the diabetes is getting worse.) Generally, two or more types of insulin are mixed together and given more than once a day to approximate the times when insulin would normally be present in the bloodstream.

Activity reduces insulin needs. Exercise has an insulin-like effect in lowering blood glucose levels. Insulin needs increase during stress, such as pregnancy, surgery, and infection and other illnesses. (You may recall that hyperglycemia results from the catabolic stress response, so it makes sense that insulin needs would increase.) Even psychological stress may precipitate periods of hyperglycemia.[5]

Insulin must be injected because, since it is a protein, it would be digested and thus ineffective if taken by mouth. Although insulin is always necessary for type I diabetics, it may also be required by some type II diabetics, often as a temporary measure to control hyperglycemia.

The hypoglycemia that occurs when blood glucose gets too low is called an insulin reaction or insulin shock. An insulin reaction can result from taking an overdose of insulin, engaging in excessive physical activity, skipping meals, or eating too little food. Diabetics should learn to recognize the symptoms of hypoglycemia; if it becomes severe, they can lapse into coma and die. For mild symptoms, the diabetic should immediately eat some form of readily absorbed glucose (fruit juice, hard candies, sugar, or glucose solutions). In severe cases, glucose is administered intravenously. Sometimes glucagon is given to counteract an insulin reaction.

[5]Forsham, 1982.

Table 3. Actions of Various Insulin Types

Type	Duration of activity	Peak of action
Rapid acting		
Regular crystalline	5-7 hr	2-4 hr
Semilente	12-16 hr	2-8 hr
Intermediate acting		
Globin	12-18 hr	6-8 hr
NPH/lente	18-24 hr	8-14 hr
Long acting		
Protamine zinc	24-30 hr	16-24 hr
Ultralente	30-36 hr	18-29 hr

Individuals suffering from insulin shock may appear to be intoxicated. This is especially tragic if the true problem is not recognized, because the person can die. To prevent such a mistake, the diabetic is often advised to wear identification in the form of a bracelet or necklace. A card in the wallet may not be adequate, since a wallet might not be checked immediately. In addition, type I diabetics should always carry sugar cubes or hard candy with them so that they can act immediately when hypoglycemic symptoms occur.

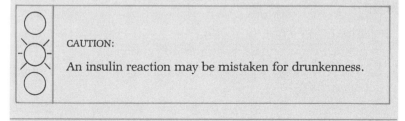

CAUTION:

An insulin reaction may be mistaken for drunkenness.

Hyperglycemia can result from excessive secretion of insulin antagonists (glucagon, epinephrine, glucocorticoids) in response to excessive administration of insulin. This is called **rebound hyperglycemia** or the **Somogyi** (so-MOHG-yee) **effect**.

Symptoms of hypoglycemia:

Nervousness
Weakness
Sweating
Shallow breathing
Double vision
Dizziness

Symptoms of hyperglycemia:

Glycosuria
Intense thirst
Confusion
Nausea
Vomiting
Labored breathing
Acetone breath

Hyperglycemia and the possibility of diabetic coma have already been discussed. The diabetic should learn to distinguish between the symptoms of hypoglycemia and hyperglycemia, because the treatments are different. The symptoms of hyperglycemia can be precipitated by stress (infection), too little insulin, too much food, or large amounts of concentrated sweets. The treatment involves administering rapid-acting insulin and correcting fluid and electrolyte imbalance by use of IV fluids. Extreme care must be exercised to avoid giving too much insulin, which can result in severe hypoglycemia.

The Diet in IDDM The diet is the mainstay of therapy in all types of diabetes. In the type I diabetic the diet must mesh with insulin therapy and exercise. The planning of a diabetic diet is a several-step process that has been well worked out.

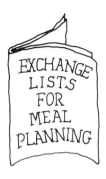

The first concern is to provide kcalories adequate to achieve or maintain ideal body weight. In the juvenile diabetic this means giving enough kcalories to support growth. The kcalories required by the type I diabetic are the same as for the general population. Therefore, the RDA can be used as a guide to determining kcalorie needs. To determine exact need, the diabetic is reassessed regularly to see if height and weight are appropriate and the diet is then adjusted if necessary. (See box "How to Individualize a Diabetic Diet Using Exchange Lists.")

How to Individualize a Diabetic Diet Using Exchange Lists

The task of planning a diabetic diet is most often the responsibility of the dietitian, who must look closely at the diabetic's diet history to determine how to best adjust the diet to the individual's lifestyle. The first few times you use exchange lists to plan such a diet, the procedure may take hours. However, with only a little practice you can learn to work out the whole plan in a matter of minutes. Here are the steps that go into planning the diet:

1. Determine ideal body weight.

Males: Allow 106 lb for the first 5 ft, then add 6 lb for each inch over 5 ft.

Females: Allow 100 lb for the first 5 ft, then add 5 lb for each inch over 5 ft.

Adjustment: Add 10 percent for large-framed individuals; subtract 10 percent for small-framed individuals.

Children: Varies with height for age; refer to growth chart (Appendix E).

As an example, let's take an adult male who is 5 ft 7 in tall and weighs 145 lb. He is of medium frame and is moderately active.

$$\text{Ideal weight} = 106 \text{ lb} + (6 \text{ lb} \times 7) = 148 \text{ lb}$$

This person will not need to lose or gain weight.

2. Calculate kcalorie needs. Multiply ideal body weight by 10 to get the basal kcaloric requirement. Add kcalories for activity: for sedentary people, add 30 percent; for moderately active people, add 50 percent; for people who engage in strenuous activity, add 100 percent. Children under 12 require about 1,000 kcal plus 100 kcal per year of age. For weight loss, subtract 500 kcal per pound of desired weight loss per week. For weight gain, add 500 kcal per pound of desired weight gain per week. Adjust kcalories as necessary based on the individual's response.

Our client would need the following number of kcalories:

$$148 \text{ lb} \times 10 \text{ kcal/lb} = 1{,}480 \text{ kcal (basal)}$$
$$1{,}480 \times 50\% = \underline{ 740 \text{ kcal (activity)}}$$
$$\text{Total} \quad 2{,}220 \text{ kcal*}$$

*This figure would be rounded off to 2,200 kcal.

If he needed to lose weight, we could subtract 500 kcal and plan on 1,700 kcal per day so that he could lose one pound per week.

3. Determine the grams of protein (12 to 20 percent of kcal), carbohydrate (50 to 60 percent of kcal), and fat (maximum 38 percent of kcal) to be included in the meal plan.

For our client, this would be translated as follows:

Protein:
$$2{,}200 \times 12\% = 264 \text{ kcal} \div 4 \text{ kcal/g} = 66 \text{ g}$$
$$2{,}200 \times 20\% = 440 \text{ kcal} \div 4 \text{ kcal/g} = 110 \text{ g}$$

Carbohydrate:
$$2{,}200 \times 50\% = 1{,}100 \text{ kcal} \div 4 \text{ kcal/g} = 275 \text{ g}$$
$$2{,}200 \times 60\% = 1{,}320 \text{ kcal} \div 4 \text{ kcal/g} = 330 \text{ g}$$

Fat:
$$2{,}200 \times 38\% = 836 \text{ kcal} \div 9 \text{ kcal/g} = 93 \text{ g}$$

His diet should contain 66-110 g protein, 275-330 g carbohydrate, and a maximum of 93 g fat.

4. Translate the diet prescription into a meal plan. (The Self-Study at the end of Chapter 8 shows how to convert amounts of grams into exchanges.) A sample 2,200 kcal meal plan is given below:

Exchange group	Number of Exchanges	Carbo-hydrate (g)	Protein (g)	Fat (g)
Milk, nonfat	3	36	24	—
Vegetables	4	20	8	—
Fruit	6	60	—	—
Bread	11	165	22	—
Meat, low fat	7	—	49	21
Fat	11	—	—	55
Total		281	103	76

5. The final step is to divide the kcalories and carbohydrate into tenths and determine the distribution of the meals. For example, let's say our client needs three meals and two snacks (one midmorning and one before bed). A typical distribution might go like this:

$$2{,}200 \text{ kcal} \div 10 = 220 \text{ kcal}$$
$$281 \text{ g carbohydrate} \div 10 = 28 \text{ g carbohydrate}$$

(continued)

	Breakfast (2/10)	Mid-morning snack (1/10)	Lunch (3/10)	Supper (3/10)	Bed-time snack (1/10)
Energy (kcal)	440	220	660	660	220
Carbohydrate (g)	56	28	84	84	28

These figures are approximations. Chances are you will not be able to divide meals so that the kcalories and carbohydrate are distributed exactly as you would wish. (See sample 2,200-kcal diabetic diet menu.)

The next step is to determine protein, carbohydrate, and fat needs (see box). The American Diabetes Association recommends that of the total kcalories allowed, 12 to 20 percent should be from protein, 50 to 60 percent from carbohydrate, and a maximum of 38 percent from fat.[6] The fat kcalories should be derived mainly from polyunsaturated sources (see Chapter 2), which may help protect against atherosclerosis. Highlight 25 discusses the basis for these recommendations in more detail.

You may already have started to wonder whether you should plan diet therapy around the insulin schedule or tailor insulin injections to the diet plan. In the hospital setting and in many physicians' practices, insulin therapy is recommended and the diet is planned around it. But this may not be an ideal approach. It may be much easier for the diabetic to follow the total treatment plan if he doesn't have to alter all his eating habits. It is probably preferable to determine eating habits, plan a diet within those habits, and then determine how insulin should be fitted into the plan. Minor dietary modifications can then be made, if necessary. When the insulin schedule has been planned first and you don't think your patient will be able to stay on the diet that has been planned around it, talk with the physician about the problem. You may be able to help work out a more acceptable diet and insulin plan.

[6]B. R. B. El-Beheri Burgess, Rationale for changes in the dietary management of diabetes, *Journal of the American Dietetic Association* 81 (1982):258-261.

After the kcaloric, protein, carbohydrate, and fat needs have been calculated, the division of the nutrients into meals is determined. Because the diet must be coordinated with the insulin dosage, it is important that the timing and composition of meals be consistent from day to day, with meals and snacks eaten at about the same time each day. Insulin dependent diabetics may be able to maintain better blood glucose control if they eat smaller meals with two or three snacks. Carbohydrate is included in every meal and snack, roughly in proportion to total kcalories. Each meal usually contains from 20 to 40 percent of the total kcalories and carbohydrate, and each snack about 10 percent. The distribution often consists of three meals, a bedtime snack, and sometimes a midafternoon or midmorning snack, depending on the individual's blood glucose levels. (See "How to Individualize a Diabetic Diet Using Exchange Lists.")

The diet for the diabetic is based on the exchange system (see Chapter 1, pp. 39-42, and Appendix L). Food is divided into groups based on contents of kcalories, carbohydrate, protein, fat, and other nutrients. The diabetic learns that foods on any one list can be "exchanged" freely for each other. However, food from one list cannot be exchanged for foods on another list. Appendix L lists the exchange systems used in the United States and Canada. Each list shows which foods are allowed on the diabetic diet. Low fat and nonfat milks, lean meats, and polyunsaturated fats should be emphasized to reduce the diet's saturated fat content.

In the past, diabetics were often advised to weigh their foods on gram scales so that portion sizes would be exact. This is called a **weighed diet**. It is no longer considered necessary to weigh foods. Instead, foods can be measured with common household measuring utensils. This is referred to as a **measured diet**.

Sample diabetic diet menu (2,200 kcal)

Breakfast
  1 soft cooked egg (1M, ½F)
  ½ c oatmeal (1B)
  1 slice whole wheat toast (1B)
  1½ tsp margarine (1½F)
  1 small banana (2Fr)
  1 cup skim milk (1Mk)
Kcal: 445   CHO: 62 g

Midmorning Snack
  ½ c orange juice (1Fr)
  6 saltine crackers (1B)
  1 oz cheddar cheese (1M, 1F)
Kcal: 210 CHO: 25 g

Lunch
  Ham sandwich
    with 2 tsp mayonnaise (2M, 2B, 2F)
  ¼ c baked beans (1B)
  ½ c carrots (1V)
  ½ c broccoli (1V)
  1 tsp margarine (1F)
  1 large apple (2Fr)
  1 cup skim milk (1Mk)
Kcal: 665 CHO: 87 g

Supper
  3 oz chicken (3M)
  ½ c sweet potatoes (2B)
  ½ c green beans (1V)
  2 tsp margarine (2F)
  Salad (1V)
  Salad dressing, 2 tsp (1F)
  2 whole wheat rolls (2B)
  ¼ cantaloupe (1Fr)
Kcal: 670 CHO: 80 g

Bedtime Snack
  1 cup skim milk (1Mk)
  3 cups popcorn (1B)
    with 2 tsp margarine (2F)
Kcal: 240 CHO: 27 g

Exchange abbreviations

B = bread F = fat Fr = fruit M = meat

Mk = milk V = vegetable

CHO = carbohydrate

The exchange lists were devised to permit the diabetic to choose from a wide selection of normal foods and yet stay within a diet plan. They work so well that they have been adopted for many other uses — for example, they are used extensively for weight reduction and fat-controlled diets (Chapters 8 and 26). Exchange lists can be used to calculate the nutrient composition of any person's diet (Chapter 19). It is well worth the time and energy to become familiar with the energy, protein, carbohydrate, and fat content and the foods included on each list.

Exchange lists can be used to tailor a diet to an individual's preferences. However, most dietitians use standard exchange patterns that have already been calculated. Appendix M contains examples of different diet plans, or standard patterns. The patterns provide such a healthful balance of energy nutrients, and the lists offer such a variety of wholesome foods to choose from, that many authorities believe the diabetic diet is the healthiest diet anyone can follow: Everyone should adopt a diabetic diet. This is comforting news to diabetics who can share their diets with their families to everyone's benefit.

Using standard patterns can save time, but they should always be adjusted to the individual. Some shortcuts to adjusting the patterns can be used. For example, the planner can substitute one bread exchange (70 kcal, 15 g carbohydrate) for one and one-half fruit exchanges (60 kcal, 15 g carbohydrate). If the client doesn't drink milk (80 kcal, 10 g carbohydrate), the planner can substitute a serving of fruit and 1 oz of lean meat (95 kcal, 10 g carbohydrate).

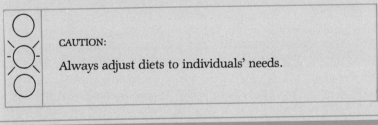

CAUTION:

Always adjust diets to individuals' needs.

In most cases, concentrated sweets are excluded from the diabetic diet (except to reverse hypoglycemia). However, some physicians allow some concentrated sweets, particularly to juvenile diabetics on occasion. Additionally, concentrated sweets may be allowed before vigorous exercise or during illness (see below).

Exercise and IDDM   During periods of unusually intense exercise, the type I diabetic will need more food, since exercise has an insulin-like effect. The following can serve as a general guide:

- No extra food is required for exercise of short duration and modest intensity (walking one-half mile at a moderate pace).

- 10 to 15 g of carbohydrate are allowed per hour of moderate exercise (hunting or playing golf).
- 20 to 30 g of carbohydrate are allowed per hour of vigorous exercise (digging or playing basketball).[7]

Delayed Meals and Illness   The type I diabetic, like all normal persons, must occasionally miss a meal. When this happens, some carbohydrate should be taken to protect against hypoglycemia. Usually 15 to 30 g of carbohydrate will forestall hypoglycemia for one to two hours on these occasions.

The insulin dependent diabetic who is in the hospital may also have problems with missing meals. The hospitalized diabetic may be N.P.O. (allowed nothing by mouth) for tests, following surgery, or if GI problems prevent food intake. Every hospital should have a standard procedure for dealing with this problem. One method is to replace at least half the prescribed carbohydrate and kcalories within three hours after the missed meal. If this cannot be done, the physician is notified and may decide that some other measure is necessary (changing the insulin schedule or giving IV dextrose). Sometimes diet prescriptions are changed so that more simple carbohydrates (which are easy to eat or drink) are included.

Concentrated carbohydrates also may be allowed when the diabetic has a poor appetite because of illness. Soft drinks are often given. The main concern is to prevent starvation and vomiting. During stress, however, it may be desirable to reduce intake somewhat, because insulin requirements increase during stress. Reducing total kcalorie and carbohydrate intake helps limit the need for extra insulin.

A source of sugar sometimes overlooked is certain drugs. The diabetic should be warned that both over-the-counter and prescription drugs may contain sugar. Members of the health care team, too, should be alert to this possibility.

Diabetics can receive central TPN or commercial tube feedings that contain considerable amounts of simple sugars. However, extra care must be taken in monitoring diabetic patients so that insulin dosage can be adjusted to meet the higher simple carbohydrate loads. Some patients may not be able to tolerate the higher levels of carbohydrate in TPN even when insulin is increased. In these persons, the concentration of glucose may have to be reduced and additional kcalories provided by IV fat emulsions (see Chapter 20). For diabetics who cannot tolerate simple carbohydrates from tube feedings, blenderized feedings that do not contain simple sugars can be devised.

[7]K. M. West, Diabetes mellitus, in *Nutritional Support of Medical Practice*, ed. H. A. Schneider, C. E. Anderson, and D. B. Coursin (Hagerstown, Md.: Harper & Row, 1977); pp. 278-296.

Treating the Non-insulin Dependent Diabetic

In many ways the treatment of the non-insulin dependent diabetic is the same as that of the insulin dependent diabetic. The main goals of therapy are the same. But because type II diabetes results from a resistance to insulin rather than from lack of insulin, there are some important differences. Many type II diabetics' blood glucose levels can be controlled by diet alone. Others have to use drugs in addition to diet.

The Diet in NIDDM The primary goal of diet therapy in NIDDM (type II) is weight reduction, if it is necessary — and the majority of type II diabetics are obese. Obese diabetics with severe hyperglycemia may have to fast or follow diets very low in kcalories (600 kcal/day) until blood glucose levels are under control. Weight reduction diets higher in kcalories (1,000 to 1,200 kcal/day) may then be given until the desired weight is reached. The type II diabetic's glucose tolerance may show marked improvement with a weight loss of as few as 5 to 10 pounds.[8] Weight loss should begin immediately, or else these diabetics may begin to require insulin. One group of investigators has reported that response to diet therapy in type II diabetes of longer duration (more than five years) was significantly poorer than in type II diabetes of shorter duration (two years or less). This difference occurred despite a similar degree of weight loss and duration of diet therapy in the two groups.[9]

The timing and distribution of meals for the type II diabetic is not critical, provided that concentrated sweets are avoided and that the total number of kcalories is consistent with the diet plan. Usually, only three meals a day are recommended. This helps prevent excessive snacking and possible weight gain. Table 4 compares the key components of diet therapy in type I and type II diabetes.

The exchange list system provides the basis for the diet in type II diabetes. If the person is already at ideal weight, a diet excluding concentrated sweets may be recommended. Table 5 lists the foods that should be avoided on such a diet.

Oral Hypoglycemic Agents Some type II diabetics cannot achieve blood glucose control by diet alone. When control is inadequate because of stress, failure to lose weight, or other factors, oral hypoglycemic agents are often prescribed.

There are two groups of oral hypoglycemic agents — the biguanides and the sulfonylureas. The biguanides were found to have undesirable side effects and were removed from the market in 1977. However, they are still used on an experimental basis. No one knows exactly how the

[8]Forsham, 1982.

[9]M. Nagulesparan, P. J. Savage, L. J. Bennion, R. H. Unger, and P. H. Bennett, Diminished effect of caloric restriction on control of hyperglycemia with increasing known duration of type II diabetes mellitus, *Journal of Clinical Endocrinology and Metabolism* 53 (1981):560-568.

Table 4. **Comparison of Type I and Type II Diabetic Diets***

Diet Approach	Type I	Type II
Reduce kcalories	Usually not necessary	Yes
Keep ratio of carbohydrate, protein, and fat consistent for each feeding	Yes	No
Eat meals at regular times	Yes	Not necessary
Eat more frequent meals	Yes	No
Use food to treat or prevent hypoglycemia	Yes	No
Replace carbohydrate when appetite is poor or meals are missed	Yes	No
Provide extra food for intense exercise	Yes	No

*Philosophies vary. Not every diet therapist would follow these guidelines in every case.

Table 5. **Foods Avoided on a Diet That Excludes Concentrated Sweets**

Cakes	Fruit ices	Milkshakes
Candy	Fruit juices, sweetened	Molasses
Cookies	Gelatin, sweetened	Pastries
Cranberry sauce	Honey	Pies
Doughnuts	Ice cream	Popsicles
Frappes	Jam	Pudding
Fruits, canned, frozen or cooked with sugar	Jelly	Sweet rolls
Fruits, glazed	Marmalade	Sugar
Fruit drinks	Milk, chocolate or condensed	Syrup
		Vegetables, glazed

sulfonylureas work, although part of their effect is to stimulate the release of insulin from the pancreas. Their major effect may be to increase the number and activity of insulin receptors in the peripheral tissue.[10]

The use of oral hypoglycemic agents has been controversial because of the findings of the University Group Diabetes Program (UGDP) study. This study, conducted by competent professionals over an eight-year period, found that tolbutamide (one type of sulfonylurea) was associated with a significant increase in deaths from heart attacks.

[10]M. N. Feinglos and H. E. Lebovitz, Sulfonylurea treatment of insulin-independent diabetes mellitus, *Metabolism* 29 (1980):488-494; Forsham, 1982.

However, there has been a great deal of criticism regarding the way the study was conducted. It has been suggested that oral hypoglycemic agents are harmful only if blood glucose levels are not adequately controlled.[11] Some physicians refuse to prescribe oral hypoglycemics; if their patients' blood glucose levels cannot be controlled by diet alone, insulin is used. Others try oral hypoglycemics in the type II diabetic when diet therapy alone fails. However, there is agreement that oral hypoglycemics do not replace dieting. The diet should be continued, even when these drugs are used.

Fiber, Alcohol, and Dietetic Foods

Fiber

You may have noticed that the carbohydrate content recommended for the diabetic's diet is fairly high (see the meal pattern in "How to Individualize a Diabetic Diet Using Exchange Lists," the sample menu, and Highlight 25). One reason that a fair amount of carbohydrate is encouraged is to provide fiber in the diet. It has been shown that a diet high in both carbohydrate and fiber helps keep blood glucose levels from rising sharply after a meal.[12]

The dietary fiber content of the diabetic diet can be increased to 25 to 35 g per 1,000 kcal by incorporation of foods high in fiber. Dried beans and peas, vegetables, whole grain breads and cereals, and fruits can be used to increase fiber content. Guar, a type of dietary fiber found in legumes, seems to be the type most beneficial in preventing sharp rises in blood glucose after a meal.[13] Type II diabetics may be able to decrease the dosage or discontinue the use of medication while on high-fiber diets. Type I diabetics may be able to reduce their insulin dosage.

The use of higher levels of carbohydrate in the diabetic diet has been promising. But there is a practical problem. In order to get in more carbohydrate, the intake of protein from meat must be reduced considerably. This can be difficult for the person who likes to eat large amounts of meat. You can probably help this person most by pointing out the advantages of the high-fiber diet. Keep in mind, too, that the high-fiber diet should be introduced little by little to help prevent abdominal discomfort and flatulence.

[11]A. M. Sackler, The unsettling UGDP controversy, *Journal of the American Medical Association* 243 (1980):1435-1436.

[12]T. G. Kiehm, J. W. Anderson, and K. Ward, Beneficial effects of high carbohdrate, high fiber diet on hyperglycemic diabetic men, *American Journal of Clinical Nutrition* 29 (1976):895-899.

[13]P. A. Crapo, J. Insel, M. Sperling, and O. G. Kolterman, Comparison of serum glucose, insulin, and glucagon responses to different types of complex carbohydrate in noninsulin-dependent diabetic patients, *American Journal of Clinical Nutrition* 34 (1981):184-190.

A question commonly asked by the diabetic is "Can I have alcohol?" The diabetic whose blood glucose is well controlled can usually include some alcohol with the consent of the physician. However, some points must be considered when alcohol is incorporated into the diet.

Alcohol

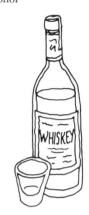

In the diabetic, alcohol may precipitate a hypoglycemic reaction, especially when the diabetic hasn't eaten for some time. This happens because alcohol inhibits the liver's output of glucose. The hypoglycemia may be overlooked because the person may appear intoxicated. Therefore, alcohol should be taken only with meals or shortly before or after meals.

Another consideration is the fact that alcohol is high in kcalories and low in nutritional value. Therefore, alcohol should be used sparingly, and the kcalories from alcohol must be calculated into the daily kcalorie allowance. Fat kcalories are most often traded for alcohol kcalories. Drinks that contain carbohydrate (drinks made with mixers, sweet wines, liqueurs) should be avoided, or their carbohydrate should be considered in the diet calculation. Whiskey, gin, vodka, and rum do not contain carbohydrate.

The combination of alcohol and oral hypoglycemic agents may cause flushing of the skin and a rapid heartbeat. People should be forewarned of this possible reaction.

Dietetic foods

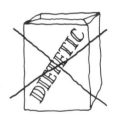

Another common concern is how to replace sugar and foods that contain sugar in the diet. In general, special "dietetic" foods are not necessary in the diabetic diet. People often misinterpret *dietetic* to mean "no kcalories," but this is not the case. Some dietetic foods may be low in sodium instead of sugar, or they may have reduced but still significant numbers of kcalories.

Some dietetic foods may be helpful, however. These include artificially sweetened soft drinks, artificial sweeteners, and water-packed canned fruits. kCalorie-free soft drinks and beverages (such as artificially sweetened tea) can be used freely and are often well liked. Artificial sweeteners that do not contain significant kcalories can help make the diet more acceptable. Two such sweeteners currently available in the United States are saccharin and aspartame. In Canada, saccharin has been banned; but another sweetener, cyclamate, is still on the market. While the use of saccharin became controversial following reports that large doses of saccharin had caused bladder tumors in rats, the effect of saccharin in humans ingesting normal amounts has not been determined. The fear that saccharin might be banned spurred research into other possible artificial sweeteners; the recent approval of aspartame by the FDA resulted from such research.

Sweeteners used to take the place of sugar (sucrose) are called **alternative sweeteners**. **Nonnutritive sweeteners** (saccharin, aspartame) do not contain appreciable kcalories; they are also called **artificial sweeteners**. **Nutritive sweeteners** (fructose, sorbitol, xylitol) contain the same number of kcalories as an equivalent amount of sugar.

Diabetes throughout the Life Cycle

The overall approach to diabetes is the same throughout life, but special problems may become apparent at different stages. Treatment will be more effective if these needs are recognized and dealt with.

Consider some of the special problems of the child diabetic. In the child, growth is sporadic. It is difficult to predict how many kcalories a child will need at any one point in time. Appetite is also variable. Furthermore, activity varies widely from day to day; a child may be quite active after school when the sun is shining but may be planted in front of the TV on a rainy day.

For these reasons, it is often recommended that a flexible diet be provided for the diabetic child. This is not to say that the diet is unrestricted, however. Meals should be balanced and provide a wide variety of foods. Concentrated sweets are only given at times of vigorous physical activity or to treat hypoglycemia. The child is not forced to finish a meal, but meals should not be skipped, since hypoglycemia can result. If the child finishes a meal and wants more, seconds can be provided. Meals should be planned for approximately the same time each day, and the child should be served the same foods as the rest of the family. Snacks are usually given two or three times a day.

Special considerations also apply to diabetes in pregnancy. The nutrient needs of the pregnant diabetic are the same as those of any pregnant woman. Hypoglycemia may occur early in pregnancy because of transfer of glucose to the fetus, vomiting, or decreased food intake resulting from nausea. Occasionally, insulin dosage must be reduced in early pregnancy. However, insulin requirements increase in the last half of pregnancy because the placenta begins secreting hormones that are antagonistic to insulin.

The geriatric diabetic may find it difficult to afford the foods called for on the diabetic diet. Furthermore, some elderly people have trouble chewing foods. Others have medical conditions that may require additional dietary modifications. Still others have sensitive digestive systems and irregular bowel habits that may be aggravated (or helped) by changing the diet.

Education for Diabetics

Educating the diabetic is best accomplished by the team approach. Both group and individual counseling can be used. The diabetic should understand the objectives of diet (and other) therapy and also must understand how the exchange system works. The teaching-learning process takes time; a person just getting over the shock of being told the diagnosis is diabetes may find the new information difficult to grasp.

The individual will be better able to adjust to therapy if it is planned with his lifestyle in mind and if he himself is active in the planning process. He must be able to learn how to manage complications of the disease. He should be seen regularly to insure that he understands the treatment plan. It helps greatly if not only the diabetic but also everyone he lives with is involved in the learning process. The best adjustment may occur if the whole family attends live-in training sessions for a week. In the case of a child, a summer camp especially for diabetic children offers the chance to "live" the diabetic lifestyle under supervision until it is accepted and automatic.

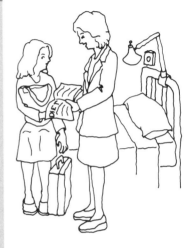

A typical occurrence in the hospital goes like this. The dietitian is paged to instruct a patient on a diabetic diet. There sits the patient, suitcase packed, dressed to go home. Generally, this dietitian will never see the person again.

There is very little chance that a diabetic diet instruction will be successful when given under these circumstances. The patient is anxious to get home and may not be able to concentrate. Even if she weren't eager to leave, one counseling session would be inadequate for teaching this type of diet.

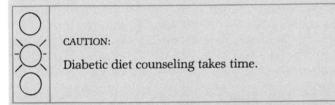

CAUTION:

Diabetic diet counseling takes time.

How can this situation be prevented? Usually, physicians are responsible for ordering a diet instruction. But if they fail to do so, reminding them when a patient hasn't been instructed yet may help. The diet advisor should be aware of patients on special diets, should be instructing them throughout their hospitalization, and should follow through either with home visits or with referrals to agencies or individuals that can provide continued help.

What to Look for in the Future

Many fascinating research efforts in diabetes are under way. For example, investigators are working diligently to produce synthetic human insulin, which would prevent problems with allergic reactions and might work more effectively than the insulins presently available. Human insulin can be synthesized from amino acids or through modification of pig insulin, but the process is too impractical to be useful at this time.

Another way that human insulin has been produced is by using recombinant DNA technology. Bacteria that contain the gene for human insulin are constructed, and the bacteria act as minifactories to manufacture human insulin. Right now this process is not practical for producing large amounts of insulin, but the FDA has approved the use of the amounts now available, and the future of this procedure looks quite promising.

Recombinant DNA

Somatostatin

Somatostatin   Another approach to controlling diabetes that is currently being researched is use of the hormone somatostatin. This approach centers around the theory that diabetes is caused not only by an insulin deficiency but also by a glucagon excess. Since glucagon acts as an antagonist to insulin, it aggravates the diabetic state. Glucagon's release from the pancreas is inhibited by somatostatin. Preliminary studies in which mixtures of insulin and somatostatin were given showed that these mixtures helped control blood glucose levels better than insulin alone.[14] However, some problems must be worked out before this type of therapy can be used.

Glucose tolerance factor

Chromium and Glucose Tolerance Factor   Some researchers believe that a marginal deficiency of chromium is an important cause of type II diabetes in developed countries. They believe that chromium-rich foods may be useful for treating the disease. One type of chromium complex, the glucose tolerance factor (GTF), is believed to enhance the action of insulin, probably by acting on insulin receptors in the cell membrane (see page 460). This is also the form of chromium that is best absorbed by the body. Refined diets that are low in whole grain breads and cereals are often also low in chromium, and such diets are typical of industrialized societies. Currently, the supplementation of the diabetic's diet with chromium remains controversial.

Artificial pancreas

closed-loop system: a type of artificial pancreas consisting of a glucose sensing device, a minicomputer, and a pump.

open-loop system: a type of artificial pancreas in which a pump (worn on the diabetic's back) constantly delivers a basal level of insulin between meals and during the night. More insulin is delivered during meals, provided the wearer presses a button.

The Artificial Pancreas   Several types of systems have been designed to work like the diabetic's defective endocrine pancreas. One mechanical approach, the closed-loop system, involves three major components: a sensor that determines the amount of glucose in the blood; a minicomputer that calculates how much insulin (or sometimes glucose) needs to be administered; and a pump that delivers the insulin or glucose intravenously. The closed-loop system responds immediately to changes in blood glucose concentration. The many drawbacks of these systems make their use impractical at the moment, but they may be useful in the future.

Another approach is the open-loop system. With an open-loop system, the glucose sensor and minicomputer are omitted. A reservoir of insulin and a pump are attached to the patient's back. The machine pumps insulin at a basal flow rate between meals and during the night. Before a meal, the patient presses a button and insulin is delivered eight times faster. The use of this system is controversial, because it is not known to work any better than an appropriately designed insulin injection schedule.

Beta cell transplants

beta cells: the pancreatic cells that synthesize insulin.

Another type of artificial pancreas uses living beta cells encapsulated in a protective membrane consisting of semipermeable fibers. The fibers allow the insulin that is synthesized by the beta cells to diffuse

[14]J. E. Gerich, M. Lorenzi, D. M. Bier, V. Schneider, E. Tsalikian, J. H. Karam, and P. H. Forsham, Prevention of human diabetic ketoacidosis by somatostatin: Evidence for an essential role of glucagon, *New England Journal of Medicine* 292 (1975):985-989.

out, but don't let antibodies or lymphocytes get in. This prevents the body from rejecting the foreign beta cells. Glucose and other nutrients can also pass through the fibers so that the cells can produce insulin as needed by the body.

If and when a system is devised that perfectly mimics the physiologic action of insulin, diabetic therapy will change drastically. Diet, now the cornerstone of therapy, will be far less important if insulin becomes available to the diabetic in the same way that it is available to the nondiabetic.

semipermeable: describes a membrane that will allow some substances to pass through, but not others.

Hypoglycemia

Like diabetes, hypoglycemia results from an imbalance of glucose homeostasis. The two major types of hypoglycemia are fasting and postprandial hypoglycemia. Their major distinguishing characteristics are shown in Table 6. Hypoglycemia is diagnosed when plasma glucose levels fall below 50 mg/100 ml during a five-hour glucose tolerance test, and when this fall is accompanied by the symptoms of hypoglycemia — shakiness, weakness, and dizziness.

Hypoglycemia should not occur except very transiently in the normal person, because hormones (insulin, glucagon, and others) should continuously adjust blood glucose levels to keep them within the normal range. However, in some individuals, it does occur.

The first main type of hypoglycemia, fasting hypoglycemia, arises after 8 to 12 hours of not eating and frequently signifies a serious

postprandial (post-PRAN-dee-ul): after a meal.

prandium = breakfast or lunch

Table 6.   Characteristics of Fasting and Postprandial Hypoglycemia

	Fasting	Postprandial
Onset of symptoms	Gradual; occurs after fasting	Sudden; occurs 2-5 hours after meals
Type of symptoms	Headache, mental dullness, fatigue, confusion, amnesia, seizures, unconsciousness	Anxiety, irritability, sweating, intense heartbeat, hunger, trembling
Duration of symptoms	Persistent	Transient
Possible causes	Hormonal imbalance, drugs, tumors	Early type II diabetes, gastric surgery, TPN
Clinical course	Can be serious; treat underlying problems	Less serious; treat with diet
Other names	—	Alimentary, reactive, idiopathic, functional

Guidelines for diet therapy in hypoglycemia:

1. Give kcalories appropriate to achieve or maintain ideal body weight.
2. Protein (20%), carbohydrate (40-45%), and fat (35-40%) supply the kcalories.
3. Avoid all concentrated sweets.
4. Eat 6 small meals.
5. Avoid alcohol.

Functional hypoglycemia is sometimes called **idiopathic hypoglycemia**, suggesting that the cause is unknown.

idio = peculiar, individual

People who think they have hypoglycemia when they do not are sometimes said to have **nonhypoglycemia**!

problem. Fasting hypoglycemia can be the result of pancreatic beta cell tumors or other tumors not associated with the pancreas. Drugs such as insulin, oral hypoglycemic agents, and alcohol can also cause fasting hypoglycemia. The treatment is to deal with the underlying medical problem so that the body will again regulate its blood glucose level as it should. In an emergency, this type of hypoglycemia may be treated by giving IV glucose.

The second main type of hypoglycemia, postprandial or reactive hypoglycemia, occurs several hours after eating. Postprandial hypoglycemia is usually caused by a relative or absolute oversecretion of insulin in response to food. Normally, when carbohydrates are absorbed, blood glucose rises, and insulin is secreted in amounts above the basal level so that blood glucose falls back to normal. However, in postprandial hypoglycemia, insulin is oversecreted, and blood glucose falls too low. The typical symptoms — rapid heartbeat, trembling, sweating, weakness, and anxiety — usually are mild, appear suddenly, and resolve fairly quickly. We have already discussed some causes of this type of hypoglycemia in previous chapters — gastric surgery and stopping central TPN solutions too quickly. Postprandial hypoglycemia also occurs in some inborn metabolic disorders and sometimes in early type II diabetes.

In true postprandial hypoglycemia, diet is the mainstay of therapy. The diet is similar to the diabetic diet, and the exchange lists are often used for instruction. The person is advised to avoid all concentrated sweets and to eat six small meals a day. kCalories appropriate to achieve or maintain ideal body weight should be given, with 40 to 45 percent of them coming from carbohydrate, 20 percent from protein, and the remainder from fat. Alcohol should be omitted or restricted because it may make hypoglycemia worse.

One type of postprandial hypoglycemia, functional hypoglycemia, is poorly understood. It is the most frequently misdiagnosed type of hypoglycemia. Part of the problem is that hypoglycemia has been widely discussed in the lay press, causing some people to diagnose themselves as having hypoglycemia without seeing a physician. Other people have been misdiagnosed by a physician.

Nutrition Assessment of Diabetic and Hypoglycemic Patients

A main concern in the nutrition assessment of the new diabetic is to accurately assess appropriate weight. This is the basis for calculating the total kcalories in the diet. On reassessment, kcalories may need to be readjusted frequently, particularly in the young person who is growing.

A good bit of time should be spent getting an accurate diet history from the new diabetic. This step will be instrumental in planning an acceptable diet as well as noting possible nutrient deficiencies. During reassessment, the diet history is useful to monitor compliance with the treatment plan. In the type I diabetic, the history is important for seeing if the individual understands how to adjust the diet for unusually strenuous exercise, missed meals, or illness or to prevent or treat hypoglycemia.

Arm anthropometrics may be difficult to obtain and interpret in some type I diabetics. This is true when the midarm area has hypertrophied from repeated insulin injections.

Summing Up

Diabetes mellitus and hypoglycemia are two metabolic disorders that result in an imbalance of blood glucose homeostasis. Patients with diabetes have high blood glucose levels; people with hypoglycemia have low levels.

There are two major types of diabetes: insulin dependent and non insulin dependent. The underlying causes and, therefore, the treatments of these disorders differ.

Type I diabetes is frequently associated with a viral infection and occurs most often in childhood. The cells of the pancreas that produce insulin are destroyed in this type of diabetes. The type II diabetic is often older and obese. In this type of diabetes, insulin secretion may be normal or even high, but the cells are less sensitive to insulin.

Diabetics are frequently prone to complications of the cardiovascular system, circulation, kidneys, eyes, and nerves. These complications can be responsible for earlier death. The weight of evidence suggests controlling blood glucose levels may help prevent complications.

The goals of diet therapy are to achieve and maintain optimal nutrition status, to maintain acceptable blood glucose levels, to prevent or delay the onset of complications, and to allow the individual to resume normal activities. In type I diabetes, diet therapy must be balanced with insulin therapy and exercise. Providing adequate kcalories for growth or maintenance of ideal weight is a major goal. Important aspects of the diet include consistent timing of meals; consistent intake of protein, carbohydrate, and fat; and provision of added carbohydrate for unusually intense exercise or to prevent hypoglycemia.

In type II diabetes, the main goal is weight loss, when necessary. Weight loss should begin as soon as possible after diagnosis.

Meal planning in diabetes centers around the exchange lists. Concentrated sweets are restricted, and the diabetic is encouraged to follow a high-fiber diet. Dietetic foods are unnecessary, although one may vary the diet by using artificial sweeteners, diet (no-kcalorie) soft drinks, and water-packed fruits.

The person with postprandial hypoglycemia also may benefit from a diabetic-type diet. He or she is often advised to eat six small meals high in protein and moderate in carbohydrate and to avoid concentrated sweets and alcohol.

To Explore Further

In addition to the references listed in the chapter notes, the following articles provide good reviews.

An article describing the new classification of diabetes is:

- Whitehouse, F. W. Classification and pathogenesis of the diabetes syndrome: A historical perspective. *Journal of the American Dietetic Association* 81 (1982):243-246.

Articles discussing diabetes and the appropriate treatment of diabetics include:

- Richardson, B. A tool for assessing the real world of diabetic noncompliance. *Nursing*, January 1982, pp. 68-70.

- Cahill, G. F., and McDevitt, H. O. Insulin-dependent diabetes mellitus: The initial lesion. *New England Journal of Medicine* 304 (1981):1454-1465. (This article contains over 175 references.)

- Flood, T. M. Diet and diabetes mellitus. *Hospital Practice*, February 1979, pp. 61-69.

- Podolsky, S., and El-Beheri, B. The principles of a diabetic diet. *Geriatrics*, December 1980, pp. 73-78.

- Malone, J. I. Nutrition and childhood diabetes. *Journal of the Florida Medical Association* 66 (1979):414-416.

- Tattersall, R. B., and Lowe, J. Diabetes in adolescence. *Diabetologia* 20 (1981):517-523.

- Cook, K. A. Diabetics can be vegetarians. *Nursing*, October 1979, pp. 70-73.

- West, K. M., Erdreich, L. J., and Stober, J. A. A detailed study of risk factors for retinopathy and nephropathy in diabetes. *Diabetes* 29 (1980):501-508.

- Stolinsky, D. C. Sugar and saccharin content of antacids. *New England Journal of Medicine* 305 (1981):166-167.

- McDonald, J. Alcohol and diabetes. *Diabetes Care* 3 (1980):629-637.

- Martin, F. I. R., Higginbotham, L., and DeLuise, M. Common errors in the treatment of diabetes mellitus. *Drugs* 19 (1980):59-62.

- Pelczynski, L., and Reilly, A. Helping your diabetic patients help themselves. *Nursing*, May 1981, pp. 76-81.

- Jackson, C. Diabetes: How your patient looks at it. *Nursing*, May 1981, pp. 82-83.

An article that provides more details of current research in diabetes is:

- Maurer, A. C. The therapy of diabetes. *American Scientist* 67 (1979):422-431.

Several well written articles on hypoglycemia include:

- Permutt, M. A. Is it really hypoglycemia? If so, what should you do? *Medical Times*, April 1980, pp. 35-43.

- Lavine, R. L. How to recognize and what to do about hypoglycemia. *Nursing*, April 1979, pp. 52-55.

- Cataland, S. Hypoglycemia: A spectrum of problems. *Heart and Lung* 7 (1978):455-462.

The American Dietetic Association (see Appendix J) offers a 90- minute cassette ($13 to members, $18 to others):

● Thorp, F. K., and Peirce, P. *Nutritional Aspects of Counseling the Child with Insulin Dependent Diabetes Mellitus*.

Additional information on diabetes for professionals and diabetics is available from the American Diabetic Association, 1 West 48th Street, New York, NY 10020.

Kathy is a 12-year-old girl who was diagnosed as having type I diabetes about a year ago, after she and her parents became worried when she began losing weight, urinating excessively, and always complaining of thirst. Kathy's grandfather also has diabetes. Recently, Kathy was admitted to the emergency room. She was nauseated and vomiting, was complaining of intense thirst, showed confusion, and was breathing hard. The physician could smell acetone on her breath. Urine tests were positive for glycosuria and ketonuria, and the blood glucose level was 400 mg/100 ml. The diagnosis was diabetic ketoacidosis. Kathy is 5 feet tall and weighs 75 pounds.

Study Questions

1. Explain the appearance of the symptoms that eventually led to the initial diagnosis of diabetes.

2. How does diabetes lead to ketoacidosis? Were Kathy's physical symptoms and laboratory tests consistent with this diagnosis? How would the ketoacidosis be managed? How can you distinguish between diabetic ketoacidosis and insulin shock?

3. When Kathy recovers, what information will she need in order to prevent future incidents of keto-acidosis? What dietary advice would you want to reinforce?

4. Assume that Kathy has never been instructed on a diabetic diet. What dietary modifications are important for her to follow? How do these recommendations contrast with those suggested for a type II diabetic?

5. Think about and discuss the influence of Kathy's age on her outlook and ability to cope with diabetes. What problems does her age pose? Consider some ways you might help her deal with these problems.

6. Discuss the possible role of diet in preventing the vascular complications of diabetes.

Carbohydrates for Diabetics: Starch, Fiber, Nutritive Sweeteners

Breakfast, 1 1/2 pints of milk and 1/2 pint of lime water, mixed together; bread and butter. For noon, plain blood puddings, made of blood and suet only. Dinner, game or old meats which have been long kept; and so far as the stomach may bear, fat and rancid old meats, as pork, to eat in moderation. Supper, the same as breakfast. — [*Dietary advice to the diabetic*]

DR. JOHN ROLLO, 1797

The dietary management of diabetes has come a long way since Dr. Rollo first recommended a low-carbohydrate diet in 1797. Before insulin was discovered in 1921, the treatment of diabetes was dependent on very low-carbohydrate diets and virtual starvation. Can you imagine what it would have been like to be a diabetic when insulin first became available? The availability of insulin made it possible to increase the carbohydrate and energy content of the diet considerably. The types and amounts of foods allowed as well as the quality of the diabetic's diet and life improved dramatically.

Even after insulin use became widespread, however, carbohydrate was still restricted in the diet. This restriction stemmed from the belief that too much carbohydrate would raise blood glucose levels. The defect in diabetes was viewed as an inability to use glucose rather than as a broader problem affecting metabolism in general. Even though the understanding of diabetes eventually changed, the carbohydrate restricted diet held its place without question for many years.

Changing Views As more investigators began to study the effect of diet on diabetes, an important concept arose. Total energy consumption appeared to play a bigger role in inducing hyperglycemia than any individual dietary component. When total kcaloric intake was appropriate, carbohydrate was well tolerated by the diabetic. Carbohydrate restrictions were gradually relaxed to approximate the amounts eaten by the normal population.

More than one benefit arose from this new approach to diet. It made it easier for the diabetic to adjust to a new way of living. Another important benefit was that the diabetic could now substantially reduce their fat intake.

Although it remains controversial whether a high-fat (particularly saturated fat) diet plays a role in atherosclerosis (see also Chapter 26), a lower-fat diet certainly cannot hurt. And since the diabetic is at increased risk of developing atherosclerosis, it seems wise to try everything possible to minimize the risk. Diabetics who have lower cholesterol levels and who often eat foods high in starch are less likely to develop atherosclerosis.[1] Figure 1 compares the different ratios of protein, carbohydrate, and fat in traditional and current diabetic diets.

Newer Recommendations The American Diabetic Association currently recommends an even higher proportion of carbohydrate in the diabetic diet. The recommendations are as follows: 50 to 60 percent of the kcalories from carbohydrate, 10 to 20 percent from protein, and 30 to 38 percent from fat. As far as possible, unsaturated fats should replace saturated fats. A reduction in cholesterol intake is also recommended.

Why increase the carbohydrate even further? Well, for one thing, several studies

[1] G. Steiner, Diabetes and atherosclerosis: An overview, *Diabetes*, Supplement 2, 1981, pp. 1-7.

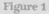

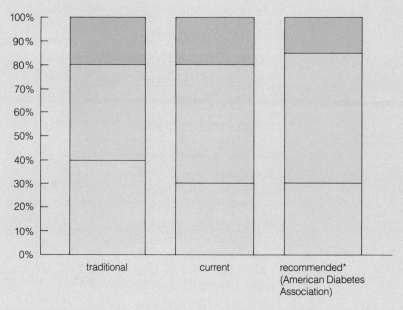

*Modified from K. West, Diabetes Mellitus, H.A. Schneider, C.E. Anderson, D.B. Coursin, eds., Nutritional Support of Medical Practice (Hagerstown: Harper and Row, 1977) p 285.

have shown that glucose tolerance actually improves as a result of higher carbohydrate intakes in diabetics as well as in normal subjects.[2] The mechanism for this improvement is unclear. But it seems that carbohydrate increases the cells' sensitivity to either endogenous or exogenous insulin.[3] Although it has been recommended that the total carbohydrate of the diet be increased, most authorities continue to recommend that diabetics avoid refined sugars.

Giving more total carbohydrate has another advantage. It is easier to plan a diet high in fiber when total carbohydrate is high. For example, good fiber sources include whole grain breads and cereals, lentils and other dried beans and peas, vegetables, and fruit; they are found in the exchange lists that contain carbohydrate (bread, vegetable, and fruit exchanges).

What's so important about fiber in the diabetic diet? The answer is that we really don't know for sure. But studies have shown that when diabetics are fed high-carbohydrate, high-fiber diets, blood glucose levels remain lower.[4] The effect of fiber on blood glucose levels is believed to be due to delayed digestion and absorption in the GI tract.

Whatever the mechanism, some investigators have been able to withdraw oral hypoglycemic agents from type II diabetics by giving a high-carbohydrate, high-fiber diet.[5] The American Diabetes

[2]R. Arky, J. Wylie-Rosett, and B. El-Beheri, Examination of current dietary recommendations for individuals with diabetes mellitus, *Diabetes Care* 5 (1982):59-63.

[3]J. D. Brunzell, R. L. Lerner, D. Porte, and E. L. Bierman, Effect of a fat free, high carbohydrate diet on diabetic subjects with fasting hyperglycemia, *Diabetes* 23 (1974):138-142.

[4]D. J. A. Jenkins, D. V. Goff, A. R. Leeds, K. G. M. M. Alberti, T. M. S. Wolever, M. A. Gassull, and T. D. R. Hockady, Unabsorbable carbohydrates and diabetes: Decreased post-prandial hyperglycemia, *Lancet* 2 (1976):172-174.

[5]T. G. Kiehm, J. W. Anderson, and K. Ward, Beneficial effects of a high carbohydrate, high fiber diet on hyperglycemic diabetic men, *American Journal of Clinical Nutrition* 29 (1976):895-899.

Association has stated that a high fiber intake is desirable. When incorporated into the diabetic diet, high-fiber foods help protect against hyperglycemia.

Critics of the High-Carbohydrate Diet Theory

Fortunately for all of us, there are investigators who look critically at study results and try to point out areas of illogical thinking or lack of evidence. Even though we may not agree with the critic, it is always important to know the other side of the story.

For example, there are some valid criticisms of the study cited earlier, in which high-carbohydrate, high-fiber diets protected against hyperglycemia. For one thing, it seems that the people studied experienced a significant weight loss during the study. The results could have been the effect of weight loss alone. Another point is that the dosages of insulin and oral hypoglycemics the people were getting may have been unnecessarily high to start with. This could have been detected by putting the subjects back on their original diets after their medication was discontinued or reduced. However, this was not done.

You may be thinking "So what? Even if the study did lack important controls, can a high-carbohydrate, high-fiber diet hurt?" Popular opinion is that, no, it won't

hurt. But opponents fear that high-carbohydrate diets may reduce metabolic control of diabetes and increase the likelihood of cardiovascular complications. Further, the studies of high-carbohydrate, high-fiber diets have only been short term. What will be shown when the long term results are available?

There also are practical drawbacks to high-carbohydrate, high-fiber diets. They represent a major change in eating habits for many people. The intake of protein from meat and meat alternates must be substantially reduced to accommodate the higher intake of carbohydrate. Fat intake is also reduced considerably. In addition, high-fiber food may be filling and difficult for some people to consume. (Take a closer look at the sample 2,200 kcalories menu in Chapter 25 and see what you think.)

A final thought is that critics of high-carbohydrate diets *do not* recommend going back to low carbohydrate intakes either. Rather, they believe that until more information is available, the diabetic diet should be similar to that of the general population.

Now you know some of the reasons why the current recommendations for the diabetic diet are not accepted by all authorities. As more research becomes available, these recommendations may (and should) change if appropriate.

Nutritive Sweeteners

Not only starch and fiber but also sugars are concerns in diet planning. The person with diabetes may miss the sweet taste of refined sugars. Several solutions to this problem are available.

Some practitioners believe that the diabetic should adjust to the new diet and learn to live without sugar. They feel that the urge for sweetness will disappear with time.

However, many diabetics would like to include alternative sweeteners in their diets. One choice is to use nonnutritive sweeteners such as saccharin, cyclamate, and aspartame. These substances were discussed in Chapter 25. They can be used to add sweetness to foods and beverages without adding kcalories or other nutrients.

The possible banning of saccharin stimulated interest in looking at other sweeteners that might be appropriate for the diabetic. Three such sweeteners are fructose, xylitol, and sorbitol. In equal amounts, table sugar (sucrose), fructose, xylitol, and sorbitol have the same number of kcalories. The three alternative sweeteners do not cause blood glucose levels to rise as high as sucrose does. However, when diabetes is poorly controlled, all of these sweeteners can be converted to glucose, aggravating hyperglycemia.

Fructose occurs naturally in honey, plants, fruits, and berries. It makes up 50 percent of the disaccharide sucrose. Since it is sweeter than sucrose, it can provide the same degree of sweetness, with fewer kcalories. However, the difference is only minor, and fructose is not an effective aid for losing weight.

Xylitol is another palatable sweetener similar in sweetness to fructose. However, when taken in large amounts, it can cause osmotic diarrhea. Furthermore

animal studies have shown that it may cause tumors. For this reason, food manufacturers have voluntarily curtailed the production of foods sweetened with xylitol.

Sorbitol is only half as sweet as sucrose. Sugar-free gums and candies are generally made with sorbitol. Like xylitol, however, it can cause osmotic diarrhea when used in large amounts.

Before these nutritive sweeteners can be recom-

mended in significant quantities, more research will be needed to see what their long-term metabolic effects are. However, in small quantities it appears they do have some value provided that these guidelines are followed: First, they should not be recommended for poorly controlled or overweight diabetics; second, they must be calculated into the diet, since they are a source of kcalories and carbohydrate.

CHAPTER 26

CONTENTS

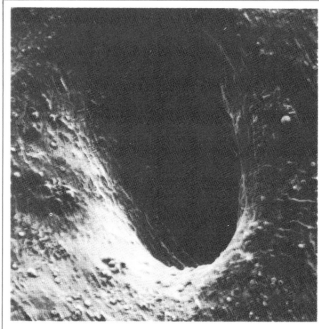

A healthy artery provides an open passage for the flow of blood.

Plaques along an artery narrow its diameter and obstruct blood flow. Clots can form, aggravating the problem.

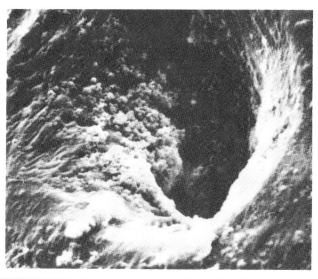

Reproduced by permission. Original material provided by Abel L. Robertson, M.D., Ph.D., University of Illinois at Chicago, Dept. of Pathology, College of Medicine, Chicago, IL 60612.

DISEASES OF THE HEART AND BLOOD VESSELS

We should consider ourselves lucky: heart disease is still our number-one killer, but nine of its 11 major risk factors are within our power to control.

EXECUTIVE FITNESS NEWSLETTER

With red light flashing and siren screaming, another ambulance races toward the hospital. The victim is one of many people who will suffer from a heart attack this year. In 1979 more than half of all deaths in the United States were due to cardiovascular diseases.[1] Of these, over 200,000 struck people were younger than 65; another 200,000 victims were between 65 and the average life expectancy of 69 for men and 77 for women. The cost to our nation is enormous; over 12 million potential years of life are lost each year from these premature deaths. Despite these grim statistics, mortality from cardiovascular disease (CVD) has been declining in recent years. Although this news gives us a reason to be optimistic, there is still a good deal to be done.

The most common cardiac disorder is coronary artery disease, which accounts for as many as 1.5 million heart attacks every year. Over 5 million people in the United States are affected by coronary artery disease.

Diseases of the heart and blood vessels are grouped together and termed **cardiovascular disease (CVD)**. When the blood supply to the heart is obstructed, **coronary artery disease (CAD)** or **coronary heart disease (CHD)** results. In **ischemic** (iss-SHEE-mic) **heart disease (IHD)** the blood supply to any organ or tissue may be cut off.

Atherosclerosis

The most common type of coronary artery disease, atherosclerosis, is characterized by an accumulation of lipid plaque within the arterial wall. Since the arteries carry blood away from the heart, they are more responsive than veins to the beat of the heart as it pumps blood outward. They must expand as a large volume of blood rushes by and then contract so that a steady blood pressure is maintained.

A general term used to describe thickening and hardening of the arteries is **arteriosclerosis**. When this process is due to the accumulation of lipid plaques within the arterial wall, the condition is **atherosclerosis**.

[1]U. S. Department of Health and Human Services, *Ninth Report of the National Heart, Lung, and Blood Advisory Council*, NIH publication no. 81-2334 (Bethesda, Md.: National Heart and Lung Institute, 1981).

plaque: lipid deposits in the arterial wall.

When the blood supply to a tissue is cut off, **gangrene** (death of tissue) follows.

thrombosis: the development of a clot (**thrombus**) which plugs a blood vessel. If such a clot breaks loose, it is an **embolus**, and when this traveling clot lodges in a blood vessel, the result is an **embolism**.

angina (an-JIGH-nuh, AN-juh-nuh): transient pain in the region of the heart caused by lack of oxygen.

aneurysm (AN-you-rism): the ballooning out of an artery wall at a point where it has been weakened by deterioration.

As an atherosclerotic plaque invades the artery and enlarges, it narrows the lumen, thus increasing the pressure of the blood against the wall (much as water pressure increases in a garden hose that has been pinched). The increased pressure can damage the artery wall as well as all the organs in the body. The plaque also causes the wall to lose its elasticity so that it cannot expand in response to the beat of the heart; so the blood pressure rises further. (This is also why atherosclerosis is sometimes called "hardening of the arteries.")

If the plaque narrows the lumen enough, it can completely block the flow of blood. The result is death to all tissues depending on that artery for nutrients and oxygen. However, before that happens, it is more likely that a clot will form, plugging the artery. This event is known as a thrombosis. If the blood supply to the heart muscle is cut off, angina or a heart attack can result. When a critical supply of blood to the brain is involved, the result is a stroke. The kidneys, lungs, and peripheral arteries can also be affected.

As pressure builds up in an artery, the arterial wall may become weakened and balloon out in places. The dilated part of the blood vessel is called an aneurysm. Aneurysms can burst, and when they occur in a major blood vessel such as the aorta, they can lead to massive bleeding and death. Hemorrhaging in the brain can also lead to stroke (discussed below). Figure 1 shows the interrelationships among various cardiovascular disorders.

The reason an atherosclerotic plaque begins to form is obscure, although a number of theories have been proposed.[2] There seems to be general agreement that some type of injury to the lining of the artery allows the invasion of smooth muscle cells, which then proliferate. For some reason these cells are unable to reach a balance between the cholesterol coming into the cell and that being carried away. As a consequence, more and more free cholesterol accumulates at the place of injury, and a plaque is born.

Figure 1 Interrelationships of various cardiovascular diseases.

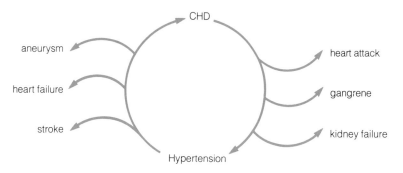

[2]D. M. Small, Cellular mechanisms for lipid deposition in atherosclerosis, part 2, *New England Journal of Medicine* 297 (1977):924-929; E. P. Benditt, The origin of atherosclerosis, *Scientific American*, February 1977, pp. 74-85.

Risk Factors in Atherosclerosis   There is widespread agreement that atherosclerosis is a multifactorial disease; that is, more than one factor appears to be involved in its development. Several risk factors appear to be associated with atherosclerosis. The major ones include high blood cholesterol levels, high blood pressure, cigarette smoking, diabetes mellitus (see Chapter 25), and obesity. Lack of exercise, certain personality traits, high levels of triglycerides in the blood, and a family history of atherosclerosis also appear to play a role. Age and gender (being male) may also be risk factors. The risk of atherosclerosis increases with age, although advanced atherosclerosis has been detected in 18-year-olds.[3] The risk is higher in men than in premenopausal women, but this advantage to women is lost after menopause. To determine your risk of developing atherosclerosis, take the quiz on p. 978.

Some of the risk factors, such as high blood cholesterol and triglycerides, high blood pressure, obesity, and smoking, are controllable. Others, such as sex and heredity, are not. It is hoped that by controlling as many risk factors as possible, people can reduce their risk of developing atherosclerosis. Unfortunately, no one can prove conclusively that this is the case, but it does not seem unreasonable to try this approach while more evidence is being collected.

Some researchers have associated CHD with what they call the Type A personality. Type A people are described as competitive, restless, driving, impatient, ambitious, discontented with their level of achievement, and tending to regard themselves as failures. The opposite personality (easy-going, untroubled), called Type B, is supposed not to be at risk for CHD. The medical community is sharply divided on its acceptance of this theory.

> The war against atherosclerosis is being waged on a battleground littered with millions of numbers generated by study of thousands of human beings. Such a battle can be fought only with statistics and computers, not with pencil-and-paper calculations. When a number of factors operate to produce human disease, it becomes nearly impossible to design a single study that will give clear-cut answers. In animal testing, all variables but one can be controlled. However, the results are merely pointers and not valid for humans until they are tested in humans.

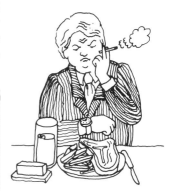

Can you identify the risk factors for CHD?

Can Diet Help?   As is true for the other risk factors, we don't really know if we can prevent atherosclerosis by reducing serum cholesterol levels through dieting. It is only fair to point out that many professionals do not believe diet plays an important part. However, most professionals (including the Nutrition Committee of the American Heart Association) do believe that diet is important.

In the early research into atherosclerosis, it was determined by chemical analysis that plaques are largely composed of lipid, particularly cholesterol. Currently, few experts doubt that high plasma cholesterol is a major risk factor in the development of atherosclerosis.

Serum, plasma, and *blood* cholesterol levels are virtually the same. See p. 690 for definitions.

[3]J. E. Corey, Dietary factors and atherosclerosis: Prevention should begin early, *Journal of School Health* **44** (1974):511-513.

	H	**E**	**A**	**R**	**T**
	1	**2**	**3**	**4**	**6**
Heredity	No known history of heart disease	One relative with heart disease over 60 years	Two relatives with heart disease over 60 years	One relative with heart disease under 60 years	Two relatives with heart disease under 60 years
	1	**2**	**3**	**5**	**6**
Exercise	Intensive exercise, work, and recreation	Moderate exercise, work, and recreation	Sedentary work and intensive recreational exercise	Sedentary work and moderate recreational exercise	Sedentary work and light recreational exercise
	1	**2**	**3**	**4**	**6**
Age	10-20	21-30	31-40	41-50	51-65
	0	**1**	**2**	**4**	**6**
Lbs.	More than 5 lbs below standard weight	± 5 lbs standard weight	6-20 lbs overweight	21-35 lbs overweight	36-50 lbs overweight
	0	**1**	**2**	**4**	**6**
Tobacco	Nonuser	Cigar or pipe	10 cigarettes or fewer per day	20 cigarettes or more per day	30 cigarettes or more per day
	1	**2**	**3**	**4**	**5**
Habits of eating fat	0% No animal or solid fats	10% Very little animal or solid fats	20% Little animal or solid fats	30% Much animal or solid fats	40% Very much animal or solid fats

Everyone plays the game of health whether he wants to or not. What is your score? Add up the numbers in each category that most nearly describe you.*

Your risk of heart attack:

4-9 Very remote	16-20 Average	26-30 Dangerous
10-15 Below average	21-25 Moderate	31-35 Urgent danger—reduce score

Other conditions—such as stress, high blood pressure, and increased blood cholesterol—detract from heart health and should be evaluated by your physician.

*Courtesy of Loma Linda University

You may recall that cholesterol is transported in the blood wrapped in a protein coat. Most plasma cholesterol is transported in the low density lipoproteins (VLDL and LDL). VLDL and LDL are also associated with atherosclerosis. High density lipoproteins (HDL), which transport the remainder of the cholesterol, do not seem to be associated with atherosclerosis. In fact, the opposite appears to be the case.[4] Studies suggest that LDL supply cholesterol to cells while HDL remove it.[5] (The reader is advised to review lipoproteins, saturated fats, and polyunsaturated fats in Chapter 6.)

lipoproteins: see pp. 182-183.

Can diet alter plasma cholesterol? The answer is yes. The level of circulating LDL is directly related to the consumption of cholesterol and saturated fats.[6] Furthermore, when either monounsaturated or polyunsaturated fats are substituted for saturated fats, cholesterol levels decrease.[7]

saturated, unsaturated fats: see pp. 60-61.

The effect of carbohydrates on cholesterol also has been studied. Currently, there is no clear evidence that an intake of sucrose increases the risk of CHD. The effect of fiber is also uncertain. It seems that some types of fiber (pectin, guar) consistently lower plasma cholesterol and LDL but that others (wheat bran) do not.[8]

The role of obesity in atherosclerosis also deserves attention. In overweight people, VLDL are usually high, LDL are moderately high, and HDL are low. Lipid levels often decrease when weight loss occurs, and HDL increase.[9] Furthermore, obesity is associated with other risk factors, including high blood pressure and diabetes. A low-sodium diet may be beneficial in that it may prevent high blood pressure in some individuals (see below).

When used in moderation, alcohol does not seem to increase the risk of CHD. In fact, it has been found that alcohol increases HDL and, in this sense, moderate usage may be beneficial.[10] However, alcohol also raises blood pressure and VLDL, possibly negating any benefit.

Many more dietary factors have been postulated to play a role in the development of atherosclerosis, including vitamins, minerals, trace elements, and individual foods. Two of the more popular theories have been that vitamin E could prevent heart disease and that coffee drinking was associated with heart disease. Some of these theories have

[4]W. B. Kannel, W. P. Castelli, and T. Gordon, Cholesterol in the prediction of atherosclerotic disease, *Annals of Internal Medicine* 90 (1979): 85-91.

[5]D. M. Small, Cellular mechanisms for lipid deposition in atherosclerosis, part 1, *New England Journal of Medicine* 297 (1977):873-877.

[6]American Heart Association Nutrition Committee, Rationale of the diet-heart statement of the American Heart Association, *Arteriosclerosis* 4 (1982):177-191.

[7]American Heart Association Nutrition Committee, 1982.

[8]M. F. Oliver, Diet and coronary heart disease, *British Medical Bulletin* 37 (1981):49-58.

[9]R. N. Wolf and S. M. Grundy, Effects of caloric restriction on plasma lipids and lipoproteins, *Clinical Research* 28 (1980):55A.

[10]American Heart Association, *Risk Factors and Coronary Disease, a Statement for Physicians* (Dallas: American Heart Association, 1980), p. 3.

been disproved; to date, there is not adequate evidence to determine the role played by the others. Table 1 lists some of the nutrients that have been mentioned in this regard. The reader is referred to the article by A. S. Truswell for more information about many of these substances (see To Explore Further).

The questions that remain with regard to diet and atherosclerosis are:

- Can atherosclerosis be prevented by the lowering of cholesterol levels through diet?
- Should the general public (including many who may not need to) be advised to modify their diets?

The general consensus is that it won't hurt to try either of these approaches.

Other Factors That Change Lipid Levels   Diet is not the only factor that can change lipid levels. For example, oral contraceptives that contain estrogen can raise LDL and lower HDL. Physical exercise may increase HDL, and smoking may lower them. Drugs also can change blood lipid levels (see below). Furthermore, people with some diseases may have high blood lipid levels.

A promising new method of lowering serum cholesterol involves replacing ordinary oils and margarines with oils and margarines made from an artificial fat, sucrose polyester (SPE), a compound composed of fatty acids linked to sucrose in a configuration that the body can't absorb. Cholesterol eaten in a meal together with SPE is carried out of the body in the feces. More importantly, the cholesterol the body itself makes and secretes into the intestine as bile is also carried out, lowering the body's total cholesterol. SPE appears to lower serum cholesterol by up to 10 to 20 percent in hypercholesterolemic subjects, while affecting normocholesterolemic subjects very little. SPE does not affect absorption of dietary fats other than cholesterol. An added benefit was inadvertently discovered: Because SPE has no available kcalories, it may be a useful substitute for oil for a person wishing to lose weight. SPE has only one known side effect: It may prevent absorption of vitamins A and D, but this problem can be dealt with by means of vitamin supplementation.

Controlling Blood Lipids

The best treatment of atherosclerosis is prevention. All attempts should be made to control the risk factors of atherosclerosis, whenever possible. As one means to this end the "prudent diet" has been recommended by the American Heart Association (AHA).[11] To follow the prudent diet:

---

[11]American Heart Association Nutrition Committee, 1982.

Table 1. Substances Other Than Fat and Carbohydrate That Have Been Linked to Blood Lipid Levels or Atherosclerosis*

Vitamins

Vitamin C	Vitamin E	Folacin

Minerals

Calcium	Magnesium

Trace elements

Iron	Zinc:copper	Vanadium
Chromium	ratio	Silicon

Other

Coffee	Garlic	Bovine milk
Tea	Onions	xanthine oxidase

*Some of these substances have been shown to be ineffective in altering blood lipid levels or changing the course of atherosclerosis; evidence on others is lacking.

- Adjust kcalorie intake to achieve or maintain ideal body weight.
- Reduce the total kcalories from fat to 30 percent of kcalories (10 percent monounsaturated fats, 10 percent polyunsaturated fats, and 10 percent saturated fats).
- Replace fat kcalories with carbohydrate. Carbohydrate should account for 45 to 55 percent of the total kcalories. The majority of these kcalories should come from complex carbohydrate.
- Reduce cholesterol intake to less than 300 mg per day.
- Limit the intake of salt. (The current statement does not set a precise limit.)

Appendixes G and H contain information about the cholesterol and fat content of various foods.

The amount of polyunsaturated fats in proportion to saturated fats can be expressed as the **P:S ratio**. A P:S ratio of 1:1 (one to one) is consistent with the AHA guidelines for a prudent diet. A diet in which the types of fats are altered is a **fat-controlled diet**.

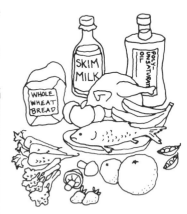

Some foods to enjoy on a prudent diet.

There is a big difference between low-fat and fat-controlled diets, although these terms are often confused in the clinical setting. A low-fat diet is low in total fat and there is no particular concern for the type of fat given. On the other hand, a fat-controlled diet generally allows more total fat but prescribes the type of fat to be used.

CAUTION:

A low-fat diet is different from a fat-controlled diet.

For most Americans this means eating less meat, eggs, and dairy products (except those made of skimmed milk); changing the type of fat used; and eating more starches, fruits, and vegetables (see Table 2). The diet may be difficult for many people to follow, and drastic changes cannot be expected overnight. The development of many new products that fit the prudent diet meal plan (cholesterol-free eggs, special cheeses, and polyunsaturated margarines) can help considerably. The AHA has many pamphlets and recipe booklets available to both professionals and the public to help them make the suggested dietary changes. Some of these publications are listed in Appendix C.

A dietary approach to prevention and therapy of cardiovascular disease that people often ask about is the Pritikin Diet. Its creator, Dr. Nathan Pritikin, has taken the principles espoused by the AHA to an extreme. His diet allows only 10 percent of kcalories from fat, for example, versus the AHA's 30 percent. Foods high in fats and sugars, as well as caffeine and alcohol, are forbidden. He also recommends vigorous daily activity, pushing the heart rate to 70 or 80 percent of its capacity for half an hour or more twice a day. Some former heart patients swear by his regimen, but authorities are cautious: It may be too low in fat, may be deficient in vitamins and minerals, has not yet been adequately tested in long-term studies. It is fairly well agreed, however, that the kinds of dietary changes Pritikin recommends, perhaps not so extreme, are more likely to help than to hurt the person wishing to avoid heart trouble; and certainly the exercise is beneficial.

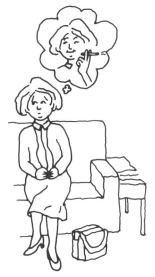

Sugar-free gum or mints can help satisfy the smoker's urge to have something in her mouth.

Another nutrition-related problem may come up when a person decides to eliminate another risk factor — smoking. People who stop smoking often gain weight. However, weight gain can be prevented. The AHA has a brochure that describes many behavior modification techniques to help eliminate this problem (see Appendix C.)

hyperlipidemia: elevated blood lipids. This term is used interchangeably with **hyperlipoproteinemia**, or elevated blood lipoproteins.

Diet and Hyperlipidemia   Diet is also used to treat people who already have elevated blood lipids, or hyperlipidemia. Cholesterol, triglycerides, or both may be elevated. Since these lipids are carried through the blood in the lipoproteins, different lipoproteins are also elevated. For example, when cholesterol levels are high, this means the LDL are elevated; and when triglycerides are high, the VLDL or chylomicrons are elevated. (The chylomicron, another lipoprotein, transports fat from the intestine through the lymph and eventually to the liver where it is metabolized; see Chapter 6). An elevation of any lipoprotein is called hyperlipoproteinemia. Table 3 summarizes the dietary modifications useful for controlling various lipoprotein elevations.

Table 2. General Guidelines for a Prudent Diet

1. Limit egg yolks to not more than three a week, including those used in cooking.
2. Limit use of shrimp, organ meats, luncheon meats, bacon, and sausage.
3. Use fish, chicken, turkey, and veal most often. Moderate-sized portions of beef, lamb, pork, and ham can be used less frequently.
4. Use lean meats trimmed of all visible fat and discard fat that cooks out of meat.
5. Avoid frying foods.
6. Use liquid vegetable oils and margarine rich in polyunsaturated fats instead of butter, shortening, or lard.
7. The label on margarine should list *liquid* vegetable oil as the first ingredient and one or more partially hydrogenated vegetable oils as additional ingredients.
8. Use skim milk and skim milk cheeses.

Adapted from American Heart Association, *The Way to a Man's Heart* (Dallas: American Heart Association, 1972).

Table 3. Lowering Blood Lipids with Diet

Lipoprotein	Major fat involved	Dietary approach
Chylomicron	Dietary triglycerides	Total fat restriction
VLDL	Triglycerides	Weight reduction Carbohydrate restriction No concentrated sweets
LDL	Cholesterol	Cholesterol restriction Saturated fat reduction Polyunsaturated fat increase

There are six basic types of hyperlipoproteinemias: types I, IIa, IIb, III, IV, and V. Types II and IV are by far the most common, and they are associated with an increased risk of CHD. Table 4 shows which lipoproteins are abnormal in each type of hyperlipoproteinemia. In each type the abnormalities are different. For our purposes here, however, we are not concerned with specific types of hyperlipoproteinemias as much as with how we can use the diet to change abnormal lipoprotein patterns.

Weight loss is especially useful in bringing VLDL back to normal. Sometimes, though, total carbohydrate may have to be restricted to reduce VLDL further. The type of carbohydrate is also important; concentrated sweets are avoided. Cholesterol and saturated fats are often moderately restricted when VLDL are high because cholesterol also may be in the high or high normal range.

Table 4. Treatment in Hyperlipoproteinemias

	Type I	Type IIa	Type IIb	Type III	Type IV	Type V
Lipid abnormality	⇑ chylomicrons ⇑ TG and C	⇑ LDL, ⇑ C	⇑ LDL, ⇑ VLDL, ⇑ C, ⇑ TG	⇑ VLDL, ⇑ C, ⇑ TG	⇑ VLDL, Normal or ⇑ C, ⇑ TG	⇑ Chylomicrons, ⇑ VLDL, ⇑ TG ⇑ C
Possible drugs	None available	Cholestyramine, Colestipol, Clofibrate, Nicotinic acid, Probucol, Gemfibrozil	Cholestyramine, Colestipol, Clofibrate, Nicotinic acid, Probucol, Gemfibrozil	Clofibrate, Nicotinic acid, Women — estrogens	Clofibrate, Nicotinic acid	Clofibrate, Nicotinic acid Women — Norethindrone acetate
Diet* Carbohydrate	Not restricted	Not restricted	40% kcal, restrict concentrated sweets	(Same as IIb)	45% kcal, restrict concentrated sweets	50% kcal, restrict concentrated sweets
Fat	25-35 g; type not restricted	⇑ polyunsaturated, ⇓ saturated	40% kcal, ⇑ polyunsaturated, ⇓ saturated	(Same as IIb)	⇑ polyunsaturated, ⇓ saturated	30% kcal, ⇑ polyunsaturated, ⇓ saturated
Cholesterol	Not restricted	Less than 300 mg	Less than 300 mg	(Same as IIb)	300-500 mg	300-500 mg
Alcohol	Avoid	Physician's discretion	Physician's discretion	(Same as IIb)	Physician's discretion	Avoid

Legend:

⇑ — Elevated or increase   TG — Triglycerides
C — Cholesterol   VLDL — Very low density lipoproteins
LDL — Low density lipoproteins

*For every type, achieve and maintain ideal body weight.

It is harder to reduce elevated cholesterol levels than triglycerides. Generally, a diet low in cholesterol, low in saturated fat, and high in polyunsaturated fat is recommended. Extremely high cholesterol levels may reflect an inherited defect of cholesterol metabolism. Often, drugs must be used along with diet to lower cholesterol levels.

When chylomicrons are elevated (as in types I and V hyperlipoproteinemia) the total amount of fat (not the type) is restricted. This makes sense, since chylomicrons are made to transport dietary fat. MCT oil can be used as a source of fat in type I hyperlipoproteinemia, because medium-chain triglycerides are not transported in the chylomicron (see p. 882). However, MCT is not used in type V, because it may cause an even greater increase in VLDL, which are elevated already.

Alcohol is not recommended in types I and V hyperlipoproteinemia. Alcohol may cause hypertriglyceridemia. Furthermore, types I and V hyperlipoproteinemia may occur secondary to alcoholism or pancreatitis, both of which require that alcohol be avoided (see Chapter 24).

Lists of foods quite similar to the diabetic exchange lists are available from the National Institutes of Health for use by people with hyperlipoproteinemia (see To Explore Further). However, for most people it is easy to adapt the diabetic exchange lists for this use. Attention must be paid to correctly adjusting the cholesterol and saturated fats in the diet by limiting the use of medium-fat and high-fat meats, whole milk, saturated fats, and bread exchanges high in fat.

Drug Treatment   As a rule, drugs are not used to treat hyperlipoproteinemia unless diet therapy has been unsuccessful. A trial period on diet alone for about three months is recommended.[12]

Drugs that lower serum lipids have two sites of action. Some work in the GI tract by preventing the absorption of cholesterol. Others work in the body after they are absorbed by different and often unknown mechanisms. Some drugs are mainly effective in lowering triglycerides; others more effectively lower cholesterol. All of these drugs can adversely affect nutrition status by interfering with food intake. The drugs, their effects, and associated nutrition problems are summarized in Table 5.

Drugs that lower blood lipids are **antilipemic agents**.

Hypertension

Hypertension is believed to affect some 60 million Americans.[13] It is arbitrarily defined as an arterial pressure of 140/90 millimeters of

hypertension: elevated blood pressure. **Secondary hypertension** has a known cause. In **essential hypertension** (also called primary or idiopathic hypertension) the cause is unknown.

---

[12]W. F. Cathcart-Rake and C. A. Dujovne, The treatment of hyperlipoproteinemias, *Rational Drug Therapy* 13 (1979):1-4.

[13]E. D. Frohlich, Physiological observations in essential hypertension, *Journal of the American Dietetic Association* 80 (1982):18-20.

In a blood pressure reading, the first figure is the **systolic** blood pressure; and the second, the **diastolic** blood pressure. The systolic pressure represents arterial pressure caused by the contraction of the left ventricle of the heart. The diastolic pressure is the arterial pressure when the heart is between beats.

When the body fluids have more trouble getting through the smaller diameter of the arteries, the condition that results is called **increased peripheral resistance**.

Any substance that helps enlarge the diameter of the arteries is a **vasodilator**; a **vasoconstrictor** reduces the diameter of the arteries.

The enzyme **kallikrein** normally splits a specific blood protein to form **kinins**. Kinins are vasodilators themselves and they also stimulate the release of a prostaglandin (see p. 88) that helps counteract vasoconstriction.

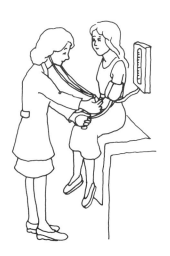

mercury (mm Hg) or greater. Above this level the incidence of cardiovascular disease increases more rapidly.

Hypertension can occur secondary to kidney diseases and various hormonal imbalances. However, such causes can be identified in only about 5 percent of cases. The other 95 percent of the time the cause of hypertension is unknown.

Hypertension can result when the diameter of the arterioles is decreased (as in atherosclerosis) or when the volume of the blood moving through the arteries is increased. (The first case is like pinching off a garden hose to cause water pressure to increase; the second is like turning the water on all the way to increase pressure.) Increased pressure caused by reduced diameter of the arteries appears to play a greater role in hypertension.

Although we don't know what causes peripheral resistance, most investigators believe that the kidneys are involved, because they play a major role in blood pressure regulation through the enzyme renin and the hormone aldosterone (see also Highlight 2 and Chapter 27). Norepinephrine, which constricts arterioles and increases the rate and strength of the heartbeat, also may be involved. Additionally, a predisposition to hypertension appears to be inherited. Kallikrein and prostaglandins may also be implicated.

Whatever the cause of hypertension, eventually peripheral resistance increases. This makes it harder for the left ventricle of the heart to pump blood through the system. If hypertension goes unchecked, eventually the left ventricle becomes enlarged and finally cannot handle the load. The result is heart failure (which will be discussed below). Hypertension is the major cause of heart failure, either alone or in combination with atherosclerosis. Increased pressure also can lead to a stroke, and the kidneys can be damaged when the heart is unable to adequately pump blood through these vital organs.

People with hypertension may be unaware that they have a problem. A major national effort has been made to identify and treat them. Even mild hypertension (diastolic pressure of 90 to 104 mm Hg) can be dangerous, and individuals with mild hypertension benefit from treatment.[14] These findings suggest an urgent need to find ways of preventing and safely treating hypertension.

Diet in Hypertension   The debate about the role of diet in preventing and treating hypertension is almost as heated as the diet-heart controversy. The biggest area of debate is whether a high-sodium diet causes hypertension, and conversely, whether following a diet moderately restricted in sodium can prevent hypertension.

The basic explanation for how sodium might contribute to hypertension goes like this: Ingestion of excess salt causes an increase in

[14]W. T. Friedewald, Current nutrition issues in hypertension, *Journal of the American Dietetic Association* 80 (1982):17.

sodium in the extracellular fluids. Water is drawn from cells through the osmotic effect, expanding the volume of the extracellular fluid, so blood pressure increases. Normally, the kidneys would rid the body of the sodium, thus normalizing the extracellular fluid volume. However, the ability to excrete excess sodium varies among individuals (this is where a hereditary factor may play a role). If the kidneys cannot perform this function over time, chronic hypertension results. Damage to the heart and kidneys then follows, and this makes the hypertension worse.

The evidence as to whether a moderately low sodium intake can prevent hypertension is inconclusive. However, many professionals and agencies (including the Food and Drug Administration) believe that enough evidence is available to warrant a recommendation to the general public to moderately restrict their sodium intake. They reason that at worst, such a diet cannot be harmful.

In this chapter we have seen two instances in which dietary changes have been suggested to the general public although evidence as to the effectiveness of the changes is not conclusive. The basic justification for both the prudent diet and the diet moderately restricted in sodium is that while they may not prove to be helpful, they will do no harm.

This may be the case for most people, but some subgroups within the population may be adversely affected. For example, diets high in polyunsaturated fats have been associated with an increased incidence of gallstones and cancer.[15] (The AHA cautiously recommends that only 10 percent of fat kcalories come from polyunsaturated fats.) Furthermore, you may recall from Chapter 23 that changes in the sodium content of infant foods may have adverse effects on children with cystic fibrosis if their diets are not supplemented with sodium. It is probably naive to think that a change in diet can be recommended for everyone without some adverse effects, even though taking that risk may be well worth the benefit.

CAUTION:

Changing the dietary patterns of a whole population can have adverse effects on subgroups within that population.

[15]American Heart Association Nutrition Committee, 1982.

Table 5.   Drugs Used in Hyperlipoproteinemia

Drug	Lipid lowered	Nutrition-related side effects
Cholestyramine	Cholesterol	Nausea, vomiting, abdominal discomfort, constipation; ⇓ vitamin B_{12} absorption; malabsorption of fat-soluble vitamins and calcium
Colestipol	Cholesterol	(same as above)
Clofibrate	Triglycerides, cholesterol	Nausea, vomiting, abdominal discomfort, loose stools; ⇓ absorption of carotene, glucose, iron, vitamin B_{12}, and electrolytes
Nicotinic acid	Triglycerides, cholesterol	Nausea, vomiting, abdominal discomfort, decreased glucose tolerance
Probucol	Cholesterol	Nausea, vomiting, abdominal discomfort, diarrhea
Gemfibrozil	Triglycerides, cholesterol	Nausea, vomiting, abdominal discomfort

The sodium-restricted diet is presented in Chapter 24.

There is less debate about the value of incorporating a low-sodium diet in the treatment of established hypertension. Studies have shown that even mild restriction of sodium can produce a modest but definite fall in blood pressure.[16] More recently, it has been shown that weight is also important in hypertension. The overweight hypertensive person can reduce blood pressure simply by losing weight. The beneficial effects can be seen even when the person does not achieve ideal body weight. The authors of one study concluded that weight loss could help reduce the dosage of medication needed to control hypertension or eliminate the need for medication altogether.[17]

A diet consisting of rice, sugar, and fruit was introduced in 1944 and found to be effective for the treatment of hypertension. It was later learned that the **Kempner rice diet** worked because it was very low in sodium.

Other factors in the diet also have been associated with hypertension, including potassium, caffeine, and alcohol. Some studies have suggested that potassium can help lower blood pressure and that it may protect against excess sodium intake.[18] Studies regarding caffeine have been contradictory. One study found that caffeine can increase

---

[16]J. A. Wilber, The role of diet in the treatment of high blood pressure, *Journal of the American Dietetic Association* 80 (1982):25-29.

[17]E. Reisin, R. Abel, M. Modan, D. S. Silverberg, H. E. Eliahou, and B. Modan, Effect of weight loss without salt restriction on the reduction of blood pressure in overweight hypertensive patients, *New England Journal of Medicine* 298 (1978):1-6.

[18]G. R. Meneely and H. D. Battarbee, High sodium-low potassium environment and hypertension, *American Journal of Cardiology* 38 (1976):768-785.

blood pressure by about 10 mm Hg in some people.[19] However, in another study, blood pressure did not change in men drinking up to six cups of coffee per day.[20] Alcohol also may elevate blood pressure.[21]

Drug Therapy of Hypertension   Two general groups of drugs are used to treat hypertension: diuretics and adrenergic blockers. Drug therapy has contributed substantially to controlling hypertension.

Diuretics are generally tried first. They work in different ways, but the net result is the same: They increase fluid loss and thus lower blood pressure. Some diuretics cause large amounts of potassium to be lost in the urine.[22] The more sodium people on these diuretics ingest, the more potassium they lose; therefore, a low-sodium, high-potassium diet is recommended for patients on potassium-wasting diuretics. Many times a potassium supplement is recommended, but often potassium intake can be greatly increased just by eating the right foods. Most people who are motivated to know the potassium contents of foods have learned that bananas, potatoes, tomatoes, and fruit juices are high in potassium. Chapter 27 presents a list of foods high in potassium, and Appendix I lists the actual potassium contents of these and other foods.

Other diuretics spare potassium.[23] They are sometimes used in combination with potassium-wasting diuretics to improve potassium balance.

Adrenergic blocking agents work by interfering with norepinephrine. These substances affect many different body tissues and therefore are generally reserved for someone not responding to diuretics.

Diet Therapy   You can help the hypertensive person most by advising on weight loss, if necessary, and on lowering sodium intake. Usualy, sodium is restricted to 2 to 4 g per day. Oftentimes, the person can achieve this level of intake by avoiding foods high in salt and adding no salt at the table (see Table 6). Prior to the availability of modern diuretics, diets very low in sodium were recommended. However, they are hard to follow and no longer appear warranted. (Chapter 24 listed foods to be allowed and avoided on more severe sodium-restricted diets.)

Recommend food high in potassium, particularly for people on potassium-wasting diuretics. Watch out for signs of hypokalemia, such

Principles of diet for hypertension:

1. Lose weight, if appropriate.
2. Limit sodium (to 2-4 g/day).
3. Include potassium-rich foods.
4. Follow the prudent diet.

[19]J. M. Richie, Central nervous system stimulants, in *Pharmacological Basis of Therapeutics*, ed. L. S. Goodman and A. Gilman (New York: Macmillan, 1975), pp. 368-378.

[20]T. R. Dawber, W. B. Kannel, and T. Gordon, Coffee and cardiovascular disease: Observations from the Framingham study, *New England Journal of Medicine* 291 (1974):871-874.

[21]American Heart Association, 1980.

[22]These include thiazide, chlorthalidone, furosemide, and ethacrynic acid.

[23]These include spironolactone and triamterine.

Table 6. No-Added-Salt Diet

● You may lightly salt foods during cooking, but do not add salt at the table.

● Avoid foods high in sodium, including:

Meats — bacon; bologna; cold cuts; chipped or corned beef; frankfurters; smoked meats; sausage; salt pork or codfish; canned, salted, or smoked fish

Sauces, seasonings, and condiments — Regular catsup; celery, garlic, and onion salt; regular chili sauce; commercial meat extracts; meat tenderizers; monosodium glutamate; olives; pickes; prepared mustard; soy and Worchestershire sauce

Other — Regular canned or frozen soups; regular bouillon; soup mixes; salted pretzels; popcorn, crackers, nuts, or other salted snack foods; potato chips; sauerkraut; regular cheese; regular peanut butter

● Low-sodium products can be substituted for regular foods.

Hints for the diet advisor:

Reduce sodium gradually.

See client regularly.

Experiment with spices and herbs.

Sodium-free spices and flavorings include:
  Allspice
  Almond extract
  Bay leaves
  Caraway seeds
  Cinnamon
  Curry powder
  Garlic
  Ginger
  Lemon extract
  Mace
  Maple extract
  Marjoram
  Mustard powder
  Nutmeg
  Paprika
  Parsley
  Pepper
  Peppermint extract
  Pimiento
  Rosemary
  Sage
  Sesame seeds
  Thyme
  Turmeric
  Vanilla extract
  Vinegar
  Walnut extract

as weakness (particularly of the legs), unexplained numbness or tingling sensation, cramps, irregular heartbeat, and excessive thirst and urination. Blood levels of potassium should be monitored regularly to prevent hypokalemia.

Many professionals also advise the hypertensive person to follow a fat-controlled prudent diet (see Table 2). This is because hypertensive people are at greater than normal risk for developing CHD.

Recently, an interdisciplinary group of health professionals identified ten steps involved in making dietary changes for hypertension control.[24] According to them, the person with hypertension should:

1. Acknowledge that he or she has hypertension.

2. Consider diet as a sole or supportive method to help control hypertension.

3. Participate in assessing his or her dietary pattern, social environment, thoughts, beliefs, and feelings.

4. Acknowledge that successful dietary change will require an extended commitment.

5. Participate in developing plans and in setting long-term blood pressure and dietary goals.

6. Participate in planning each step in dietary change.

7. Make each dietary change.

8. Participate in assessing the success of each dietary change.

9. Participate in assessing the attainment of blood pressure goals.

10. Participate in devising a plan for maintaining the changes as dietary and blood pressure goals are reached.

[24]U.S. Department of Health and Human Services, *Report of the Working Group on Critical Patient Behaviors in the Dietary Management of High Blood Pressure*, NIH publication no. 81-2269, 1981.

Hopefully, by using these steps, professionals will help their clients achieve successful management of hypertension.

It may be difficult for people to drastically change their sodium intake. Foods eaten without salt may taste unpalatable to the person who normally uses it liberally. (Have you ever tried scrambled eggs or fried potatoes without salt?) Diet compliance is most unlikely when a person is merely handed an instruction sheet with no additional encouragement or guidance.

Several things can help. For one thing, reduce sodium gradually so that the person can adjust gradually to the flavor of unsalted foods. (This implies that you will see the person regularly for followup, which also is important.) Encourage people to experiment with other spices and herbs that can help replace salt. Several cookbooks that help in this regard are available (see Appendix C).

Teach your clients to read labels, too. Table 7 lists sources of sodium to look for on labels. Local water supplies may have a high sodium content, and when this water is used in food products, they may contribute significantly to sodium intake.

Read labels.

Help people to realize that processed foods, milk, and dairy products are high in sodium. Most people are surprised to learn that a serving of cornflakes contains more sodium than a serving of cocktail peanuts — and that a serving of chocolate pudding contains still more.[25] Medications such as antacids, antibiotics, cough medicines, laxatives, pain relievers, and sedatives may contain sodium. Some toothpastes and mouthwashes also contain large amounts of sodium; recommend that people rinse thoroughly after brushing their teeth or using a mouthwash and also avoid swallowing these compounds.

Look out for sodium in food, water, medicines, toothpastes, and mouthwashes.

Low-Sodium Products   Many low-sodium products are available for use with low-sodium diets. In general, a palatable diet can be planned without the use of low-sodium products. However, some people (particularly those on diets very low in sodium) like to use these items to add variety. It is important for you and your client to recognize that many of these products are not sodium-free, so the amount of sodium they contain must be calculated into the diet.

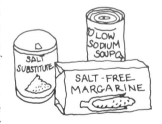

The sodium in salt substitutes is generally relaced by potassium. Most people don't like the taste of salt substitutes; some find food more acceptable without any salt at all. The use of a potassium-containing salt substitute, though, serves the dual purpose of increasing potassium intake while reducing sodium. However, salt substitutes containing potassium should not be used by people with renal insufficiency. Some products contain a combination of half regular table salt and half salt substitute. While these products may be more palatable, they also can contribute a significant amount of salt in the diet.

[25]Salt and high blood pressure, *Consumer Reports*, March 1979, reprint.

Table 7. Substances in Foods That Contain Sodium

Baking powder	Monosodium glutamate	Sodium benzoate
Baking soda	Salt	Sodium hydroxide
Brine	Sodium alginate	Sodium propionate
Disodium phosphate		

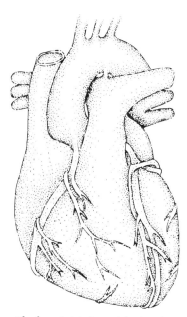

The heart gets its nutrient and oxygen not from inside its chambers but from arteries that lie on its surface. These are the coronary arteries.

myocardial infarction (MI): death of heart tissue caused by reduced blood flow to that tissue.

Surgery to provide a blood supply to tissue affected by occluded coronary arteries is called **coronary artery bypass surgery**.

Heart Attacks

The heart gets its nutrients and oxygen not from inside its chambers but from arteries that lie on its surface. A myocardial infarction (MI), or heart attack, occurs when the supply of blood to the heart muscle is cut off, resulting in tissue death. Atherosclerosis is the most common contributor to heart attacks, but they also can be caused by spasms of the coronary arteries, infection of the membrane covering the heart, rheumatic heart disease, and other conditions. As an area of heart tissue dies, enzymes that are associated with heart cells leak out into the general circulation. (This situation is similar to the leaking out of digestive enzymes in patients with pancreatitis.) A raised level of these enzymes in the blood is often used in diagnosing heart attacks.

The heart attack victim, like an accident victim, is in shock at first. In shock, fluid leaves the vascular compartment and moves temporarily to the interstitial space. The person experiences this fluid shift as if it came from dehydration, and complains of extreme thirst. But the body does not need water, and in fact increasing its fluid load at such a time would be unwise. The only fluid the person in shock should be given is ice chips, to relieve the sensation of thirst without adding much water to the system.

Immediately after an MI, a person is usually nauseated; don't give him or her anything to eat. If, as shock resolves, the person still remains nauseated, IV infusions are started to prevent dehydration.

After several hours of observation, you can usually give the patient foods orally. You want to give food that minimizes the work the heart must do; the first foods should be liquids or soft, bland foods given in frequent, small feedings.[26] Small feedings help prevent abdominal distention, which can cause the diaphragm to be pushed up toward the heart.

Be sure you serve foods that are neither too hot nor too cold. Temperature extremes can stimulate the vagus nerve, slowing the heart rate. At first, the diet is low in kcalories (1,000-1,200), with more kcalories added as the patient improves.

The diet should be moderately restricted in sodium (about 2 g) and, in most cases, should be fat controlled (see the prudent diet). Many

[26]N. K. Wenger, Guidelines for dietary management after myocardial infarction, *Geriatrics*, August 1979, pp. 75-83.

hospitals restrict caffeinated coffee and tea during the first few days after an MI, although there is little scientific evidence to support such a restriction.[27] Indeed, denying coffee to a person who really enjoys it may do more harm than good.

After the patient is out of immediate danger (in about five to ten days), tailor the diet to his or her own needs — for example, to deal with hyperlipidemia, hypertension, obesity, diabetes, or the like. Oftentimes, a diet to reduce weight, control fat, and moderately restrict sodium is appropriate and can be planned to include only three meals a day.

People that continue to have chest pain after an MI may benefit from eating small, frequent meals. Tell them to try eating slowly and resting before and after meals.

Diet principles for MI:

1. Immediately after MI:
   Nothing by mouth.
   IV fluids, if necessary.
   Ice chips for thirst.
2. After several hours:
   Liquids or soft, bland foods.
   Frequent feedings.
   Moderate-temperature foods.
   Sodium-restricted, low-kcal diet.
3. After 5 to 10 days:
   3 meals a day.
   Diet adjusted for individual.

Probably all of us know at least one person that seems destined for a heart attack. He is the overweight, hard-driving executive with hypertension who only jokes about exercising and dieting. Then one day it happens. When you visit him in the hospital, you can hardly believe your ears.

Overnight, it seems, your friend's attitude has changed dramatically. He now realizes he is mortal and begins to value his life. He suddenly respects any advice the health care team can offer him. He wants to take positive steps toward changing his lifestyle and improving his chances for survival.

Your friend is a typical MI victim. He is like a sponge trying to soak up any advice that may help him. This person is one of the most enjoyable patients to work with because he listens to what you say and will do his best to follow your advice.

Be sure to seize the opportunity afforded to you by giving sound and useful counsel. Your patient will benefit from your suggestions and you will be rewarded by your patient's interest and appreciation.

Congestive Heart Failure

Many diseases — cardiovascular disease, hypertension, and kidney disease — can lead to congestive heart failure (CHF). In CHF, the heart can no longer pump enough blood through the circulatory system. Because the heart is not adequately pumping, blood flow to the kidneys is reduced. This change signals the kidneys to retain fluid. The retained fluid increases the load on the heart and further weakens it. Since blood

congestive heart failure (CHF): a syndrome in which the heart can no longer adequately pump blood through the circulatory system.

[27]Wenger, 1979.

pulmonary edema: fluid in the lungs.

Enlargement of the heart is **cardiomegaly** (CAR-dee-oh-MEG-uh-lee).

mega = big

A rapid heart rate is **tachycardia** (TACK-ee-CAR-dee-uh).

tachys = rapid

Drugs frequently used to increase the strength of the heart's contractions are **digitalis glycosides**.

Principles of diet for CHF:

1. Lose weight, if appropriate.
2. Restrict sodium and (sometimes) fluids.
3. Use food that is easy to chew and digest.
4. Eat small, frequent meals.

Heart disease can cause protein-kcalorie malnutrition (PCM), usually marasmus; the tissues fail to receive enough nutrients if the heart is weak. This PCM is called **cardiac cachexia**.

cerebrovascular accident or incident (CVA, CVI): a stroke.

entering the heart from the veins cannot be pumped out effectively, peripheral and sometimes pulmonary edema results. The patient becomes "congested" with excess fluids. The heart enlarges and begins to beat more rapidly to try to compensate for its inability to pump. CHF is life threatening, particularly when it is accompanied by pulmonary edema.

Diuretics and drugs that increase the strength of heart muscle contractions are important in the treatment of CHF. Bed rest helps to reduce the work load on the heart. Generally, diet therapy includes measures to reduce the work required of the damaged heart and to alleviate edema.

The level of sodium restriction is determined by the individual's tolerance. The amount permitted may be as low as 250 to 500 mg; however, many physicians would rather give more sodium (about 2 g) and use diuretics as needed. This approach is generally preferred by the person on the diet as well.

Fluid restriction, although usually unnecessary, may sometimes help. It is indicated when sodium restriction is unsuccessful in relieving edema. The level of fluid restriction depends on the patient's condition.

Protein, vitamins, and minerals should be adequate to prevent nutrient deficiencies, which can further tax the heart. Small feedings help prevent abdominal distention and displacement of the diaphragm toward the heart. Foods that are easy to chew and digest and do not form gas are generally recommended.

Some people with chronic CHF develop malnutrition, probably because of anorexia, unappealing diets, long-term use of medications, and the inability of the heart to adequately pump oxygen and nutrients to the cells. Undernutrition in these people often goes unnoticed because edema masks their underweight condition.

Nutrition and the Stroke Victim

When blood flow to the brain is insufficient or when blood vessels burst and blood flows into the brain, a stroke or cerebrovascular accident (CVA) results. A stroke is actually a cerebrovascular rather than a cardiovascular disorder. Recovery for some stroke victims is unremarkable. The optimal diet for these patients is based on their underlying medical condition (hyperlipidemia, hypertension, obesity).

However, many stroke victims have either temporary or permanent problems with chewing, swallowing, and the physical process of eating. The care of people with difficulties in chewing and swallowing was discussed in Chapter 23. Tube feedings often are indicated initially. Many patients who have problems with the physical aspects of eating can be helped a great deal through the use of special feeding devices. Several of these devices are shown in Figure 2.

Nutrition Assessment of Patients with Cardiovascular Disorders

To help you pinpoint areas of particular concern in the nutrition assessment of individuals with cardiovascular diseases, consider the following:

1. In taking a diet history, pay particular attention to the total kcaloric intake and to the sodium, cholesterol, saturated fat, and polyunsaturated fat content of the diet. This will help you determine how significant recommended diet changes will be if they are necessary. You must also determine through the history if there are other medical conditions, such as diabetes, that may alter nutrient needs. Additionally, check to see if the person intends to give up smoking or has recently done so.

2. Generally, you should not encounter problems in taking anthropometric measurements in most people with cardiovascular diseases. The exception is the patient with edema (such as in CHF).

3. Standard lab values such as albumin and transferrin may be abnormal in people with either hypertension or CHF if they are retaining fluids. The serum cholesterol and triglyceride levels should be monitored in people with hyperlipidemia. Monitoring serum potassium levels in people on diuretics is essential.

Regardless of the type of person you are assessing, look for factors in their history that place them at risk for CHD. Based on this information, you may be able to suggest a prudent diet and other relevant lifestyle changes before the problem of CHD becomes evident.

Figure 2   Special feeding devices.

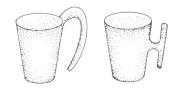

These cups can be used by people who cannot grasp handles well

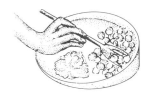

Using a plate with a built up side allows food to be pushed onto a spoon or fork with one hand

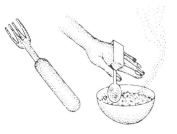

Utensils with built up handles or cuffs are also useful for people who cannot grasp well.

Summing Up

Cardiovascular diseases are among the major causes of death in the United States. The principle cause of coronary heart disease (CHD) is atherosclerosis. CHD can lead to hypertension, heart failure, heart attacks, strokes, aneurysms, and death.

The role of diet in the prevention of atherosclerosis is widely debated. However, evidence is sufficient to prompt the American Heart Association to recommend a fat-controlled, low- salt diet to the general public. Once a person has already developed one of several types of hyperlipidemia, the dietary treatment depends on which lipids are elevated.

Elevated triglyceride levels can often be reduced through weight loss and sometimes carbohydrate restriction (particularly restriction of concentrated sweets). Reducing elevated cholesterol levels through diet is more difficult, but the following measures may help: Lose weight, reduce cholesterol intake, reduce total fat intake, reduce saturated fat intake, and increase polyunsaturated fats in the diet.

Many but not all professional groups also recommend reducing sodium intake for the general public. Advice to restrict sodium in established hypertension has more support. Sodium restriction can augment the effectiveness of diuretic therapy. Weight loss alone also can have a considerable impact on reducing hypertension.

Following a heart attack, the patient's diet generally progresses from N.P.O. to a low-kcalorie, easily digestible, sodium-restricted liquid or soft diet of bland foods given in frequent small feedings. After the patient is out of danger, the diet is tailored to his or her medical status.

In congestive heart failure (CHF), a diet restricted in kcalories, sodium, and sometimes fluid is prescribed to reduce the work load of the heart. Small, frequent feedings of foods that are easy to chew and digest are given. People with CHF may develop malnutrition, which often goes unnoticed, since weight may appear normal because of edema.

The stroke victim may develop temporary or permanent problems with chewing, swallowing, or other physical aspects of eating. These people can often be helped when the consistency of the diet is altered or when special feeding equipment adapted to their needs is used.

To Explore Further

Many excellent references are available on diet and cardiovascular disease. Two important and highly recommended references are:

● American Heart Association Nutrition Committee. Rationale of the diet-heart statement of the American Heart Association. *Arteriosclerosis* 4 (1982):177-191.

● American Heart Association. *Risk Factors and Coronary Disease, a Statement for Physicians*. Dallas: American Heart Association, 1980.

Publications that discuss the role of diet in the development of atherosclerosis include:

● Oliver, M. F. Diet and coronary heart disease. *British Medical Bulletin* 37 (1981):49-58.

This well-balanced article provides a lot of information.

● Truswell, A. S. Diet and plasma lipids — a reappraisal. *American Journal of Clinical Nutrition* 31 (1978):977-989.

This article reviews dietary factors associated with altering plasma lipids.

Articles suggesting a positive association between diet and atherosclerosis include:

● Feldman, E. B. Does nutrition play a role in cardiovascular disease? *Geriatrics*, July 1980, pp. 65-85.

● Zilversmit, D. B. Diet and heart disease, prudence, probability, and proof. *Arteriosclerosis* 2 (1982):83-84.

Two articles which suggest that there is no association between diet and heart disease are given below. The first sparked considerable controversy.

- Mann, G. V. Diet-heart: end of an era. *New England Journal of Medicine* 297 (1977):644-649.

- Ahrens, E. H. Diet and heart disease, shaping public perceptions when proof is lacking. *Arteriosclerosis* 2 (1982):85-86.

Articles of interest in specific areas of CHD include:

- Oster, P., Schlierf, G., Heuck, C. C., Hahn, S., Szymanski, H., and Schellenberg, B. Diet and high density lipoproteins. *Lipids* 16 (1981):93-97.

- Zukel, W. J., Oglesby, P., and Schnaper, H. W. The multiple risk factor intervention trial (MRFIT): I. Historical perspectives. *Preventive Medicine* 10 (1981):387-401.

The second article describes a major clinical trial to determine if an intervention program aimed at reducing serum cholesterol levels, blood pressure, and smoking could reduce the risk of death from CHD in high-risk men.

An interesting article describes the unsupported theory that bovine milk xanthine oxidase plays an important role in the development of atherosclerosis:

- Oster, K. A. Atherosclerosis, conjectures, data and facts. *Nutrition Today*, November/December 1981, pp. 28-29.

An article that includes more than 250 references is:

- Voller, R. D., and Strong, W. B. Pediatric aspects of atherosclerosis. *American Heart Journal* 101 (1981):815-836.

Important articles on managing hyperlipoproteinemias include the following. The booklet listed first contains dietary instructions and food lists for each type of hyperlipidemia.

- National Heart and Lung Institute. *Dietary Management of Hyperlipoproteinemia*. DHEW publication no. (NIH) 7-110. Bethesda, Md.: National Heart and Lung Institute, 1974.

- Lees, R. S., and Lees, A. M. Therapy of hyperlipidemias. *Postgraduate Medicine*, September 1976, pp. 99-107.

- Cathcart-Rake, W. F., and Dujovne, C. A. The treatment of hyperlipoproteinemias. *Rational Drug Therapy*, July 1979, pp. 1-4.

Several articles of interest regarding hypertension appeared on pp. 17-48 of the *Journal of the American Dietetic Association* 80 (1982). Articles dealing with current issues, physiology, pediatric concerns, and the role of diet in hypertension as well as the position of the Food and Drug Administration on dietary sodium and sodium in food processing are included.

Excellent suggestions for managing diet therapy in hypertension are found in:

- U.S. Department of Health and Human Services. *Report of the Working Group on Critical Patient Behaviors in the Dietary Management of High Blood Pressure*. NIH publication no. 81-2269. Bethesda, Md.: National Heart and Lung Institute, 1981.

Several other articles dealing with hypertension and diet include the following. The first article outlines the general approach to hypertension management:

- Moser, M. Hypertension, how therapy works. *American Journal of Nursing* 80 (1980):937-941.

● Pleuss, J., and Kochar, M. S. Dietary considerations in hypertension. *Postgraduate Medicine*, June 1981, pp. 34-43.

● Kent, S. How dietary salt contributes to hypertension. *Geriatrics*, June 1981, pp. 14-20.

● Kolata, G. Value of low sodium diets questioned. *Science* 216 (1982):38-39.

Other references on cardiovascular diseases include:

● Wenger, N. K. Guidelines for dietary management after myocardial infarction. *Geriatrics*, August 1979, pp. 75-83.

● Heymsfield, S. B., Smith, J., Redd, S., and Whitworth, H. B. Nutritional support in cardiac failure. *Surgical Clinics of North America* 61 (1981):635-652.

Hyperlipo-proteinemia, Hypertension

Mr. Garrett, age 45, has just been diagnosed to have type IV hyperlipoproteinemia. He is 5 ft 7 in tall and weighs 200 lb. Mr. Garrett has a family history of CHD. His diet is high in kcalories, cholesterol, total fat, and saturated fats. He smokes a pack of cigarettes a day and his lifestyle leaves him little room for exercise. Mr. Garrett also has hypertension, for which diuretics have been prescribed. He frequently forgets to take his pills, though, and his blood pressure is often quite high.

Study Questions

1. Name the risk factors for CHD in Mr. Garrett's history.
Which of them can he control? Which can be helped by diet? What complications can result from CHD?

2. What type of diet, if any, would you recommend for Mr. Garrett's type of hyperlipidemia? Explain the rationale for each diet change. How will his current diet change? What types of foods should he eat?

3. What type of diet, if any, would you recommend for Mr. Garrett's hypertension? What suggestions might you give to help him make the necessary diet changes? What blood value should be monitored regularly? Why?

4. Name at least three ways in which Mr. Garrett could benefit from losing weight. How can exercise fit into a weight loss plan? If Mr. Garrett decides to quit smoking, how might his weight be affected?

5. Discuss nutrition considerations if Mr. Garrett should have a heart attack, congestive heart failure, or a stroke.

Nutrition and the Lungs

The knowledge ... is relatively recent [of the] intimate relationship, probably a causal one, between nutritional deficiency and infection.

R. K. CHANDRA

Nutrition for people with diseases of the lungs is a neglected area of clinical nutrition today. This is unfortunate, because mortality from obstructive lung diseases is increasing more rapidly than from cancer. (At the same time mortality from cardiovascular and cerebrovascular diseases is actually decreasing; see Figure 1.) The cost of obstructive lung diseases in terms of health care, wages, and time lost from work exceeds $15 billion per year.[1]

Like heart disease, chronic obstructive pulmonary disease (COPD) appears to be multifactorial. Efforts have been underway to identify the risk factors for COPD and to clarify the disease process itself. Researchers are also looking for ways to improve the length and quality of life for people with COPD. Can nutrition play a role? Research in this area is scant, although some information is available.

A Word about COPD The two major types of COPD are emphysema and chronic bronchitis. The primary risk factor for COPD is smoking. Other risk factors that may play a role include exposure to environmental pollution (including exposure of nonsmokers to cigarette smoke), alcohol consumption, family history of respiratory disorders and, possibly, repeated respiratory tract infections in young children.

In emphysema the small passages and air sacs within the lungs lose their elasticity. The victim has trouble exhaling to remove air taken in during inspiration. Stale air containing an excess of carbon dioxide becomes trapped in the lung, and the lung enlarges to accommodate the increased air volume. As they expand, the lung walls thin out; then they tend to collapse during exhalation. Emphysema is believed to be caused by the destruction of elastin, the major structural protein in the normal lung.

The individual with chronic bronchitis suffers

[1]U.S. Department of Health and Human Services, *Ninth Report of the National Heart, Lung, and Blood Advisory Council*, NIH publication no. 81-2334 (Bethesda, Md.: National Heart and Lung Institute, 1981).

Miniglossary

alveoli: air sacs in the lungs.

bronchioles: the air passages from the trachea to the lungs.

bronchitis (bronk-EYE-tiss): clogging of the lung's air passages by mucus and inflammation.

chronic obstructive pulmonary disease (COPD): diseases that cause blockage of the lung's air passages and thus interfere with the exchange of gases between the air and the body. Also called chronic obstructive lung disease (COLD) and chronic obstructive airways diseases (COAD).

elastin: a structural protein in the lung.

emphysema (em-phi-ZEE-muh): a type of COPD in which the lungs lose their elasticity and the victim has trouble exhaling.

intercostal muscles: the muscles between the ribs.

mechanical ventilator: a machine that "breathes" for the person who can't.

Pickwickian syndrome: inadequate ventilation of the lungs caused by obesity.

pulmonary: relating to the lung.

respiratory failure: severe lung dysfunction.

from a different problem. This person produces excessive mucus, which clogs the air passages. These passages also become inflamed, which contributes to the obstruction.

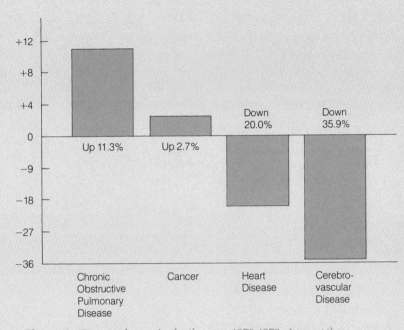

Figure 1 Percent change in death rates, 1970-1979. Among these leading causes of death in the United States, COPD is increasing most rapidly. (Data are adjusted for the aging of the population.)

From U.S. Department of Health and Human Services, *Ninth Report of the National Heart, Lung, and Blood Advisory Council,* NIH publication no. 81-2334, 1981.

Regardless of the type of COPD, eventually the exchange of gases (oxygen and carbon dioxide) between the atmosphere and the body becomes impaired. It becomes more difficult for the oxygen necessary for metabolism to reach the tissues, and removal of carbon dioxide (a waste product from metabolism) is also incomplete. There is no cure for COPD. Treatment is aimed at relieving the symptoms.

Nutrition Risk Factors in the Development of COPD
At present no known risk factors for the development of COPD are directly related to nutrition. However, there is a possibility that nutrition

plays an indirect role. For example, poor nutrition status in children has been associated with a high incidence of pulmonary infections.[2] (See also Highlight 22). Investigators have also noticed a tendency toward emphysema-like changes in starving children and adults.[3]

[2]J. W. James, Longitudinal study of the morbidity of diarrheal and respiratory infections in malnourished children, *American Journal of Clinical Nutrition* 25 (1972):690-694.

[3]A. Braude-Heller, J. Ratbalsam, and R. Elbinger, Clinique de la famine chez les enfants, as cited in J. Askanazi, C. Weissman, S. H. Rosenbaum, A. I. Hyman, J. Milic-Emili, and J. M. Kinney, Nutrition and the respiratory system, *Critical Care Medicine* 10 (1982):163-172.

The ability to clear the lungs of bacteria appears to be impaired by semistarvation.[4] The more weight lost, the greater the impairment. Since repeated respiratory infections may be a risk factor for COPD, nutrition can have an indirect role in its development.

Nutrition Status in COPD
Once a person has developed COPD, two nutrition related problems are frequently noted — weight loss and infection. People with COPD, particularly those with emphysema, frequently lose weight.[5] As COPD advances, weight loss progresses. Since the lungs are muscles, they lose mass and strength as body weight decreases, which in turn negatively affects lung function. Investigators have noted that the incidence of heart failure and mortality are higher in people with COPD who lose weight.[6]

[4]G. M. Green and E. H. Kass, Factors influencing the clearance of bacteria by the lung, *Journal of Clinical Investigation* 43 (1964):769-776.

[5]P. d'A Semple, W. S. Watson, G. H. Beastall, M. I. F. Bethel, J. K. Grant, and R. Hume, Diet, absorption, and hormone studies in relation to body weight in obstructive airways disease, *Thorax* 34 (1979):783-788.

[6]E. Vandenbergh, K. P. van de Woestijne, and A. Gyselen, Weight changes in the terminal stages of chronic obstructive pulmonary disease, relation to respiratory function and prognosis, *American Review of Respiratory Disease* 95 (1967):556-566.

Some factors that have been proposed to explain why many individuals with COPD lose weight include:

● Decreased food intake.

● Malabsorption.

● Increased energy expenditure associated with labored breathing.

● Hormonal influences.

Loss of appetite has commonly been thought to be the main reason for weight loss in COPD, but many investigators have concluded that neither poor intake nor impaired absorption accounts for the weight loss.[7] Nutrient requirements may be increased by the disease process itself and possibly mediated through hormonal changes.

The frequent respiratory infections seen in COPD also can contribute to malnutrition. As we discussed in Chapter 22, infection increases nutrient needs, and nutrient deficiencies in turn can increase the likelihood of infection. The severe weight loss which can occur in COPD may create a vicious

[7]P. d'A Semple and co-authors, 1979; A. M. Hunter, M. A. Carey, and H. W. Larsh, The nutritional status of patients with chronic obstructive pulmonary disease, *American Review of Respiratory Disease* 124 (1981):376-381.

cycle of malnutrition and infection. Furthermore, if weakened by malnutrition, the lungs cannot expel bacteria as they normally do.

It is to be hoped that the exact mechanisms of weight loss in COPD will be more clearly delineated in the future. With this knowledge, the best approach to helping people with COPD maintain weight can be defined and used in the clinical setting.

Before leaving the subject of nutrition and the lung, we will briefly discuss two other areas that deserve consideration. These areas are obesity and pulmonary function and nutrition in respiratory failure.

The Effect of Obesity on Pulmonary Function

The exchange of gases in the lungs is impaired in severe obesity, which interferes with the ability of the intercostal muscles and the diaphragm to ventilate the lung. The result is a condition in which the body can't retain enough oxygen; also, carbon dioxide levels remain high. This condition, called the Pickwickian syndrome, is characterized by lethargy and an uncontrolled tendency to sleep. In severe cases, death can result.

Even in less severe obesity, more work is required of the

lungs when extra weight is carried on the chest wall. As a result, obese people may have trouble breathing when they exercise or when they develop respiratory infections.

Nutrition and Respiratory Failure

In today's intensive care units, respiratory failure is a frequent cause of morbidity and mortality. Malnutrition in this setting can help precipitate respiratory failure in several ways. We have already discussed the fact that the lung muscle mass can decrease as a result of malnutrition; this makes it harder for malnourished patients to carry on forceful respiratory movements and increases the likelihood of their developing pulmonary infections. Furthermore, when patients are being maintained on mechanical ventilators, it may take longer to wean them from support if their lungs are weak. Therefore, careful attention must be paid to meeting nutrition needs in people under intensive care.

Patients with respiratory failure spend more energy, especially during attempts to wean them from mechanical ventilation. The type of nutrients used to provide energy needs appears to be important for these people. They are usually candidates for TPN, and most TPN solutions are high in glucose. However, glucose (and protein) generate more carbon dioxide when metabolized than does fat. Thus, the TPN solution chosen should perhaps derive half of its nonprotein kcalories from fat and half from glucose, based on what little is known at present.

Much work remains to be done regarding nutrition and the lung. The presentations here are very brief and are only intended to call your attention to these neglected subjects.

CHAPTER 27

CONTENTS

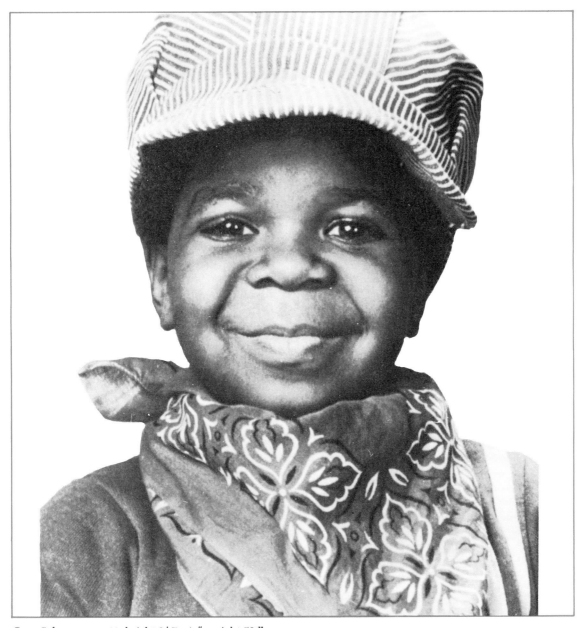

Gary Coleman, age 11, height 3′ 7 1/2″, weight 50 lb.

NUTRITION AND KIDNEY DISEASES

*The internal environment must be suitable for the life of all the cells it touches.
... the final, most delicate regulation of [internal fluid] composition is in the
kidney.*

G. G. SIMPSON

The kidneys certainly illustrate the old adage that good things come in small packages. Although each kidney is only about the size of a fist, together, they comprise the key organ in maintaining chemical homeostasis in the body.

Probably the best way to appreciate the kidneys' vast importance is to see what happens when they aren't working properly. Kidney failure can be a devastating, and sometimes fatal, disease. However, the management of persons with renal disease has improved greatly, and today they can often enjoy a full, high-quality life.

What the Kidneys Do

The kidneys are two bean-shaped organs located just above the waist on each side of the spinal column. The working unit of the kidney is called the nephron (see Figure 1). Each nephron consists of a tuft of capillaries, enclosed by a cup-shaped membrane called the glomerulus, and an associated series of tubules. The kidneys' job is to filter out substances that the body doesn't need and eliminate them in the urine. In so doing, these organs serve many important homeostatic functions: they maintain fluid, electrolyte, and acid-base balance, and they rid the body of metabolic waste products.

Some 1,200 ml of blood passes through the kidneys every minute — about one quarter of the heart's total output. Blood rushes through the glomerulus at about 650 ml per minute, and from this blood, 120 ml of fluid filters through the glomerulus and enters the tubules. The fluid that enters the tubules, called the filtrate, is watery looking because it is devoid of red blood cells. The rate at which filtrate is formed (normally about 120 ml per minute), known as the glomerular filtration rate (GFR), is an index of kidney function.

The **nephron**, the working unit of the kidney, consists of the glomerulus and a series of tubules. The **glomerulus** is a cup-shaped membrane enclosing a tuft of capillaries. The first part of the **tubule** surrounds the glomerulus. A pressure gradient between the glomerulus and the tubule drives fluid into the tubule, and filtration begins. As the filtrate moves along, the tubules return needed materials to the blood and send wastes to the bladder.

The kidney:
1. Maintains fluid, electrolyte, and acid-base balance.
2. Eliminates metabolic waste products.
3. Secretes renin, responds to aldosterone, and produces erythropoietin.
4. Activates vitamin D.

glomerular filtration rate (GFR): the rate at which filtrate is formed. Normally, GFR is 120 ml/min.

Figure 1 One of the kidney's many nephrons. Blood enters the glomerulus, and some of its fluid, with dissolved substances, is filtered into the tubules (1). Then the blood passes alongside the tubules, which return fluid and substances needed by the body (2). The tubule passes waste materials (urine) on to the bladder (3).

The cleansing of blood in the nephron is roughly analogous to the way you might have your car cleaned up at the service station. First you remove all your possessions and trash so that the car can be vacuumed (1). Then you put what you want to keep back in the car (2) and throw away the trash (3).

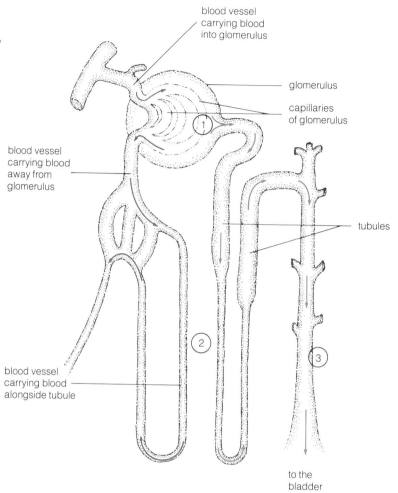

blood vessel carrying blood into glomerulus

glomerulus

capillaries of glomerulus

blood vessel carrying blood away from glomerulus

tubules

blood vessel carrying blood alongside tubule

to the bladder

As the filtrate travels down the tubules, its composition is continually changing. In the end, substances the body needs are returned to the general circulation, and waste products (including excess metabolites) are eliminated in the urine. Thus the kidneys maintain chemical homeostasis.

The work of the kidneys doesn't end here. They help regulate blood pressure by secreting the enzyme renin and by responding to the hormone aldosterone (see Figure 2 and Highlight 2). The kidneys also produce another hormone, erythropoietin, which stimulates red blood cell production. Finally, the kidney is the site where vitamin D is converted to its final, active form. Active vitamin D plays an essential role in normal calcium absorption, calcium and phosphorus metabolism, and bone maintenance.

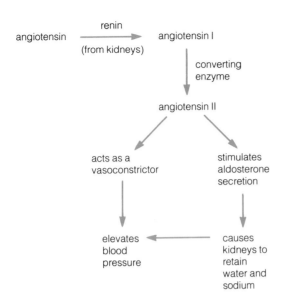

Figure 2   The renin-angiotensin mechanism. Renin from the kidney splits the plasma protein angiotensin to form angiotensin I; in the presence of another enzyme, angiotensin I is activated to angiotensin II, which acts as a vasoconstrictor and also stimulates aldosterone secretion. The net effect is to raise blood pressure.

Renal Failure

With all these important functions there is little doubt that renal failure can have serious consequences. Renal failure can occur suddenly (acute renal failure) or over a period of time (chronic renal failure). It occurs when the nephrons lose sufficient function that they cannot maintain normal homeostatic and hormonal mechanisms. Oftentimes acute renal failure is only temporary. Chronic renal failure is usually irreversible.

Renal disease may be caused by damage to the kidneys themselves, as in nephritis, renal artery obstruction, nephrotic syndrome (see below), kidney stones (see below), and renal tubular disorders. Renal failure can also result from other diseases, such as diabetic nephropathy, hypertension, atherosclerosis, and septic shock.

As the nephrons fail, the normal composition of the blood and urine is altered. Therefore, laboratory tests using these fluids are useful for evaluating renal function. Clearance tests measure the GFR, which decreases as renal failure progresses. Blood urea nitrogen (BUN), creatinine, and uric acid are the body's principal nitrogen-containing metabolic waste products. They accumulate in the blood when renal function is impaired.

As renal failure progresses to a severe stage, a complex of symptoms, the uremic syndrome, develops, precipitated by a buildup of toxic waste products in the blood. The uremic patient experiences a wide array of symptoms in virtually every body system. Some of the more common symptoms include fatigue, weakness, decreased mental alertness, muscular twitches, muscle cramps, anorexia, nausea, vomiting, stomatitis, and an unpleasant taste in the mouth. The skin may itch uncomfortably. In later stages, gastrointestinal ulcers and bleeding are common.

renal failure: failure of the nephrons to maintain normal function.

An inflammation of the kidney is **nephritis**. **Pyelonephritis** is an inflammation of the kidney and bladder. Inflammation of the glomerular capillaries is **glomerulonephritis**.

nephrosclerosis: impairment of renal blood flow because of renal artery damage. It can be caused by hypertension or atherosclerosis.

uremic syndrome: a complex of symptoms seen late in renal disease, caused by the buildup of toxic waste products in the blood.

When urea (which can be excreted through sweat) crystallizes and becomes visible on the skin, it is called **uremic frost**.

The overall goal of dietary management of renal failure is to achieve or maintain optimal nutrition status while preventing the buildup of toxic waste products. The actual diet must be tailored to each individual; the dietary constituents that must usually be controlled include total kcalories, protein, sodium, potassium, phosphorus, and fluids.

Chronic Renal Disease

The capacity of the kidney to function despite loss of some nephrons is referred to as **renal reserve**.

In chronic renal disease the nephrons are gradually and progressively destroyed. The remaining nephrons get bigger in an attempt to maintain normal functioning. The hypertrophied nephrons work so efficiently that about 80 percent of them can be destroyed before renal function is seriously affected. The GFR may decrease to one-tenth of the normal rate, 10 to 12 ml per minute, before symptoms appear. You can see, then, why renal disease may be advanced before it is even detected.

The severe stage of renal disease in which diet alone is no longer effective in maintaining normal functions is called **end-stage renal disease (ESRD)**.

The early stages of renal disease generally involve no dietary restrictions. However, as nitrogenous waste products build up in the blood (azotemia) and the GFR decreases, the person with renal disease benefits from dietary restrictions aimed at preventing hypertension, edema, congestive heart failure, and uremia. The diet is prescribed and regularly adjusted based on the degree of renal insufficiency.

azotemia: abnormal accumulation of nitrogenous substances in the blood.

Eventually, if renal failure progresses far enough, diet alone cannot prevent uremia. At this point, dialysis has to be used or else the patient will die. (See box "Dialysis and Kidney Transplants.")

The metabolism of nutrients and their end products are significantly affected by renal failure for many reasons. Some of these include:

- Failure to excrete toxic waste products.
- Inability of the renal tubules to reabsorb many needed nutrients.
- Reduced GI absorption of some nutrients.
- Reduced inactivation of many hormones, including insulin, parathyroid hormone, glucagon, and thyrotropin.
- Reduced synthesis of other important substances, such as erythropoietin and active vitamin D.
- Alteration of nutrient needs by other medical therapy (drugs and dialysis).
- Decreased food intake because of GI distress, depression, superimposed illnesses, or restrictive or unpalatable diets.

wasting syndrome: the pattern of poor growth and weight loss frequently seen in patients with chronic renal disease.

Because of these difficulties, the nutrition status of people with chronic renal disease is often compromised. The child with renal disease often fails to grow normally, and people of any age with renal disease may have reduced muscle mass, fat tissue, and visceral protein levels. These characteristics are frequently called the wasting syndrome. Special attention to the patient's nutrient needs can help prevent this problem.

Dialysis and Kidney Transplants

The kidneys are virtually irreplaceable. There are no perfect substitutes for kidneys that have failed. However, although they may not be as good as the real thing, dialysis and kidney transplants can be life saving for the end-stage renal failure patient.

Let's first take a look at dialysis. Dialysis works on the principle of simple diffusion and osmosis through a semipermeable membrane. When the membrane that covers the abdominal organs (the peritoneum) serves as the semipermeable membrane, then the procedure is called **peritoneal dialysis**. A synthetic semipermeable membrane also can be used. In this case, blood leaves the person's artery through tubing that passes the semipermeable membrane. The blood returns through the person's vein after passing the membrane. This procedure is called **hemodialysis**.

The way dialysis works is actually very simple. A solution similar in composition to normal blood plasma, called the dialysate, is placed on one side of the semipermeable membrane; the patient's blood flows by on the other side. The blood has a higher concentration of urea and electrolytes than the dialysate, so these substances diffuse from the blood into the dialysate. The dialysate also contains glucose; the higher the concentration of glucose in the dialysate, the more fluid will move from the blood into the dialysate by osmosis.

In hemodialysis the blood is returned to the patient's body after it has passed through the machine that houses the semipermeable membrane and dialysate. Oftentimes chronic renal failure patients on hemodialysis get four- to eight-hour treatments, three times a week.

In peritoneal dialysis, the dialysate is infused directly through a tube into the patient's abdomen. The fluid is kept in the abdomen for about 30 minutes, then drained from the peritoneal cavity by gravity. One complete exchange takes about an hour. The total treatment takes from 24 to 72 hours.

The use of hemodialysis as the preferred method of treatment became widespread in the 1960s. However, recently there has been a trend toward using peritoneal dialysis, because the technique has improved. Both methods can be adapted for home use. Recently, continuous ambulatory peritoneal dialysis (CAPD) has become popular. Using this technique, the person on dialysis completes one exchange using the procedure discussed above three to five times each day, seven days a week. Thus, dialysis is continuous.

Dialysis takes over two important functions of the kidney: waste removal and fluid removal. In so doing, dialysis reduces the symptoms of uremia, hypertension, and edema and the risk of congestive heart failure. But the hormonal functions of the kidney are not restored. Anemia is still a problem. (Actually, blood loss

Miniglossary of Dialysis and Kidney Transplant Terms

arteriovenous shunt: surgically made access to the circulation of the person on hemodialysis.

Cushingoid appearance: a characteristic appearance seen in people who take large doses of corticosteroids. The face becomes puffy and the body looks obese, with extra fat deposited on the upper back or shoulders (sometimes called a "buffalo hump").

dialysate: a solution used during dialysis to draw off extra fluids and wastes from the blood.

dialysis: a system based on the principles of diffusion and osmosis across a semipermeable membrane and used to remove excess fluids and wastes from the blood. In **hemodialysis**, a synthetic semipermeable membrane is used. The peritoneum serves as the semipermeable membrane in **peritoneal dialysis**. (The **peritoneum** is the body cavity containing the intestines.) **Chronic ambulatory peritoneal dialysis (CAPD)** is a method of providing continuous dialysis at home.

diffusion: flow of particles from an area where they are more concentrated to an area where they are less concentrated.

histocompatibility: the compatibility between donor and recipient that enables cells from a donor's tissue to survive in a recipient without being rejected.

osmosis: flow of water from an area of high concentration of solute to one of low concentration.

during hemodialysis compounds this problem.) Hypertension may still persist, and hypotension can be a problem if too much fluid is removed during dialysis. (See also "Nutrition in Dialysis.")

An alternative to dialysis in end-stage renal failure is a kidney transplant. Many kidney transplants successfully restore kidney function and normal growth. For this reason, transplants are particularly desirable in children. The only patients who are not considered candidates for kidney transplants are the very old, patients with other life-threatening conditions, or patients who prefer dialysis. Many would prefer transplants; however, a suitable kidney donor can't always be found.

Finding a suitable kidney donor is of paramount importance. Once a kidney has been transplanted, it will be rejected and treated as a foreign protein (see Highlight 22) unless the cells of the donor and recipient are properly matched. Without such a match, a transplant cannot take place.

After the new kidney is in place, the patient must take very large doses of corticosteroids to prevent rejection. Because of this medical therapy, the patient can develop muscular weakness, GI bleeding, carbohydrate intolerance, sodium retention and hypertension, and a characteristic puffy-faced appearance. Infections and increased susceptibility to malignant tumors are also common. (People who have had kidney transplants have a 35-times-greater risk of developing malignant tumors, especially lymphomas and skin and lip cancers.[1] The kidney may be rejected or fail to function, in which case dialysis must be reinstituted or a new transplant performed. (See also "Nutrition and the Renal Transplant Patient.")

[1]J. B. Reckling, Safeguarding the renal transplant patient, *Nursing*, February 1982, pp. 47-49.

The next several sections are written as if they were addressed to the diet planner. "You" must reduce protein in this condition, increase kcalories in that. In fact you, the reader, may not be the diet planner, but it is important for you to understand what that person has to do. As you read the following sections, notice how complex the diet for renal disease often has to be. Notice how critical the control of certain nutrients is. Notice what those nutrients are, and keep in mind how food choices will be affected by restrictions placed on those nutrients.

When you communicate with someone who has renal disease, or with a member of his or her family, or with another person on the health care team, it may not be necessary for you to know that the person is allowed exactly 20 g of protein a day, but it is important to know *why* protein must be restricted. Whatever your place on the team, you are most effective if you truly understand and can communicate the necessity of the renal diet.

Energy and Protein   Providing the right amount of protein to the renal failure patient is like walking a tightrope. Too little protein and the person develops malnutrition. Too much protein and you increase blood urea levels (the toxic waste product of protein metabolism).

Ideally, you want to provide a diet with enough essential amino acids to support normal nitrogen balance without increasing the BUN. You can use the guidelines in Table 1 to calculate protein needs in renal failure. Notice that protein is adjusted to the kidneys' ability to excrete wastes as measured by the GFR. Just as important as the amount of protein in the diet is the quality of the protein. Sources of protein with high biological value, such as eggs, milk, meat, poultry, and fish, are given the greatest emphasis.

Clinicians disagree about when a low-protein diet becomes too low to maintain nutrition status. Some investigators believe that once the GFR falls below 4 to 5 ml per minute, dialysis is needed so that protein intake can be adequate without precipitating uremia. However, others continue to give diets very low in protein (about 20 g) to avoid the need for dialysis. Virtually all of the protein in this type of diet must be of high quality.

The concept of supplying a low-protein diet high in essential amino acids to people with renal failure was first introduced by Giordano, Giovannetti, and Maggiore.[2] The rationale of the diet (often called the G-G or Giordano-Giovannetti diet) is that excess urea in the blood together with essential amino acids in the diet can be used by the body to synthesize nonessential amino acids. In theory, by using urea in this way you can reduce blood urea levels and supply adequate protein at the same time. Unfortunately, it appears that the use of endogenous urea for protein synthesis is limited.[3]

Furthermore, these diets are very restrictive and unpalatable. It is often difficult to get people to consume adequate kcalories on a very-low-protein diet; without enough kcalories, protein will be used for energy.

However, researchers have been expanding on this concept, and new approaches to diet may be commonly used in the future. Very-low-protein diets supplemented with either essential amino acids or essential amino acids and keto acid analogues of essential amino acids have been shown to be effective in maintaining acceptable nitrogen balance while reducing the symptoms of uremia.[4] More recently, a

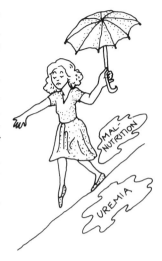

Urea is the waste product, normally excreted, into which many of the body's unused amino groups (NH_2) are collected:

urea

$$\underset{(H_2N)}{} \overset{\displaystyle O}{\underset{\displaystyle C}{\|}} \underset{(NH_2)}{}$$ amino groups

When you replace the amino group (NH_2) of an amino acid with a hydroxy group (OH), you have made a keto acid analogue. For example, pyruvic acid is the keto acid analogue of alanine:

pyruvic acid
$$\begin{array}{c} COOH \\ | \\ HC - \boxed{OH} \\ | \\ CH_3 \end{array}$$

alanine
$$\begin{array}{c} COOH \\ | \\ HC - \boxed{NH_2} \\ | \\ CH_3 \end{array}$$

In renal failure it is hoped that the body will draw upon its unexcreted urea to put NH_2 back on the keto acid analogues, making the amino acids it needs.

[2]C. Giordano, Use of exogenous and endogenous urea for protein synthesis in normal and uremic subjects, *Journal of Laboratory and Clinical Medicine* 62 (1963):231-246; S. Giovanneti and Q. Maggiore, A low-nitrogen diet with proteins of high biological value for severe chronic uraemia, *Lancet* 1 (1964):1000-1003.

[3]A. R. Varcoe, D. Halliday, E. R. Carson, P. Richards, and A. S. Travill, Anabolic role of urea in renal failure, *American Journal of Clinical Nutrition* 31 (1978):1601-1607.

[4]P. Fürst, M. Ahlberg, A. Alvestrand, and J. Bergström, Principles of essential amino acid therapy in uremia, *American Journal of Clinical Nutrition* 31 (1978):1744-1755; M. Walser, Principles of keto acid therapy in uremia, *American Journal of Clinical Nutrition* 31 (1978):1756-1760.

E.H., an adult with chronic renal failure, is on peritoneal dialysis. At 155 lb, she has the following protein and energy needs:

Protein:

1.2 g/kg × 70 kg = 85 g
1.5 g/kg × 71 kg = 106 g

Protein intake should be from 85 to 106 g (notice that this is not a low protein intake).

Energy:

35 kcal/kg × 71 kg = 2,485 kcal

For comparison, a 12-year-old child who weighs only 75 lb would require more than 2,500 kcal/day for optimal growth.

study has suggested that the combination of essential amino acids and keto acid analogues actually reduces the rate of renal deterioration as compared with conventional low-protein diets or dialysis treatments.[5]

Once the decision has been made to use dialysis, protein intake is less restrictive. Individuals on hemodialysis require 1.0 to 1.2 g protein per kg of body weight (compare with the normal adult RDA of 0.8 g/kg). The patient on peritoneal dialysis requires even more protein (from 1.2 to 1.5 g/day). (See box "Dialysis and Kidney Transplants.")

Regardless of the protein allowance, all people with renal failure need adequate kcalories to maintain or achieve ideal body weight and to prevent protein catabolism. For adults, at least 35 kcal/kg per day should be given. For children, 100 or even more kcal/kg per day is often desirable, and about 80 kcal/kg is considered a realistic intake. Below 40 kcal/kg per day, a child can't grow at all.

Because the renal diet often is low in protein, kcalories from nonprotein sources are very important. Frequently, fats (margarine, cream, butter) and concentrated sweets (hard candy, jelly) can be used to increase intake. However, concentrated sweets are not recommended if the renal patient is also diabetic.

The little girl beams with pleasure when Charlie, the nurse, comes into the room. This is one of the high points of her day. "Do you have a lollipop for me?" she asks.

"Yep," says Charlie, reaching into his pocket. "Your favorite color, red. Eat it all up and I'll bring you another one."

Why is this nurse feeding the child candy? Because the child has renal disease and has a hard time getting enough kcalories to protect the protein she eats, the staff has been instructed to keep giving her sugar in whatever form she will accept it. A lollipop is like a clear liquid, because it melts in the mouth; it contains no protein or electrolytes to burden the kidney; but it offers sugar to help spare protein. Nothing could be more appropriate for this growing child's health.

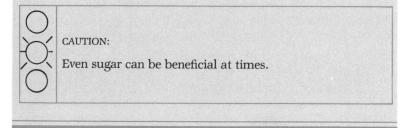

CAUTION:

Even sugar can be beneficial at times.

[5]G. Barsotti, A. Guiducci, F. Ciardella, and S. Giovanneti, Effects on renal function of a low-nitrogen diet supplemented with essential amino acids and ketoanalogues and of hemodialysis and free protein supply in patients with chronic renal failure, *Nephron* 27 (1981):113-117.

Table 1.   Guidelines for Protein Intake in Chronic
Renal Failure Patients not on Dialysis

GFR (ml/min)	Protein (g)
>25	No restriction
20-25	60-90
15-20	50-70
10-15	40-55
4-10	Men: 40; women: 35

Adapted from J. D. Kopple, Nutritional therapy in kidney failure, *Nutritional Reviews* 39
(1981):193-206.

Many patients with chronic renal failure develop type IV hyperlipoproteinemia and atherosclerosis. For these individuals, diets lower in
carbohydrate and higher in fat with a high ratio of polyunsaturated to
saturated fat may help lower serum triglycerides and reduce the risk or
progression of atherosclerosis.[6]

Fluid and Electrolytes   Renal disease causes disturbances in the sea
of fluid and electrolytes that bathes the cells. Early in renal failure, the
kidneys lose the ability to reabsorb sodium as normal kidneys do.
Therefore, even though renal volume may be decreased somewhat, the
patient can maintain sodium balance on a moderate sodium intake.
However, as end-stage renal disease approaches, less urine is excreted,
and the patient cannot handle normal amounts of sodium. He or she
can thus develop hypertension, edema, and heart failure. At this point,
sodium and water are restricted. A typical diet will contain from 1 to 3
g of sodium and 1,500 to 3,000 ml of fluid daily. A person on dialysis
who is excreting little or no urine may need to restrict sodium and
fluids further. Foods that are considered part of the fluid allowance are
listed in Table 2.

When urine volume is decreased,
oliguria exists; **anuria** means
that no urine at all is being excreted.

Since individual needs vary, you must carefully monitor each patient's weight, blood pressure, and urine output to determine exact
needs. Body weight and blood pressure will increase if sodium (and
fluid) is being retained and will decrease if sodium intake is too low.
(Urine output is also useful as a basis for estimating daily fluid needs.
Simply add 500 ml — for insensible water loss — to 24-hour urine
output.)

[6]M. L. Sanfelippo, R. S. Swenson, and G. M. Reaven, Reduction of plasma triglycerides by
diet in subjects with chronic renal failure, *Kidney International* 11 (1977):54-61.

Table 2. Substances Controlled on Fluid Restricted Diets

Beverages

Alcoholic beverages	Milk
Carbonated beverages	Tea
Coffee	Water
Juices	Any other

Foods*

Ice cream (melts to 1/2 initial volume)	Popsicles
Ice milk (melts to 1/2 initial volume)	Sherbet (melts to 2/3 initial volume)
Jello	Soup

Other

Cream	Ice (melts to 9/10 initial volume)

*Although all foods contain some water, these are the foods considered part of the fluid allowance on a fluid restricted diet.

Most people with renal failure do not have problems handling typical intakes of potassium. However, hyperkalemia can occur, and if it does, it can be fatal. Therefore, potassium is moderately restricted to about 1.5 to 2.8 g per day. Table 3 lists food high in potassium that should be avoided. Again, individuals' needs vary.

If your patient is also on potassium-wasting diuretics (see Chapter 26), then potassium intake may need to be increased. The sodium and potassium contents of many foods are listed in Appendix I.

Phosphorus, Calcium, and Vitamin D Normally, our bodies maintain a balance of phosphorus and calcium in the blood. When phosphorus levels rise, calcium falls, and vice versa. The parathyroid hormone (PTH) and active vitamin D play essential roles in maintaining this balance (see Highlight 2). The balance of calcium and phosphorus is extremely important in maintaining the structure of our bones. Bone disease (renal osteodystrophy) frequently occurs in the person with chronic renal failure. In recent years, the mechanisms involved in bone disease have been studied extensively but have not been clearly defined. Several factors seem to interact in causing bone disease.

First of all, phosphorus is normally excreted in the urine when serum levels are elevated. But in kidney disease, phosphorus is retained. As serum phosphorus levels rise, serum calcium levels fall. The low serum calcium concentration triggers the release of PTH, which works to increase calcium levels by increasing the renal excretion of phosphorus.

renal osteodystrophy: bone disorders (osteomalacia and osteitis fibrosis) resulting from calcium and phosphorus imbalances in renal disease.

Table 3. Foods High in Potassium

Vegetables

Artichokes*	Rhubarb*
Broccoli	Rutabagas
Brussels sprouts	Tomatoes
Parsnips*	Tomato juice*
Pinto beans	Vegetable juice*
Pumpkins*	Winter squash*
Potatoes, baked* or pared and boiled	Yams

Fruits

Apricots*	Oranges
Apricot nectar	Orange juice
Avocadoes*	Papayas*
Bananas*	Peaches*
Cantaloupes*	Pears
Dates*	Pineapples
Figs	Pineapple juice
Grapefruit	Prunes*
Grapefruit juice	Prune juice*
Honeydew melons*	Raisins*
Nectarines*	Tangerines

Other

Bran cereal	Molasses, dark* and light
Chocolate	Peanuts*
Cocoa	Walnuts*
Meat*	Wheat germ
Milk*	Whole grain bread

*Typical serving contains more than 250 mg potassium.

For a while, this helps maintain lower serum phosphorus and higher serum calcium levels, but every time the GFR falls, more parathyroid hormone is needed to maintain effectiveness. Hyperparathyroidism develops. Finally, as the GFR continues to drop, parathyroid hormone becomes ineffective in lowering serum phosphorus levels.

These problems are compounded by the fact that the diseased kidney makes little or no active vitamin D. Under normal conditions, active vitamin D works with PTH to help mobilize calcium from bone and increase serum calcium levels. With less active vitamin D available, PTH has to work harder to maintain normal serum calcium levels. Calcium absorption in the GI tract is also impaired, further lowering serum calcium. Additionally, diets that are restricted in protein and phosphorus tend to be low in calcium as well.

Figure 3 Events leading to renal osteodystrophy.

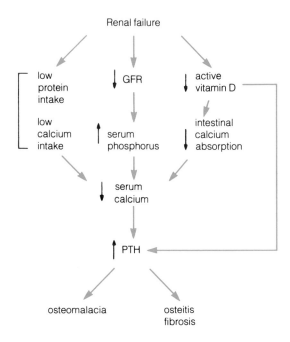

osteomalacia: softening of the bones.

osteitis fibrosis: disturbance of calcium and phosphorus metabolism caused by hyperparathyroidism. The disorder is characterized by kidney stones, decalcification and softening of bones, and sometimes, formation of cysts and tumors.

The deposition of phosphorus and calcium salts in soft tissue is called **metastatic calcification**.

The net result is that the normal bone matrix is disrupted. The bones become soft (demineralized) and fracture easily. Growth retardation is common. The person with renal bone disease may experience bone pain related to the hyperparathyroidism. The high levels of ineffective PTH can cause the total amount of phosphorus to stay high. When this happens, phosphorus and calcium may form a salt that is deposited in soft tissues and blood vessels. Figure 3 summarizes the events that lead to renal osteodystrophy.

Every day the renal team sees a group of adults and children, many of whom are small for their age. Many of the adults have had renal transplants, and their kidneys are now functioning well; but before they received the transplants, they had already suffered irreversible growth failure. The children are suffering growth failure now, and the team must seize the chance to make up the deficit before the end of puberty.

The cycle of events leading to renal osteodystrophy is largely preventable through dietary control. Phosphorus levels are maintained in the low normal range (2 to 3 mg per 100 ml) by reduction of phosphorus intake. The amount of phosphorus given depends on the degree of renal function. (Generally, a low-protein diet is low in phosphorus anyway.) Table 4 lists foods high in phosphorus. If diet

Table 4.   Foods High in Phosphorus

Chocolate	Milk products
Cocoa	Nuts
Dried beans and peas	Organ meats
Dried fruit	Peanut butter
Fish, canned	Whole grain breads
Game	Whole grain cereals
Milk	

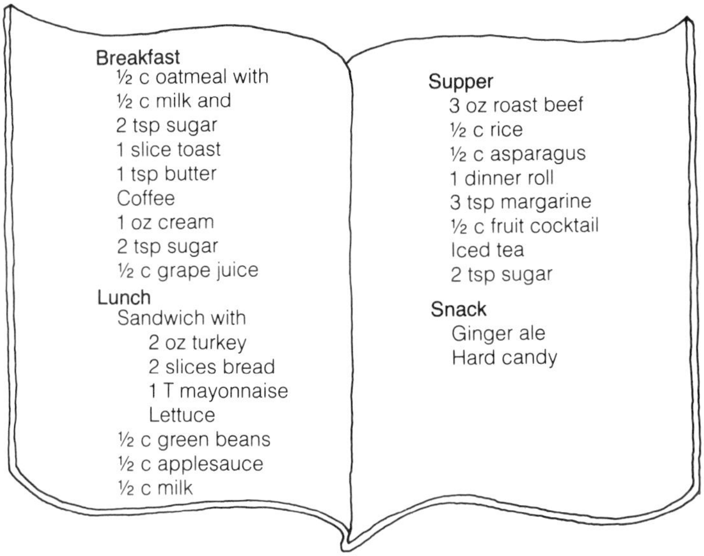

Breakfast
½ c oatmeal with
½ c milk and
2 tsp sugar
1 slice toast
1 tsp butter
Coffee
1 oz cream
2 tsp sugar
½ c grape juice

Lunch
Sandwich with
2 oz turkey
2 slices bread
1 T mayonnaise
Lettuce
½ c green beans
½ c applesauce
½ c milk

Supper
3 oz roast beef
½ c rice
½ c asparagus
1 dinner roll
3 tsp margarine
½ c fruit cocktail
Iced tea
2 tsp sugar

Snack
Ginger ale
Hard candy

Sample renal diet menu (60 g protein; sodium and potassium controlled). You can increase the kcalories in this diet by preparing food with oil or unsalted margarine (regular margarine, if allowed) and by using additional sugar or syrup whenever possible. For example, eating canned fruit packed in heavy syrup rather than in juice can help.

alone fails to keep phosphorus levels in check, the patient is given phosphate binders, aluminum-containing antacids that work by binding phosphorus in the GI tract, thus making it unavailable for absorption.

Most renal patients receive 1,200 to 1,600 mg of calcium in supplement form each day to help prevent bone disease. Large doses of vitamin D (50,000 to 200,000 IU daily) can be given to improve the absorption and utilization of calcium. Recently, the active form of vitamin D has become available commercially, and its use is on the rise. Much smaller doses of active vitamin D or synthetic analogues can achieve the desired effect. The dose must be carefully tailored to the individual to prevent hypercalcemia. (Active vitamin D is not given if serum phosphorus levels are high.)

Renal failure patients should never take antacids, laxatives, or enemas that are high in magnesium; serious hypermagnesemia can result.

A deranged mental state seen in some people on dialysis and characterized by abnormal speech, muscular jerks, and convulsions, **dialysis encephalopathy**, has been associated with aluminum toxicity.

In a person with renal failure, true weight is measured immediately after dialysis when excess fluid has been removed.

Other Nutrients   Renal patients frequently develop vitamin deficiencies. The restrictive diet may be partly responsible, since diets low in potassium also are low in water-soluble vitamins. Vitamins can also be lost during dialysis, and drug therapy can change nutrient needs. The metabolism of nutrients also may be affected in people with uremia. Generally, generous amounts of vitamin B_6 (5 mg), vitamin C (70 to 100 mg), and folacin (1 mg) are given along with the RDA of the remaining water-soluble vitamins. People on dialysis have higher needs for vitamin B_6 (10 mg) and vitamin C (100 mg). Other than vitamin D, supplementation of the fat-soluble vitamins is usually not necessary.

Iron deficiency anemia is frequently seen in chronic renal failure patients, and they often receive iron supplements. There are many reasons why iron may be lost. For one thing, the patient may lose blood (and iron) because blood is drawn frequently for testing. Additionally, GI bleeding is fairly common. People on hemodialysis can lose some blood during dialysis. Finally, the intestinal absorption of iron may be impaired in people with uremia. Anemia unrelated to iron deficiency also can occur. The decreased production of erythropoietin leads to decreased synthesis of red blood cells to carry oxygen. The toxins that accumulate in renal failure can shorten the life span of the existing red blood cells, compounding the problem.

Zinc may be deficient in people on dialysis. They frequently complain of anorexia and altered taste perceptions (dysgeusia); these features are typical of zinc deficiency. In one study, researchers showed that supplemental zinc improved taste sensitivity and appetite.[7]

Aluminum also may be a problem for dialysis patients. Contamination of the dialysate with aluminum has been linked to mental disturbances, bone fractures, and a severe anemia.[8] The nutrient needs of renal patients are summarized in Table 5.

Nutrition in Dialysis   Dialysis solves some of the problems of the renal patient. He or she doesn't have to be as careful to restrict nutrients when they can be dialyzed away.

A more liberal protein intake is allowed because some blood proteins and amino acids are lost in the dialysate. Fluid intake is controlled to allow a weight gain of about 2 to 2 1/2 pounds between dialysis treatments. Water-soluble vitamins also can be lost during dialysis, and therefore additional vitamins are given, as described earlier.

[7]E. Atkin-Thor, B. W. Goddard, J. O'Nion, R. L. Stephen, and W. J. Kolff, Hypogeusia and zinc depletion in chronic dialysis patients, *American Journal of Clinical Nutrition* 31 (1978):1948-1951.

[8]A. M. Pierides, W. G. Edwards, U. X. Cullum, J. T. McCall, and H. A. Ellis, Hemodialysis encephalopathy with osteomalacic fractures aand muscle weakness, *Kidney International* 18 (1980):115-124.

Table 5.   Typical Nutrient Needs in Chronic Renal Failure*

	Predialysis	Hemodialysis	Peritoneal dialysis
Energy (kcal/kg)	35-50	35-50	35-50
Protein (g/kg)	(See Table 1)	1.0-1.2	1.2-1.5
Fluid (ml)	1,500-3,000	750-1,500	750-1,500
Sodium (g)	1.0-3.0	1.0-1.5	1.0-1.5
Potassium (g)	1.5-2.8	1.5-2.8	3.0-3.5
Phosphorus (mg)	600-1,200	600-1,200	600-1,200
Supplements			
Calcium (mg)	1,200-1,600	1,000	1,200-1,600
Folacin (mg)	1	1	1
Vitamin B_6 (mg)	5	10	10
Vitamin C (mg)	70-100	100	100
Other water-soluble			
vitamins	RDA	RDA	RDA
Vitamin D	As appropriate	As appropriate	As appropriate

*The actual amounts of these nutrients in the diet must be highly individualized based on each person's responses.

Adapted from J. D. Kopple, Nutritional therapy in kidney failure, *Nutrition Reviews* 39 (1981):193-206; D. J. Rodriguez and V. M. Hunter, Nutritional intervention in chronic renal failure, *Nursing Clinics of North America* 16 (1981):573-585.

Peritoneal dialysis poses some additional problems. The person on this type of dialysis is asked to watch sodium intake, because sodium is not as effectively removed in peritoneal dialysis. (Table 5 summarizes nutrient recommendations for patients on dialysis.)

Nutrition and the Renal Transplant Patient   The renal transplant patient is allowed a much freer choice of foods than the person on dialysis, provided that renal function is normal; but the drugs that must be taken can cause some nutrition problems. Depending on the patient's medical status, the following measures may be necessary:

● Restrict kcalories to avoid excessive weight gain. (Corticosteroids can cause the appetite to increase.)

● Increase protein intake. (Corticosteroids can increase protein catabolism and lead to negative nitrogen balance.)

● Restrict sodium. (Hypertension and edema often accompany corticosteroid treatment.)

● Increase potassium. (Many of these patients are on potassium-wasting diuretics.)

● Avoid concentrated sweets. (Glucose intolerance can develop in patients taking corticosteroids.)

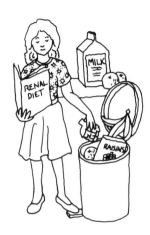

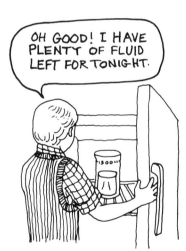

Renal transplant patients may develop temporary periods of kidney rejection or they may permanently reject their new kidney. Often they must go back on a renal failure diet during these times. This may be very difficult to accept, and patients should be prepared for this possibility before it occurs.

Helpful Hints   If you think a renal diet is difficult to plan, think of what it must be like to follow. The shock of finding out you have renal disease would be quite enough. Being told about the restrictive diet would make matters worse. People who have just been told they have renal disease must cope with many things. Don't expect them to understand instructions (including diet instructions) in one session. Explain the concept of the diet several times and evaluate the patient's compliance frequently.

Many patients can comply with a sodium restriction by following a no-added-salt diet (see Chapter 26), but renal failure patients can't use many low-sodium products and salt substitutes because they contain potassium. Potassium can be kept in check if foods high in potassium are avoided (see Table 3). Similarly, phosphorus intake can be controlled (see Table 4). Caution your clients to measure foods and to be sure kcaloric intake is adequate.

The severe thirst experienced by many people with renal failure makes compliance with fluid restriction extremely difficult. One method for helping patients monitor their fluid intake is to have them fill a container of water with their total fluid allowance at the start of each day. For example, they can fill a jar with 1,500 ml of water if this is their fluid allowance. Every time they use a liquid food or drink, an equivalent amount of water is discarded from the container, and they can look at the jar to get an idea of how much fluid they have left for the day. Remind the patient to save some of the fluid allowance for taking medications.

Other hints for controlling thirst: Freeze fluids (they take longer to eat), add lemon juice to water to make it more refreshing, and gargle with refrigerated mouthwash when thirsty.[9] Sometimes chewing gum or sucking on hard candy can relieve thirst.

The renal failure diet can be extremely restrictive, unappealing, and monotonous. Try to provide exciting and appetizing changes. Special renal cookbooks can be a big help (see Appendix C). Incorporate favorite foods whenever possible (this is especially important with children). Encourage renal patients and their families to eat together and eat the same kinds of foods. Many times only the portion sizes will need to be adjusted. Spices and seasonings such as garlic and onion powder, chili, curry, oregano, pepper, and lemon juice can add zest to many foods.

[9]D. J. Rodriguez and V. M. Hunter, Nutritional intervention in the treatment of chronic renal failure, *Nursing Clinics of North America* 16 (1981):573-585.

No doubt you have long since arrived at the conclusion that designing renal diets is a task for a specialist. The complexities pile up: The diet planner must raise/lower intakes of sodium, potassium, protein, kcalories, liquids, lipids, vitamins, minerals. Not only that, he must find food combinations that will deliver the necessary amounts of these nutrients. And not only that, he must find foods to deliver these nutrients that *the individual on the diet will accept and enjoy*. The renal dietitian faces these challenges every day.

With all that hard work to do, the diet planner has still another task — communicating with, and especially listening to, the patient. Inside that tangled web of grossly altered metabolic processes, dialysis lines, and toxic waste products is a person — often, a frightened or discouraged one. One patient will say he dreams of ice cream sodas, forbidden for their high sodium content; he needs at least to feel understood. Another says she feels guilty because her mother spends so much time preparing special foods for her; she, too, needs support. Another is fighting guilt and resentment because repeatedly, in spite of the rules he knows he should follow, he sneaks forbidden foods high in protein. If you have ever been "on a diet," even though it wasn't a renal diet, you will appreciate some of the problems these patients face.

The life the person with renal disease has to live involves many frustrations. Successful treatment often hinges on compliance with diet and drug orders. All the members of the health care team need to know what is involved, if they are to offer the most effective possible support.

Acute Renal Failure

One author described the difference between chronic and acute renal failure very nicely when she stated, "If you can think of chronic renal failure as a downhill course for your patient, acute renal failure is like seeing him go over a cliff no one quite knew was there." [10] The typical victim of acute renal failure is hypercatabolic and has some major illness such as an infection or a burn or has suffered a cardiac arrest. Suddenly, the GFR drops, urine output decreases, blood pressure shoots up, and toxic waste products begin to build up in the blood. Acidosis is common. As the body's cells break down, potassium is released from the intracellular fluid and the kidneys are unable to excrete it. Blood potassium levels rise sharply. Hiccups, anorexia, nausea, and vomiting

[10]J. L. Stark, How to succeed against acute renal failure, *Nursing*, July 1982, pp. 26-33.

Reduced blood flow can lead to acute renal failure; this is said to be a **prerenal** cause.

A urinary tract obstruction can lead to acute renal failure; this is a **postrenal** cause. (The kidney can make urine but the urine can't get outside the body.)

Damage to the kidney cells themselves is an **intrarenal** cause of acute renal failure.

The early phase of acute renal failure, when urine volume is decreased, is the **oliguric phase**; the phase characterized by large fluid and electrolyte losses in the urine is the **diuretic phase**; the gradual return of renal function marks the **recovery phase**.

are common clinical symptoms of acute renal failure. GI bleeding and diarrhea sometimes occur. Drowsiness, agitation, and confusion are frequently seen.

What went wrong? Many times acute renal failure is caused by problems outside the kidney. For example, acute renal failure can develop when blood flow to the kidney is reduced. This can occur for many reasons, including heart failure, shock, or severe blood loss after trauma (surgery, accident). As less blood reaches the nephron, the pressure gradient between the glomerulus and the tubules decreases. The body can't make normal amounts of urine.

Another cause of acute renal failure that originates outside the kidney is a urinary tract obstruction. In this case, the kidney can make urine but the urine can't get out of the body.

Damage to the kidneys themselves can also cause acute renal failure; infections, toxins, some drugs, and environmental pollutants can damage kidney cells. Death of kidney cells from lack of blood flow to them, ischemia, can also lead to acute renal failure.

In the early stages of acute renal failure, urine volume often diminishes markedly. (Sometimes, though, too much urine is produced.) Later, the kidneys are unable to conserve water and the patient begins excreting large amounts of urine and electrolytes. After this period, kidney function gradually improves over a 3 to 12 month period, provided that the patient recovers.

In some cases, acute renal failure is reversible. In others, it progresses into chronic renal failure. About half of all people with acute renal failure die.

The primary concern in acute renal failure is to treat the underlying disorder to prevent permanent or further damage to the kidneys. For example, if severe blood loss is the problem, a blood transfusion is given to restore blood volume.

Other measures must be taken to restore fluid and electrolyte balance and minimize levels of toxic waste products. In addition to the nutrition factors discussed below, diuretics are often used to mobilize fluids in the oliguric phase of acute renal failure. Dialysis (either peritoneal dialysis or hemodialysis) is necessary when blood urea, creatinine, or potassium is very high.

Energy and Protein   As mentioned, the patient in acute renal failure is often hypercatabolic and suffering from some other major illness. Add to these conditions nausea, vomiting, and confusion, and you have a person who really needs kcalories but is unable to eat. It is particularly important for this patient to receive adequate kcalories to reverse the hypercatabolic state. The breakdown of protein contributes to the rising blood urea and potassium levels. The patient's actual kcaloric needs depend on the rate of catabolism; usually 35 to 50 kcal/kg of body weight are needed.

Protein needs also vary, depending on the catabolic rate. The protein requirement of people with acute renal failure is unknown. Generally, their diet is restricted to about 30 to 40 g of protein per day. However, impaired wound healing, infection, muscular wasting, and very negative nitrogen balance are commonly seen in these patients. They often die. It has been suggested that they might benefit from a higher protein intake, even though this might necessitate dialysis.[11] Once dialysis is instituted, protein intake is not so critical, and 70 to 85 g may be given.[12]

Fluid and Electrolytes   The total amount of fluid is carefully controlled to avoid overhydration or dehydration. You can determine fluid requirements by carefully measuring urine output. To the volume of urine, add about 400 to 500 ml for water lost through the skin, lungs, and perspiration. The patient who is vomiting, has diarrhea, or has a high fever needs extra water. In the oliguric stage the patient will get small volumes of fluids. But in the diuretic stage up to 3 liters of urine may be lost daily, and large amounts of fluids will have to be given.

Likewise, sodium may be very restricted (500 to 1,000 mg) in the oliguric phase but may change as the patient enters the diuretic phase. Pay special attention to potassium in the patient with acute renal failure — hyperkalemia can be life threatening. In the oliguric phase potassium may be restricted to less than 2 g per day; however, potassium may have to be supplemented during the diuretic phase.

Drugs called exchange resins must sometimes be used to treat severe hyperkalemia. These drugs, which are placed rectally, cause sodium to be exchanged for potassium in the colon, and the potassium is then excreted in the stool. Another method that can temporarily reduce high potassium levels is to give IV dextrose and insulin. Potassium moves into the cells with glucose. However, this is only a temporary measure.

Enteral and Parenteral Nutrition

When patients with either acute or chronic renal failure are hypercatabolic or for other reasons are unable to eat adequately, then special nutrition support is in order. As discussed in Chapter 20, first you can try supplementing the diet or offering a liquid diet. Offer the patient supplements between meals to increase the amount of energy he or she consumes. Table 6 lists some supplements useful for this purpose. But remember, the person with renal failure who is only allowed a certain amount of fluid has to derive the maximum energy

[11]M. J. Blumenkrantz, J. D. Kopple, A. Koffler, A. K. Kamdar, M. D. Healy, E. I. Feinstein, and S. G. Massry, Total parenteral nutrition in the management of acute renal failure, *American Journal of Clinical Nutrition* 31 (1978):1831-1840.

[12]W. P. Steffee, Nutritional support in renal failure, *Surgical Clinics of North America* 61 (1981):661-670.

Table 6. Special Nutrition Products for Use in Renal Failure

Product	Use
Amin-Aid (McGaw)	Provides essential amino acids and kcalories
Controlyte (Doyle)	Provides 2 kcal/ml in the form of carbohydrate
Microlipid (Organon)	Provides 4.5 kcal/ml in the form of fat
Moducal (Mead Johnson)	Provides 2 kcal/ml in the form of carbohydrate
Polycose (Ross)	Provides 2 kcal/ml in the form of carbohydrate
Sumacal (Organon)	Provides 4 kcal/g in the form of carbohydrate
Travasorb Renal (Travenol)	Provides essential and nonessential amino acids, kcalories, and water-soluble vitamins

from a small volume: Use products with more than 1 kcal/ml. Some products that are specially formulated for renal patients are available, and they can be taken orally or by tube (see Table 6). Other formulas also can be adapted for the renal patient. Remember to notice the amounts of vitamins and minerals delivered by these products, however; with some of them, added vitamin and mineral supplements are needed. The composition of some vitamin and mineral supplements is given in Appendix O.

There has been a growing interest in the use of TPN for people in renal failure. Early studies using essential amino acid solutions when this method was used.[13] The original study compared the essential amino acid solution with a glucose solution. Since then, other studies have suggested that using mixtures of both nonessential and essential amino acids (at lower concentrations than in standard TPN solutions) was comparable to using essential amino acids alone.[14]

To prevent fluid overload during TPN, 70 percent rather than 50 percent glucose solutions are used. This way more kcalories are provided in a smaller volume. Electrolytes are monitored closely and adjusted as necessary. Glucose intolerance and insulin resistance are common in both uremia and catabolic illnesses, so insulin must often be given with the TPN solution.

[13]R. M. Abel, C. H. Beck, W. M. Abbott, J. A. Ryan, G. O. Barnett, and J. E. Fischer, Improved survival from acute renal failure after treatment with intravenous essential L-amino acids and glucose, *New England Journal of Medicine* 288 (1973):695-699.

[14]J. M. Mirtallo, P. J. Schneider, K. Mavko, R. L. Ruberg, and P. J. Fabri, A comparison of essential and general amino acid infusions in the nutritional support of patients with compromised renal function, *Journal of Parenteral and Enteral Nutrition* 6 (1982):109-113; M. J. Blumenkrantz et al., 1978.

Nephrotic Syndrome

The nephrotic syndrome is not a disease, but rather a complex of symptoms caused by the loss of plasma protein into the urine. Many disorders can lead to nephrotic syndrome — glomerulonephritis, diabetes mellitus, infections, and renal vein thrombosis are some associated disorders.

Normally, only small plasma proteins pass through the glomerulus into the filtrate. These proteins are then reabsorbed in the tubules and returned to the blood. But in the nephrotic syndrome, the permeability of the glomerular capillaries increases and very large amounts of plasma protein are lost in the urine. Since albumin is the major plasma protein, it is also the major protein lost in the urine.

The excretion of protein in the urine is **proteinuria**.

As plasma proteins are lost, the blood levels of proteins fall sharply. This together with other factors causes fluid to move into the interstitial space, and edema develops. As the protein loss continues, lean body mass breaks down. Losses of other plasma proteins such as immuno-globulins render the person with nephrotic syndrome prone to infections, which can compromise nutrition status further. The loss of transferrin (the iron-carrying protein) may lead to anemia (see Figure 4). Serum lipid levels rise markedly for unknown reasons.

The treatment of the nephrotic syndrome depends largely on the underlying cause. Sometimes corticosteroids are used. Diet is always important in preventing protein malnutrition and alleviating edema.

A diet high in kcalories (50 to 60 kcal/kg of body weight), and high in protein (about 120 g per day) is prescribed. The more protein the person can eat, the better.

In the hospital you may find some physicians who believe that a normal protein diet is better than a high-protein diet for the person with nephrotic syndrome. This is because, as protein intake increases, so does the level of protein in the urine. This observation has led some physicians to believe that high-protein diets lead to a deterioration of renal function. However, people on normal protein diets may be unable to maintain nitrogen balance.

Restricting sodium is very important, since sodium is avidly retained by the body in nephrotic syndrome. In the early treatment, a diet very low in sodium (250 mg) is used to help mobilize the fluid which has accumulated in the interstitial space. Diuretics also are used for this purpose. Once the patient is free of edema and sodium balance has been achieved, the sodium restriction is liberalized to about 1,500 mg per day. (See Chapters 24 and 26 for more information on low-sodium diets.) If potassium-wasting diuretics are prescribed, foods high in potassium become important in the diet.

Figure 4 The nephrotic syndrome.

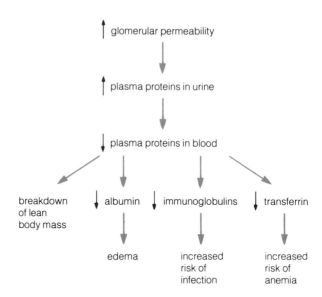

Patients with nephrotic syndrome often have hyperlipidemia — most commonly, type II or V (see Chapter 26). These patients also are at high risk for atherosclerosis. Therefore, it is often recommended that they follow the diet appropriate for the type of hyperlipoproteinemia they have.

Kidney Stones

The occurrence of kidney stones, or nephrolithiasis, is quite common throughout the world. Ninety percent of kidney stones contain calcium phosphate, calcium oxalate, or both. Less common stones are composed of uric acid, cystine, or magnesium ammonium phosphate. All of the stone constituents are relatively insoluble in urine. When their concentrations get high, they form crystals that eventually precipitate and get larger. (This is a simplified version of the complex and incompletely understood mechanism by which kidney stones form.)

The causes of kidney stones vary depending on the type of stone. But a condition that interferes with urinary flow (such as a urinary tract infection) or increases blood and urine levels of the stone former (such as dietary excesses) can favor stone formation.

The role of diet in preventing and treating kidney stones has been debated, and some physicians do not consider diet a part of treatment. But there are situations where diet may be helpful and should be considered along with other treatments.

One cornerstone of therapy important in managing all types of kidney stones is fluid intake. Advise the patient with kidney stones to drink from 3 to 4 liters of fluids each day so that urine will be dilute.

Emphasize the importance of drinking water before bed and during the night, since the urine becomes concentrated overnight.

Calcium Oxalate and Calcium Phosphate Stones   Unknown causes or hyperparathyroidism are usually responsible for calcium stones. Small bowel disease (see Chapter 23), immobilization, excessive intake of vitamin D or calcium (in susceptible people), and alkali abuse can also result in calcium stones.

In some people who have calcium stones, normal mechanisms for controlling dietary calcium absorption in the intestine are altered. We usually respond to excess dietary calcium by decreasing calcium absorption in the intestine. But people in whom this mechanism is not working absorb more calcium and develop hypercalciuria. For these people, reducing dietary calcium by avoiding foods high in calcium is useful. They also benefit from avoiding vitamin D supplements and vitamin D fortified foods.

Calcium oxalate stones caused by enteric hyperoxaluria (see Chapter 23) can sometimes be helped by diet. Normally, most dietary oxalate forms an unabsorbable complex with calcium in the GI tract and is excreted in the feces. But in individuals with bowel diseases and steatorrhea, calcium is lost with fatty acids, permitting the absorption of oxalate. (The malabsorption of bile acids also changes the permeability of the colon; this change allows the absorption of oxalate which is normally excreted.) Eventually, the oxalate is found in excess amounts in the urine and can precipitate with calcium to form calcium oxalate stones. Dietary oxalate is reduced by elimination of foods high in oxalate (see Table 7). Not all people with enteric hyperoxaluria respond to a low-oxalate diet; it appears that some people produce oxalate endogenously from some unknown source.[15]

Megadoses of vitamin C also have been reported to cause hyperoxaluria. Vitamin C can be metabolized to oxalate in some people. Therefore, vitamin C supplements should be avoided by patients with hyperoxaluria.

Other Kidney Stones   Magnesium ammonium phosphate stones can precipitate when the urine becomes alkaline. This most often occurs when the urinary tract is infected with organisms that release ammonia. Sometimes an acid forming diet (see Chapters 14 and 21) can help acidify the urine.

Uric acid stones can form when the urine is consistently acid or when excess uric acid is present in the urine. A base forming diet (see Chapters 14 and 21) along with medication can help make the urine more basic. At one time, low-purine diets were commonly prescribed to reduce uric acid in the urine. However, these diets are quite

Diseases that occur without apparent cause are said to be **idiopathic**.

alkali abuse: excessive use of alkalinizing agents such as antacids.

A metabolic disorder that results in excess uric acid in the blood and sometimes in the urine is **gout**. The low-purine diet helps reduce the excess of purines (part of DNA and the principal source of uric acid). (For a reference on gout see To Explore Further.)

[15]A. F. Hofmann, Enteric hyperoxaluria, *Nutrition and the MD*, September 1979.

Table 7. Foods High in Oxalate

Vegetables

Baked beans canned in tomato sauce	Kale
	Leeks
Beans, green, wax, or dried	Mustard greens
Beets	Okra
Celery	Parsley
Chard, Swiss	Peppers, green
Chive	Potatoes, sweet
Collards	Rutabagas
Dandelion greens	Spinach
Eggplant	Summer squash
Escarole	Watercress

Fruits

Blackberries	Lemon peel
Blueberries	Lime peel
Currants, red	Orange peel
Dewberries	Raspberries
Fruit cocktail	Rhubarb
Gooseberries	Strawberries
Grapes, Concord	Tangerines

Other

Chocolate	Pepper (more than 1 tsp/day)
Cocoa	Soybean crackers
Draft beer	Soybean curd (tofu)
Fruit cake	Tea
Grits	Tomato soup
Peanut butter	Vegetable soup
	Wheat germ

Adapted from D. M. Ney, A. F. Hofmann, C. Fischer, and N. Stubblefield, *The Low Oxalate Diet Book* (San Diego: University of California, 1981).

A metabolic disorder in which large amounts of the amino acids cystine, lysine, arginine, and ornithine are excreted in the urine is **cystinuria**.

restrictive. Medications are now available which are very effective in reducing uric acid levels; they are commonly used instead of diet for this purpose.

Cystine stones form as a result of a genetic disorder. Dietary treatment of these stones involves using a base forming diet that is low in methionine.

Urinary Tract Infections

People with urinary tract infections should be encouraged to eat a well-balanced diet and to drink plenty of fluids. Fluids will help prevent stagnation and the growth of bacteria and also help deliver antibiotics to the urinary tract where they are needed. Many antibiotics used for urinary tract infections work better in an acid urine; therefore, people with such infections may be encouraged to use acid producing juices and foods (see Chapter 21).

> The person with a urinary tract infection is typically told to drink plenty of cranberry juice. This suggestion stems from the widespread belief that cranberry juice can lower urinary pH more effectively than other food and drinks. Also, cranberry juice contains a precursor of an acid which has an antibacterial action in the urine.
>
> Unfortunately, it is impractical to use cranberry juice for these purposes. Although cranberry juice has a high acidity, it is not dependable for consistently lowering urinary pH. Furthermore, the antibacterial potential of cranberry juice is never achieved because the antibacterial product is not concentrated enough to be effective.[16]

Nutrition Assessment of Renal Patients

As we have seen, the renal failure patient is at high risk for malnutrition. It becomes essential that nutrition assessments be made frequently and that problems be prevented or immediately corrected before nutrient stores are depleted. Some things you should consider carefully include the following:

1. The diet history is extremely important. For the new renal failure patient just ready to begin a restricted diet, try to determine the usual intake of kcalories, protein, sodium, potassium, phosphorus, calcium, and vitamin D. This will help you in adjusting the patient's current eating habits for better compliance. A careful diet history for the patient already following a renal diet is important for assessing his or her understanding of and compliance with the diet. For the person with kidney stones, the diet history can be used to identify foods high in calcium, vitamin D, oxalate, or vitamin C, as appropriate.

2. Anthropometric measurements in renal failure patients will be significantly influenced by the state of hydration. Weights taken immediately after dialysis treatments will more accurately reflect true weight. When the patient isn't on dialysis, weight may be deceptively normal or high because of water retention. Likewise, arm measurements are affected by edema. The person with nephrotic syndrome may be dehydrated; anthropometic measurements also are affected by dehydration.

---

[16]Cranberries and urinary infections, *Nutrition and the MD*, August 1982.

3. Weight changes are actually more useful in assessing the state of hydration than in determining body weight in renal failure patients. Increases in weight and blood pressure suggest fluid retention. Weight loss and low blood pressure suggest dehydration.

4. Weight and height in children must be routinely assessed to insure that their diets are adequate for growth. Remember that growth failure is common in children with renal failure. Weight loss often occurs in renal failure. Wasting is common in people with nephrotic syndrome who are not eating enough protein.

5. Albumin and transferrin levels may be extremely low in patients with nephrotic syndrome. Levels rise when protein intake is adequate. People with renal failure also have lower transferrin levels than the healthy population; these are even lower when malnutrition accompanies renal disease.

6. Serum electrolytes, BUN, and creatinine must be carefully monitored in all renal failure patients.

7. Serum lipids are frequently elevated in both chronic renal failure and nephrotic syndrome.

Renal patients must be carefully monitored to prevent growth failure and renal osteodystrophy. Anemia also may be a problem that can be partially corrected by diet.

Summing Up

The kidneys play a vital role in maintaining chemical homeostasis, controlling blood pressure, converting vitamin D to its active form, and producing a hormone that stimulates the formation of red blood cells. When the kidneys fail, toxic waste products and electrolytes build up, acid-base balance is upset, blood pressure may rise, and bone disorders and anemia may develop.

Because renal failure causes multiple problems, the diet of the renal patient must be carefully controlled. The diet prescription is based on the remaining kidney function and the careful monitoring of serum electrolytes, BUN, and creatinine. The diet prescription often must specify the intake of kcalories, protein, sodium, potassium, phosphorus, and fluids. Calcium, vitamin D, and water-soluble vitamins are given in supplemental form.

As renal function deteriorates to a critical level, diet alone cannot prevent the symptoms of uremia. At this point, dialysis is introduced, and a kidney transplant may be considered. Dialysis changes dietary needs. Most significantly, protein intake can be liberalized.

People in acute renal failure are frequently hypercatabolic. Serum potassium levels may rise sharply, and deterioration of renal function appears rapidly. Acute renal failure can take three courses: it can be reversed; it can progress into chronic renal failure; or it can be fatal.

The patient with nephrotic syndrome is particularly vulnerable to protein malnutrition because large amounts of protein are lost in the urine. As a consequence, edema and muscle wasting occur. Lipids are frequently elevated. The diet of the nephrotic patient should be high in kcalories and protein to maintain nitrogen balance. Sodium must be carefully restricted to avoid water retention and edema. A fat-controlled diet is indicated if the person has hyperlipidemia.

The value of diet in preventing or treating kidney stones is widely debated. An important guideline for people with kidney stones is to drink plenty of fluids — at least 3 to 4 liters daily. Drinking water before going to bed and during the night is especially important. Depending on the type of stone, benefit may be derived from restricting dietary calcium and vitamin D, restricting oxalate and vitamin C, or consuming foods which tend to alkalinize or acidify the urine.

People with urinary tract infections should be encouraged to eat a well-balanced diet. Like people with kidney stones, they benefit by drinking plenty of fluids.

To Explore Further

Two highly recommended articles dealing with nutrient requirements in chronic renal failure are:

- Kopple, J. D. Nutritional therapy in kidney failure. *Nutrition Reviews* 39 (1981):193-206.

- Rodriguez, D. J., and Hunter, V. M. Nutritional intervention in the treatment of chronic renal failure. *Nursing Clinics of North America* 16 (1981):573-585.

Other articles of interest dealing with specific aspects of chronic renal disease include:

- Hetrick, A., Frauman, A. C., and Gilman, C. M. Nutrition in renal disease: When the patient is a child. *American Journal of Nursing* 79 (1979):2152-2154.

- Barsotti, G., Guiducci, A., Ciardella, F., and Giovannetti, S. Effects on renal function of a low-nitrogen diet supplemented with essential amino acids and ketoanalogues and of hemodialysis and free protein supply in patients with chronic renal failure. *Nephron* 27 (1981):113-117.

- Walser, M. Principles of keto acid therapy in uremia. *American Journal of Clinical Nutrition* 31 (1978):1756-1760.

- Fürst, P., Ahlberg, M., Alvestrand, A., and Bergström, J. Principles of essential amino acid therapy in uremia. *American Journal of Clinical Nutrition* 31 (1978):1744-1755.

- Cochran, M. Aspects of renal bone disease. *Australian and New Zealand Journal of Medicine* 11 (1981):33-37.

- Stark, J. L. BUN/creatinine: Your keys to kidney function. *Nursing*, May 1980, pp. 33-38.

Two worthwhile references on acute renal failure are:

- Stark, J. L. How to succeed against acute renal failure. *Nursing*, July 1982, pp. 26-33.

- Evans, D. B. Acute renal failure. *Practitioner* 220 (1978):893-900.

Additional information on dialysis and transplants can be found in:

- Luke, B. Nutrition in renal disease: The adult on dialysis. *American Journal of Nursing* 79 (1979):2155-2157.

- Madden, M. A., Zimmerman, S. W., and Simpson, D. P. Longitudinal comparison of intermittent versus continuous ambulatory peritoneal dialysis, in the same patients. *Clinical Nephrology* 16 (1981):293-299.

- Bodnar, D. M. Rationale for nutritional requirements for patients on continuous ambulatory peritoneal dialysis. *Journal of the American Dietetic Association* 80 (1982):247-249.

- Gahl, G. M., Baeyer, H. V., Averdunk, R., Riedinger, H., Borowzak, B., Schurig, R., Becker, H., and Kessel, M. Outpatient evaluation of dietary intake and nitrogen removal in continuous ambulatory peritoneal dialysis. *Annals of Internal Medicine* 94 (1981):643-646.

- Reckling, J. B. Safeguarding the renal transplant patient. *Nursing*, February 1980, pp. 47-49.

The article by B. Luke contains an excellent flow chart which depicts the abnormalities and clinical symptoms seen in renal failure. The article by G. M. Gahl and associates suggests that we may be overestimating protein requirements in CAPD patients.

Kidney stones are discussed in more detail in the following articles:

- Smith, L. H., Van Den Berg, C. J., and Wilson, D. M. Nutrition and urolithiasis. *New England Journal of Medicine* 298 (1978):87-89.

- Broadus, A. E., and Thier, S. O. Metabolic basis of renal-stone disease. *New England Journal of Medicine* 300 (1979):839-845.

Various aspects of hyperoxaluria are discussed in:

- *Nutrition and the MD*, September 1979.

An excellent reference on oxalate is:

- Ney, D. M., Hofmann, A. F., Fischer, C., and Stubblefield, N. *The Low Oxalate Diet Book*. San Diego: University of California, 1981.

This booklet is available for about $2 from: General Clinical Research Center, University Hospital, 225 Dickinson Street, San Diego, CA 92103.

In this text we have not discussed gout because it is most often treated with drugs rather than diet. If you would like more information on gout, the following article provides a good review:

- Khachadurian, A. K. Hyperuricemia and gout: An update. *American Family Physician*, December 1981, pp. 143-148.

Renal Failure

S.M. was 35 when she started having kidney problems. At that time, she sustained many injuries in an auto accident and lost so much blood that she almost died before reaching the hospital. She developed acute renal failure that gradually progressed into chronic renal failure. S.M. is 5 ft 3 in tall and weighs 100 lb. Her GFR is 15 ml/min, and her BUN, creatinine, and electrolytes have been well controlled.

Study Questions

1. Describe the most probable reason that S.M. developed acute renal failure. What other problems can cause acute renal failure?

2. Describe the phases of acute renal failure. What are S.M.'s dietary needs in each phase? What waste products and electrolytes are of greatest concern? Why? What factors would you have kept in mind when determining

S.M.'s kcaloric and protein needs during her episode of acute renal failure?

3. Consider the diet of the patient with chronic renal failure. What nutrients are of particular concern? What factors determine the diet of each person with renal failure? How does the presence of glucose intolerance or diabetes, hyperlipidemia, anemia, or bone disease affect the diet?

4. Consider S.M.'s diet. Calculate her energy and protein needs. How does her current weight affect her kcaloric needs? What other information would you need to de-

cide if S.M.'s diet should be further restricted? Which vitamins and minerals shoud be supplemented? Why?

5. What options will be available to S.M. once her GFR drops below 4 ml/min and she can no longer forestall uremia by diet alone? How would each of these options change her nutrient needs?

6. Write down everything you ate yesterday. Now see which foods you could not have eaten if you were on a diet in which sodium, phosphorus, and potassium were restricted (use Tables 3 and 4 in this Chapter and the no-added-salt diet in Chapter 26). Finally, add to these restrictions a limit of 40 g of protein. How does this alter the types of food and the portion sizes you ate? Is your diet still adequate in kcalories? If not, how can you increase your kcalorie intake and still stay within the diet?

Therapeutic Diets in Perspective

There are some remedies worse than the disease.

PUBLILIUS SYRUS, 1st century B.C.

Of all the Highlights we have written for this book, this one contains the most opinion and the fewest facts. Its purpose is to help you sort out the pros and cons of therapeutic diets and learn how to develop a set of priorities to decide when a diet is of critical importance, when it is only slightly helpful, and when it may even be contraindicated.

Such a decision should first be based on all the available facts. What are the proven benefits of the diet in question? What are its negative effects? What are the proven risks of *not* following the diet? When all the pros and cons have been added up, however, some crucial ingredients have to be added: the intangible, human factors of real life situations. You have to exercise your clinical judgment in deciding how hard to "push" a diet. It is a matter of opinion, and opinions differ. Three examples follow.

Ted   Ted is a busy executive who leads a hectic life. Last year he found out that he had a peptic ulcer. His doctor prescribed a traditional bland diet with six small meals a day and told Ted to drink plenty of milk and to take antacids between meals.

You have been asked to talk to Ted about the diet. You have gotten to know him pretty well during his hospital stay. You know that he barely has time to eat three meals a day, let alone six. He hates milk. The only thing he likes about the diet is that he can still have his usual bedtime snack. After the doctor briefly told him about the diet, Ted confided in you that he has no intention of sticking to it. He was outraged

when the nurses refused to bring him his morning coffee.

What should you say to Ted? First of all, consult the facts: The traditional bland diet is of little proven value. Eating frequent meals and drinking milk may actually increase gastric acid secretion (see Chapter 23). Couple these facts with your knowledge that Ted won't follow the diet anyway, and you have several major factors weighing against it.

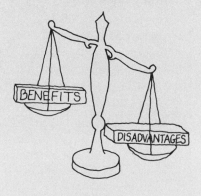

And what about coffee? True, coffee, even if decaffeinated, increases gastric acid secretion. But will Ted's stomach secrete even more acid if he gets worked up about *not* having coffee? You can't know the answer to this question, but you do know Ted, so your opinion has to be given some weight. All in all, it seems to you that the minuses outweigh the pluses in this case.

You decide to discuss your concerns with Ted's doctor and suggest an alternative

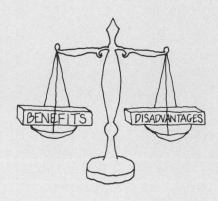

approach. With the doctor's approval, you present Ted with a liberal bland diet instruction. You tell him three meals a day is fine. As for coffee, you tell him it's not recommended, and you tell him why. But you add that, if he does drink coffee, he should limit it to his one favorite cup in the morning and not drink it on an empty stomach.

The situation changes if the diagnosis is different. Suppose that Ted doesn't have an ulcer, but rather a hiatal hernia. This time the doctor prescribes a liberal bland diet with five small meals and no eating before bedtime. Ted does not see how he can squeeze in two extra meals, and he does not want to give up his bedtime snack. Should you suggest to the doctor that Ted doesn't need this diet? Let's look at how the ratio of benefits to disadvantages has changed.

This time the diet is more justifiable. Smaller feedings will help prevent stomach distention, which can aggravate the hiatal hernia. Furthermore, heartburn can result if the diet is not followed and it can be quite painful. Coffee lowers the cardiac sphincter pressure, which also aggravates the problem.

The major drawback of the diet is that Ted will have to change his lifestyle somewhat. He will have to find time to squeeze in extra feedings and to live without a

bedtime snack.

This time the benefits of the diet outweigh the disadvantages. If Ted wishes to avoid the pain of heartburn and the possible complications of hiatal hernia, he will have to find a way to make the necessary adjustments. You can help him by suggesting foods that are quick and easy to prepare and eat.

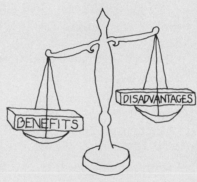

Jennifer   Jennifer is an animated, healthy young woman of 25. She was born with phenylketonuria (PKU), but it was diagnosed within three days' time, and her parents instituted the PKU diet immediately to promote Jennifer's normal development. The diet was discontinued when Jennifer was six years old, and she has led a quite normal life since then. Now she is pregnant, and her doctor has told her she must go back on the PKU diet. She is expressing resentment to you at the necessity of following the diet's myriad rules and using its expensive special products. She remembers

that the diet cramped her lifestyle and prevented her participating fully in many social activities even when she was only five.

What should you say to Jennifer? First, consult the facts. Obviously (as Highlight 3 made clear), to evade the doctor's orders would in this case pose considerable risks, not to Jennifer herself but to her unborn infant. Although following the diet will not insure that Jennifer's baby will not be mentally and physically disabled, such an outcome is inevitable if she does not follow the diet. You owe it to her to present her with the facts, and to make sure that she receives meticulous instruction about all the intricacies of the diet. Jennifer will make her own decision, but you can't in good conscience support her in a choice not to comply with the doctor's orders. (We discussed some of the subtleties involved in an area similar in some ways — the use of alcohol in pregnancy — in a digression in Chapter 15.)

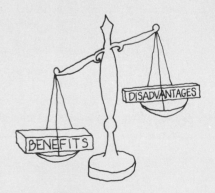

Other diets for which the pros strongly outweigh the cons are those that bring about life-sustaining changes in metabolism. Among these diets are those for liver failure, for renal failure, and for insulin-dependent diabetes. All of your efforts should be directed at insuring compliance with these diets. A patient's complaint that such a diet is restrictive is not a cue for you to tell the person "never mind, it's all right not to follow the diet." Rather, remember that no diet is so rigid that it cannot be planned to some extent around the individual's lifestyle and preferences. There are no foods that can't be worked into most diets on occasion with careful planning. The key is that "forbidden" foods should be used on occasion only, in limited amounts, and only when their inclusion in the diet is planned. An occasional lapse from the diet rules will not be fatal, but the better the compliance with a metabolism-normalizing diet, the better supported is the patient's recovery and health.

Martha   Martha's case illustrates another set of considerations that enter into decision making about therapeutic diets. You have seen Martha in the hospital several times over the last few years. She is a sweet, elderly lady (70 years old) with several problems:

- Obesity.
- Non-insulin-dependent diabetes.
- A hiatal hernia.
- Type IV hyperlipoproteinemia.
- Chronic constipation.

For the first time, her doctor is recommending that she be put on a diet. Considering her multiple problems, the diet that might be appropriate for Martha would be:

- Low in kcalories.
- Low in total fat, saturated fat, and cholesterol and high in polyunsaturated fat.
- Low in concentrated sweets.
- Restricted in foods that cause gastric acid secretion.
- High in fiber.

But several problems are entailed by all these changes.

For one thing, these are quite a few changes to inflict on someone who has already lived 70 years. For another, to try to obey all those rules at once would be very confusing. You'd better analyze the pros and cons and establish priorities before deciding what kind of diet instruction to present to Martha.

To make the diet low in kcalories would help with four of Martha's five problems. It would help to: bring about weight loss; normalize blood glucose; bring down her high triglycerides; and reduce abdominal pressure to improve her hernia. Three of these four advantages would also be gained by making the diet low in concentrated sweets: weight loss, blood glucose control, and lowering of triglycerides. It would seem advisable, then, to help Martha at least to work out a low-kcalorie, low-concentrated-sweets diet, and it would not be difficult to do so.

To make Martha's diet high in fiber as well would help with her constipation problem, would facilitate weight loss by displacing kcalorie-rich foods, and might improve her blood glucose control, three of the five goals chosen for her. Martha could probably understand this diet and, with help, might incorporate these changes into her eating habits, especially if you gave her reason to hope that she would notice an improvement in her health.

What about all the proposed changes in the kinds and amounts of fat proposed for Martha's diet? A review of the facts on similar cases suggests that a fat-controlled diet for a woman Martha's age might not significantly reduce the risk of

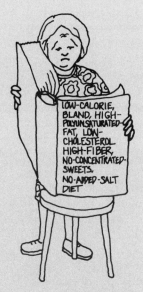

atherosclerosis. In this case, asking her to change menus she has used for years might not be worth the trouble. As for the matter of eliminating irritating foods to help with the hiatal hernia, perhaps you should discuss this with her. What you and Martha might work out together might be a low-kcalorie diet in which high-fiber foods are emphasized and concentrated sweets are discouraged. You might make Martha aware of the foods likely to irritate her hiatal hernia, and leave the use of those foods to her discretion.

If you care enough to provide the best nutrition care for your clients, you will work hard to develop skill in giving diet advice. You won't simply hand the same sheet of instructions to everyone who has the same "label." Furthermore, because research in diet therapy is an active and fast-moving area, you will keep your eyes and ears open for new information on the benefits and risks of alternatives in diet. You will be willing to form opinions — carefully, while also being careful not to become opinionated. You will develop your clinical judgment as all good judges do, by allowing each new fact and each new case to find its proper place in the making of your decisions.

CHAPTER 28

CONTENTS

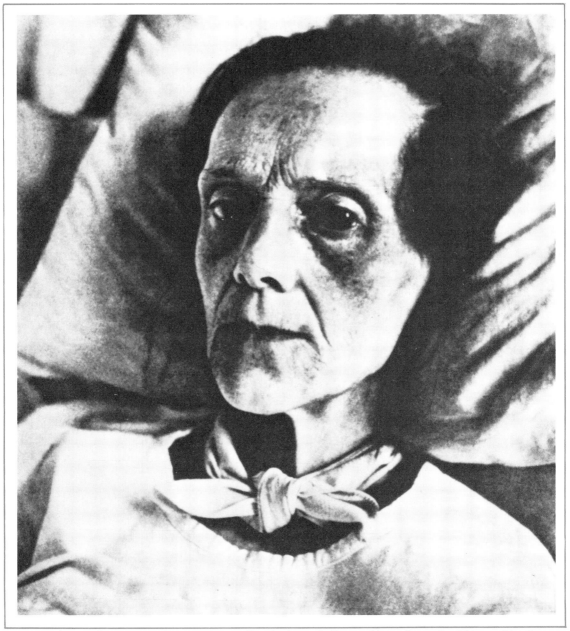

Cancer cachexia. The cancer patient experiences disturbed metabolism and loss of appetite. This combination makes nutrition care urgent.

Reproduced with permission of Nutrition Today magazine, P.O. Box 1828, Annapolis, Maryland 21404, May/June 1981.

NUTRITION FOR PEOPLE WITH CANCER

"In the future cancer will be the way of dying for more and more people. . . .
Such a trend will certainly impose new obligations on physicians, dietitians,
and other health professionals to gain a better understanding of the very
special nutrition requirements of the cancer patient."

M. E. SHILS

Alfred finally found the nerve to look at himself in the mirror again. In the few short months since he had begun therapy for cancer he had seen himself literally waste away. He remembered how proud he always had been of his physically fit body and, at the sight of his emaciated reflection in the mirror, he sank back into depression.

The loss of appetite and the wasting frequently seen in people with cancer is called the cancer-cachexia syndrome. In this chapter we will be looking at the factors that contribute to this syndrome and at ways to deal with the nutrition problems associated with it. We will not be discussing how diet might cause cancer; this is considered in Highlight 28.

What is Cancer?

Cancer is not a single disease. There are cancers — plural. The word *cancer* refers to any growths, tumors, or neoplasms that grow wild. It is correct to speak of cancers in the plural because there are different kinds of tumors, many of which are specific to certain parts of the body. When a neoplasm grows, it interferes with the normal functioning of an organ or tissue. The growth seemingly has no built-in brakes, as normal growth does. Furthermore, cancerous cells are alive, and as they grow they take nutrients from the host's diet or body reserves.

Full-blown cancer develops from some initiating event. That event may be radiation, either the general radiation that is always present or medical or industrial radiation. Or the event may be the intrusion of a chemical — a carcinogen — into the cell.

The radiation or carcinogen may alter the protein-making machinery of the cell, so that the DNA produces a new "foreign" protein. Since this is an unfamiliar protein, the cell has no built-in feedback mechanism to tell the DNA to halt its production. The words *neoplasm*, *malignant tumor*, and *cancer* are often used interchangeably to describe the unchecked growth of foreign cells.

tumor: a growth of new tissue with no function; **benign** tumors usually do not cause problems; **malignant** tumors (cancers) are serious. A **carcinoma** is a cancer that affects epithelial tissue. A **sarcoma** is a cancer arising from the muscle, bone, or connective tissue. A **hematopoietic** (hee-MAT-oh-poy-ET-ic) **neoplasm** is a malignant tumor of the blood and immune system. A cancer that spreads to another area is said to **metastasize** (met- ASS-tuh-size).

oma = tumor

neoplasm: a tumor; often used to denote a malignant tumor or cancer.

neo = new

initiating event: an event caused by radiation or chemical reaction that can give rise to cancer.

carcinogen: a cancer-causing substance.

carcin = cancer
gen = give rise to

The incidence of cancer is expected to increase.[1] This is because more and more people are living longer and death from heart disease is declining.

Cancer Cachexia

cancer cachexia: a syndrome induced by many cancers; major symptoms are anorexia with inadequate food intake; speeded-up metabolism and wasting; and general ill health associated with cancer.

About two-thirds of all people with cancer develop cachexia.[2] These people get caught in a downward spiral. They lose their appetites (anorexia), which leads to muscle wasting and poor health (cachexia), which further contributes to the inadequate intake of nutrients. Malnutrition interferes with their quality of life and contributes to the morbidity and mortality associated with the disease process.[3]

Like cancer itself, cancer cachexia is a multifactorial problem. It can be caused by decreased intake of food, increased energy needs, or both. Inadequate intake can result from both decreased appetite and impaired digestion and absorption of nutrients.

Different factors may be at work in different patients to cause anorexia and cachexia. At one time it was believed that the wasting that accompanies cancer was an inevitable part of the disease process. However, we now know that nutrition intervention can be successful in preventing or improving this syndrome. No doubt much more will be learned about the causes of cancer cachexia in the future, and indeed, a good deal has already been learned.

What Causes Anorexia?

Anorexia is widely recognized as the most significant cause of malnutrition in people with cancer. The factors that cause anorexia are many and, in some cases, not clearly understood. Some of the known causes are summarized in Figure 1.

Psychological stress

Psychological stresses can be an important factor in decreasing the patient's appetite. Just finding out you have cancer can cause so much anxiety that eating becomes totally unimportant. People with terminal cancer may feel that eating simply isn't worth the effort. In addition, poor self image may result from some treatments for cancer (from a colostomy to treat colon cancer or from the hair loss that follows chemotherapy, for example). The depression that follows interferes with food intake. As weight loss continues, depression may grow worse.

Never underestimate the importance of the patient's feelings.

[1]M. E. Shils, How to nourish the cancer patient, *Nutrition Today*, May/June 1981, pp. 4-15.

[2]M. Groër and M. Pierce, Guarding against cancer's hidden killer: Anorexia-cachexia, *Nursing*, June 1981, pp. 39-43.

[3]K. B. Harvey, A. Bothe, and G. L. Blackburn, Nutritional assessment and patient outcome during oncological therapy, *Cancer* 43 (1979):2065-2069.

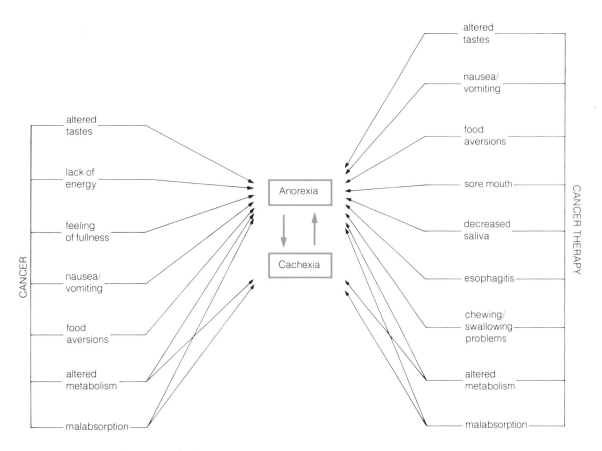

Figure 1   Causes of cancer cachexia.

Acknowledge and respect them, and try to help the patient deal with them. Above all else, treat each person as an individual.

Anorexia Caused by Cancer Itself   Anorexia and weight loss may occur before a person even realizes that he or she has cancer. In some cases, these complaints are what bring the person to visit the doctor. No one knows what precipitates anorexia. One hypothesis is that peptides and other metabolites produced by the tumor cause anorexia by acting on nerve cells and the hypothalamus.[4] (The hypothalamus is believed to be the appetite control center of the brain.)

Tumor-produced anorexia

Another problem in the person with cancer is a premature feeling of fullness. "I feel so hungry, but I take a few bites and I'm full." Sometimes the patient feels full for a good reason. For example, the tumor may be pushing against the stomach to cause fullness. But for the most part, the reason for this complaint is unknown.

Early satiety

[4]A. Theologides, Anorexia-producing intermediary metabolites, *American Journal of Clinical Nutrition* 29 (1976):552-558.

Fatigue

Loss of strength is sometimes called **asthenia** (ass-THEE-nee-uh).

The person with cancer often tires easily. This may interfere with his or her ability to prepare and eat a meal. Many hospitalized cancer patients have the most energy and feel the least full in the morning. As the day progresses, they become drained and feel full rapidly. The situation may be different for some people at home. One author reports that women homemakers with cancer may eat breakfast poorly and eat more for dinner.[5]

Obstructions

Some types of cancer can result in anorexia because they cause an obstruction in the GI tract. For example, a tumor of the esophagus may cause a partial or complete obstruction; the person with such a tumor will be unable to eat or will have difficulty swallowing. A tumor obstructing the lower GI tract may cause nausea and vomiting.

But cancer itself is not the only factor that interferes with food intake. The treatment the patient gets for cancer generally has many detrimental effects.

Anorexia Caused by Cancer Therapy   The treatment for cancer often involves radiation therapy, chemotherapy, surgery, or any combination of the three. Through their use, cancer can sometimes be arrested and nutrition problems corrected on a long-term basis.[6] But ironically, any of these treatments can also cause major nutrition problems. In this section we will be discussing how these therapies cause anorexia. The ways they affect digestion, absorption, and metabolism are discussed later.

chemotherapy: the use of drugs to arrest or destroy cancer cells (see also Chapter 21).

chemo = chemical

Radiation therapy works by disrupting the chemical bonds necessary to form DNA. This is why radiation works best on cells that are actively dividing and making new DNA, like tumor cells. It is also why radiation damages normal body cells that divide actively, such as the cells of the GI tract. The cancer cells divide fastest, so they are the most affected by radiation, but other actively dividing cells are also susceptible.

The nutrition (and other) side effects of radiation depend on many factors. Some of them are the type of radiation, the area of the body being irradiated, the size of the area, the dose, and the clinical status of the person in therapy.

Many chemotherapeutic drugs work the same way as radiation — they destroy dividing cells by interfering with DNA or RNA synthesis. Among the types of chemotherapeutic agents are: antibiotics, alkaloids, alkylating agents, antimetabolites, steroids, and others. Like radiation, these drugs also affect normal cells, and those that divide most frequently are most likely to be affected. The current trend in chemotherapy is to use high doses of several chemotherapeutic agents together in cycles. This helps assure that malignant cells will be killed. Although these treatments are more effective in many cases, they also intensify undesirable side effects.

Radiation and chemotherapy can cause anorexia, nausea, and vomiting. All of these symptoms, of course, tend to reduce food intake.

[5]Shils, 1981.

[6]Shils, 1981.

Table 1 summarizes the possible effects of radiation and chemotherapy on nutrition status.

Patients receiving radiation therapy to the head and neck can develop other problems interfering with food intake. They may have altered taste sensations or decreased taste sensitivity. As a result of this "mouth blindness," foods they once liked may become unpleasant to them. Many patients develop an intolerance for meat, especially red meat. For some, food is just not sweet enough, and for others, many foods are too sweet.

Mouth blindness

Radiation to the head and neck area also can cause the amount of saliva to decrease, and the saliva that remains is often thick. The patient with this condition may have a lot of problems swallowing. The bones of the jaws and the teeth can also be damaged, further interfering with the ability to chew and swallow.

Dry mouth

Radiation to the esophagus can cause esophagitis (see Chapter 23). Many times this problem resolves itself when radiation therapy is stopped. But some people develop fibrosis and sometimes strictures, resulting in permanent swallowing problems.

Esophagitis

Table 1.   Possible Effects of Radiation and Chemotherapy on Nutrition Status

Radiation	Chemotherapy
Decreased intake	
Anorexia	Anorexia
Nausea	Nausea
Vomiting	Vomiting
Taste alterations	Taste alterations
⇓ Salivary secretions	Abdominal pain
Thick salivary secretions	Intestinal ulcers
Damage to teeth and bone	
Esophagitis	
Increased nutrient losses	
Diarrhea	Diarrhea
Intestinal obstructions	Malabsorption
Malabsorption	
Fistula formation	
Chronic blood loss from intestine and bladder	
Altered metabolism	
(Secondary to malnutrition)	Fluid and electrolyte imbalance
	Negative nitrogen and calcium balance
	Hyperglycemia
	Interference with vitamins or other metabolites

Stomatitis

Mouth ulcers

Food aversions

Chemotherapeutic drugs also are called **antineoplastic agents**.

Radical surgery

Like radiation, chemotherapy can cause problems in addition to anorexia, nausea, and vomiting. It can inflame the lining of the mouth (stomatitis) and sometimes cause mouth ulcers, making chewing and swallowing painful. The person on chemotherapy may also experience abdominal pain or develop intestinal ulcers which interfere with food intake. Finally, people on chemotherapy may develop a strong dislike for certain foods, tastes, and odors (see "Food Aversions").

Surgery can affect food intake in people with cancer as in people having surgery for any other reason (see Chapters 22 and 23). It can cause anorexia, nausea, and vomiting. In addition, some types of surgery used almost exclusively in the treatment of cancer have special effects on food intake. Radical surgery of the head and neck falls in this category. Partial or total removal of the tongue, resection of the muscles and salivary glands, and removal of the lower jaw invariably create extensive problems with chewing and swallowing; patients with these kinds of surgery may have to be maintained on tube feeding or TPN. Table 2 summarizes how surgery for cancer can affect nutrition status.

Excess Nutrient Losses

The nutrition status of the person with cancer can be impaired not only because intake decreases but also because nutrients may be lost excessively. These losses can be the result of the cancer itself or the treatment for it.

Depending on the location and type of cancer, maldigestion or malabsorption of nutrients can occur. For example, there may be a deficiency of pancreatic enzymes (cancer of the pancreas) or bile salts (cancer of the liver). In the Zollinger-Ellison syndrome (see Chapter 23), hypersecretion of gastric acid inactivates digestive enzymes. Tumors of the small bowel can lead to malabsorption, too. Malabsorption caused by blind loop syndrome (see Chapter 23) can occur when a tumor obstructs the upper small intestine.

Malabsorption

Fluid and electrolyte imbalance

The changes in the small intestine caused by radiation therapy are collectively called **radiation enteritis**.

Cancers that cause severe vomiting, diarrhea, or both can result in electrolyte imbalances and dehydration. For example, a tumor obstructing the small bowel may cause vomiting, and some tumors that secrete hormones can produce severe diarrhea.

Radiation to the small bowel often interferes with normal intestinal function, causing diarrhea and vomiting. Many times intestinal function returns after radiation therapy ends. But for some patients, changes may be permanent. After radiation therapy to the intestine, the structure of the intestine changes. The intestinal wall becomes thick and fibrotic, and the small intestinal arteries may become so inflamed that blood flow to some sections of the bowel is cut off. The intestine may narrow and become obstructed, or a fistula may form. Malabsorption and chronic blood loss from the intestine and bladder can result in malnutrition as well as fluid and electrolyte imbalance.

The patient on chemotherapy also may develop diarrhea and malabsorption. This is because the cells of the intestine cannot

Food Aversions

For many years, researchers have looked for physiologic causes to explain the anorexia which frequently accompanies cancer. Today, an interesting new insight shows promise of having a major impact on the understanding and prevention of anorexia.

Cancer patients frequently develop strong dislikes (aversions) to certain foods, tastes, and odors. These aversions seem to develop when certain foods, tastes, or odors are associated with unpleasant symptoms such as nausea and vomiting.[7] For example, if a person eats a certain food before receiving a treatment that makes him nauseated (such as chemotherapy), he learns to dislike that food.

If you think about it, this would normally be an adaptive reaction. An animal "learns" to avoid foods that make it sick by developing just such an aversion. Unfortunately, however, the person with cancer may be led to avoid foods that could help to make him well. Learning to hate his favorite foods because of their association with unpleasant body sensations worsens his anorexia.

Experiments in both humans and animals have shown that food aversions can develop in association with chemotherapy. In one experiment, children were served an unusually flavored ice cream before receiving chemotherapy.[8] After one to four weeks, they were offered a choice between eating the same flavor of ice cream and playing a game. These children were one-third as likely to choose the ice cream as control children who had received the ice cream without a simultaneous chemotherapy treatment. Another set of children received chemotherapy but not ice cream; they were not averse to eating the ice cream later. The experiment showed clearly that food aversions could develop in people undergoing chemotherapy.

Animal studies have shown that radiation therapy and unpleasant symptoms caused by tumor growth itself can also cause food aversions.[9] More research will be needed to determine if similar reactions occur in humans.

The idea of learned food aversions raises several important questions: What is the best way to prevent aversions? What foods are most likely to become aversive? Are food aversions permanent? How much influence do food aversions have on anorexia? While research into this new area of investigation continues, it seems wise to let people know that they may develop food aversions and to suggest that they "save" their favorite foods for periods when they are feeling relatively well and not eat within an hour or two (either before or after) scheduled radiation therapy or chemotherapy treatments.

[7] I. L. Bernstein and R. A. Sigmundi, Tumor anorexia: A learned food aversion? *Science* 209 (1980):416-418.

[8] I. L. Bernstein, Physiological and psychological mechanisms of cancer anorexia, *Cancer Research* 42 (1982):715s-720s.

[9] Bernstein, 1982.

Table 2. Possible Effects of Surgery on Nutrition Status

Head and neck resection

Difficulty in chewing/swallowing
Inability to chew/swallow

Esophageal resection

Decreased stomach motility	Steatorrhea
Decreased gastric acid production	Fistula formation
Diarrhea	Stenosis

Stomach resection

Dumping syndrome	Vitamin B_{12} malabsorption
Hypoglycemia	General malabsorption
Lack of gastric acid	

Intestinal resection

General malabsorption	Hyperoxaluria
Steatorrhea	Fluid and electrolyte imbalance
Diarrhea	Blind loop syndrome

Pancreatic resection

General malabsorption
Diabetes mellitus

regenerate as they normally do, and nutrient absorption is impaired. As we saw in Chapter 23, surgery to the GI tract also can have many ill effects on nutrition status. (These effects were summarized in Table 2.)

Thus, all these forms of treatment for cancer, as well as cancer itself, point in the same direction: malnutrition. In fact, it has been estimated that more than half of all the deaths attributed to cancer are actually caused by starvation.

Metabolic Consequences of Cancer

So far we have seen how decreased intake and increased losses of nutrients can contribute to cancer cachexia. Now let's look at how metabolic changes in cancer may further aggravate this syndrome.

Although research has not revealed the underlying reasons, it appears that people with cancer have increased energy expenditure.[10] In other words, they use more energy than healthy persons do. The tumor demands some energy, but the metabolic needs of the host are increased as well, sometimes even before the tumor is large enough to

[10]I. Warnold, K. Lundholm, and T. Scherstén, Energy balance and body composition in cancer patients, *Cancer Research* 38 (1978):1801-1807.

be detected. (This is one reason why, in preventive medicine, an important question in the dietary interview is "Have you experienced any recent changes in appetite or body weight?")

If decreased intake were the only problem in people with cancer, then weight loss would largely occur at the expense of body fat. But in cancer, muscle wasting is extreme. This wasting is accounted for, in part, by metabolic changes that occur in cancer.

In normal cells, energy is derived through the cycle that uses oxygen (the TCA cycle; see Highlight 7A) rather than through the pathway that involves no oxygen (the glycolytic pathway). The TCA cycle is the more efficient of the two, and can metabolize either glucose or fat for energy. But tumor cells use the glycolytic pathway to make energy. This pathway produces less energy and relies on glucose as an energy substrate. Therefore, the tumor cells must use glucose as their primary energy source. After the host's glycogen stores are depleted, muscle catabolism occurs to provide the amino acids necessary to make new glucose.

As the tumor metabolizes glucose by way of glycolysis, lactic acid (lactate) is produced. This lactate is then returned to the liver, where it is reconverted to glucose in an energy-requiring process. Thus, a demand is placed on the host to provide this energy. Accumulated lactate also may contribute to nausea.[11] (Sensations of nausea have even been experienced by healthy volunteers given an infusion of lactate.)

Another problem is that many people with cancer are hyperglycemic, probably for two reasons. For one thing, they tend to be insulin resistant; for another, they display decreased insulin release in response to a glucose load. Hunger generally corresponds to a return of blood glucose to fasting levels, and in the person with cancer this return may be delayed — hence the person's lack of appetite.

One author postulates that people with cancer produce excessive body heat after a meal.[12] The excess heat produces an unpleasant sensation that they learn to avoid by eating less. This theory ties in well with the idea that cancer patients develop learned food aversions.

The energy needs of people with cancer may be high for other reasons — emotional or physiological stress or surgery, for example. Both chemotherapy and radiation can interfere with the immune system, and infections can easily occur, again increasing energy and nutrient needs (see Chapter 22).

Chemotherapy using vitamin antagonists (see Chapter 21) can result in nutrient deficiencies and block normal metabolic pathways. This further interferes with nutrition status; anemias caused by a variety of vitamin deficiencies are frequently seen in cancer patients.

[11]W. D. DeWys, Pathophysiology of cancer cachexia: Current understanding and areas for future research, *Cancer Research* 42 (1982):721s-726s.

[12]DeWys, 1982.

Some tumors produce hormones that can affect normal body functions. For example, as previously discussed, the Zollinger-Ellison syndrome is caused by tumors that secrete gastrin; the gastrin triggers the production of excess gastric acid, and digestive enzymes become inactivated.

Obviously, the person with cancer is at extremely great risk for poor nutrition status. Nutrition care is often crucial to recovery.

Nutrition Care of the Patient with Cancer

For many years the deteriorating nutrition status that accompanies cancer was largely ignored. Many practitioners believed that emaciation and physical debilitation were an inevitable result of cancer. Others believed that if you fed the host, you also fed the tumor and that you should therefore starve the patient. Another problem was the state of the art of how patients could be fed. (Remember that the widespread use of tube feedings and TPN has been a recent advance.)

Today, attitudes regarding the benefits of nutrition for the cancer patient have changed dramatically. Attention to the diet can prevent or reverse poor nutrition status, and the advantages of maintaining optimal nutrition status are recognized. The patient in good nutrition status:

- Enjoys a better quality of life. (The malnourished person is less active and becomes weak, eats less, becomes weaker, and goes into a downward spiral.)
- Is less susceptible to infections (see Chapter 22).
- Probably, tolerates cancer therapies better (surgery, chemotherapy, and radiation therapy).

In animal studies, it has been shown that improved nutrition can result in increased tumor growth. However, in humans, tumor growth is generally not accelerated markedly by improved nutrition.[13] Furthermore, it has been suggested that accelerated tumor growth may be beneficial for people receiving chemotherapy or radiation, since these treatments are more effective in rapidly dividing cells. Do not allow your clients with cancer to starve themselves in the mistaken belief that they will be starving their cancer.

[13]Shils, 1981.

Finally, in considering the value of nutrition support in cancer, it is important to remember that cancer cachexia rather than cancer itself can actually be the cause of death sometimes.[14] In cancer, extreme malnutrition is a sign of impending death.[15] Therefore, feeding the cancer patient before he or she becomes depleted is particularly important.

Oral Diets during Therapy   There are a few general measures to help the patient maintain nutrition status during radiation or chemotherapy. For one thing, you can encourage patients to overeat between chemotherapy treatments, to compensate for weight loss during treatments. For another, you can minimize the likelihood of learned food aversions by having patients fast for several hours before radiation therapy or chemotherapy.[16]

People with cancer, particularly those who feel they cannot be helped by therapy, are easy targets for peddlers of nutrition "cures." They may take massive doses of vitamins and/or minerals, some of which may be toxic. Generally, people will not volunteer information about their use of vitamin supplements. Be sure to find out what supplements, and what amounts of them, your clients may be taking.

Tube Feedings and Parenteral Nutrition   Whenever possible, people with cancer should be encouraged to eat regular foods to meet nutrient needs. But often, this is very difficult. Sometimes giving liquid supplements between or with meals can be very helpful. However, when anorexia persists, particularly during and immediately after treatment, then tube feedings or parenteral nutrition may be indicated (see Chapter 20). Begin these measures before severe malnutrition sets in.

Although the use of enteral and parenteral nutrition may be beneficial for many patients, there are some additional considerations. These measures may cause some people to gain fat and water weight rather than lean body mass. Further, since the tumor also may grow as a consequence of better nutrition, enteral and parenteral nutrition should only be used when the patient is on some type of anticancer therapy.

[14]Groër and Pierce, 1981.

[15]J. van Eys, Effect of nutritional status on response to therapy, *Cancer Research* 42 (1982):747s-753s.

[16]W. D. DeWys, Nutritional care of the cancer patient, *Journal of the American Medical Association* 244 (1980):374-376.

There are some important questions (in addition to those mentioned above) that must be answered before aggressive measures are taken to provide the cancer patient with nutrition support. Is the person a candidate for other anticancer therapy? Providing nutrition support to a person with terminal cancer who cannot be given other treatments is usually contraindicated. But sometimes another question comes up. If aggressive support will help maintain the quality of life, should it be encouraged? This question is harder to answer. On the one hand, the person who is dying should be as comfortable as possible. On the other hand, TPN is expensive, and it may prolong life unnecessarily. The patient may have false hopes about what TPN might accomplish. The terminal cancer patient who is a candidate for TPN should be given the facts on which to base his or her decision. This decision must be respected.

Give the patient a reason to eat.

Eat during best times.

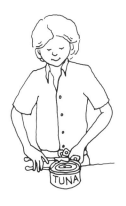

Use foods that are easy to prepare, and easy to eat.

Eat smaller meals.

Don't drink with meals.

Use nutritious liquids.

Empty kcalorie foods: foods that contain kcalories but contain few nutrients.

Use time-saving appliances.

Improving Appetite   When working with an anorectic cancer patient, always remember to give them a good reason to eat. Explain that they may be better able to tolerate their treatment if they eat well and that they will stay stronger and be more able to maintain their activity level.

Counsel them to take advantage of times when they feel best to eat more and to prepare foods that can be eaten when they simply don't have the energy to prepare a meal. For many people, morning is the best time of the day. For them, eating a high-kcalorie, high-protein breakfast will help. As the day wears on and they begin to tire easily, they can eat foods that were prepared earlier or that are easy to prepare and eat. Canned, frozen, or convenience foods are good alternatives. Encourage these patients to let friends and family help with meals whenever possible.

People who complain of fullness can eat smaller meals more often. Chewing foods slowly and saving liquids for after meals can also help. Replace empty kcalorie liquids with juices, milk, milkshakes, instant breakfast drinks, or liquid supplements that add nutrients to the diet. Recommend that greasy, high-fat foods be avoided, because they slow down gastric motility.

Find out what appliances clients have that can help reduce the time it takes them to fix a meal. Blenders, electric frying pans, toaster-ovens, microwave ovens, and dishwashers are very useful. Patients who do not have these appliances may be able to purchase them.

You can also give your clients hints on how they can add kcalories and protein to their diets. Some suggestions are given in Table 3.

People with cancer frequently complain of a bitter or metallic taste in their mouths. Because of this taste alteration, they frequently dislike red meat, and they may prefer to use fish, poultry, eggs, or dairy products in its place. Meat casseroles or soups and sauces added to

Table 3.   Suggestions for Increasing kCalories and Protein in the Diet

- Add 2 T of milk powder to the milk that you drink, use in recipes, or add to soups, puddings, and cereals.
- Add ground meats, chicken, fish, or grated cheese to sauces, soups, casseroles, or vegetables.
- Use extra butter, margarine, or cream cheese on bread.
- Eat peanut butter on fruit, celery, or crackers.
- Use butter or margarine whenever possible (on bread, potatoes, vegetables, pasta, and rice).
- Use yogurt, sour cream, or a sour cream dip with vegetables.
- Use mayonnaise as a salad dressing and on sandwiches.
- Add whipping cream to desserts and hot chocolate or use it to lighten coffee.
- Have snacks available at all times.
- Add nuts and dried fruits such as raisins to desserts or cereals.
- Use cream instead of milk with cereal.

meat may be more appealing than meat served alone, and meats served at room temperature or cold meats may taste better than hot meats. Suggest marinating poultry and meats in sweet wines, Italian dressing, or sweet-sour sauces. Using strong seasonings such as oregano, basil, mint, or tarragon can help. And you can suggest that clients use a mouthwash or brush their teeth before eating, to start with a fresher, more pleasant feeling.

Use eggs, fish, poultry.

Add sauces and seasonings to meat.

Serve meat cold or at room temperature.

Controlling Nausea and Vomiting   Nausea and vomiting are common complaints of people on chemotherapy. Some patients get so sick that they decide to discontinue the therapy. Standard drugs normally used to control nausea and vomiting are frequently ineffective in cancer patients (see Highlight 21).

Some diet guidelines may help. Advise the patient to eat smaller meals and avoid high-fat foods. Save liquids for between meals. When the patient is nauseated, slowly sipping clear beverages such as ginger ale or sucking popsicles or ice cubes made from a favorite liquid may help. Encourage patients to use liquids to prevent dehydration when vomiting is a problem. For nausea, suggest that patients lie down with head elevated after eating. Loosening the clothing and getting fresh air can also help relieve nausea.

Avoid high-fat foods.

Lie down, loosen clothing, and get fresh air.

If the smell of certain foods causes nausea, they should be avoided. It may be best to let someone else do the cooking or use foods that can be eaten without cooking.

Avoid smells that cause nausea.

Take a brief history to determine if the patient becomes nauseated or vomits at about the same time each day. If so, have the patient avoid favorite foods near that time to prevent the development of learned food aversions.

Use softer foods.

Drink with a straw.

Overcoming Chewing and Swallowing Problems   We have already discussed the general guidelines for handling problems with chewing and swallowing (see Chapter 23). These same principles apply to people with cancer who have mouth sores, decreased salivary secretions, or resections that interfere with chewing and swallowing.

People with chewing and swallowing difficulties may need softer foods to which sauces and gravies have been added. They may tolerate casseroles well. Spicy, acidic, or coarse foods should be avoided by patients with mouth sores. Suggest that the patient who has trouble swallowing try tilting his or her head back or forward to see if this helps. Using a straw makes drinking easier. Smoking and alcoholic beverages can irritate the throat. Liquid supplements or tube feedings may sometimes be necessary.

Patients who have decreased saliva may feel better if they rinse their mouths frequently. One author recommends swabbing the mouth with meat tenderizer to help relieve dry mouth, because it contains an enzyme (papain) that helps break up thick mucous secretions.[17] Artificial saliva is available to help reduce irritation and ease chewing and swallowing. In people with little saliva, special attention should be paid to oral hygiene, because they are more susceptible to dental caries. Concentrated sweets should be avoided.

Relieving Other GI Discomforts   Patients with cancer may complain of diarrhea, constipation, heartburn, or gas. Others, particularly those who have had radiation therapy to the small bowel, develop lactose intolerance. The nutrition recommendations for these problems were discussed in Chapter 23.

As you read about ways of handling nutrition related problems in the cancer patient, you may be deceived into thinking that it's not that hard to get the person to eat. For example, if you want someone to get more kcalories, you recommend adding fats to the diet. But think again. What if the person is nauseated and feels full after taking a few bites? For this person, a low-fat diet is recommended. That cuts out many ways for increasing kcaloric intake. A similar problem occurs in the lactose intolerant person who needs to add more protein to his or her diet: Milkshakes are the ideal way to add nourishment, but this patient gets sick from drinking milk.

So you see, getting a person with cancer to eat is a lot harder than it appears. The health professional has to work very closely with the individual to find acceptable food choices that provide for a well-balanced diet.

[17]G. L. Larsen, Rehabilitation for the patient with head and neck cancer, *American Journal of Nursing* 82 (1982):119-121.

Nutrition Assessment of Cancer Patients

The nutrition assessment of the cancer patient is particularly important in preventing severe malnutrition. Some areas that deserve special consideration include the following:

1. Look closely at the patient's diet history. Look for the adequacy of the diet and any foods that cause problems.

2. Check to see what type of therapy the patient has been receiving or will receive to determine how nutrition status may be affected.

3. Check the patient's weight history, noting any weight loss which has occurred unintentionally as a result of cancer or its treatment.

4. Ask the patient about special diets and vitamin and mineral supplements.

5. Record anthropometric measurements regularly. This will help you determine if the patient's energy and protein needs are being met. Step in to correct problems early, before they become severe.

6. Edema may be present in certain types of cancer, and can affect anthropometric measurements.

7. Patients with severe vomiting or diarrhea may be dehydrated. Biochemical parameters in dehydrated people may falsely appear to be normal.

The person with cancer is frequently at high risk for malnutrition. The health care team should be alert to the possibility of malnutrition and should take corrective measures to avoid the problem.

Summing Up

Cancer cachexia is frequently seen in people with cancer. Although the mechanisms of this syndrome are not fully understood, an interplay of several factors seems to be involved. Cancer cachexia can be caused by inadequate availability of nutrients (from either poor intake or increased nutrient losses) or by increased metabolic needs.

Anorexia can result from cancer itself, from cancer therapy, or from psychological stresses and learned food aversions caused by cancer or its therapy. People with anorexia typically complain of nausea, vomiting, a feeling of fullness, and being too tired to eat. Cancers obstructing the GI tract can also cause anorexia.

Cancer therapy can affect food intake by causing nausea, vomiting, taste alterations, mouth sores, or decreased saliva. Surgery can also interfere with the ability to chew and swallow.

Therapy for cancer and cancer itself can increase nutrient losses. Malabsorption can result from obstructions, fistulas, radiation enteritis, blind loop syndrome, and GI resections.

Metabolism also is altered in cancer. The tumor preferentially uses glycolysis to generate energy; when glucose is depleted, then the body must break down lean tissue for energy. Lactate and high blood glucose levels in the host may contribute to nausea and decreased appetite, respectively. The host catabolizes muscle protein to make glucose and to supply the tumor with amino acids for protein synthesis. This contributes to cachexia.

Oral, tube, and parenteral feedings can be used to support the patient with cancer; specific recommendations depend on the individual's eating problems. Every avenue should be pursued that will facilitate maintaining or restoring good nutrition status.

To Explore Further

The increased awareness of the role of nutrition in cancer has generated much research and many review articles.

A supplemental issue of *Cancer Research* published in February 1982 compiled presentations made at the Pediatric Cancer and Nutrition Workshop, held in Bethesda, Maryland. Many topics pertinent to both children and adults were included. Another issue of *Cancer Research* published in July 1977 contains presentations made at the Conference on Nutrition and Cancer Therapy, held in Key Biscayne, Florida.

A good general review article on the interrelationship between nutrition and cancer is:

- Bulter, J. H. Nutrition and cancer: A review of the literature. *Cancer Nursing*, April 1980, pp. 131-136.

Recently, several excellent articles have been published on the practical aspects of feeding cancer patients. They include:

- Shils, M. E. How to nourish the cancer patient. *Nutrition Today*, May/June 1981, pp. 4-15.
- Bloch, A. S. Practical hints for feeding the cancer patient. *Nutrition Today*, November/December 1981, pp. 23-25.
- DeWys, W. D. Nutritional care of the cancer patient. *Journal of the American Medical Association* 244 (1980):374-376.
- DeWys, W. D., and Kubota, T. T. Enteral and parenteral nutrition in the care of the cancer patient. *Journal of the American Medical Association* 246 (1981):1725-1727.
- Groër, M., and Pierce, M. Guarding against cancer's hidden killer: Anorexia-cachexia. *Nursing*, June 1981, pp. 39-43.

An article reviewing several important aspects of care for the person with head and neck cancer is:

- Larsen, G. L. Rehabilitation for the patient with head and neck cancer. *American Journal of Nursing* 82 (1982):119-121.

Two worthwhile articles that discuss how people with cancer deal with their nutrition problems are:

● Thompson, E. S. Personal nutrition experiences of two cancer patients . . . Thanks, but no spare ribs! *Nutrition Today*, May/June 1981, pp. 22-23.

● Oser, J. An unusual diet for an unusual handicap. *Nutrition Today*, May/June 1981, pp. 24-25.

A teaching aid by M. E. Shils titled *How to Nourish the Cancer Patient* is available from the Nutrition Today Society (address in Appendix J).

Several publications are available free of charge through Ross Laboratories (address in Appendix J):

● Nursing care of the cancer patient with nutritional problems. *Ross Roundtable on Oncology Nursing*, Columbus, Ohio: Ross Laboratories, 1981.

● Cancer. *Dietary Modifications in Disease. Columbus, Ohio: Ross Laboratories, 1978.*

● Shils, M.E., ed. Nutritional problems in cancer patients, *Nutrition in Disease.* Columbus, Ohio: Ross Laboratories, 1976.

An interesting article that presents a speech made by one doctor who believes that diet can "cure" cancer can be found in:

● Gerson, M. The cure of advanced cancer by diet therapy: A summary of 30 years of clinical experimentation. *Physiological Chemistry and Physics* 10 (1978):449-464.

(A note to the reader: Dr. Gerson's diet does not have support in the general medical community; its value is unproven.)

An article about a problem of people with cancer that affects their food intake is:

● Goldberg, R. J. Management of depression in the patient with advanced cancer. *Journal of the American Medical Association* 246 (1981):373-376.

Mr. Wayne first came to see his doctor when he noticed that he was losing weight rapidly and that he seemed to be drained of energy. He also had a lesion in his mouth that wouldn't heal. Mr. Wayne has a history of alcohol and cigarette abuse. After being admitted to the hospital, tests confirmed a diagnosis of cancer of the mouth. The doctor would like to prepare Mr. Wayne nutritionally before proceeding with radiation therapy. Radical surgery is a possibility. A thorough nutrition assessment revealed that Mr. Wayne was suffering from severe protein-kcalorie malnutrition which was classified as kwashiorkor-marasmus mix. His height and weight are 5 ft 10 in and 125 lb.

Study Questions

1. What is Mr. Wayne's ideal weight? His % IBW? What other anthropometric measurements would you expect to see depleted? Will serum protein levels be low?

2. How might Mr. Wayne's past history have affected his nutrition status before he developed cancer? In what ways can cancer affect his nutrition status? How can radiation therapy affect his nutrition status? Discuss the possible impact of radical head and neck surgery on his nutrition status.

3. Describe cancer cachexia. What are some of its causes? What are the benefits of preventing or correcting it?

4. Discuss the possible feeding routes for replenishing Mr. Wayne's nutrient stores prior to treatment. How might radiation therapy or radical surgery narrow the choice of feeding routes?

5. If Mr. Wayne is able to take food by mouth, what suggestions will you give him for dealing with poor appetite, nausea and vomiting, dry and sore mouth, and chewing and swallowing problems? Is he likely to develop lactose intolerance or radiation enteritis? Why or why not?

Can Nutrition Prevent Disease?

In the way we live our daily lives, we either enhance our health or diminish it.

JOHN W. FARQUHAR

Before 1980, textbooks of diet therapy gave little or no space to the subject of nutrition for people with cancer. In this book, the whole of Chapter 28 deals with diet therapy for cancer, reflecting a recent burst of new knowledge. Similarly, in the late 1970s, there were many offerings of diet advice to the public, but they included little or no information on *prevention* of cancer; they aimed their dietary recommendations primarily at prevention of atherosclerosis, hypertension, and diabetes. This Highlight brings you up to date on how much more is now known about the ways in which a good diet may help prevent cancer. In doing so, it presents a long-neglected example of a "yes" answer to the question asked in the title. The Highlight concludes with some statements about other diseases.

First, a word about the sources of available information. Epidemiology — the study of whole populations in different areas of the world — provides one means of gathering information on diet and cancer. Another approach is to conduct case control studies — studies of people who have cancer and of other people as closely matched as possible in age, occupation, and other key variables, to see what differences in their lifestyles may account for the differing cancer incidences. Still another approach is to test

possible causes of cancer on animals under controlled laboratory conditions in which all other variables can be ruled out. Each type of study has its limitations and has to be interpreted with an awareness of those limitations.

Epidemiological Studies

A thought-provoking finding from epidemiological study comes from the comparison of high-risk and low-risk areas. If only 10 people out of 1,000 get a certain kind of cancer in location X, while 100 out of 1,000 get that same kind of cancer in location Y, researchers are inclined to conclude that 90 percent of the cancers in location Y are caused by some environmental factor and are therefore, in theory, preventable. In fact, comparison of high- and low-risk areas suggests that 80 to 90 percent of human cancers may in-

deed be preventable.[1] There are aspects of our environment over which we have little or no control, but we can certainly control our food choices. Hence the great challenge to researchers is to discover what dietary differences might exist between people who do and don't get cancer.

Early epidemiological studies showed that the incidence of certain cancers varied by geographic area and by racial group.[2] Japanese immigration to the United States after World War I provided an especially interesting opportunity for such study. The Japanese living in Japan develop more stomach cancers and fewer colon cancers than people in the United States and other Western countries. However, when Japanese come to the United States, their children develop both stomach and colon cancers at a rate like that of Americans. What changes the susceptibility of Japanese immigrants? It probably isn't pollution, because Japan and the United States are both industrial countries. However, something in the environment has changed, and an obvious candidate is diet.

[1]B. S. Reddy, L. A. Cohen, G. D. McCoy, P. Hill, J. H. Weisburger, and E. L. Wynder, Nutrition and its relationship to cancer, *Advances in Cancer Research* 32 (1980):238-345.

[2]D. Burkitt, Epidemiology of cancer of the colon and rectum, *Cancer* 28 (1971):3-13.

Some other interesting questions arise from this comparison. Curiously, even though the incidence of colon cancer rises in the immigrants, Japanese women of the second generation retain the same rate of breast cancer as women in Japan; a change in breast cancer rates doesn't show up until the third generation.[3] This is in contrast to the fact that, worldwide, breast and colon cancer correlate, rising and falling together in the same population. Does the rate of breast cancer in adulthood reflect the food intakes of childhood so that it takes more than one generation to bring about a change? Answering one question only raises more questions.

Other population studies provide additional clues for the cancer detectives. Some of these studies show that Seventh-Day Adventists have a remarkably lower death rate from cancers of all kinds than the general population of the United States. This religious sect has rules against smoking, using alcohol, and using hot condiments and spices. It encourages a lacto-ovo-vegetarian diet and especially forbids pork, which is spoken of in the Bible as "unclean meat." Even Seventh-Day Adventists who do not strictly obey all these rules eat meat very sparingly. Even after cancers linked to smoking and alcohol are discounted, Seventh-

Day Adventists still have a mortality rate from cancer about one-half to two-thirds that of the rest of the population.

In this case, as with all epidemiological studies, many questions have to be raised. Is the group's low cancer mortality rate due to its low consumption of meat and high consumption of vegetables and cereal grains? Or is there some factor other than diet that makes this group unique? The Seventh-Day Adventists are of a higher-than-average socioeconomic level, and more are college-educated; what influence might these factors have on their incidence of cancer?[4]

In order to track down the factors that are associated with cancers in some populations, B. S. Drasar and D. Irving studied the diets of people in 37 countries. They documented the food available per person per day, as well as other indicators of lifestyle, such as possession of radio receivers and motor vehicles. They found many correlations, but one of the most interesting showed both breast and colon cancer to be strongly associated "with indicators of affluence, such as a high-fat diet rich in animal protein and the availability of motor vehicles. However, the

correlation with fat and animal protein was higher than for the other factors."[5] Other investigators have reported similar findings.[6]

Any attempt to link dietary components with disease should be approached with caution. An increase in one component of the diet causes increases or decreases in others.[7] If a close correlation is shown between a disease and, say, the consumption of animal protein, how can you be sure that the critical factor is the animal protein? It may be increased fat consumption; fat goes with animal protein in foods. Or the disease may occur because of what is crowded out: the vitamins, minerals, or fiber contained in the missing fruits, vegetables, and cereals.

Another problem inherent in epidemiological studies is that they depend on dietary recall. People tend to have trouble remembering how much of each food they have eaten.[8] And in the case of cancer studies, the need is not so much to know what the diet is like now as to

[3] Reddy and co-authors, 1980.

[4] R. L. Phillips, Role of life-style and dietary habits in risk of cancer among Seventh Day Adventists, *Cancer Research* 35 (1975):3513-3522.

[5] B. S. Drasar and D. Irving, Environmental factors and cancer of the colon and breast, *British Journal of Cancer* 27 (1973):167-172.

[6] K. K. Carroll, Experimental evidence of dietary factors and hormone-dependent cancers, *Cancer Research* 35 (2) (1975):3374-3383.

[7] Carroll, 1975; B. Modan, Role of diet in cancer etiology, *Cancer* 40 (1977):1887-1891.

[8] Modan, 1977.

know what it was like at an earlier time, say, 30 years ago, when the initiating event may have taken place.[9] In this connection, study of the Seventh-Day Adventists offers hope of clarifying the relationship between animal protein and cancer. Most of them can tell you exactly when they quit eating meat — they quit when they joined the church.

Case Control Studies

Case control studies have generally pointed the same way as epidemiological studies: they implicate diet in cancer causation. When 179 Hawaiian Japanese colon cancer cases were carefully matched with 357 Hawaiian Japanese controls, the cancer cases were seen to engage in strikingly higher consumption of meat, especially beef. An Israeli study showed fiber consumption to be lower in colon cancer cases than in controls. A study of U.S. blacks with colon cancer showed them to be eating less fiber and more saturated fat than controls. A study of people in Minnesota and in Norway found less frequent use of vegetables in people with colon cancer; a New York study found specifically

[9]A. B. Miller, Role of nutrition in the etiology of breast cancer, *Cancer* 39 (1977):2704-2708; B. Armstrong and R. Doll, Environmental factors and cancer incidence and mortality in different countries, with special reference to dietary practices, *International Journal of Cancer* 15 (1975):617-631.

less use of cabbage, broccoli, and Brussels sprouts in colon cancer victims. These studies have led reviewers to the view that, at least in colon cancer, a diet "high in total fat, low in fiber, and high in beef [is] associated with an increased incidence of large-bowel cancer in man."[10]

Animal Studies: Fat and Cancer

After epidemiological and case control studies have tentatively identified a dietary factor, researchers often turn to experiments with laboratory animals. Animal researchers can control many variables while manipulating only the diet.

Laboratory studies using animals confirmed suspicions that fat, of all the dietary components, is uniquely correlated with cancer. For example, K. K. Carroll found that he could increase the number of mammary tumors in rats if he raised their dietary fat.[11] The fat was not initiating the cancers, however; to get the tumors started, Carroll had to expose the animals to a known carcinogen. After that exposure, the high-fat diet made more cancers develop and made them develop earlier than did low-fat diets.

From these and many other such studies, the conclusion has been reached that people wishing to employ dietary means to reduce the

[10]Reddy and co-authors, 1980.

[11]Carroll, 1975.

> **Miniglossary**
>
> **case control study:** an epidemiological study that matches groups with respect to all variables except the one of interest.
>
> **promoter:** a substance that does not initiate cancer, but that favors its development once the initiating event has taken place.

risk of contracting cancer would do well to curtail their fat intake. The recommendations for avoiding heart and artery disease also include fat restriction, so cancer prevention and heart disease prevention can be aided by the same means. There would appear to be no harm in reducing fat kcalories to the point where they contribute a maximum of 30 percent of total kcalories, and many cancer researchers suggest a stricter limit: 20 percent of total kcalories. For the "average American" to accomplish this degree of fat restriction in practice means drastically reducing the amount of fat used in food preparation.

People who have suspected and feared food additives as carcinogens (Highlight 13) are often surprised to learn that fat may be far more significant in cancer causation. Fat is not a cancer initiator but is thought rather to be a promoter, somehow enhancing the process by which cancer gets established in a cell or tissue once the first events have taken place. A high-fat diet may promote cancer in any of a number of ways:

● By causing the body to secrete more of certain hormones (for example, estrogen), thus creating a climate favorable to development of certain cancers (for example, breast cancer).

● By promoting the secretion of bile into the intestine; bile may then be converted by organisms in the colon into compounds that cause cancer.

● By being incorporated into cell membranes and changing them so that they offer less defense against cancer-causing invaders.

It may not be fat in general, but certain forms of fat, that have these effects. Importantly, it seems that polyunsaturated fat is as responsible as, or even more responsible than, saturated fat for promoting cancer, so the person wishing to apply this information should reduce consumption of *all* forms of fat.[12]

Fiber and Cancer In general, wherever the diet is high in fat-rich foods, it is simultaneously low in vegetable fiber. There is a possibility that the absence of fiber promotes cancer independently of the presence of fat, although these two possibilities are difficult to separate in studies of humans, and the association of fat with cancer is stronger than that of fiber-lack with cancer. Still, fiber might help protect against some cancer — for example, by promoting the excretion of bile from the body, or by speeding up the transit time of all materials through the colon so that the colon walls are not exposed for long to cancer-causing substances. That fiber does have an independent protective effect of some kind is supported by evidence from Finland. The Finns eat a high-fat diet, but unlike other such diets, theirs is very high in fiber as well. Their colon cancer rate is low, suggesting that fiber has a protective effect even in the presence of a high-fat diet.[13]

If fat and/or a meat-rich diet are implicated in causation of certain cancers, and if fiber and/or a vegetable-rich diet are associated with pre-

vention, then vegetarians should have a lower incidence of those cancers. They do. The Seventh-Day Adventists have already been mentioned; other vegetarian women also have less breast cancer than do omnivores. A possible explanation is suggested by the finding that vegetarian women excrete more estrogens in their feces, so they probably have lower total body estrogen contents than meat eaters do.[14]

Vegetables and Cancer A number of studies have suggested other relationships between cancer and the intake of vegetables, especially certain kinds of vegetables. A case control study has already been mentioned that places cabbage and its relatives in a favorable light. Similarly, careful comparisons of stomach cancer victims' diets with those of case controls show less use of vegetables in the cancer group — in one case, vegetables in general; in another, fresh vegetables; in others, lettuce and other fresh greens; or vegetables containing vitamin C.[15] One of the suspects for the causation of stomach cancer is nitrosamines, produced in the stomach from

[12]It may not, in fact, be polyunsaturated fat but *processed* polyunsaturated fat containing *trans*-fatty acids that is ultimately incriminated in cancer promotion. We have offered a discussion of this possibility elsewhere: E. N. Whitney and E. M. N. Hamilton, Highlight 2: Dietary fat and cancer, in *Understanding Nutrition*, 2nd ed. (St. Paul, Minn.: West, 1981), pp. 84-93.

[13]E. L. Wynder, Dietary habits and cancer epidemiology, *Cancer* 43 (1979):1955-1961, as cited by S. H. Brammer and R. L. DeFelice, Dietary advice in regard to risk for colon and breast cancer, *Preventive Medicine* 9 (1980):544-549.

[14]B. R. Goldin, H. Adlercreutz, J. T. Dwyer, L. Swenson, J. H. Warram, and S. L. Gorbach, Effect of diet on excretion of estrogens in pre- and postmenopausal women, *Cancer Research* 41 (1981):3771-3773.

[15]Reddy and co-authors, 1980.

nitrites. The vegetables may help keep nitrosamines from forming by contributing vitamin C, which inhibits the conversion of nitrites to nitrosamines (Highlight 14).

When environmental causes of another kind of cancer — that of the head and neck — have been sought, the overwhelmingly major factor has appeared not to be diet but rather to be alcohol and tobacco consumption. Again, however, some dietary factors have turned up here and there, again pointing to a low intake of fruits and raw vegetables in cancer cases, but this time specifically to the fruits and vegetables that contribute vitamin A and riboflavin. Vitamin A and its relatives the retinoids are also important in preventing cancers of epithelial origin, including skin cancer.[16]

Among the known actions of vitamin A are the important roles it plays in maintaining the immune function. A strong immune system may be able to prevent cancers from gaining control even after they have gotten started in the body. The steps in cancer development are thought to be:

1. Exposure to a carcinogen.

2. Entry of the carcinogen into a cell.

3. Initiation, probably by the carcinogen's altering the cellular DNA somehow.

4. Tumor formation, probably involving several more steps before the cell begins to multiply out of control.

Immunity can work even after the fourth step, blocking tumor formation after initiation has taken place. Some studies suggest that this may be where vitamin A makes its contribution. In Norway, a five-year prospective study showed lung cancer incidence to be 60 to 80 percent lower in men with a high vitamin A intake than in those with a low intake; in Japan, a study of 280,000 persons showed lung cancer rates to be 20 to 30 percent lower in smokers who ate yellow or green vegetables daily than in those who did not. In ex-smokers who ingested yellow or green vegetables daily the reduction was much greater, as if the repair of damage done by smoking (initiation of cancer) was enhanced by something in the vegetables.[17] A reviewer, impressed by abundant evidence along these lines, says "No human population at risk for the development of cancer should be allowed to remain in a vitamin A deficient state."[18]

Green vegetables have also been seen to have a protective effect beyond those already discussed for vitamin A, vitamin C, and fiber. The effects of the members of the cabbage family, for example, may be due to their containing substances known as indoles, which may act by inducing an enzyme in the host that destroys carcinogens.[19]

Cancer Prevention The foregoing sections have revealed some of the major known connections between diet and cancer, and have, we hope, made clear that much remains to be learned about these connections. Still, many people working in cancer research believe that we already know enough to take some tentative preventive steps. One reviewer says, "The public is looking for answers regarding this diet:cancer link and will look to anyone willing to provide answers, regardless of his/her qualifications. . . . The recommendations offered here constitute no risk and may help lower the incidence of . . . cancers." The recommendations she gives

[16]J. L. Werther, Food and cancer, *New York State Journal of Medicine*, August 1980, pp. 1401-1408.

[17]Werther, 1980.

[18]M. B. Sporn, Retinoids and carcinogenesis, *Nutrition Reviews* 35 (1977):65-69.

[19]L. W. Wattenberg, W. D. Loub, L. K. Lam, and J. L. Speier, Dietary constituents altering the responses to chemical carcinogens, *Federation Proceedings* 35 (1976):1327-1331; L. W. Wattenberg and W. D. Loub, Inhibition of polycyclic aromatic hydrocarbon-induced neoplasia by naturally occurring indoles, *Cancer Research* 38 (1978):1410-1413.

are to reduce total fat and kcalorie intake and to ingest more complex carbohydrates, both starch and fiber — advice in agreement with recommendations made to the public for promotion of health in many other respects.[20]

Nutrition and Disease

This Highlight has focused on cancer to compensate for the neglect it has received until the recent past, but it is fitting to end this book with a statement about the relationships between nutrition and disease prevention in general. Since the late 1970s the government and the media have expressed more and more emphatically the conviction that nutrition has the potential to help prevent the modern "killer diseases" — diabetes, atherosclerosis, hypertension, and others, as well as cancer. Reflecting this conviction, a variety of government agencies have offered dietary goals and guidelines to the public:

- *Dietary Goals for the United States*, 1977 (see Chapter 1).
- *Dietary Guidelines for Americans*, 1979 (see Chapter 1).
- *Healthy People*, the Surgeon General's report, 1979,

which included a set of recommendations on diet.[21]

Each of these made reference to the fact that today's most prevalent diseases are lifestyle diseases — diseases that we bring upon ourselves — and offers advice that we bolster our defenses against them by avoiding monotony in our food choices, by practicing moderation in our use of fat, saturated fat, sugar, salt, and alcohol, and by maintaining ideal weight.

If you have read the preceding chapters you will be familiar with all these guidelines and many more. Table 1 restates the many preventive contributions for which nutrition can reasonably claim credit. Obviously, nutrition has an important place in disease prevention.

The Place of Preventive Nutrition
Nutrition quackery is largely based on the notion that certain foods and nutrients have almost miraculous power to promote health. Table 1, too, displays an impressive list of health-promoting effects of good nutrition, but there is a difference. It does not advocate the use of specific foods — and certainly not of nutrient supplements — nor does it imply that even the most

scrupulous attention to nutrition will guarantee freedom from disease. Taken together, the recommendations of Table 1 simply add up to an adequate, balanced, and varied diet composed of nutritious foods — a quiet, sensible prescription for good nutritional health.

Table 1 does not tell the whole story, however. Nutrition shares with other lifestyle factors the responsibility for maintaining health. A complete prescription for good health might read as follows:

- Get regular sleep.
- Eat regular meals.
- Maintain desirable weight.
- Don't smoke.
- Drink alcohol moderately or not at all.
- Get regular exercise.[22]

Nutrition is represented by two of the six items in this list.

Even a person who abides by all six of these health practices has no guarantee of immunity from disease. Chance elements cannot be eliminated, no matter how scrupulously a person eats right, avoids "vices," and practices moderation in all things. Sometimes life just isn't fair: someone who has cultivated all the right health habits may be struck down

---

[20]Brammer and DeFelice, 1980.

[21]*Healthy People*, the Surgeon General's Report on Health Promotion and Disease Prevention, DHEW (PHS) publication no. 79-55071 (Washington, D.C.: Government Printing Office, 1979).

[22]N. B. Belloc and L. Breslow, Relationship of physical health status and health practices, *Preventive Medicine* 1 (1972):409-421.

Table 1.   Examples of Preventive Effects of Good Nutrition*

Adequate intake of protein, kcalories, essential nutrients (during pregnancy)	*helps prevent*	birth defects mental/physical retardation low birth weight poor resistance to disease
(in infancy, childhood)		growth deficits poor resistance to disease
(in adulthood, old age)		malnutrition poor resistance to disease
Moderation in kcaloric intake (throughout life)	*helps prevent*	obesity and related diseases such as diabetes and hypertension
Adequate intake of any essential nutrient (at any time in life)	*prevents*	deficiency diseases such as cretinism, scurvy, and folacin-deficiency anemia
Adequate calcium intake (throughout life)	*helps prevent*	adult bone loss
Adequate iron intake (during pregnancy)	*helps prevent*	maternal anemia
(in childhood)		anemia, poor school performance
Adequate fluoride intake (in childhood)	*helps prevent*	dental caries
Moderation in sodium intake (from childhood or beginning at any time)	*helps prevent*	hypertension and related diseases of the heart and kidney
Adequate fiber intake (from childhood or beginning at any time)	*helps prevent*	digestive malfunctions such as constipation and diverticulosis possibly colon or other cancer
Adequate vitamin A intake (throughout life)	*helps prevent*	susceptibility to epithelial cancer
Moderation in fat intake (beginning in childhood)	*helps prevent*	hyperlipidemia, susceptibility to some cancers
Moderation in sugar intake (beginning in childhood)	*helps prevent*	dental caries
Moderation in alcohol intake (beginning in childhood)	*helps prevent*	liver disease malnutrition
Moderation in intake of all essential nutrients (throughout life)	*prevents*	toxicity states

*Relationships shown are not exclusive; that is, in all but two instances the nutrition variable does not by itself prevent, but is known to contribute to prevention of, the conditions.

by a disease or accident that he in no way "deserved." One aspect of disease causation that no one can control is the genetic side; Figure 1 shows that some diseases are purely hereditary (sickle-cell anemia, for example) while others are caused solely by poor nutrition (deficiency disease), and many fall along the spectrum between the extremes.

The statement that wise food choices and other life-style habits promote good health has to be qualified in still another way. Lewis Thomas puts it this way: "We are paying too little attention, and respect, to the built-in durability and sheer power of the human organism. . . . It is a distortion . . . to picture the human being as a teetering, fallible contraption, always needing watching and patching, always on the verge of flapping to pieces . . . ."[23] Everyone is familiar with the occasional oldster who smokes, drinks, and cusses his or her way into great old age with no at-

[23]L. Thomas, Your very good health, *Nutrition Today*, July/August 1978, pp. 30-31.

Figure 1   Not all diseases are equally influenced by diet. Some are purely hereditary, like sickle cell anemia. Some may be inherited (or the tendency to them may be inherited) but may be influenced by diet, like some forms of diabetes. Some are purely dietary, like the vitamin- and mineral-deficiency diseases.

Some authorities are concerned that the offering of dietary advice to the public may seem to exaggerate the power of nutrition in preventing disease. Nutrition alone is certainly not enough to prevent many diseases.

Adapted from R. E. Olson, Are professionals jumping the gun in the fight against chronic disease? *Journal of the American Dietetic Association* 74 (1979):543-550, Figure 2.

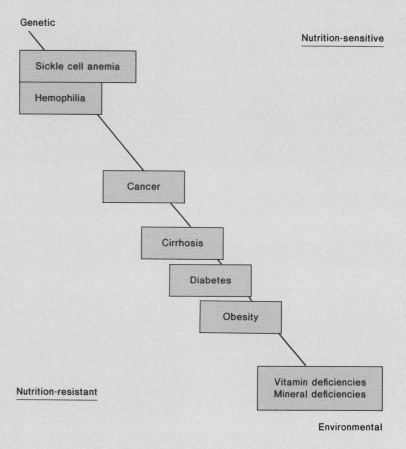

tention to good health habits — providing proof of Thomas's point. This book began with a celebration of the wisdom and resiliency of the body (Highlights 1 and 2) and ends by repeating that theme. The body has tremendous stability and self-correcting ability. We can trust the body to take care of itself magnificiently amidst many fluctuations imposed on it.

Finally, because the body and the mind work together to maintain health (Highlight 6), we will do well to cultivate a healthy mental attitude as well as healthy physical habits. Expecting to be well is oftentimes half the battle. Having learned all we can about nutrition and food choices, and having practiced for a time to develop the desired habits, we need not continue to spend many hours daily on that task. Just as riding a bicycle or driving a car takes much concentration at first and then becomes automatic, so too does the adoption of healthful food habits require study and effort at first and then become integrated with the other aspects of life to make a whole in which no part has undue emphasis. Ultimately, the obtaining and delivery of good nutrition are not ends in themselves, but serve a higher purpose, the celebration of life and the service of humankind.

To Explore Further

An issue not discussed here is the possible connection of coffee with pancreatic cancer. One careful study showed that there was such an association:

● MacMahon, B., Yen, S., Trichopoulos, D., Warren, K., and Nardi, G. Coffee and cancer of the pancreas, *New England Journal of Medicine* 304 (1981):630-633.

A critique of that study suggests that there is no such association after all:

● Feinstein, A. R., Horwitz, R. I., Spitzer, W. O., and Battista, R. N. Coffee and pancreatic cancer, the problems of etiologic science and epidemiologic case-control research (commentary). *Journal of the American Medical Association* 246 (1981):957.

Books Not Recommended

The following list was compiled from several sources, two of which deserve special mention. The Chicago Nutrition Association has for many years been reviewing books on nutrition and diet and providing information about them to the public in its *Nutrition References and Book Reviews* (the 5th edition was published in 1981). All books marked with an asterisk (*) have been on their "not recommended" lists; their booklet gives the reasons why. They also list books that contain valid nutrition information, and provide a "how to choose a book" section for evaluating other nutrition references you may come across. This valuable reference is available for $8 a copy; consult Appendix J for the address. The American Council on Science and Health, since 1979, has been performing a similar service. *ACSH News and Views* is published every two months and carries several thoughtful reviews of new books on health in each issue. Consumers Union, which publishes *Consumer Reports*, and the Nutrition Foundation, which publishes *Nutrition Reviews*, also serve the public by sifting valid from misleading nutrition information. Books reviewed by these reviewers are identified by numbered footnotes.

Inclusion in this list does not necessarily mean we dislike these books or think they are badly written. We have many of them in our own libraries; some offer good ideas and inspiration; and some are very well written indeed — but they do not provide reliably valid nutrition information. Many of the claims they make are groundless and much of the advice they offer is unfounded and even downright dangerous.

For books we recommend to provide the core of a professional library, turn to Appendix J; for pamphlets and booklets to share with friends and clients, scan Appendix C.

Abrahamson, E. M., and Pezet, A. W. *Body, Mind & Sugar.*[1]

Adams, C. *Eat Well Diet Book.*[*]

Adams, R. *Miracle Medicine Foods.*[*]

Air Force Diet.[2]

Alexander, D. D. *Arthritis and Common Sense.*[*]

Altman, N. *Eating for Life — A Book About Vegetarianism.*[*]

Anchell, M. *How I Lost 36,000 Pounds.*[*]

Arnow, I. *Food Power: A Doctor's Guide to Commonsense Nutrition.*[*]

Ashley, R., and Duggal, H. *Dictionary of Nutrition.*[*]

Atkins, R. *Dr. Atkins' Diet Revolution.*[*]

Atkins, R. *Dr. Atkins' Nutrition Breakthrough.*[3]

Bailey, H. *Your Key to a Healthy Heart.*[*]

Barnes, B., and Barnes, C. *Solved: Riddle of Heart Attacks.*[*]

Bassler, T., and Burger, R. *Whole Life Diet.*[*]

Blaine, T. R. *Goodbye Allergies.*[1]

Blaine, T. R. *Mental Health Through Nutrition.*[*]

Boody, S., and Clausen, M. *High-Energy, Low-Budget, Weight-Loss Diet.*[*]

Breneman, J. *Basics of Food Allergy.*[*]

Cantor, A. J. *How to Lose Weight the Doctor's Way.*[*]

Cantor, A. J. *Dr. Cantor's Longevity Diet.*[*]

Carey, R. L., Vyhmeister, I. B., and Hudson, J. S. *Common-Sense Nutrition.*[*]

Carkin, G. *Today's Manna.*[*]

Clark, L. *Be Slim and Healthy (How to Have a Trimmer Body the Natural Way).*[*]

Clark, L. *Stay Young Longer.*[*]

Cooper, J., and Hagen, P. *Dr. Cooper's Fabulous Fructose Diet.*[*]

Cousins, N. *Anatomy of an Illness: Reflections on Healing and Regeneration.*[4]

Cummings, B. *Stay Young and Vital.*[*]

Davis, A. *Let's Cook It Right.*[*]

Davis, A. *Let's Eat Right to Keep Fit.**

Davis, A. *Let's Get Well.**

Davis, A. *Let's Have Healthy Children.**

Davis, A. *Vitality Through Planned Nutrition.**

Davis, A. *You Can Stay Well.**

Dean, M. *Complete Gourmet Nutrition Cookbook.**

DeGroot, R. *How I Reduced with the Rockefeller Diet.**

Dong, C. M., and Banks, J. *Arthritis Cookbook.*[1]

Dufty, W. *Sugar Blues.*

Edelstein, B. *Woman Doctor's Diet for Women.**

Eiteljorg, S. *Sweet Way to Diet.**

Elwood, C. *Feel Like a Million.**

Feingold, B., and Feingold, H. *Feingold Cookbook for Hyperactive Children.**

Ferguson, J., and Taylor, C. *A Change for Heart.**

Fiore, E. L. *Low Carbohydrate Diet.**

Fredericks, C. *Carlton Fredericks Cookbook for Good Nutrition.**

Fredericks, C. *Eat, Live and be Merry.**

Fredericks, C. *Eat Well, Get Well, Stay Well.*[5]

Fredericks, C. *Food Facts and Fallacies.**

Fredericks, C. *Low Blood Sugar and You.**

Fredericks, C. *New and Complete Nutrition Handbook.**

Fredericks, C. *Nutrition: Your Key to Good Health.**

Fredericks, C. *Psycho-Nutrition.**

Fredericks, C., and Bailey, H. *Food Facts and Fallacies.**

Friedman, M., and Rosenman, R. *Type A Behavior and Your Heart.**

Glass, J. *Live to Be 180.**

Harvey, W. *On corpulence in relation to disease.*[2]

Hatfield, A., and Stanton, P. *Right! It's Fun to Eat: How to Help Your Child Eat Cookbook and Guide to Better Nutrition.**

Hauser, G. *Be Happier, be Healthier.**

Hauser, G. *Look Younger, Live Longer.**

Hauser, G. *Mirror, Mirror on the Wall.**

Hauser, G. *New Diet Does it.**

Hauser, G. *New Guide to Intelligent Reducing.**

Hunter, B. *Natural Food Cookbook.**

Hunter, B. *Great Nutrition Robbery.**

Hunter, K. *Health Foods and Herbs.**

Hurd, F. J., and Hurd, R. *Ten Talents.**

Jacobson, M. *Eaters Digest: Consumer's Factbook of Food Additives.**

Jacobson, M., and Center for Science in the Public Interest. *Nutrition Scoreboard: Your Guide to Better Eating.**

Jameson, G., and Williams, E. *Drinking Man's Diet.*[1]

Jarvis, D. C. *Folk Medicine — A Vermont Doctor's Guide to Good Health.**

Kaplan, R., Saltzman, B., Ecker, L., and Williams, P. *Wholly Alive.**

Kirschnerr, H. E. *Life Food Juices.**

Kloss, J. *Back to Eden.**

Kordel, L. *Cook Right — Live Longer.**

Kordel, L. *Eat and Grow Younger.*

Kordel, L. *Eat Your Troubles Away.**

Kordel, L. *Live to Enjoy the Money you Make.**

Lasky, M. *Complete Junk Food Book.**

Lederman, M. *Slim Gourmet or The Joys of Eating.**

Leinwoll, S. *Low Cholesterol, Lower Calorie French Cooking.**

Leonard, J. N., Hofer J. L., and Pritikin, N. *Live Longer Now.*

Levitt, E. *Wonderful World of Natural-Food Cookery.**

Levy, J., and Bach-y-Rita, P. *Vitamins: Their Use and Abuse.**

Lewis, C. *Nutrition, Nutritional Considerations for the Elderly.**

Linn, R., and Stuart, S. L. *Last Chance Diet.*

Living Better, Recipes for a Healthy Heart.

MacKarness, R. *Eat Fat and Grow Slim.**

Maislen, R., Kadish, T., and Lerner, N. *Eat, Think and Be Thinner the Weigh of Life Way.**

Malone, F. *Bees don't get arthritis.*[1]

Mazel, J. *Beverly Hills Diet.*[6]

Martin, C. G. *How to Live to Be 100.**

Miller, S., and Miller, J. *Food for Thought.**

Mulhauser, R. *More Vitamins and Minerals with Fewer Calories.**

Munro, D. C. *Man Alive — You're Half Dead.**

Murray, F. *Program Your Heart for Health.**

*"National Health Federation Bulletin."**

Newbold, H. *Vitamin C Against Cancer.**

Newton, M. *New Life Cook Book: Based on the Health and Nutritional Philosophy of the Edgar Cayce Readings.**

Null, G., and Null, S. *Complete Handbook of Nutrition.**

Null, G. *Body Pollution*, now retitled: *How to Get Rid of the Poisons in Your Body.**

*Nutrition Almanac.**

O'Brian, L. H. *Forget About Calories.**

Oski, F., and Bell, J. *Don't Drink Your Milk!**

Passwater, R. *Easy No-Flab Diet.**

Patrick, L. *How to Eat Well and Live Longer.**

Pauling, L. *Vitamin C and the Common Cold.*

Pelstring, L., and Hauck, J. *Food to Improve Your Health.**

Petrie, S., and Stone, R. *Fat Destroyer Foods: Magic Metabolic Diet.**

Pfeiffer, C. *Zinc and Other Micro-Nutrients.**

Philpott, W., and Kalita, D. K., *Brain Allergies: The Psychonutrient Connection.*[7]

Pim, L. *Invisible Additives.*[8]

*"Prevention" Magazine.**

Pritikin, N., and McGrady, P. *Pritikin Program for Diet and Exercise.**

Reuben, D. *Everything You Always Wanted to Know About Nutrition.**

Righter, C. *Your Astrological Guide to Health and Diet.**

Rodale, J. I. *Complete Book of Food and Nutrition.**

Rodale, J. I. *Complete Book of Vitamins.**

Rodale, J. I. *Happy People Rarely Get Cancer.*[2]

Rodale, J. I. *How to Grow Vegetables and Fruits by the Organic Method.**

Rodale, J. I. *Live to Eighty, Feel Like Forty.**

Rodale, J. I. *My Own Technique of Eating for Health.**

Rodale, J. I. *Our Poisoned Earth.**

Rodale, J. I. *Prostate.*[2]

Ronsard, N. *Cellulite — Those Lumps, Bumps and Bulges You Couldn't Lose Before.**

Rose, I. F. *Faith, Love and Seaweed.**

Rosenberger, A. *Eat Your Way to Better Health.**

Rosenvold, L., and Rosenvold, D. *Nutrition for Life.**

Roth, J. *Cooking for the Hyperactive Child.**

Roth, J. *Food/Depression Connection.**

Roty, J., and Philips, N. N. *Bio-Organics: Your Food and Your Health.**

Schiff, M. *Doctor Schiff's Miracle Weight Loss Guide.**

Schneour, E. *Malnourished Mind.**

Shefferman, M. *Food for Longer Living.**

Sheinkin, D., Schachter, M., and Hutton, R. *Food Connection.**

Simmons, R. *Never Say Diet Book.*

Smith, L. *Feed Your Kids Right.*[9]

Solomon, N. *Truth About Weight Control.**

Stillman, I. M., and Baker, S. S. *Doctor's Quick Inches-Off Diet.**

Stillman, I. M., and Baker, S. S. *Doctor's Quick Teenage Diet.**

Stillman, I. M., and Baker, S. S. *Doctor's Quick Weight Loss Diet.**

Stone, I. *Healing Factor, "Vitamin C" Against Disease.**

Taller, H. *Calories Don't Count.**

Tarnower, H., and Baker, S. *Complete Scarsdale Medical Diet.**

Tobe, J. H. *"No-Cook" Book.**

Toms, A. *Eat Drink and Be Healthy — The Joy of Eating Natural Foods.**

Top, J. D. *You Don't Have to be Sick.**

Turchetti, R., and Morella, J. *New Age Nutrition.**

Verrett, J., and Carper, J. *Eating May be Hazardous to Your Health: The Case Against Food Additives.**

Vitamin E for Ailing and Healthy Hearts.[1]

Vitamin E: Key to Sexual Satisfaction.[1]

Vitamin E: Your Key to a Healthy Heart.[1]

Wade, C. *Arthritis, Nutrition and Natural Therapy.*[1]

Walczak, M. *Nutrition — Applied Personally.**

Watson, G. *Nutrition and Your Mind.**

West, R. *Stop Dieting! Start Losing!**

West, R. *Teen-age Diet Book.**

Williams, R. *Nutrition Against Disease.**

Williams, R. *Nutrition in a Nutshell.**

Williams, R. *Wonderful World Within You: Your Inner Nutritional Environment.**

Wilson, M. *Double Your Energy and Live Without Fatigue.**

A

Winter, R. *A Consumer's Dictionary of Food Additives.**

Wood, H. C. *Overfed But Under-Nourished — Nutritional Aspects of Health and Disease.**

Yntema, S. *Vegetarian Baby.*

Yudkin, J. *Sweet and Dangerous.**

[1]This book was reviewed by Consumers Union and found to contain misleading information as reported in: *Health Quackery* (New York: Consumers Union, 1980).

[2]This book was reviewed and found to contain misinformation as reported in: *Nutrition Reviews*, *Special Supplement on Misinformation and Food Faddism*, July 1974.

[3]F. J. Stare and V. Aronson, Book review, in *ACSH News and Views*, November/December 1981, pp. 6-7.

[4]T. Smith, Book review, in *ACSH News and Views*, April 1980, p. 7.

[5]M. A. Cassese and F. J. Stare, Book review, in *ACSH News and Views*, January/February 1981, pp. 7, 10.

[6]E. McDowell, Behind the best sellers, *New York Times*, 23 August 1981, as reprinted in *ACSH Media Update*, Fall 1981, p. 26.

[7]B. McPherrin, Book review, in *ACSH News and Views*, May/June 1981, pp. 7, 10.

[8]D. Roll, Book review, in *ACSH News and Views*, May/June 1982, p. 14.

[9]M. Kroger, Book review, in *ACSH News and Views*, February 1980, p. 6.

APPENDIX B

Basic Chemistry Concepts

CONTENTS

This appendix is intended to provide the background in basic chemistry that you need to understand the nutrition concepts presented in this book.

Chemistry is the branch of natural science that is concerned with the description and classification of matter, with the changes that matter undergoes, and with the energy associated with these changes. **Matter** is anything that takes up space and has mass. **Energy** is the ability to do work.

Matter: The Properties of Atoms

Every substance has characteristics or properties that distinguish it from all other substances and thus give it a unique identity. These properties are both physical and chemical. The physical properties include such characteristics as color, taste, texture, and odor, as well as the temperatures at which a substance changes its state (changes from a solid to a liquid or from a liquid to a gas) and the weight of a unit volume (its density). The chemical properties of a substance have to do with how it reacts with other substances or responds to a change in its environment so that new substances with different sets of properties are produced.

A physical change is one that does not change a substance's chemical composition. For example, when ice changes to liquid water and to steam, two hydrogen atoms and one oxygen atom remain bound together in all three states. However, a chemical change does occur if an electric current is passed through water. The water disappears, and two different substances are formed: hydrogen gas, which is flammable, and oxygen gas, which supports life. Chemical changes are also referred to as **chemical reactions**.

Substances: Elements and Compounds

Molecules are the smallest particles of a substance that retain all the properties of that substance. If the molecules of a substance are composed of atoms that are all alike, the substance is an **element.** If the molecules are composed of two or more different kinds of atoms, the substance is a **compound**.

Just over 100 elements are known, and these are listed in Table 1. A familiar example is hydrogen, whose molecules are composed only of hydrogen atoms linked together in pairs (H_2). On the other hand, over a million compounds are known. An example is the sugar glucose: Each of its molecules is composed of 6 carbon, 6 oxygen, and 12 hydrogen atoms linked together in a specific arrangement (as described in Chapter 1).

The Nature of Atoms   Atoms themselves are made of smaller particles. The atomic nucleus contains **protons** (positively charged particles);

B

Table 1   Chemical Symbols for the Elements

Number of protons (atomic number)	Element	Number of electrons in outer shell	Number of protons (atomic number)	Element	Number of electrons in outer shell
1	Hydrogen (H)	1	52	Tellurium (Te)	6
2	Helium (He)	2	53	Iodine (I)	7
3	Lithium (Li)	1	54	Xenon (Xe)	8
4	Beryllium (Be)	2	55	Cesium (Cs)	1
5	Boron (B)	3	56	Barium (Ba)	2
6	Carbon (C)	4	57	Lanthanum (La)	2
7	Nitrogen (N)	5	58	Cerium (Ce)	2
8	Oxygen (O)	6	59	Praseodymium (Pr)	2
9	Fluorine (F)	7	60	Neodymium (Nd)	2
10	Neon (Ne)	8	61	Promethium (Pm)	2
11	Sodium (Na)	1	62	Samarium (Sm)	2
12	Magnesium (Mg)	2	63	Europium (Eu)	2
13	Aluminum (Al)	3	64	Gadolinium (Gd)	2
14	Silicon (Si)	4	65	Terbium (Tb)	2
15	Phosphorus (P)	5	66	Dysprosium (Dy)	2
16	Sulfur (S)	6	67	Holmium (Ho)	2
17	Chlorine (Cl)	7	68	Erbium (Er)	2
18	Argon (Ar)	8	69	Thulium (Tm)	2
19	Potassium (K)	1	70	Ytterbium (Yb)	2
20	Calcium (Ca)	2	71	Lutetium (Lu)	2
21	Scandium (Sc)	2	72	Hafnium (Hf)	2
22	Titanium (Ti)	2	73	Tantalum (Ta)	2
23	Vanadium (V)	2	74	Tungsten (W)	2
24	Chromium (Cr)	1	75	Rhenium (Re)	2
25	Manganese (Mn)	2	76	Osmium (Os)	2
26	Iron (Fe)	2	77	Iridium (Ir)	2
27	Cobalt (Co)	2	78	Platinum (Pt)	1
28	Nickel (Ni)	2	79	Gold (Au)	1
29	Copper (Cu)	1	80	Mercury (Hg)	2
30	Zinc (Zn)	2	81	Thallium (Tl)	3
31	Gallium (Ga)	3	82	Lead (Pb)	4
32	Germanium (Ge)	4	83	Bismuth (Bi)	5
33	Arsenic (As)	5	84	Polonium (Po)	6
34	Selenium (Se)	6	85	Astatine (At)	7
35	Bromine (Br)	7	86	Radon (Rn)	8
36	Krypton (Kr)	8	87	Francium (Fr)	1
37	Rubidium (Rb)	1	88	Radium (Ra)	2
38	Strontium (Sr)	2	89	Actinium (Ac)	2
39	Yttrium (Y)	2	90	Thorium (Th)	2
40	Zirconium (Zr)	2	91	Protactinium (Pa)	2
41	Niobium (Nb)	1	92	Uranium (U)	2
42	Molybdenum (Mo)	1	93	Neptunium (Np)	2
43	Technetium (Tc)	1	94	Plutonium (Pu)	2
44	Ruthenium (Ru)	1	95	Americium (Am)	2
45	Rhodium (Rh)	1	96	Curium (Cm)	2
46	Palladium (Pd)	—	97	Berkelium (Bk)	2
47	Silver (Ag)	1	98	Californium (Cf)	2
48	Cadmium (Cd)	2	99	Einsteinium (Es)	2
49	Indium (In)	3	100	Fermium (Fm)	2
50	Tin (Sn)	4	101	Mendelevium (Md)	2
51	Antimony (Sb)	5	102	Nobelium (No)	2

and **electrons** (negatively charged particles) surround the nucleus. Because opposite charges attract, the number of protons (+) in the nucleus of an atom determines the number of electrons (−) around it. The positive charge on a proton is equal to the negative charge on an electron, so that the charges cancel each other out and leave the atom neutral.

The nucleus may also include **neutrons**, subatomic particles that have no charge. Protons and neutrons are of equal mass, and together they give an atom its weight. Electrons are of negligible mass but represent the atom's chemical energy.

Each type of atom has a characteristic number of protons in its nucleus. The hydrogen atom (symbol H) is the simplest of all. It possesses a single proton, with a single electron associated with it:

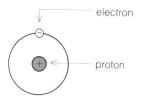

Hydrogen atom (H), atomic number 1.

Just as hydrogen always has one proton, helium always has two, lithium three, and so on. The **atomic number** of each type of atom represents the number of protons it contains. The atomic number never changes; it gives the atom its identity. All of the known atomic elements are listed in Table 1, and their atomic numbers are shown.

All atoms except hydrogen also have neutrons in their nuclei, and these contribute to their atomic weight. Helium, for example, has two neutrons in its nucleus in addition to its two protons, for a total of four nuclear particles and an atomic weight of 4. However, only the two protons are charged, and these determine the number of electrons the atom has. The number of electrons determines how the atom will chemically react with other atoms. Hence the

atomic number, not the weight, is what gives an atom its chemical nature.

Besides hydrogen, the atoms most common in living things are carbon (C), nitrogen (N), and oxygen (O), whose atomic numbers are 6, 7, and 8 respectively. Their structures are more complicated than that of hydrogen. Each possesses a number of electrons equal to the number of protons in its nucleus. These electrons have two energy levels, symbolized in the following diagrams as two orbits, or shells:

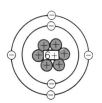

Carbon atom (C), atomic number 6.

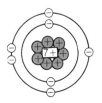

Nitrogen atom (N), atomic number 7.

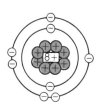

Oxygen atom (O), atomic number 8.

In this and all diagrams of atoms that follow, only the protons and electrons are shown. The neutrons, which contribute only to atomic weight, not to charge, are omitted.

The shells closest to the nucleus are occupied by electrons of lesser energy. Thus the two electrons in the first shells of carbon, nitrogen, and oxygen have less energy than the electrons in their second or outer shells. Also, the first shell can hold only two electrons; when it is full, it is in a very stable energy state, or a state of lowest energy.

The most important structural feature of an atom for determining its chemical behavior is the number of electrons in its outer shell. The first shell is full when it is occupied by two electrons, so an atom with three protons has a filled first shell. Its third electron posssesses greater energy and has a greater probability of being farther from the nucleus. In other words, the third electron is not so tightly bound as the first two and has a high probability of flying off to join other substances in chemical reactions. As a matter of fact, lithium, atomic number 3, is just such a highly reactive element.

The second shell is completely full when it has eight electrons. A substance that has a full outer shell tends to enter into no chemical reactions. Atomic number 10, neon, is a chemically inert substance, because its outer shell is complete. Fluorine, atomic number 9, has a great tendency to draw an electron from other substances to complete its outer shell and thus is highly reactive. Carbon has a half-full outer shell, which helps explain its great versatility; it can combine with other elements in a great variety of ways to form a large number of compounds.

Atoms seek to reach a state of maximum stability or of lowest energy in the same way that a ball will roll down a hill until it reaches the lowest place. An atom achieves a state of maximum stability by two means:

- By having a filled outer shell (occupied by the maximum number of electrons it can hold)
- By being electrically neutral

In order to achieve this stability, an atom may become bonded to other atoms.

Chemical Bonding

Atoms often complete their outer shells by sharing electrons with other atoms. In order to complete its outer shell, a carbon atom requires four electrons. A hydrogen atom requires one. Thus when a carbon atom shares electrons with four hydrogen atoms, each completes its outer shell:

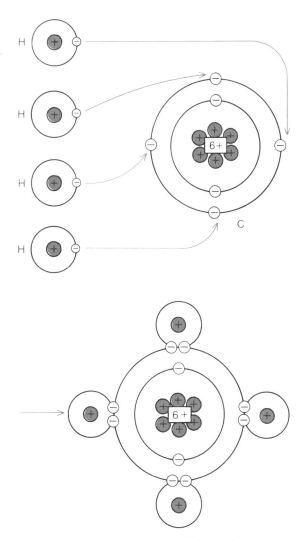

Methane molecule. The **chemical formula** for methane is CH_4. (Note that with the sharing of electrons, every atom has a filled outer shell.)

This electron sharing binds the atoms together and satisfies the conditions of maximum stability for the molecule: The outer shell of each atom is complete, since hydrogen effectively has the required two electrons in its first and outer shell and carbon has eight electrons in its second and outer shell; and the molecule is electrically neutral, with a total of ten protons and ten electrons.

Bonds that involve the sharing of electrons, like the bond between carbon and hydrogen, are the most stable kind of association that atoms can form with one another. They are sometimes called **covalent bonds**, and the resulting combinations of atoms are called molecules. A single pair of shared electrons forms a **single bond**. A simplified way to represent a single bond is with a single line. Thus the structure of methane could be represented (ignoring the inner-shell electrons that do not participate in bonding):

$$
\begin{array}{c}
\text{H} \\
| \\
\text{H} - \text{C} - \text{H} \\
| \\
\text{H}
\end{array}
$$

Methane (**chemical structure**).

Similarly, one nitrogen atom and three hydrogen atoms can share electrons to form one molecule of ammonia:

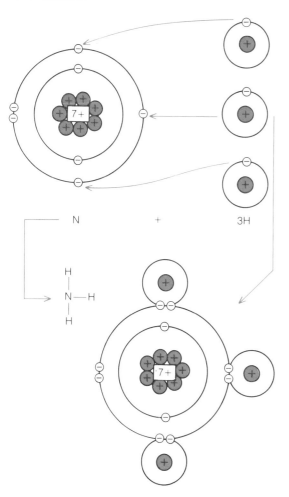

Ammonia molecule (NH_3). (Count the electrons in each atom's outer shell.)

Similarly, one oxygen atom may be bonded to two hydrogen atoms to form one molecule of water:

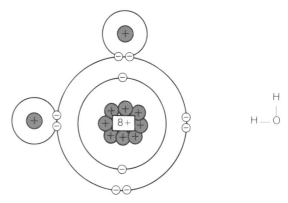

Water molecule (H_2O).

When two oxygen atoms form a molecule of oxygen, they must share two pairs of electrons. This **double bond** may be represented as two single lines:

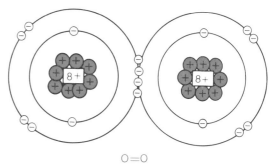

O=O

Oxygen molecule (O_2).

Small atoms form the tightest, most stable bonds. H, O, N, and C are the smallest atoms capable of forming one, two, three, and four electron-pair bonds (respectively). This fact is the basis for the simple statement in Chapter 1 that when you draw compounds containing these atoms, hydrogen must always have one, oxygen two, nitrogen three, and carbon four lines radiating to other atoms:

B

H—   —O—   N—   —C

The stability of the associations between these small atoms and the versatility with which they can combine make them very common in living things. Interestingly, all cells, whether they come from animals, plants, or bacteria, contain the same elements in very nearly the same proportions.[1] The atomic elements found in living things are shown in Table 2.

Formation of Ions

An atom such as sodium (Na, atomic number 11) is more likely to lose an electron than to share electrons. Sodium possesses a filled inner shell of two electrons and a filled second shell of eight; there is only one electron in its outermost shell:

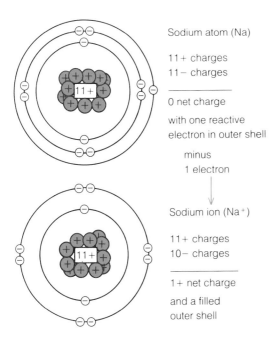

Sodium atom (Na)

11+ charges
11− charges
—————
0 net charge
with one reactive
electron in outer shell

minus
1 electron

Sodium ion (Na⁺)

11+ charges
10− charges
—————
1+ net charge
and a filled
outer shell

If sodium loses this electron, it satisfies one condition for stability: a filled outer shell (now its second shell counts as the outer shell). However, it is not electrically neutral. It has 11 protons (positive) and only 10 electrons (negative). It therefore is positively charged. Such a structure is called an **ion**—an atom or molecule that has lost or gained one or more electrons and so is electrically charged.

An atom such as chlorine (Cl, atomic number 17) is likely to gain an electron for a similar reason. It possesses filled inner shells of two and eight electrons and has seven electrons in its outermost shell. Gaining one electron makes its outer shell complete and thus makes it a negatively charged ion:

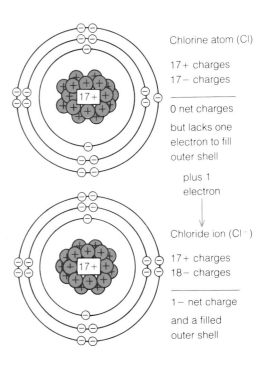

Chlorine atom (Cl)

17+ charges
17− charges
—————
0 net charges

but lacks one
electron to fill
outer shell

plus 1
electron

Chloride ion (Cl⁻)

17+ charges
18− charges
—————
1− net charge
and a filled
outer shell

A positively charged ion such as a sodium ion (Na⁺) is a **cation**; a negatively charged ion such as chloride ion (Cl⁻) is an **anion**. Cations and anions attract one another to form **salts**:

[1]V. Rodwell, Appendix: Organic chemistry (a brief review), in *Review of Physiological Chemistry*, ed. H. Harper (Los Altos, Calif.: Lange Medical Publications, 1971), p. 499.

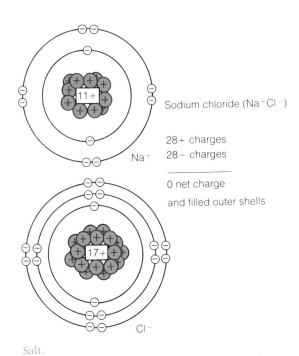

Sodium chloride (Na⁺Cl⁻)

28+ charges
28− charges
_____
0 net charge

and filled outer shells

Salt.

Table 2   Elemental Composition of Living Cells

Element	Chemical symbol	Composition by weight (%)
Oxygen	O	65
Carbon	C	18
Hydrogen	H	10
Nitrogen	N	3
Calcium	Ca	1.5
Phosphorus	P	1.0
Sulfur	S	0.25
Sodium	Na	0.15
Magnesium	Mg	0.05
TOTAL		99.30*

*The remaining 0.70 percent by weight is contributed by the trace elements: copper (Cu), zinc (Zn), selenium (Se), molybdenum (Mo), fluorine (F), chlorine (Cl), iodine (I), manganese (Mn), cobalt (Co), iron (Fe). There are also variable traces of some of the following in cells: lithium (Li), strontium (Sr), aluminum (Al), silicon (Si), lead (Pb), vanadium (V), arsenic (As), bromium (Br), and others.

With all its electrons, sodium is a shiny, highly reactive metal; chlorine is the poisonous greenish-yellow gas that was used in World War I. But after they have transferred electrons, they form the harmless white salt familiar to you as table salt, or sodium chloride (Na⁺Cl⁻). The dramatic difference illustrates how profoundly the electron arrangement can influence the nature of a substance. The wide distribution of salt in nature attests to the stability of the union between the ions. Each meets the other's needs (a good marriage).

When dry, salt exists as crystals; its ions are stacked very regularly into a lattice, with positive and negative ions alternating in a sort of three-dimensional checkerboard structure. In water, however, the salt quickly dissolves, and its ions separate from each other, forming an electrolyte solution in which they move about freely. Covalently bonded molecules do not dissociate like this in water solution. Molecules and ion pairs (salts) behave very differently in many ways.

An ion can also be a group of atoms bound together in such a way that the group has a charge and enters into reactions as a single unit. Many such groups are active in the fluids of the body: The bicarbonate ion is composed of five atoms—one H, one C, and three Os—and has a net charge of -1 (HCO_3^-). Another important ion of this type is a phosphate ion with one H, one P, and four Os, and a net charge of -2 (HPO_4^{-2}). (For a description of the behavior of salts in water, electrolytes, and osmosis, which follows from this, see Chapter 14.)

Whereas many elements have only one configuration in the outer shell and thus only one way they can bond with other elements, some elements have the possibility of varied configurations. Iron is such an element. Under some conditions iron has two electrons in its outer shell, and under other circumstances it has three. If iron has two electrons in its outer shell and loses them, it then has a net charge of $+2$, and we call it ferrous iron. If it has three electrons in its outer shell and donates them, it becomes the $+3$ ion, or ferric iron.

(Note: It is important to remember that a positive charge on an ion means that negative charges—electrons—have been lost and not that positive charges have been added. If you could add two protons to an iron atom, they would go to the nucleus, adding 2 to its atomic number. Then it would no longer be iron, atomic number 26, but nickel, atomic number 28—and it would gain two more electrons to balance its positive charges.)

Ferrous iron.

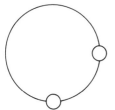 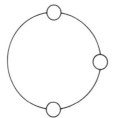

Ferrous iron (Fe^{++}) (had 2 outer-shell electrons but has lost them)

26+ charges
24− charges
_____
2+ net charge

Ferric iron (Fe^{+++}) (had 3 outer-shell electrons but has lost them)

26+ charges
23− charges
_____
3+ net charge

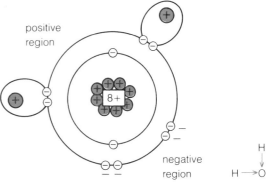

positive region

negative region

A polar molecule

H
↓
H—→O

The arrows show displacement of electrons toward the O nucleus, so the negative region is near the O, the positive region near the Hs.

Water (H$_2$O).

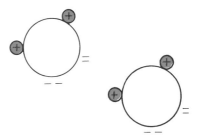

Water, Acids, and Bases

The water molecule is electrically neutral, having an equal number of protons and electrons. However, if the hydrogen atom is to share its one electron with oxygen, that electron must spend most of its time near the large positively charged oxygen nucleus on the oxygen side of the hydrogen atom. This leaves the positive proton (nucleus of the hydrogen atom) exposed on the outer part of the water molecule. We know, too, that the two hydrogens both bond toward the same side of the oxygen. These two ideas explain the fact that water molecules are **polar**: They have regions of more positive and more negative charge.

Polar molecules like water are drawn to one another by the attractive forces between the positive polar areas of one and the negative poles of another. These attractive forces, sometimes known as polar or **hydrogen bonds**, occur

among many molecules and also within the different parts of single large molecules. Although very weak in comparison to covalent bonds, polar bonds may occur in such abundance that they become exceedingly important in determining the structure of such large molecules as proteins and DNA.

Water molecules have a slight tendency to ionize, separating into positive and negative ions. In any given amount of pure water, a small but constant number of these ions is present, and the number of positive ions exactly equals the number of negative ions.

An **acid** is a substance that releases H$^+$ ions (protons) in water solution. Hydrochloric acid (HCl) is such a substance, because it dissociates in water solution into H$^+$ and Cl$^-$ ions. Acetic acid is also an acid, because it ionizes in water to acetate ions and free H$^+$:

```
    H   O                    H   O
    |   ||                   |   ||
H—C—C—O—H  ——>  H—C—C—O⁻   +   H⁺
    |                        |
    H                        H
```

Acetic acid dissociates into an acetate ion and a hydrogen ion.

The more H^+ ions free in a water solution, the stronger the acid.

Chemists define degrees of acidity by means of the **pH scale.** The pH scale runs from 0 to 14. A pH of 1 is extremely acidic, 7 is neutral, and 13 is very basic. There is a tenfold difference between points on this scale. A solution with pH 3, for example, has *ten times* as many H^+ ions as a solution with pH 4. At pH 7, the concentrations of free H^+ and OH^- are exactly the same, 1/10,000,000 moles per liter (10^{-7} moles per liter).[2] At pH 4, the concentration of free H^+ ions is 1/10,000 (10^{-4}) moles per liter. This is a higher concentration of H^+ ions, and the solution is therefore acidic.

A **base** is a substance that can soak up or combine with H^+ ions, thus reducing the acidity of a solution. The compound ammonia is such a substance. The ammonia molecule has two electrons that are not shared with any other atom; a hydrogen ion (H^+) is just a naked proton with no shell of electrons at all. Thus the proton readily combines with the ammonia molecule to form an ammonium ion and so is withdrawn from the solution as a free proton and no longer contributes to its acidity. Many

```
    H                             H
    |                             |
 :N—H      +   H⁺  ——>   H—N⁺—H
    |                             |
    H                             H
```

The two dots here represent the two electrons not shared with another atom. These are ordinarily not shown in chemical structure drawings. Compare this with the earlier diagram of an ammonia molecule.

Ammonia captures a hydrogen ion from water.

[2] A mole is a certain number (about 6×10^{23}) molecules. The pH of a solution is defined as the negative logarithm of the hydrogen ion concentration of the solution. Thus if the concentration is 10^{-2} (moles per liter), the pH is 2; if 10^{-8}, the pH is 8; and so on.

compounds containing nitrogen are important bases in living systems. Acids and bases neutralize each other to produce substances that are neither acid nor base.

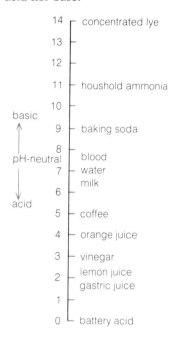

Note: Each step is ten times as concentrated in base (1/10 as acid) as the one below it.

Chemical Reactions

A chemical reaction or chemical change is one that results in the disappearance of substances and the formation of new ones. Almost all such reactions involve a change in the bonding of atoms: Old bonds are broken, and new ones are formed. The nuclei of atoms are never involved in chemical reactions—only their outer-shell electrons. At the end of a reaction there is always the same number of atoms of each type as there was at the beginning. For example, two hydrogen molecules can react with one oxygen molecule to form two water molecules. In this reaction two substances (hydrogen and oxygen) disappear, and a new one (water) is formed, but at the end of the reaction there are still four H atoms and two O atoms, just as there were at the beginning. The only difference is in how they are linked.

B

Hydrogen and oxygen react to form water:

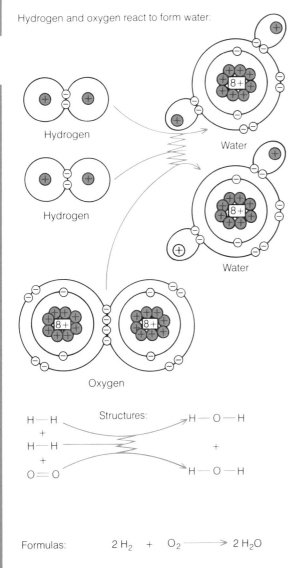

In a few instances chemical reactions involve not the relinking of atoms but the exchanging of electrons among atoms. The transfer of an electron from one molecule to another is known as an **oxidation-reduction reaction**. The loss of an electron is known as **oxidation**, and the compound that loses the electron is said to be oxidized. (The reason for the name is that many substances—such as carbohydrates—lose electrons only when oxygen is available to accept them.) **Reduction** is the gain of an electron. Oxidation and reduction take place simultaneously, because an electron that is lost by one atom is accepted by another.

Sometimes an electron travels in company with a proton as part of a hydrogen atom. In that case, oxidation involves the removal of the hydrogen ion (proton) and its electron from one substance; reduction involves the transfer of both a hydrogen ion and an electron to another substance. (The reduction of oxygen—the addition of hydrogen atoms—thus results in the formation of water.)

If a reaction results in a net increase in chemical bond energy, it is referred to as a reduction reaction. For example, the chief result of photosynthesis is the reduction of carbon (from carbon dioxide to the carbon in sugar). Conversely, if there is a net decrease in chemical bond energy (with a release of energy as heat or light), the reaction is often referred to as an oxidation process. For example, sugar is oxidized in the body to carbon dioxide and water.

Chemical reactions tend to occur spontaneously if the end products are in a lower energy state (are more stable) than the reacting compounds were. These reactions give off energy, often in the form of heat, as they occur. The generation of heat by wood burning in a fireplace and the maintenance of human body warmth both depend on energy-yielding chemical reactions. They are "downhill" reactions: They occur easily, although they may require some activation energy to get them started, just as a ball requires a push to get started rolling downhill (see Highlight 7).

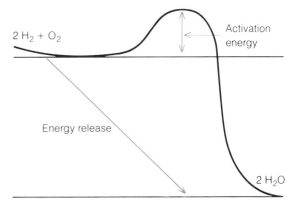

"Uphill" reactions, in which the products contain more energy than the reacting compounds started with, do not occur until an energy source is provided. An example of such an energy source is the sunlight used in photosynthesis, where carbon dioxide and water (low-energy compounds) are combined to form the sugar glucose (a higher-energy compound). Another example is the use of the energy in glucose to combine two low-energy compounds in the body into the high-energy compound ATP (see Highlight 7). The energy in ATP may be used to power many other energy-requiring, "uphill" reactions. Clearly, any of many different molecules can be used as a temporary storage place for energy.

Neither downhill nor uphill reactions occur until something sets them off (activation) or until a path is provided for them to follow. The body uses enzymes as a means of providing paths and controlling its chemical reactions (see Chapter 3). By controlling the availability and the action of its enzymes, the body can "decide" which chemical reactions to prevent and which to promote.

APPENDIX C

Patient/Client Education Materials

The following is a collection of free and inexpensive booklets, pamphlets, and films that you might like to recommend to clients and friends. (For references from which to build yourself a professional library, see Appendix J; for books *not* recommended, Appendix A.) Addresses and prices are subject to change.

General references on diet include:

● Stare, F. J. and Whelan, E. M. *Eat OK — Feel OK: Food Facts & Your Health*. North Quincy, Mass.: Christopher Publishing House, 1978 ($9.75).

● White, P. L. and Selvey, N. *Let's Talk about Food*. Littleton, Mass.: P. F. G., Inc., 1977 ($6.95 cloth, $5.00 paper).

● *Nutrition Source Book*. Rosemont, Ill.: National Dairy Council, 1978 (free).

● *A Diet for Today*, a booklet available from Dept. X, P.O. Box 307, Coventry, CT 06238 (free).

● *Sensible Eating Can Be Delicious* (booklet). Fleischmann's Margarines, 1976 (address in Appendix J).

Suggestions for controlling dietary fat can be found in:

● *Planning Fat-Controlled Meals* (booklet). General Mills, Nutrition Department, 1972.

● *Fats in Food and Diet* (booklet). Agriculture Information Bulletin: #361. Washington, D.C.: Government Printing Office, 1974 ($.30).

● *Dietary Control of Cholesterol* (booklet). Fleischmann's Margarines, 1969 (address in Appendix J).

Check the references at the end of Chapter 2, too.

For vegetarians, some references are listed at the end of Highlight 4.

Strategies for dealing with stress (not only related to diet) are offered at the end of Highlight 6.

Some good books on weight control are listed at the end of Chapter 8; a few shorter references are:

● *Healthy Approach to Slimming*. Monroe, Wisc.: American Medical Association, 1978 ($1.00).

● *Obesity*. Washington, D.C.: Nutrition Foundation, Office of Education, undated (free).

● Jordan, H. A. *Eating is Okay!* New York, N.Y.: New American Library, 1978 ($1.50 paper).

For information and referrals on alcohol (not only nutrition-related), look up *Alcohol* in the telephone book, or write to the National Council on Alcoholism or to the Clearinghouse for Alcohol Information (both addresses are in Appendix J). A recommended reference is:

● *Alcoholism* (pamphlet). Metropolitan Life Insurance Company (local offices in many cities).

To help clients control high blood pressure, suggest:

● *What you should know about ... The National Program to Control High Blood Pressure* (leaflet). NIH publication no. 80-632. Bethesda, Md.: Public Health Service, National Heart, Lung, and Blood Institute, 1979.

● *High Blood Pressure Facts and Fiction* (leaflet). NIH publication no. 80-1218. Bethesda, Md.: Public Health Service, National Heart, Lung, and Blood Institute, undated.

• *Sensible Ways to Cut Down on Sodium* (leaflet), available from Adolph's, Ltd., Consumer Services Dept., 33 Benedict Place, Greenwich, CT 06830.

• *Special Recipes for Low Sodium Diets* (booklet). White Plains, N.Y.: General Foods, undated.

There's a reference at the end of Chapter 12, too. Additional information can be obtained from the American Heart Association (address in Appendix J).

To help the new ex-smoker not to gain weight, offer these references from the American Heart Association (address in Appendix J):

• *Guidelines for a Weight Control Component in a Smoking Cessation Program* (booklet).

• *Weight Control Guidance in Smoking Cessation* (leaflet).

For people with physical disabilities:

• *Mealtime Manual for People with Disabilities and the Aging*. Camden, N.J.: Campbell Soup Co., undated ($3.25).

• *Adaptation and Techniques for the Disabled Homemaker*. Minneapolis, Minn.: Sister Kenny Institute, undated ($2.95).

• *Do It Yourself Again — Self-Help Devices for the Stroke Patient*. Dallas, Texas: American Heart Association, undated (free).

• *A Manual on Food and Nutrition for the Disabled*. Toronto, Ontario: Ryerson Polytechnical Institute, undated ($4.95; $4.00 prepaid).

For cancer patients and their families:

• *Chemotherapy and you, a guide to self-help during treatment* (booklet). NIH publication no. 81-1136, Bethesda, Md.: U.S. Department of Health and Human Services, Public Health Service, National Cancer Institute, 1980 (free).

• *Diet and Nutrition, a resource for parents of children with cancer* (booklet). NIH publication no. 80-2038, Bethesda, Md.: U.S. Department of Health and Human Services, Public Health Service, National Cancer Institute, 1979 (free).

• *Eating Hints, Recipes and Tips for Better Nutrition During Cancer Treatment* (spiral bound booklet). Bethesda, Md.: Office of Cancer Communications, National Cancer Institute, 1980.

• *Nutrition for Patients receiving Chemotherapy and Radiation Treatments* (booklet). American Cancer Society, 1974.

Several booklets available for patients with allergies include:

• American Dietetic Association. *Allergy Recipes*. Chicago: ADA, 1969. Address in Appendix J.

• U.S. Department of Agriculture. *Baking for People with Food Allergies*, Home and Garden Bulletin No. 146, rev. ed. Washington, D.C.: USDA, 1975.

• Sheedy, C. H., and Keifetz, N. *Cooking for Your Celiac Child*. New York: Dial, 1969.

• Wood, N. M. *Gourmet Food on a Wheat Free Diet*. Springfield: Charles C. Thomas, 1972.

• Frazier, C. A. *Coping with Food Allergy*. New York: New York Times Co., 1974.

• Sainsbury, I. S. *The Milk-Free and Milk-Free, Egg-Free Cookbook*. Springfield: Charles C. Thomas, 1974.

• *Wheat, Milk and Egg Free Recipes*. Consumer Services Department, Quaker Oats Company, Chicago, IL 60654.

On pregnancy —

• *Inside My Mom*, a set of about 80 slides with a cassette, prepared by the March of Dimes.

Inside My Mom is a delightful description of pregnancy from the fetus's point of view, intended to motivate the pregnant woman to eat right. It is available from the local March of Dimes office or from the National Foundation, March of Dimes, PO Box 2000, White Plains, NY 1060. The March of Dimes has been very active in working to prevent birth defects, and you might inquire what other materials they have available.

A booklet on nutrition for pregnant women and parents that you can recommend with confidence is:

● Alfin-Slater, R. B., Aftergood, L., and Ashley, J. *Nutrition and Motherhood*. Available from PO Box 2160, 6931 Van Nuys Blvd., Van Nuys, CA 91405, for $2.95.

For the breastfeeding mother, the USDHEW makes available a short (twenty-two-page) how-to booklet:

● Breast feeding. DHEW publication no. (HSA) 79-5109. Write to the U.S. Government Printing Office (see Appendix J).

An international organization of women who believe in breastfeeding and who help each other is the LaLeche League, 9616 Minneapolis Avenue, Franklin Park, IL 60131.

About infants —

● *First Foods*, a 14-minute color film on feeding babies during their first year, excellent for showing in clinics, prenatal classes, etc., is available from the Society for Nutrition Education (address in Appendix J).

● A handy 50-page record-keeping booklet with month-by-month instructions to parents on infant feeding, *What Shall I Feed My Baby?* is available from USDA. Ask for Program Aid no. 1281 (June 1981).

● Heslin, J. A., and Natow, A. F. *No-Nonsense Nutrition: For Your Baby's First Year*. Boston: CBI Publishing, 1978. This is a good paperback on infant feeding for healthy babies.

Small items that we have also found useful are:

● *Food: From Birth to Birthday*, a 19-page pamphlet available from the National Dairy Council, Rosemont, IL 60018. Publication number B205 (2), 1977.

● *Food with Love*, a 56-page booklet available free from the Pennsylvania Department of Education, Division of Food Service, 8 South 13th Street, Pittsburgh, PA 15203.

Parents Magazine makes available $58 worth of excellent filmstrip-cassette sets mostly for parental education. Write Department F, 52 Vanderbilt Avenue, New York, NY 10017.

On teaching children to resist the allure of television commercials:

● *Seeing through Commercials: A Children's Guide to TV Advertising* is a 1976 film available (for $220) from Vision Films, PO Box 48896, Los Angeles, CA 90048.

● A booklet, *Buy and Buy*, to help 9- to 13-year-olds learn to see through cereal commercials, is available for $.55 from MVR Hall, Cornell University, Ithaca, NY 14853.

● A 12-page foldout, *Children and Television*, by Action for Children's Television (ACT), can be obtained for $.50 by writing to ACT, 46 Austin Street, Newtonville, MA 02160. You might want to inquire what other resources they have.

For people concerned with the nutrition education of children, the national Nutrition Education Clearing House puts out a listing of reference materials. For example:

● *Secondary Teaching Materials and Teacher References*, rev. ed. Nutrition Education Resource Series 4. Berkeley, Calif.: Society for Nutrition Education, 1977 (address in Appendix J).

For people who feed children:

● Goodwin, M. T., and Pollen, G. *Creative Food Experiences for Children*. Washington, D.C.: Center for Science in the Public Interest, 1974 (paperback). Available from Box 3099, Washington, D.C. 20010. This paperback encourages children to participate in the preparation of healthful foods.

● Lansky, V. *The Taming of the C.A.N.D.Y.*

Monster. Wayzata, Minn.: Meadowbrook Press, 1978 (paperback). This is an unusual cookbook that encourages creativity in the kitchen and helps to solve such problems as what-to-put-in-the-lunchbox.

● Williams, J., and Smith, M. *Middle Childhood: Behavior and Development*, 2nd ed. New York: Macmillan, 1980.

For the parents of a child with insulin-dependent diabetes there are many pointers of value in a series of three articles that appeared in *Nutrition Today*.

● Jackson, R. L. Insulin-dependent diabetes in children and young adults. *Nutrition Today*, November/December 1979, pp. 26-32.

● Jackson, R. L. Management and treatment of the child with diabetes. *Nutrition Today*, March/April 1980, pp. 6-12, 27-29.

● Jackson, R. L. Education of the parents of a child with diabetes. *Nutrition Today*, May/June 1980, pp. 30-34.

The A.D.A. Forecast is a bimonthly magazine for diabetics available through the American Diabetes Association (address in Appendix J). See also Appendix A (Books Not Recommended) and Appendix J (Recommended Nutrition References).

Books and booklets of special interest to the athlete are:

● Katch, F. I.; McArdle, W. D.; and Boylan, B. R. *Getting in Shape, an Optimum Approach to Fitness and Weight Control*. Boston: Houghton Mifflin, 1979.

● Smith, N. J. *Food for Sport*. Palo Alto, Calif.: Bull Publishing, 1976.

● Williams, M. H. *Nutritional Aspects of Human Physical and Athletic Performance*. Springfield, Ill.: Charles C. Thomas, 1976.

● *Nutrition for Athletes*, available from the American Alliance for Health, Physical Education, and Recreation, 1201 16th Street NW, Washington, DC 20036.

Four excellent articles on nutrition for the athlete appeared in Nutrition Today, November/December 1979:

● Hanley, D. F., Jr., Athletic training — and how diet affects it; Vitousek, S. H., Is more better?; Hursh, L. M., Practical hints about feeding athletes; and Hanley, D. F., Jr., Basic diet guidance for athletes.

Practical pointers on buying, preparing, and cooking food can be found in:

● Peterkin, B. *Your Money's Worth in Foods*.

This 29-page pamphlet is available for $.60 from Home and Garden Bulletin, U.S. Government Printing Office, Washington, DC 20402.

● Nidetch, J. *Weight Watchers Program Cookbook*. Great Neck, N.Y.: Hearthside Press, 1973.

Although originally intended for dieters, the Weight Watchers book is useful for older people. Many of the recipes are for one or two servings. Nidetch has experimented with standard "down home" recipes to lower saturated fat and sugar content, thus enhancing their value for someone trying to eat in line with the *Dietary Guidelines*. Her dessert recipes using dry skimmed milk are especially recommended.

For help in detecting and avoiding fraudulent products and claims, see U.S. Senate, Special Committee on Aging, *Frauds and Deceptions Affecting the Elderly*, a publication available from the U.S. Government Printing Office, Washington, DC 20402.

For help in finding all the retirement communities in your area, contact Retirement, Research, and Welfare Association, Andrus Building, 215 Long Beach Boulevard, Long Beach, CA 90802.

APPENDIX D

Aids to Calculation

CONTENTS

D

This appendix gives examples of solutions to each type of mathematical problem encountered in the text. The steps toward the solutions are especially adapted for the use of pocket calculators.

Conversion Factors and Cancellation of Units

Conversion factors are useful mathematical tools in everyday calculations, especially as we move from the British system of measurement to the metric system. (Both systems are described at the end of this appendix.)

A conversion factor is a fraction in which the numerator and the denominator use different units for the same quantity. For example, 4 c and 1 qt (U.S.) are equivalent amounts.[1] The conversion factor would be either:

$$\frac{4\ c}{1\ qt} \quad or \quad \frac{1\ qt}{4\ c}$$

Since both fractions equal one, measurements can be multiplied by either factor without changing the value of the measurement.

[1] The imperial quart, used in Canada, is equal to 5 c. The Canadian student should adjust the following calculations accordingly.

For example, how many cups are in 2 qt?

$$2\ qt\ \times\ \frac{4\ c}{1\ qt}\ =\ 8\ c$$

(The Canadian student should get an answer of 10 c.) The factor used in this example was chosen because we wanted the answer to be in cups; thus cups had to be in the numerator of the factor.

A way of confirming that the problem is stated correctly is to cancel the units in the same manner that numerals are canceled in a problem involving multiplication of fractions. The unit that cannot be canceled is the one that will appear in the answer. For example:

$$\cancel{qts}\ \times\ \frac{cups}{\cancel{qts}}\ =\ cups$$

Following are two examples of problems commonly encountered in a nutrition course; they illustrate the use of conversion factors and cancellation of units.

Example 1   Convert your weight in pounds to kilograms (see the inside back cover for conversion factors). Say that you weigh 130 pounds. Because the answer you are seeking should be in kilograms, kilograms must remain uncanceled and in the numerator.

$$130\ \cancel{lb}\ \times\ \frac{1\ kg}{2.2\ \cancel{lb}}\ =\ \frac{130\ kg}{2.2}\ =\ \square$$

This calculation would be fed into a calculator as 130 ÷ 2.2; the number you would get is 59.09. However, this answer is unacceptable, because 59.09 denotes an accuracy of measurement not present in the original measurement (130 pounds). A more acceptable answer is either 59 or 60 kilograms.[2]

Example 2   Determine how many grams of protein you should consume each day in order to meet the recommended intake for protein (see Appendix O). The conversion factor would be either:

$$\frac{.8 \text{ g protein}}{1 \text{ kg ideal body weight}}$$

or

$$\frac{1 \text{ kg ideal body weight}}{.8 \text{ g protein}}$$

For this example, say that your ideal weight is 115 pounds (see the inside back cover). Thus:

$$\frac{115 \text{ lb}}{\text{ideal weight}} \times \frac{1 \text{ kg}}{2.2 \text{ lb}} \times \frac{.8 \text{ g protein}}{1 \text{ kg ideal weight}} = \square$$

Note that cancellation of units "kg," "lb," "ideal weight," leaves "grams protein" uncancelled and in the numerator.

The actual calculation: $\frac{115 \times .8 \text{ g protein}}{2.2} = \square$

For a 115 pound adult 42 g protein per day would meet the recommended intake.

---

[2]The degree of accuracy of a measurement is reflected in the recording of that measurement and is not altered by any subsequent calculations. The measurement 130 pounds denotes to the reader that the person's weight is about 130 pounds. If the person's weight had been very accurately determined and if that degree of accuracy had been considered necessary, the weight would have been recorded as 130.0, signifying that the weight was exactly 130.0 pounds, correct to a tenth of a pound. Any mathematical calculation with a measurement does not improve the accuracy of the original measurement, and the recording of answers should reflect this. In this example, 59.09 kilograms would indicate that the weight is correct to a hundredth of a kilogram, which is impossible given the fact that the original measurement was not that accurate. Either 59 kg or 60 kg would more properly reflect the truth.

Ratio and Proportion

Some students find the ratio and proportion method convenient in many calculations in nutrition courses (as when seeking the amount of saturated fat in a 4-oz broiled hamburger although Appendix H gives the amount in a 3-oz hamburger). A proportion statement is a statement that a ratio, say 2:3, is equal to another ratio, say 4:6. If one of the four numbers in a proportion is unknown and the other three are known, the unknown number can be calculated using simple algebra. Suppose that the number 6 is unknown in the above proportion but that 2, 3, and 4 are known. You would think, "2 is to 3 as 4 is to what number?" This would be written:

$$\frac{2}{3} = \frac{4}{x}$$

The simple algebra:

$$2x = 4 \times 3$$
$$x = \frac{4 \times 3}{2}$$
$$x = 6$$

When stating a problem using ratio and proportion, be sure that the units of measure are the same on both sides of the equation.

Example 3   How many grams of saturated fat are contained in a 4-oz broiled hamburger? By consulting Appendix H, you can find out that a 3-oz broiled hamburger contains 8 g saturated fat. Thus:

$$\frac{3 \text{ oz hamburger}}{8 \text{ g saturated fat}} = \frac{4 \text{ oz hamburger}}{x \text{ g saturated fat}}$$
$$3x = 4 \times 8$$
$$x = \frac{4 \times 8}{3}$$

Note: $\frac{oz}{g} = \frac{oz}{g}$. The units of measure are the same on both sides of the equation.

$$\frac{4 \times 8}{3} = \square$$

Answer: There are 11 g saturated fat in a 4-oz broiled hamburger.

Example 4   Calculate the P:S ratio of a diet that contains 80 g of saturated fatty acid and 32 g of linoleic acid.

$$\frac{\text{32 g polyunsaturated fatty acid}}{\text{80 g saturated fatty acid}} = \frac{32}{80} = \square$$

The P:S ratio in this case is 0.4, which denotes a diet relatively high in saturated fat. For every gram of saturated fat, this person is consuming 0.4 g of polyunsaturated fat, a ratio of 0.4:1.0.

Finding Percent

To find what percentage a part is of a whole, express the relationship of the part to the whole as a fraction, multiply by 100, and reduce to the simplest terms. In the fraction, the figure that represents the whole amount goes into the denominator, and the figure representing the part of the whole that you are concerned with becomes the numerator.

Example 5   Calculate what percentage of your carbohydrate kcalories come from sweets. Say that you normally consume 850 kcal from carbohydrates and 175 kcal from sweets.

$$\frac{\text{175 kcal from sweets}}{\text{850 kcal from all carbohydrates}} \times 100 =$$

$$\frac{175 \times 100}{850} = \square$$

Answer: 21 percent of the kcalories from carbohydrates are derived from sweets.

Systems of Measurement

There are and have been many systems of measurement, but the most important to us are the metric system and the British system.

The Metric System   The metric system is a uniform, international system of measure. It is simple to use since, like the monetary system in the United States and Canada, it is a decimal system.

● *Length units.*
  1 meter (m) = 100 centimeters (cm)
  1,000 meters = 1 kilometer (km)
● *Weight units.*
  1 kilogram (kg) = 1,000 grams (gm or g)
  1 g = 1,000 milligrams (mg)
  1 mg = 1,000 micrograms (μg)
● *Volume units.*
  1 liter (l) = 1,000 milliliters (ml)
  1 milliliter = 1 cubic centimeter (cc)
● *Temperature units.* The Celsius thermometer scale is based on 100 equal divisions between the point at which pure water turns to ice ($0°$ C) and the point at which it boils ($100°$ C) at standard atmospheric pressure. Temperatures recorded in this system are recorded as degrees Celsius ($°$ C). This scale, also known as the centigrade scale, is used for all scientific work.
● *Energy units.* The Committee on Nomenclature of the American Institute of Nutrition in 1970 recommended that the term kilojoule (kJ) replace the kilocalorie (kcal) as soon as practicable. A kilocalorie is the amount of energy required to raise a kilogram of pure water one degree on the Celsius scale. A kilojoule is the amount of energy expended when a kilogram is moved one meter by a force of one Newton.

$$1 \text{ kcal} = 4.184 \text{ kJ}$$

Further information on the metric system can be obtained by writing to the Metric Information Office of the National Bureau of Standards, Washington, D.C. 20234.

The British System   The British system is not a decimal system.

● *Length units.*
  1 foot (ft) = 12 inches (in)
  1 yard (yd) = 3 feet
● *Weight units.*
  1 pound (lb) = 16 ounces (oz)
● *Volume units.*
  3 teaspoons (tsp) = 1 tablespoon (tbsp)
  16 tbsp = 1 cup (c)
  1 c = 8 fluid ounces (fl oz)
  4 c = 1 quart (qt)
  5 c = 1 imperial quart (qt), Canada

● *Temperature units.* The Fahrenheit thermometer scale is based on 180 divisions between the point at which pure water turns to ice (32° F) and the point at which pure water boils (212° F) at standard atmospheric pressure. This scale is commonly used in the United States and Canada for everyday household use but is not used for scientific measurements.

Conversions between Measurement Systems

● *Length.*

$$1 \text{ in} = 2.54 \text{ cm}$$
$$1 \text{ ft} = 30.48 \text{ cm}$$
$$39.37 \text{ in} = 1 \text{ m}$$

● *Weight.*

$$1 \text{ oz} = 28.35 \text{ g (nutritionists usually use either 28 or 30 g)}$$
$$2.2 \text{ lb} = 1 \text{ kg}$$

● *Volume.*

$$1.06 \text{ qt} = 1 \text{ l}$$
$$0.85 \text{ imperial qt} = 1 \text{ l}$$

● *Temperature.*

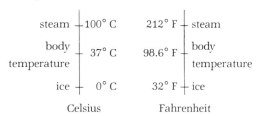

The symbol t_F in the following conversion equations represents the numerical value of a temperature on the Fahrenheit scale; t_C represents that of the Celsius scale.

$$t_F = 9/5 \ t_C + 32$$
$$t_C = 5/9 \ (t_F - 32)$$

APPENDIX E

Assessment Standards and Tools

Chapter 18 provides the basic information needed to evaluate a subject's nutrition status. Tables in Chapter 18 include:

1. Determining Frame Size from Height-Wrist Circumference Ratio — for use in obtaining a person's ideal body weight range.

2. Relationship between Degree of Undernutrition and % IBW — for use in determining the severity (stage of advancement) of malnutrition in non-obese people.

3. Relationship between Degree of Undernutrition and % UBW — for use in determining the severity of malnutrition in overweight hospitalized people.

4. Selected Laboratory Tests and Physical Findings Useful for Assessing Some Vitamin and Mineral Deficiencies — a quick reference guide.

5. Relationship between Degree of Undernutrition and Serum Proteins — for use in assessing severity of protein malnutrition.

6. Summary of Body Compartments Assessed by Biochemical and Anthropometric Measurements — a quick reference to identify tests for various facets of a person's protein-kcalorie nutrition status.

7. Physical Findings Associated with Various Nutrient Imbalances — a guide to help interpret the physical signs which may be observed in advanced cases of undernutrition.

8. Risk Factors for Poor Nutrition Status — a list of events and conditions which may contribute to nutrition imbalances in people who are experiencing one or more of these factors.

In Chapter 15, ways of assessing a child's growth

in height and weight were discussed. This appendix contains additional information useful in assessing nutrition status. First are the charts used to assess growth in children.

Growth Charts

Figures 1, 2, 3, and 4 are standards used to identify how a particular child's growth indices compare with the indices of a population of children selected by the National Center for Health Statistics. The following steps are useful for evaluating growth:

1. Select the appropriate chart based on age and sex. For example, for a 3-month-old female infant weighing 12 lb with a length of 23 in, you would use the chart for girls, birth to 36 months (Figure 1A).

2. Locate the child's age on bottom or top of chart (in our example, 3 months).

3. Locate the child's weight in lb or kg on the lower left or right side of the chart (in our example, 12 lb.)

4. Mark the chart where the age and weight lines intersect. (In our example, this is just above the 50th percentile. Note where we marked the chart.)

5. To find the child's percentile for length or height and age, start by locating the child's age on the top of the chart and the length on the upper right or left side. Proceed as you did when you were comparing age and weight. (Note the mark on the chart for the baby in our example.)

Figures 1a and 1b are useful for comparing infants' length and weight gain to those of the sample population.

Use Figures 2a and 2b to determine the percentile of head circumference development, and for assessing weight for length.

Children's growth in height and weight may be compared to the standards on Figures 3a and 3b.

Figures 4a and 4b omit the age factor when comparing the heights and weights of prepubescent children to the standards and are useful for determining if weight is appropriate for height.

Figure 5 is a grid for use in assessing a pregnant woman's weekly weight gain per week of gestation.

Other Standards and Tools

In addition to the information just given and in Chapters 15 and 18, the person evaluating nutrition status often uses other standards and tools:

- Standards for triceps skinfold. These standards are useful in comparing a person's fatfold to a reference population, in this case, a population of white males and females age one to 75 years tested in the Health and Nutritional Examination Survey I of the United States (see Table 1).
- Standards for midarm muscle circumference. The derived midarm muscle circumference (p. 689) can be compared to those compiled in the Health and Nutritional Examination Survey I (see Table 2).
- Standards for midarm circumference. The midarm circumference can also be compared to data collected in the Health and Nutritional Examination Survey I (see Table 3).
- A nomogram used to derive a person's midarm muscle circumference without calculations. One of two nomograms can be used for any midarm circumference between 8.0 cm and 40.0 cm (see Figures 6A and 6B).
- Tables showing the expected urinary creatinine excretion of men and women (see Tables 3A and 3B). In Chapter 18, creatinine excretion was described as a metabolite of energy breakdown in skeletal muscle. It is considered to be a reflection of the amount of skeletal muscle present in a person's body. Another useful aspect of the 24 hour creatinine output is that it can be used as a standard against which to compare the urinary output of the water-soluble vitamins that are involved in energy metabolism, such as riboflavin and thiamin. Creatinine is a reflection of actively metabolizing muscle tissue and is a value which remains relatively constant from day to day. Use Tables 4A and 4B as standards of 24 hour creatinine excretion for height and sex to calculate a person's creatinine height index (CHI).

E

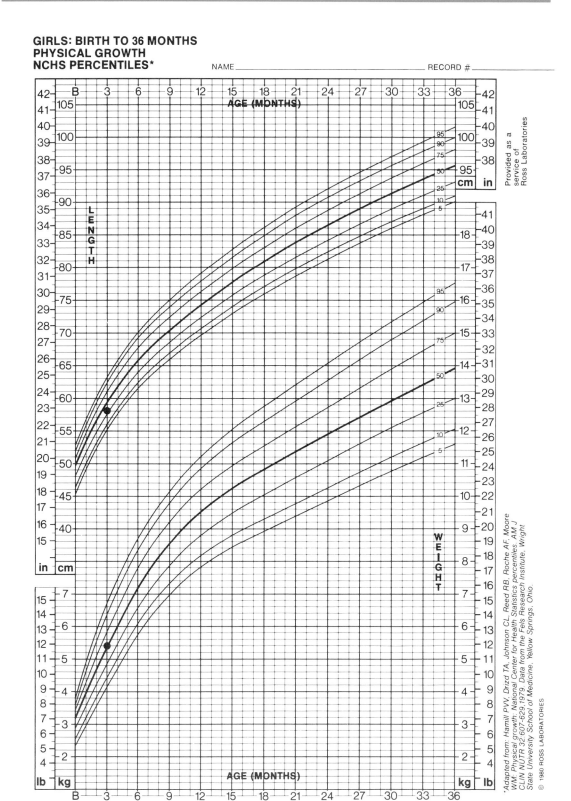

**GIRLS: BIRTH TO 36 MONTHS
PHYSICAL GROWTH
NCHS PERCENTILES***

NAME _____   RECORD # _____

Figure 1a   Girls: Birth to 36 months physical growth NCHS percentiles — length and weight for age.

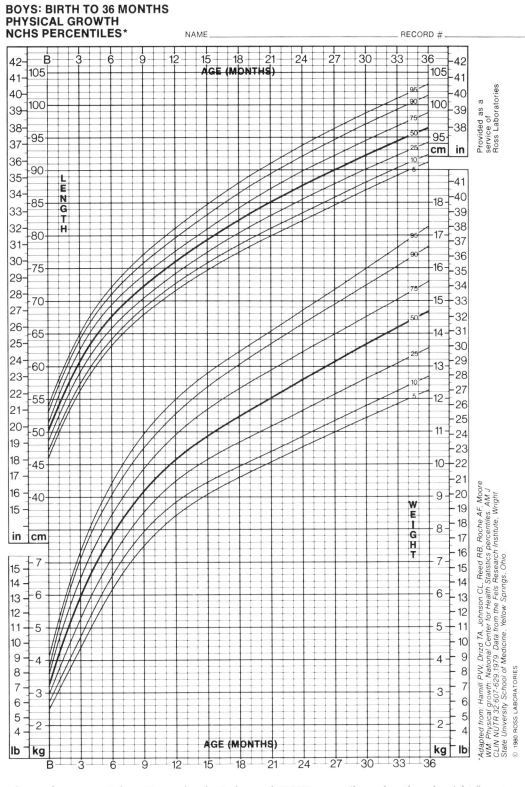

BOYS: BIRTH TO 36 MONTHS PHYSICAL GROWTH NCHS PERCENTILES*

NAME _____   RECORD # _____

Figure 1b   Boys: Birth to 36 months physical growth NCHS percentiles — length and weight for age.

E

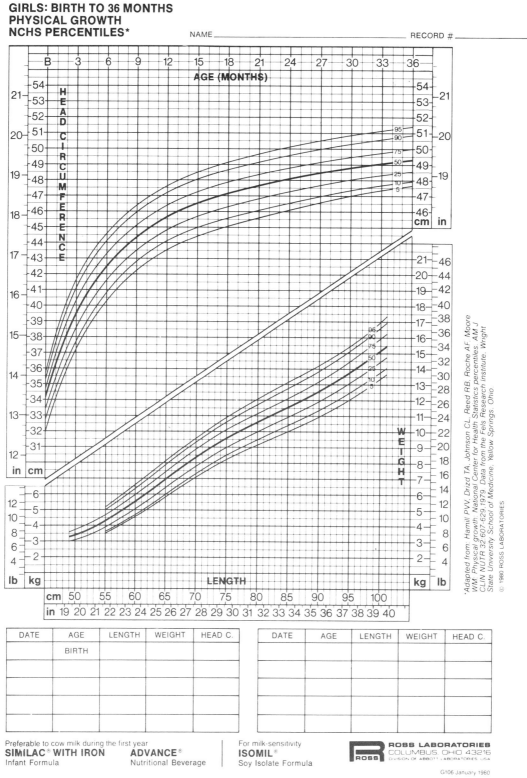

Figure 2a   Girls: Birth to 36 months physical growth NCHS percentiles — head circumference for age; and weight for length.

**BOYS: BIRTH TO 36 MONTHS
PHYSICAL GROWTH
NCHS PERCENTILES***

NAME _____   RECORD # _____

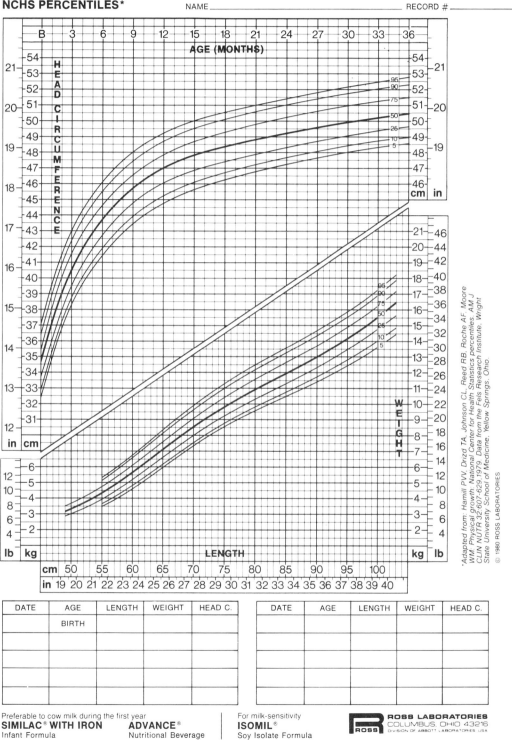

DATE	AGE	LENGTH	WEIGHT	HEAD C.
	BIRTH			

DATE	AGE	LENGTH	WEIGHT	HEAD C.

Preferable to cow milk during the first year
SIMILAC® WITH IRON   ADVANCE®
Infant Formula   Nutritional Beverage

For milk-sensitivity
ISOMIL®
Soy Isolate Formula

ROSS LABORATORIES
COLUMBUS, OHIO 43216
DIVISION OF ABBOTT LABORATORIES, USA

G105 January 1980

Figure 2b   Boys: Birth to 36 months physical growth NCHS percentiles — head circumference for age; and weight for length.

E

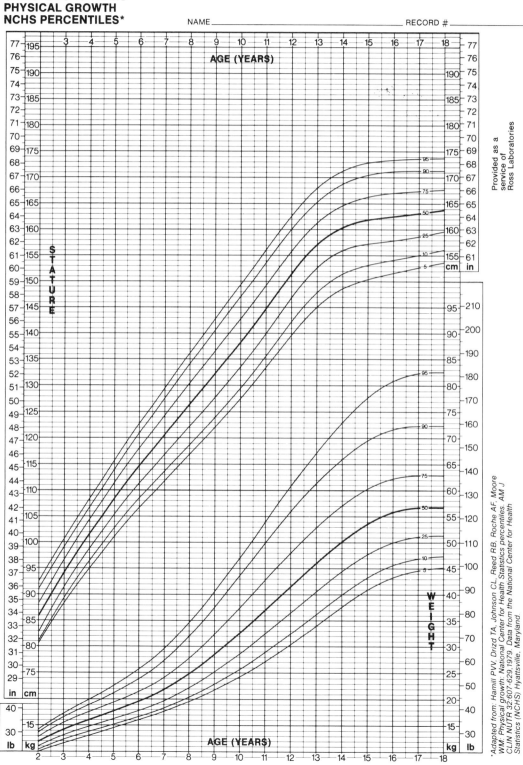

**GIRLS: 2 TO 18 YEARS
PHYSICAL GROWTH
NCHS PERCENTILES***

NAME _____ RECORD # _____

*Adapted from: Hamill PVV, Drizd TA, Johnson CL, Reed RB, Roche AF, Moore WM: Physical growth: National Center for Health Statistics percentiles. AM J CLIN NUTR 32:607-629,1979. Data from the National Center for Health Statistics (NCHS) Hyattsville, Maryland.

Provided as a service of Ross Laboratories

© 1980 ROSS LABORATORIES

Figure 3a   Girls: 2 to 18 years physical growth NCHS percentiles — height and weight for age.

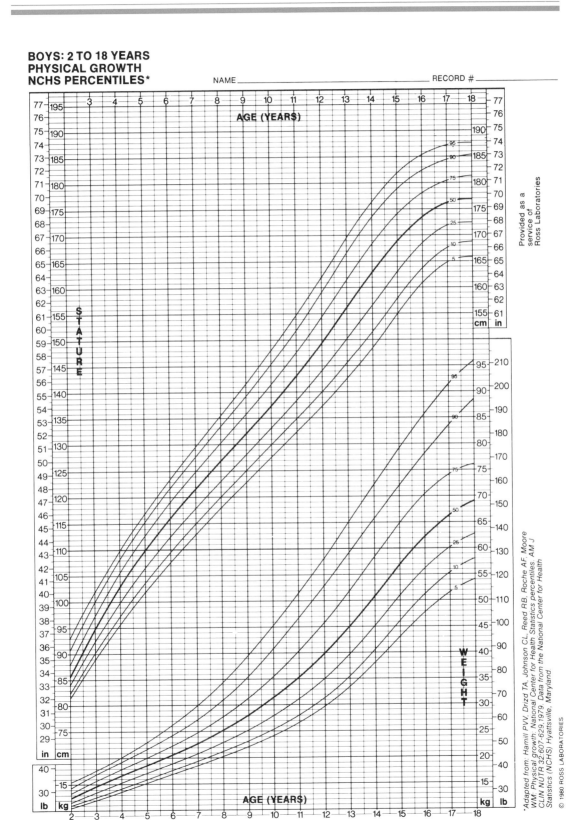

Figure 3b   Boys: 2 to 28 years physical growth NCHS percentiles — height and weight for age.

E

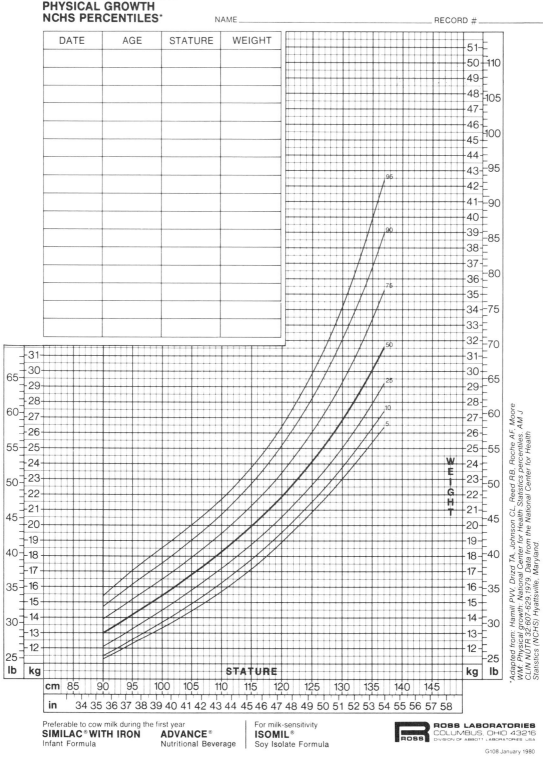

Figure 4a   Girls: Prepubescent physical growth NCHS percentiles — weight for height.

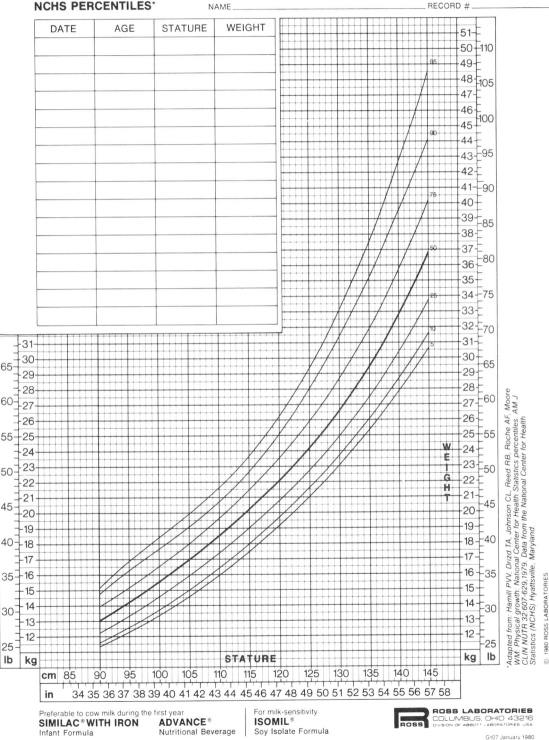

Figure 4b   Boys: Prepubescent physical growth NCHS percentiles — weight for height.

E

Prenatal weight gain grid.

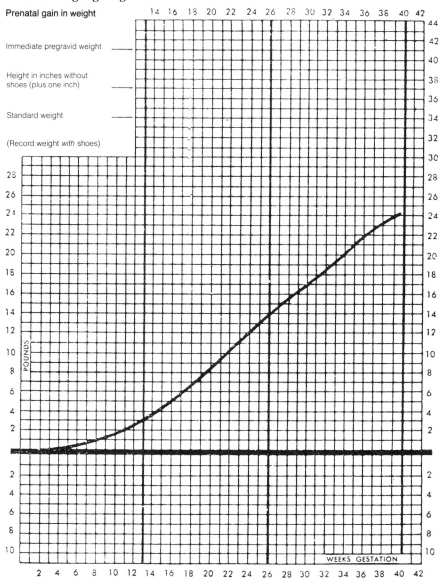

Figure 5   Prenatal gain in weight.

Table 1.   Triceps Skinfold Percentiles (millimeters)

Age	Male					Female				
	5th	25th	50th	75th	95th	5th	25th	50th	75th	95th
1- 1.9	6	8	10	12	16	6	8	10	12	16
2- 2.9	6	8	10	12	15	6	9	10	12	16
3- 3.9	6	8	10	11	15	7	9	11	12	15
4- 4.9	6	8	9	11	14	7	8	10	12	16
5- 5.9	6	8	9	11	15	6	8	10	12	18
6- 6.9	5	7	8	10	16	6	8	10	12	16
7- 7.9	5	7	9	12	17	6	9	11	13	18
8- 8.9	5	7	8	10	16	6	9	12	15	24
9- 9.9	6	7	10	13	18	8	10	13	16	22
10-10.9	6	8	10	14	21	7	10	12	17	27
11-11.9	6	8	11	16	24	7	10	13	18	28
12-12.9	6	8	11	14	28	8	11	14	18	27
13-13.9	5	7	10	14	26	8	12	15	21	30
14-14.9	4	7	9	14	24	9	13	16	21	28
15-15.9	4	6	8	11	24	8	12	17	21	32
16-16.9	4	6	8	12	22	10	15	18	22	31
17-17.9	5	6	8	12	19	10	13	19	24	37
18-18.9	4	6	9	13	24	10	15	18	22	30
19-24.9	4	7	10	15	22	10	14	18	24	34
25-34.9	5	8	12	16	24	10	16	21	27	37
35-44.9	5	8	12	16	23	12	18	23	29	38
45-54.9	6	8	12	15	25	12	20	25	30	40
55-64.9	5	8	11	14	22	12	20	25	31	38
65-74.9	4	8	11	15	22	12	18	24	29	36

Adapted from A. R. Frisancho, New norms of upper limb fat and muscle areas for assessment of nutritional status, *American Journal of Clinical Nutrition* 34 (1981):2540-2545.

E

Table 2.   Midupper Arm Muscle Circumference (centimeters)

	Male					Female				
Age	5th	25th	50th	75th	95th	5th	25th	50th	75th	95th
1- 1.9	11.0	11.9	12.7	13.5	14.7	10.5	11.7	12.4	13.9	14.3
2- 2.9	11.1	12.2	13.0	14.0	15.0	11.1	11.9	12.6	13.3	14.7
3- 3.9	11.7	13.1	13.7	14.3	15.3	11.3	12.4	13.2	14.0	15.2
4- 4.9	12.3	13.3	14.1	14.8	15.9	11.5	12.8	13.6	14.4	15.7
5- 5.9	12.8	14.0	14.7	15.4	16.9	12.5	13.4	14.2	15.1	16.5
6- 6.9	13.1	14.2	15.1	16.1	17.7	13.0	13.8	14.5	15.4	17.1
7- 7.9	13.7	15.1	16.0	16.8	19.0	12.9	14.2	15.1	16.0	17.6
8- 8.9	14.0	15.4	16.2	17.0	18.7	13.8	15.1	16.0	17.1	19.4
9- 9.9	15.1	16.1	17.0	18.3	20.2	14.7	15.8	16.7	18.0	19.8
10-10.9	15.6	16.6	18.0	19.1	22.1	14.8	15.9	17.0	18.0	19.7
11-11.9	15.9	17.3	18.3	19.5	23.0	15.0	17.1	18.1	19.6	22.3
12-12.9	16.7	18.2	19.5	21.0	24.1	16.2	18.0	19.1	20.1	22.0
13-13.9	17.2	19.6	21.1	22.6	24.5	16.9	18.3	19.8	21.1	24.0
14-14.9	18.9	21.2	22.3	24.0	26.4	17.4	19.0	20.1	21.6	24.7
15-15.9	19.9	21.8	23.7	25.4	27.2	17.5	18.9	20.2	21.5	24.4
16-16.9	21.3	23.4	24.9	26.9	29.6	17.0	19.0	20.2	21.6	24.9
17-17.9	22.4	24.5	25.8	27.3	31.2	17.5	19.4	20.5	22.1	25.7
18-18.9	22.6	25.2	26.4	28.3	32.4	17.4	19.1	20.2	21.5	24.5
19-24.9	23.8	25.7	27.3	28.9	32.1	17.9	19.5	20.7	22.1	24.9
25-34.9	24.3	26.4	27.9	29.8	32.6	18.3	19.9	21.2	22.8	26.4
35-44.9	24.7	26.9	28.6	30.2	32.7	18.6	20.5	21.8	23.6	27.2
45-54.9	23.9	26.5	28.1	30.0	32.6	18.7	20.6	22.0	23.8	27.4
55-64.9	23.6	26.0	27.8	29.5	32.0	18.7	20.9	22.5	24.4	28.0
65-74.9	22.3	25.1	26.8	28.4	30.6	18.5	20.8	22.5	24.4	27.9

Adapted from A. R. Frisancho, New norms of upper limb fat and muscle areas for assessment of nutritional status, *American Journal of Clinical Nutrition* 34 (1981):2540-2545.

Table 3.   **Midupper Arm Circumference (centimeters)**

	Male					Female				
Age	5th	25th	50th	75th	95th	5th	25th	50th	75th	95th
1- 1.9	14.2	15.0	15.9	17.0	18.3	13.8	14.8	15.6	16.4	17.7
2- 2.9	14.1	15.3	16.2	17.0	18.5	14.2	15.2	16.0	16.7	18.4
3- 3.9	15.0	16.0	16.7	17.5	19.0	14.3	15.8	16.7	17.5	18.9
4- 4.9	14.9	16.2	17.1	18.0	19.2	14.9	16.0	16.9	17.7	19.1
5- 5.9	15.3	16.7	17.5	18.5	20.4	15.3	16.5	17.5	18.5	21.1
6- 6.9	15.5	16.7	17.9	18.8	22.8	15.6	17.0	17.6	18.7	21.1
7- 7.9	16.2	17.7	18.7	20.1	23.0	16.4	17.4	18.3	19.9	23.1
8- 8.9	16.2	17.7	19.0	20.2	24.5	16.8	18.3	19.5	21.4	26.1
9- 9.9	17.5	18.7	20.0	21.7	25.7	17.8	19.4	21.1	22.4	26.0
10-10.9	18.1	19.6	21.0	23.1	27.4	17.4	19.3	21.0	22.8	26.5
11-11.9	18.6	20.2	22.3	24.4	28.0	18.5	20.8	22.4	24.8	30.3
12-12.9	19.3	21.4	23.2	25.4	30.3	19.4	21.6	23.7	25.6	29.4
13-13.9	19.4	22.8	24.7	26.3	30.1	20.2	22.3	24.3	27.1	33.8
14-14.9	22.0	23.7	25.3	28.3	32.3	21.4	23.7	25.2	27.2	32.2
15-15.9	22.2	24.4	26.4	28.4	32.0	20.8	23.9	25.4	27.9	32.2
16-16.9	24.4	26.2	27.8	30.3	34.3	21.8	24.1	25.8	28.3	33.4
17-17.9	24.6	26.7	28.5	30.8	34.7	22.0	24.1	26.4	29.5	35.0
18-18.9	24.5	27.6	29.7	32.1	37.9	22.2	24.1	25.8	28.1	32.5
19-24.9	26.2	28.8	30.8	33.1	37.2	21.1	24.7	26.5	29.0	34.5
25-34.9	27.1	30.0	31.9	34.2	37.5	23.3	25.6	27.7	30.4	36.8
35-44.9	27.8	30.5	32.6	34.5	37.4	24.1	26.7	29.0	31.7	37.8
45-54.9	26.7	30.1	32.2	34.2	37.6	24.2	27.4	29.9	32.8	38.4
55-64.9	25.8	29.6	31.7	33.6	36.9	24.3	28.0	30.3	33.5	38.5
65-74.9	24.8	28.5	30.7	32.5	35.5	24.0	27.4	29.9	32.6	37.3

Adapted from A. R. Frisancho, New norms of upper limb fat and muscle areas for assessment of nutritional status, *American Journal of Clinical Nutrition* 34 (1981):2540-2545.

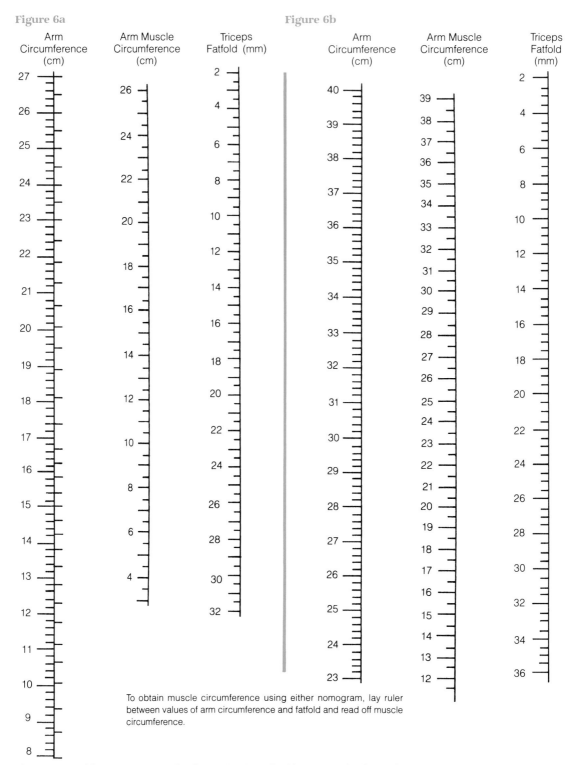

Figure 6a

Figure 6b

To obtain muscle circumference using either nomogram, lay ruler between values of arm circumference and fatfold and read off muscle circumference.

Figure 6a and b   Nomograms for determination of midarm muscle circumference.

Reproduced with permission from Gurney, J., and Jelliffe, D., Arm anthropometry in nutritional assessment; nomogram for rapid calculation of muscle circumference and cross-sectional muscle and fat areas. *American Journal of Clinical Nutrition*. 26: 912, 1973, as adapted by Grant, A. *Nutritional Assessment Guidelines* (available from P.O. Box 25057, Northgate Station, Seattle, WA 98125), 2nd ed., 1979.

Table 4A.   Expected 24-Hour Urinary Creatinine Excretion for Men

Height		Small frame		Medium frame		Large frame	
in.	cm.	Ideal weight (kg)	Creatinine (mg per 24 hr)	Ideal weight (kg)	Creatinine (mg per 24 hr)	Ideal weight (kg)	Creatinine (mg per 24 hr)
61	154.9	52.7	1212	56.1	1290	60.7	1396
62	157.5	54.1	1244	57.7	1327	62.0	1426
63	160.0	55.4	1274	59.1	1359	63.6	1463
64	162.5	56.8	1306	60.4	1389	65.2	1500
65	165.1	58.4	1343	62.0	1426	66.8	1536
66	167.6	60.2	1385	63.9	1470	68.9	1585
67	170.2	62.0	1426	65.9	1516	71.1	1635
68	172.7	63.9	1470	67.7	1557	72.9	1677
69	175.3	65.9	1516	69.5	1598	74.8	1720
70	177.8	67.7	1557	71.6	1647	76.8	1766
71	180.3	69.5	1599	73.6	1693	79.1	1819
72	182.9	71.4	1642	75.7	1741	81.1	1865
73	185.4	73.4	1688	77.7	1787	83.4	1918
74	187.9	75.2	1730	80.0	1846	85.7	1971
75	190.5	77.0	1771	82.3	1893	87.7	2017

Table 4B.   Expected 24-Hour Urinary Creatinine Excretion for Women

Height		Small frame		Medium frame		Large frame	
in.	cm.	Ideal weight (kg)	Creatinine (mg per 24 hr)	Ideal weight (kg)	Creatinine (mg per 24 hr)	Ideal weight (kg)	Creatinine (mg per 24 hr)
56	142.2	43.2	778	46.1	830	50.7	913
57	144.8	44.3	797	47.3	851	51.8	932
58	147.3	45.4	817	48.6	875	53.2	958
59	149.8	46.8	842	50.0	900	54.5	981
60	152.4	48.2	868	51.4	925	55.9	1006
61	154.9	49.5	891	52.7	949	57.3	1031
62	157.5	50.9	916	54.3	977	58.9	1060
63	160.0	52.3	941	55.9	1006	60.6	1091
64	162.5	53.9	970	57.9	1042	62.5	1125
65	165.1	55.7	1003	59.8	1076	64.3	1157
66	167.6	57.5	1035	61.6	1109	66.1	1190
67	170.2	59.3	1067	63.4	1141	67.9	1222
68	172.7	61.4	1105	65.2	1174	70.0	1260
69	175.2	63.2	1138	67.0	1206	72.0	1296
70	177.8	65.0	1170	68.9	1240	74.1	1334

From Grant, A., *Nutritional Assessment Guidelines*, 2nd ed. (available from P.O. Box 25057, Northgate Station, Seattle, WA 98125), 2nd ed., 1979.

APPENDIX F

SUGAR

Miniglossary

Terms used to mean "sugar" and sugar substitutes on labels include the following. In terms of nutritional value, most of these are very much the same. Those marked by an asterisk (*) have a low energy value, and are added to foods as low-kcalorie sugar substitutes. Fructose is included here because it is sometimes used as a sweetener when a lower-kcalorie product is desired. Other monosaccharides are discussed in Chapter 1.

aspartame* (aspartyl-phenylalanine methyl ester): a dipeptide that tastes remarkably like sugar, but is 200 times sweeter than sucrose. The compound turns sour if it is heated and so cannot be used for cooking or baking. Aspartame, called "Nutra Sweet" by the G. O. Searle Company, is blended with lactose and with an anticaking agent and is sold commercially as "Equal." Individuals who must restrict phenylalanine (as in PKU children) cannot use this sweetener, because in the body it is enzymatically hydrolyzed into the amino acids phenylalanine and aspartic acid from which it was formulated.

brown sugar: sugar crystals contained in molasses syrup with natural flavor and color, 91 to 96 percent pure sucrose. (Some refiners add syrup to refined white sugar to make brown sugar.)

corn sweeteners: a term that refers to corn syrup and sugars derived from corn.

corn syrup: a syrup produced by the action of enzymes on cornstarch. High-fructose corn syrup may contain as little as 42 percent or as much as 90 percent fructose; dextrose makes up the balance.

cyclamate: a zero-kcalorie sweetener used in Canada, but not in the U.S.

dextrose: the technical name for glucose.

fructose*: a monosaccharide, about twice as sweet as sucrose, so that less of it can be added to foods in order to obtain the desired intensity of sweetness, while avoiding some kcalories.

honey: invert sugar formed by an enzyme from nectar gathered by bees. Composition and flavor vary, but honey usually contains fructose, glucose, maltose, and sucrose.

invert sugar: a mixture of glucose and fructose formed by the splitting of sucrose in a chemical process. Sold only in liquid form, sweeter than sucrose, invert sugar is used as an additive to help preserve food freshness and prevent shrinkage.

levulose: the technical name for fructose.

maple sugar: although once a common sweetener, this sugar is rarely added to foods and is commonly replaced by sucrose and artificial maple flavoring. The only source of true maple sugar is the concentrated sap of the sugar maple trees, and it is expensive when compared with other sweeteners.

molasses: a thick, brown syrup, which tastes bitter and sour as well as sweet, created during cane sugar production. Molasses contains a few minerals.

natural sweeteners: a term that refers to any of the sugars listed here.

raw sugar: the residue of evaporated sugar cane juice, tan or brown in color. Raw sugar can only be sold in the U.S. if the impurities (dirt, insect fragments, and the like) have been removed.

saccharin (sodium saccharine): discovered in 1879, and used in the U.S. since that time, a zero-kcalorie sweetener that is at least 200 times sweeter than sucrose. Individuals who must restrict sodium intake should avoid saccharin-containing products.

sorbitol, mannitol, maltitol, xylitol: sugar alcohols, that can be derived from fruits or produced from dextrose; not utilizable by ordinary mouth bacteria, so do not promote tooth decay.

sucrose: table sugar or powdered (confectioner's) sugar, 99.9 percent pure.

Table 1 presents the amount of refined sugar in common foods measured in teaspoons. No one will be surprised to see that soft drinks contain a large quantity of refined sugar, but it may be a surprise to learn that sugar is added to dried fruits, hamburger buns, and other items.

Table 1. Refined Sugar in Common Foods[1]

Food	Portion size	Approximate sugar content (tsp)*	Food	Portion size	Approximate sugar content (tsp)*
Beverages			Lifesavers	1	$1/3$
Cola drinks	12 oz	9	Peanut brittle	1 oz	$3 1/2$
Ginger ale	12 oz	7	Marshmallow	1	$1 1/2$
Lemon soda	12 oz	11			
Orange soda	12 oz	$11 1/2$	**Fruits and canned juices**		
Orangeade	8 oz	5	Raisins	1/2 c	4
Root beer	10 oz	$4 1/2$	Currants, dried	1 tbsp	4
Seven-Up	12 oz	9	Prunes, dried	3-4 medium	4
Soda pop	8 oz	5	Apricots, dried	4-6 halves	4
Soda water	8 oz	0	Dates, dried	3-4 stoned	$4 1/2$
Sweet cider	1 c (8 oz)	$4 1/2$	Figs, dried	$1 1/2$-2 small	4
Tonic water	8 oz	$5 1/2$	Fruit cocktail	1/2 c	5
			Rhubarb, stewed, sweetened	1/2 c	8
Jams and jellies			Canned apricots	4 halves and 1 tbsp syrup	$3 1/2$
Apple butter	1 tbsp	1			
Jelly	1 tbsp	4-6	Applesauce, sweetened	1/2 c	2
Orange marmalade	1 tbsp	4-6			
Peach butter	1 tbsp	1	Prunes, stewed, sweetened	4-5 medium and 2 tbsp juice	8
Strawberry jam	1 tbsp	4			
			Canned peaches	2 halves and 1 tbsp syrup	$3 1/2$
Candies					
Milk chocolate bar (Hershey bar)	$1 1/2$ oz	$2 1/2$	Fruit salad	1/2 c	$3 1/2$
Chewing gum	1 stick	$1/2$	Fruit syrup	2 tbsp	$2 1/2$
Chocolate cream	1 piece	2	Orange juice	1/2 c	2
Chocolate mints	1 piece	2	Pineapple juice unsweetened	1/2 c	$2 3/5$
Fudge	1 oz square	$4 1/2$			
Gum drop	1	2			
Hard candy	4 oz	20			

*Measured in teaspoon equivalents of granulated sugar.
†Actual sugar content.
‡For the total carbohydrate content, add about 3% lactose. Value reflects only sucrose, glucose, and fructose.

All of the values in Table 1 were adapted from: Hidden sugars in foods (a three-page typescript), Department of Pedodontics, College of Dentistry, University of Iowa, Iowa City, Iowa, March 1974. Developed by Arthur J. Nowak, D.M.D., professor, College of Dentistry, Department of Pedodontics, University of Iowa, and reprinted with his permission; D. A. T. Southgate, A. A. Paul, A. C. Dean, and A. A. Christie, Free sugars in foods, *Journal of Human Nutrition* 32 (1978): 335-347; and M. C. Martin-Villa, C. Vidal-Valverde, and E. Rojas-Hidalgo, Soluble sugars in soft drinks, *American Journal of Clinical Nutrition* 34 (1981): 2151- 2153.

F

Table 1.   Refined Sugar in Common Foods (cont'd)

Food	Portion size	Approximate sugar content (tsp)*	Food	Portion size	Approximate sugar content (tsp)*
Grape juice, commercial	1/2 c	$3_2/5$	Eggnog, all milk	1 (8 oz)	$4_1/2$
Canned fruit juices, sweetened	1/2 c	2	Ice cream soda	1	5
			Cocoa, all milk	1 c (5 oz milk)	4
			Ice cream sundae	1	7
Breads and cereals			Chocolate, all milk	1 c (5 oz milk)	6
White bread	1 slice	1/2	Malted milk shake	1 (10 oz)	5
Cornflakes, Wheaties, Krispies, etc.	1 bowl and 1 tbsp sugar	4-8	Sherbet	1/2 c	9
			Yogurt,‡ sweetened fruit	1 c	9
Hamburger bun	1	3			
Hot dog bun	1	3	**Desserts**		
			Apple cobbler	1/2 c	3
Cakes and cookies			Custard	1/2 c	2
Angel food cake	4 oz	7	French pastry	1 (4 oz)	5
Applesauce cake	4 oz	$5_1/2$	Jello	1/2 c	$4_1/2$
Banana cake	2 oz	2	Apple pie	1 slice (average)	7
Cheesecake	4 oz	2	Junket	1/2 c	3
Chocolate cake, plain	4 oz	6	Berry pie	1 slice	10
Chocolate cake, iced	4 oz	10	Cherry pie	1 slice	10
Coffeecake	4 oz	$4_1/2$	Cream pie	1 slice	4
Cupcake, iced	1	6	Custard pie	1 slice	10
Fruitcake	4 oz	5	Coconut pie	1 slice	10
Jelly-roll	2 oz	$2_1/2$	Lemon pie	1 slice	7
Orange cake	4 oz	4	Peach pie	1 slice	7
Pound cake	4 oz	5	Pumpkin pie	1 slice	5
Sponge cake	1 oz	2	Rhubarb pie	1 slice	4
Strawberry shortcake	1 serving	4	Raisin pie	1 slice	13
Brownies, unfrosted	1 (3/4 oz)	3	Banana pudding	1/2 c	2
Molasses cookies	1	2	Bread pudding	1/2 c	$1_1/2$
Chocolate cookies	1	$1_1/2$	Chocolate pudding	1/2 c	$1_1/2$
Fig newtons	1	5	Plum pudding	1/2 c	4
Ginger snaps	1	3	Rice pudding	1/2 c	5
Macaroons	1	6	Tapioca pudding	1/2 c	3
Nut cookies	1	$1_1/2$	Brown betty	1/2 c	3
Oatmeal cookies	1	2	Plain pastry	1 (4 oz)	3
Sugar cookies	1	$1_1/2$			
Chocolate eclair	1	7	**Sugars and syrups**		
Cream puff	1	2	Brown sugar	1 tbsp	3†
Donut, plain	1	3	Granulated sugar	1 tbsp	3†
Donut, glazed	1	6	Corn syrup	1 tbsp	3†
Snail	1 (4 oz)	$4_1/2$	Karo syrup	1 tbsp	3†
			Honey	1 tbsp	3†
Dairy products			Molasses	1 tbsp	$3_1/2$†
Ice cream	1/3 pint ($3_1/2$ oz)	$3_1/2$	Chocolate sauce	1 tbsp	$3_1/2$†
Ice cream bar	1 (depending on size)	1-7	**Wines**		
			Wine, medium rosé	$3_1/2$ oz	3/4
Ice cream cone	1	$3_1/2$	Wine, dry white	$3_1/2$ oz	trace
			Wine, medium sherry	$3_1/2$ oz	1
			Vermouth, dry	$3_1/2$ oz	$1_1/2$
			Vermouth, sweet	$3_1/2$ oz	$4_1/2$

*Measured in teaspoon equivalents of granulated sugar.

†Actual sugar content.

‡For the total carbohydrate content, add about 3% lactose. Value reflects only sucrose, glucose, and fructose.

Table 2 shows which brands of ready-to-eat cereals have the most and which have the least refined sugar. The percentages of sugar per cereal weight were arranged in rank order, from lowest to highest. The dentist who published most of this information suggested, tentatively, that to avoid promoting the development of dental decay, the consumer should choose cereals containing less than 20 percent refined sugar.

Table 2. Refined Sugar (Sucrose) in Breakfast Cereals

Cereal	Sucrose (percent)	Cereal	Sucrose (percent)
Less than 10 percent sucrose*		**20 to 29 percent sucrose**	
Shredded Wheat, large biscuit	1.0	All Bran	20.0
Shredded Wheat, spoon-size biscuit	1.3	Heartland, coconut	21.2
Cheerios	2.2	C. W. Post, plain	21.0
Puffed Rice	2.4	Granola, with almonds and filberts	21.4
Uncle Sam Cereal	2.4	Quaker 100% Natural, with apples	21.9
Wheat Chex	2.6	and cinnamon	
Grape Nut Flakes	3.3	Fortified Oat Flakes	22.2
Puffed Wheat	3.5	Familia	22.4
Alpen	3.8	Vita Crunch, regular	22.7
Post Toasties	4.1	Heartland	23.1
Product 19	4.1	C. W. Post, with raisins	24.3
Corn Total	4.4	Nature Valley Granola, with cinnamon	24.0
Special K	4.4	and raisins	
Wheaties	4.7	Super Sugar Chex	24.5
Corn Flakes, Kroger	5.1	Heartland, with raisins	24.7
Peanut Butter	5.2	Quaker 100% Natural, with raisins	25.0
Grape Nuts	6.6	and dates	
Corn Flakes, Food Club	7.0	Country Morning	25.8
Crispy Rice	7.3	Vita Crunch, with raisins	26.0
Corn Chex	7.5	Vita Crunch, with almonds	26.5
Corn Flakes, Kellogg	7.8	Nature Valley Granola, with fruit	28.0
Total	8.1	and nuts	
Rice Chex	8.5	Sugar Frosted Flakes	29.0
Crisp Rice	8.8		
Raisin Bran, Skinner	9.6	**30 to 39 percent sucrose**	
Concentrate	9.9	Bran Buds	30.2
		Sugar Sparkled Corn Flakes	32.2
10 to 19 percent sucrose		Frosted Mini Wheats	33.6
Rice Krispies, Kellogg	10.0	Sugar Pops	37.8
Raisin Bran, Kellogg	10.6		
Buck Wheat	13.6	**40 to 49.5 percent sucrose**	
Life	14.5	Alpha Bits	40.3
Granola, with dates	14.5	Sir Grapefellow	40.7
Granola, with raisins	14.5	Super Sugar Crisp	40.7
Sugar-Frosted Corn Flakes	15.6	Cocoa Puffs	43.0
40% Bran Flakes, Post	15.8	Cap'n Crunch	43.3
Team	15.9	Crunch Berries	43.4
Brown Sugar-Cinnamon Frosted Mini	16.0	Kaboom	43.8
Wheats		Frankenberry	44.0
40% Bran Flakes, Kellogg	16.2	Frosted Flakes	44.0
Quaker 100% Natural, with	18.2	Count Chocula	44.2
brown sugar and honey		Orange Quangeroos	44.7
100% Bran	18.4		

*The glucose content of these cereals is less than 5 percent, except for Special K and Kellogg Corn Flakes (6.4 percent), Kellogg Raisin Bran (14.1 percent), and Heartland, with raisins (5.6 percent). Other sugars, such as fructose, were not analyzed.

Table 2.   Refined Sugar (Sucrose) in Breakfast Cereals (cont'd)

Cereal	Sucrose (percent)	Cereal	Sucrose (percent)
Quisp	44.9	**50 to 59 percent sucrose**	
Boo Berry	45.7	Cinnamon Crunch	50.3
Vanilly Crunch	45.8	Lucky Charms	50.4
Baron Von Redberry	45.8	Cocoa Pebbles	53.5
Cocoa Krispies	45.9	Apple Jacks	55.0
Trix	46.6	Fruity Pebbles	55.1
Froot Loops	47.4	King Vitamin	58.5
Honeycomb	48.8		
Pink Panther	49.2	**More than 60 percent sucrose**	
		Sugar Smacks	61.3
		Super Orange Crisp	68.0

*Measured in teaspoon equivalents of granulated sugar.

†Actual sugar content.

‡For the total carbohydrate content, add about 3% lactose. Value reflects only sucrose, glucose, and fructose.

B. W. Li and P. J. Schuhmann, Gas chromatographic analysis of sugars in granola cereals, *Journal of Food Science* 46 (1981): 425-427; I. L. Shannon, Sucrose and glucose in dry breakfast cereals, *Journal of Dentistry for Children*, September/October 1974, pp. 17-20. The reader who wants to pursue the subject further might find another article interesting: I. L. Shannon and W. B. Wescott, Sucrose and glucose concentrations of frequently ingested foods, *Journal of the Academy of General Dentistry*, May/June 1975, pp. 37-43, which presents sucrose and glucose contents for diet soft drinks (less than 0.1 percent); commercially available cheeses (less than 2.0 percent); fresh fruits and vegetables (from 0 to about 5 percent); commercially available luncheon meats (less than 1 percent for those analyzed); commercially available crackers and wafers (from about 1 to 10 percent, except for graham crackers, Cinnamon Treats, Cinnamon Crisp, and glazed Sesame Crisp, which contained from 10 to 30 percent); commercially available breads (less than 1 percent for those analyzed, except for old-fashioned cinnamon loaf); and commercially available snack foods (from 0 to 3 percent except for Morton's Kandi-roos, which contained almost 50 percent sucrose). Dr. Shannon's data are used here with his permission and that of the publisher.

Sugar amounts in Country Morning, C. W. Post, Familia, Heartland, Nature Valley, Quaker Natural, and Vita Crunch were estimated from sugar amounts in dry weights of cereal, assuming the cereals were 5 percent water (in fact, 10 other cereals ranged from 2 to 8 percent water).

To Explore Further

A more extensive analysis of the sugar content of foods has been published by D. A. T. Southgate, A. A. Paul, A. C. Dean, and A. A. Christie, Free sugars in foods, *Journal of Human Nutrition* 32 (1978): 335-347. This reference shows the breakdown for each food into glucose, fructose, lactose, maltose, and sucrose, for about 150 foods including some unusual ones such as rose hips syrup.

APPENDIX G

Fats: Cholesterol and P:S Ratios

To adopt a "prudent diet," you are advised to control kcalories and salt intake; to avoid empty-kcalorie foods, especially those high in concentrated sugars; and to make sure that fat intake is kept in line. To manage fat consumption, three measures are recommended: (1) cut total fat; (2) reduce cholesterol intake; and (3) adjust the ratio of polyunsaturated to saturated fat so that it balances in favor of the polyunsaturates.

For the first objective, total fat intake can be calculated using Appendix H, as suggested in the Self-Study following Highlight 2.

For the second objective, cholesterol intake can be estimated using Table 1 in this appendix.

The U.S. dietary goals suggested a cholesterol intake of 300 mg a day or less, although there is some disagreement about this recommendation (see Highlight 6).

As for the third objective, nutritionists tend to think in terms of the P:S ratio (the ratio of polyunsaturated to saturated fat). In general, according to present thinking, a high P:S ratio is desirable. The P:S ratio of a day's food intake or menu can be calculated precisely (as explained in the Self-Study following Highlight 2), but you can get a general idea of the fat quality of common fat-containing foods and vegetable oils from Tables 2 and 3.

Table 1   Cholesterol Content of Foods[1]

Food	Serving size	Cholesterol (mg)	Food	Serving size	Cholesterol (mg)
Meat, fish, poultry			sweetbreads	3 oz	396
Beef, cooked, lean, trimmed			brain	3 oz	1,810
of separable fat	3 oz	77	kidney	3 oz	690
Lamb, lean, cooked	3 oz	83	Fish		
Pork, cooked, lean, trimmed	3 oz	77	caviar (fish roe)	1 tbsp	48
Veal, cooked, lean	3 oz	86	cod	3 oz	72
Chicken, dark meat	3 oz	76	haddock	3 oz	51
Chicken, light meat	3 oz	54	halibut	3 oz	51
Turkey, dark meat	3 oz	86	flounder	3 oz	43
Turkey, light meat	3 oz	65	herring	3 oz	83
Rabbit, domestic	3 oz	52	salmon, cooked	3 oz	40
Variety meats			trout	3 oz	47
liver (beef, calf, lamb),			tuna, packed in oil	3 oz	56
cooked	3 oz	372	sardines	1 can	
chicken liver	3 oz	480		(3 3/4 oz)	109
heart	3 oz	274			

[1]Adapted from the booklet by the Greater Los Angeles Affiliate of the American Heart Association, *Consumers Guide to Fat: Cholesterol-Controlled Food Products* (Los Angeles: American Heart Association, 1978); and from E. N. Whitney and E. M. N. Hamilton, *Understanding Nutrition*, 1st ed. (St. Paul, Minn.: West, 1977), pp. 537-538.

Table 1 Cholesterol Content of Foods (cont'd)

Food	Serving size	Cholesterol (mg)
Shellfish		
abalone	3 oz	120
crab	3 oz	85
clams	3 oz	55
lobster	1/2 c	57
oysters	3 oz	40
scallops	1/2 c (scant)	45
shrimp	3 oz	96
Eggs		
Yolk	1 medium	240
White		0
Dairy products		
Milk, whole	1 c (8 oz)	34
Milk, low-fat (2%)	1 c	22
Milk, nonfat (skim)	1 c	5
Buttermilk	1 c	14
Yogurt, low-fat plain	1 c	17
Yogurt, low-fat flavored	1 c	14
Sour cream	1 tbsp	8
Whipped cream	1 tbsp	20
Half and half	1 tbsp	6
Ice milk	1 c	26

Food	Serving size	Cholesterol (mg)
Ice cream	1 c	56
Butter	1 tsp	12
Cheese		
American	1 oz	26
Blue or roquefort	1 oz	25
Camembert	1 oz	28
Cheddar, mild or sharp	1 oz	28
Cottage		
creamed (4% fat)	1 c	48
uncreamed	1 c	13
Cream cheese	1 tbsp	16
Mozzarella, low moisture, part skim	1 oz	18
Muenster	1 oz	25
Parmesan	1 oz	27
Ricotta, part skim	1 oz	14
Swiss	1 oz	28
Nondairy fats		
Lard or other animal fat	1 tsp	5
Margarine, all vegetable		0
Margarine, 2/3 animal fat, 1/3 vegetable fat	1 tsp	3

Table 2 P:S Ratios of Foods

Relative P:S ratio	Foods	Relative P:S ratio	Foods
High (more than 2 1/2 times as much polyunsaturated as saturated fat)	Almonds Corn oil Cottonseed oil Linseed oil Margarine, soft Mayonnaise (made with any of the oils in this group) Safflower oil Sesame oil Soybean oil Sunflower oil Walnuts	Medium (about equal amounts of poly-unsaturated and saturated fat)	Beef, heart and liver Chicken heart Hydrogenated or hardened vegetable oils Pecans Peanut butter Solid margarines
		Low (about a tenth to a half as much polyunsaturated as saturated fat)	Chicken liver Lard Olive oil Palm oil Pork Veal
Medium-high (about twice as much polyunsaturated as saturated fat)	Chicken breast, skin, thigh Freshwater fish Peanut oil Semisolid margarines	Very low (less than a tenth as much polyunsaturated as saturated fat)	Beef, both lean and fat Butter Coconut oil Egg yolk Milk and milk products Mutton, both lean and fat

Table 3   Percent Fatty Acid Composition of Commonly Used Cooking and Salad Oils*

Oil	Saturated %	Mono-unsaturated %	Poly-unsaturated %
Coconut	86	6	2
Corn	13	25	58
Cottonseed	26	19	51
Olive	14	72	9
Palm	48	38	9
Palm kernel	81	11	1
Peanut	19	46	30
Safflower	9	12	74
Sesame	15	40	40
Soybean (partially hydrogenated)	13	47	40
Soybean (unhydrogenated)	15	23	58
Sunflower	10	21	64
Vegetable, P:S >1	15	47	34
Walnut	11	15	66
Wheat germ	17	16	61

G

*You may notice that the total percent fatty acids in the oils listed do not add up to 100. Other substances such as sterols, vitamins, phospholipids, and water that are present in the oils make up the unmeasured fraction.

Table 3 adapted from H. B. Brown, Current focus on fat in the diet, White Paper, *ADA* (1977):25.

APPENDIX H

Table of Food Composition

The following table is the standard table found in all nutrition textbooks and references. It presents the kcalorie content, energy-nutrient composition, and vitamin and mineral contents of 615 common foods by household measure.[1] It can be purchased from the U.S. Government Printing Office (address in Appendix J) as a handy softcover booklet. Canadian users may prefer to use *Nutrient Value of Some Common Foods* (Health and Welfare Canada) which has the advantage of being metricated.

Of the minerals, only calcium and iron are included in this table. You might also be curious about zinc, but we have chosen not to present information here on the zinc contents of foods. A few references are available that do.[2]

Of the vitamins, vitamin A, thiamin, riboflavin, niacin, and vitamin C (ascorbic acid) are included. An expanded version of this table, presently being published in installments by the U.S. Department of Agriculture, Agricultural Research Service, includes folacin and other vitamin information, as well as the amino acid analysis of foods.[3]

Fast foods are not listed in this table, but we have included a separate appendix (Appendix N) listing the nutrient contents of foods sold in the most popular fast-food restaurants. The nutrient content of brand-name products—cookies, snack foods, cookie mixes, canned fruits, TV dinners, condiments, and so on—can be obtained from Consumer Guide.[4] The composition of foods used by various ethnic groups, which are also not found in this table, can be requested from the U.S. Department of Agriculture.[5] Finally, because new information on the composition of foods is coming out monthly, a useful reference is the looseleaf notebook available from a group of Boston-area dietitians, which lists many other references for nutrients and data that are often difficult to locate.[6]

---

[1]U.S. Department of Agriculture, Nutritive values of the edible parts of foods, *Nutritive Value of Foods*, Home and Garden Bulletin no. 72 (Washington, D.C.: Government Printing Office, 1971), table 1.

[2]K. A. Haeflein and A. I. Rasmussen, Zinc content of selected foods, *Journal of the American Dietetic Association* 70 (1977):610-616; E. W. Murphy, B. W. Willis, and B. K. Watt, Provisional tables of the zinc content of foods, *Journal of the American Dietetic Association* 66 (1975):345-355; and J. H. Freeland and R. J. Cousins, Zinc content of selected foods, *Journal of the American Dietetic Association* 68 (1976):526-529.

[3]A table of the folacin contents of 299 foods has also been published: B. P. Perloff and R. R. Butrum, Folacin in selected foods, *Journal of the American Dietetic Association* 70 (1977):161-172.

[4]*Food: The Brand Name Game* (Skokie, Ill.: Consumer Guide, 1974).

[5]*Composition of Foods Used by Ethnic Groups: Selected References to Sources of Data* can be requested from Dr. Louise Page, Food and Diet Appraisal Group, Consumer and Food Economics Institute, U.S. Department of Agriculture, Agricultural Research Service, Hyattsville MD 20782. For Japanese-American food equivalents, a reprint is available from the American Dietetic Association (address in Appendix J).

[6]*Nutrient Composition of Foods: Selected References and Tables*, available from the Boston Area Research Dietitians Special Practice Group, Massachusetts Dietetic Association (1978).

TABLE 2.—NUTRITIVE VALUES OF THE EDIBLE PART OF FOODS
(Dashes (—) denote lack of reliable data for a constituent believed to be present in measurable amount)

Item No. (A)	Foods, approximate measures, units, and weight (edible part unless footnotes indicate otherwise) (B)		Grams	Water (C) Percent	Food energy (D) Calories	Protein (E) Grams	Fat (F) Grams	Fatty Acids Saturated (total) (G) Grams	Unsaturated Oleic (H) Grams	Linoleic (I) Grams	Carbohydrate (J) Grams	Calcium (K) Milligrams	Iron (L) Milligrams	Vitamin A value (M) International units	Thiamin (N) Milligrams	Riboflavin (O) Milligrams	Niacin (P) Milligrams	Ascorbic acid (Q) Milligrams
	DAIRY PRODUCTS (CHEESE, CREAM, IMITATION CREAM, MILK; RELATED PRODUCTS)																	
	Butter. See Fats, oils; related products, items 103-108																	
	Cheese:																	
	Natural:																	
1	Blue	1 oz	28	42	100	6	8	5.3	1.9	0.2	1	150	0.1	200	0.01	0.11	0.3	0
2	Camembert (3 wedges per 4-oz container)	1 wedge	38	52	115	8	9	5.8	2.2	.2	Trace	147	.1	350	.01	.19	.2	0
	Cheddar:																	
3	Cut pieces	1 oz	28	37	115	7	9	6.1	2.1	.2	Trace	204	.2	300	.01	.11	Trace	0
4		1 cu in	17.2	37	70	4	6	3.7	1.3	.1	Trace	124	.1	180	Trace	.06	Trace	0
5	Shredded	1 cup	113	37	455	28	37	24.2	8.5	.7	1	815	.8	1,200	.03	.42	.1	0
	Cottage (curd not pressed down):																	
	Creamed (cottage cheese, 4% fat):																	
6	Large curd	1 cup	225	79	235	28	10	6.4	2.4	.2	6	135	.3	370	.05	.37	.3	Trace
7	Small curd	1 cup	210	79	220	26	9	6.0	2.2	.2	6	126	.3	340	.04	.34	.3	Trace
8	Low fat (2%)	1 cup	226	79	205	31	4	2.8	1.0	.1	8	155	.4	160	.05	.42	.3	Trace
9	Low fat (1%)	1 cup	226	82	165	28	2	1.5	.5	.1	6	138	.3	80	.05	.37	.3	Trace
10	Uncreamed (cottage cheese dry curd, less than ½% fat)	1 cup	145	80	125	25	1	.4	.1	Trace	3	46	.3	40	.04	.21	.2	0
11	Cream	1 oz	28	54	100	2	10	6.2	2.4	.2	1	23	.3	400	Trace	.06	Trace	0
	Mozzarella, made with—																	
12	Whole milk	1 oz	28	48	90	6	7	4.4	1.7	.2	1	163	.1	260	Trace	.08	Trace	0
13	Part skim milk	1 oz	28	49	80	8	5	3.1	1.2	.1	1	207	.1	180	.01	.10	Trace	0
	Parmesan, grated:																	
14	Cup, not pressed down	1 cup	100	18	455	42	30	19.1	7.7	.3	4	1,376	1.0	700	.05	.39	.3	0
15	Tablespoon	1 tbsp	5	18	25	2	2	1.0	.4	Trace	Trace	69	Trace	40	Trace	.02	Trace	0
16	Ounce	1 oz	28	18	130	12	9	5.4	2.2	.1	1	390	.3	200	.01	.11	.1	0
17	Provolone	1 oz	28	41	100	7	8	4.8	1.7	.1	1	214	.1	230	.01	.09	Trace	0
	Ricotta, made with—																	
18	Whole milk	1 cup	246	72	430	28	32	20.4	7.1	.7	7	509	.9	1,210	.03	.48	.3	0
19	Part skim milk	1 cup	246	74	340	28	19	12.1	4.7	.5	13	669	1.1	1,060	.05	.46	.2	0
20	Romano	1 oz	28	31	110	9	8	5.0	—	—	1	302	—	160	—	.11	Trace	0
21	Swiss	1 oz	28	37	105	8	8	5.0	1.7	.2	1	272	Trace	240	.01	.10	Trace	0
	Pasteurized process cheese:																	
22	American	1 oz	28	39	105	6	9	5.6	2.1	.2	Trace	174	.1	340	.01	.10	Trace	0
23	Swiss	1 oz	28	42	95	7	7	4.5	1.7	.1	1	219	.2	230	Trace	.08	Trace	0
24	Pasteurized process cheese food, American	1 oz	28	43	95	6	7	4.4	1.7	.1	2	163	.2	260	.01	.13	Trace	0
25	Pasteurized process cheese spread, American	1 oz	28	48	80	5	6	3.8	1.5	.1	2	159	.1	220	.01	.12	Trace	0
	Cream, sweet:																	
26	Half-and-half (cream and milk)	1 cup	242	81	315	7	28	17.3	7.0	.6	10	254	.2	260	.08	.36	.2	2
27		1 tbsp	15	81	20	Trace	2	1.1	.4	Trace	1	16	Trace	20	.01	.02	Trace	Trace
28	Light, coffee, or table	1 cup	240	74	470	6	46	28.8	11.7	1.0	9	231	.1	1,730	.08	.36	.1	2
29		1 tbsp	15	74	30	Trace	3	1.8	.7	.1	1	14	Trace	110	Trace	.02	Trace	Trace

NUTRIENTS IN INDICATED QUANTITY

H

H

TABLE 2.—NUTRITIVE VALUES OF THE EDIBLE PART OF FOODS - Continued
(Dashes (—) denote lack of reliable data for a constituent believed to be present in measurable amount)

Item No.	Foods, approximate measures, units, and weight (edible part unless footnotes indicate otherwise)			Water	Food energy	Pro-tein	Fat	Fatty Acids			Carbo-hydrate	Calcium	Iron	Vitamin A value	Thiamin	Ribo-flavin	Niacin	Ascorbic acid
								Satu-rated (total)	Unsaturated Oleic	Lino-leic								
(A)	(B)		Grams	Per-cent	Cal-ories	Grams	Grams	Grams	Grams	Grams	Grams	Milli-grams	Milli-grams	Inter-national units	Milli-grams	Milli-grams	Milli-grams	Milli-grams
				(C)	(D)	(E)	(F)	(G)	(H)	(I)	(J)	(K)	(L)	(M)	(N)	(O)	(P)	(Q)
	DAIRY PRODUCTS (CHEESE, CREAM, IMITATION CREAM, MILK; RELATED PRODUCTS)—Con.																	
	Cream, sweet—Continued																	
	Whipping, unwhipped (volume about double when whipped):																	
30	Light	1 cup	239	64	700	5	74	46.2	18.3	1.5	7	166	0.1	2,690	0.06	0.30	0.1	1
31		1 tbsp	15	64	45	Trace	5	2.9	1.1	.1	Trace	10	Trace	170	Trace	.02	Trace	Trace
32	Heavy	1 cup	238	58	820	5	88	54.8	22.2	2.0	7	154	.1	3,500	.05	.26	.1	1
33		1 tbsp	15	58	80	Trace	6	3.5	1.4	.1	Trace	10	Trace	220	Trace	.02	Trace	Trace
34	Whipped topping, (pressurized)	1 cup	60	61	155	2	13	8.3	3.4	.3	7	61	Trace	550	.02	.04	Trace	0
35		1 tbsp	3	61	10	Trace	1	.4	.2	Trace	Trace	3	Trace	30	Trace	Trace	Trace	0
36	Cream, sour	1 cup	230	71	495	7	48	30.0	12.1	1.1	10	268	.1	1,820	.08	.34	.2	2
37		1 tbsp	12	71	25	Trace	3	1.6	.6	.1	1	14	Trace	90	Trace	.02	Trace	Trace
	Cream products, imitation (made with vegetable fat):																	
	Sweet:																	
	Creamers:																	
38	Liquid (frozen)	1 cup	245	77	335	2	24	22.8	.3	Trace	28	23	.1	¹220	0	0	0	0
39		1 tbsp	15	77	20	Trace	1	1.4	Trace	0	2	1	Trace	¹10	0	0	0	0
40	Powdered	1 cup	94	2	515	5	33	30.6	.9	Trace	52	21	.1	¹190	0	¹.16	0	0
41		1 tsp	2	2	10	Trace	1	.7	Trace	0	1	Trace	Trace	¹Trace	0	¹Trace	0	0
	Whipped topping:																	
42	Frozen	1 cup	75	50	240	1	19	16.3	1.0	.2	17	5	.1	¹650	0	0	0	0
43		1 tbsp	4	50	15	Trace	1	.9	.1	Trace	1	Trace	Trace	¹30	0	0	0	0
44	Powdered, made with whole milk	1 cup	80	67	150	3	10	8.5	.6	.1	13	72	Trace	¹290	.02	.09	Trace	1
45		1 tbsp	4	67	10	Trace	Trace	.4	Trace	Trace	1	4	Trace	¹10	Trace	Trace	Trace	Trace
46	Pressurized	1 cup	70	60	185	1	16	13.2	1.4	.2	11	4	Trace	¹330	0	0	0	0
47		1 tbsp	4	60	10	Trace	1	.8	.1	Trace	1	Trace	Trace	¹20	0	0	0	0
48	Sour dressing (imitation sour cream) made with nonfat dry milk.	1 cup	235	75	415	8	39	31.2	4.4	1.1	11	266	.1	¹20	.09	.38	.2	2
49		1 tbsp.	12	75	20	Trace	2	1.6	.2	.1	1	14	Trace	¹Trace	.01	.02	Trace	Trace
	Ice cream. See Milk desserts, frozen (items 75-80).																	
	Ice milk. See Milk desserts, frozen (items 81-83).																	
	Milk:																	
	Fluid:																	
50	Whole (3.3% fat)	1 cup	244	88	150	8	8	5.1	2.1	.2	11	291	.1	²310	.09	.40	.2	2
	Lowfat (2%):																	
51	No milk solids added	1 cup	244	89	120	8	5	2.9	1.2	.1	12	297	.1	500	.10	.40	.2	2
	Milk solids added:																	
52	Label claim less than 10 g of protein per cup.	1 cup	245	89	125	9	5	2.9	1.2	.1	12	313	.1	500	.10	.42	.2	2

¹Vitamin A value is largely from beta-carotene used for coloring. Riboflavin value for items 40-41 apply to products with added riboflavin.
²Applies to product without added vitamin A. With added vitamin A, value is 500 International Units (I.U.).

(A)	(B)		(C)	(D)	(E)	(F)	(G)	(H)	(I)	(J)	(K)	(L)	(M)	(N)	(O)	(P)	(Q)
53	Label claim 10 or more grams of protein per cup (protein fortified)	1 cup	88	135	10	5	3.0	1.2	.1	14	352	.1	500	.11	.48	.2	3
	Lowfat (1%):																
54	No milk solids added	1 cup	90	100	8	3	1.6	.7	.1	12	300	.1	500	.10	.41	.2	2
55	Milk solids added Label claim less than 10 g of protein per cup	1 cup	90	105	9	2	1.5	.6	.1	12	313	.1	500	.10	.42	.2	2
56	Label claim 10 or more grams of protein per cup (protein fortified)	1 cup	89	120	10	3	1.8	.7	.1	14	349	.1	500	.11	.47	.2	3
	Nonfat (skim):																
57	No milk solids added	1 cup	91	85	8	Trace	.3	.1	Trace	12	302	.1	500	.09	.34	.2	2
58	Milk solids added Label claim less than 10 g of protein per cup	1 cup	90	90	9	1	.4	0.1	Trace	12	316	0.1	500	0.10	0.43	0.2	2
59	Label claim 10 or more grams of protein per cup (protein fortified)	1 cup	89	100	10	1	.4	.1	Trace	14	352	.1	500	.11	.48	.2	3
60	Buttermilk	1 cup	90	100	8	2	1.3	.5	Trace	12	285	.1	380	.08	.38	.1	2
	Canned. Evaporated, unsweetened																
61	Whole milk	1 cup	74	340	17	19	11.6	5.3	0.4	25	657	.5	[3]610	.12	.80	.5	5
62	Skim milk	1 cup	79	200	19	1	.3	.1	Trace	29	738	.7	[4]1,000	.11	.79	.4	3
63	Sweetened, condensed	1 cup	27	980	24	27	16.8	6.7	.7	166	868	.6	[4]1,000	.28	1.27	.6	8
	Dried.																
64	Buttermilk	1 cup	3	465	41	7	4.3	1.7	.2	59	1,421	.4	[5]260	.47	1.90	1.1	7
	Nonfat instant																
65	Envelope, net wt. 3.2 oz[7]	1 envelope	4	325	32	1	.4	.1	Trace	47	1,120	.3	[6]2,160	.38	1.59	.8	5
66	Cup[5]	1 cup	4	245	24	Trace	.3	.1	Trace	35	837	.2	[6]1,610	.28	1.19	.6	4
	Milk beverages. Chocolate milk (commercial):																
67	Regular	1 cup	82	210	8	8	5.3	2.2	.2	26	280	.6	[3]300	.09	.41	.3	2
68	Lowfat (2%)	1 cup	84	180	8	5	3.1	1.3	.1	26	284	.6	500	.10	.42	.3	2
69	Lowfat (1%)	1 cup	85	160	8	3	1.5	.7	.1	26	287	.6	500	.10	.40	.2	2
70	Eggnog (commercial)	1 cup	74	340	10	19	11.3	5.0	.6	34	330	.5	890	.09	.48	.3	4
71	Malted milk, home-prepared with 1 cup of whole milk and 2 to 3 heaping tsp of malted milk powder (about 3/4 oz): Chocolate	1 cup of milk plus 3/4 oz of powder	81	235	9	9	5.5	—	—	29	304	.5	330	.14	.43	.7	2
72	Natural	1 cup of milk plus 3/4 oz of powder	81	235	11	10	6.0	—	—	27	347	.3	380	.20	.54	1.3	2
	Shakes, thick[8]																
73	Chocolate, container, net wt. 10.6 oz.	1 container	72	355	9	8	5.0	2.0	.2	63	396	.9	260	.14	.67	.4	0
74	Vanilla, container, net wt. 11 oz.	1 container	74	350	12	9	5.9	2.4	.2	56	457	.3	360	.09	.61	.5	0

[3]Applies to product without vitamin A added
[4]Applies to product with added vitamin A. Without added vitamin A, value is 20 International Units (I.U.).
[5]Yields 1 qt of fluid milk when reconstituted according to package directions
[6]Applies to product with added vitamin A.
[7]Weight applies to product with label claim of 1 1/3 cups equal 3.2 oz.
[8]Applies to products made from thick shake mixes and that do not contain added ice cream. Products made from milk shake mixes are higher in fat and usually contain added ice cream.

H

TABLE 2.—NUTRITIVE VALUES OF THE EDIBLE PART OF FOODS - Continued
(Dashes (—) denote lack of reliable data for a constituent believed to be present in measurable amount)

Item No (A)	Foods, approximate measures, units, and weight (edible part unless footnotes indicate otherwise) (B)	Grams	Water (C) Percent	Food energy (D) Calories	Protein (E) Grams	Fat (F) Grams	Fatty Acids Saturated (total) (G) Grams	Unsaturated Oleic (H) Grams	Unsaturated Linoleic (I) Grams	Carbohydrate (J) Grams	Calcium (K) Milligrams	Iron (L) Milligrams	Vitamin A value (M) International units	Thiamin (N) Milligrams	Riboflavin (O) Milligrams	Niacin (P) Milligrams	Ascorbic acid (Q) Milligrams
	DAIRY PRODUCTS (CHEESE, CREAM, IMITATION CREAM, MILK; RELATED PRODUCTS)—Con.																
	Milk desserts, frozen:																
	Ice cream:																
	Regular (about 11% fat):																
75	Hardened ½ gal	1,064	61	2,155	38	115	71.3	28.8	2.6	254	1,406	1.0	4,340	.42	2.63	1.1	6
76	1 cup	133	61	270	5	14	8.9	3.6	.3	32	176	.1	540	.05	.33	.1	1
77	3-fl oz container	50	61	100	2	5	3.4	1.4	.1	12	66	Trace	200	.02	.12	.1	Trace
78	Soft serve (frozen custard) 1 cup	173	60	375	7	23	13.5	5.9	.6	38	236	.4	790	.08	.45	.2	1
79	Rich (about 16% fat), hardened ½ gal	1,188	59	2,805	33	190	118.3	47.8	4.3	256	1,213	.8	7,200	.36	2.27	.9	5
80	1 cup	148	59	350	4	24	14.7	6.0	.5	32	151	.1	900	.04	.28	.1	1
	Ice milk:																
81	Hardened (about 4.3% fat) ½ gal	1,048	69	1,470	41	45	28.1	11.3	1.0	232	1,409	1.5	1,710	.61	2.78	.9	6
82	Hardened (about 4.3% fat) 1 cup	131	69	185	5	6	3.5	1.4	.1	29	176	.1	210	.08	.35	.1	1
83	Soft serve (about 2.6% fat) 1 cup	175	70	225	8	5	2.9	1.2	.1	38	274	.3	180	.12	.54	.2	1
84	Sherbet (about 2% fat) ½ gal	1,542	66	2,160	17	31	19.0	7.7	.7	469	827	2.5	1,480	.26	.71	1.0	31
85	1 cup	193	66	270	2	4	2.4	1.0	.1	59	103	.3	190	.03	.09	.1	4
	Milk desserts, other:																
86	Custard, baked 1 cup	265	77	305	14	15	6.8	5.4	.7	29	297	1.1	930	.11	.50	.3	1
	Puddings:																
	From home recipe:																
	Starch base:																
87	Chocolate 1 cup	260	66	385	8	12	7.6	3.3	.3	67	250	1.3	390	.05	.36	.3	1
88	Vanilla (blancmange) 1 cup	255	76	285	9	10	6.2	2.5	.2	41	298	Trace	410	.08	.41	.3	2
89	Tapioca cream 1 cup	165	72	220	8	8	4.1	2.5	.5	28	173	.7	480	.07	.30	.2	2
	From mix (chocolate) and milk:																
90	Regular (cooked) 1 cup	260	70	320	9	8	4.3	2.6	.2	59	265	.8	340	.05	.39	.3	2
91	Instant 1 cup	260	69	325	8	7	3.6	2.2	.3	63	374	1.3	340	.08	.39	.3	2
	Yogurt:																
	With added milk solids:																
	Made with lowfat milk:																
92	Fruit-flavored[9] 1 container, net wt., 8 oz	227	75	230	10	3	1.8	.6	.1	42	343	.2	[10]120	.08	.40	.2	1
93	Plain 1 container, net wt., 8 oz	227	85	145	12	4	2.3	.8	.1	16	415	.2	[10]150	.10	.49	.3	2
94	Made with nonfat milk 1 container, net wt., 8 oz	227	85	125	13	Trace	.3	.1	Trace	17	452	.2	[10]20	.11	.53	.3	2
95	Made with whole milk 1 container, net wt., 8 oz	227	88	140	8	7	4.8	1.7	.1	11	274	.1	280	.07	.32	.2	1
	EGGS																
	Eggs, large (24 oz per dozen):																
	Raw:																
96	Whole, without shell 1 egg	50	75	80	6	6	1.7	2.0	.6	Trace	28	1.0	260	.04	.15	Trace	0
97	White 1 white	33	88	15	3	Trace	0	0	0	Trace	4	Trace	0	Trace	.09	Trace	0
98	Yolk 1 yolk	17	49	65	3	6	1.7	2.1	.6	1	26	.9	310	.04	.07	Trace	0
	Cooked:																
99	Fried in butter 1 egg	46	72	85	5	6	2.4	2.2	.6	1	26	.9	290	.03	.13	Trace	0

9 Content of fat, vitamin A, and carbohydrate varies. Consult the label when precise values are needed for special diets.
10 Applies to product made with milk containing no added vitamin A.

(A)	(B)	(C)	(D)	(E)	(F)	(G)	(H)	(I)	(J)	(K)	(L)	(M)	(N)	(O)	(P)	(Q)
100	Hard-cooked, shell removed .... 1 egg	50	80	6	6	1.7	2.0	.6	1	28	1.0	260	.04	.14	Trace	0
101	Poached .... 1 egg	50	80	6	6	1.7	2.0	.6	1	28	1.0	260	.04	.13	Trace	0
102	Scrambled (milk added) in butter. Also omelet. 1 egg	64	95	6	7	2.8	2.3	.6	1	47	.9	310	.04	.16	Trace	0
	FATS, OILS; RELATED PRODUCTS															
	Butter:															
	Regular (1 brick or 4 sticks per lb):															
103	Stick (½ cup) .... 1 stick	113	815	1	92	57.3	23.1	2.1	Trace	27	.2	3,470[a]	.01	.04	Trace	0
104	Tablespoon (about ⅛ stick) .... 1 tbsp	14	100	Trace	12	7.2	2.9	.3	Trace	3	Trace	430[a]	Trace	Trace	Trace	0
105	Pat (1 in square, ⅓ in high; 90 per lb) .... 1 pat	5	35	Trace	4	2.5	1.0	.1	Trace	1	Trace	150[a]	Trace	Trace	Trace	0
	Whipped (6 sticks or two 8-oz containers per lb):															
106	Stick (½ cup) .... 1 stick	76	540	1	61	38.2	15.4	1.4	Trace	18	.1	2,310[a]	Trace	.03	Trace	0
107	Tablespoon (about ⅛ stick) .... 1 tbsp	9	65	Trace	8	4.7	1.9	.2	Trace	2	Trace	290[a]	Trace	Trace	Trace	0
108	Pat (1 ¼ in square, ⅓ in high; 120 per lb) .... 1 pat	4	25	Trace	3	1.9	.8	.1	Trace	1	Trace	120[a]	0	Trace	Trace	0
109	Fats, cooking (vegetable shortenings) .... 1 cup	200	1,770	0	200	48.8	88.2	48.4	0	0	0	—	0	0	0	0
110	.... 1 tbsp	13	110	0	13	3.2	5.7	3.1	0	0	0	0	0	0	0	0
111	Lard .... 1 cup	205	1,850	0	205	81.0	83.8	20.5	0	0	0	0	0	0	0	0
112	.... 1 tbsp	13	115	0	13	5.1	5.3	1.3	0	0	0	0	0	0	0	0
	Margarine:															
	Regular (1 brick or 4 sticks per lb):															
113	Stick (½ cup) .... 1 stick	113	815	1	92	16.7	42.9	24.9	Trace	27	.2	3,750[b]	.01	.04	Trace	0
114	Tablespoon (about ⅛ stick) .... 1 tbsp	14	100	Trace	12	2.1	5.3	3.1	Trace	3	Trace	470[b]	Trace	Trace	Trace	0
115	Pat (1 in square, ⅓ in high; 90 per lb) .... 1 pat	5	35	Trace	4	.7	1.9	1.1	Trace	1	Trace	170[b]	Trace	Trace	Trace	0
116	Soft, two 8-oz containers per lb .... 1 container	227	1,635	1	184	32.5	71.5	65.4	Trace	53	.4	7,500[b]	.01	.08	1	0
117	.... 1 tbsp	14	100	Trace	12	2.0	4.5	4.1	Trace	3	Trace	470[b]	Trace	Trace	Trace	0
	Whipped (6 sticks per lb):															
118	Stick (½ cup) .... 1 stick	76	545	Trace	61	11.2	28.7	16.7	Trace	18	.1	2,500[b]	Trace	.03	Trace	0
119	Tablespoon (about ⅛ stick) .... 1 tbsp	9	70	Trace	8	1.4	3.6	2.1	Trace	2	Trace	310[b]	Trace	Trace	Trace	0
	Oils, salad or cooking:															
120	Corn .... 1 cup	218	1,925	0	218	27.7	53.6	125.1	0	0	0	—	0	0	0	0
121	.... 1 tbsp	14	120	0	14	1.7	3.3	7.8	0	0	0	—	0	0	0	0
122	Olive .... 1 cup	216	1,910	0	216	30.7	154.4	17.7	0	0	0	—	0	0	0	0
123	.... 1 tbsp	14	120	0	14	1.9	9.7	1.1	0	0	0	—	0	0	0	0
124	Peanut .... 1 cup	216	1,910	0	216	37.4	98.5	67.0	0	0	0	—	0	0	0	0
125	.... 1 tbsp	14	120	0	14	2.3	6.2	4.2	0	0	0	—	0	0	0	0
126	Safflower .... 1 cup	218	1,925	0	218	20.5	25.9	159.8	0	0	0	—	0	0	0	0
127	.... 1 tbsp	14	120	0	14	1.3	1.6	10.0	0	0	0	—	0	0	0	0
128	Soybean oil, hydrogenated (partially hardened) .... 1 cup	218	1,925	0	218	31.8	93.1	75.6	0	0	0	—	0	0	0	0
129	.... 1 tbsp	14	120	0	14	2.0	5.8	4.7	0	0	0	0	0	0	0	0
130	Soybean-cottonseed oil blend, hydrogenated .... 1 cup	218	1,925	0	218	38.2	63.0	99.6	0	0	0	0	0	0	0	0
131	.... 1 tbsp	14	120	0	14	2.4	3.9	6.2	0	0	0	0	0	0	0	0

[a] Based on year-round average.

[b] Based on average vitamin A content of fortified margarine. Federal specifications for fortified margarine require a minimum of 15,000 International Units (I.U.) of vitamin A per pound.

TABLE 2.—NUTRITIVE VALUES OF THE EDIBLE PART OF FOODS - Continued
(Dashes (—) denote lack of reliable data for a constituent believed to be present in measurable amount)

NUTRIENTS IN INDICATED QUANTITY

Item No. (A)	Foods, approximate measures, units, and weight (edible part unless footnotes indicate otherwise) (B)	Grams	Water Percent (C)	Food energy Calories (D)	Protein Grams (E)	Fat Grams (F)	Saturated (total) Grams (G)	Unsaturated Oleic Grams (H)	Unsaturated Linoleic Grams (I)	Carbohydrate Grams (J)	Calcium Milligrams (K)	Iron Milligrams (L)	Vitamin A value International units (M)	Thiamin Milligrams (N)	Riboflavin Milligrams (O)	Niacin Milligrams (P)	Ascorbic acid Milligrams (Q)
	FATS, OILS; RELATED PRODUCTS—Con.																
	Salad dressings:																
	Commercial																
	Blue cheese:																
132	Regular . . . 1 tbsp	15	32	75	1	8	1.6	1.7	3.8	1	12	Trace	30	Trace	.02	Trace	Trace
133	Low calorie (5 Cal per tsp) . . . 1 tbsp	16	84	10	Trace	1	.5	.3	Trace	1	10	Trace	30	Trace	.01	Trace	Trace
	French:																
134	Regular . . . 1 tbsp	16	39	65	Trace	6	1.1	1.3	3.2	3	2	.1	—	—	—	—	—
135	Low calorie (5 Cal per tsp) . . . 1 tbsp	16	77	15	Trace	1	.1	.1	.4	2	2	.1	—	—	—	Trace	—
	Italian:																
136	Regular . . . 1 tbsp	15	28	85	Trace	9	1.6	1.9	4.7	1	2	Trace	Trace	Trace	Trace	Trace	—
137	Low calorie (2 Cal per tsp) . . . 1 tbsp	15	90	10	Trace	1	.1	.1	.4	Trace	Trace	Trace	Trace	Trace	Trace	Trace	—
138	Mayonnaise . . . 1 tbsp	14	15	100	Trace	11	2.0	2.4	5.6	Trace	3	.1	40	Trace	.01	Trace	—
	Mayonnaise type:																
139	Regular . . . 1 tbsp	15	41	65	Trace	6	1.1	1.4	3.2	2	2	Trace	30	Trace	Trace	Trace	—
140	Low calorie (8 Cal per tsp) . . . 1 tbsp	16	81	20	Trace	2	.4	.4	1.0	2	3	Trace	40	Trace	Trace	Trace	—
141	Tartar sauce, regular . . . 1 tbsp	14	34	75	Trace	8	1.5	1.8	4.1	1	3	.1	30	Trace	Trace	Trace	Trace
	Thousand Island:																
142	Regular . . . 1 tbsp	16	32	80	Trace	8	1.4	1.7	4.0	2	2	.1	50	Trace	Trace	Trace	Trace
143	Low calorie (10 Cal per tsp) . . . 1 tbsp	15	68	25	Trace	2	.4	.4	1.0	2	2	.1	50	Trace	Trace	Trace	Trace
	From home recipe:																
144	Cooked type[13] . . . 1 tbsp	16	68	25	1	2	.5	.6	.3	2	14	.1	80	.01	.03	Trace	Trace
	FISH, SHELLFISH, MEAT, POULTRY, RELATED PRODUCTS																
	Fish and shellfish:																
145	Bluefish, baked with butter or margarine . . . 3 oz	85	68	135	22	4	—	—	—	0	25	0.6	40	.09	.08	1.6	—
	Clams:																
146	Raw, meat only . . . 3 oz	85	82	65	11	1	0.2	Trace	Trace	2	59	5.2	90	.08	.15	1.1	8
147	Canned, solids and liquid . . . 3 oz	85	86	45	7	1	.6	.4	.1	2	47	3.5	—	.01	.09	.9	—
148	Crabmeat (white or king), canned, not pressed down . . . 1 cup	135	77	135	24	3	—	—	—	1	61	1.1	—	.11	.11	2.6	—
149	Fish sticks, breaded, cooked, frozen (stick, 4 by 1 by ½ in) . . . 1 fish stick or 1 oz	28	66	50	5	3	—	—	—	2	3	.1	0	.01	.02	.5	—
150	Haddock, breaded, fried[14] . . . 3 oz	85	66	140	17	5	1.4	2.2	1.2	5	34	1.0	—	.03	.06	2.7	2
151	Ocean perch, breaded, fried[14] . . . 1 fillet	85	59	195	16	11	2.7	4.4	2.3	6	28	1.1	—	.10	.10	1.6	—
152	Oysters, raw meat only (13-19 medium Selects) . . . 1 cup	240	85	160	20	4	1.3	.2	.1	8	226	13.2	740	.34	.43	6.0	—
153	Salmon, pink, canned, solids and liquid . . . 3 oz	85	71	120	17	5	.9	.8	.1	0	[15]167	.7	60	.03	.16	6.8	—

[13] Fatty acid values apply to product made with regular-type margarine.
[14] Dipped in egg, milk or water, and breadcrumbs; fried in vegetable shortening.
[15] If bones are discarded, value for calcium will be greatly reduced.

H

(A)	Food	(B)	(C)	(D)	(E)	(F)	(G)	(H)	(I)	(J)	(K)	(L)	(M)	(N)	(O)	(P)	(Q)
154	Sardines, Atlantic, canned in oil, drained solids.	3 oz	85	175	20	9	3.0	2.5	.5	0	372	2.5	190	.02	.17	4.6	—
155	Scallops, frozen, breaded, fried, reheated.	6 scallops	90	175	16	8	—	—	—	9	—	.5					—
156	Shad, baked with butter or margarine, bacon.	3 oz	85	170	20	10	—	—	—	0	20	.5	30	.11	.22	7.3	—
	Shrimp:																
157	Canned meat	3 oz	85	100	21	1	.1	.1	Trace	1	98	2.6	50	.01	.03	1.5	—
158	French fried[16]	3 oz	85	190	17	9	2.3	3.7	2.0	9	61	1.7	—	.03	.07	2.3	—
159	Tuna, canned in oil, drained solids.	3 oz	85	170	24	7	1.7	1.7	.7	0	7	1.6	70	.04	.10	10.1	—
160	Tuna salad[17]	1 cup	205	350	30	22	4.3	6.3	6.7	7	41	2.7	590	.08	.23	10.3	2
	Meat and meat products:																
161	Bacon, (20 slices per lb, raw), broiled or fried, crisp	2 slices	15	85	4	8	2.5	3.7	.7	Trace	2	.5	0	.08	.05	.8	—
	Beef,[18] cooked:																
	Cuts braised, simmered or pot roasted:																
162	Lean and fat (piece, 2 1/2 by 2 1/2 by 3/4 in)	3 oz	85	245	23	16	6.8	6.5	.4	0	10	2.9	30	.04	.18	3.6	—
163	Lean only from item 162	2.5 oz	72	140	22	5	2.1	1.8	.2	0	10	2.7	10	.04	.17	3.3	—
	Ground beef, broiled:																
164	Lean with 10% fat	3 oz or patty 3 by 5/8 in	85	185	23	10	4.0	3.9	.3	0	10	3.0	20	.08	.20	5.1	—
165	Lean with 21% fat	2.9 oz or patty 3 by 5/8 in	82	235	20	17	7.0	6.7	.4	0	9	2.6	30	.07	.17	4.4	—
	Roast, oven cooked, no liquid added																
	Relatively fat, such as rib:																
166	Lean and fat (2 pieces, 4 1/8 by 2 1/4 by 1/4 in)	3 oz	85	375	17	33	14.0	13.6	.8	0	8	2.2	70	.05	.13	3.1	—
167	Lean only from item 166	1.8 oz	51	125	14	7	3.0	2.5	.3	0	6	1.8	10	.04	.11	2.6	—
	Relatively lean, such as heel of round:																
168	Lean and fat (2 pieces, 4 1/8 by 2 1/4 by 1/4 in)	3 oz	85	165	25	7	2.8	2.7	.2	0	11	3.2	10	.06	.19	4.5	—
169	Lean only from item 168	2.8 oz	78	125	24	3	1.2	1.0	0.1	0	10	3.0	Trace	0.06	0.18	4.3	—
	Steak:																
	Relatively fat-sirloin, broiled:																
170	Lean and fat (piece, 2 1/2 by 2 1/2 by 3/4 in)	3 oz	85	330	20	27	11.3	11.1	.6	0	9	2.5	50	.05	.15	4.0	—
171	Lean only from item 170	2.0 oz	56	115	18	4	1.8	1.6	.2	0	7	2.2	10	.05	.14	3.6	—
	Relatively lean-round, braised:																
172	Lean and fat (piece, 4 1/8 by 2 1/4 by 1/2 in)	3 oz	85	220	24	13	5.5	5.2	.4	0	10	3.0	20	.07	.19	4.8	—
173	Lean only from item 172	2.4 oz	68	130	21	4	1.7	1.5	.2	0	9	2.5	10	.05	.16	4.1	—
	Beef, canned:																
174	Corned beef	3 oz	85	185	22	10	4.9	4.5	.2	0	17	3.7	—	.01	.20	2.9	—
175	Corned beef hash	1 cup	220	400	19	25	11.9	10.9	.5	24	29	4.4	—	.02	.20	4.6	—

[16] Dipped in egg, breadcrumbs, and flour or batter.
[17] Prepared with tuna, celery, salad dressing (mayonnaise type), pickle, onion, and egg.
[18] Outer layer of fat on the cut was removed to within approximately 1/2 in of the lean. Deposits of fat within the cut were not removed

H

H

TABLE 2.—NUTRITIVE VALUES OF THE EDIBLE PART OF FOODS - Continued
(Dashes (—) denote lack of reliable data for a constituent believed to be present in measurable amount)

NUTRIENTS IN INDICATED QUANTITY

Item No. (A)	Foods, approximate measures, units, and weight (edible part unless footnotes indicate otherwise) (B)	Grams	Water Percent (C)	Food energy Calories (D)	Protein Grams (E)	Fat Grams (F)	Fatty Acids Saturated (total) Grams (G)	Unsaturated Oleic Grams (H)	Unsaturated Linoleic Grams (I)	Carbohydrate Grams (J)	Calcium Milligrams (K)	Iron Milligrams (L)	Vitamin A value International units (M)	Thiamin Milligrams (N)	Riboflavin Milligrams (O)	Niacin Milligrams (P)	Ascorbic acid Milligrams (Q)
	FISH, SHELLFISH, MEAT, POULTRY; RELATED PRODUCTS—Con.																
	Meat and meat products:—Continued																
176	Beef, dried, chipped ... 2½-oz jar	71	48	145	24	4	2.1	2.0	.1	0	14	3.6	—	.05	.23	2.7	0
177	Beef and vegetable stew ... 1 cup	245	82	220	16	11	4.9	4.5	.2	15	29	2.9	2,400	.15	.17	4.7	17
178	Beef potpie (home recipe), baked[19] (piece, ⅓ of 9-in diam. pie) ... 1 piece	210	55	515	21	30	7.9	12.8	6.7	39	29	3.8	1,720	.30	.30	5.5	6
179	Chili con carne with beans, canned ... 1 cup	255	72	340	19	16	7.5	6.8	.3	31	82	4.3	150	.08	.18	3.3	—
180	Chop suey with beef and pork (home recipe) ... 1 cup	250	75	300	26	17	8.5	6.2	.7	13	60	4.8	600	.28	.38	5.0	33
181	Heart, beef, lean, braised ... 3 oz	85	61	160	27	5	1.5	1.1	.6	1	5	5.0	20	.21	1.04	6.5	1
	Lamb, cooked: Chop, rib (cut 3 per lb with bone), broiled:																
182	Lean and fat ... 3.1 oz	89	43	360	18	32	14.8	12.1	1.2	0	8	1.0	—	.11	.19	4.1	—
183	Lean only from item 182 ... 2 oz	57	60	120	16	6	2.5	2.1	.2	0	6	1.1	—	.09	.15	3.4	—
	Leg, roasted:																
184	Lean and fat (2 pieces, 4⅛ by 2¼ by ¼ in) ... 3 oz	85	54	235	22	16	7.3	6.0	.6	0	9	1.4	—	.13	.23	4.7	—
185	Lean only from item 184 ... 2.5 oz	71	62	130	20	5	2.1	1.8	.2	0	9	1.4	—	.12	.21	4.4	—
	Shoulder, roasted:																
186	Lean and fat (3 pieces, 2½ by 2½ by ¼ in) ... 3 oz	85	50	285	18	23	10.8	8.8	.9	0	9	1.0	—	.11	.20	4.0	—
187	Lean only from item 186 ... 2.3 oz	64	61	130	17	6	3.6	2.3	.2	0	8	1.0	—	.10	.18	3.7	—
188	Liver, beef, fried[20] (slice, 6½ by 2⅜ by ⅜ in ... 3 oz	85	56	195	22	9	2.5	3.5	.9	5	9	7.5	[21]45,390	.22	3.56	14.0	23
	Pork, cured, cooked:																
189	Ham, light cure, lean and fat, roasted (2 pieces, 4⅛ by 2¼ by ¼ in)[22] ... 3 oz	85	54	245	18	19	6.8	7.9	1.7	0	8	2.2	0	.40	.15	3.1	—
	Luncheon meat:																
190	Boiled ham, slice (8 per 8-oz pkg.) ... 1 oz	28	59	65	5	5	1.7	2.0	.4	0	3	.8	0	.12	.04	.7	—
	Canned, spiced or unspiced:																
191	Slice, approx. 3 by 2 by ½ in. ... 1 slice	60	55	175	9	15	5.4	6.7	1.0	1	5	1.3	0	.19	.13	1.8	—
	Pork, fresh,[18] cooked: Chop, loin (cut 3 per lb with bone), broiled:																
192	Lean and fat ... 2.7 oz	78	42	305	19	25	8.9	10.4	2.2	0	9	2.7	0	.75	.22	4.5	—
193	Lean only from item 192 ... 2 oz	56	53	150	17	9	3.1	3.6	.8	0	7	2.2	0	.63	.18	3.8	—

[19]Crust made with vegetable shortening and enriched flour.
[18]Outer layer of fat on the cut was removed to within approximately ½ in. of the lean. Deposits of fat within the cut were not removed.
[22]About one-fourth of the outer layer of fat on the cut was removed. Deposits of fat within the cut were not removed.
[20]Regular-type margarine used
[21]Value varies widely.

H

(A)	(B)	(C)	(D)	(E)	(F)	(G)	(H)	(I)	(J)	(K)	(L)	(M)	(N)	(O)	(P)	(Q)
	Roast, oven cooked, no liquid added:															
194	Lean and fat (piece, 2 ½ by 2 ½ by ¾ in), 3 oz	85	310	21	24	8.7	10.2	2.2	0	9	2.7	0	.78	.22	4.8	—
195	Lean only from item 194, 2.4 oz	68	175	20	10	3.5	4.1	.8	0	9	2.6	0	.73	.21	4.4	—
	Shoulder cut, simmered:															
196	Lean and fat (3 pieces, 2 ½ by 2 ½ by ¼ in), 3 oz	85	320	20	26	9.3	10.9	2.3	0	9	2.6	0	.46	.21	4.1	—
197	Lean only from item 196, 2.2 oz	63	135	18	6	2.2	2.6	.6	0	8	2.3	0	.42	.19	3.7	—
	Sausages (see also Luncheon meat (items 190-191)):															
198	Bologna, slice (8 per 8-oz pkg), 1 slice	28	85	3	8	3.0	3.4	.5	Trace	2	.5	—	.05	.06	.7	—
199	Braunschweiger, slice (6 per 6-oz pkg), 1 slice	28	90	4	8	2.6	3.4	.8	1	3	1.7	1,850	.05	.41	2.3	—
200	Brown and serve (10-11 per 8-oz pkg), browned, 1 link	17	70	3	6	2.3	2.8	.7	Trace	—	—	—	—	—	—	—
201	Deviled ham, canned, 1 tbsp	13	45	2	4	1.5	1.8	.4	0	1	.3	0	.02	.01	.2	—
202	Frankfurter (8 per 1-lb pkg), cooked (reheated), 1 frankfurter	56	170	7	15	5.6	6.5	1.2	1	3	.8	0	.08	.11	1.4	—
203	Meat, potted (beef, chicken, turkey), canned, 1 tbsp	13	30	2	2	—	—	—	0	—	—	0	Trace	.03	.2	—
204	Pork link (16 per 1-lb pkg), cooked, 1 link	13	60	2	6	2.1	2.4	.5	Trace	1	.3	0	.10	.04	.5	—
	Salami:															
205	Dry type, slice (12 per 4-oz pkg), 1 slice	10	45	2	4	1.6	1.6	.1	Trace	1	.4	—	.04	.03	.5	—
206	Cooked type, slice (8 per 8-oz pkg), 1 slice	28	90	5	7	3.1	3.0	.2	Trace	3	.7	—	.07	.07	1.2	—
207	Vienna sausage (7 per 4-oz can), 1 sausage	16	40	2	3	1.2	1.4	.2	Trace	1	.3	—	.01	.02	.4	—
	Veal, medium fat, cooked, bone removed:															
208	Cutlet (4 ⅛ by 2 ¼ by ½ in), braised or broiled, 3 oz	85	185	23	9	4.0	3.4	.4	0	9	2.7	—	.06	.21	4.6	—
209	Rib (2 pieces, 4 ⅛ by 2 ¼ by ¼ in), roasted, 3 oz	85	230	23	14	6.1	5.1	.6	0	10	2.9	—	.11	.26	6.6	—
	Poultry and poultry products:															
	Chicken, cooked:															
210	Breast, fried,[23] bones removed, ½ breast (3.3 oz with bones), 2.8 oz	79	160	26	5	1.4	1.8	1.1	1	9	1.3	70	.04	.17	11.6	—
211	Drumstick, fried,[23] bones removed (2 oz with bones), 1.3 oz	38	90	12	4	1.1	1.3	.9	Trace	6	.9	50	.03	.15	2.7	—
212	Half broiler, broiled, bones removed (10.4 oz with bones), 6.2 oz	176	240	42	7	2.2	2.5	1.3	0	16	3.0	160	.09	.34	15.5	—
213	Chicken, canned, boneless, 3 oz	85	170	18	10	3.2	3.8	2.0	0	18	1.3	200	.03	.11	3.7	3
214	Chicken a la king, cooked (home recipe), 1 cup	245	470	27	34	12.7	14.3	3.3	12	127	2.5	1,130	.10	.42	5.4	12
215	Chicken and noodles, cooked (home recipe), 1 cup	240	365	22	18	5.9	7.1	3.5	26	26	2.2	430	.05	.17	4.3	Trace
	Chicken chow mein:															
216	Canned, 1 cup	250	95	7	Trace	—	—	—	18	45	1.3	150	.05	.10	1.0	13
217	From home recipe, 1 cup	250	255	31	10	2.4	3.4	3.1	10	58	2.5	280	.08	.23	4.3	10

[19]Crust made with vegetable shortening and enriched flour.
[23]Vegetable shortening used

TABLE 2.—NUTRITIVE VALUES OF THE EDIBLE PART OF FOODS - Continued
(Dashes (—) denote lack of reliable data for a constituent believed to be present in measurable amount)

Item No. (A)	Foods, approximate measures, units, and weight (edible part unless footnotes indicate otherwise) (B)	Grams	Water (C) Percent	Food energy (D) Calories	Protein (E) Grams	Fat (F) Grams	Fatty Acids Saturated (total) (G) Grams	Unsaturated Oleic (H) Grams	Unsaturated Linoleic (I) Grams	Carbohydrate (J) Grams	Calcium (K) Milligrams	Iron (L) Milligrams	Vitamin A value (M) International units	Thiamin (N) Milligrams	Riboflavin (O) Milligrams	Niacin (P) Milligrams	Ascorbic acid (Q) Milligrams
	FISH, SHELLFISH, MEAT, POULTRY; RELATED PRODUCTS—Con.																
	Poultry and poultry products — Continued																
218	Chicken potpie (home recipe), baked,[19] piece (⅓ or 9-in diam. pie) . . . . 1 piece	232	57	545	23	31	11.3	10.9	5.6	42	70	3.0	3,090	.34	.31	5.5	5
	Turkey, roasted, flesh without skin:																
219	Dark meat, piece, 2½ by 1⅝ by ¼in. . . . 4 pieces	85	61	175	26	7	2.1	1.5	1.5	0	—	2.0	—	.03	.20	3.6	—
220	Light meat, piece, 4 by 2 by ¼ in. . . . 2 pieces	85	62	150	28	3	.9	.6	.7	0	—	1.0	—	.04	.12	9.4	—
	Light and dark meat:																
221	Chopped or diced . . . . 1 cup	140	61	265	44	9	2.5	1.7	1.8	0	11	2.5	—	.07	.25	10.8	—
222	Pieces (1 slice white meat, 4 by 2 by ¼in with 2 slices dark meat, 2½ by 1⅝ by ¼ in). . . . 3 pieces	85	61	160	27	5	1.5	1.0	1.1	0	7	1.5	—	.04	.15	6.5	—
	FRUITS AND FRUIT PRODUCTS																
	Apples, raw, unpeeled, without cores:																
223	2¾-in diam. (about 3 per lb with cores) . . . . 1 apple	138	84	80	Trace	1	—	—	—	20	10	.4	120	.04	.03	.1	6
224	3¼ in diam. (about 2 per lb with cores) . . . . 1 apple	212	84	125	Trace	1	—	—	—	31	15	.6	190	.06	.04	.2	8
225	Applejuice, bottled or canned[24] . . . . 1 cup	248	88	120	Trace	Trace	—	—	—	30	15	1.5	—	.02	.05	.2	[25]2
	Applesauce canned:																
226	Sweetened . . . . 1 cup	255	76	230	1	Trace	—	—	—	61	10	1.3	100	.05	.03	.1	[25]3
227	Unsweetened . . . . 1 cup	244	89	100	Trace	Trace	—	—	—	26	10	1.2	100	.05	.02	.1	[25]2
	Apricots:																
228	Raw, without pits (about 12 per lb with pits). . . . 3 apricots	107	85	55	1	Trace	—	—	—	14	18	.5	2,890	.03	.04	.6	11
229	Canned in heavy sirup (halves and sirup) . . . . 1 cup	258	77	220	2	Trace	—	—	—	57	28	.8	4,490	.05	.05	1.0	10
	Dried:																
230	Uncooked (28 large or 37 medium halves per cup). . . . 1 cup	130	25	340	7	1	—	—	—	86	87	7.2	14,170	.01	.21	4.3	16
231	Cooked, unsweetened, fruit and liquid. . . . 1 cup	250	76	215	4	1	—	—	—	54	55	4.5	7,500	.01	.13	2.5	8
232	Apricot nectar, canned . . . . 1 cup	251	85	145	1	Trace	—	—	—	37	23	.5	2,380	.03	.03	.5	[26]36
233	Avocados, raw, whole, without skins and seeds: California, mid- and late- winter (with skin and seed, 3⅛-in diam.; wt., 10 oz). . . . 1 avocado	216	74	370	5	37	5.5	22.0	3.7	13	22	1.3	630	.24	.43	3.5	30

[24]Also applies to pasteurized apple cider.
[25]Applies to product without added ascorbic. For value of product with added ascorbic acid, refer to label.
[26]Based on product with label claim of 45% of U.S. RDA in 6 fl oz.

(A)	(B)	(C)	(D)	(E)	(F)	(G)	(H)	(I)	(J)	(K)	(L)	(M)	(N)	(O)	(P)	(Q)
234	Florida, late summer and fall (with skin and seed, 3⅝-in diam. wt. 1 lb) — 1 avocado	304	390	4	33	6.7	15.7	5.3	27	30	1.8	880	.33	.61	4.9	43
235	Banana without peel (about 2.6 per lb with peel) — 1 banana	119	100	1	Trace	—	—	—	26	10	.8	230	.06	.07	.8	12
236	Banana flakes — 1 tbsp	6	20	Trace	Trace	—	—	—	5	2	.2	50	.01	.01	.2	Trace
237	Blackberries, raw — 1 cup	144	85	2	1	—	—	—	19	46	1.3	290	.04	.06	.6	30
238	Blueberries, raw — 1 cup	145	90	1	1	—	—	—	22	22	1.5	150	.04	.09	.7	20
	Cantaloup. See Muskmelons (item 271).															
	Cherries:															
239	Sour (tart), red, pitted, canned, water pack — 1 cup	244	105	2	Trace	—	—	—	26	37	.7	1,660	.07	.05	.5	12
240	Sweet, raw, without pits and stems — 10 cherries	68	45	1	Trace	—	—	—	12	15	.3	70	.03	.04	.3	7
241	Cranberry juice cocktail, bottled, sweetened — 1 cup	253	165	Trace	Trace	—	—	—	42	13	.8	Trace	.03	.03	.1	[27]81
242	Cranberry sauce, sweetened, canned, strained — 1 cup	277	405	Trace	1	—	—	—	104	17	.6	60	.03	.03	.1	6
	Dates:															
243	Whole, without pits — 10 dates	80	220	2	Trace	—	—	—	58	47	2.4	40	.07	.08	1.8	0
244	Chopped — 1 cup	178	490	4	1	—	—	—	130	105	5.3	90	.16	.18	3.9	0
245	Fruit cocktail, canned, in heavy sirup — 1 cup	255	195	1	Trace	—	—	—	50	23	1.0	360	.05	.03	1.0	5
	Grapefruit:															
	Raw, medium, 3¾-in diam. (about 1 lb 1 oz):															
246	Pink or red — ½ grapefruit with peel[28]	241	50	1	Trace	—	—	—	13	20	.5	540	.05	.02	.2	44
247	White — ½ grapefruit with peel[28]	241	45	1	Trace	—	—	—	12	19	.5	10	.05	.02	.2	44
248	Canned, sections with sirup — 1 cup	254	180	2	Trace	—	—	—	45	33	.8	30	.08	.05	.5	76
	Grapefruit juice:															
249	Raw, pink, red, or white — 1 cup	246	95	1	Trace	—	—	—	23	22	.5	(²⁹)	.10	.05	.5	93
	Canned, white:															
250	Unsweetened — 1 cup	247	100	1	Trace	—	—	—	24	20	1.0	20	.07	.05	.5	84
251	Sweetened — 1 cup	250	135	1	Trace	—	—	—	32	20	1.0	30	.08	.05	.5	78
	Frozen concentrate, unsweetened:															
252	Undiluted, 6-fl oz can	207	300	4	1	—	—	—	72	70	.8	60	.29	.12	1.4	286
253	Diluted with 3 parts water by volume — 1 cup	247	100	1	Trace	—	—	—	24	25	.2	20	.10	.04	.5	96
254	Dehydrated crystals, prepared with water (1 lb yields about 1 gal) — 1 cup	247	100	1	Trace	—	—	—	24	22	.2	20	.10	.05	.5	91
	Grapes, European type (adherent skin), raw:															
255	Thompson Seedless — 10 grapes	50	35	Trace	Trace	—	—	—	9	6	.2	50	.03	.02	.2	2
256	Tokay and Emperor, seeded types — 10 grapes[30]	60	40	Trace	Trace	—	—	—	10	7	.2	60	.03	.02	.2	2
	Grapejuice:															
257	Canned or bottled — 1 cup	253	165	1	Trace	—	—	—	42	28	.8	—	.10	.05	.5	[25]Trace
	Frozen concentrate, sweetened:															
258	Undiluted, 6-fl oz can	216	395	1	Trace	—	—	—	100	22	.9	40	.13	.22	1.5	[31]32
259	Diluted with 3 parts water by volume — 1 cup	250	135	1	Trace	—	—	—	33	8	.3	10	.05	.08	.5	[31]10

[27]Based on product with label claim of 100% of U.S. RDA in 6 fl oz.

[28]Weight includes peel and membranes between sections. Without these parts, the weight of the edible portion is 123 g for item 246 and 118 g for item 247.

[29]For white-fleshed varieties, value is about 20 International Units (I.U.) per cup; for red-fleshed varieties, 1,080 I.U.

[30]Weight includes seeds. Without seeds, weight of the edible portion is 57 g.

[31]Applies to product without added ascorbic acid. With added ascorbic acid, based on claim that 6 fl oz of reconstituted juice contain 45% or 50% of the U.S. RDA, value in milligrams is 108 or 120 for a 6-fl oz can (item 258), 36 or 40 for 1 cup of diluted juice (item 259).

H

TABLE 2.—NUTRITIVE VALUES OF THE EDIBLE PART OF FOODS - Continued
(Dashes (—) denote lack of reliable data for a constituent believed to be present in measurable amount)

Item No (A)	Foods, approximate measures, units, and weight (edible part unless footnotes indicate otherwise) (B)	Grams	Water (C) Percent	Food energy (D) Calories	Protein (E) Grams	Fat (F) Grams	Fatty Acids Saturated (total) (G) Grams	Unsaturated Oleic (H) Grams	Linoleic (I) Grams	Carbohydrate (J) Grams	Calcium (K) Milligrams	Iron (L) Milligrams	Vitamin A value (M) International units	Thiamin (N) Milligrams	Riboflavin (O) Milligrams	Niacin (P) Milligrams	Ascorbic acid (Q) Milligrams
	FRUITS AND FRUIT PRODUCTS—Con.																
260	Grape drink, canned — 1 cup	250	86	135	Trace	Trace	—	—	—	35	8	.3	—	[32].03	[32].03	.3	[38]
261	Lemon, raw, size 165, without peel and seeds (about 4 per lb with peels and seeds) — 1 lemon	74	90	20	1	Trace	—	—	—	6	19	.4	10	.03	.01	.1	39
	Lemon juice:																
262	Raw — 1 cup	244	91	60	1	Trace	—	—	—	20	17	.5	50	.07	.02	.2	112
263	Canned, or bottled, unsweetened — 1 cup	244	92	55	1	Trace	—	—	—	19	17	.5	50	.07	.02	.2	102
264	Frozen, single strength, unsweetened, 6-fl oz can — 1 can	183	92	40	1	Trace	—	—	—	13	13	.5	40	.05	.02	.2	81
	Lemonade concentrate, frozen:																
265	Undiluted, 6-fl oz can — 1 can	219	49	425	Trace	Trace	—	—	—	112	9	.4	40	.05	.06	.7	66
266	Diluted with 4 1/3 parts water by volume — 1 cup	248	89	105	Trace	Trace	—	—	—	28	2	.1	10	.01	.02	.2	17
	Limeade concentrate, frozen:																
267	Undiluted, 6-fl oz can — 1 can	218	50	410	Trace	Trace	—	—	—	108	11	.2	Trace	.02	.02	.2	26
268	Diluted with 4 1/3 parts water by volume — 1 cup	247	89	100	Trace	Trace	—	—	—	27	3	Trace	Trace	Trace	Trace	Trace	6
	Limejuice:																
269	Raw — 1 cup	246	90	65	1	Trace	—	—	—	22	22	.5	20	.05	.02	.2	79
270	Canned, unsweetened — 1 cup	246	90	65	1	Trace	—	—	—	22	22	.5	20	.05	.02	.2	52
271	Muskmelons, raw, with rind, without seed cavity. Cantaloup, orange-fleshed (with rind and seed cavity, 5-in diam., 2 1/3 lb) — 1/2 melon with rind[33]	477	91	80	2	Trace	—	—	—	20	38	1.1	9,240	.11	.08	1.6	90
272	Honeydew (with rind and seed cavity, 6 1/2-in diam. 5 1/4 lb) — 1/10 melon with rind[33]	226	91	50	1	Trace	—	—	—	11	21	.6	60	.06	.04	.9	34
	Oranges, all commercial varieties, raw:																
273	Whole, 2 5/8-in diam., without peel and seeds (about 2 1/2 per lb with peel and seeds) — 1 orange	131	86	65	1	Trace	—	—	—	16	54	.5	260	.13	.05	.5	66
274	Sections without membranes — 1 cup	180	86	90	2	Trace	—	—	—	22	74	.7	360	.18	.07	.7	90
	Orange juice:																
275	Raw, all varieties — 1 cup	248	88	110	2	Trace	—	—	—	26	27	.5	500	.22	.07	1.0	124
276	Canned, unsweetened — 1 cup	249	87	120	2	Trace	—	—	—	28	25	1.0	500	.17	.05	.7	100
	Frozen concentrate:																
277	Undiluted, 6-fl oz can — 1 can	213	55	360	5	Trace	—	—	—	87	75	.9	1,620	.68	.11	2.8	360
278	Diluted with 3 parts water by volume — 1 cup	249	87	120	2	Trace	—	—	—	29	25	.2	540	.23	.03	.9	120
279	Dehydrated crystals, prepared with water (1 lb yields about 1 gal) — 1 cup	248	88	115	1	Trace	—	—	—	27	25	.5	500	.20	.07	1.0	109

[32] For products with added thiamin and riboflavin but without added ascorbic acid, values in milligrams would be 0.60 to thiamin, 0.80 for riboflavin, and trace for ascorbic acid. For products with only ascorbic acid added, value varies with the brand. Consult the label.

[33] Weight includes rind. Without rind, the weight of the edible portion is 272 g for item 271 and 149 g for item 272.

H

H

(A)	(B)	(C)	(D)	(E)	(F)	(G)	(H)	(I)	(J)	(K)	(L)	(M)	(N)	(O)	(P)	(Q)
	Orange and grapefruit juice:															
	Frozen concentrate:															
280	Undiluted, 6-fl oz can	59	330	4	1	—	—	—	78	61	.8	800	.48	.06	2.3	302
281	Diluted with 3 parts water by volume	88	110	1	Trace	—	—	—	26	20	.2	270	.15	.02	.7	102
282	Papayas, raw, ½-in cubes	89	55	1	Trace	—	—	—	14	28	.4	2,450	.06	.06	.4	78
	Peaches:															
283	Raw. Whole, 2½-in diam., peeled, pitted (about 4 per lb with peels and pits)	89	40	1	Trace	—	—	—	10	9	.5	1,330[34]	.02	.05	1.0	7
284	Sliced	89	65	1	Trace	—	—	—	16	15	.9	2,260[34]	.03	.09	1.7	12
	Canned, yellow-fleshed, solids and liquid (halves or slices):															
285	Sirup pack	79	200	1	Trace	—	—	—	51	10	.8	1,100	.03	.05	1.5	8
286	Water pack	91	75	1	Trace	—	—	—	20	10	.7	1,100	.02	.07	1.5	7
	Dried:															
287	Uncooked	25	420	5	1	—	—	—	109	77	9.6	6,240	.02	.30	8.5	29
288	Cooked, unsweetened, halves and juice	77	205	3	1	—	—	—	54	38	4.8	3,050	.01	.15	3.8	5
	Frozen, sliced, sweetened:															
289	10-oz container	77	250	1	Trace	—	—	—	64	11	1.4	1,850	.03	.11	2.0	116[35]
290	Cup	77	220	1	Trace	—	—	—	57	10	1.3	1,630	.03	.10	1.8	103[35]
	Pears:															
	Raw, with skin, cored:															
291	Bartlett, 2½-in diam. (about 2½ per lb with cores and stems)	83	100	1	1	—	—	—	25	13	.5	30	.03	.07	.2	7
292	Bosc, 2½-in diam. (about 3 per lb with cores and stems)	83	85	1	1	—	—	—	22	11	.4	30	.03	.06	.1	6
293	D'Anjou, 3-in diam. (about 2 per lb with cores and stems)	83	120	1	1	—	—	—	31	16	.6	40	.04	.08	.2	8
294	Canned, solids and liquid, sirup pack, heavy (halves or slices)	80	195	1	1	—	—	—	50	13	.5	10	.03	.05	.3	3
	Pineapple:															
295	Raw, diced	85	80	1	Trace	—	—	—	21	26	.8	110	.14	.05	.3	26
296	Canned, heavy sirup pack, solids and liquid: Crushed, chunks, tidbits	80	190	1	Trace	—	—	—	49	28	.8	130	.20	.05	.5	18
	Slices and liquid:															
297	Large	80	80	Trace	Trace	—	—	—	20	12	.3	50	.08	.02	.2	7
	1 slice; 2¼ tbsp liquid															
298	Medium	80	45	Trace	Trace	—	—	—	11	6	.2	30	.05	.01	.1	4
	1 slice; 1¼ tbsp liquid															
299	Pineapple juice, unsweetened, canned	86	140	1	Trace	—	—	—	34	38	.8	130	.13	.05	.5	80[27]
	Plums:															
	Raw, without pits:															
300	Japanese and hybrid (2 1/8-in diam., about 6½ per lb with pits)	87	30	Trace	Trace	—	—	—	8	8	.3	160	.02	.02	.3	4
301	Prune-type (1½-in diam., about 15 per lb with pits)	79	20	Trace	Trace	—	—	—	6	3	.1	80	.01	.01	.1	1

[34]Represents yellow-fleshed varieties. For white-fleshed varieties, value is 50 International Units (I.U.) for 1 peach, 90 I.U. for 1 cup of slices.
[35]Value represents products with added ascorbic acid. For products without added ascorbic acid, value in milligrams is 116 for a 10-oz container, 103 for 1 cup.
[27]Based on product with label claim of 100% of U.S. RDA in 6 fl oz.

TABLE 2.—NUTRITIVE VALUES OF THE EDIBLE PART OF FOODS - Continued
(Dashes (—) denote lack of reliable data for a constituent believed to be present in measurable amount)

H

| | | | | | | | Fatty Acids | | | | | | | | | | |
| | | | | | | | | Unsaturated | | | | | | | | | |
Item No. (A)	Foods, approximate measures, units, and weight (edible part unless footnotes indicate otherwise) (B)		Water (C)	Food energy (D)	Protein (E)	Fat (F)	Saturated (total) (G)	Oleic (H)	Linoleic (I)	Carbohydrate (J)	Calcium (K)	Iron (L)	Vitamin A value (M)	Thiamin (N)	Riboflavin (O)	Niacin (P)	Ascorbic acid (Q)
		Grams	Percent	Calories	Grams	Grams	Grams	Grams	Grams	Grams	Milligrams	Milligrams	International units	Milligrams	Milligrams	Milligrams	Milligrams
	FRUITS AND FRUIT PRODUCTS—Con.																
	Plums—Continued																
	Canned, heavy sirup pack (Italian prunes), with pits and liquid:																
302	Cup	1 cup[36]	272	77	215	1	Trace	—	—	—	56	23	2.3	3,130	.05	.05	1.0	5
303	Portion	3 plums; 2¾ tbsp liquid[36]	140	77	110	1	Trace	—	—	—	29	12	1.2	1,610	.03	.03	.5	3
	Prunes, dried, "softenized," with pits:																
304	Uncooked	4 extra large or 5 large prunes[36]	49	28	110	1	Trace	—	—	—	29	22	1.7	690	.04	.07	.7	1
305	Cooked, unsweetened, all sizes, fruit and liquid	1 cup[36]	250	66	255	2	1	—	—	—	67	51	3.8	1,590	.07	.15	1.5	2
306	Prune juice, canned or bottled	1 cup	256	80	195	1	Trace	—	—	—	49	36	1.8	—	.03	.03	1.0	5
	Raisins, seedless:																
307	Cup, not pressed down	1 cup	145	18	420	4	Trace	—	—	—	112	90	5.1	30	.16	.12	.7	1
308	Packet, ½ oz (1½ tbsp)	1 packet	14	18	40	Trace	Trace	—	—	—	11	9	.5	Trace	.02	.01	.1	Trace
	Raspberries, red:																
309	Raw, capped, whole	1 cup	123	84	70	1	1	—	—	—	17	27	1.1	160	.04	.11	1.1	31
310	Frozen, sweetened, 10-oz container	1 container	284	74	280	2	1	—	—	—	70	37	1.7	200	.06	.17	1.7	60
311	Rhubarb, cooked, added sugar: From raw	1 cup	270	63	380	1	Trace	—	—	—	97	211	1.6	220	.05	.14	.8	16
312	From frozen, sweetened	1 cup	270	63	385	1	1	—	—	—	98	211	1.9	190	.05	.11	.5	16
	Strawberries:																
313	Raw, whole berries, capped	1 cup	149	90	55	1	1	—	—	—	13	31	1.5	90	0.04	0.10	0.9	88
	Frozen, sweetened:																
314	Sliced, 10-oz container	1 container	284	71	310	1	1	—	—	—	79	40	2.0	90	.06	.17	1.4	151
315	Whole, 1-lb container (about 1¾ cups)	1 container	454	76	415	2	1	—	—	—	107	59	2.7	140	.09	.27	2.3	249
316	Tangerine, raw, 2⅜-in diam., size 176, without peel (about 4 per lb with peels and seeds)	1 tangerine	86	87	40	1	Trace	—	—	—	10	34	.3	360	.05	.02	.1	27
317	Tangerine juice, canned, sweetened	1 cup	249	87	125	1	Trace	—	—	—	30	44	.5	1,040	.15	.05	.2	54
318	Watermelon, raw, 4 by 8 in wedge with rind and seeds[37] (1/16 of 32⅔-lb melon, 10 by 16 in)	1 wedge with rind and seeds[37]	926	93	110	2	1	—	—	—	27	30	2.1	2,510	.13	.13	.9	30
	GRAIN PRODUCTS																
	Bagel, 3-in diam.:																
319	Egg	1 bagel	55	32	165	6	2	0.5	0.9	0.8	28	9	1.2	30	.14	.10	1.2	0
320	Water	1 bagel	55	29	165	6	1	.2	.4	.6	30	8	1.2	0	.15	.11	1.4	0
321	Barley, pearled, light, uncooked	1 cup	200	11	700	16	2	.3	.2	.8	158	32	4.0	0	.24	.10	6.2	0
	Biscuits, baking powder, 2-in diam. (enriched flour, vegetable shortening):																
322	From home recipe	1 biscuit	28	27	105	2	5	1.2	2.0	1.2	13	34	.4	Trace	.08	.08	.7	Trace
323	From mix	1 biscuit	28	29	90	2	3	.6	1.1	.7	15	19	.6	Trace	.09	.08	.8	Trace

[36]Weight includes pits. After removal of the pits, the weight of the edible portion is 258 g for item 302, 133 g for item 303, 43 g for item 304, and 213 g for item 305.
[37]Weight includes rind and seeds. Without rind and seeds, weight of the edible portion is 426 g.

(A)	(B)	(g)	(C)	(D)	(E)	(F)	(G)	(H)	(I)	(J)	(K)	(L)	(M)	(N)	(O)	(P)	(Q)
324	Breadcrumbs (enriched)[38]																
	Dry, grated ... 1 cup	100	7	390	13	5	1.0	1.6	1.4	73	122	3.6	Trace	.35	.35	4.8	Trace
	Soft. See White bread (items 349–350).																
	Breads:																
325	Boston brown bread, canned, slice, 3 1/4 by 1/2 in.[38] ... 1 slice	45	45	95	2	1	.1	.2	.2	21	41	.9	390[39]	.06	.04	.7	0
	Cracked-wheat bread (3/4 enriched wheat flour, 1/4 cracked wheat):[38]																
326	Loaf, 1 lb	454	35	1,195	39	10	2.2	3.0	3.9	236	399	9.5	Trace	1.52	1.13	14.4	Trace
327	Slice (18 per loaf)	25	35	65	2	1	.1	.2	.2	13	22	.5	Trace	.08	.06	.8	Trace
	French or vienna bread, enriched:[38]																
328	Loaf, 1 lb	454	31	1,315	41	14	3.2	4.7	4.6	251	195	10.0	Trace	1.80	1.10	15.0	Trace
	Slice:																
329	French (5 by 2 1/2 by 1 in)	35	31	100	3	1	.2	.4	.4	19	15	.8	Trace	.14	.08	1.2	Trace
330	Vienna (4 3/4 by 4 by 1/2 in)	25	31	75	2	1	.2	.3	.3	14	11	.6	Trace	.10	.06	.8	Trace
	Italian bread, enriched:																
331	Loaf, 1 lb	454	32	1,250	41	4	.6	.3	1.5	256	77	10.0	0	1.80	1.10	15.0	0
332	Slice, 4 1/2 by 3 1/4 by 3/4 in.	30	32	85	3	Trace	Trace	Trace	.1	17	5	.7	0	.12	.07	1.0	0
	Raisin bread, enriched:[38]																
333	Loaf, 1 lb	454	35	1,190	30	13	3.0	4.7	3.9	243	322	10.0	Trace	1.70	1.07	10.7	Trace
334	Slice (18 per loaf)	25	35	65	2	1	.2	.3	.2	13	18	.6	Trace	.09	.06	.6	Trace
	Rye bread:																
	American, light (2/3 enriched wheat flour, 1/3 rye flour):																
335	Loaf, 1 lb	454	36	1,100	41	5	.7	.5	2.2	236	340	9.1	0	1.35	.98	12.9	0
336	Slice (4 3/4 by 3 3/4 by 7/16 in)	25	36	60	2	Trace	Trace	Trace	.1	13	19	.5	0	.07	.05	.7	0
	Pumpernickel (2/3 rye flour, 1/3 enriched wheat flour):																
337	Loaf, 1 lb	454	34	1,115	41	5	.7	.5	2.4	241	381	11.8	0	1.30	.93	8.5	0
338	Slice (5 by 4 by 3/8 in)	32	34	80	3	Trace	Trace	Trace	.2	17	27	.8	0	.09	.07	.6	0
	White bread, enriched:[38]																
	Soft-crumb type:																
339	Loaf, 1 lb	454	36	1,225	39	15	3.4	5.3	4.6	229	381	11.3	Trace	1.80	1.10	15.0	Trace
340	Slice (18 per loaf)	25	36	70	2	1	.2	.3	.3	13	21	.6	Trace	.10	.06	.8	Trace
341	Slice, toasted	22	25	70	2	1	.2	.3	.3	13	21	.6	Trace	.08	.06	.8	Trace
342	Slice (22 per loaf)	20	36	55	2	1	.2	.2	.2	10	17	.5	Trace	.08	.05	.7	Trace
343	Slice, toasted	17	25	55	2	1	.2	.2	.2	10	17	.5	Trace	.06	.05	.7	Trace
344	Loaf, 1 1/2 lb	680	36	1,835	59	22	5.2	7.9	6.9	343	571	17.0	Trace	2.70	1.65	22.5	Trace
345	Slice (24 per loaf)	28	36	75	2	1	.2	.3	.3	14	24	.7	Trace	.11	.07	.9	Trace
346	Slice, toasted	24	25	75	2	1	.2	.3	.3	14	24	.7	Trace	.09	.07	.9	Trace
347	Slice (28 per loaf)	21	36	65	2	1	.2	.3	.3	12	20	.6	Trace	.10	.06	.8	Trace
348	Slice, toasted	21	25	65	3	1	.2	.3	.3	12	20	.6	Trace	.08	.06	.8	Trace
349	Cubes ... 1 cup	30	36	80	3	1	.2	.3	.3	15	25	.8	Trace	.12	.07	1.0	Trace
350	Crumbs ... 1 cup	45	36	120	4	1	.3	.5	.5	23	38	1.1	Trace	.18	.11	1.5	Trace
	Firm-crumb type:[38]																
351	Loaf, 1 lb	454	35	1,245	41	17	3.9	5.9	5.2	228	435	11.3	Trace	1.80	1.10	15.0	Trace
352	Slice (20 per loaf)	23	35	65	2	1	.2	.3	.3	12	22	.6	Trace	.09	.06	.8	Trace
353	Slice, toasted	20	24	65	2	1	.2	.3	.3	12	22	.6	Trace	.07	.06	.8	Trace
354	Loaf, 2 lb	907	35	2,495	82	34	7.7	11.8	10.4	455	871	22.7	Trace	3.60	2.20	30.0	Trace
355	Slice (34 per loaf)	27	35	75	2	1	.2	.3	.3	14	26	.7	Trace	.11	.06	.9	Trace
356	Slice, toasted	23	24	75	2	1	.2	.3	.3	14	26	.7	Trace	.09	.06	.9	Trace

[38]Made with vegetable shortening.
[39]Applies to product made with white cornmeal. With yellow cornmeal, value is 30 International Units (I.U.).
[38]Made with vegetable shortening.

H

TABLE 2.—NUTRITIVE VALUES OF THE EDIBLE PART OF FOODS - Continued
(Dashes (—) denote lack of reliable data for a constituent believed to be present in measurable amount)

NUTRIENTS IN INDICATED QUANTITY

Item No (A)	Foods, approximate measures, units, and weight (edible part unless footnotes indicate otherwise) (B)	Grams	Water (C) Percent	Food energy (D) Calories	Protein (E) Grams	Fat (F) Grams	Fatty Acids Saturated (total) (G) Grams	Unsaturated Oleic (H) Grams	Linoleic (I) Grams	Carbohydrate (J) Grams	Calcium (K) Milligrams	Iron (L) Milligrams	Vitamin A value (M) International units	Thiamin (N) Milligrams	Riboflavin (O) Milligrams	Niacin (P) Milligrams	Ascorbic acid (Q) Milligrams
	GRAIN PRODUCTS—Con.																
	Breads:—Continued																
	Whole-wheat bread:																
	Soft-crumb type:[38]																
357	Loaf, 1 lb	454	36	1,095	41	12	2.2	2.9	4.2	224	381	13.6	Trace	1.37	.45	12.7	Trace
358	Slice (16 per loaf)	28	36	65	3	1	.1	.2	.2	14	24	.8	Trace	.09	.03	.8	Trace
359	Slice, toasted	24	24	65	3	1	.1	.2	.2	14	24	.8	Trace	.07	.03	.8	Trace
	Firm-crumb type:[38]																
360	Loaf, 1 lb	454	36	1,100	48	14	2.5	3.3	4.9	216	449	13.6	Trace	1.17	.54	12.7	Trace
361	Slice (18 per loaf)	25	36	60	3	1	.1	.2	.3	12	25	.8	Trace	.06	.03	.7	Trace
362	Slice, toasted	21	24	60	3	1	.1	.2	.3	12	25	.8	Trace	.05	.03	.7	Trace
	Breakfast cereals:																
	Hot type, cooked:																
	Corn (hominy) grits, degermed:																
363	Enriched ... 1 cup	245	87	125	3	Trace	Trace	Trace	.1	27	2	.7	[40]Trace	.10	.07	1.0	0
364	Unenriched ... 1 cup	245	87	125	3	Trace	Trace	Trace	.1	27	2	.2	[40]Trace	.05	.02	.5	0
365	Farina, quick-cooking, enriched ... 1 cup	245	89	105	3	Trace	Trace	Trace	.1	22	147	([42])	0	.12	.07	1.0	0
366	Oatmeal or rolled oats ... 1 cup	240	87	130	5	2	.4	.8	.9	23	22	1.4	0	.19	.05	.2	0
367	Wheat, rolled ... 1 cup	240	80	180	5	1	—	—	—	41	19	1.7	0	.17	.07	2.2	0
368	Wheat, whole-meal ... 1 cup	245	88	110	4	1	—	—	—	23	17	1.2	0	.15	.05	1.5	0
	Ready-to-eat:																
369	Bran flakes (40% bran), added sugar, salt, iron, vitamins ... 1 cup	35	3	105	4	1	—	—	—	28	19	5.6	1,540	.46	.52	6.2	0
370	Bran Flakes with raisins, added sugar, salt, iron, vitamins ... 1 cup	50	7	145	4	1	—	—	—	40	28	7.9	[43]2,200	(44)	(44)	(44)	0
	Corn flakes:																
371	Plain, added sugar, salt, iron, vitamins ... 1 cup	25	4	95	2	Trace	—	—	—	21	(44)	(44)	(44)	(44)	(44)	(44)	[45]13
372	Sugar-coated, added salt, iron, vitamins ... 1 cup	40	2	155	2	Trace	—	—	—	37	1	(44)	1,760	.53	.60	7.1	[45]21
373	Corn, oat flour, puffed, added sugar, salt, iron, vitamins ... 1 cup	20	4	80	2	1	—	—	—	16	4	5.7	880	.26	.30	3.5	11
374	Corn, shredded, added sugar, salt, iron, thiamin, niacin ... 1 cup	25	3	95	2	Trace	—	—	—	22	1	.6	0	.33	.05	4.4	13
375	Oats, puffed, added sugar, salt, minerals, vitamins ... 1 cup	25	3	100	3	1	—	—	—	19	44	4.0	1,100	.33	.38	4.4	13
	Rice, puffed:																
376	Plain, added iron, thiamin, niacin ... 1 cup	15	4	60	1	Trace	—	—	—	13	3	.3	0	.07	.01	.7	0

[40]Applies to white varieties. For yellow varieties, value is 150 International Units (I.U.).
[42]Value may range from less than 1 mg to about 8 mg depending on the brand. Consult the label.
[43]Applies to product with added nutrient. Without added nutrient, value is trace.
[44]Value varies with the brand. Consult the label.
[45]Applies to product with added nutrient. Without added nutrient, value is trace.

(A)	(B)	(C)	(D)	(E)	(F)	(G)	(H)	(I)	(J)	(K)	(L)	(M)	(N)	(O)	(P)	(Q)
377	Presweetened, added salt, iron, vitamins. 1 cup	28	115	1	0	—	—	—	26	3	(44)	[45]1,240	(44)	(44)	(44)	[45]515
378	Wheat flakes, added sugar, salt, iron, vitamins. 1 cup	30	105	3	Trace	—	—	—	24	12	4.8	1,320	.40	.45	5.3	16
	Wheat, puffed:															
379	Plain, added iron, thiamin, niacin. 1 cup	15	55	2	Trace	—	—	—	12	4	.6	0	.08	.03	1.2	0
380	Presweetened, added salt, iron, vitamins. 1 cup	38	140	3	Trace	—	—	—	33	7	(44)	1,680	.50	.57	6.7	[45]20
381	Wheat, shredded, plain. 1 oblong biscuit or 1/2 cup spoon-size biscuits.	25	90	2	1	—	—	—	20	11	.9	0	.06	.03	1.1	0
382	Wheat germ, without salt and sugar, toasted. 1 tbsp	6	25	2	1	0.2	0.4	0.4	3	3	.5	10	.11	.05	.3	1
383	Buckwheat flour, light, sifted. 1 cup	98	340	6	1	—	—	—	78	11	1.0	0	.08	.04	.4	0
384	Bulgur, canned, seasoned 1 cup	135	245	8	4	—	—	—	44	27	1.9	0	.08	.05	4.1	0
	Cake icings. See Sugars and Sweets (items 532–536).															
	Cakes made from cake mixes with enriched flour.[46]															
	Angelfood:															
385	Whole cake (9 3/4-in diam. tube cake) 1 cake	635	1,645	36	1	—	—	—	377	603	2.5	0	.37	.95	3.6	0
386	Piece, 1/12 of cake. 1 piece	53	135	3	Trace	—	—	—	32	50	.2	0	.03	.08	.3	0
	Coffeecake:															
387	Whole cake (7 3/4 by 5 5/8 by 1 1/4 in). 1 cake	430	1,385	27	41	11.7	16.3	8.8	225	262	6.9	690	.82	.91	7.7	1
388	Piece, 1/6 of cake. 1 piece	72	230	5	7	2.0	2.7	1.5	38	44	1.2	120	.14	.15	1.3	Trace
	Cupcakes, made with egg, milk, 2 1/2-in diam.:															
389	Without icing. 1 cupcake	25	90	1	3	.8	1.2	7	14	40	.3	40	.05	.05	4	Trace
390	With chocolate icing. 1 cupcake	36	130	2	5	2.0	1.6	.6	21	47	.4	60	.05	.06	4	Trace
	Devil's food with chocolate icing:															
391	Whole, 2 layer cake (8- or 9-in diam.) 1 cake	1,107	3,755	49	136	50.0	44.9	17.0	645	653	16.6	1,660	1.06	1.65	10.1	1
392	Piece, 1/16 of cake. 1 piece	69	235	3	8	3.1	2.8	1.1	40	41	1.0	100	.07	.10	6	Trace
393	Cupcake, 2 1/2-in diam. 1 cupcake	35	120	2	4	1.6	1.4	.5	20	21	.5	50	.03	.05	.3	Trace
	Gingerbread:															
394	Whole cake (8-in square). 1 cake	570	1,575	18	39	9.7	16.6	10.0	291	513	8.6	Trace	0.84	1.00	7.4	Trace
395	Piece, 1/9 of cake. 1 piece	63	175	2	4	1.1	1.8	1.1	32	57	.9	Trace	.09	.11	.8	Trace
	White, 2 layer with chocolate icing:															
396	Whole cake (8- or 9-in diam.) 1 cake	1,140	4,000	44	122	48.2	46.4	20.0	716	1,129	11.4	680	1.50	1.77	12.5	2
397	Piece, 1/16 of cake. 1 piece	71	250	3	8	3.0	2.9	1.2	45	70	.7	40	.09	.11	.8	Trace
	Yellow, 2 layer with chocolate icing:															
398	Whole cake (8- or 9-in diam.) 1 cake	1,108	3,735	45	125	47.8	47.8	20.3	638	1,008	12.2	1,550	1.24	1.67	10.6	2
399	Piece, 1/16 of cake. 1 piece	69	235	3	8	3.0	3.0	1.3	40	63	.8	100	.08	.10	.7	Trace
	Cakes made from home recipes using enriched flour:[47]															
	Boston cream pie with custard filling:															
400	Whole cake (8-in diam.) 1 cake	825	2,490	41	78	23.0	30.1	15.2	412	553	8.2	1,730	1.04	1.27	9.6	2
401	Piece, 1/12 of cake. 1 piece	69	210	3	6	1.9	2.5	1.3	34	46	.7	140	.09	.11	.8	Trace

[44] Value varies with the brand. Consult the label.
[45] Applies to product with added nutrient. Without added nutrient, value is trace.
[46] Excepting angelfood cake, cakes were made from mixes containing vegetable shortening; icings, with butter.
[47] Excepting spongecake, vegetable shortening used for cake portion; butter, for icing. If butter or margarine used for cake portion, vitamin A values would be higher.

TABLE 2.—NUTRITIVE VALUES OF THE EDIBLE PART OF FOODS - Continued
(Dashes (—) denote lack of reliable data for a constituent believed to be present in measurable amount)

| | | | | | | | Fatty Acids | | | | | | | | | | |
| | | | | | | | | Unsaturated | | | | | | | | | |
Item No. (A)	Foods, approximate measures, units, and weight (edible part unless footnotes indicate otherwise) (B)	Grams	Water Percent (C)	Food energy Calories (D)	Protein Grams (E)	Fat Grams (F)	Saturated (total) Grams (G)	Oleic Grams (H)	Linoleic Grams (I)	Carbohydrate Grams (J)	Calcium Milligrams (K)	Iron Milligrams (L)	Vitamin A value International units (M)	Thiamin Milligrams (N)	Riboflavin Milligrams (O)	Niacin Milligrams (P)	Ascorbic acid Milligrams (Q)
	GRAIN PRODUCTS—Con.																
	Cakes made from home recipes using enriched flour[47]																
	Fruitcake, dark:																
402	Loaf, 1-lb (7½ by 2 by 1½ in) ... 1 loaf	454	18	1,720	22	69	14.4	33.5	14.8	271	327	11.8	540	.72	.73	4.9	2
403	Slice, 1/30 of loaf ... 1 slice	15	18	55	1	2	.5	1.1	.5	9	11	.4	20	.02	.02	.2	Trace
	Plain, sheet cake:																
	Without icing:																
	Whole cake (9-in square)																
404	... 1 cake	777	25	2,830	35	108	29.5	44.4	23.9	434	497	8.5	1,320	1.21	1.40	10.2	2
405	Piece, 1/9 of cake ... 1 piece	86	25	315	4	12	3.3	4.9	2.6	48	55	.9	150	.13	.15	1.1	Trace
	With uncooked white icing:																
	Whole cake (9-in square)																
406	... 1 cake	1,096	21	4,020	37	129	42.2	49.5	24.4	694	548	8.2	2,190	1.22	1.47	10.2	2
407	Piece, 1/9 of cake ... 1 piece	121	21	445	4	14	4.7	5.5	2.7	77	61	.8	240	.14	.16	1.1	Trace
	Pound:[49]																
408	Loaf, 8½ by 3½ by 3¼ in ... 1 loaf	565	16	2,725	31	170	42.9	73.1	39.6	273	107	7.9	1,410	.90	.99	7.3	0
409	Slice, 1/17 of loaf ... 1 slice	33	16	160	2	10	2.5	4.3	2.3	16	6	.5	80	.05	.06	.4	0
	Spongecake:																
410	Whole cake (9¾-in diam. tube cake) ... 1 cake	790	32	2,345	60	45	13.1	15.8	5.7	427	237	13.4	3,560	1.10	1.64	7.4	Trace
411	Piece, 1/12 of cake ... 1 piece	66	32	195	5	4	1.1	1.3	.5	36	20	1.1	300	.09	.14	.6	Trace
	Cookies made with enriched flour:[50,51]																
	Brownies with nuts:																
	Home-prepared, 1¾ by 1¾ by ⅞ in:																
412	From home recipe ... 1 brownie	20	10	95	1	6	1.5	3.0	1.2	10	8	.4	40	.04	.03	.2	Trace
413	From commercial recipe ... 1 brownie	20	11	85	1	4	.9	1.4	1.3	13	9	.4	20	.03	.02	.2	Trace
414	Frozen, with chocolate icing,[52] 1½ by 1¾ by ⅞ in ... 1 brownie	25	13	105	1	5	2.0	2.2	.7	15	10	.4	50	.03	.03	.2	Trace
	Chocolate chip:																
415	Commercial, 2¼-in diam., ⅜ in thick ... 4 cookies	42	3	200	2	9	2.8	2.9	2.2	29	16	1.0	50	.10	.17	.9	Trace
416	From home recipe, 2⅓-in diam. ... 4 cookies	40	3	205	2	12	3.5	4.5	2.9	24	14	.8	40	.06	.06	.5	Trace
417	Fig Bars, square (1⅝ by 1⅝ by ⅜ in) or rectangular (1½ by 1¾ by ½ in) ... 4 cookies	56	14	200	2	3	.8	1.2	.7	42	44	1.0	60	.04	.14	.9	Trace
418	Gingersnaps, 2-in diam., ¼ in thick ... 4 cookies	28	3	90	2	2	.7	1.0	.6	22	20	.7	20	.08	.06	.7	0
419	Macaroons, 2¾-in diam., ¼ in thick ... 2 cookies	38	4	180	2	9	—	—	—	25	10	.3	0	.02	.06	.2	0

[47]Excepting spongecake, vegetable shortening used for cake portion; butter, for icing. If butter or margarine used for cake ortion, vitamin A valkues would be higher.
[48]Equal weights of flour, sugar, eggs, and vegetable shortening.
[49]Products are commercial unless otherwise specified
[50]Made with enriched flour and vegetable shortening except for macaroons which do not contain flour or shortening.
[51]Icing made with butter.

H

(A)	(B)	(C)	(D)	(E)	(F)	(G)	(H)	(I)	(J)	(K)	(L)	(M)	(N)	(O)	(P)	(Q)
420	Oatmeal with raisins, 2 5/8-in diam., 1/4 in thick. 4 cookies	52	235	3	8	2.0	3.3	2.0	38	11	1.4	30	.15	.10	1.0	Trace
421	Plain, prepared from commercial chilled dough, 2 1/2-in diam., 1/4 in thick. 4 cookies	48	240	2	12	3.0	5.2	2.9	31	17	0.6	30	0.10	0.08	0.9	0
422	Sandwich type (chocolate or vanilla), 1 3/4-in diam., 3/8 in thick. 4 cookies	40	200	2	9	2.2	3.9	2.2	28	10	.7	0	.06	.10	.7	0
423	Vanilla wafers, 1 3/4-in diam., 1/4 in thick. 10 cookies	40	185	2	6	—	—	—	30	16	.6	50	.10	.09	.8	0
	Cornmeal:															
424	Whole-ground, unbolted, dry form. 1 cup	122	435	11	5	.5	1.0	2.5	90	24	2.9	[53]620	.46	.13	2.4	0
425	Bolted (nearly whole-grain), dry form. 1 cup	122	440	11	4	.5	.9	2.1	91	21	2.2	[53]590	.37	.10	2.3	0
	Degermed, enriched:															
426	Dry form. 1 cup	138	500	11	2	2	.4	.9	108	8	4.0	[53]610	.61	.36	4.8	0
427	Cooked. 1 cup	240	120	3	Trace	Trace	.1	.2	26	2	1.0	[53]140	.14	.10	1.2	0
	Degermed, unenriched:															
428	Dry form. 1 cup	138	500	11	2	2	.4	.9	108	8	1.5	[53]610	.19	.07	1.4	0
429	Cooked. 1 cup	240	120	3	Trace	Trace	.1	.2	26	2	.5	[53]140	.05	.02	.2	0
	Crackers:[38]															
430	Graham, plain, 2 1/2-in square. 2 crackers	14	55	1	1	.3	.5	.3	10	6	.5	0	.02	.08	.5	0
431	Rye wafers, whole-grain, 1 7/8 by 3 1/2 in. 2 wafers	13	45	2	Trace	—	—	—	10	7	.5	0	.04	.03	.2	0
432	Saltines, made with enriched flour. 4 crackers or 1 packet	11	50	1	1	.3	.5	.4	8	2	.5	0	.05	.05	.4	0
	Danish pastry (enriched flour), plain without fruit or nuts:[54]															
433	Packaged ring, 12 oz. 1 ring	340	1,435	25	80	24.3	31.7	16.5	155	170	6.1	1,050	.97	1.01	8.6	Trace
434	Round piece, about 4 1/4-in diam. by 1 in. 1 pastry	65	275	5	15	4.7	6.1	3.2	30	33	1.2	200	.18	.19	1.7	Trace
435	Ounce. 1 oz	28	120	2	7	2.0	2.7	1.4	13	14	.5	90	.08	.08	.7	Trace
	Doughnuts, made with enriched flour:[38]															
436	Cake type, plain, 2 1/2-in diam., 1 in high. 1 doughnut	25	100	1	5	1.2	2.0	1.1	13	10	.4	20	.05	.05	.4	Trace
437	Yeast-leavened, glazed, 3 3/4-in diam., 1 1/4 in high. 1 doughnut	50	205	3	11	3.3	5.8	3.3	22	16	.6	25	.10	.10	.8	0
	Macaroni, enriched, cooked (cut lengths, elbows, shells):															
438	Firm stage (hot). 1 cup	130	190	7	1	—	—	—	39	14	1.4	0	.23	.13	1.8	0
	Tender stage:															
439	Cold macaroni. 1 cup	105	115	4	Trace	—	—	—	24	8	.9	0	.15	.08	1.2	0
440	Hot macaroni. 1 cup	140	155	5	1	—	—	—	32	11	1.3	0	.20	.11	1.5	0
	Macaroni (enriched) and cheese:															
441	Canned.[55] 1 cup	240	230	9	10	4.2	3.1	1.4	26	199	1.0	260	.12	.24	1.0	Trace
442	From home recipe (served hot).[56] 1 cup	200	430	17	22	8.9	8.8	2.9	40	362	1.8	860	.20	.40	1.8	Trace
	Muffins made with enriched flour.[38] From home recipe:															
443	Blueberry, 2 3/8-in diam., 1 1/2 in high. 1 muffin	40	110	3	4	1.1	1.4	.7	17	34	.6	90	.09	.10	.7	Trace
444	Bran. 1 muffin	40	105	3	4	1.2	1.4	.8	17	57	1.5	90	.07	.10	1.7	Trace

[38]Made with vegetable shortening.
[53]Applies to yellow varieties; white varieties contain only a trace.
[54]Contains vegetable shortening and butter.
[55]Made with corn oil.
[56]Made with regular margarine.
[38]Made with vegetable shortening.

H

TABLE 2.—NUTRITIVE VALUES OF THE EDIBLE PART OF FOODS - Continued
(Dashes (—) denote lack of reliable data for a constituent believed to be present in measurable amount)

Item No. (A)	Foods, approximate measures, units, and weight (edible part unless footnotes indicate otherwise) (B)		Water (C)	Food energy (D)	Protein (E)	Fat (F)	Fatty Acids Saturated (total) (G)	Unsaturated Oleic (H)	Unsaturated Linoleic (I)	Carbohydrate (J)	Calcium (K)	Iron (L)	Vitamin A value (M)	Thiamin (N)	Riboflavin (O)	Niacin (P)	Ascorbic acid (Q)
		Grams	Percent	Calories	Grams	Grams	Grams	Grams	Grams	Grams	Milligrams	Milligrams	International units	Milligrams	Milligrams	Milligrams	Milligrams
	GRAIN PRODUCTS—Con.																
	Muffins made with enriched flour [56]—Continued																
	From home recipe: —Continued																
445	Corn (enriched degermed cornmeal and flour), 2 3/8-in diam., 1 1/2 in high. 1 muffin	40	33	125	3	4	1.2	1.6	.9	19	42	.7	[57]120	.10	.10	.7	Trace
446	Plain, 3-in diam., 1 1/2 in high. 1 muffin	40	38	120	3	4	1.0	1.7	1.0	17	42	0.6	40	0.09	0.12	0.9	Trace
	From mix, egg, milk:																
447	Corn, 2 3/8-in diam., 1 1/2 in high.[58] 1 muffin	40	30	130	3	4	1.2	1.7	.9	20	96	6	[57]100	.08	.09	.7	Trace
448	Noodles (egg noodles), enriched, cooked. 1 cup	160	71	200	7	2	—	—	—	37	16	1.4	110	.22	.13	1.9	0
449	Noodles, chow mein, canned. 1 cup	45	1	220	6	11	—	—	—	26	—	—	—	—	—	—	—
450	Pancakes, (4-in diam.).[58] Buckwheat, made from mix (with buckwheat and enriched flours), egg and milk added. 1 cake	27	58	55	2	2	.8	.9	.4	6	59	.4	60	.04	.05	.2	Trace
	Plain:																
451	Made from home recipe using enriched flour. 1 cake	27	50	60	2	2	.5	.8	.5	9	27	.4	30	.06	.07	.5	Trace
452	Made from mix with enriched flour, egg and milk added. 1 cake	27	51	60	2	2	.7	.7	.3	9	58	.3	70	.04	.06	.2	Trace
	Pies, piecrust made with enriched flour, vegetable shortening (9-in diam.):																
	Apple:																
453	Whole. 1 pie	945	48	2,420	21	105	27.0	44.5	25.2	360	76	6.6	280	1.06	.79	9.3	9
454	Sector, 1/7 of pie. 1 sector	135	48	345	3	15	3.9	6.4	3.6	51	11	.9	40	.15	.11	1.3	2
	Banana cream:																
455	Whole. 1 pie	910	54	2,010	41	85	26.7	33.2	16.2	279	601	7.3	2,280	.77	1.51	7.0	9
456	Sector, 1/7 of pie. 1 sector	130	54	285	6	12	3.8	4.7	2.3	40	86	1.0	330	.11	.22	1.0	1
	Blueberry:																
457	Whole. 1 pie	945	51	2,285	23	102	24.8	43.7	25.1	330	104	9.5	280	1.03	.80	10.0	28
458	Sector, 1/7 of pie. 1 sector	135	51	325	3	15	3.5	6.2	3.6	47	15	1.4	40	.15	.11	1.4	4
	Cherry:																
459	Whole. 1 pie	945	47	2,465	25	107	28.2	45.0	25.3	363	132	6.6	4,160	1.09	.84	9.8	Trace
460	Sector, 1/7 of pie. 1 sector	135	47	350	4	15	4.0	6.4	3.6	52	19	.9	590	.16	.12	1.4	Trace
	Custard:																
461	Whole. 1 pie	910	58	1,985	56	101	33.9	38.5	17.5	213	874	8.2	2,090	.79	1.92	5.6	0
462	Sector, 1/7 of pie. 1 sector	130	58	285	8	14	4.8	5.5	2.5	30	125	1.2	300	.11	.27	.8	0
	Lemon meringue:																
463	Whole. 1 pie	840	47	2,140	31	86	26.1	33.8	16.4	317	118	6.7	1,430	.61	.84	5.2	25
464	Sector, 1/7 of pie. 1 sector	120	47	305	4	12	3.7	4.8	2.3	45	17	1.0	200	.09	.12	.7	4
	Mince:																
465	Whole. 1 pie	945	43	2,560	24	109	28.0	45.9	25.2	389	265	13.3	20	.96	.86	9.8	9

[57] Applies to product made with yellow cornmeal.
[58] Made with enriched degermed cornmeal and enriched flour.

(A)	(B)		(C)	(D)	(E)	(F)	(G)	(H)	(I)	(J)	(K)	(L)	(M)	(N)	(O)	(P)	(Q)
466	Sector, 1/7 of pie	1 sector	135	43	365	3	16	4.0	6.6	3.6	56	38	1.9	Trace	.14	.12	1.4	1
	Peach:																	
467	Whole	1 pie	945	48	2,410	24	101	24.8	43.7	25.1	361	95	8.5	6,900	1.04	.97	14.0	28
468	Sector, 1/7 of pie	1 sector	135	48	345	3	14	3.5	6.2	3.6	52	14	1.2	990	.15	.14	2.0	4
	Pecan:																	
469	Whole	1 pie	825	20	3,450	42	189	27.8	101.0	44.2	423	388	25.6	1,320	1.80	.95	6.9	Trace
470	Sector, 1/7 of pie	1 sector	118	20	495	6	27	4.0	14.4	6.3	61	55	3.7	190	.26	.14	1.0	Trace
	Pumpkin:																	
471	Whole	1 pie	910	59	1,920	36	102	37.4	37.5	16.6	223	464	7.3	22,480	.78	1.27	7.0	Trace
472	Sector, 1/7 of pie	1 sector	130	59	275	5	15	5.4	5.4	2.4	32	66	1.0	3,210	.11	.18	1.0	Trace
473	Piecrust (home recipe) made with enriched flour and vegetable shortening, baked	1 pie shell, 9-in diam.	180	15	900	11	60	14.8	26.1	14.9	79	25	3.1	0	.47	.40	5.0	0
474	Piecrust mix with enriched flour and vegetable shortening, 10-oz pkg. prepared and baked	Piecrust for 2-crust pie, 9-in diam.	320	19	1,485	20	93	22.7	39.7	23.4	141	131	6.1	0	1.07	.79	9.9	0
475	Pizza (cheese) baked, 4 3/4-in sector; 1/8 of 12-in diam. pie.[19]	1 sector	60	45	145	6	4	1.7	1.5	0.6	22	86	1.1	230	0.16	0.18	1.6	4
	Popcorn, popped:																	
476	Plain, large kernel	1 cup	6	4	25	1	Trace	Trace	.1	.2	5	1	.2	—	—	.01	.1	0
477	With oil (coconut) and salt added, large kernel	1 cup	9	3	40	1	2	1.5	.2	.2	5	1	.2	—	—	.01	.2	0
478	Sugar coated	1 cup	35	4	135	2	1	.5	.2	.4	30	2	.5	—	—	.02	.4	0
	Pretzels, made with enriched flour:																	
479	Dutch, twisted, 2 3/4 by 2 5/8 in.	1 pretzel	16	5	60	2	1	—	—	—	12	4	.2	0	.05	.04	.7	0
480	Thin, twisted, 3 1/4 by 2 1/4 by 1/4 in.	10 pretzels	60	5	235	6	3	—	—	—	46	13	.9	0	.20	.15	2.5	0
481	Stick, 2 1/4 in long	10 pretzels	3	5	10	Trace	Trace	—	—	—	2	1	Trace	0	.01	.01	.1	0
	Rice, white, enriched:																	
482	Instant, ready-to-serve, hot	1 cup	165	73	180	4	Trace	Trace	Trace	Trace	40	5	1.3	0	.21	(59)	1.7	0
	Long grain:																	
483	Raw	1 cup	185	12	670	12	1	.2	.2	.2	149	44	5.4	0	.81	.06	6.5	0
484	Cooked, served hot	1 cup	205	73	225	4	Trace	.1	.1	.1	50	21	1.8	0	.23	.02	2.1	0
	Parboiled:																	
485	Raw	1 cup	185	10	685	14	1	.2	.1	.2	150	111	5.4	0	.81	.07	6.5	0
486	Cooked, served hot	1 cup	175	73	185	4	Trace	.1	.1	.1	41	33	1.4	0	.19	.02	2.1	0
	Rolls, enriched:[38]																	
	Commercial:																	
487	Brown-and-serve (12 per 12-oz pkg.), browned	1 roll	26	27	85	2	2	.4	.7	.5	14	20	.5	Trace	.10	.06	.9	Trace
488	Cloverleaf or pan, 2 1/2-in diam., 2 in high	1 roll	28	31	85	2	2	.4	.6	.4	15	21	.5	Trace	.11	.07	.9	Trace
489	Frankfurter and hamburger (8 per 11 1/2-oz pkg.)	1 roll	40	31	120	3	2	.5	.8	.6	21	30	.8	Trace	.16	.10	1.3	Trace
490	Hard, 3 3/4-in diam., 2 in high.	1 roll	50	25	155	5	2	.4	.6	.5	30	24	1.2	Trace	.20	.12	1.7	Trace
491	Hoagie or submarine, 11 1/2 by 3 by 2 1/2 in.	1 roll	135	31	390	12	4	.9	1.4	1.4	75	58	3.0	Trace	.54	.32	4.5	Trace
	From home recipe:																	
492	Cloverleaf, 2 1/2-in diam., 2 in high.	1 roll	35	26	120	3	3	.8	1.1	.7	20	16	.7	30	.12	.12	1.2	Trace
	Spaghetti, enriched, cooked:																	
493	Firm stage, "al dente," served hot	1 cup	130	64	190	7	1	—	—	—	39	14	1.4	0	.23	.13	1.8	0
494	Tender stage, served hot	1 cup	140	73	155	5	1	—	—	—	32	11	1.3	0	.20	.11	1.5	0

[19]Crust made with vegetable shortening and enriched flour
[59]Product may or may not be enriched with riboflavin. Consult the label.
[38]Made with vegetable shortening.

TABLE 2.—NUTRITIVE VALUES OF THE EDIBLE PART OF FOODS - Continued
(Dashes (—) denote lack of reliable data for a constituent believed to be present in measurable amount)

Item No. (A)	Foods, approximate measures, units, and weight (edible part unless footnotes indicate otherwise) (B)		Water Per cent (C)	Food energy Cal- ories (D)	Pro- tein Grams (E)	Fat Grams (F)	Fatty Acids Satu- rated (total) Grams (G)	Unsaturated Oleic Grams (H)	Unsaturated Lino- leic Grams (I)	Carbo- hydrate Grams (J)	Calcium Milli- grams (K)	Iron Milli- grams (L)	Vitamin A value Inter- national units (M)	Thiamin Milli- grams (N)	Ribo- flavin Milli- grams (O)	Niacin Milli- grams (P)	Ascorbic acid Milli- grams (Q)
		Grams															
	GRAIN PRODUCTS—Con.																
	Spaghetti (enriched) in tomato sauce with cheese:																
495	From home recipe	1 cup	250	77	260	9	9	2.0	5.4	.7	37	80	2.3	1,080	.25	.18	2.3	13
496	Canned	1 cup	250	80	190	6	2	.5	.3	.4	39	40	2.8	930	.35	.28	4.5	10
	Spaghetti (enriched) with meat balls and tomato sauce:																
497	From home recipe	1 cup	248	70	330	19	12	3.3	6.3	.9	39	124	3.7	1,590	.25	.30	4.0	22
498	Canned	1 cup	250	78	260	12	10	2.2	3.3	3.9	29	53	3.3	1,000	.15	.18	2.3	5
499	Toaster pastries	1 pastry	50	12	200	3	6	—	—	—	36	60[54]	1.9	500	.16	.17	2.1	(60)
	Waffles, made with enriched flour, 7-in diam.[38]																
500	From home recipe	1 waffle	75	41	210	7	7	2.3	2.8	1.4	28	85	1.3	250	.17	.23	1.4	Trace
501	From mix, egg and milk added	1 waffle	75	42	205	7	8	2.8	2.9	1.2	27	179	1.0	170	.14	.22	.9	Trace
	Wheat flours: All-purpose or family flour, enriched:																
502	Sifted, spooned	1 cup	115	12	420	12	1	0.2	0.1	0.5	88	18	3.3	0	0.74	0.46	6.1	0
503	Unsifted, spooned	1 cup	125	12	455	13	1	.2	.1	.5	95	20	3.6	0	.80	.50	6.6	0
504	Cake or pastry flour, enriched, sifted, spooned	1 cup	96	12	350	7	1	.1	.1	.3	76	16	2.8	0	.61	.38	5.1	0
505	Self-rising, enriched, unsifted, spooned	1 cup	125	12	440	12	1	.2	.1	.5	93	331	3.6	0	.80	.50	6.6	0
506	Whole-wheat, from hard wheats, stirred	1 cup	120	12	400	16	2	.4	.2	1.0	85	49	4.0	0	.66	.14	5.2	0
	LEGUMES (DRY), NUTS, SEEDS; RELATED PRODUCTS																
	Almonds, shelled:																
507	Chopped (about 130 almonds)	1 cup	130	5	775	24	70	5.6	47.7	12.8	25	304	6.1	0	.31	1.20	4.6	Trace
508	Slivered, not pressed down (about 115 almonds)	1 cup	115	5	690	21	62	5.0	42.2	11.3	22	269	5.4	0	.28	1.06	4.0	Trace
	Beans, dry: Common varieties as Great Northern, navy, and others: Cooked, drained:																
509	Great Northern	1 cup	180	69	210	14	1	—	—	—	38	90	4.9	0	.25	.13	1.3	0
510	Pea (navy)	1 cup	190	69	225	15	1	—	—	—	40	95	5.1	0	.27	.13	1.3	0
	Canned, solids and liquid: White with—																
511	Frankfurters (sliced)	1 cup	255	71	365	19	18	—	—	—	32	94	4.8	330	.18	.15	3.3	Trace
512	Pork and tomato sauce	1 cup	255	71	310	16	7	2.4	2.8	.6	48	138	4.6	330	.20	.08	1.5	5
513	Pork and sweet sauce	1 cup	255	66	385	16	12	4.3	5.0	1.1	54	161	5.9	—	.15	.10	1.3	—
514	Red kidney	1 cup	255	76	230	15	1	—	—	—	42	74	4.6	10	.13	.10	1.5	—
515	Lima, cooked, drained	1 cup	190	64	260	16	1	—	—	—	49	55	5.9	—	.25	.11	1.3	—

[60]Value varies with the brand. Consult the label.

(A)	(B)	(C)	(D)	(E)	(F)	(G)	(H)	(I)	(J)	(K)	(L)	(M)	(N)	(O)	(P)	(Q)
516 Blackeye peas, dry, cooked (with residual cooking liquid)	1 cup	250	190	13	1	—	—	—	35	43	3.3	30	.40	.10	1.0	—
517 Brazil nuts, shelled (6-8 large kernels)	1 oz	28	185	4	19	4.8	6.2	7.1	3	53	1.0	Trace	.27	.03	.5	—
518 Cashew nuts, roasted in oil	1 cup	140	785	24	64	12.9	36.8	10.2	41	53	5.3	140	.60	.35	2.5	—
Coconut meat, fresh:																
519 Piece, about 2 by 2 by ½ in	1 piece	45	155	2	16	14.0	.9	.3	4	6	.8	0	.02	.01	.2	1
520 Shredded or grated, not pressed down	1 cup	80	275	3	28	24.8	1.6	.5	8	10	1.4	0	.04	.02	.4	2
521 Filberts (hazelnuts), chopped (about 80 kernels)	1 cup	115	730	14	72	5.1	55.2	7.3	19	240	3.9	40	.53	—	1.0	Trace
522 Lentils, whole, cooked	1 cup	200	210	16	Trace	—	—	—	39	50	4.2	—	.14	.12	1.2	0
523 Peanuts, roasted in oil, salted (whole, halves, chopped)	1 cup	144	840	37	72	13.7	33.0	20.7	27	107	3.0	—	.46	.19	24.8	0
524 Peanut butter	1 tbsp	16	95	4	8	1.5	3.7	2.3	3	9	.3	0	.02	.02	2.4	0
525 Peas, split, dry, cooked	1 cup	200	230	16	1	—	—	—	42	22	3.4	80	.30	.18	1.8	—
526 Pecans, chopped or pieces (about 120 large halves)	1 cup	118	810	11	84	7.2	50.5	20.0	17	86	2.8	150	1.01	.15	1.1	2
527 Pumpkin and squash kernels, dry, hulled	1 cup	140	775	41	65	11.8	23.5	27.5	21	71	15.7	100	.34	.27	3.4	—
528 Sunflower seeds, dry, hulled	1 cup	145	810	35	69	8.2	13.7	43.2	29	174	10.3	70	2.84	.33	7.8	—
Walnuts:																
Black:																
529 Chopped or broken kernels	1 cup	125	785	26	74	6.3	13.3	45.7	19	Trace	7.5	380	.28	.14	.9	—
530 Ground (finely)	1 cup	80	500	16	47	4.0	8.5	29.2	12	Trace	4.8	240	.18	.09	.6	—
531 Persian or English, chopped (about 60 halves)	1 cup	120	780	18	77	8.4	11.8	42.2	19	119	3.7	40	.40	.16	1.1	2

SUGARS AND SWEETS

(A)	(B)	(C)	(D)	(E)	(F)	(G)	(H)	(I)	(J)	(K)	(L)	(M)	(N)	(O)	(P)	(Q)
Cake icings:																
Boiled, white:																
532 Plain	1 cup	94	295	1	0	0	0	0	75	2	Trace	0	Trace	.03	Trace	0
533 With coconut	1 cup	166	605	3	13	11.0	.9	Trace	124	10	.8	0	.02	.07	.3	0
Uncooked:																
534 Chocolate made with milk and butter	1 cup	275	1,035	9	38	23.4	11.7	1.0	185	165	3.3	580	.06	.28	.6	1
535 Creamy fudge from mix and water	1 cup	245	830	7	16	5.1	6.7	3.1	183	96	2.7	Trace	.05	.20	.7	Trace
536 White	1 cup	319	1,200	2	21	12.7	5.1	.5	260	48	Trace	860	Trace	.06	Trace	Trace
Candy:																
537 Caramels, plain or chocolate	1 oz	28	115	1	3	1.6	1.1	.1	22	42	.4	Trace	.01	.05	.1	Trace
Chocolate:																
538 Milk, plain	1 oz	28	145	2	9	5.5	3.0	.3	16	65	.3	80	.02	.10	.1	Trace
539 Semisweet, small pieces (60 per oz)	1 cup or 6-oz pkg	170	860	7	61	36.2	19.8	1.7	97	51	4.4	30	.02	.14	.9	0
540 Chocolate-coated peanuts	1 oz	28	160	5	12	4.0	4.7	2.1	11	33	.4	Trace	.10	.05	2.1	Trace
541 Fondant, uncoated (mints, candy corn, other)	1 oz	28	105	Trace	1	.1	.3	.1	25	4	.3	0	Trace	Trace	Trace	0
542 Fudge, chocolate, plain	1 oz	28	115	1	3	1.3	1.4	.6	21	22	.3	Trace	.01	.03	.1	Trace
543 Gum drops	1 oz	28	100	Trace	Trace	—	—	—	25	2	.1	0	0	Trace	Trace	0
544 Hard	1 oz	28	110	0	Trace	—	—	—	28	6	.5	0	0	0	0	0
545 Marshmallows	1 oz	28	90	1	Trace	—	—	—	23	5	.5	0	0	Trace	Trace	0
Chocolate-flavored beverage powders (about 4 heaping tsp per oz):																
546 With nonfat dry milk	1 oz	28	100	5	1	.5	.3	Trace	20	167	.5	10	.04	.21	.2	1
547 Without milk	1 oz	28	100	1	1	.4	.2	Trace	25	9	.6	—	.01	.03	.1	0
548 Honey, strained or extracted	1 tbsp	21	65	Trace	0	0	—	0	17	1	.1	0	Trace	.01	.1	Trace
549 Jams and preserves	1 tbsp	20	55	Trace	Trace	—	—	—	14	4	.2	Trace	Trace	.01	Trace	Trace
550	1 packet	14	40	Trace	Trace	—	—	—	10	4	.1	Trace	Trace	Trace	Trace	Trace
551 Jellies	1 tbsp	18	50	Trace	Trace	—	—	—	13	4	.3	Trace	Trace	.01	Trace	Trace
552	1 packet	14	40	Trace	Trace	—	—	—	10	3	.2	Trace	Trace	Trace	Trace	1

H

TABLE 2.—NUTRITIVE VALUES OF THE EDIBLE PART OF FOODS - Continued
(Dashes (—) denote lack of reliable data for a constituent believed to be present in measurable amount)

Item No. (A)	Foods, approximate measures, units, and weight (edible part unless footnotes indicate otherwise) (B)		Weight (Grams)	Water (C) Percent	Food energy (D) Calories	Protein (E) Grams	Fat (F) Grams	Fatty Acids Saturated (total) (G) Grams	Unsaturated Oleic (H) Grams	Unsaturated Linoleic (I) Grams	Carbohydrate (J) Grams	Calcium (K) Milligrams	Iron (L) Milligrams	Vitamin A value (M) International units	Thiamin (N) Milligrams	Riboflavin (O) Milligrams	Niacin (P) Milligrams	Ascorbic acid (Q) Milligrams
	SUGARS AND SWEETS—Con.																	
	Sirups:																	
	Chocolate-flavored sirup or topping:																	
553	Thin type	1 fl oz or 2 tbsp	38	32	90	1	1	.5	.3	Trace	24	6	.6	Trace	.01	.03	.2	0
554	Fudge type	1 fl oz or 2 tbsp	38	25	125	2	5	3.1	1.6	.1	20	48	.5	60	.02	.08	.2	Trace
	Molasses, cane:																	
555	Light (first extraction)	1 tbsp	20	24	50	—	—	—	—	—	13	33	.9	—	.01	.01	Trace	—
556	Blackstrap (third extraction)	1 tbsp	20	24	45	—	—	—	—	—	11	137	3.2	—	.02	.04	.4	—
557	Sorghum	1 tbsp	21	23	55	—	—	—	—	—	14	35	2.6	—	—	.02	Trace	—
558	Table blends, chiefly corn, light and dark	1 tbsp	21	24	60	0	0	0	0	0	15	9	.8	0	0	0	0	0
	Sugars:																	
559	Brown, pressed down	1 cup	220	2	820	0	0	0	0	0	212	187	7.5	0	.02	.07	.4	0
	White:																	
560	Granulated	1 cup	200	1	770	0	0	0	0	0	199	0	.2	0	0	0	0	0
561		1 tbsp	12	1	45	0	0	0	0	0	12	0	Trace	0	0	0	0	0
562		1 packet	6	1	23	0	0	0	0	0	6	0	Trace	0	0	0	0	0
563	Powdered, sifted, spooned into cup	1 cup	100	1	385	0	0	0	0	0	100	0	.1	0	0	0	0	0
	VEGETABLE AND VEGETABLE PRODUCTS																	
	Asparagus, green:																	
	Cooked, drained:																	
	Cuts and tips, 1 1/2- to 2-in lengths:																	
564	From raw	1 cup	145	94	30	3	Trace	—	—	—	5	30	.9	1,310	.23	0.26	2.0	38
565	From frozen	1 cup	180	93	40	6	Trace	—	—	—	6	40	2.2	1,530	.25	.23	1.8	41
	Spears, 1/2-in diam. at base:																	
566	From raw	4 spears	60	94	10	1	Trace	—	—	—	2	13	.4	540	.10	.11	.8	16
567	From frozen	4 spears	60	92	15	2	Trace	—	—	—	2	13	.7	470	.10	.08	.7	16
568	Canned, spears, 1/2-in diam. at base	4 spears	80	93	15	2	Trace	—	—	—	3	15	1.5	640	.05	.08	.6	12
	Beans:																	
	Lima, immature seeds, frozen, cooked, drained:																	
569	Thick-seeded types (Fordhooks)	1 cup	170	74	170	10	Trace	—	—	—	32	34	2.9	390	.12	.09	1.7	29
570	Thin-seeded types (baby limas)	1 cup	180	69	210	13	Trace	—	—	—	40	63	4.7	400	.16	.09	2.2	22
	Snap:																	
	Green:																	
	Cooked, drained:																	
571	From raw (cuts and French style)	1 cup	125	92	30	2	Trace	—	—	—	7	63	.8	680	.09	.11	.6	15
	From frozen:																	
572	Cuts	1 cup	135	92	35	2	Trace	—	—	—	8	54	.9	780	.09	.12	.5	7
573	French style	1 cup	130	92	35	2	Trace	—	—	—	8	49	1.2	690	.08	.10	.4	9
574	Canned, drained solids (cuts)	1 cup	135	92	30	2	Trace	—	—	—	7	61	2.0	630	.04	.07	.4	5

H

(A)	Food	(B)	g	(C)	(D)	(E)	(F)	(G)	(H)	(I)	(J)	(K)	(L)	(M)	(N)	(O)	(P)	(Q)
	Yellow or wax. Cooked, drained.																	
575	From raw (cuts and French style).	1 cup	125	93	30	2	Trace	—	—	—	6	63	.8	290	.09	.11	.6	16
576	From frozen (cuts).	1 cup	135	92	35	2	Trace	—	—	—	8	47	.9	140	.09	.11	.5	8
577	Canned, drained solids (cuts).	1 cup	135	92	30	2	Trace	—	—	—	7	61	2.0	140	.04	.07	.4	7
	Beans, mature. See Beans, dry (items 509-515) and Blackeye peas, dry (item 516).																	
	Bean sprouts (mung):																	
578	Raw	1 cup	105	89	35	4	Trace	—	—	—	7	20	1.4	20	.14	.14	.8	20
579	Cooked, drained	1 cup	125	91	35	4	Trace	—	—	—	7	21	1.1	30	.11	.13	.9	8
	Beets: Cooked, drained, peeled:																	
580	Whole beets, 2-in diam.	2 beets	100	91	30	1	Trace	—	—	—	7	14	.5	20	.03	.04	.3	6
581	Diced or sliced	1 cup	170	91	55	2	Trace	—	—	—	12	24	.9	30	.05	.07	.5	10
	Canned, drained solids:																	
582	Whole beets, small	1 cup	160	89	60	2	Trace	—	—	—	14	30	1.1	30	.02	.05	.2	5
583	Diced or sliced	1 cup	170	89	65	2	Trace	—	—	—	15	32	1.2	30	.02	.05	.2	5
584	Beet greens, leaves and stems, cooked, drained.	1 cup	145	94	25	2	Trace	—	—	—	5	144	2.8	7,400	.10	.22	.4	22
	Blackeye peas, immature seeds, cooked and drained:																	
585	From raw	1 cup	165	72	180	13	1	—	—	—	30	40	3.5	580	.50	.18	2.3	28
586	From frozen	1 cup	170	66	220	15	1	—	—	—	40	43	4.8	290	.68	.19	2.4	15
	Broccoli, cooked, drained: From raw:																	
587	Stalk, medium size	1 stalk	180	91	45	6	1	—	—	—	8	158	1.4	4,500	.16	.36	1.4	162
588	Stalks cut into ½-in pieces	1 cup	155	91	40	5	Trace	—	—	—	7	136	1.2	3,880	.14	.31	1.2	140
	From frozen:																	
589	Stalk, 4 ½ to 5 in long	1 stalk	30	91	10	1	Trace	—	—	—	1	12	.2	570	.02	.03	.2	22
590	Chopped	1 cup	185	92	50	5	1	—	—	—	9	100	1.3	4,810	.11	.22	.9	105
	Brussels sprouts, cooked, drained:																	
591	From raw, 7-8 sprouts (1 ¼- to 1 ½-in diam.)	1 cup	155	88	55	7	1	—	—	—	10	50	1.7	810	.12	.22	1.2	135
592	From frozen	1 cup	155	89	50	5	Trace	—	—	—	10	33	1.2	880	.12	.16	.9	126
	Cabbage: Common varieties: Raw:																	
593	Coarsely shredded or sliced	1 cup	70	92	15	1	Trace	—	—	—	4	34	0.3	90	0.04	0.04	0.2	33
594	Finely shredded or chopped	1 cup	90	92	20	1	Trace	—	—	—	5	44	.4	120	.05	.05	.3	42
595	Cooked, drained	1 cup	145	94	30	2	Trace	—	—	—	6	64	.4	190	.06	.06	.4	48
596	Red, raw, coarsely shredded or sliced	1 cup	70	90	20	1	Trace	—	—	—	5	29	.6	30	.06	.04	.3	43
597	Savoy, raw, coarsely shredded or sliced	1 cup	70	92	15	2	Trace	—	—	—	3	47	.6	140	.04	.06	.2	39
598	Cabbage, celery (also called pe-tsai or wongbok), raw, 1-in pieces.	1 cup	75	95	10	1	Trace	—	—	—	2	32	.5	110	.04	.03	.5	19
599	Cabbage, white mustard (also called bokchoy or pakchoy), cooked, drained.	1 cup	170	95	25	2	Trace	—	—	—	4	252	1.0	5,270	.07	.14	1.2	26
	Carrots: Raw, without crowns and tips, scraped:																	
600	Whole, 7 ½ by 1 ⅛ in, or strips, 2 ½ to 3 in long.	1 carrot or 18 strips	72	88	30	1	Trace	—	—	—	7	27	.5	7,930	.04	.04	.4	6
601	Grated	1 cup	110	88	45	1	Trace	—	—	—	11	41	.8	12,100	.07	.06	.7	9

H

TABLE 2.—NUTRITIVE VALUES OF THE EDIBLE PART OF FOODS - Continued
(Dashes (—) denote lack of reliable data for a constituent believed to be present in measurable amount)

H

Item No. (A)	Foods, approximate measures, units, and weight (edible part unless footnotes indicate otherwise) (B)	Grams	Water (C) Percent	Food energy (D) Calories	Protein (E) Grams	Fat (F) Grams	Fatty Acids Saturated (total) (G) Grams	Unsaturated Oleic (H) Grams	Linoleic (I) Grams	Carbohydrate (J) Grams	Calcium (K) Milligrams	Iron (L) Milligrams	Vitamin A value (M) International units	Thiamin (N) Milligrams	Riboflavin (O) Milligrams	Niacin (P) Milligrams	Ascorbic acid (Q) Milligrams
	VEGETABLE AND VEGETABLE PRODUCTS—Con.																
	Carrots—Continued																
602	Cooked (crosswise cuts), drained . . . . . 1 cup	155	91	50	1	Trace	—	—	—	11	51	.9	16,280	.08	.08	.8	9
	Canned:																
603	Sliced, drained solids . . . . 1 cup	155	91	45	1	Trace	—	—	—	10	47	1.1	23,250	.03	.05	.6	3
604	Strained or junior (baby food) . . . . 1 oz (1¾ to 2 tbsp)	28	92	10	Trace	Trace	—	—	—	2	7	.1	3,690	.01	.01	.1	1
	Cauliflower:																
605	Raw, chopped . . . . 1 cup	115	91	31	3	Trace	—	—	—	6	29	1.3	70	.13	.12	.8	90
	Cooked, drained:																
606	From raw (flower buds) . . . . 1 cup	125	93	30	3	Trace	—	—	—	5	26	.9	80	.11	.10	.8	69
607	From frozen (flowerets) . . . . 1 cup	180	94	30	3	Trace	—	—	—	6	31	.9	50	.07	.09	.7	74
	Celery, Pascal type, raw:																
608	Stalk, large outer, 8 by 1½ in, at root end . . . . 1 stalk	40	94	5	Trace	Trace	—	—	—	2	16	.1	110	.01	.01	.1	4
609	Pieces, diced . . . . 1 cup	120	94	20	1	Trace	—	—	—	5	47	.4	320	.04	.04	.4	11
	Collards, cooked, drained:																
610	From raw (leaves without stems) . . . . 1 cup	190	90	65	7	1	—	—	—	10	357	1.5	14,820	.21	.38	2.3	144
611	From frozen (chopped) . . . . 1 cup	170	90	50	5	1	—	—	—	10	299	1.7	11,560	.10	.24	1.0	56
	Corn, sweet:																
	Cooked, drained:																
612	From raw, ear 5 by 1¾ in . . . . 1 ear[61]	140	74	70	2	1	—	—	—	16	2	.5	[62]310	.09	.08	1.1	7
	From frozen:																
613	Ear, 5 in long . . . . 1 ear[61]	229	73	120	4	1	—	—	—	27	4	1.0	[62]440	.18	.10	2.1	9
614	Kernels . . . . 1 cup	165	77	130	5	1	—	—	—	31	5	1.3	[62]580	.15	.10	2.5	8
	Canned:																
615	Cream style . . . . 1 cup	256	76	210	5	2	—	—	—	51	8	1.5	[62]840	.08	.13	2.6	13
	Whole kernel:																
616	Vacuum pack . . . . 1 cup	210	76	175	5	1	—	—	—	43	6	1.1	[62]740	.06	.13	2.3	11
617	Wet pack, drained solids . . . . 1 cup	165	76	140	4	1	—	—	—	33	8	.8	[62]580	.05	.08	1.5	7
	Cowpeas. See Blackeye peas. (Items 585-586).																
	Cucumber slices, ⅛ in thick (large, 2⅛-in diam.; small, 1¾-in diam.):																
618	With peel . . . . 6 large or 8 small slices	28	95	5	Trace	Trace	—	—	—	1	7	.3	70	.01	.01	.1	3
619	Without peel . . . . 6½ large or 9 small pieces	28	96	5	Trace	Trace	—	—	—	1	5	.1	Trace	.01	.01	.1	3
620	Dandelion greens, cooked, drained . . . . 1 cup	105	90	35	2	1	—	—	—	7	147	1.9	12,290	.14	.17	—	19
621	Endive, curly (including escarole), raw, small pieces . . . . 1 cup	50	93	10	1	Trace	—	—	—	2	41	.9	1,650	.04	.07	.3	5
	Kale, cooked, drained:																
622	From raw (leaves without stems and midribs) . . . . 1 cup	110	88	45	5	1	—	—	—	7	206	1.8	9,130	.11	.20	1.8	102
623	From frozen (leaf style) . . . . 1 cup	130	91	40	4	1	—	—	—	7	157	1.3	10,660	.08	.20	.9	49

NUTRIENTS IN INDICATED QUANTITY

[61]Weight includes cob. Without cob, weight is 77 g for item 612, 126 g for item 613
[62]Based on yellow varieties. For white varieties, value is trace.

(A)	(B)	(C)	(D)	(E)	(F)	(G)	(H)	(I)	(J)	(K)	(L)	(M)	(N)	(O)	(P)	(Q)
	Lettuce, raw:															
	Butterhead, as Boston types:															
624	Head, 5-in diam — 1 head[63] — 220	95	25	2	Trace	—	—	—	4	57	3.3	1,580	.10	.10	5	13
625	Leaves — 1 outer or 2 inner or 3 heart leaves — 15	95	Trace	Trace	Trace	—	—	—	Trace	5	.3	150	.01	.01	Trace	1
	Crisphead, as Iceberg:															
626	Head, 6-in diam — 1 head[64] — 567	96	70	5	1	—	—	—	16	108	2.7	1,780	.32	.32	1.6	32
627	Wedge, ¼ of head — 1 wedge — 135	96	20	1	Trace	—	—	—	4	27	.7	450	.08	.08	.4	8
628	Pieces, chopped or shredded — 1 cup — 55	96	5	Trace	Trace	—	—	—	2	11	.3	180	.03	.03	.2	3
629	Looseleaf (bunching varieties including romaine or cos), chopped or shredded pieces — 1 cup — 55	94	10	1	Trace	—	—	—	2	37	.8	1,050	.03	.04	.2	10
630	Mushrooms, raw, sliced or chopped — 1 cup — 70	90	20	2	Trace	—	—	—	3	4	.6	Trace	.07	.32	2.9	2
631	Mustard greens, without stems and midribs, cooked, drained — 1 cup — 140	93	30	3	1	—	—	—	6	193	2.5	8,120	.11	.20	.8	67
632	Okra pods, 3 by ⅝ in, cooked — 10 pods — 106	91	30	2	Trace	—	—	—	6	98	.5	520	.14	.19	1.0	21
	Onions:															
	Mature:															
	Raw:															
633	Chopped — 1 cup — 170	89	65	3	Trace	—	—	—	15	46	.9	[65]Trace	.05	.07	.3	17
634	Sliced — 1 cup — 115	89	45	2	Trace	—	—	—	10	31	.6	[65]Trace	.03	.05	.2	12
635	Cooked (whole or sliced), drained — 1 cup — 210	92	60	3	Trace	—	—	—	14	50	.8	[65]Trace	.06	.06	.4	15
636	Young green, bulb (⅜ in diam.) and white portion of top — 6 onions — 30	88	15	Trace	Trace	—	—	—	3	12	.2	Trace	.02	.01	.1	8
637	Parsley, raw, chopped — 1 tbsp — 4	85	Trace	Trace	Trace	—	—	—	Trace	7	.2	300	Trace	.01	Trace	6
638	Parsnips, cooked (diced or 2-in lengths) — 1 cup — 155	82	100	2	1	—	—	—	23	70	.9	50	.11	.12	.2	16
	Peas, green:															
	Canned:															
639	Whole, drained solids — 1 cup — 170	77	150	8	1	—	—	—	29	44	3.2	1,170	.15	.10	1.4	14
640	Strained (baby food) — 1 oz (1 ¾ to 2 tbsp) — 28	86	15	1	Trace	—	—	—	3	3	.3	140	.02	.03	.3	3
641	Frozen, cooked, drained — 1 cup — 160	82	110	8	Trace	—	—	—	19	30	3.0	960	.43	.14	2.7	21
642	Peppers, hot, red, without seeds, dried (ground chili powder, added seasonings) — 1 tsp — 2	9	5	Trace	Trace	—	—	—	1	5	.3	1,300	Trace	.02	.2	Trace
	Peppers, sweet (about 5 per lb, whole), stem and seeds removed:															
643	Raw — 1 pod — 74	93	15	1	Trace	—	—	—	4	7	.5	310	.06	.06	.4	94
664	Cooked, boiled, drained — 1 pod — 73	95	15	1	Trace	—	—	—	3	7	.4	310	.05	.05	.4	70
	Potatoes, cooked:															
645	Baked, peeled after baking (about 2 per lb, raw) — 1 potato — 156	75	145	4	Trace	—	—	—	33	14	1.1	Trace	.15	.07	2.7	31
	Boiled (about 3 per lb, raw):															
646	Peeled after boiling — 1 potato — 137	80	105	3	Trace	—	—	—	23	10	.8	Trace	.12	.05	2.0	22
647	Peeled before boiling — 1 potato — 135	83	90	3	Trace	—	—	—	20	8	.7	Trace	.12	.05	1.6	22
	French-fried, strip, 2 to 3 ½ in long:															
648	Prepared from raw — 10 strips — 50	45	135	2	7	1.7	1.2	3.3	18	8	.7	Trace	.07	.04	1.6	11
649	Frozen, oven heated — 10 strips — 50	53	110	2	4	1.1	.8	2.1	17	5	.9	Trace	.07	.01	1.3	11
650	Hashed brown, prepared from frozen — 1 cup — 155	56	345	3	18	4.6	3.2	9.0	45	28	1.9	Trace	.11	.03	1.6	12

[63] Weight includes refuse of outer leaves and core. Without these parts, weight is 163 g

[64] Weight includes core. Without core, weight is 539 g

[65] Value based on white-fleshed varieties. For yellow-fleshed varieties, value in International Unite (I.U.) is 70 for item 633, 50 for item 634, and 80 for item 635

H

TABLE 2. — NUTRITIVE VALUES OF THE EDIBLE PART OF FOODS - Continued
(Dashes (—) denote lack of reliable data for a constituent believed to be present in measurable amount)

H

Item No. (A)	Foods, approximate measures, units, and weight (edible part unless footnotes indicate otherwise) (B)		Water (C) Per cent	Food energy (D) Calories	Protein (E) Grams	Fat (F) Grams	Fatty Acids Saturated (total) (G) Grams	Unsaturated Oleic (H) Grams	Linoleic (I) Grams	Carbohydrate (J) Grams	Calcium (K) Milligrams	Iron (L) Milligrams	Vitamin A value (M) International units	Thiamin (N) Milligrams	Riboflavin (O) Milligrams	Niacin (P) Milligrams	Ascorbic acid (Q) Milligrams
	VEGETABLE AND VEGETABLE PRODUCTS—Con.	Grams															
	Potatoes, cookes—Continued																
	Mashed, prepared from—																
	Raw:																
651	Milk added	1 cup .. 210	83	135	4	2	.7	.4	Trace	27	50	.8	40	.17	.11	2.1	21
652	Milk and butter added	1 cup .. 210	80	195	4	9	5.6	2.3	.2	26	50	.8	360	.17	.11	2.1	19
653	Dehydrated flakes (without milk), water, milk, butter, and salt added	1 cup .. 210	79	195	4	7	3.6	2.1	.2	30	65	.6	270	.08	.08	1.9	11
654	Potato chips, 1 ¾ by 2 ½ in oval cross section	10 chips .. 20	2	115	1	8	2.1	1.4	4.0	10	8	.4	Trace	.04	.01	1.0	3
655	Potato salad, made with cooked salad dressing	1 cup .. 250	76	250	7	7	2.0	2.7	1.3	41	80	1.5	350	.20	.18	2.8	28
656	Pumpkin, canned	1 cup .. 245	90	80	2	1	—	—	—	19	61	1.0	15,680	.07	.12	1.5	12
657	Radishes, raw (prepackaged) stem ends, rootlets cut off	4 radishes .. 18	95	5	Trace	Trace	—	—	—	1	5	.2	Trace	.01	.01	.1	5
658	Sauerkraut, canned, solids and liquid	1 cup .. 235	93	40	2	Trace	—	—	—	9	85	1.2	120	.07	.09	.5	33
	Southern peas. See Blackeye peas (items 585-586).																
	Spinach:																
659	Raw, chopped	1 cup .. 55	91	15	2	Trace	—	—	—	2	51	1.7	4,460	.06	.11	.3	28
	Cooked, drained:																
660	From raw	1 cup .. 180	92	40	5	1	—	—	—	6	167	4.0	14,580	.13	.25	.9	50
	From frozen:																
661	Chopped	1 cup .. 205	92	45	6	1	—	—	—	8	232	4.3	16,200	.14	.31	.8	39
662	Leaf	1 cup .. 190	92	45	6	1	—	—	—	7	200	4.8	15,390	.15	.27	1.0	53
663	Canned, drained solids	1 cup .. 205	91	50	6	1	—	—	—	7	242	5.3	16,400	.04	.25	.6	29
	Squash, cooked:																
664	Summer (all varieties), diced, drained	1 cup .. 210	96	30	2	Trace	—	—	—	7	53	.8	820	.11	.17	1.7	21
665	Winter (all varieties), baked, mashed	1 cup .. 205	81	130	4	1	—	—	—	32	57	1.6	8,610	.10	.27	1.4	27
	Sweetpotatoes:																
	Cooked (raw, 5 by 2 in, about 2 ½ per lb):																
666	Baked in skin, peeled	1 potato .. 114	64	160	2	1	—	—	—	37	46	1.0	9,230	.10	.08	.8	25
667	Boiled in skin, peeled	1 potato .. 151	71	170	3	1	—	—	—	40	48	1.1	11,940	.14	.09	.9	26
668	Candied, 2 ½ by 2-in piece	1 piece .. 105	60	175	1	3	2.0	.8	.1	36	39	.9	6,620	.06	.04	.4	11
	Canned:																
669	Solid pack (mashed)	1 cup .. 255	72	275	5	1	—	—	—	63	64	2.0	19,890	.13	.10	1.5	36
670	Vacuum pack, piece 2 ¾ by 1 in	1 piece .. 40	72	45	1	Trace	—	—	—	10	10	.3	3,120	.02	.02	.2	6
	Tomatoes:																
671	Raw, 2 ⅗-in diam. (3 per 12 oz pkg.)	1 tomato[66] .. 135	94	25	1	Trace	—	—	—	6	16	.6	1,110	.07	.05	.9	[67]28
672	Canned, solids and liquid	1 cup .. 241	94	50	2	Trace	—	—	—	10	[68]14	1.2	2,170	.12	.07	1.7	41
673	Tomato catsup	1 cup .. 273	69	290	5	1	—	—	—	69	60	2.2	3,820	.25	.19	4.4	41
674		1 tbsp .. 15	69	15	Trace	Trace	—	—	—	4	3	.1	210	.01	.01	.2	2

[66] Weight includes cores and stem ends. Without these parts, weight is 123 g.

[67] Based on year-round average. For tomatoes marked from November through May, value is about 12 mg; from June through October, 32 mg.

[68] Applies to product without calcium salts added. Value for products with calcium salts added may be as much as 63 mg for whole tomatoes, 241 mg for cut forms.

(A)	(B)	(C)	(D)	(E)	(F)	(G)	(H)	(I)	(J)	(K)	(L)	(M)	(N)	(O)	(P)	(Q)
	Tomato juice, canned:															
675	Cup . . . . 1 cup	243	45	2	Trace	—	—	—	10	17	2.2	1,940	.12	.07	1.9	39
676	Glass (6 fl oz) . . . . 1 glass	182	35	2	Trace	—	—	—	8	13	1.6	1,460	.09	.05	1.5	29
677	Turnips, cooked, diced . 1 cup	155	35	1	Trace	—	—	—	8	54	.6	Trace	.06	.08	.5	34
	Turnip greens, cooked, drained:															
678	From raw (leaves and stems) 1 cup	145	30	3	Trace	—	—	—	5	252	1.5	8,270	.15	.33	.7	68
679	From frozen (chopped) . 1 cup	165	40	4	Trace	—	—	—	6	195	2.6	11,390	.08	.15	.7	31
680	Vegetables, mixed, frozen, cooked . . . . . . 1 cup	182	115	6	1	—	—	—	24	46	2.4	9,010	.22	.13	2.0	15

APPENDIX I

Sodium and Potassium

The following tables are reprinted from the second edition of the U.S. Dietary Goals.[1] The Goals recommended restricting salt intake to about 5 g a day, which effectively means reducing sodium intake to about 2 g (2,000 mg).

[1]Select Committee on Nutrition and Human Needs, *Dietary Goals for the United States*, 2nd ed. (Washington, D.C.: Government Printing Office, 1977), pp. 80-83. The Senate's tables are taken from information in U.S. Department of Agriculture, Agricultural Research Service, Composition of foods: Raw, processed, prepared, *Agricultural Handbook No. 8* (Washington, D.C.: Government Printing Office, 1963).

(This salt excludes that present in the natural food before processing.) The goals have been superseded by a more relaxed recommendation from the USDA that we should be moderate in our use of salt, but the specific amounts of sodium in foods may still be of interest to those who wish to compare one food with another. No recommendation was made for the daily consumption of potassium, but people taking diuretics, instructed by their physicians to eat foods high in potassium to replace losses, may be interested to see what foods contain large amounts of this mineral.

I

Table 1   Average Sodium and Potassium Contents of Common Foods*

Food	Weight (g)	Sodium (mg)	Potassium (mg)	Food	Weight (g)	Sodium (mg)	Potassium (mg)
Meat, fish, or poultry, cooked without added salt				Scallops, fresh	100	265	476
				Shrimp, raw	100	140	220
Average	30	33	125	Shrimp, frozen or canned	100	140	200-312
Clams, soft	100	36	239	Sweet breads	100	116	433
Clams, hard	100	205	311	Tuna, canned	100	800	240
Crab, canned	100	1,000	110	Tuna, salt-free, canned	100	46	382
Crab, steamed	100	456	271				
Flounder	100	237	587	**Cheese**			
Frankfurters (2)	100	1,100	220	American cheese	30	341	25
Frozen fish (cod)	100	400	400	Cream cheese	30	75	22
Haddock	100	177	348	Cottage cheese	30	76	28
Kidneys, beef	100	253	324	Cottage cheese, unsalted	30	6	—
Lobster, canned	100	210	180	Low-sodium cheese (cheddar)	30	3	120
Lobster, fresh	100	325	258				
Oysters, raw	100	73	121	**Egg**			
Salmon, canned	100	522	349	Whole, fresh and frozen (1)	50	61	65
Salmon, salt-free, canned	100	48	391				

*Fresh fruits and fruit juices are naturally very low in sodium and thus are not listed individually in this table.

Table 1   Average Sodium and Potassium Contents of Common Foods (cont'd)

Food	Weight (g)	Sodium (mg)	Potassium (mg)
Whites, fresh and frozen	50	73	70
Yolks, fresh	50	26	49
Milk			
Buttermilk, cultured	120	135	192
Condensed sweetened milk	120	135	377
Evaporated milk, undiluted	120	142	364
Powdered milk, skim	30	160	544
Low-sodium milk, canned	120	6	288
Whole	240	120	346
Yogurt (skim milk)	100	51	143
Potato			
White, baked in skin	100	4	323
White, boiled	100	2	285
Instant, prepared with water, milk, fat	100	256	290
Sweet (canned solid pack)	100	48	200
Breads			
Bakery, white	25	127	26
Bakery, whole-wheat	25	132	68
Bakery, rye	25	139	36
Low-sodium (local)	25	4	25
Plain muffin	40	132	38
English muffin	57	215	57
A-proten rusk (1)	11	4	5
Graham crackers (2)	14	93	53
Low-sodium crackers (2)	9	10	11
Vanilla wafers (5)	14	35	10
Yeast doughnut	30	70	24
Cake doughnut	.35	160	32
Cereal, dry			
Kellogg's Corn Flakes	30	282	15
Puffed Rice	15	trace	7
Rice Krispies	30	267	15
Special K	30	244	17
Puffed Wheat	15	trace	21
Shredded Wheat	20	1	52

Food	Weight (g)	Sodium (mg)	Potassium (mg)
Kellogg's Sugar Frosted Flakes	30	200	19
Sugar Pops	30	67	22
Bran Flakes	30	118	151
Cereal, cooked without added salt			
Corn grits, enriched, regular	100	1	11
Farina, enriched, regular	100	2	9
Farina, instant cooking	100	7	13
Farina, quick cooking	100	190	10
Oatmeal or Rolled Oats	100	2	61
Pettijohn's Wheat	100	trace	84
Rice	100	5	28
Rice, instant	100	trace	trace
Wheat, rolled	100	trace	84
Wheatena	100	trace	84
Fat			
Bacon (1 strip)	7	73	17
Butter	5	49	3
Margarine	5	49	1
Mayonnaise	15	90	5
Mayonnaise, low-sodium	15	17	1
Low-sodium butter	15	1	3
Unsalted margarine (Fleischmann's)	5	1	1
Vegetable oil	15	0	0
Cream			
Coffee Mate	1[†]	4	27
Half-and-half	30	14	39
Heavy whipping cream (30%)	30	10	27
Poly-perx	30	—	11
Sour cream (Sealtest)	30	13	43
Table cream (18%)	30	13	37
Whipped topping	30	4	6

I

[†]In teaspoons.

Table 1 Average Sodium and Potassium Contents of Common Foods (cont'd)

Food	Weight (g)	Sodium (mg)	Potassium (mg)
Gravy			
Low-sodium	30	10	25
Regular	30	210	28
Peanut butter			
Cellu, Salt-free	15	1	100
Regular, made with small amounts of added fat and salt	15	91	100
Desserts			
Baked custard (Delmark)	120	128	174
D'zerta	120	35	0
Gelatin	120	51	1
Ice cream (4-oz cup)	60	23	49
Sherbet	60	6	14
Water ice	60	trace	2
Cakes			
All varieties except gingerbread and fruit cakes (both mixes and recipes)	50[‡]	123	50
With low-sodium shortening and baking powder	50[‡]	10-20	75-150
Pies			
All varieties except raisin, mince (1/8 of 9-inch pie)	320[‡]	375	180
Candy			
Hard candy (1 equals 5 g)	100	32	4
Gum drops (8 small equals 10 g)	100	35	5
Jelly beans	100	12	1
Salt			
(1 g NaCl—1 packet salt)	—	400	—
(5 g NaCl—1 tsp)	—	2,000	—
Salt substitutes			
Diamond Crystal	500[§]	1	220
Co-salt	500[§]	0	185

Food	Weight (g)	Sodium (mg)	Potassium (mg)
Adolph's	500[§]	0	241
McCormick's	500[§]	0	234
Morton	500[§]	0	250
Sugar substitutes			
Saccharine (1/4-grain tablet)	1	1	0
Sucaryl	500[§]	0	0
Sweet-10	500[§]	0	0
Adolph's	500[§]	0	0
Morton	500[§]	0	0
Diamond Crystal	500[§]	0	0
Beverages			
Beer	100	7	25
Chocolate syrup (2 tsp)	10	5	29
Coca-Cola	100	4	1
Coffee, instant (beverage)	—	1	50
Cranberry juice	100	1	10
Diet Seven-Up	100	10	0
Egg nog, reconstituted	240	250	630
Fresca	100	18	0
Frozen lemonade, reconstituted	100	trace	16
Gingerale	100	6	2
Hot chocolate (Carnation, 1 pack 6 oz water)	100 —	104	190
Kool-Aid, reconstituted	240	trace	0
Meritene, reconstituted	240	250	740
Pepsi Cola	100	2	4
Royal Crown Cola	100	3	trace
Seven-Up	100	9	0
Sprite	100	16	0
Tab	100	5	0
Tea, instant (beverage)	—	trace	25

[‡]Average serving.

[§]In milligrams.

Table 2   Sodium Content of Vegetables*

Vegetable	Sodium (mg)
Group I (0-20 mg/100 g,† average 7.4 mg)	
Asparagus	7
Broccoli	12
Brussels sprouts	14
Cabbage, common	14
Cauliflower	9
Chicory	7
Collards	16
Corn	2
Cow peas	1
Cucumbers	6
Eggplant	1
Endive	14
Escarole	14
Green peppers	13
Kohlrabi	6
Leeks	5
Lentils	3
Lettuce	9
Lima beans, not frozen	1
Mushrooms, raw	15
Mustard green	10
Navy beans	7
Okra	2
Onions	7
Parsnips	8
Peas, dried, split, cooked	13
Peas, green	1
Potatoes, baked in skin	4

Vegetable	Sodium (mg)
Potatoes, boiled, pared before cooking	3
Radishes	18
Rutabagas	4
Squash, summer or winter	1
String beans	2
Sweet potato	10
Tomatoes	4
Turnip greens	17
Wax beans	2
Yams	4
Group II (23-60 mg/100 g,† average 40 mg)	
Artichoke	30
Beets	43
Black-eyed peas, frozen only	39
Carrots	33
Chinese cabbage	23
Dandelion greens	44
Kale	43
Parsley	45
Red cabbage	26
Spinach	50
Turnips	34
Watercress	52
Group III (75-126 mg/100 g,† average 81 mg)	
Beet greens	76
Celery	88
Chard, Swiss	86

*This table assumes the use of fresh vegetables without salt added in cooking. The amount of salt added to canned and frozen vegetables can vary. *Agricultural Handbook No. 8* from the USDA estimates that canned vegetables average 235 mg sodium per 100 g edible portion. Frozen vegetables range from almost no sodium to as high as 125 mg sodium per 100 g edible portion.

†A 100-g portion for most vegetables is about a 1/2-c to 1-c serving.

I

APPENDIX J

Recommended Nutrition References

The To Explore section at the end of the Introduction to Part One suggests places to go for nutrition information, and the references at the end of each chapter and highlight offer many references on the topics treated there. Appendix A is devoted to Books Not Recommended, and Appendix C to books and booklets you might like to recommend to clients. This appendix offers some recommended general references for the person interested in building a library on nutrition.

Books

Nutrition Reviews' Present Knowledge in Nutrition, 4th ed. (Washington, D.C.: Nutrition Foundation, 1976), 605 pages (paperback $12) will bring you up to date on fifty-three topics, including energy, obesity, twenty-nine nutrients, diabetes, coronary heart disease, fiber, renal disease, parenteral nutrition, malnutrition, growth and its assessment, brain development, immunity, alcohol, fiber, milk intolerances, dental health, drugs, and toxins. The only major omissions seem to be nutrition and food intake and national nutrition status surveys. Watch for an update; these come out about every five or six years.

A tidy paperback volume containing thirteen thought-provoking articles from the *New England Journal of Medicine*, each about ten pages long, is *Current Concepts in Nutrition* (Massachusetts Medical Society, 1979). A scholarly volume from the *Journal of Nutrition*, five times larger than *Current Concepts*, is *Nutritional Requirements of Man, a Conspectus of Research* (New York and Washington, D.C.: Nutrition Foundation, 1980). The *Conspectus* has a major review article on human requirements for each

of the following: protein, amino acids, vitamin A, calcium, zinc, vitamin C, iron, folacin, and copper.

R. S. Goodhart and M. E. Shils, eds., *Modern Nutrition in Health and Disease*, 6th ed. (Philadelphia: Lea and Febiger, 1980), 1153 pages (about $50) is a major technical reference book on nutrition topics, containing forty encyclopedic articles on the nutrients, foods, the diet, metabolism, malnutrition, age-related needs, and nutrition in disease, with twenty-eight appendixes. We also recommend *Human Nutrition and Dietetics*, 7th ed., by S. Davidson, R. Passmore, J. F. Brock, and A. S. Truswell (New York: Churchill Livingstone, 1979).

Many students also like to have a separate copy of the Table of Food Composition (Appendix H in this book), which is available in softcover from the Government Printing Office (address below). Another more comprehensive book of food composition, which also gives foods in household measures, is *Bowes and Church's Food Values of Portions Commonly Used*. The twelfth edition was available from J. B. Lippincott Company, Philadelphia, as of 1975.

Many excellent publications are available on the important subject of food faddism and misinformation. A whole issue of *Nutrition Reviews* was devoted to this topic and includes a list of suggested readings to help the reader identify faddists, quacks, and promoters: *Nutrition Reviews/Supplement: Nutrition Misinformation and Food Faddism*, July 1974. R. Deutsch has recently revised his entertaining and revealing book on food faddism under the title *The New Nuts among the Berries: How Nutrition Nonsense Captured America* (Palo Alto, Calif.: Bull Publishing, 1977). V. Herbert's latest book, with S. Barrett, *Vitamins and Health Foods: The Great American Hustle* (Philadelphia: Stickley,

1981, $12) is highly recommended. To see what other books are reliable references, send for the Chicago Nutrition Association's *Nutrition References and Book Reviews*, address below.

The syndicated column on nutrition by J. Mayer and J. Dwyer, which appears in many newspapers, presents well-researched, reliable answers to current questions. The column by R. Alfin-Slater and Jelliffe is also accurate and trustworthy.

One of the most readable, entertaining, and relevant books of readings in nutrition to come out in recent years is L. Hofmann, ed., *The Great American Nutrition Hassle* (Palo Alto, Calif.: Mayfield, 1978). This book would make an excellent discussion-topic source for a course in which *Nutrition: Concepts and Controversies* is assigned. *Hassle* includes articles by recognized authorities on the RDA, fast foods, additives, infant nutrition, fad diets, sugar, alcohol, and most of the other topics treated in this book's Highlights.

Another book that readers may wish to add to their libraries is the latest edition of *Recommended Dietary Allowances*, available from the National Academy of Sciences (address below).

We also recommend our own book, E. M. N. Hamilton and E. N. Whitney, *Nutrition: Concepts and Controversies*, 2nd ed. (St. Paul, Minn.: West, 1981), which explores current nutrition topics other than those treated here. *Concepts* is also available in a hardcover, trade edition.

Journals

Nutrition Today, the publication of the Nutrition Today Society, is an excellent magazine for the interested layperson. It makes a point of raising controversial issues and providing a forum for conflicting opinions. References are seldom printed in the magazine but are available on request. The articles are written by recognized authorities and are entertaining and thought-provoking. Six issues per year, $12.50 ($6.25 for dietetics students), from Director of Membership Services, Nutrition Today Society, P.O. Box 773, Annapolis, MD 21404.

The *Journal of the American Dietetic Association*, the official publication of the ADA, contains articles of interest to dietitians and nutritionists, news of legislative action on food and nutrition, and a very useful section of abstracts of articles from many other journals of nutrition and related areas. Twelve issues per year, $24 ($12 for dietetics students), from the American Dietetic Association (address below).

Nutrition Reviews, a publication of The Nutrition Foundation, Inc., does much of the work for the library researcher, compiling recent evidence on current topics and presenting extensive bibliographies. Twelve issues per year, $12 ($6 for students), from the Nutrition Foundation, Inc., 489 Fifth Avenue, New York, NY 10017.

Nutrition and the MD is a monthly newsletter that provides up to date, easy to read, and practical information on nutrition for health care providers. It is available for $34/year from PM, Inc. (address below).

Other journals that deserve mention here are the *Journal of Nutrition*, *Food Technology*, the *American Journal of Clinical Nutrition*, and the *Journal of Nutrition Education*. FDA Consumer, a government publication with many articles of interest to the consumer, is available from the Food and Drug Administration (address below). Many other journals of value are referred to throughout this book.

Catalogs, Publication Lists, Free and Inexpensive Materials

Lists of publications can be obtained from the following organizations.

ADA catalog (free) from:

> The American Dietetic Association
> 430 North Michigan Avenue
> Chicago, IL 60611

Publications list (free) from:

> The American Medical Association
> 535 North Dearborn Street
> Chicago, IL 60610

J

Nutrition References and Book Reviews (54 pages, $2) from:

> The Chicago Nutrition Association
> 8158 Kedzie Avenue
> Chicago, IL 60652

The "Know How" catalog from

> Cooperative Extension
> N.Y. State
> College of Agriculture and Life Sciences
> Cornell University
> Ithaca, NY 14853

A guide to free health materials, listing over 2,000 items, can be obtained for $15 from:

> Educators Progress Service, Inc.
> 214 Center Street
> Randolph, WIS 53956

A catalog of nutrition education material is available from *Family Circle Magazine*, good for more listings of free and inexpensive literature:

> Family Circle
> 488 Madison Avenue
> New York, NY 10022

Other free and inexpensive materials can be obtained from the following addresses:

U.S. government:

Consumer Nutrition Center
Human Nutrition Information Service
Federal Center Building
Hyattsville, MD 20782

Human Nutrition Research Division
Agricultural Research Center
Beltsville, MD 20705

Department of the Interior
Fish and Wildlife Services
Bureau of Commercial Fisheries
Washington, DC 20240

Extension Service, USDA
Room 6007, 3.South Building
Washington, DC 20250

Food and Nutrition Service, USDA
Washington, DC 20250

Food and Drug Administration (FDA)
5600 Fishers Lane
Rockville, MD 20852

The Food and Nutrition Information Education Resources Center (FNIERC)
National Agriculture Library
10301 Baltimore Boulevard, Room 304
Beltsville, MD 20705
Tel: (301) 344-3719

Information Division
Agricultural Marketing Service, USDA
Washington, DC 20250

National Academy of Sciences/National Research Council (NAS/NRC)
2101 Constitution Avenue NW
Washington, DC 20418

Office of Child Development
Office of Education
Public Health Service
Washington, DC 20204

U.S. Government Printing Office
The Superintendent of Documents
Washington, DC 20402

Consumer and advocacy groups:

> Center for Science in the Public Interest (CSPI)
> 1755 S Street, NW
> Washington, DC 20009

> Children's Foundation
> 1420 New York Avenue, NW
> Suite 800
> Washington, DC 20005

> Community Nutrition Institute
> 1146 19th Street NW
> Washington, DC 20036

> Food Research and Action Center (FRAC)
> 2011 I Street, NW
> Washington, DC 20006

Professional and service organizations:

> American Academy of Pediatrics
> PO Box 1034
> Evanston, IL 60204

> American College of Nutrition
> 100 Manhattan Avenue #1606
> Union City, NJ 07087

> American Dental Association
> 211 East Chicago Avenue
> Chicago, IL 60611

> American Dietetic Association
> 620 North Michigan Avenue
> Chicago, IL 60611

American Heart Association
7320 Greenville Avenue
Dallas, TX 75231

American Home Economics Association
2010 Massachusetts Avenue NW
Washington, DC 20036

American Institute of Nutrition
9650 Rockville Pike
Bethesda, MD 20014

American Medical Association
Section of Nutrition Information
535 North Dearborn Street
Chicago, IL 60610

The American National Red Cross
Food and Nutrition Consultant
National Headquarters
Washington, DC 20006

American Public Health Association
1015 Fifteenth Street NW
Washington, DC 20005

American Society for Clinical Nutrition
9650 Rockville Pike
Bethesda, MD 20014

The Canadian Diabetes Association
1491 Yonge Street
Toronto, Ontario M4T 1Z5 Canada

The Canadian Dietetic Association
123 Edward Street, Suite 601
Toronto, Ontario M5G 1E2 Canada

Institute of Food Technologists
221 North La Salle Street
Chicago, IL 60601

LaLeche League International, Inc.
9616 Minneapolis Avenue
Franklin Park, IL 60131

March of Dimes Birth Defects Foundation
173 West Madison Street
Chicago, IL 60602

Meals for Millions/Freedom from Hunger
Foundation
1800 Olympic Boulevard
PO Drawer 680
Santa Monica, CA 90406

National Council on Alcoholism
733 Third Avenue
New York, NY 10017

National Nutrition Consortium
1635 P Street NW, Suite 1
Washington, DC 20036

Nutrition Foundation
888 Seventeenth Street NW
Washington, DC 20036

Nutrition Today Society
101 Ridgely Avenue
PO Box 465
Annapolis, MD 21404

PM, Inc. (Publisher of *Nutrition and the MD*)
14349 Victory Boulevard, #204
Van Nuys, CA 91401

Rice Council
P.O. Box 22802
Houston, TX 77027

Society for Nutrition Education
1736 Franklin Street
Oakland, CA 94612

Soy Protein Council
1800 M Street NW
Washington, DC 20036

Trade organizations produce many excellent free materials that promote nutritional health. Naturally, they also promote their own products. The student must learn to differentiate between "slanted" and valid information. We find the brief reviews in *Contemporary Nutrition* (put out by General Mills), the Dairy Council Digest, Ross Laboratories' *Dietetic Currents*, and R. A. Seelig's reviews from the United Fresh Fruit and Vegetable Association to be generally reliable and very useful.

American Meat Institute
59 Van Buren Street
Chicago, IL 60605

Best Foods
Consumer Service Department
Division of CPC International
Internation Plaza
Englewood Cliffs, NJ 07623

Borden Farm Products
Division Borden Company
350 Madison Ave.
New York, NY 10017

Campbell Soup Company
Food Service Products Division
375 Memorial Avenue
Camden, NJ 08101

Cereal Institute
135 S. LaSalle St.
Chicago, IL 60603

Del Monte Kitchens
Del Monte Corporation
215 Fremont Street
San Francisco, CA 94119

Fleischmann's Margarines
Standard Brands, Inc.
625 Madison Avenue
New York, NY 10022

General Foods Consumer Center
250 North Street
White Plains, NY 10625

General Mills
PO Box 113
Minneapolis, MN 55440

Gerber Products Company
445 State Street
Fremont, MI 49412

H. J. Heinz
Consumer Relations
PO Box 57
Pittsburg, PA 15230

Hunt-Wesson Foods
Educational Services
1645 West Valencia Drive
Fullerton, CA 92634

Kellogg Company
Department of Home Economics Services
Battle Creek, MI 49016

Mead Johnson Nutritionals
2404 Pennsylvania Avenue
Evansville, IN 47721

National Commission on Egg Nutrition
205 Touvy Ave.
Park Ridge, IL 60668

National Dairy Council
111 North Canal Street
Chicago, IL 60618

Nestle Company
Home Economics Division
100 Bloomingdale Road
White Plains, NY 10605

Oscar Mayer Company
Consumer Service
PO Box 1409
Madison, WI 53701

The Potato Board
1385 South Colorado Blvd.
Suite 512
Denver, CO 80222

Poultry and Egg National Board
8 South Michigan Ave.
Chicago, IL 60603

Ross Laboratories
Director of Professional Services
Columbus, OH 43216

Sister Kenny Institute
Chicago Ave. at 27th St.
Minneapolis, MN 55407

Sunkist Growers
Consumer Service, Division BB
Box 7888
Valley Annex
Van Nys, CA 91409

VNIS (Vitamin Nutrition Information Service)
Hoffmann-LaRoche
340 Kingsland Ave.
Nutley, NJ 07110

United Fresh Fruit and Vegetable Association
777 1st St. NW
Washington, DC 20005

Vitamin Information Bureau
383 Madison Ave.
New York, NY 10017

Wheat Flour Institute
309 West Jackson Blvd.
Chicago, IL 60606

International organizations (United Nations):

Food and Agriculture Organization of the United
Nations (FAO)
North American Regional Office
1325 C Street SW
Washington, DC 20025

Food and Agriculture Organization (FAO)
Via delle Terma di Caracella
0100 Rome, Italy

World Health Organization (WHO)
1211 Geneva 27
Switzerland

APPENDIX K

Fiber

If you are attempting to evaluate your fiber intake, it is important to be aware of the distinction made in Chapter 1: The fiber in the colon is not the same as the fiber found in foods when they are analyzed in the laboratory. In the colon, the fiber that remains is whatever has resisted the action of human GI tract enzymes. This is dietary fiber. But when foods are analyzed in a laboratory, they are exposed to stronger agents—dilute acid and dilute alkali. What remains after these treatments is crude fiber. For every gram of crude fiber, there may be 2 to 3 g of dietary fiber.

Diets in the United States probably provide an average of about 4 g of crude fiber a day, as compared with about 6 g back in 1900. Some fiber enthusiasts recommend intakes higher than these, but there may be hazards in overdosing with fiber, as with any other food constituent. Even conservative authorities, however, seem to agree that there would be no harm in aiming at a crude fiber intake from foods of about 6 g a day.

Table 1 shows estimates of the crude fiber contents of foods. Table 2 shows approximations of the dietary fiber contents of foods. We recommend that you read the article it came from for an understanding of the limitations on the accuracy of the numbers in the table and for a breakdown of the fiber types into cellulose, lignin, and other sources.

Table 1   Approximate Crude Fiber Content Per Serving of Food[1]

Food	Serving size	Crude fiber (g)
Cereals	1/2-2/3 c	
All bran		3.0
Wheat bran		0.8
40% bran		0.9
Most other cooked or ready-to-eat		trace-0.3
Breads	1 slice	
Whole-wheat, pumpernickel		0.4
Raisin, rye, French, Italian, enriched white		0.05-0.2
Fruits	medium or 1/2 c	
Watermelon		1.5
Apple (with skin)		2.0
Prunes, dried peaches		1.5
Honeydew melon, banana		1.0
Berries		1.0

Food	Serving size	Crude fiber (g)
Peaches, apricots, citrus fruits, fruit cocktail		0.5
Fruit juice		0.2
Vegetables	1/2-2/3 c	
Parsnips, peas, brussels sprouts		2.0
Pork and beans		2.0
Lima beans		1.5
Kidney beans		1.0
Broccoli, carrots		1.0
Green beans, corn, celery, turnip, tomato, greens		0.5-1.0
Potato (with skin)		0.8
Potato chips, spinach		<0.5
Nuts	1/2 c	1.0-2.0
Sunflower seeds	1 c	2.0

[1]E. M. N. Hamilton and E. N. Whitney, *Nutrition: Concepts and Controversies* (St. Paul: West, 1979), pp. 499-500.

Table 2   Dietary Fiber in Selected Foods[2]

Food	Total dietary fiber (g/100 g)
Flour	
White, bread-making	3.15
Brown	7.87
Whole-meal	9.51
Bran	44.0
Breads	
White	2.72
Brown	5.11
Hovis	4.54
Whole-meal	8.50
Cereals	
All-Bran	26.7
Cornflakes	11.0
Grapenuts	7.00
Readibrek	7.60
Rice Krispies	4.47
Puffed Wheat	15.41
Sugar Puffs	6.08
Shredded Wheat	12.26
Swiss breakfast (mixed brands)	7.41
Weetabix	12.72
Biscuits	
Chocolate digestive (half-coated)	3.50
Chocolate (fully coated)	3.09
Crispbread, rye	11.73
Crispbread, wheat	4.83
Ginger biscuits	1.99
Matzo	3.85
Oatcakes	4.00
Semisweet	2.31
Short-sweet	1.60
Wafers (filled)	1.62
Leafy vegetables	
Broccoli tops (boiled)	4.10
Brussels sprouts (boiled)	2.86
Cabbage (boiled)	2.83
Cauliflower (boiled)	1.80
Lettuce (raw)	1.53
Onions (raw)	2.10
Legumes	
Beans, baked (canned)	7.27
Beans, runner (boiled)	3.35

Food	Total dietary fiber (g/100 g)
Peas, frozen (raw)	7.75
garden (canned)	6.28
processed (canned)	7.85
Root vegetables	
Carrots, young (boiled)	3.70
Parsnips (raw)	4.90
Swedes (raw)	2.40
Turnips (raw)	2.20
Potatoes	
Main crop (raw)	3.51
Chips (fried)	3.20
Crisps	11.9
Canned, drained	2.51
Other vegetables	
Peppers (cooked)	0.93
Tomatoes, fresh	1.40
canned, drained	0.85
Sweet corn, cooked	4.74
canned, drained	5.69
Fruits	
Apples, flesh only,	1.42
peel only	3.71
Bananas	1.75
Cherries (flesh and skin)	1.24
Grapefruit (canned)	0.44
Guavas (canned)	3.64
Mandarin oranges (canned)	0.29
Mangoes (canned)	1.00
Peaches (flesh and skin)	2.28
Pears, flesh only	2.44
peel only	8.59
Plums (flesh and skin)	1.52
Rhubarb (raw)	1.78
Strawberries, raw,	2.12
canned	1.00
Sultanas	4.40
Nuts	
Brazils	7.73
Peanuts	9.30
Preserves	
Jam, plum,	0.96
strawberry	1.12

[2]Adapted from D. A. T. Southgate, B. Bailey, E. Collinson, and A. F. Walker, A guide to calculating intakes of dietary fibre, *Journal of Human Nutrition* 30 (1976):303-313, with the permission of the authors and publisher.

Table 2   Dietary Fiber in Selected Foods (cont'd)

Food	Total dietary fiber (g/100 g)
Lemon curd	0.20
Marmalade	0.71
Mincemeat	3.19
Peanut butter	7.55
Pickle	1.53
Dried soups (as purchased)	
Minestrone	6.61
Oxtail	3.84
Tomato	3.32

Food	Total dietary fiber (g/100 g)
Beverages (concentrated)	
Cocoa	43.27
Drinking chocolate	8.20
Coffee and chicory essence	0.79
Instant coffee	16.41
Extracts	
Bovril	0.91
Marmite	2.69

APPENDIX L

Exchange Systems

CONTENTS

For an introduction to the use of exchange systems, see Chapter 1. Two exchange systems are presented here, for the use of U.S. and Canadian readers.

United States

The United States system divides foods into six lists—the milk, vegetable, fruit, bread, meat, and fat lists.[1] The items listed first in each group are from the standard exchange lists used in the United States. We have also listed some Chinese foods and some fast foods to show that the exchange system can be adapted to other uses. At the end of the section is a list of "unlimited" foods, which have negligible kcalories.

The exchange system can be used to plan diets at many different kcalorie levels. Six such diets, from 1,000 to 2,200 kcal/day, are shown in Appendix M, Table 6.

[1]The U.S. exchange system presented here is based on material in *Exchange Lists for Meal Planning*, prepared by committees of the American Diabetes Association and the American Dietetic Association in cooperation with the National Institute of Arthritis, Metabolism, and Digestive Diseases and the National Heart and Lung Institute, National Institutes of Health, Public Health Service, U.S. Department of Health, Education, and Welfare.

The Chinese foods listed in these tables are reprinted from *Diabetes and Chinese Food*, ©1978, with the written permission of the Canadian Dietetic Association. We have adjusted the Canadian exchanges used in these examples so that they correspond approximately in food value to the U.S. exchanges. *Diabetes and Chinese Food* is available for a nominal charge from the Canadian Diabetes Association (address in Appendix J).

The fast food data are reprinted by permission from "Nutritional Analysis of Foods Served at McDonald's" (© McDonald's, 1976).

Milk List (12 g carbohydrate, 8 g protein, 80 kcal)*

Amount	Food
Nonfat fortified milk	
1 c	Skim or nonfat milk
1 c	Buttermilk made from skim milk
1 c	Yogurt made from skim milk (plain, unflavored)
1/3 c	Powdered, nonfat dry milk, before adding liquid
1/2 c	Canned evaporated skim milk, before adding liquid
Low-fat fortified milk	
1 c	1% fat fortified milk (add 1/2 fat exchange)†
1 c	2% fat fortified milk (add 1 fat exchange)‡
1 c	Yogurt made from 2% fortified milk (plain, unflavored) (add 1 fat exchange)†
Whole milk (add 2 fat exchanges)	
1 c	Whole milk
1 c	Buttermilk made from whole milk
1 c	Yogurt made from whole milk (plain, unflavored)
1/2 c	Canned evaporated whole milk, before adding liquid
Chinese foods	
1 c	Soybean milk, unsweetened
2 blocks	Soybean curd (2 1/2 x 2 1/2 x 1 1/2 in)
2/3 c	Soybean, cooked
Fast foods §	

*A milk exchange is a serving of food equivalent to 1 c of skim milk in its energy nutrient content. One milk exchange contains substantial amounts of carbohydrate and protein and about 80 kcal.

†These milk exchanges contain more fat than skim milk. Add 1/2 fat exchange.

‡These milk exchanges contain more fat than skim milk. Add 1 fat exchange.

§These fast foods contain 1/2 milk exchange and added bread and fat: chocolate shake (3 1/2 bread, 2 fat, 365 kcal); vanilla shake (3 bread, 1 1/2 fat, 325 kcal); strawberry shake (3 1/2 bread, 1 1/2 fat, 345 kcal).

Vegetable List (5 g carbohydrate, 2 g protein, 25 kcal)*

Amount	Food
1/2 c	Asparagus
1/2 c	Bean sprouts
1/2 c	Beets
1/2 c	Broccoli
1/2 c	Brussels sprouts
1/2 c	Cabbage
1/2 c	Carrots
1/2 c	Cauliflower
1/2 c	Celery
1/2 c	Cucumbers
1/2 c	Eggplant
1/2 c	Green pepper
	Greens
1/2 c	Beet greens
1/2 c	Chards
1/2 c	Collard greens
1/2 c	Dandelion greens
1/2 c	Kale
1/2 c	Mustard greens
1/2 c	Spinach
1/2 c	Turnip greens
1/2 c	Mushrooms
1/2 c	Okra
1/2 c	Onions
1/2 c	Rhubarb
1/2 c	Rutabaga
1/2 c	Sauerkraut
1/2 c	String beans, green or yellow
1/2 c	Summer squash
1/2 c	Tomatoes
1/2 c	Tomato juice
1/2 c	Turnips
1/2 c	Vegetable juice cocktail
1/2 c	Zucchini
Chinese foods	
1/2 c	Beansprouts, soy
1/2 c	Lotus root (1/3 segment)
1/2 c	Waterchestnut
1/2 c	Yam bean root

*A vegetable exchange is a serving of any vegetable that contains a moderate amount of carbohydrate, a small but significant amount of protein, and about 25 kcal.

L

Fruit List (10 g carbohydrate, 40 kcal)*

Amount	Food
1 small	Apple
1/3 c	Apple juice
1/2 c	Applesauce (unsweetened)
2 medium	Apricots, fresh
4 halves	Apricots, dried
1/2 small	Banana
1/2 c	Blackberries
1/2 c	Blueberries
1/4 small	Cantaloupe melon
10 large	Cherries
1/3 c	Cider
2	Dates
1	Fig, fresh
1	Fig, dried
1 half	Grapefruit
1/2 c	Grapefruit juice
12	Grapes
1/4 c	Grape juice
1/8 medium	Honeydew melon
1/2 small	Mango
1 small	Nectarine
1 small	Orange
1/2 c	Orange juice
3/4 c	Papaya

Amount	Food
1 medium	Peach
1 small	Pear
1 medium	Persimmon (native)
1/2 c	Pineapple
1/3 c	Pineapple juice
2 medium	Plums
2 medium	Prunes
1/4 c	Prune juice
1/2 c	Raspberries
2 tbsp	Raisins
3/4 c	Strawberries
1 medium	Tangerine
1 c	Watermelon

Chinese foods

Amount	Food
1 medium	Guava, fresh
3 medium	Kumquats, fresh
4 medium	Lychee, fresh
1/2 small or 1/3 c	Mango
1/2 small or 1/3 c	Papaya
1/2 medium	Persimmon
1/3 medium	Pomelo

Fast foods†

*A fruit exchange is a serving of fruit that contains about 10 g of carbohydrate and 40 kcal. The protein and fat content of fruit is negligible.

†Apple and cherry pies contain 1½ exchanges of fruit but also 1 bread and 3½ fat exchanges.

Bread List (15 g carbohydrate, 2 g protein, 70 kcal)*

Amount	Food
Bread	
1 slice	White (including French and Italian)
1 slice	Whole-wheat
1 slice	Rye or pumpernickel
1 slice	Raisin
1 half	Small bagel
1 half	Small English muffin
1	Plain roll, bread
1 half	Frankfurter roll
1 half	Hamburger bun
3 tbsp	Dried bread crumbs
1 6-in	Tortilla

Amount	Food
Cereal	
1/2 c	Bran flakes
3/4 c	Other ready-to-eat cereal, unsweetened
1 c	Puffed cereal, unfrosted
1/2 c	Cereal, cooked
1/2 c	Grits, cooked
1/2 c	Rice or barley, cooked
1/2 c	Pasta, cooked (spaghetti, noodles, or macaroni)
3 c	Popcorn, popped, no fat added
2 tbsp	Cornmeal, dry
2½ tbsp	Flour
1/4 c	Wheat germ

*A bread exchange is a serving of bread, cereal, or starchy vegetable that contains appreciable carbohydrate (15 g) and a small but significant amount of protein (2 g), totaling about 70 kcal.

Bread List (15 g carbohydrate, 2 g protein, 70 kcal) (cont'd)

Amount	Food
Crackers	
3	Arrowroot
2	Graham, 2 1/2-in square
1 half	Matzoth, 4 × 6 in
20	Oyster
25	Pretzels, 3 1/8 in long × 1/8 in diameter
3	Rye wafers, 2 × 3 1/2 in
6	Saltines
4	Soda, 2 1/2-in sq
Dried beans, peas, and lentils	
1/2 c	Beans, peas, lentils, dried and cooked
1/4 c	Baked beans, no pork, canned
Starchy vegetables	
1/3 c	Corn
1 small	Corn on cob
1/2 c	Lima beans
2/3 c	Parsnips
1/2 c	Peas, green, canned, or frozen
1 small	Potato, white
1/2 c	Potato, mashed
3/4 c	Pumpkin
1/2 c	Squash (winter, acorn, or butternut)
1/4 c	Yam or sweet potato
Prepared foods†	
1	Biscuit, 2-in diameter (add 1 fat exchange)
1	Corn bread, 2 × 2 × 1 in (add 1 fat exchange)

Amount	Food
1	Corn muffin, 2-in diameter (add 1 fat exchange)
5	Crackers, round butter type (add 1 fat exchange)
1	Muffin, plain, small (add 1 fat exchange)
8	Potatoes, french fried, 2 × 3 1/2 in (add 1 fat exchange)
15	Potato chips or corn chips (add 2 fat exchanges)
1	Pancake, 5 × 1/2 in (add 1 fat exchange)
1	Waffle, 5 × 1/2 in (add 1 fat exchange)
Chinese foods	
1 small or 2/3 medium	Bow (Chinese steamed dough)
6	Chestnuts
1 c	Congee
1/4 c	Glutinous rice, cooked
2/3 c	Gruel rice, cooked
1/2 c	Noodles, cooked (shrimp, thin rice, flat rice, cellophane)
2 tbsp	Rice flour or glutinous rice flour
3 small or 1/3 c	Taro
4	Wonton wrapper (5 × 5 in)

†These foods contain more fat than bread. When calculating fat values, add fat exchanges as indicated (1 fat exchange = 5 g fat).

Meat List (7 g protein, 3 g fat + variable added fat; 55 kcal + kcalories for added fat)*

Amount	Food
Low-fat meat	
1 oz	Beef—baby beef (very lean), chipped beef, chuck, flank steak, tenderloin, plate ribs, plate skirt steak, round (bottom, top), all cuts rump, spareribs, tripe
1 oz	Lamb—leg, rib, sirloin, loin (roast and chops), shank, shoulder

Amount	Food
1 oz	Pork—leg (whole rump, center shank), ham, smoked (center slices)
1 oz	Veal—leg, loin, rib, shank, shoulder, cutlets
1 oz	Poultry—meat-without-skin of chicken, turkey, cornish hen, guinea hen, pheasant

*A meat exchange is a serving of protein-rich food that contains negligible carbohydrate but a significant amount of protein (7 g) and fat (3 g), roughly equivalent to the amounts in 1 oz of lean meat; contains about 55 kcal.

Meat List (7 g protein, 3 g fat + variable added fat; 55 kcal + kcalories for added fat) (cont'd)

Amount	Food
1 oz	Fish—any fresh or frozen
1/4 c	Canned salmon, tuna, mackerel, crab, lobster
5 (or 1 oz)	Clams, oysters, scallops, shrimp
3	Sardines, drained
1 oz	Cheese, containing less than 5% butterfat
1/4 c	Cottage cheese, dry and 2% butterfat
1/2 c	Dried beans and peas (add 1 bread exchange)[†]

Medium-fat meat (add 1/2 fat exchange)[‡]

Amount	Food
1 oz	Beef—ground (15% fat), corned beef (canned), rib eye, round (ground commercial)
1 oz	Pork—loin (all cuts tenderloin), shoulder arm (picnic), shoulder blade, Boston butt, Canadian bacon, boiled ham
1 oz	Liver, heart, kidney, sweetbreads (high in cholesterol)
1/4 c	Cottage cheese, creamed
1 oz	Cheese—mozzarella, ricotta, farmer's cheese, Neufchatel
3 tbsp	Parmesan cheese
1	Egg (high in cholesterol)

High-fat meat (add 1 fat exchange)[⊥]

Amount	Food
1 oz	Beef—brisket, corned beef (brisket), ground beef (more than 20% fat), hamburger (commercial), chuck (ground commercial), roasts (rib), steaks (club and rib)

Amount	Food
1 oz	Lamb—breast
1 oz	Pork—spare ribs, loin (back ribs), pork (ground), country-style ham, deviled ham
1 oz	Veal—breast
1 oz	Poultry—capon, duck (domestic), goose
1 oz	Cheddar-type cheese
1 slice	Cold cuts, $4_{1/2} \times 1/8$ in
1 small	Frankfurter

Peanut butter

Amount	Food
2 tbsp	Peanut butter (add $2_{1/2}$ fat exchanges)[†]

Chinese foods[‡]

Amount	Food
1/4 c	Canned or cooked abalone, crabmeat, eel, lobster, conch, cuttlefish, squid, octopus, fish maw, sea cucumbers, jellyfish, etc.
10 medium	River snails
2 medium	Frog legs
3 medium	Duck feet
1 medium or 1/2 large	Duck egg, salted
1 medium	Egg, preserved or limed
1/2 block	Soybean curd, fresh, $2_{1/2} \times 1_{1/4} \times 1_{1/2}$ in
2 pieces	Soybean curd, fried, $3 \times 6 \times 1/2$ inches

Fast foods[§]

[†]These foods contain more carbohydrate or fat than lean meat. When calculating carbohydrate or fat values, add bread or fat exchanges as indicated.

[‡]These exchanges are not separated into high-, medium-, and low-fat exchanges.

[§]Most fast-food meats are for variable numbers of exchanges and have other exchanges added: hamburger (1 high-fat meat, 2 bread, 260 kcal); cheeseburger ($1_{1/2}$ high-fat meat, 2 bread, 306 kcal); Quarter Pounder® (3 high-fat meat, 2 bread, 420 kcal); Big Mac® (3 high-fat meat, $2_{1/2}$ bread, $1_{1/2}$ fat, 540 kcal); Quarter Pounder® with cheese (4 high-fat meat, 2 bread, 520 kcal); Egg McMuffin® (2 high-fat meat, $1_{1/2}$ bread, 1 fat, 350 kcal); pork sausage (1 high-fat meat, $1_{1/2}$ fat, 185 kcal).

L

Fat List (5 g fat, 45 kcal)*

Amount	Food
Polyunsaturated fat	
1 tsp	Margarine (soft, tub, or stick)†
1/8	Avocado (4-in diameter)‡
1 tsp	Oil—corn, cottonseed, safflower, soy, sunflower
1 tsp	Oil, olive‡
1 tsp	Oil, peanut‡
5 small	Olives‡
10 whole	Almonds‡
2 large whole	Pecans‡
20 whole	Peanuts, Spanish‡
10 whole	Peanuts, Virginia‡
6 small	Walnuts
6 small	Nuts, other‡
Saturated fat	
1 tsp	Margarine, regular stick
1 tsp	Butter
1 tsp	Bacon fat

Amount	Food
1 strip	Bacon, crisp
2 tbsp	Cream, light
2 tbsp	Cream, sour
1 tbsp	Cream, heavy
1 tbsp	Cream cheese
1 tbsp	French dressing§
1 tbsp	Italian dressing§
1 tsp	Lard
1 tsp	Mayonnaise§
2 tsp	Salad dressing, mayonnaise type§
3/4-in cube	Salt pork
Chinese foods	
1 tsp	Sesame or chili oil
1 piece	Coconut meat, 1 × 1 × 1.2 in
2 1/2 tsp	Coconut, grated
2 tsp	Coconut cream (no water)
1 tbsp	Sesame seeds
1-in cube	Fatty cured Chinese pork

*A fat exchange is a serving of any food that contains negligible carbohydrate and protein but appreciable fat (5 g), totaling about 45 kcal.

†Made with corn, cottonseed, safflower, soy, or sunflower oil only.

‡Fat content is primarily monounsaturated.

§If made with corn, cottonseed, safflower, soy, or sunflower oil, can be assumed to contain polyunsaturated fat.

Unlimited Foods (negligible kcal)*

Amount	Food
	Diet kcalorie-free beverage
	Coffee
	Tea
	Bouillon without fat
	Unsweetened gelatin
	Unsweetened pickles
	Salt and pepper
	Red pepper
	Paprika
	Garlic
	Celery salt
	Parsley
	Nutmeg
	Lemon
	Mustard
	Chili powder
	Onion salt or powder
	Horseradish
	Vinegar
	Mint
	Cinnamon
	Lime
	Raw vegetables—chicory, Chinese cabbage, endive, escarole, lettuce, parsley, radishes, watercress

Amount	Food
Chinese foods	
	Plain agar-agar
	Seasonings, spices, herbs† such as soy sauce, monosodium glutamate, star anise, five-spices powder
	Chinese parsley, kelp, sea girdle, laver, and seaweed hair
1 tsp	Shrimp sauce or dried shrimp
1 tsp or 2 nuts	Gingko nuts
1/2 block	White bean curd cheese, 1 1/2 × 3/4 × 1 in
1/4 block	Red bean curd cheese, 1 × 1/4 × 1/2 in
1 c or less	Watery vegetables, including bamboo shoots, bitter melon, bottle gourd, cabbage (celery, mustard, or spoon; fresh, pickled, spiced, salted, or salted and dried), Chinese broccoli, Chinese eggplant, fungi (black, brown, or white), snow peas, turnips (Chinese or green), watercress, winter melon, wolfberry leaves

*These are "free foods" that contain negligible carbohydrate, protein, and fat and therefore negligible kcalories.

†Does not include some starchy and sugar-preserved Chinese herbs.

Canada

The Canadian system works the same way as the U.S. system, but the serving sizes and some of the foods listed are different.[2] Notable among the differences are:

● The standard serving size for milk is one half cup (not 1 c), and whole milk rather than skim is the basis for calculation.

● Vegetables are listed in two groups, the A group (7 g carbohydrate, 2 g protein) and the B group (about half as much carbohydrate and protein). Serving sizes vary. Two group B vegetable servings may be traded for one group A vegetable serving.

● Meats are not divided into low-, medium-, and high-fat categories. An ounce of any meat is considered to provide 7 g protein, 5 g fat.

[2]The Canadian exchange system is taken from *Exchange Lists for Meal Planning for Diabetics in Canada*, published by The Canadian Diabetes Association (Toronto, Ontario, 1977), and is used with their permission.

Milk List (6 g carbohydrate, 4 g protein, 4 g fat)*

Amount	Food
Whole milk	
1/2 c	Whole milk
1/4 c	Evaporated whole milk
Low-fat milk	
1/2 c	2% milk[†]
1/2 c	2% buttermilk[†]
1/2 c	Skim milk[‡]
2 tbsp	Powdered skim milk (instant)[‡]
1/2 c	Skim buttermilk[‡]
1/3 c	Yogurt (plain)[‡]

*A milk exchange is a serving of food equivalent to 1/2 c of whole milk in its energy-nutrient content.

[†]These milk exchanges contain less fat than whole milk. Subtract 1/2 fat exchange.

[‡]These milk exchanges contain less fat than whole milk. Subtract 1 fat exchange.

Vegetable List—Group A (7 g carbohydrate, 2 g protein)*

Amount	Food
1/4 c	Beans—dried navy, lima (canned or cooked)
1/4 c	Beans, green lima
1/2 c	Beets, canned or cooked
2/3 c	Beet greens, cooked
4 stalks	Broccoli, cooked
1/2 c	Brussels sprouts, cooked
3 level tbsp	Canned condensed soup (undiluted)[†]
1/2 c	Carrots, raw, diced, cooked
2½ tbsp	Corn, canned cream style or niblet[†]
1/2 c	Dandelion greens, cooked
2 slices 4 × 4 × 1 in	Eggplant, raw
2/3 c	Kohlrabi, cooked
4 or 1/3 c chopped	Onions, green
1 medium or 1/3 c chopped	Onions, mature, raw
1/3 c	Parsnips, cooked[†]
1/3 c	Peas, green, frozen[†]
1/3 c	Peas, fresh, green, cooked
1/4 c	Peas, green, canned (drained)
2 level tbsp	Potatoes, mashed[†]
1/2 small	Potato, boiled or baked
1/2 c	Pumpkin, canned
3 level tbsp	Rice, cooked[†]
3/4 c	Sauerkraut, canned
1/2 c	Squash, hubbard or pepper, baked or mashed
3/4 c	Tomatoes, canned
2/3 c	Tomato juice, no sugar added
1/2 c	Turnip, yellow or white cooked
2/3 c	Vegetable juice, mixed
1/2 c	Vegetables, mixed carrots and peas
1/3 c	Vegetables, mixed carrots, peas, green lima beans, corn

*A vegetable exchange is a serving of any vegetable that contains a moderate amount of carbohydrate and a small but significant amount of protein.

[†]These vegetables also appear on the bread list in larger servings. They are included in group A for those people whose diet is low in kcalories and to add variety in making up casserole dishes, soups, and the like for any diet.

Vegetable List—Group B*

Amount	Food
5 stalks	Asparagus
1/2 c	Beans, yellow or green, canned or cooked
1 c	Bean sprouts, raw
1/2 c	Cabbage, raw or cooked
1/2 c	Cauliflower, cooked
4 stalks or 1/2 c chopped	Celery, raw
1/2 c	Celery, cooked
1/2 c	Chard, cooked
1/2 medium or 8 slices	Cucumber
1 6-in stalk	Endive
1/2 c	Fiddleheads

Amount	Food
1/2 c	Kale
1/8 head 4 large leaves	Lettuce
2	Onions, green
1 medium	Pepper, green, raw, or cooked
3 tbsp	Pimento, canned
6	Radish
1/2 c	Spinach, cooked or canned
1/3 c	Tomato juice (no sugar added)
1 medium (2 1/4-in diameter)	Tomato, raw
1/2 c	Vegetable marrow, cooked
1/2 c	Zucchini

*Two servings of group B vegetables equal one serving of group A vegetables. One serving from group B may be taken "free" at any meal.

Fruit List (10 g carbohydrate)*

Amount	Food
1/2 medium	Apple, raw
1/3 c	Apple juice
1/2 c	Applesauce
2	Apricots, raw with stone
5 halves + 2 tbsp juice	Apricots, canned, cooked, or dried
1/2 6-in	Banana
1/3 c	Blackberries, raw
1/2 c	Blueberries, raw
1/2 5-in diameter	Cantaloupe with rind
1 c	Cantaloupe cubes or balls
10 large	Cherries, raw
1/3 c + 2 tbsp juice	Cherries, canned, red, pitted, cooked
1 average	Crabapple
2	Dates
2/3 c	Fruit cocktail, canned
1 + 1 tbsp juice	Fig, cooked
1	Fig, dried
3/4 c	Gooseberries, raw
1/2 small (3 1/2-in diameter)	Grapefruit, raw

Amount	Food
1/2 c with juice	Grapefruit sections, raw
1/2 c	Grapefruit juice
14 medium	Grapes, slipskin
14 medium	Grapes, Malaga and seedless
1/4 c	Grape juice
1/2 melon 5-in diameter	Honeydew melon with rind
3/4 c	Honeydew cubes or balls
1/2 c	Huckleberries
1/2 c	Loganberries
1 medium	Nectarine
1 medium (2 1/2 in diameter)	Orange, raw
1/2 c + juice	Orange sections
1/2 c	Orange juice
3/4 c + juice (14 sections)	Orange, mandarin sections (canned dietetic)
1 medium	Peach, raw with stone
2 large halves + 2 tbsp juice	Peaches, canned or cooked

*One fruit exchange is a serving of fruit that contains about 10 g of carbohydrate. The protein and fat content of fruit is negligible.

Fruit List (10 g carbohydrate) (cont'd)

Amount	Food
1 small	Pear, raw
2 halves + 2 tbsp juice	Pears, canned or cooked
1/2 c	Pineapple, raw, cubed
1/2 c cubes or 2 slices + 2 tbsp juice	Pineapple, canned
1/2 c	Pineapple, crushed
1/3 c	Pineapple juice
2 medium	Plums, raw with stone
2 medium + 2 tbsp juice	Plums, canned or cooked
1/2	Pomegranate
2	Prunes, cooked
1/4 c	Prune juice
2 level tbsp	Raisins
1/2 c	Raspberries, raw

Amount	Food
1/2 c	Raspberries, canned or cooked
2 c	Rhubarb, raw
1 c	Rhubarb, cooked
1/2 c	Saskatoons
1 c	Strawberries, raw
3/4 c	Strawberries, canned or cooked
1 (2 1/2-in diameter)	Tangerines
1 c	Tomato juice (no sugar added)
1 slice 1 in thick and 5 in triangle	Watermelon, with skin
1 c	Watermelon cubes
1/6-pt brick	Ice cream—plain vanilla, strawberry, chocolate (add 5 g butter or 1 fat exchange)

Bread List (15 g carbohydrate, 2 g protein)*

Amount	Food
1 slice	Bread
4 (4 1/2 in each)	Bread sticks
6 (6 in each)	Bread sticks, thin
1/2	Bagel
1/4 c	Brewis, cooked (Newfoundland)
1/2 bun	Hamburger bun (3 1/2-in)
1/2 bun	Wiener bun (6-in)
4 rectangular slices or 8 round slices	Melba toast (commercial)
1	Matzo (6-in square)
3	Arrowroots
4	Graham wafers (2-in)
1 1/2 biscuits	Holland rusks
6	Soda biscuits (2-in)
2 tbsp	Cereals, uncooked (dry weight)
1/2 c	Cereals, cooked

Amount	Food
3/4 c	Cereals, cold, flaked
1 c	Cereals, puffed
2/3 biscuit	Cereals, Shredded Wheat
2 tbsp	Cornstarch
2 1/2 tbsp	Flour
1/3 c	Beans and peas, dried, cooked
1/2 c	Corn, canned
1 cob	Corn on the cob (4 1/2 × 1 1/2 × 2 in)
1 1/4 c	Popcorn
2/3 c	Parsnips
1/2 c	Peas, canned
2/3 c	Peas, frozen
1 small or 1/3 c mashed	Potatoes
1/2 c	Macaroni, cooked
1/3 c	Rice, spaghetti, noodles (cooked)
6 tbsp	Canned condensed soup (undiluted)

*A bread exchange is a serving of bread, cereal, or starchy vegetable equivalent in energy-nutrient content to one slice of cracked or whole-wheat, white, brown, or rye bread weighing 30 g. A bread exchange contains appreciable carbohydrate and a small but significant amount of protein.

L

Meat List (7 g protein, 5 g fat)*

Amount	Food
1 medium	Egg

Meat and poultry

Amount	Food
1 slice 4 × 2 × 1/4 in	Sliced medium-fat beef, corned beef, lamb, pork, veal, ham, liver, poultry
1 piece 4 × 2 × 1/4 in	Steak
3 $1_1/2$-in cubes	Diced beef for stewing
2 tbsp or small patty (3 tbsp raw)	Minced beef
2/3 oz	Salt beef (dried)
1 small	Lamb loin chop
1/2 medium	Pork, veal chop
3 slices	Bacon, back or side (crisp)
1 slice, 1/8 in thick	Luncheon-type meats
1 slice, 1/4 in thick ($1_1/2$-2-in diameter)	Liverwurst, salami, summer sausage
$1_1/2$ (12 per lb)	Sausages†
1 piece 4 × 2 × 1/4 in	Seal
1 (12 per lb)	Wieners†

Fish

Amount	Food
1 piece 2 × 1 × 1 in	Fillets of haddock, halibut, cod, sole, whitefish‡
1 piece 2 × 1 × 1 in	Fillet of salmon
1 piece 2 × 1 × 1 in	Salmon steak
1/4 c	Canned chicken haddie, crabmeat, lobster, salmon, tuna
3 fish 3-in each	Sardines (drained)
3 medium	Clams, fresh
3 medium	Oysters
2 medium	Scallops
4 medium	Shrimps, prawns

Cheese

Amount	Food
1 cube $1_1/2$ × 1 × 1 in or 1 slice (presliced, packaged) $3_1/2$ × $3_1/2$ × 1/8 in	Cheddar or processed
$1_1/2$ sections	Gruyere
4 level tbsp	Dried, grated (Parmesan)
3 tbsp	Cottage, creamed
3 tbsp	Cottage, dry (skim)‡
1 piece $2_1/2$-in diameter and 1/4-in thick or 1 slice presliced, packaged $3_1/2$ × $3_1/2$ × 1/8-in	Skim milk, processed‡

*A meat exchange is a serving of protein-rich food that contains negligible carbohydrate but a significant amount of protein and fat, roughly equivalent to the amounts in 1 oz (30 g) of meat.

†For special sizes of sausages and wieners, check weight and number per package.

‡These items contain less fat than most meats. Subtract 1 fat exchange.

L

Fat List (5 g fat)*

Amount	Food
1/8 of 4-in avocado	Avocado pear†
1 strip	Bacon (side)
1 tsp or 1 pat (1 × 1 × 1/4 in)	Butter or margarine
1 tsp	Cooking fat or oil
3 tbsp	Cream, cereal (10%)†
2 tbsp	Cream, coffee (18%)
2 tbsp	Cream, commercial sour
1 tbsp	Cream, whipping
1 rounded tbsp	Cream, whipped
1 tbsp	Cream cheese (white)
1 tbsp	French dressing
1 tsp	Mayonnaise
10	Peanuts†
4	Cashews†
6	Almonds, filberts†
4-5 halves	Pecans, walnuts†
2	Brazil nuts†
5 small	Olives, green
3 medium	Olives, ripe with pit
1/2 tbsp	Peanut butter†

*A fat exchange is a serving of food equivalent to 1 tsp butter in its fat content. Most fat exchanges have negligible carbohydrate.

†It is advisable to limit these items to two servings per day because of the carbohydrate content.

kCalorie-Free Foods*

Food	
Artificial sweetener	Watercress
Non-kcaloric carbonated beverages (dietetic)	Food coloring
	Gelatin, plain
Clear tea or coffee	Artificially sweetened jelly powders
Bouillon	
Clear broth	Horseradish
Consomme	Mushrooms
Flavouring (vanilla, lemon extract)	Parsley
	Rennet tablets
Vinegar	

Seasoning, spices, and herbs

Cinnamon	Sage
Curry powder	Poultry seasoning
Ginger	Mixed whole spices
Nutmeg	Salt and pepper
Mint	Onion salt
Marjoram	Garlic salt

*No significant food value. These foods may be used on kcalorie-restricted diets without restriction.

kCalorie-Poor Foods*

Amount	Food
1 tsp	Cream substitute, powdered (nondairy)
1 tsp	Cocoa (plain)
1 tbsp	Cranberries, cooked without sugar
1 medium serving	Dulse
1 tsp	Fruit spread and jelly, dietetic
1 tbsp	Lemon juice
1 medium	Lemon wedge or slice
1 tsp	Catsup
1 tsp	Chili sauce
1 tsp	Steak sauce
1 tbsp	Partridge berries (Newfoundland)
1 medium	Pickle, dill, unsweetened
4	Pickles, sour, mixed
4	Pickles, sweet, mixed (dietetic)
1 tbsp	Pimento or chopped green pepper
1 tsp	Prepared mustard
1 tbsp	Whipped topping, commercial, powder

*Low in kcalories. These foods may be used in amounts up to two servings a day in kcalorie-restricted diets.

L

APPENDIX M

Food Group Plans

CONTENTS

Food group plans are designed to provide an easy way to approach diet adequacy for all nutrients. This appendix describes the U.S. and Canadian food group plans, with a critique and suggestions for use.

The U.S. Four Food Group Plan

The Four Food Group Plan is a simple and quick guideline for diet planning. But it is not a guarantee of adequacy. Individual foods vary in nutrient content, and the selection of foods within each group can make a big difference in the nutritional adequacy of a diet. However, a diet that is planned around this guide is more apt to be nutritionally adequate than one that is randomly chosen.

Each of the four food groups contains foods that are similar in origin and in nutrient content (see Table 1).

The eight nutrients named in Table 1 are used as indicator nutrients. The meat and milk groups also contribute vitamin B_{12}, important because it is found only in animal products. These two groups and the grain group help provide zinc, a nutrient whose importance is becoming better recognized. All of the other essential nutrients are also found in these foods.

The expectation of the people who devised this plan is that a diet providing adequate amounts of the eight indicator nutrients will provide

Table 1 The Four Food Groups (U.S.)

Food group	Sample foods	Main nutrient contributions
Meat and meat substitutes	Beef, pork, lamb, fish, poultry, eggs, nuts, legumes	Protein, iron, riboflavin, niacin, thiamin
Milk and milk products	Milk, buttermilk, yogurt, cheese, cottage cheese, soy milk, ice cream	Calcium, protein, riboflavin, thiamin
Fruits and vegetables	All fruits and vegetables	Vitamin A, vitamin C, thiamin, additional iron and riboflavin
Grains (bread and cereal products)	All whole-grain and enriched flours and products	Additional riboflavin, niacin, iron, thiamin

ample amounts of all the other nutrients as well. This is not an entirely safe assumption. When fortified foods are involved (to which perhaps only the eight indicator nutrients have been added), the food label may read the same as for a truly nutritious food, but the food may be

M

Table 2   Interlocking Pattern of Key Nutrients in the Food Groups (Canada)

Nutrient	Milk and milk products	Bread and cereals	Fruits and vegetables	Meat and alternates
Vitamin A	Vitamin A		Vitamin A	Vitamin A
Thiamin		Thiamin		Thiamin
Riboflavin	Riboflavin	Riboflavin		Riboflavin
Niacin		Niacin		Niacin
Folic acid			Folic acid	Folic acid
Vitamin C			Vitamin C	
Vitamin D	Vitamin D			
Calcium	Calcium			
Iron		Iron	Iron	Iron
Protein	Protein	Protein		Protein
Fat	Fat			Fat
Carbohydrate		Carbohydrate	Carbohydrate	

relatively nutrient-empty, except for the added nutrients.

The Four Food Group Plan specifies that a certain quantity of food must be consumed from each group. For the adult, the number of servings recommended is two meat, two milk, four fruits and vegetables, and four grains. For the serving sizes and recommendations for other age groups, please refer to Chapter 1, Table 3.

Canada's Food Guide

Canada's Food Guide is similar to the Four Food Group Plan and was developed with the same intent. The handbook explaining it presents the pattern of nutrient intakes shown in Table 2.[1] The Food Guide recommends, for adults, a slightly different pattern from the Four Food Group Plan, as shown in Table 3.

[1]Canadian Ministry of Health and Welfare, *Canada's Food Guide: Handbook* cat. no. H21-74/1977, Ottawa, Ontario, 1977.

Critique of the Four Food Group Plan

The Four Food Group Plan is subject to two major criticisms. One is that it does not include enough of the foods that people really eat. The other is that it encourages overeating.

Many foods that we eat don't fit into any of the four food groups. Consider butter, margarine, cream, sour cream, salad dressing, mayonnaise, jam, jelly, broth, coffee, tea, alcoholic beverages, synthetic products, and others. These items are grouped together into a miscellaneous category. Some of these items do contribute some nutrients to the day's intake. However, either they are not foods, their nutrient content is not significant in enough of the indicator nutrients characteristic of a food group, or their nutrient content has been greatly diluted by fat, sugar, or water. Other foods that we eat fail to fit because they are mixed dishes: soups, casseroles, and the like. The diet planner who relies on these dishes finds the Four Food Group Plan too rigid for his use.

Some say that diet planners undermine the health of those they plan for by insisting that people eat too much food. For all its virtues, the

Table 3   Servings in Canada's Food Guide

Food group	Recommended number of servings (adult)	Serving size
Meat and alternates	2	60-90 g (2-3 oz) cooked lean meat, poultry, liver, or fish
		60 ml (4 tbsp) peanut butter
		250 ml (1 c) cooked dried peas, beans, or lentils
		80-250 ml (1/3-1 c) nuts or seeds
		60 g (2 oz) cheddar, processed, or cottage cheese
		2 eggs
Milk and milk products	2*	250 ml (1 c) milk, yogurt, or cottage cheese
		45 g (1 1/2 oz) cheddar or processed cheese
Fruits and vegetables	4-5†	125 ml (1/2 c) vegetables or fruits
		125 ml (1/2 c) juice
		1 medium potato, carrot, tomato, peach, apple, orange, or banana
Bread and cereals	3-5‡	1 slice bread
		125-250 ml (1/2-1 c) cooked or ready-to-eat cereal
		1 roll or muffin
		125-200 ml (1/2-3/4 c) cooked rice, macaroni, or spaghetti

*Children up to 11 years, 2-3 servings; adolescents, 3-4 servings; pregnant and nursing women, 3-4 servings. Skim, 2%, whole, buttermilk, reconstituted dry, or evaporated milk may be used as a beverage or as the main ingredient in other foods. Cheese may also be chosen. In addition, a supplement of vitamin D is recommended when the milk that is consumed does not contain added vitamin D.

†Include at least two vegetables. Choose a variety of both vegetables and fruits—cooked, raw, or their juices. Include yellow or green or green, leafy vegetables.

‡Whole-grain or enriched. Whole-grain products are recommended.

Four Food Group Plan may inadvertently encourage overeating. The emphasis has been on including, not limiting, foods: "Be sure to get enough milk—enough meat—enough fruit—enough cereal. Don't forget your protein, your calcium, your B vitamins." In the process, until recently, the problem of the kcalories being consumed along the way has been largely ignored. A man going down the cafeteria line at dinner time may spot a cherry pie, say to himself "I haven't had my fruit for the day," and help himself to a slice. The cherries in the pie are indeed a fruit and are nutritious; the piecrust is made of grain and may add B vitamins and iron to his day's intake. But what if he has already exceeded his kcalorie allowance for the day? The Four Food Group Plan does state that one should adjust food choices and serving sizes to achieve and maintain ideal weight but offers no guidance for doing this. Eating well has thus become equivalent, in many people's minds, to eating a lot.

Suggestions for Use

The Four Food Group Plan appears quite rigid, but it can be used with great flexibility once its intent is understood. For example, cheese can be substituted for milk, because it supplies the same nutrients in about the same amounts. Legumes and nuts are alternative choices for meats. The Plan can be adapted to casseroles and other mixed dishes and to different national and cultural cuisines, such as the Chinese, vegetarian, and others. The exchange lists can be used with the Four Food Group Plan to obtain a great variety of menus.

Suppose you want to plan menus that are adequate but not excessive in kcalories. The Four Food Group Plan promotes adequacy, but most people (notably young college women) say, "I couldn't possibly eat all that food without getting fat!" The following demonstration shows that it can be done; it may come as a surprise that it can be done extremely well.

A person who wants to include all the nutrients but to limit consumption of excess kcalories

M

at the same time can use the Four Food Group Plan as a guide for selecting the foundation foods and the exchange lists to choose the actual items. In the example given here, the U.S. (ADA) exchange system is used (see Appendix L):

Table 4   How to Use the Four Food Group Plan and the Exchange System to Plan Diets

Four Food Group Plan	Exchange system	Example	Energy cost (kcal)
Milk—2 c	Milk list—2 exchanges	2 c skim milk	160
Meat—2 servings (2-3 oz each)	Meat list—5 exchanges*	5 oz lean meat	265
Fruits and vegetables—4 servings	Fruit and vegetable lists—4 exchanges	2 vegetable exchanges	70
		2 fruit exchanges	80
Bread and cereals—4 servings	Bread list—4 exchanges	4 bread exchanges	280
TOTAL			855

*In the Four Food Group Plan, a serving of meat is 2-3 oz. In the exchange system, a meat exchange is 1 oz.

For a total of 855 kcal, adequacy for most of the major nutrients has probably been achieved. An average adult woman would still have more than 1,000 kcal to spend. Some of these could be spent using whole milk instead of skim or higher-fat meats or larger servings. Others could be invested in fats (such as salad dressing and margarine), sugar, even alcohol. If these additions are made, they can be made by choice rather than through the unintentional use of high-kcalorie foods to begin with.

An alternative choice is to emphasize adequacy more heavily by investing the spare kcalories in iron-rich and other protective foods. With judicious selections, the diet can reach 100 percent of the RDA for all the indicator nutrients, and this will help to provide generous amounts of the unlisted nutrients as well.

The planner can also realistically aim to meet the USDA Guidelines. To the above 855-kcal foundation, the average person could add much more meat and fat. But a person who is aware of the possible hazards associated with the typical U.S. diet might instead follow the USDA's advice and eat more fruits, vegetables, and whole grains.

The final plan might be like that outlined in Table 5 (of many possible examples). The planner then could achieve variety by selecting different foods each day from the exchange lists.

The Four Food Group Plan can be used as a basis for planning diets at many different energy levels. Table 6 shows six different diets—from 1,200 to 3,000 kcal/day—designed on a Four Food Group Plan foundation, using the exchange system as the source of food items to choose in each group.

Table 5   A Sample Diet Plan*

Exchanges	Energy (kcal)
2 milk	160
5 lean meat	275
2 vegetable	50
3 fruit	120
10 bread	700
5 fat	225
TOTAL	1,530

*This diet derives about 20 percent of its kcalories from protein, about 55 percent from carbohydrate, and about 25 percent from fat.

Table 6.   Diet Plans for Different kCalorie Intakes

Number of ex-changes	Energy level (kcal)					
	1,000	1,200	1,500	1,800	2,000	2,200
Lowfat milk	1	1	2	2	3	3
Vegetable	2	2	2	2	3	4
Fruit	3	4	5	6	6	6
Bread	5	6	7	8	10	11
Lean meat	4	5	6	7	7	7
Fat	4	5	6	7	9	11

These patterns of exchanges supply 50 to 60 percent of the kcalories as carbohydrate, 12 to 20 percent as protein, and less than 38 percent as fat.

The Modified Four Food Group Plan

Since the Four Food Group Plan was originally devised, RDAs have been established for many more nutrients than were taken into account at first. A test of the Plan using real foods shows that a person following it may easily fail to meet his or her RDAs for some of these new nutrients, in particular: vitamin E, vitamin B$_6$, magnesium, and zinc. Iron is also a problem, as it has been from the beginning.

A modification of the Four Food Group Plan, devised to solve these problems, was published in 1978. It recommends:

- 2 servings milk and milk products (as before)

- 2 servings meat, fish, or poultry (serving size 3 oz, not 2-3 oz)

- 2 servings legumes and/or nuts (portion size 3/4 cup), to provide more of the five nutrients just mentioned

- 4 servings fruits and vegetables (as before)

- 4 servings whole-grain (not enriched) products, for the same five nutrients

- 1 serving fat and/or oil (for vitamin E)

Most selections of foods based on this plan would supply 100 percent of the RDA for all nutrients but iron for women, and would miss meeting the woman's iron RDA by only ten percent. The average energy content of a diet selected according to this plan is high—2,200 kcal—and the authors of the plan acknowledge that this is a disadvantage. It restricts the freedom of food choices for the person whose kcalorie allowance is limited. But they feel that this disadvantage is outweighed by the plan's virtual guarantee of dietary adequacy.[2]

[2]J. C. King, S. H. Cohenour, C. G. Corrucini, and P. Schneeman, Evaluation and modification of the basic four food guide, *Journal of Nutrition Education* 10 (1978):27-29.

M

APPENDIX N

Fast Foods

CONTENTS

The following data are reprinted from a publication by Ross Laboratories.[1] We appreciate their permission, and that of the authors, to use this information.

[1]E. A. Young, E. H. Brennan, and G. L. Irving, guest eds., Perspectives on fast foods, *Public Health Currents*, *Ross Timesaver* 21 (May/June 1981).

N

Nutritional Analysis of Fast Foods (Dashes indicate no data available. X=Less than 2% US RDA; tr=trace.)

Food item	Weight (g)	Energy (kcal)	Protein (g)	Carbohydrate (g)	Fat (g)	Calcium (mg)	Iron (mg)	Vitamin A value (IU)	Thiamin (mg)	Riboflavin (mg)	Niacin (mg)	Vitamin C (mg)
ARBY'S®												
Roast Beef	140	350	22	32	15	80	3.6	X	0.30	0.34	5	X
Beef and Cheese	168	450	27	36	22	200	4.5	X	0.38	0.43	6	X
Super Roast Beef	263	620	30	61	28	100	5.4	X	0.53	0.43	7	X
Junior Roast Beef	74	220	12	21	9	40	1.8	X	0.15	0.17	3	X
Ham & Cheese	154	380	23	33	17	200	2.7	X	0.75	0.34	5	X
Turkey Deluxe	236	510	28	46	24	80	2.7	X	0.45	0.34	8	X
Club Sandwich	252	560	30	43	30	200	3.6	X	0.68	0.43	7	X

Source: Consumer Affairs, Arby's, Inc, Altanta, Georgia. Nutritional analysis by Technological Resources, Camden, New Jersey.

Food item	Weight (g)	Energy (kcal)	Protein (g)	Carbohydrate (g)	Fat (g)	Calcium (mg)	Iron (mg)	Vitamin A value (IU)	Thiamin (mg)	Riboflavin (mg)	Niacin (mg)	Vitamin C (mg)
BURGER CHEF®												
Hamburger	91	244	11	29	9	45	2.0	114	0.17	0.16	2.7	1.2
Cheeseburger	104	290	14	29	13	132	2.2	267	0.18	0.21	2.8	1.2
Double Cheeseburger	145	420	24	30	22	223	3.2	431	0.20	0.32	4.4	1.2
Fish Filet	179	547	21	46	31	145	2.2	400	0.23	0.22	2.7	1.0
Super Shef® Sandwich	252	563	29	44	30	205	4.5	754	0.31	0.40	6.0	9.3
Big Shef® Sandwich	186	569	23	38	36	152	3.6	279	0.26	0.31	4.7	1.0
TOP Shef® Sandwich	138	661	41	36	38	194	5.4	273	0.35	0.47	8.1	0
Funmeal® Feast	—	545	15	55	30	61	2.8	123	0.25	0.21	4.6	12.8
Rancher® Platter*	316	640	32	33	42	66	5.3	1750*	0.29	0.38	8.6	23.5
Mariner® Platter*	373	734	29	78	34	63	3.3	2069*	0.34	0.23	5.2	23.5
French Fries, small	68	250	2	20	19	9	0.7	0	0.07	0.04	1.7	11.5
French Fries, large	85	351	3	28	26	13	0.9	0	0.10	0.06	2.4	16.2
Vanilla Shake (12 oz.)	336	380	13	60	10	497	0.3	387	0.10	0.66	0.5	0
Chocolate Shake (12 oz.)	336	403	10	72	9	449	1.1	292	0.16	0.76	0.4	0
Hot Chocolate	—	198	8	23	8	271	0.7	288	0.93	0.39	0.3	2.1

*Includes salad. Source: Burger Chef Systems, Inc. Indianapolis, Indiana. Nutritional analysis from *Handbook No. 8.* Washington: US Dept of Agriculture.

Food item	Weight (g)	Energy (kcal)	Protein (g)	Carbohydrate (g)	Fat (g)	Calcium (mg)	Iron (mg)	Vitamin A value (IU)	Thiamin (mg)	Riboflavin (mg)	Niacin (mg)	Vitamin C (mg)
CHURCH'S FRIED CHICKEN®												
White Chicken Portion	100	327	21	10	23	94	1.00	160	0.10	0.18	7.2	0.7
Dark Chicken Portion	100	305	22	7	21	15	1.3	140	0.10	0.27	5.3	1.0

Source: Church's Fried Chicken, San Antonio, Texas. Nutritional analysis by Medallion Laboratories, Minneapoolis, Minnesota.

N

Nutritional Analysis of Fast Foods
(Dashes indicate no data available. X=Less than 2% US RDA; tr=trace.) (Con'd)

Food item	Weight (g)	Energy (kcal)	Protein (g)	Carbo-hydrate (g)	Fat (g)	Calcium (mg)	Iron (mg)	Vitamin A value (IU)	Thiamin (mg)	Ribo-flavin (mg)	Niacin (mg)	Vitamin C (mg)
DAIRY QUEEN®												
Frozen Dessert	113	180	5	27	6	150	X	100	0.09	0.17	X	X
DQ Cone, small	71	110	3	18	3	100	X	100	0.03	0.14	X	X
DQ Cone, regular	142	230	6	35	7	200	X	300	0.09	0.26	X	X
DQ Cone, large	213	340	10	52	10	300	X	400	10.15	0.43	X	X
DQ Dip Cone, small	78	150	3	20	7	100	X	100	0.03	0.17	X	X
DQ Dip Cone, regular	156	300	7	40	13	200	0.4	300	0.09	0.34	X	X
DQ Dip Cone, large	234	450	10	58	20	300	0.4	400	0.12	0.51	X	X
DQ Sundae, small	106	170	4	30	4	100	0.7	100	0.03	0.17	X	X
DQ Sundae, regular	177	290	6	51	7	200	1.1	300	0.06	0.26	X	X
DQ Sundae, large	248	400	9	71	9	300	1.8	400	0.09	0.43	X	X
DQ Malt, small	241	340	10	51	11	300	1.8	400	0.06	0.34	0.4	2.4
DQ Malt, regular	418	600	15	89	20	500	3.6	750	0.12	0.60	0.8	3.6
DQ Malt, large	588	840	22	125	28	600	5.4	750	0.15	0.85	1.2	6
DQ Float	397	330	6	59	8	200	X	100	0.12	0.17	X	X
DQ Banana Split	383	540	10	91	15	350	1.8	750	0.60	0.60	0.8	18
DQ Parfait	284	460	10	81	11	300	1.8	400	0.12	0.43	0.4	X
DQ Freeze	397	520	11	89	13	300	X	200	0.15	0.34	X	X
Mr. Misty® Freeze	411	500	10	87	12	300	X	200	0.15	0.34	X	X
Mr. Misty® Float	404	440	6	85	8	200	X	100	0.12	0.17	X	X
"Dilly"® Bar	85	240	4	22	15	100	0.4	100	0.06	0.17	X	X
DQ Sandwich	60	140	3	24	4	60	0.4	100	0.03	0.14	0.4	X
Mr. Misty Kiss®	89	70	0	17	0	X	X	X	X	X	X	X
Brazier® Cheese Dog	113	330	15	24	19	168	1.6	—	—	0.18	3.3	—
Brazier® Chili Dog	128	330	13	25	20	86	2.0	—	0.15	0.23	3.9	11.0
Brazier® Dog	99	273	11	23	15	75	1.5	—	0.12	0.15	2.6	11.0
Fish Sandwich	170	400	20	41	17	60	1.1	tr	0.15	0.26	3.0	tr
Fish Sandwich w/Ch	177	440	24	39	21	150	0.4	100	0.15	0.26	3.0	tr
Super Brazier® Dog	182	518	20	41	30	158	4.3	tr	0.42	0.44	7.0	14.0
Super Brazier® Dog w/Ch	203	593	26	43	36	297	4.4	—	0.43	0.48	8.1	14.0
Super Brazier® Chili Dog	210	555	23	42	33	158	4.0	—	0.42	0.48	8.8	18.0
Brazier® Fries, small	71	200	2	25	10	tr	0.4	tr	0.06	tr	0.8	3.6
Brazier® Fries, large	113	320	3	40	16	tr	0.4	tr	0.09	0.03	1.2	4.8
Brazier® Onion Rings	85	300	6	33	17	20	0.4	tr	0.09	tr	0.4	2.4

Source: International Dairy Queen, Inc. Minneapolis, Minnesota. Nutritional analysis by Raltech Scientific Services, Inc. (formerly WARF), Madison, Wisconsin. (Nutritional analysis not applicable in the state of Texas.)

JACK IN THE BOX®

Hamburger	97	263	13	29	11	82	2.3	49	0.27	0.18	5.6	1.1
Cheeseburger	109	310	16	28	15	172	2.6	338	0.27	0.21	5.4	<1.1
Jumbo Jack® Hamburger	246	551	28	45	29	134	4.5	246	0.47	0.34	11.6	3.7
Jumbo Jack® Hamburger w/Ch	272	628	32	45	35	273	4.6	734	0.52	0.38	11.3	4.9
Regular Taco	83	189	8	15	11	116	1.2	356	0.07	0.08	1.8	<0.9
Super Taco	146	285	12	20	17	196	1.9	599	0.10	0.12	2.8	1.6
Moby Jack® Sandwich	141	455	17	38	26	167	1.7	240	0.30	0.21	4.5	1.4
Breakfast Jack® Sandwich	121	301	18	28	13	177	2.5	442	0.41	0.47	5.1	3.4
French Fries	80	270	3	31	15	19	0.7	—	0.12	0.02	1.9	3.7
Onion Rings	85	351	5	32	23	26	1.4	—	0.24	0.12	3.1	<1.2
Apple Turnover	119	411	4	45	24	11	1.4	—	0.23	0.12	2.5	<1.2
Vanilla Shake*	317	317	10	57	6	349	0.2		0.16	0.38	0.5	<3.2
Strawberry Shake*	328	323	11	55	7	371	0.6		0.16	0.46	0.6	<3.3
Chocolate Shake*	322	325	11	55	7	348	0.7		0.16	0.64	0.6	<3.2
Vanilla Shake	314	342	10	54	9	349	0.4	440	0.16	0.47	0.5	3.5
Strawberry Shake	328	380	11	63	10	351	0.3	426	0.16	0.62	0.5	<3.3
Chocolate Shake	317	365	11	59	10	350	1.2	380	0.16	0.60	0.6	<3.2
Ham & Cheese Omelette	174	425	21	32	23	260	4.0	766	0.45	0.70	3.0	<1.7
Double Cheese Omelette	166	423	19	30	25	276	3.6	797	0.33	0.68	2.5	1.7
Ranchero Style Omelette	196	414	20	33	23	278	3.8	853	0.33	0.74	2.6	<2.0
French Toast	180	537	15	54	29	119	3.0	522	0.56	0.30	4.4	9.2
Pancakes	232	626	16	79	27	105	2.8	488	0.63	0.44	4.6	<26.2
Scrambled Eggs	267	719	26	55	44	257	5.0	694	0.69	0.56	5.2	<12.8

Special formula for shakes sold in California, Arizona, Texas and Washington. Source: Jack-in-the-Box, Foodmaker, Inc., San Diego, California. Nutritional analysis by Raltech Scientific Services, Inc. (formerly WARF), Madison, Wisconsin.

N

Nutritional Analysis of Fast Foods (Dashes indicate no data available. X=Less than 2% US RDA; tr=trace.) (Con'd)

Food item	Weight (g)	Energy (kcal)	Protein (g)	Carbo-hydrate (g)	Fat (g)	Calcium (mg)	Iron (mg)	Vitamin A value (IU)	Thiamin (mg)	Ribo-flavin (mg)	Niacin (mg)	Vitamin C (mg)
KENTUCKY FRIED CHICKEN®												
Original Recipe® Dinner*												
Wing & Rib	322	603	30	48	32	—	—	25.5	0.22	0.19	10.0	36.6
Wing & Thigh	341	661	33	48	38	—	—	25.5	0.24	0.27	8.4	36.6
Drum & Thigh	346	643	35	46	35	—	—	25.5	0.25	0.32	8.5	36.6
Extra Crispy Dinner*												
Wing & Rib	349	755	33	60	43	—	—	25.5	0.31	0.29	10.4	36.6
Wing & Thigh	371	812	36	58	48	—	—	25.5	0.31	0.35	10.3	36.6
Drum & Thigh	376	765	38	55	44	—	—	25.5	0.32	0.38	10.4	36.6
Mashed Potatoes	85	64	2	12	1	—	—	<18	<0.01	0.02	0.8	4.9
Gravy	14	23	0	1	2	—	—	<3	0.00	0.01	0.1	<0.2
Cole Slaw	91	122	1	13	8	—	—	—	—	—	—	—
Rolls	21	61	2	11	1	—	—	<5	0.10	0.04	1.0	0.3
Corn (5.5-inch ear)	135	169	5	31	3	—	—	162	0.12	0.07	1.2	2.6
LONG JOHN SILVER'S®												
Fish w/Batter (2 pc)	136	366	22	21	22	—	—	—	—	—	—	—
Fish w/Batter (3 pc)	207	549	32	32	32	—	—	—	—	—	—	—
Treasure Chest®	143	506	30	32	33	—	—	—	—	—	—	—
Chicken Planks® (4 pc)	166	457	27	35	23	—	—	—	—	—	—	—
Peg Legs® w/Batter (5 pc)	125	350	22	26	28	—	—	—	—	—	—	—
Ocean Scallops (6 pc)	120	283	11	30	13	—	—	—	—	—	—	—
Shrimp w/Batter (6 pc)	88	268	8	30	13	—	—	—	—	—	—	—
Breaded Oysters (6 pc)	156	441	13	53	19	—	—	—	—	—	—	—
Breaded Clams	142	617	18	61	34	—	—	—	—	—	—	—
Fish Sandwich	193	337	22	49	31	—	—	—	—	—	—	—
French Fryes	85	288	4	33	16	—	—	—	—	—	—	—
Cole Slaw	113	138	1	16	8	—	—	—	—	—	—	—
Corn on the Cob (1 ear)	150	176	5	29	4	—	—	—	—	—	—	—
Hushpuppies (3)	45	153	3	20	7	—	—	—	—	—	—	—
Clam Chowder (8 oz)	170	107	5	15	3	—	—	—	—	—	—	—

*Includes two pieces of chicken, mashed potato and gravy, cole slaw, and roll. Source: Kentucky Fried Chicken, Inc. Louisville, Kentucky. Nutritional analysis by Raltech Scientific Sevices, Inc. (formerly WARF), Madison, Wisconsin.

Source: Long John Silver's Food Shoppes, Lexington, Kentucky. Nutritional analysis by L. V. Packett, PhD. The Department of Nutrition and Food Science, University of Kentucky.

McDONALD'S®

Egg McMuffin®	138	327	19	31	15	226	2.9	97	0.47	0.44	3.8	<1.4
English Muffin, Buttered	63	186	5	30	5	117	1.5	164	0.28	0.49	2.6	0.8
Hotcakes w/Butter & Syrup	214	500	8	94	10	103	2.2	257	0.26	0.36	2.3	4.7
Sausage (Pork)	53	206	9	tr	19	16	0.8	<32	0.27	0.11	2.1	0.5
Scrambled Eggs	98	180	13	3	13	61	2.5	652	0.08	0.47	0.2	1.2
Hashbrown Potatoes	55	125	2	14	7	5	0.4	<14	0.06	<0.01	0.8	4.1
Big Mac®	204	563	26	41	33	157	4.0	530	0.39	0.37	6.5	2.2
Cheeseburger	115	307	15	30	14	132	2.4	345	0.25	0.23	3.8	1.6
Hamburger	102	255	12	30	10	51	2.3	82	0.25	0.18	4.0	1.7
Quarter Pounder®	166	424	24	33	22	63	4.1	133	0.32	0.28	6.5	<1.7
Quarter Pounder® w/Ch	194	524	30	32	31	219	4.3	660	0.31	0.37	7.4	2.7
Filet-O-Fish®	139	432	14	37	25	93	1.7	42	0.26	0.20	2.6	<1.4
Regular Fries	68	220	3	26	12	9	0.6	<17	0.12	0.02	2.3	12.5
Apple Pie	85	253	2	29	14	14	0.6	<34	0.02	0.02	0.2	<0.8
Cherry Pie	88	260	2	32	14	12	0.6	114	0.03	0.02	0.4	<0.8
McDonaldland® Cookies	67	308	4	49	11	12	1.5	<27	0.23	0.23	2.9	0.9
Chocolate Shake	291	383	10	66	9	320	0.8	349	0.12	0.44	0.5	<2.9
Strawberry Shake	290	362	9	62	9	322	0.2	377	0.12	0.44	0.4	4.1
Vanilla Shake	291	352	9	60	8	329	0.2	349	0.12	0.70	0.3	3.2
Hot Fudge Sundae	164	310	7	46	11	215	0.6	230	0.07	0.31	1.1	2.5
Caramel Sundae	165	328	7	53	10	200	0.2	279	0.07	0.31	1.0	3.6
Strawberry Sundae	164	289	7	46	9	174	0.4	230	0.07	0.30	1.0	2.8

Source: McDonald's Corporation, Oak Brook, Illinois. Nutritional analysis by Raltech Scientific Services, Inc. (formerly WARF), Madison, Wisconsin.

TACO BELL®

Bean Burrito	166	343	11	48	12	98	2.8	1657	0.37	0.22	2.2	15.2
Beef Burrito	184	466	30	37	21	83	4.6	1675	0.30	0.39	7.0	15.2
Beefy Tostada	184	291	19	21	15	208	3.4	3450	0.16	0.27	3.3	12.7
Bellbeefer®	123	221	15	23	7	40	2.6	2961	0.15	0.20	3.7	10.0
Bellbeefer® w/Ch	137	278	19	23	12	147	2.7	3146	0.16	0.27	3.7	10.0
Burrito Supreme®	225	457	21	43	22	121	3.8	3462	0.33	0.35	4.7	16.0
Combination Burrito	175	404	21	43	16	91	3.7	1666	0.34	0.31	4.6	15.2
Enchirito®	207	454	25	42	21	259	3.8	1178	0.31	0.37	4.7	9.5
Pintos 'N Cheese	158	168	11	21	5	150	2.3	3123	0.26	0.16	0.9	9.3
Taco	83	186	15	14	8	120	2.5	120	0.09	0.16	2.9	0.2
Tostada	138	179	9	25	6	191	2.3	3152	0.18	0.15	0.8	9.7

Source: 1) *Menu Item Portions*, San Antonio, Texas, Taco Bell Co. July 1976. 2) Adams CF *Nutritive Value of American Foods* in common units in *Handbook No. 456*. Washington USDA Agricultural Research Service November 1975. 3) Church EF, Church HN (eds) *Food Values of Portions Commonly Used* ed 12. Philadelphia, JB Lippincott Co. 1975. 4) Valley Baptist Medical Center, Food Service Department *Descriptions of Mexican-American Foods*. Fort Atkinson, Wisconsin. NASCO.

N

Food item	Weight (g)	Energy (kcal)	Protein (g)	Carbo-hydrate (g)	Fat (g)	Calcium (mg)	Iron (mg)	Vitamin A value (IU)	Thiamin (mg)	Ribo-flavin (mg)	Niacin (mg)	Vitamin C (mg)
WENDY'S®												
Single Hamburger	200	470	26	34	26	84	5.3	94	0.24	0.36	5.8	0.6
Double Hamburger	285	670	44	34	40	138	8.2	128	0.43	0.54	10.6	1.5
Triple Hamburger	360	850	65	33	51	104	10.7	220	0.47	0.68	14.7	2.0
Single w/Cheese	240	580	33	34	34	228	5.4	221	0.38	0.43	6.3	0.7
Double w/Cheese	325	800	50	41	48	177	10.2	439	0.49	0.75	11.4	2.3
Triple w/Cheese	400	1040	72	35	68	371	10.9	472	0.80	0.84	15.1	3.4
Chili	250	230	19	21	8	83	4.4	1188	0.22	0.25	3.4	2.9
French Fries	120	330	5	41	16	16	1.2	40	0.14	0.07	3.0	6.4
Frosty	250	390	9	54	16	270	0.9	355	0.20	0.60	X	0.7

Source: Wendy's International Inc. Dublin, Ohio. Nutritional analysis by Medallion Laboratories, Minneapolis, Minnesota.

N

APPENDIX O

Recommended Nutrient Intakes

CONTENTS

A variety of organizations have developed guidelines for how much of each nutrient different age and sex groups should consume daily.

Canada

Table 1 shows nutritional guidelines established by the Canadian government.[1]

FAO/WHO

The Food and Agriculture Organization of the World Health Organization has set its own standards for nutrient intakes.[2]

Protein quality varies greatly from country to country, and the human requirement for protein depends on its quality, so the FAO/WHO standard (see Table 2) is stated in terms of high-quality milk or egg protein to avoid misinterpretation. Other tables published by FAO/WHO assume lower quality protein, and still others are stated in terms of amino acid needs.

The FAO/WHO iron recommendations (see Table 7) were based on the assumption that the upper limit of iron absorption by normal individuals would be 10 percent if they consumed less than 10 percent of their kcalories from foods of animal origin, 15 percent if 10 to 25 percent, and 20 percent if more than 25 percent.

[1]Canada, Department of National Health and Welfare, *Dietary Standards for Canada* (Ottawa, Ontario: Department of Public Printing and Stationery, 1975), pp. 70-71.

[2]FAO/WHO, *Energy and Protein Requirements*, WHO Technical Report Series no. 522 (1973), pp. 25, 31, 35, 74. Tables 2 through 7 are presented as examples for comparison with the Canadian and U.S. standards and should not be used as a basis for diet planning without reading the WHO report. Vitamin A recommendations are from FAO/WHO *Requirements of Vitamin A, Thiamine, Riboflavine, and Niacin, 1967*, as cited by R. L. Pike and M. L. Brown, *Nutrition: An Integrated Approach*, 2nd ed. (New York: Wiley, 1975), p. 929. The recommendations for the three B vitamins are from *Requirements of Vitamin A, Thiamine, Riboflavine,*

and Niacin, report of a joint FAO/WHO expert group, Rome, Italy, 6-17 September 1965, part 8, table 6. Ascorbic acid recommendations are from FAO/WHO *Requirements of Ascorbic Acid, Vitamin D, Vitamin B_{12}, Folate, and Iron, 1970* as cited in Pike and Brown, 1975, p. 929. FAO/WHO has published additional recommendations for vitamins D, B_{12}, and folate. Calcium recommendations are from FAO/WHO, *Calcium Requirements*, WHO Technical Report Series no. 230 (1962), as adapted and cited in Pike and Brown, 1975, p. 926. Iron recommendations are from FAO/WHO, *Requirements of Ascorbic Acid, Vitamin D, Vitamin B_{12}, Folate, and Iron*, FAO Nutrition Meeting Report Series no. 47 (1970), p. 54, as adapted and cited by Pike and Brown, 1975, p. 928.

O

Table 1   Dietary Standards, 1975

Age	Sex	Weight (kg)	Height (cm)	Energy (kcal)	Protein (g)	Water-soluble vitamins				
						Thiamin (mg)	Niacin (mg equiv.)	Riboflavin (mg)	Vitamin B_6* (mg)	Folate (μg)
0-6 mo	Both	6	—	kg × 117	kg × 2.2 (2.0)‡	0.3	5	0.4	0.3	40
7-11 mo	Both	9	—	kg × 108	kg × 1.4	0.5	6	0.6	0.4	60
1-3 yr	Both	13	90	1,400	22	0.7	9	0.8	0.8	100
4-6 yr	Both	19	110	1,800	27	0.9	12	1.1	1.3	100
7-9 yr	M	27	129	2,200	33	1.1	14	1.3	1.6	100
	F	27	128	2,000	33	1.0	13	1.2	1.4	100
10-12 yr	M	36	144	2,500	41	1.2	17	1.5	1.8	100
	F	38	145	2,300	40	1.1	15	1.4	1.5	100
13-15 yr	M	51	162	2,800	52	1.4	19	1.7	2.0	200
	F	49	159	2,200	43	1.1	15	1.4	1.5	200
16-18 yr	M	64	172	3,200	54	1.6	21	2.0	2.0	200
	F	54	161	2,100	43	1.1	14	1.3	1.5	200
19-35 yr	M	70	176	3,000	56	1.5	20	1.8	2.0	200
	F	56	161	2,100	41	1.1	14	1.3	1.5	200
36-50 yr	M	70	176	2,700	56	1.4	18	1.7	2.0	200
	F	56	161	1,900	41	1.0	13	1.2	1.5	200
51+ yr	M	70	176	2,300**	56	1.4	18	1.7	2.0	200
	F	56	161	1,800**	41	1.0	13	1.2	1.5	200
Pregnancy	F	—	—	+300††	+20	+0.2	+2	+0.3	+0.5	+50
Lactation	F	—	—	+500	+24	+0.4	+7	+0.6	+0.6	+50

*Recommendations are based on estimated average daily protein intake of Canadians.

**Recommended energy intake for those 66 years and over reduced to 2,000 kcal for men and 1,500 kcal for women.

†† Increased energy intake recommended during second and third trimesters. An increase of 100 kcal per day is recommended during the first trimester.

‡Recommended protein intake of 2.2 g per kilogram body weight for infants age 0 to 2 months and 2.0 g per kilogram body weight for those age 3 to 5 months. Protein recommendation for infants 0 to 11 months assumes consumption of breast milk or protein of equivalent quality.

O

	Fat-soluble vitamins				Minerals					
Vitamin B_{12} (μg)	Vitamin C (mg)	Vitamin A (RE)	Vitamin D (μg cholecalciferol)[†]	Vitamin E (mg d-α-tocopherol)	Calcium (mg)	Phosphorus (mg)	Magnesium (mg)	Iodine (μg)	Iron (mg)	Zinc (mg)
0.3	20[§]	400	10	3	500[II]	250[II]	50[II]	35[II]	7[II]	4[II]
0.3	20	400	10	3	500	400	50	50	7	5
0.9	20	400	10	4	500	500	75	70	8	5
1.5	20	500	5	5	500	500	100	90	9	6
1.5	30	700	2.5[#]	6	700	700	150	110	10	7
1.5	30	700	2.5[#]	6	700	700	150	100	10	7
3.0	30	800	2.5[#]	7	900	900	175	130	11	8
3.0	30	800	2.5[#]	7	1,000	1,000	200	120	11	9
3.0	30	1,000	2.5[#]	9	1,200	1,200	250	140	13	10
3.0	30	800	2.5[#]	7	800	800	250	110	14	10
3.0	30	1,000	2.5[#]	10	1,000	1,000	300	160	14	12
3.0	30	800	2.5[#]	6	700	700	250	110	14	11
3.0	30	1,000	2.5[#]	9	800	800	300	150	10	10
3.0	30	800	2.5[#]	6	700	700	250	110	14	9
3.0	30	1,000	2.5[#]	8	800	800	300	140	10	10
3.0	30	800	2.5[#]	6	700	700	250	100	14	9
3.0	30	1,000	2.5[#]	8	800	800	300	140	10	10
3.0	30	800	2.5[#]	6	700	700	250	100	9	9
+1.0	+20	+100	+2.5[#]	+1	+500	+500	+25	+15	+1[‡‡]	+3
+0.5	+30	+400	+2.5[#]	+2	+500	+500	+75	+25	+1[‡‡]	+7

[#] Most older children and adults receive vitamin D from the sun, but 2.5 μg daily is recommended. This intake should be increased to 5.0 μg daily during pregnancy and lactation and for those confined indoors or otherwise deprived of sunlight for extended periods.

[†] A μg cholecalciferol equals 1 μg ergocalciferol (40 IU vitamin D activity).

[‡‡] A recommended total intake of 15 mg daily during pregnancy and lactation assumes the presence of adequate stores of iron. If stores are suspected of being inadequate, additional iron as a supplement is recommended.

[§] Considerably higher levels may be prudent for infants during the first week of life.

[II] The intake of breast-fed infants may be less than the recommendation but is considered adequate.

O

Table 2   Safe Levels of Protein

Age	Body weight (kg)	Protein per kg per day (g)	Protein per person per day (g)	Adjusted level for proteins of different quality* (g per person per day)		
				Score 80	Score 70	Score 60
Infants						
6-11 mo	9.0	1.53	14	17	20	23
Children						
1-3 yr	13.4	1.19	16	20	23	27
4-6 yr	20.2	1.01	20	26	29	34
7-9 yr	28.1	0.88	25	31	35	41
Male adolescents						
10-12 yr	36.9	0.81	30	37	43	50
13-15 yr	51.3	0.72	37	46	53	62
16-19 yr	62.9	0.60	38	47	54	63
Female adolescents						
10-12 yr	38.0	0.76	29	36	41	48
13-15 yr	49.9	0.63	31	39	45	52
16-19 yr	54.4	0.55	30	37	43	50
Adult man	65.0	0.57	37	46[†]	53[†]	62[†]
Adult woman	55.0	0.52	29	36[†]	41[†]	48[†]
Pregnant woman, latter half of pregnancy			add 9	add 11	add 13	add 15
Lactating woman, first 6 mo			add 17	add 21	add 24	add 28

*Scores are estimates of the quality of the protein usually consumed relative to that of egg or milk. The safe level of protein intake is adjusted by multiplying it by 100 and dividing by the score of the food protein. For example, $100/60 = 1.67$, so for a child of 1-4 years, the safe level of protein intake would be 16×1.67, or 27 g of protein having a relative quality of 60.

[†]The correction may overestimate adult protein requirements.

Table 3   Energy Requirements of Children and Adolescents

Age (years)	Body weight (kg)	Energy per kg per day (kcal)	Energy per person per day (kcal)
Children			
1	7.3	112	820
1-3	13.4	101	1,360
4-6	20.2	91	1,830
7-9	28.1	78	2,190

Age (years)	Body weight (kg)	Energy per kg per day (kcal)	Energy per person per day (kcal)
Male adolescents			
10-12	36.9	71	2,600
13-15	51.3	57	2,900
16-19	62.9	49	3,070
Female adolescents			
10-12	38.0	62	2,350
13-15	49.9	50	2,490
16-19	54.4	43	2,310

O

Table 4   Energy Requirements of Adults

Body weight (kg)	Activity level*			
	Lightly active (kcal)	Moderately active (kcal)	Very active (kcal)	Exceptionally active (kcal)
Men				
50	2,100	2,300	2,700	3,100
55	2,310	2,530	2,970	3,410
60	2,520	2,760	3,240	3,720
65	2,700	3,000	3,500	4,000
70	2,940	3,220	3,780	4,340
75	3,150	3,450	4,050	4,650
80	3,360	3,680	4,320	4,960

Body weight (kg)	Activity level*			
	Lightly active (kcal)	Moderately active (kcal)	Very active (kcal)	Exceptionally active (kcal)
Women				
40	1,440	1,600	1,880	2,200
45	1,620	1,800	2,120	2,480
50	1,800	2,000	2,350	2,750
55	2,000	2,200	2,600	3,000
60	2,160	2,400	2,820	3,300
65	2,340	2,600	3,055	3,575
70	2,520	2,800	3,290	3,850

*The activity levels defined by FAO/WHO are as follows:

LIGHTLY ACTIVE

Men: most professional men (lawyers, doctors, accountants, teachers, architects, etc.), office workers, shop workers, unemployed men

Women: housewives in houses with mechanical household appliances, office workers, teachers, most professional women

MODERATELY ACTIVE

Men: most men in light industry, students, building workers (excluding heavy laborers), many farmworkers, soldiers not in active service, fishermen

Women: most women in light industry, housewives without mechanical household appliances, students, department store workers

VERY ACTIVE

Men: some agricultural workers, unskilled laborers, forestry workers, army recruits and soldiers in active service, mineworkers, steelworkers

Women: some farmworkers (especially in peasant agriculture), dancers, athletes

EXCEPTIONALLY ACTIVE

Men: lumberjacks, blacksmiths, rickshaw pullers

Women: construction workers

Table 5   Recommended Vitamin Intakes

Age	Vitamin A (μg retinol)	Thiamin (mg)	Riboflavin (mg)	Niacin (mg equiv.)	Ascorbic acid (mg)
0-6 mo	*	*	*	*	*
7-12 mo	300	0.4	0.6	6.6	20
1-3 yr	250	0.5-0.6	0.6-0.8	7.6-9.6	20
4-6 yr	300	0.7	0.9	11.2	20
7-9 yr	400	0.8	1.2	13.9	20
10-12 yr	575	1.0	1.4	16.5	20
13-15 yr (boys)	725	1.2	1.7	20.4	30
13-15 yr (girls)	725	1.0	1.4	17.2	30
16-19 yr (boys)	750	1.4	2.0	23.8	30
16-19 yr (girls)	750	1.0	1.3	15.8	30
Adults (men)	750	1.3	1.8	21.1	30
Adults (women)	750	0.9	1.3	15.2	30

*It is assumed that the infant will be breastfed by a well-nourished mother. The mother should have 450 additional retinol μg per day during this period.

Table 6   Recommended Intake of Calcium

Age	Practical allowance (mg/day)
0-12 mo*	500-600
1-9 yr	400-500
10-15 yr	600-700
16-19 yr	500-600
Adult	400-500

*Artificially fed only.

Table 7   Recommended Daily Intake of Iron

Age	Absorbed iron required (mg)	Recommended intake according to type of diet, proportion of animal foods		
		Below 10% of kcalories	10-25% of kcalories	Over 25% of kcalories
0-4 mo	0.5	*	*	*
5-12 mo	1.0	10	7	5
1-12 yr	1.0	10	7	5
13-16 yr (boys)	1.8	18	12	9
13-16 yr (girls)	2.4	24	18	12
Menstruating women	2.8	28	19	14
Men and nonmenstruating women	0.9	9	6	5

*It is assumed that breastfeeding will provide adequate iron

United States

Some of the U.S. recommendations appear in the RDA tables on the inside front cover. The remaining RDAs are here. For the U.S. RDA used on food labels, see page 441.

	Vitamins			Trace elements†						Electrolytes		
Age (years)	Vitamin K (µg)	Biotin (µg)	Pantothenic acid (mg)	Copper (mg)	Manganese (mg)	Fluoride (mg)	Chromium (mg)	Selenium (mg)	Molybdenum (mg)	Sodium (mg)	Potassium (mg)	Chloride (mg)
0-0.5	12	35	2	0.5-0.7	0.5-0.7	0.1-0.5	0.01-0.04	0.01-0.04	0.03-0.06	115 - 350	350 - 925	275 - 700
0.5-1	10-20	50	3	0.7-1.0	0.7-1.0	0.2-1.0	0.02-0.06	0.02-0.06	0.04-0.08	250 - 750	425-1,275	400-1,200
1-3	15-30	65	3	1.0-1.5	1.0-1.5	0.5-1.5	0.02-0.08	0.02-0.08	0.05-0.1	325 - 975	550-1,650	500-1,500
4-6	20-40	85	3-4	1.5-2.0	1.5-2.0	1.0-2.5	0.03-0.12	0.03-0.12	0.06-0.15	450-1,350	775-2,325	700-2,100
7-10	30-60	120	4-5	2.0-2.5	2.0-3.0	1.5-2.5	0.05-0.2	0.05-0.2	0.1 -0.3	600-1,800	1,000-3,000	925-2,775
11+	50-100	100-200	4-7	2.0-3.0	2.5-5.0	1.5-2.5	0.05-0.2	0.05-0.2	0.15-0.5	900-2,700	1,525-4,575	1,400-4,200
Adults	70-140	100-200	4-7	2.0-3.0	2.5-5.0	1.5-4.0	0.05-0.2	0.05-0.2	0.15-0.5	1,100-3,300	1,875-5,625	1,700-5,100

*Because there is less information on which to base allowances, these figures are not given in the main table of the RDA and are provided here in the form of ranges of recommended intakes.

†Since the toxic levels for many trace elements may be only several times usual intakes, the upper levels for the trace elements given in this table should not habitually be exceeded.

O

Table 9   Mean Heights and Weights and Recommended Energy Intake

Age (years)	Weight (kg)	Weight (lb)	Height (cm)	Height (in)	Energy needs* (kcal)	Energy needs* (MJ)†
0.0-0.5	6	13	60	24	kg × 115 (95-145)	kg × 0.48
0.5-1.0	9	20	71	28	kg × 105 (80-135)	kg × 0.44
Children						
1-3	13	29	90	35	1,300 (900-1,800)	5.5
4-6	20	44	112	44	1,700 (1,300-2,300)	7.1
7-10	28	62	132	52	2,400 (1,650-3,300)	10.1
Males						
11-14	45	99	157	62	2,700 (2,000-3,700)	11.3
15-18	66	145	176	69	2,800 (2,100-3,900)	11.8
19-22	70	154	177	70	2,900 (2,500-3,300)	12.2
23-50	70	154	178	70	2,700 (2,300-3,100)	11.3
51-75	70	154	178	70	2,400 (2,000-2,800)	10.1
76+	70	154	178	70	2,050 (1,650-2,450)	8.6
Females						
11-14	46	101	157	62	2,200 (1,500-3,000)	9.2
15-18	55	120	163	64	2,100 (1,200-3,000)	8.8
19-22	55	120	163	64	2,100 (1,700-2,500)	8.8
23-50	55	120	163	64	2,000 (1,600-2,400)	8.4
51-75	55	120	163	64	1,800 (1,400-2,200)	7.6
76+	55	120	163	64	1,600 (1,200-2,000)	6.7
Pregnant					+300	
Lactating					+500	

*The energy allowances for the young adults are for men and women doing light work. The allowances for the two older age groups represent mean energy needs over these age spans, allowing for a 2 percent decrease in basal (resting) metabolic rate per decade and a reduction in activity of 200 kcal per day for men and women between 51 and 75 years, 500 kcal for men over 75 years, and 400 kcal for women over 75. The customary range of daily energy output, shown in parentheses, is based on a variation in energy needs of ± 400 kcal at any one age, emphasizing the wide range of energy intakes appropriate for any group of people. Energy allowances for children through age 18 are based on median energy intakes of children these ages followed in longitudinal growth studies. The values in parentheses are tenth and ninetieth percentiles of energy intake, to indicate the range of energy consumption among children of these ages.

†MJ stands for megajoules (1 MJ = 1,000 kJ).

O

APPENDIX P

Vitamin/Mineral Supplements Compared

The following tables are useful for comparing the essential vitamin and mineral contents of supplements commonly available in the United States. Notice that blank columns have been provided for the addition of locally available products you may wish to compare with those shown here.

Not all ingredients in vitamin/mineral preparations are of proven benefit. To facilitate meaningful comparison, the table lists only the nutrients known to be needed in supplement form on occasion. Other nutrients and compounds found on the labels of these supplements are listed in the table notes.

When a supplement is needed that supplies certain particular nutrients, this table will ease the task of selecting an appropriate one. Notice, for example, that many preparations marketed for the elderly are composed largely of alcohol, with few vitamins or minerals. These are "tonics," not vitamin/mineral supplements. A tonic may be useful if the only need is for comfort and the benefit of the placebo effect, but if an elderly person needs a balanced assortment of vitamins and minerals and cannot easily take pills, it may be advisable to suggest a liquid preparation designated for infants.

Notice the very low levels of calcium present in some of these preparations. A product that supplies 20 mg of calcium provides only 2 percent of an adult's RDA for calcium and would have no significant impact on a person's calcium nutrition. For further discussion of this point, see page 416.

Table 1. Supplements for Infants and Children

Company	Lederle	Miles Laboratories	Mead-Johnson	Mead Johnson	Radiance
Product	Centrum Jr.	Flintstones plus Iron	Poly-Vi-Sol with Iron (drops)	Poly-Vi-Sol with Iron (chewable)	Chewable for Children
Intended Users	Children over 4	Children 1 to 12	Infants	Children and adults	Children 2 to 12
Recommended Daily Dose	1 tablet	1 tablet	1 ml	1 tablet	1 tablet
Vitamins					
Vitamin A (IU)	5,000	2,500	1,500	2,500	4,000
Vitamin D (IU)	400	400	400	400	400
Vitamin E (IU)	15	15	5	15	3.4
Vitamin C (mg)	60	60	35	60	60
Thiamin (B_1) (mg)	1.5	1.05	0.5	1.05	2.0
Riboflavin (B_2) (mg)	1.7	1.2	0.6	1.2	2.4
Vitamin B_6 (mg)	2.0	1.05	0.4	1.05	2.0
Vitamin B_{12} (μg)	6.0	4.5	—	4.5	10.0
Niacin (mg)	20.0	13.5	8.0	13.5	10.0
Folacin (mg)	0.4	0.3	—	0.3	—
Minerals					
Calcium (mg)	—	—	—	—	19
Phosphorus (mg)	—	—	—	—	0.0
Iron (mg)	18	15	10	12	12
Potassium (mg)	1.6	—	—	—	4
Magnesium (mg)	25	—	—	—	22
Zinc (mg)	10	—	—	—	—
Copper (mg)	2	—	—	—	0.2
Iodine (μg)	—	—	—	—	—
Manganese (mg)	1	—	—	—	—
Cost per day*					

Radiance Chewables also contain 2 mg pantothenic acid, 10 mg biotin, 2 mg inositol, and 2 mg of a choline compound.

Neo-life Chewables also contain 10 mg pantothenic acid, 0.075 mg inositol, and 0.05 mg of a choline compound.

Williams Chewables also contain 2.5 mg pantothenic acid, and 37.5 mg biotin.

Amway Chewables also contain 5 mg pantothenic acid.

Shaklee Chewables also contain 5 mg pantothenic acid, 150 mg biotin, and 0.2 mg inositol.

Table 1.   Supplements for Infants and Children (continued)

Chocks	Neolife	J. B. Williams	Upjohn	Amway Nutrilite	Shaklee	Other
Bugs Bunny plus Iron	Chewable New-Jr.	Chewable Popeye with Mins/Iron	Unicap Chewable	Chewables	Vita-lea Chewables	
Children 1 to 12	Children 2 and up	Children	Children	Children	Children	
1 tablet	3 tablets	1 tablet	1 tablet	1 tablet	2 tablets	
2,500	3,000	2,500	5,000	2,500	2,500	
400	300	400	400	400	200	
15	9	15	15	10	15	
60	60	60	60	40	45	
1.05	1.5	1.05	1.5	0.7	1.05	
1.2	1.5	1.2	1.7	0.8	1.2	
1.05	1.2	1.05	2.0	0.7	1.0	
4.5	3.0	4.5	6.0	3.0	4.5	
13.5	10.0	13.5	20.0	9.0	10.0	
0.3	—	0.3	0.4	0.2	0.2	
—	—	—	—	—	160	
—	—	—	—	—	125	
15	3	15	—	5	10	
—	—	40	—	—	100	
—	—	40	—	—	8	
—	—	12	—	—	1	
—	0.002	1.5	—	—	1	
—	75	105	—	—	75	
—	1	—	—	—	—	

*Since product costs varies so widely by location (and local prices have changed dramatically in the last two years), the computation of cost/day is left for the reader to complete. To compute this value, divide the total retail price by the number of doses per container. For example: XYZ vitamins are sold in bottles of 100 tablets. The recommended dose is 2 tablets per day, therefore there are 50 doses in the bottle. At $5.00 per bottle, XYZ Vitamins cost $.10 per day.

P

Table 2.   Supplements for Adults

Company	Lederle	Lederle	Parke-Davis	Squibb	Miles Lab
Product	Stress Tabs 600	Centrum A to Zinc	Myadec	Theragram M	One-A-Day plus Iron
Recommended Daily Dose	1 tablet	1 tablet	1 tablet	1 tablet	1 tablet
Vitamins					
Vitamin A (IU)	—	5,000	10,000	10,000	5,000
Vitamin D (IU)	—	400	400	400	400
Vitamin E (IU)	30	30	30	15	15
Vitamin C (mg)	600	90	250	200	60
Thiamin (B_1) (mg)	15.0	2.25	10.0	10.3	1.5
Riboflavin (B_2) (mg)	15.0	2.6	10.0	10.0	1.7
Vitamin B_6 (mg)	5.0	3.0	5.0	4.1	2.0
Vitamin B_{12} (μg)	12	9	6	5	6
Niacin (mg)	100	20	100	100	20
Folacin (mg)	—	0.4	0.4	—	0.4
Minerals					
Calcium (mg)	—	162	—	20	—
Phosphorus (mg)	—	125	—	—	—
Iron (mg)	—	27	20	12	18
Potassium (mg)	—	7.5	—	—	—
Magnesium (mg)	—	100	100	65	—
Zinc (mg)	—	22.5	20	1.5	100
Copper (mg)	—	3	2	2	—
Iodine (μg)	—	150	150	150	—
Manganese (mg)	—	7.5	1.25	1.0	—

Cost per day*

Lederle Centrum A to Zinc also contains 10 mg pantothenic acid, and 45 μg biotin.

Radiance Nutri-Mega also contains 50 mg pantothenic acid, 50 μg biotin, 50 mg inositol, 50 mg PABA, 50 mg choline compound, and 80 mg lecithin.

Neo-Life Formula IV also contains 12 mg pantothenic acid, 65 mg inositol, 30 mg PABA, 30 mg lecithin, 40 mg diastase, 40 mg lipase (pancreatin), and 168 mg linoleic acid.

Origin Multivitamins also contains 20 mg pantothenic acid, 25 μg biotin, 10 mg inositol, and 20 mg of a choline compound.

Amway Nutrilite Double X also contains 10 mg pantothenic acid, 5 μg chromium, and 5 μg selenium.

J. B. Williams Vitabank also contains 18 mg pantothenic acid and 25 μg selenium.

Miles Labs One-A-Day plus Minerals also contains 10 mg pantothenic acid, 10 μg chromium, 10 μg selenium, and 10 μg molybdenum.

Lederle Stress-Tabs 600, Centrum A to Zinc, Parke-Davis Myadec, and Squibb Theragram M, also contain pantothenic acid: 20 mg, 20 mg, 18.4 mg, and 10 mg respectively.

P

Table 2.   Supplements for Adults (continued)

Radiance	Neo-Life	Amway Nutrilite	J. B. Williams	Origin	Miles Lab	Other
Nutri-mega	Formula IV	Double X	Vitabank	Multi-vitamin	One-A-Day plus Minerals	
2 tablets	2 capsules	9 tablets	1 tablet	1 tablet	1 tablet	
10,000	4,000	15,000	5,000	10,000	5,000	
400	400	400	400	400	400	
300	10	30	30	30	30	
300	90	500	90	250	60	
50	10	15	2.25	20	1.5	
50	10	15	2.6	20	1.7	
50	10	15	3.0	5.0	2.0	
50	10	9	9	6	6	
50	50	35	20	150	20	
0.4	0.1	0.4	0.4	0.4	0.4	
200	—	900	170	100	130	
50	—	450	130	—	100	
18	25	18	18	30	18	
30	—	—	7.5	5	5	
50	35	300	100	50	100	
15	—	15	15	7.5	15	
2	2	2	2	1	2	
150	100	150	150	150	150	
30	—	5.0	2.5	1.5	2.5	

*Since product costs varies so widely by location (and local prices have changed dramatically in the last two years), the computation of cost/day is left for the reader to complete. To compute this value, divide the total retail price by the number of doses per container. For example: XYZ vitamins are sold in bottles of 100 tablets. The recommended dose is 2 tablets per day, therefore there are 50 doses in the bottle. At $5.00 per bottle, XYZ Vitamins cost $.10 per day.

P

Table 3. **Supplements and Tonics for the Elderly**

Company	Ross Labs	Lederle	J. B. Williams	Upjohn	Other
Product	Vi-Daylin plus Iron	Gevrabon	Geritol	Unicap Senior	
Recommended Daily Dose	1 tsp	1 oz	1 oz	1 tablet	
Vitamins					
Vitamin A (IU)	2,500	—	—	5,000	
Vitamin D (IU)	400	—	—	—	
Vitamin E (IU)	15	—	—	15	
Vitamin C (mg)	60	—	—	60	
Thiamin (B_1) (mg)	1.05	5.0	5.0	1.2	
Riboflavin (B_2) (mg)	1.2	2.5	5.0	1.7	
Vitamin B_6 (mg)	1.05	1.0	1.0	2.0	
Vitamin B_{12} (μg)	4.5	1.0	1.5	6.0	
Niacin (mg)	13.5	50	100	14.0	
Folacin (mg)	—	—	—	0.4	
Minerals					
Calcium (mg)	—	—	2	—	
Phosphorus (mg)	—	—	—	—	
Iron (mg)	10	15	100	10	
Potassium (mg)	—	—	—	5	
Magnesium (mg)	—	2	—	—	
Zinc (mg)	—	2	—	15	
Copper (mg)	—	—	—	2	
Iodine (μg)	—	100	—	150	
Manganese (mg)	—	2	—	1	
Alcohol (%)	0.5	18	12	—	

Cost per day*

Lederle Gevrabon also contains 100 mg inositol and 100 mg of a choline compound.

J. B. Williams Geritol also contains 100 mg of a choline compound and 50 mg methionine.

*Since product costs varies so widely by location (and local prices have changed dramatically in the last two years), the computation of cost/day is left for the reader to complete. To compute this value, divide the total retail price by the number of doses per container. For example: XYZ vitamins are sold in bottles of 100 tablets. The recommended dose is 2 tablets per day, therefore there are 50 doses in the bottle. At $5.00 per bottle, XYZ Vitamins cost $.10 per day.

INDEX

Numbers in bold face refer to pages where definitions or major discussions appear.

Numbers in italics refer to illustrations, diagrams, or chemical structures.

A number followed by a 't' (e.g., 356t) refers to a table.

Letters A, B, C, etc., refer to Appendixes.

A

AAA (aromatic amino acid), **937**
AAP. *See* American Academy of Pediatrics
Abdomen. *See* GI disorders, disease names
Abortion, 499, 503
Absorption. *See* nutrient names
Abstract, 371
Ac, **801**
Accent, 419
Acetaldehyde, 339, 340, 342, 344
Acetic acid, 59, 62
Acetone, 212, 946, 949
Acetyl CoA, 70, **202**, 234-237, 314-316, 339-340, 343
Acetylcholine, 166, 167, 169
Achalasia, **859**, 860
Achlorhydria, **865**
Acid, **59**, 96, 98, 154-155, 160, 343, B
  -base balance, **127**, 310, 343, 359, 410, 421, 490, 779
  former, 490-492, 811
  gastric, 644, 865, 866, 926
  indigestion, 154
  see also Acidosis, Diets (acid ash), Fatty acid, Ulcer, Vitamin C
Acidophilus milk. *See* Milk
Acidosis, **127**, 422, 494, 946, 1021
Acne, 388, 455, 618
Acres (to grow food). *See* Land
Acrilonitrile, 504
Acromial process, **687**
ACSH News and Views, A

ACTH, 82, 83, 84, *192*
Actin (of muscle), 241
Active site (of enzyme), 314
Active transport, 178, 187
Activity (muscular). *See* Exercise
Acute (disease/symptom), **863**
Adaptation, 246-251, 608, 677, 827, 828, 886, 910; *see also* Formula, Tube feeding
Addict (addiction, addictive), **627**, **910**
  alcohol, 598, 907-910
  marihuana and, 600
  sugar, 617-627
  see also Alcoholism, Pregnancy
Additives, 4, 466-477, **468**, 479, 496, F
  cancer and, 454, 1059
  contaminants as, 503-510
  incidental/indirect/intentional, 467, **468**, 503, **506**
  on labels, 429
  sugar and salt as, 432
  see also Pollution
Addresses (for nutrition information), J
Adenosine triphosphate. *See* ATP
ADH (antidiuretic hormone), **84**, *192*, **344**, 347, **486**, 830t; *see also* Vasopressin
Adipose cell, **56**; *see also* Fat (in body)
Adolescence (Adolescents, Teenagers), 591-612
  anorexia nervosa in, 286
  diabetes in, 942
  growth in, 285, 517, 518, 581
  nutrition problems of, 676
  obesity in, 267, 268, 285
  pregnancy in, 528, 533, 536, 538, 539, 557
  sexual development in, 519
  vitamin C intakes, 357
  see also Acne, Erikson
Adrenal gland, **20**, 82, **492**
  alcohol and, 913
  cortex, 82, 84, 85, 86, *192*
  medulla, 82, 85, *192*

stress and, 356
vitamin A and, 381
vitamin C and, 356
water retention and, 486-487
Adrenaline, 20, 85, 191, 356
Adrenergic blocker, 989
Adrenocortical hormone, 70
Adrenocorticotropin, 82
Advertising (food), 427, 621
Aerobic, **231**, 234, **605**; *see also* Exercise
Afebrile, **836**
Africa(n), 639, 711, 712
Age, 222-224, 253, 266, 357, 414, 694; *see also* Atherosclerosis, Older adult
Ageusia, **728**
Aging. *See* Older adult
Ague (frauds), **404**
AHA. *See* American Heart Association
Air embolism, 779
Alanine, 96, 1011
Alarm signal/reaction (of stress), 190, *192*
Albumin, **412**, 691
  assessment of, 690, 693t, 695t
  binding of tryptophan to, 167
  buffering action, 127
  calcium regulation, 412
  diarrhea and, 765
  low levels, 839, 843, 893, 932, 1025, 1030
  TPN solution of, 776
  see also Protein
Alcohol, 23, 30, 134, 181, 339-348, C, F, M
  adaptation to, 246-248
  appetite and, 797t
  dehydrogenase (ADH), 339-341, 344, 911
  Dietary Guidelines and, 32-33
  diseases and, 959, 964, 979, 982-985, 988, 1000, 1061
  effects on nutrients, 324-327, 330, 339-348, 447, 802t, 812
  kcalories in, 9, 280t
  preventive nutrition and, 1058, 1062, 1063t